Geriatric Medicine

Geriatric Medicine

Second Edition

Dennis Jahnigen, M.D.

Goodstein Professor of Geriatrics
University of Colorado School of Medicine
Director, Center on Aging
University of Colorado Health Sciences Center
Denver, Colorado

Robert Schrier, M.D.

Professor and Chairman, Department of Medicine
University of Colorado School of Medicine
Denver, Colorado

**Blackwell
Science**

Blackwell Science

Editorial offices:

238 Main Street, Cambridge, Massachusetts 02142, USA

Osney Mead, Oxford OX2 0El, England

25 John Street, London WC1N 2BL, England

23 Ainslie Place, Edinburgh EH3 6AJ, Scotland

54 University Street, Carlton, Victoria 3053, Australia

Other Editorial Offices:

Arnette Blackwell SA, 224, Boulevard Saint Germain, 75007 Paris, France

Blackwell Wissenschafts-Verlag GmbH Kurfürstendamm 57, 10707 Berlin, Germany

Zehetnergasse 6, A-1140 Vienna, Austria

Distributors:

USA

  Blackwell Science, Inc.

  238 Main Street

  Cambridge, Massachusetts 02142

  (Telephone orders: 800-215-1000 or 617-876-7000; Fax orders: 617-492-5263) °

Canada

  Copp Clark, Ltd.

  2775 Matheson Blvd. East

  Mississauga, Ontario

  Canada, L4W 4P7

  (Telephone orders: 800-263-4374 or 905-238-6074)

Australia

  Blackwell Science Pty., Ltd.

  54 University Street

  Carlton, Victoria 3053

  (Telephone orders: 03-9347-0300; fax orders 03-9349 3016)

Outside North America and Australia

  Blackwell Science, Ltd.

  c/o Marston Book Services, Ltd.

  P.O. Box 269

  Abingdon

  Oxford OX14 4YN

  England

  (Telephone orders: 44-01235-465500; fax orders 44-01235-465555)

Acquisitions: Jim Krosschell

Development: Kathleen Broderick

Production: Karen Feeney

Manufacturing: Lisa Flanagan

Typeset by Best-set Typesetter Ltd., Hong Kong

Printed and bound by Braun-Brumfield, Inc.

© 1996 by Blackwell Science, Inc.

Printed in the United States of America

96 97 98 99 5 4 3 2 1

Contents

Contents

Foreword

Dennis W. Jahnigen, M.D., a nationally known leader in geriatrics, has been invited to be a coeditor of this edition of *Geriatric Medicine*. His experience has led to improved organization and coverage of the growing field of geriatrics in this edition.

It is estimated that by the year 2000, 60 percent of the internist's work will involve care of the elderly. There is rapid growth in nonhospital care settings for the elderly, and the number of nursing home beds are projected to double by the year 2000. In order to meet these changing demands, it is essential that primary care physicians become increasingly proficient as acute and chronic care providers of the elderly population. In the present edition we have organized the material into basic subjects; general geriatric care, geriatric syndromes, and common diseases. We have added specific chapters on emergency department care, home care, and nursing home care. We have addressed the problems of confusional states, falls, and fractures. Other new chapters include perioperative care and geriatric rehabilitation, as well as more coverage on ethical concerns in geriatric care. Ethnic issues, gynecology, and thermoregulation are covered by the foremost leaders in the field. It is our hope that the material covered in this edition of *Geriatric Medicine* brings state-of-the-art information to primary care physicians and geriatric specialists alike.

Robert W. Schrier, M.D.

Preface

My wife's grandmother was virtually blind for the last several years of her life prior to her death at age 104; yet she enjoyed flowers, trees, and all of nature in a manner as to enrich the lives of those around her. In such a relationship, it is clear that there are strengths in many of our aged population that we must strive to reveal and nurture. Our society has become so enamored of youth and physical beauty that old age is feared by many. This fear must not allow us to forget the grace, wisdom, and humanity that can only be imbued in our spirits by the experiences accrued from the passing of the years. It is likely that these spiritual qualities of older age allowed Grandma Moses to paint her famous *Christmas Eve* at the age of 100 and Michelangelo to finish his *Last Judgment* in the Sistine Chapel at age 66. George Bernard Shaw continued to write when he was in his eighties, and one of his inspirational quotations from *Back to Methuselah*, which has meant much to me, is "You see things; and you may say, Why? But I dream things that never were; and I say Why not?" The old as well as the young have the spiritual gift to dream and ask why not. As physicians, we must commit ourselves to preserve the function and health of our older citizens so that their dreams can enrich future generations.

In the play *The Elephant Man*, the physician, Mr. Frederick Treves, tells John Merrick, the patient suffering from neurofibromatosis, "We cannot cure you but we can care for you." Out of that caring emerged a kindly and creative spirit that endeared John Merrick to London society, although physical beauty and good health were not his to possess. As physicians, we may be able to cure the diseases of the elderly only infrequently, but we can always project a feeling of caring to our aged patients. We must encourage our aged citizens to share with us their wisdom, courage, and spiritual strength, because these should be ingredients of the basic moral fiber of any society.

A lesson that physicians and nonphysicians alike must remember was stated by Samuel Johnson in *The Rambler*: "He that would pass the latter part of life with honor and decency, must when he is young, consider that he shall one day be old and remember when he is old that he was once young."

D.W.J.
R.W.S.

Acknowledgments

We want to acknowledge the excellent support of Ginger Vaughn and Cheri Burge in the organization and preparation of the manuscripts, and Shirley Artese who assisted with the editing process. The quotations throughout the book were chosen by Barbara Schrier. In this endeavor, as in everything we undertake, the support of our spouses has been a critical and constant source of inspiration.

Dennis W. Jahnigen, M.D.
Robert W. Schrier, M.D.

DEDICATION

To our parents,
whose courage, wisdom, and humanity
have enriched our lives.

It is too late! Ah, nothing is too late
Till the tired heart shall cease to palpitate.
Cato learned Greek at eighty; Sophocles
Wrote his grand Odeipus, and Simonides
Bore off the prize of verse from his compeers,
When each had numbered more than four-score years, . . .
Chaucer, at Woodstock with the nightingales,
At sixty wrote the Canterbury Tales;
Goeth at Weimar, toiling to the last,
Completed Faust when eighty years were past.
These are indeed exceptions; but they show
How far the gulf-stream of our youth may flow
Into the arctic regions of our lives . . .
For age is opportunity no less
Than youth itself, though in another dress,
And as the evening twilight fades away
The sky is filled with stars, invisible by day.

Longfellow, Morituri Salutamus, 1.238

Contributors

Jerome G. Alpiner, PhD
Coordinator of Audiology, Auchology, and Speech
  Pathology Service
Veterans Administration Medical Center
Denver, Colorado

Steven W. Andresen, D.O.
Staff Physician Hematology/Medical Oncology
The Cleveland Clinic Foundation
Cleveland, Ohio

William P. Arend, MD
Professor of Medicine
Head, Division of Rheumatology
University of Colorado School of Medicine
Denver, Colorado

Jeffrey Astroth, DDS
Associate Professor of Dentistry
University of Colorado School of Dentistry
Director of Dentistry
Division of Geriatrics
University Hospital
Denver, Colorado

Richard R. Augspurger, MD
Associate Clinical Professor of Surgery
University of Colorado School of Medicine
Denver, Colorado

Hugh R.K. Barber, MD
Professor of Clinical Obstetrics and Gynecology
Cornell University Medical College
Director, Department of Obstetrics and Gynecology
Lennox Hill Hospital
New York, New York

Douglas B. Berkey, DMD, MPH, MS
Associate Professor and Chair
Department of Applied Dentistry
University of Colorado School of Dentistry
Denver, Colorado

Robert H. Binstock, PhD
Professor of Aging, Health, and Society
Department of Epidemiology and Biostatistics
Case Western Reserve School of Medicine
Cleveland, Ohio

Raymond A. Borazanian, BS
Technical Editor
Cleveland Journal of Medicine
The Cleveland Clinic Foundation
Cleveland, Ohio

Walter M. Bortz, MD
Clinical Associate Professor of Medicine
Stanford University
Stanford, California
Physician
Palo Alto Medical Foundation
Palo Alto, California

William R. Brown, MD
Professor of Medicine
Division of Gastroenterology and Hepatology
Department of Medicine
University of Colorado School of Medicine
Chief, Gastroenterology
Veterans Administration Medical Center
Denver, Colorado

Kenneth Brummel-Smith, MD
Associate Professor of Medicine and Family Medicine
Oregon Health Sciences University
Acting Chief, Section of Geriatrics
Portland Veterans Administration Medical Center
Portland, Oregon

Gordon J. Chelune, PhD, ABPP
Head, Section of Neuropsychology
Department of Neurology and Psychiatry and
    Psychology
The Cleveland Clinic Foundation
Cleveland, Ohio

Ronnie Chernoff, MhD, RD
Professor of Nutrition and Dietetics
University of Arkansas for Medical Science
Associate Director, GRECC
John L. McMellan Memorial Veterans Hospital
Little Rock, Arkansas

David H. Collier, MD
Associate Professor of Medicine
University of Colorado School of Medicine
Chief of Rheumatology
Denver Health Medical Center
Denver, Colorado

E. David Crawford, MD
Professor and Chairman
Division of Urology
University of Colorado School of Medicine
Denver, Colorado

Michael D. Cressman, DO
Associate Professor for Clinical Pharmacology
University of Pittsburgh Medical Center
Pittsburgh, Pennsylvania

Marilyn Davis, RN, MS
Senior Project Manager
Integrated Therapeutics
Schering-Plough
Kenworth, New Jersey

Robert Donahue, MD
Professor of Surgery
Division of Urology
University of Colorado School of Medicine
Denver, Colorado

Christopher M. Filley, MD
Associate Professor of Neurology and Psychiatry
University of Colorado School of Medicine
Staff Neurologist
Veterans Administration Medical Center
Denver, Colorado

James E. Fitzpatrick, MD, COL, MC
Associate Clinical Professor, Department of
    Dermatology
University of Colorado School of Medicine
Denver, Colorado
Chief, Department of Dermatology
Fitzsimmons Army Medical Center
Aurora, Colorado

David S. Geldmacher, MD
Assistant Professor of Neurology
Case Western Reserve University
Clinical Director, Alzheimer Center
University Hospitals of Cleveland
Cleveland, Ohio

John G. Gerber, MD
Professor of Medicine and Pharmacology
Division of Clinical Pharmacology and Toxicology, and
    Division of Infectious Diseases
University of Colorado School of Medicine
Department of Medicine
University Hospital
Denver, Colorado

Ray W. Gifford, MD
Professor of Internal Medicine
Ohio State University College of Medicine
Columbus, Ohio
Consultant, Department of Nephrology and
    Hypertension
The Cleveland Clinic Foundation
Cleveland, Ohio

Martin J. Gorbien, MD
Assistant Professor of Medicine
University of Chicago Pritzker School of Medicine
Section of Internal Medicine
University of Chicago Hospitals
Chicago, Illinois

William R. Hiatt, MD
Professor of Medicine
University of Colorado School of Medicine
Denver, Colorado

Fred D. Hofeldt, MD
Professor of Medicine
University of Colorado School of Medicine
Denver, Colorado
Acting Director of Medicine
Denver Health Medical Center
Denver, Colorado

Alan S. Hollister, MD, PhD
Associate Professor of Medicine and Pharmacology
University of Colorado School of Medicine
Denver, Colorado

Thomas Hornick, MD
Assistant Professor of Medicine
Case Western Reserve University
Cleveland Veterans Administration Medical Center
Cleveland, Ohio

Richard L. Hughes, MD
Director, University of Colorado Affiliated Hospitals'
    Stroke Project
Department of Neurology
Denver Health Medical Center
Denver, Colorado

Evelyn Hutt, MD
Assistant Clinical Professor
University of Colorado School of Medicine
Clinical Geriatrician
Swedish Medical Center
Denver, Colorado

Dennis W. Jahnigen, MD
Goodstein Professor of Geriatrics
University of Colorado School of Medicine
Director, Center on Aging
University of Colorado Health Sciences Center
Denver, Colorado

Fran E. Kaiser, MD
Professor of Medicine
St. Louis University Medical School
Associate Director, Division of Geriatric Medicine
Director, Sexual Dysfunction Clinic
Director, Menopause Clinic
St. Louis University Health Sciences Center
St. Louis, Missouri

Paul R. Katz, MD
Associate Professor of Medicine
University of Rochester School of Medicine and
    Dentistry
Medical Director
Monroe Community Hospital
Rochester, New York

Timothy Keay, MD, MA
Assistant Professor of Geriatrics
Department of Family Medicine
University of Maryland School of Medicine
Baltimore, Maryland

Talmadge E. King, Jr. MD
Executive Vice President for Clinical Affairs
National Jewish Center for Immunology and
    Respiratory Medicine
Vice Chairman for Clinical Affairs
University of Colorado School of Medicine
Professor of Medicine
Division of Pulmonary Sciences and Critical Care
    Medicine
University of Colorado School of Medicine
Denver, Colorado

Deborah C. Koltai, PhD
Bryan Alzheimer's Disease Research Center
Duke University Medical Center
Durham, North Carolina

Kenneth J. Koval, MD
Chief, Fracture Service
Hospital for Joint Disease
New York, New York

Jerome Kowal, MD
Professor of Medicine
Case Western Reserve University
Attending Physician-Medical
University Hospitals of Cleveland
Cleveland, Ohio

Andrew M. Kramer, MD
Associate Professor of Geriatric Medicine
Director of Research, Division of Geriatrics
University of Colorado Health Sciences Center
Denver, Colorado

F. Marc LaForce, MD
Professor of Medicine
University of Rochester School of Medicine and
    Dentistry
Rochester, New York
Physician-in-Chief, Department of Medicine
The Genesee Hospital
Rochester, New York

Roger H.S. Langston, MD, CM, FACS
Cornea Services, Division of Ophthalmology
The Cleveland Clinic Foundation
Cleveland, Ohio

Randall E. Lee, MD
Assistant Professor of Medicine
University of California, Davis
Staff Gastroenterologist
Veterans Affairs Northern California
David Grant USAF Medical Center
Travis AFB, California

Moshe Levi, MD
Professor of Medicine
The University of Texas Southwestern Medical School
Chief, Renal Section
Dallas Veterans Affairs Medical Center
Dallas, Texas

JoAnn Lindenfeld, MD
Professor of Medicine
University of Colorado School of Medicine
Director, Heart Failure and Transplant Clinic
University Hospital
Denver, Colorado

Scott L. Mader, MD
Assistant Professor of Medicine
Oregon Health Sciences Center
ACOS/Extended Care
Veterans Affairs Medical Center
Portland, Oregon

David E. Mann, MD
Associate Professor of Medicine
University of Colorado School of Medicine
Director, Cardiac Electrophysiology Laboratory
University Hospital
Denver, Colorado

Spero Manson, PhD
Professor of Psychiatry
University of Colorado School of Medicine
Director, National Center for American and Alaska
    Natives
Mental Health Research
Denver, Colorado

Frank H. Marsh, JD, PhD
Professor, Center for Applied and Professional Ethics
University of Tennessee College of Medicine
Professor of Medicine
University of Tennessee Medical Center
Knoxville, Tennessee

Lynn Mason, PhD
Assistant Dean, Graduate School
University of Colorado Health Sciences Center
Denver, Colorado

Kevin McCully, PhD
Assistant Professor of Medicine
Medical College of Pennsylvania and Hahnemann
    University School of Medicine
Philadelphia, Pennsylvania

Lawrence A. Meredith, MD
Clinical Assistant Professor of Neurology
Behavioral Neurology Section
University of Colorado School of Medicine
Denver, Colorado

Donna L. Miller, D.O.
Department of Internal Medicine
The Cleveland Clinic Foundation
Cleveland, Ohio

Paul D. Miller, MD
Clinical Professor of Medicine
University of Colorado School of Medicine
Medical Director
Colorado Center for Bone Research
Lakewood, Colorado

Alison A. Moore, MD, MPH
Assistant Professor of Medicine
UCLA School of Medicine
UCLA Medical Center
Los Angeles, California

Michael G. Moran, MD
Associate Professor of Psychiatry
University of Colorado School of Medicine
Director of Psychiatry
National Jewish Center for Immunology and
    Respiratory Medicine
Denver, Colorado

Nora E. Morgenstern, MD
Associate Professor
Stanford Medical School
Stanford, California
Department of Medicine, Division of Geriatrics
University Hospital
Denver, Colorado

John E. Morley, MD
Dammeet Professor of Gerontology
Division Director, Geriatric Medicine
St. Louis University School of Medicine
St. Louis University Hospital
St. Louis, Missouri

Laura Mosqueda, MD
Assistant Professor and Chair of Geriatrics
Department of Family Medicine
University of Southern California School of Medicine
Los Angeles, California

Kenneth B. Newman, MD
Associate Professor of Medicine
Pulmonary and Critical Care Medicine
University of Cincinnati College of Medicine
Cincinnati, Ohio

Sylvia K. Oboler, MD
Associate Professor of Medicine
University of Colorado Health Sciences Center
Denver, Colorado
Assistant Chief, Ambulatory Care
Veterans Administration Medical Center
Denver, Colorado

Biff F. Palmer, MD
Associate Professor of Internal Medicine
University of Texas Southwestern Medical Center
Director of Chronic Dialysis Unit & Peritoneal Dialysis
    Program
Parkland Memorial Hospital
Dallas, Texas

Robert M. Palmer, MD
Head, Section of Geriatric Medicine
Department of Internal Medicine
The Cleveland Clinic Foundation
Cleveland, Ohio

Joel Posner, MD
Professor of Medicine
Medical College of Pennsylvania and Hahnemann
    University School of Medicine
Philadelphia, Pennsylvania

Stephen G. Post, PhD
Associate Professor
Center for Biomedical Ethics
Case Western Reserve University School of Medicine
Cleveland, Ohio

Karyn P. Prochoda, MD
Instructor, Department of Medicine
University of Colorado School of Medicine
Denver Veterans Affairs Medical Center
Denver, Colorado

Judith G. Regensteiner
Associate Professor of Medicine
University of Colorado School of Medicine
Denver, Colorado

David B. Reuben, MD
Associate Professor of Medicine
University of California, Los Angeles, School of
    Medicine
University of California, Los Angeles Medical Center
Los Angeles, California

Terri Richardson, MD
Assistant Professor
University of Colorado School of Medicine
Medical Director
Eastside Health Center, Denver Health Medical Center
Denver, Colorado

Jeffrey M. Robbins, DPM
Chairman, Department of Community Medicine
Professor, Podiatric Medicine
Ohio College of Podiatric Medicine
Chief, Podiatry Section
Cleveland Veterans Affairs Medical Center
Cleveland, Ohio

Laurence J. Robbins, MD
Associate Professor of Medicine
University of Colorado School of Medicine
Associate Chief of Staff
Geriatrics and Extended Care
Veterans Administration Medical Center
Denver, Colorado

Vivyenne Roche, MB
Clinical Instructor
Section of Geriatric Medicine
Veterans Administration Medical Center
Denver, Colorado

Matthew Rydberg, MD
Medical Officer
Kayenta Public Health Service
Kayenta, Arizona

Arthur B. Sanders, MD, FACP
Professor, Section of Emergency Medicine
Department of Surgery
University of Arizona College of Medicine
Attending Physician
Emergency Medicine
University Medical Center
Tuscon, Arizona

Milton J. Schleve, MD
Dermatologic Surgeon
Sorkin Dermatology Associates
Staff Physician
St. Joseph Hospital
Denver, Colorado

Robert W. Schrier, MD
Professor and Chairman, Department of Medicine
University of Colorado School of Medicine
Denver, Colorado

Paul A. Seligman, MD
Professor of Medicine
University of Colorado School of Medicine
Staff Physician
University Hospital
Denver, Colorado

John F. Steiner, MD, MPH
Associate Professor of Medicine
University of Colorado School of Medicine
Attending Physician
University Hospital
Denver, Colorado

George Taler, MD
Assistant Professor
Family Medicine
University of Maryland School of Medicine
Baltimore, Maryland

Peter J. Whitehouse, MD, PhD
Professor of Neurology
Division of Geriatric Neurology
Case Western Reserve University
Director, Alzheimer Center
University Hospitals of Cleveland
Cleveland, Ohio

Margaret-Mary G. Wilson, MCRP (UK)
Subspecialty Resident
Department of Internal Medicine
Division of Geriatric Medicine
St. Louis University Medical Sciences Center
The Geriatric Research, Education and Clinical Center
Veterans Admisistration Center
St. Louis, Missouri

Eugene E. Wolfel, MD
Associate Professor of Medicine
Division of Cardiology
University of Colorado School of Medicine
Denver, Colorado

Joseph D. Zuckerman, MD
Associate Professor of Orthopaedic Surgery
New York University School of Medicine
Chairman, Department of Orthopaedic Surgery
Hospital for Joint Diseases
New York, New York

Part I   Principles of Aging

Chapter 1
Human Aging—Normal and Abnormal

Walter M. Bortz

To know how to grow old is the master work of wisdom, and one of the most difficult chapters in the great art of living.

Henri Frederic Amiel (1821–1881)
L.J. Peter, Peter's Quotations: Ideas for Our Time

Geriatrics is the richest domain in the field of medicine. This fact has been wonderfully captured by Steel and Williams in their article "Geriatrics—The Fruition of the Clinician" (1). Geriatric medicine ordains that the whole person is the object for study and care, not just his or her parts. Further, the person is viewed not at a singular moment, but over time. The encounter, then, is not an isolated point, but the area under the curve, otherwise known as continuity of care.

Geriatric medicine is even more than the care of the whole person over a period of time. It is the care of a whole person over a period of time in a rich environmental matrix that presents a complex set of psychosocial and economic realities. The patient is shaped by the matrix and, in turn, shapes the environment to a large extent. This shifting, reciprocal relationship is constantly challenging.

Geriatric medicine evokes from the practitioner the best of clinical, psychological, and social skills. It evokes—indeed demands—an integrated approach by the physician to the patient. The physician-patient interface is augmented by allied health professionals. In no other branch of medicine is the concept of teamwork as important to patient care.

Geriatrics' symmetric, professional relative is pediatrics, which has appropriately emphasized developmental processes in its study domain. Recently, geriatrics has also included developmental biology in its reach. The work of Baltes (2) and of Schaie and Willis (3) has documented how competence can continue to grow into old age. In fact, geriatrics can be viewed as mainly developmental *and* undevelopmental (frailty), no longer constrained by hereditable features central in pediatrics. Recognition of developmental and undevelopmental forces in geriatrics encourages a conceptual framework that emphasizes function over form, becoming over being, dynamics over stasis. The framework becomes not "What diseases does the patient have?" so much as "What can the patient do?"

Yates has coined the phrase "homeodynamics" to describe the ongoing, interreactive relationship of the aging person with the environment (4). Homeodynamics represents a more insightful term than Cannon's "homeostasis" (5) in that it reveals an awareness of the constantly integrating complexity of the machinery of life. Geriatric medicine encompasses a newly evolved, richly descriptive framework. Care of older people mandates a continuous identification of the participation of time in people's lives. Similarly, it is sensitive to the subjective participation of the patient in the clinical encounter. Standard practice parameters such as blood pressure and cholesterol levels become freely mixed with the patient's highly personal perception of health or illness. The lack of congruity between the patient's rating of wellness-illness and the physician's rating of those conditions has been noted.

We are fortunate that Stewart and others have developed a new descriptive system known as *outcomes technology* at the same time that geriatrics identifies its defining parameters (6). Outcomes technology encompasses all previous clinical domains and enriches them by factoring in subjective and temporal components. Outcomes technology is particularly powerful when applied to problems of geriatric medicine.

Outcomes technology acknowledges that the quality of life has a priority equal to or greater than length of life. As quality is acknowledged, active life expectancy as proposed by Katz et al becomes a validated concept (7). The proposition of active life expectancy asserts that not all life is of equal quality. Clearly, life that is functional has higher personal value than its reciprocal. The activities of daily living (ADLs) and instrumental activities of daily living (IADLs) of Katz et al (8) and Fillenbaum (9) evolved as measurement tools to quantitate active life.

Geriatric medicine is even more precious because it involves caring stewardship at the end of a person's life. Moral and ethical dimensions are the daily business of geriatrics. Issues bearing on the meaning and relevance of being alive are intrinsic to the practice of geriatric medicine. The breadth, depth, and intensity of the experience of being a physician charged with the care of older patients should attract the brightest and the best of our profession. It is our fruition.

Redefining Medicine

Geriatric medicine is new. Its science base is now just emerging. Until now, the student of the illnesses of older persons has been confused by the inadvertent, nonrigorous admixture of conditions that are not strictly attributable to the passage of time. Most biomarkers for aging proposed before now have been wrong (10). Human aging is being redefined (11,12).

One hundred years ago, tuberculosis was thought to indicate aging because mostly older people had the disease. Fifty years ago, arteriosclerosis was thought to indicate aging—an assertion of God's will—"A man is as old as his arteries" (13). These mislabelings appear naive today, but the remnant of too facile categorization of conditions seen in older persons as occurring simply because a person is old is still too prevalent.

As a geriatrician applies discipline in the assay of ailments encountered along the lifespan, a new and simplified description of medicine emerges. Such a derivative

insight may seem presumptuous as a proposition for a new paradigm. Common sense dictates, however, that it is impossible to grasp the wholeness of a play or novel or ball game if the last act or chapter or innings are obscure. Now, as the elements of the last of life become illumined, we are newly able to conceptualize a description of the whole. Pursuit of the basic principles of geriatric medicine leads to derivative conclusions that spread beyond mere consideration of the medical care of older persons. As geriatricians focus more rigorously on the clinical presentations of their patients, it is critical to identify those elements that are preventable, or curable, or immutable.

Without question, medical care for people beyond retirement age has been infiltrated by fatalism that, on closer inspection, is inappropriate. The old punch line, "But Doc, the other leg is just as old and it's fine," still applies to innumerable decision points involving diagnostic and therapeutic issues. As the knowledge base expands, we are newly capable of proposing an organized format that applies not only to persons in the latter part of their lives, but to the entire lifespan of human existence.

Table 1.1 presents a formulation that represents a conceptual framework on which the entirety of medicine can be described. Textbooks of medicine are often organized as a mix of chapter headings: offending agent (tuberculosis); tissue response (allergy); organ or system problems (coronary artery disease, electrolyte imbalance); diagnostic headings (lymphoma); behavioral anomalies (depression); and the like. Such erratic groupings lead to nonconsecutive, nonlinear, ad hoc approaches to illness. Assumption of the newly proposed conceptual framework lends emphasis not only to pathogenic mechanisms but, more important, leads directly to consistent themes of therapy. Further, this format implies increased emphasis on function without cost to diagnosis of disease. This is

Table 1.1. Categories of Human Illness.

Category	Example	Solution
Type I: Blueprint Error	Hereditable diseases	Genetic engineering, eugenics
Type II: Extrinsic Agency	Infection, trauma, malignancy, allergy, toxins	Antibiotics, surgery
Type III: Intrinsic Agency	Heart disease, stroke, musculoskeletal fragility	Behavior modification
Type IV: Aging		Philosophy, ? antioxidants

of more than theoretical value because the domains of remedy that derive from this formulation provide focus to public policy efforts that address the many disjunctions in medical care as it is now provided. As now constituted, too much effort and too many resources are being dedicated to curative efforts; prevention is clearly the appropriate strategy. The immensity of faulty resource allocation can scarcely be overestimated.

Too much pathology has been assigned to the chronology of living. This mechanism is undeniably a participating agency, but it is inappropriately incorporated into major decision making. Rationing by age is rampant (14). Entry into intensive care units, transplant availability, and diagnostic and therapeutic vigor are all prejudiced by chronology, the validity of which is highly suspect (15,16).

One can derive much clarity of insight by dividing human illness into four basic categories: 1) blueprint errors, 2) conditions of external agency, 3) conditions of internal agency, and 4) aging. This framework is similar in many ways to that of the epidemiologist who groups human conditions into three general categories of host, environment, and interaction of host and environment. The current proposition includes the dimension of time. In like fashion, McKeown divided human disease into prenatal disease, diseases of deficiency and poverty, and diseases of maladaptation and affluence (17).

Blueprint errors are nearly exclusively confined to the first part of life. Type I conditions, genetic diseases, comprise the relatively rare and tragic illnesses seen early in life, such as sickle cell disease and cystic fibrosis. These types of diseases result from the unfortunate disruption of the union of healthy or flawed chromosomes from the two parents. The bad seed results. Substantial progress is being made in our understanding of the basic problems inherent in this blueprint error and leads logically to the evolution of strategies that can counteract the basic flaws in the design. This recognition is critical to our conceptualization of all human illness, especially geriatric medicine. An almost universally accepted axiom is that if a person wants to achieve longevity, the most important action to take is to select long-lived ancestors. Innumerable evidence shows that correlation of the lifespan of a parent and child is weak, and that any correlation virtually disappears for advanced ages. A recent paper reviewing a large collection of twin records from Denmark

reported that monozygotic twins (average age of death, 72 years) died 14.1 years apart, dizygotic twins 18.5 years apart, and a control group of nonrelated pairs of similar ages died 19.2 years apart. The authors concluded, as had others before them, that genetic influence on longevity, although present, is relatively minor and that environmental influences predominate (18). The basic implication of this knowledge is that one cannot assume that just because one's ancestors lived long, or short, this factor is hereditable and, therefore, immutable. Longevity derives primarily from the individual, not from the family tree. For older persons, it is not the hardware of life that is predominantly at issue, it is the software.

The second category, conditions of external agency, is the area that has occupied the bulk of medical experience and involvement to date. This is the domain in which the environment plays the principal role. The host, the patient, plays the second, passive role. Infections, toxins, accidents, carcinogens, allergens, and violence are the main inciting agents. Direct counteractive strategies emerge – avoidance, immunization, and the magic bullet of antibiotics and antitoxins to abet surgical efforts to neutralize or reverse environmental assaults on the organism. Without question, much of the success and glory of medical science of the past 50 years emerges from this category. At the start of this century, eight of the top 10 killers were of category 2, and all eight of them have been eliminated or drastically controlled (19). These diseases tend to be episodic, are mostly unpredictable, and often lack a time component. A large percentage of malignancies has been attributed to environmental causes (20). Unfortunately, the conditions that are killing people now do not yield to the conceptually simple, direct proximate cause and proximate remedy approaches inherent in category 2 conditions.

In conditions of category 3, those of internal agency, the environment does not constitute a hostile, affecting force. In the normally functioning individual, the environment acts as the mechanism that assures anabolic form and function, which guarantees the integrity and vitality of the organism. Category 3 illnesses result from an inappropriate interfacing of the host person with the environment – either too much (stress) or too little (disuse). Category 3 conditions now dominate the medical arena. The chronic degenerative conditions of vascular compromise, musculoskeletal disorders, and several affective conditions are grouped in category 3. The conditions of internal agency have time as an integral participant; they occur after protracted, inappropriate interfacing of the individual with the environment. Broadly observed stress, as an excessive energetic burden, and disuse, as an insufficient workload, are operative in category 3 when an improperly modulated interaction of the individual with his or her lifestyle prevails.

Because category 3 conditions have their origin within the organism, they must also have their primary correction within the organism. Sixty years ago, Selye proposed the *general adaptation syndrome*, a set of conditions commonly found together that were the result not of a singular acute assault on the organism, but the result of the end product of a series of noxious and oppressive attacks (i.e., stress) (21). Selye's conceptualization of this constellation of findings included ulcer, diabetes, hypertension, and kidney changes. These conditions had as their root mechanism the excess production of corticosteroids, which was, in turn, a response to an overly stimulated autonomic nervous system. Sapolsky has extended Selye's seminal studies (22).

But, just as the organism reacts adversely to excessive energetic throughput, it also suffers (in my judgment, even more quantitatively) from insufficient interaction with the environment. As Boswell wrote, "Acute diseases are from Heaven and chronical from ourselves: the dart of death, indeed, falls from heaven, but we poison it by our own misconduct: to die is the fate of man; but to die with lingering anguish is generally his folly" (23). Whereas drugs and surgery are often employed in category 3 conditions, their use is ancillary and thereby less effective. We do not cure heart attacks, strokes, emphysema, diabetes, arthritis, and other such conditions by magic bullets. Category 2 remedies merely palliate category 3 conditions. If success is to be forthcoming with conditions of internal agency, preventive strategies that use behavioral modifications are directly appropriate. These strategies connote design of life activities that are neither too frenetic (stress) nor too lax (disuse). Each part of our bodies achieves and maintains optimal function when the appropriate energetic stimulus is applied. Too much or too little leads to disordered function and structure that, over time, becomes pathologic in degree. Further, preventive strategies carry with them the advantages of low cost, accessibility, and safety—elements that are generally lacking in category 2 remedies.

Figure 1.1 represents the time appearance of the four illness categories. Aside from extrinsic forces that occur randomly throughout life, such as accidents, the middle years are relatively immune from deterioration. However, at midlife, the condition secondary to intrinsic agencies, those caused by inappropriate interfacing of the host and environment, become clinically apparent. The latent period between the initiation of the maladaptation (usually around 30 years of age) and the clinical appearance of illness secondary to the failure of homeodynamic

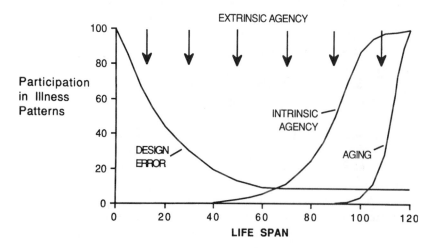

Figure 1.1. Life calendar of offending agencies.

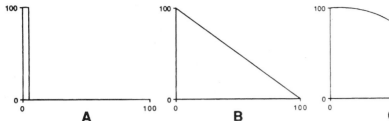
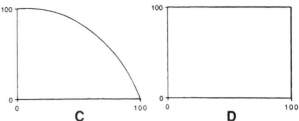

Figure 1.2. Four theoretical survival graphs.

process is a result of our redundant capacities and to the slow pace of loss.

To illustrate this formulation, one could imagine analogous the scenarios that could occur when 100 new coffee cups appear in a new restaurant. Four possible survival experiences would occur (Figure 1.2). In model A, in which all cups break on the first day of business, design error is likely. The cups' construction was simply not up to the rigors of normal existence. Model B indicates that each day one cup breaks; at the end of 100 days, all 100 cups are gone. This rate of loss conforms to category 2 of the medical reformulation model above and closely mirrors the human survival curves seen in America at the end of the 1800s. Model C shows that nearly all cups last for 50 days, but then a marked breakage occurs. A few cups endure to old age, but only a few. This is our present human survival curve and conforms to category 3 conditions in which breakage appears as a result of accumulated assaults for which self-corrective efforts are insufficient to prevent damage. Model D represents the ideal, rectangularized curve in which all cups last the full 100-day survival range, at which time they all break secondary to onboard physicochemical decay (system failure).

It is evident that many illnesses exhibit several participating agencies. Malignancies often show a genetic tendency, an environmental provocation, and a host responsiveness. Immune disorders and osteoarthritis also have multiple origins, yet the emphasis on primary agency, although not specific in these cases, is nonetheless helpful in assigning appropriate analytic strategies.

Much has been written about the heterogeneity of older persons. In my view, the heterogeneity springs not from the nature of aging itself, but from the fact that older persons exhibit infinite combination of disease, stress, and disuse mingled with their chronologic change. As we become increasingly competent in the prevention and reversibility of type II and type III conditions, we will have a pure model of aging. Now we die of component failure. Eventually we will die of systems failure. The "one hoss shay" will become real, "all at once and nothing first just as bubbles when they burst" (24).

Redefining Aging

What is aging? As mentioned above, human aging has lacked a theoretical access. Geriatric textbooks are full of the many changes seen in older people, but it is evident that most of the changes previously ascribed to aging are not thus ascribable. In fact, the list of somatic changes that can be strictly ascribable to chronologic decay is short. Yates proposed that senescence, which he describes as a set of age-driven catabolic events, begins at maturity (4). Like the biologist's halting efforts to describe life, medicine has had trouble defining aging. It has lacked critical insight into the basic nature of aging, mainly because of its rootedness in the first categories of illness. The theoretical thermophysicists, most notably Prigogine (25) and coworkers from Brussels and Austin, produced a format derived from a deeper probe into the nature of the second law of thermodynamics, which enables access to a conceptual framework for aging. The three basic components of any analysis of aging are energy, matter, and time. A terse and rigorous definition of aging to encompass these three elements would be: *aging is the effect of an energy flow on matter over time.* The second law of thermodynamics asserts that any isolated system tends inevitably to a less orderly state caused by the irreversible loss of energy, usually as heat, to the environment. The progressive tendency to disorder is termed *entropy*. Death is the final entropic event. Yet life exists as an apparent contradiction to this law. Atkins wrote, "coherence is intrinsically transient and crumbles into incoherence when the structure ceases to be driven by a flow of energy" (26). The final answer to the question of whether mankind can uncover some strategy to offset the catabolic arrows of nonlinear, nonequilibrium thermodynamics and thereby prolong life and export death is unknown, but at least we are starting to know how to ask the important questions. Yates believes that humans as self-organizing systems are ultimately beholden to senescence and mortality, because, after maturity, those forces that originally give us form and function reach their limits and thereby cause death (4). Metabolism and time cause death.

Despite its limitations and exceptions, the rate-of-living theory proposed by Rubner (27) and refined by Pearl (28) provides a rationale for conforming the lifespan of various species. Walford calculated that each gram of animal protoplasm processes 10,000 calories per lifetime. "A mouse in its two- or three-year lifetime processes the same amount of energy as does an elephant in its lifetime of 55 or 60 years" (29). Only the mouse does it faster.

The two important experimental maneuvers used to manipulate lifespan are cooling and restricted feeding. The cooling technique, first discovered early in this century at the Rockefeller Institute, is applicable only to invertebrates (fruit flies) and cold-blooded animals (fish). The length of life of these creatures can be dialed precisely by raising or lowering the temperature of their environment. The length of life is doubled or halved for every 10° Centigrade lowered or raised. This is strikingly similar to the kinetic properties of chemical reactions. The relevance of this basic observation to the wear-and-tear theory of longevity is evident.

The mechanism of the restricted feeding model of life extension, first demonstrated by McCay 50 years ago, is less clear (30). Superficially, one might presume that a similar slowdown secondary to reduced caloric availability should result in a lowered metabolic rate, and thereby conform to the rate-of-living theory. However, Masoro has meticulously demonstrated that restricted feeding does not result in a lowered metabolic rate (31). Nevertheless, Gavrilov and Gavrilova projected that the lessened

substrate availability and metabolic throughput could result in less wear and tear without altering the basic metabolic rate (32). Clarification of this area is anticipated.

If one accepts that aging is an example of the second law of thermodynamics at work and that its ultimate entropic event, death, represents a sum total of damage scores that overcome the body's compensatory abilities (33), it is logical to assay which bodily alterations in structure and function appear to be time driven, category 4, conditions.

Mechanism of Aging

Metabolism has a cost. Its cost, paradoxically, occurs because our metabolism is oxygen driven. Oxygen is toxic to many inanimate objects. It rusts, and it supports catabolic conflagration. Dean has called oxygen a "molecular terrorist" (Dean C, personal communication, 1995). Coincident to its intimate participation in all oxidative biochemical reactions is the by-product generation of several forms of highly toxic chemically reactive oxygen atoms. These supercharged, free radical particles serve to create various forms of mischief and result in denaturation of protein, disruption of DNA, breakage of mitochondrial elements, creation of adverse cross-linkages, and stiffening of membranes—all as a result of our immersion in an oxygen-rich atmosphere. Ames et al calculated that oxygen free radicals are responsible for 10,000 DNA modifications per cell per day (34). Wei et al found a linear decrease of 0.61 percent per year of DNA repair capacity in skin samples (35). It has also been suggested that the finite number of cell replications observable in the Hayflick phenomenon (36) may ultimately be the result of oxidative damage to DNA.

It is important to note that the human organism, like all life, is not an isolated system. It is in active interchange with the environment. Schrodinger's description of life as "sucking orderliness from its environment" is memorable (37). This interchange enables repair mechanisms and a degree of respite from the oxidative havoc discussed above. Three enzyme classes—glutathione reductase, catalase, and superoxide dismutase—catalyze a number of biochemical reactions that scavenge the free radicals. Similarly, a number of compounds including ascorbic acid, vitamin E, and beta carotene have antioxidant effects. Studies that have shown correlation between life span and DNA repair mechanisms and levels of superoxide dismutase are highly notable (38). The contribution of these studies to the overall question of human longevity is, however, unestablished at present. Several years ago, Schneider and Reed concluded, "The available evidence at this time does not support recommending diet supplements for either life extension or prevention of cancer" (39).

The issue of physical exercise and peroxidative reactions is interesting. Hypothetically, exercise, by virtue of its increase of oxidative performance, would hasten free radical damage. Indeed, there are numerous reports that indicate that a bout of exercise does generate increased levels of toxic compounds (40). But this reality is immediately challenged by other reports that indicate that antioxidative enzyme levels are also increased by exercise, so that the net effect of physical exercise and peroxidative damage is damped or eliminated. Such a proposition is kindred to the proposition that all creatures possess the same number of heartbeats per lifetime. Exercise would be presumed to use up the allotment more precociously; however, it is well recognized that the pulse rate of a conditioned person not exercising is substantially slower than that of the unfit person; thus, the gross effect is offset.

Yates proposes that senescence occurs as the result of the changes produced by damage and that exceed repair capacity (4). Similarly, Gavrilov and Gavrilova suggest that age changes occur as the result of "signal to noise" deterioration (32). Life, at the present time, is an incurable condition.

Rate of Aging

How fast do we age? Shock, in a frequently referenced figure first presented in 1960, recorded declines of 15 to 90 percent in the following functional capacities — renal, cardiac, respiratory, basal metabolic rate (BMR), conduction velocity, and cell water — in subjects from 35 to 90 years of age (41). These percentages, however, were contaminated by inadvertent inclusion in the study samples of individuals with subclinical disease. Nevertheless, in my view, the feature of disuse has been at least as great a confounder of our understanding of the rate of true chronologically determined age change (42). Mooradian (43) and Evans and Rosenberg (10) have emphasized that all previous

biomarkers of aging have been in error. In fact, until now, almost everything we have thought about aging has been wrong.

To discuss the actual rate of age changes, it is necessary to place functionality in a quantitative form. Humans are blessed with much redundant function. We have two eyes, two ears, two lungs, two kidneys, two testicles or ovaries — one of any of these would serve just as well. This means that we can sacrifice 50 percent of original capacity with no apparent decline in performance. We can run a marathon with one lung, excrete all our waste materials with one kidney, or perfuse our tissues with 50 percent arterial luminal obstruction. It is not until 70 percent of maximal capacity is surrendered that clinical dysfunction appears (44). When another 10 percent is lost and only 20 percent remains, death lurks. This means that the standard contact point between physician and patient usually occurs when the patient experiences 20 to 30 percent of maximal function. The morbidity zone is the point at which most encounters occur and most expenses accrue. Compression or expansion of morbidity occurs in the 20 to 30 percent margin. For example, by analogy, if a person has $150,000 in a checking account, the person can accommodate a free-wheeling lifestyle. If the person has only $15 in the account, however, the person must be vigilant about how large a check can be drawn. Of course, we all have a much better idea of how much money is in our checking accounts than we have about how much health is in our vitality accounts. Small withdrawals over time add up; at a critical moment, black ink turns to red, vitality becomes frailty, and frailty's close cousin, death, appears.

To establish the true rate of age change one must insure that the population under study is free of the two major contaminating conditions of disease and disuse. A study of the Master's athlete best illustrates this criterion. Performance records for running, rowing, and swimming were surveyed and plotted by age groups from 35 years (the age at which most Master's records begin) to beyond 70 years (Bortz W IV, Bortz W II, personal communication, 1995). It is striking to observe that for all endurance and sprint events, the annual rate of decline was approximately 0.5 percent per year. Because participation in such exertion involves maximal participation for most of the body's major systems — circulatory, respiratory,

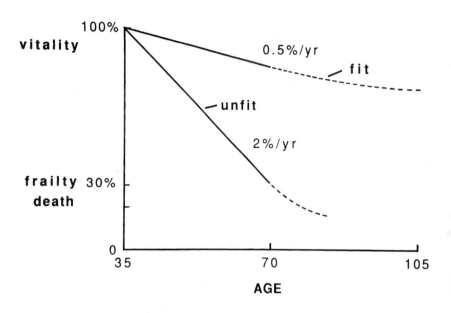

Figure 1.3. Time effect of fitness/ unfitness on vitality. (Reproduced by permission from Blair S, et al. Physical fitness and all-cause mortality: a prospective study of healthy men and women. JAMA 1989;262:2395–2401.)

neuromuscular, metabolic, and thermoregulatory—it is argued that no one of these systems or its components can decay functionally at a rate faster than 0.5 percent per year. In my view, however, 0.5 percent per year represents the maximum rate of deteriorative change that can occur in any and all the systems involved in heavy exercise performance. Kasch et al reported that maximum oxygen consumption (VO_2max) declines at 0.5 percent per year in a group of fit individuals followed longitudinally for 25 years from ages 44 to 79 years (45). Kasch's 0.5 percent per year figure is similar to the earlier VO_2max data of Rogers et al (46), and close to the 0.6 percent figure noted above for DNA damage in skin biopsies (35). These data are derived from fit athletes, but that is not believed to preclude extension of these figures to other fit individuals. The absolute level of performance will be less, but the rate of change is likely the same.

Conversely, the work of Kasch et al reported a decline of 2 percent per year in VO_2max performance in a group of untrained individuals (45). This rate is believed to be sensitive to the degree of lack of fitness. Moreover, absolute bedrest or the casting of a limb results in rates of deterioration in excess of 2 percent per year. Casting a limb for only a few weeks results in a 77 percent fall in the oxidative capacity of the muscles, 2 percent per day (47). Figure 1.3 shows these rates superimposed on the previously established parameters of vitality and frailty. At an aging decay rate of 0.5 percent per year, no threat to vitality occurs until advanced years. It is unknown whether the linearity of changes from ages 35 to 70 is sustainable. The progressive improvement in the athletic records of Master's athletes at the upper ages seems to indicate that further improvement is potentially possible, but a cascade effect may lead to a crescendo through additive effects. In any case, the picture until age 70 is clear. On the other hand, if an unfit individual progressively accumulates 2 percent losses per year, the marker of frailty, 30 percent, will be penetrated by age 70, and morbidity will be evident.

Defining Frailty

In thermophysical terms, frailty is the predictable result of an organism losing contact with its environment (48). The reciprocal of frailty, vitality, can be seen in an analysis of the mechanisms of growth. All living tissues are shaped by their environment to a major degree. This plasticity is generally not recognized. Medical fashion reaches first to genetic codings for causative mechanisms. In my view, particularly with regard to geriatric medicine, a greater appreciation of the effect of environmental-individual interreactivity on structure and function would serve us

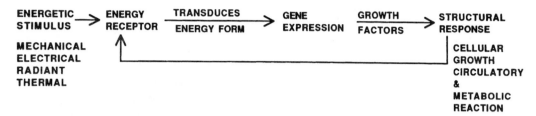

Figure 1.4. Conversion of energetic stimulus to structure. (Reproduced by permission from Bortz W. The physics of frailty. J Am Geriatr Soc 1993;41:1004–1008.)

better. D'Arcy Thompson wrote, "organisms are shaped directly by forces acting upon them: optima of forces are nothing more than the natural states of plastic matter in the presence of appropriate physical forces" (frailty) (49). Ninety-eight percent of the molecules of our body are different from one year to the next. The form of this year's molecules depends on the shaping forces acting on them. Braam and Davis showed that the mere touching of a plant's leaves and stem results in a 100-fold increase in messenger RNA levels within 10 to 30 minutes (50). Trees and shrubs demonstrate vividly by their forms their interreactivity with the sun, wind, and rain of their environments. Humans do the same.

Figure 1.4 displays a representation of the positive feedback loop by which an organism conforms its structures to its environment. Quanta of energy of numerous types—mechanical, radiant, thermal, and electric—confront the body, which is elaborately equipped with batteries of antennae, that capture energy and transduce it to a biologically useful form, mainly through the processes of oxidative phosphorylation. The repackaged energy has two functions—to conduct the business of metabolism and to alert and endow the genic mechanisms with energy for appropriate reactive response. The resulting structural adaptations render the tissue more appropriate to its environment and thus abet the evolutionary process. Only those genes that are directly impacted by the stimulus are expressed. According to Carter et al, "Physical forces act to push/pull cells and their matrix into different juxtapositions, thereby facilitating chemical gradients and physical patterns. These gradients involve growth factors, cytokines, and circulatory, and metabolic adaptations" (51).

Frailty results when anabolic interreactive processes are interrupted (48). The rate of development of frailty depends on the degree of isolation from energetic input, but the rate can be precocious. Frailty can result from the process of aging itself, but is mostly the result of disuse. The composite effects of organismic insulation apply to every aspect of the body, from the subcellular to the whole. No part is immune from the adage "Use it or lose it." The form of use varies according to the function of the particular part. On the basis of the whole body, movement is quantitatively the most important use, since on a mass base alone much of the body is dedicated to the purpose of movement. Yet each cell, tissue, organ, and system has its tasks, and as they perform the task, they conform their structures to that task, brain cells no less than muscle cells, the intestine no less than bones. Positron emission tomography scans show vividly how parts of the brain challenged by an environmental task react with increased circulation and metabolic activity. Diamond's work showed that rats raised in both enriched and deprived circumstances grew (or atrophied) brain cell dendrites to conform to the challenge (52).

Disuse

Aging has as one of its principal threats the potential of disuse. Disuse, in turn, is the principal type of pathogenetic mechanism of category 3 conditions. Numerous expectations provide seeming justification for a withdrawal process as humans age. Changes in the state of health, career status, and family responsibilities all give signals that life holds less challenge and zest. Diminished biologic and social roles create self-fulfilling result. By

Table 1.2. The Disuse Syndrome.

Cardiovascular vulnerability
Musculoskeletal fragility
Immunologic susceptibility
Obesity
Depression
Precocious aging

analogous example, a grandfather's clock, "in arrest," has three diagnoses: it is broken, worn out, or needs to be wound up (11). The same parameters hold for older persons. Repair by winding up may result in a 40-year recapture of earlier vitality.

Table 1.2 incorporates the pathologies of disuse so pervasive in clinical medicine into a single rubric called *the disuse syndrome* (53), similar to the conditions of back pain, heart disease, obesity, and mental disorders grouped by Kraus and Raab (54).

Cardiovascular vulnerability is linked intimately to disuse. Innumerable studies now confirm this connection. Cardiodynamic features, vessel anatomy, blood lipids, and coagulability all participate in vulnerability. A fundamental treatment for hypertension is physical exercise by which the vascular bed is enlarged. Of note is the fact that domesticated animals have smaller heart sizes relative to body weight than do wild animals. The human heart weight to body weight ratio is particularly low (55). Thus, the smaller the heart, the smaller the coronary vessels. Both the coronary vessel diameter and, particularly, the vessel's distensibility resulting from heightened endothelial relaxing factor correlate with fitness levels (55). Poiseuille's Law asserts that the flow through any vessel is proportional to the radius of the vessel to the fourth power. Smaller vessels, such as in women and smaller individuals, are at increased risk for occlusion. The participation of disuse in serum lipid abnormalities is clearly defined. Wood et al demonstrated that one of the major determinants of high-density lipoprotein cholesterol levels is degree of physical activity (57). Of corollary importance is the fact that the fibrinolytic activity of blood also correlates with fitness levels (58). Restated, inactivity leads to stagnant blood, and clot formation soon follows. The three components of vascular disease—vessel corru-

gation and occlusion, lipid abnormality, and blood coagulability—all derive from disuse.

Musculoskeletal fragility is a clear statement of disuse. The classic study of Fiatarone et al presents an impressive discussion of how nonagenarians increased their muscle bulk and strength after a few weeks of pumping iron (59). Space medicine provides further proofs (42). Sex hormones and dietary calcium without exercise are not sufficient to offset osteopenia. Evans coined the term "sarcopenia" to emphasize the major pathologic role that muscle wasting plays in hip and vertebral fractures (10). Obviously, osteopenia and sarcopenia do not have their sole presentation in older people, but they are clearly more common in older persons as small decrements begin to exceed the threshold of structural loss.

Nearly every geriatrics text includes as a change of aging the increase in body fat. That diminished physical activity produces fat accumulation is clear. Mayer repeatedly demonstrated in animal models and humans that there is a progression from lessened activity to fat accumulation to lessened sequence of activity (60). Therapeutically, it is now a consensus that any successful weight loss program must include increased exercise as an integral part of its regimen (61). Caloric restriction alone is futile. Insulin insensitivity and the cascade of pathologies that attend it are clearly related to disuse (62).

Immunologic susceptibility is part of the disuse syndrome. Participation of physical fitness in numerous host to resistance mechanisms is clear (63). As in other areas, however, when exercise is extreme, the benefit of improved immune responsiveness is lost and decreased resistance to infection is apparent. Moderation is apparently the key to beneficial results. Improved T-cell function, cytokine production, cytotoxic protection, and immunoglobulin levels have been documented in fit persons.

Disuse may also participate in tumor formation. Fewer colon (64), lung (65), breast, ovarian, and prostate (66) malignancies are reported in fit persons. How much the decreased incidence of cancer is the result of associated behavioral advantage or of the aspects of fitness itself is uncertain.

There may also be a relationship between allergies and fitness levels (67). The reciprocal relationship between histamine and the catecholamines appears to be tilted favorably by an exercise protocol.

Many psychiatrists regularly suggest a running program in their therapy for depression. Johnsgaard stated, "No depression is severe enough to endure a ten mile run" (68). The validity of this claim is not substantiated, but the sensitivity of the neurotransmitters involved in depression, the catechols and endorphins, certainly is linked to physical activity (69). The pharmacologic employ of antidepressant agents, like other classes of drugs, may be considered to be proxies for a fitness program. The establishment of a walking program for persons aged 85 has been shown to have a marked benefit in measures of quality of life (70). Self-esteem and independence are obviously abetted by an exercise protocol.

Taken in the aggregate, the predictable results of disuse contribute to precocious aging. Satchel Paige's renowned query, "How old would you be if you didn't know how old you were?" reflects sensitivity to degrees of physical fitness. Figure 1.3 shows the functional offset of a fitness protocol to many decades of chronologic decay. Blair et al, in a study of 13,000 individuals with an eight-year follow-up, showed that Darwin was right after all, the fittest survived (71). But within this simple observation, two critical qualifiers stand out. First, the difference between those who do nothing and those who do a little makes the largest quantitative impact. In other words, the first step is the most meaningful. Second, the older we become, the more fitness becomes increasingly powerful as a predictor for survival. Stated in another fashion, fitness for a younger person is optional; fitness for an older person is imperative.

Disengagement

Aligned with and kindred to the biologic catabolic products of disuse are the psychological and sociologic patterns that follow disengagement. For 30 years, psychologists have developed the theory of disengagement (72). It is proposed that a decrease in social interactivity is normal and inevitable with aging. Disengagement connotes lessened social roles and withdrawal from active life. Diminished sexuality for men and women is a further symbol of decline and of lessened quality of life. Such an involutional proposition serves to feed on itself—the more older people retire from the adventures of life, the more the social environment and stimulation retires from them, resulting in an abandonment motif such as is notable in aboriginal cultures. Loss of useful social roles follows disengagement; interactive living becomes contracted.

Carstensen, however, challenges the notion that disengagement is the normative psychosocial course of aging and proposes instead that it represents retreat before an anticipated death (73). To assess this, Carstensen surveyed the gay community and found it to be at least as socially engaged as the straight community—unless members became positive for human immunodeficiency virus (HIV), at which time a marked social retrenchment was noted. When an HIV-positive individual developed clinical acquired immunodeficiency syndrome (AIDS), the individual withdrew and prepared to die.

Therefore, disengagement is shown not to be sensitive to age, but rather to be an active option that is exercised before proximate death. But what if the older individual disengages in his or her sixties, with several decades of potential vital life expectancy ahead? Setting an expectation for a long life helps to fulfill that expectation. Social withdrawal and active aging are incompatible (74). Loss of self-efficacy leads to dependence and a lowered quality of life.

Bandura has done most to enlarge our understanding of self-efficacy (75). Having a sense of control over one's life is clearly a major determinant of satisfaction, and this sense becomes progressively more important as we age. Langer and Rodin wrote, "Control is more likely to affect health than health is to affect control" (76). Aging, with its series of losses, can lead to the helpless-hopeless syndrome proposed by Seligman (77). Losses are real, but of greater importance is the individual's capacity to deal with loss. This is why self-efficacy is so central to successful aging.

Bandura wrote a prescription for self-efficacy much as the physician writes one for penicillin. The components of building self-efficacy are four: first, creation of small steps of mastery; second, provision of peer examples; third, social persuasion by use of knowledge concerning the perceived loss; and fourth, diminishment of supposed cues of failure, such as dyspnea or discomfort when embarking on a walking program.

Maintenance of a high degree of self-efficacy is also central to successful aging. The work of Csikszentmihaly on "flow" is pertinent (78). Flow is described as the process of total involvement with life. Csikszentmihaly studied flow experimentally. Using what he calls the "experience sampling method," Csikszentmihaly asked his subjects to wear an electronic paging device for a week. When a beeper went off randomly, the subjects recorded what they were doing and rated their "flow quotient." The results of this study are challenging. Across cultures, ages, and genders, in thousands of studies, most persons reported high flow states when they were at work, but only one-third as much flow during leisure activities. The higher the professional position, the higher the at-work flow percentage, but even blue collar workers preferred work to leisure at a 2:1 ratio. Television viewing was rated as a particularly low-flow experience. Mastery of adversity appears to be the central theme in the state of flow; individuals not only value mastering of adversity for themselves but also find it praiseworthy in others. Having a sense of control over experience is counterentropic because it requires the active investment of energy. Therefore, disuse and disengagement are seen to be twin pathologies particularly evident and pernicious in older persons. Identification of this pervasive assault on the structural and functional intactness in aging is the central vantage point that can be developed into a comprehensive program of geriatric medicine.

Further extension of the competency of aging has been a central focus of the work of Baltes (2). Baltes identified the ancient dream of excellence, "wisdom," as his experimental domain. He subjected wisdom to the empiric method, much as Csikszentmihaly did with flow. Wisdom was identified as "dealing in the important and difficult matters associated with the conduct of and meaning of life that is directed to the well-being of mankind." Wisdom reflected a maturity of knowledge, judgment, and advice with unusual depth of perspective and tolerance. Specifically, wisdom was defined "as an expert knowledge system in the fundamental pragmatics of life, permitting excellent judgment and advice involving important and uncertain matters of life." Baltes' method consisted of posing of complex social problems and rating the answers on several scales that reflect factual and strategic knowledge, appreciation of context, uncertainty, and tolerance. With this approach, Baltes showed that there is, in general, a scarcity of wisdom across the life

span. However, unlike the results from cognitive performance tests, there was no decline in wisdom with time. Of greater importance, however, was the observation that all of the highest raters were old. In other words, not all old people were wise, but all very wise people were old.

Aggregated experience appears to be the essential component of wisdom. Diamond depicted this graphically; Figure 1.5 reflects her work on enrichment (52). Schaie and Willis, in many studies, showed that a cognitive training program can affect the commonly observed declines in intellectual abilities (3). Carstensen wrote, "It is an illusion that irremedial psychological deterioration is the modal course of old age" (74). Therefore, it appears that the brain, like other organs of the body, like other features of the universe, is optimally conformed to the business of life when energized by a flow of activity. Disuse and disengagement abort full life vitality. Aging can bring gain as well as loss.

Summary and Conclusions

As the dimension of time is applied to the human condition, a central truth emerges. Biologic, psychological and sociologic integrity across the life span is assured by one single, consistent strategy. This strategy is the regular, modulated flow of an energetic stimulus on the body and lifestyle. Too much energy as stress or too little enery as disuse renders the individual at risk so that extrinsic threats that would otherwise be damped and neutralized are rendered pathogenic. Stress and disuse are incremental and are thereby time dependent, but they are not aging because they are preventable and their changes are reversible by reordering the energy level. Changes secondary to stress and disuse are distinct from time-dependent age changes that have the perioxidative debris of metabolism as the inciting agent. The rate of functional decline caused solely by age is less than previously proposed and is likely to be in the range of 0.5 percent per year.

Justice Marie Garibaldi of the New Jersey Supreme Court wrote in *In re* Farrell that "Matters of Fate have become matters of Choice" (79). This powerful summary statement applies wonderfully to the field of geriatric medicine, indeed to medicine as a whole. Until the present knowledge base was established, physicians commonly retired with fatalism when confronted by the con-

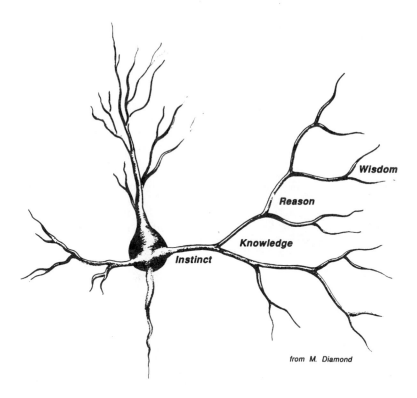

Wisdom

Reason

Knowledge

Instinct

from M. Diamond

Figure 1.5. Structural representation of brain cell complexity. (Reproduced by permission from Diamond M. Extensive cortical depth measurement and neuron size increase in the cortex of environmentally enriched rats. J Comp Neurol 1967;131:357–364.)

ditions encountered in older persons. These problems are always complex, seldom susceptible to a simplistic solution, and thereby often frustrating to professionals accustomed to singular presentations capable of simple description and simple solution. The dimension of time is a further complexity.

What now permits choice and, thereby, an approach to the idealized life design is knowledge. We are newly empowered to sort out the agency of the disorders of older persons. Fortunately, most of the disorders are actively susceptible to prevention and reversal. Major functional improvement is nearly always possible. Yet, there remain true age changes that at the present time are immutable. Yates believes these changes are deeply inscribed and represent the ultimate inability of an organism, once fully developed, to rid itself of the disorderly states inherent in metabolism after maturity has been achieved.

Whether the processes of aging described herein as conforming largely to a 0.5 percent yearly rate will someday be approachable is unknown, but, for the time being, we have enough work to do to insure that our maximal lifespan is approached individually and collectively in as energized, functional capacity as possible. The dying of the light should come late and be abrupt, a consummation rendered possible by the new knowledge brought by geriatric medicine.

References

1. Steel K, Williams KF. Geriatrics: the fruition of the clinician. Arch Intern Med 1974;134:1125–1126.
2. Baltes P. The aging mind: potential and limits. Gerontologist 1993;33:580–594.
3. Schaie KW, Willis S. Can decline in adult intellectual functioning be reversed? Dev Psychol 1986;22:223–30.
4. Yates FE, Benton L. Loss of integration and stability with age: theories and conjectures. In: Masoro E, ed. Handbook of Physiology: aging. Oxford: Oxford University, 1993.
5. Cannon W. Organization for physiologic homeostasis. Physiol Rev 1929;9:399–431.
6. Stewart A, Ware S, eds. Measuring functioning and well being: the medical outcomes study approach. Durham: Duke University Press, 1992.

7. Katz S, Branch LG, Branson MH, et al. Active life expectancy. N Engl J Med 1983;309:1218–1223.

8. Katz S, Ford A, Moskowitz R, et al. Studies of illness in old age and the index of ADL: a standardized measure of biologic and psychosocial function. JAMA 1983;185:94–100.

9. Fillenbaum GE. Screening the elderly: a brief instrumental activities of daily living measure. J Am Geriatr Soc 1985;33:698–701.

10. Evans W, Rosenberg I. Biomarkers. New York: Simon & Schuster, 1991.

11. Bortz W. Redefining human aging. J Am Geriatr Soc 1987;37:1092–1096.

12. Rowe J, Kahn R. Human aging: usual and successful. Science 1987;273:143–149.

13. Cazalis.

14. Avorn J. Benefit and cost analysis in geriatric care. N Engl J Med 1984;310:1294–1295.

15. Sage WM, Hurst CR, Silverman JF, Bortz W. Intensive care for the elderly: outcomes of elective and non-elective admissions. J Am Geriatr Soc 1987;35:312–318.

16. Manton K. Changing concepts of morbidity and mortality in the elderly population. Milbank Q, 1982.

17. McKeown T. The origin of human disease. Cambridge, MA: Basil Blackwood, 1988.

18. McGue M, Vaupel J, Holm N, Harvald B. Longevity is moderately heritable in a sample of Danish twins born in 1870–1880. J Gerontol Biol Sci 1993;48:B237–B244.

19. Sagan L. The health of nations. New York: Basic Books, 1987.

20. Henderson B, Ross R, Pike M. Toward the primary prevention of cancer. Science 1991;254:1081–1268.

21. Selye H. The story of the adaptation syndrome. Acta Montreal, 1952.

22. Sapolsky R, Armanini M, Packard D, Tombaugh G. Stress and glucocorticoids in aging. Endocrinol Metab Clin North Am 1987;16:965–980.

23. Boswell J. In: Chapman R, ed. Life of Johnson. World Classics. Oxford: Oxford University Press, 1983.

24. Holmes OW. The deacon's masterpiece: or the wonderful one hoss shay. From The Autocrat of the Breakfast-Table. In: The Complete Poetical Works of O.W. Holmes, Boston: Houghton Mifflin, 1908.

25. Prigogine I, Stenger I. Order out of chaos. NY: Bantam, 1988.

26. Atkins P. The Second Law. Freeman, NY: Scientific American Books, 1984.

27. Rubner M. Das Problem des Lebensdauer. Munich: Oldenbourg, 1908.

28. Pearl RA. The rate of living: being an account of some experimental studies on the biology of life duration. NY: Knopf, 1928.

29. Walford R. Maximum life span. NY: Norton, 1983.

30. McCay C. The effect of retarded growth on life span and upon the ultimate body size. J Nutr 1935;10:63–75.

31. Masoro E. Dietary restrictions and aging. J Am Geriatr Soc 1993;41:994–999.

32. Gavrilov LA, Gavrilova NS. The biology of lifespan: a quantitative approach. Chur, Switzerland: Hamarand Academic Publishers, 1991.

33. Bortz W. Aging as entropy. Exp Gerontol 1986;21:321–328.

34. Ames B, Shinenaga MK, Park EM. In: Davies KJA, ed. Oxidative damage and repair: clinical, biological and medical aspects. Elmsford NY: Pergamon, 1985:193–204.

35. Wei Q, Matonoski GM, Farme ER, et al. DNA repair and aging in basal cell carcinoma: a molecular epidemiologic study. Proc Natl Acad Sci USA 1993;90:1614–1618.

36. Hayflick L. Aging under glass. In: Maramorosh K, ed. Advances in cell culture. Orlando: Academic Press, 1988.

37. Schrodinger E. What is life: the physical aspects of living cells. NY: Cambridge University Press, 1967.

38. Adelman R, Saul RL, Ames BN. Oxidative damage to DNA. Relation to species, metabolic rate and life span. Proc Natl Acad Sci USA 1988;88:2706–2708.

39. Schneider E, Reed J. Life extension. N Engl J Med 1985; 312:1159–1168.

40. Sumida S. Exercise-induced lipid peroxidation and leakage of enzymes before and after vitamin E supplementation. Int J Biochem 1989;21:835–838.

41. Shock N. Mortality and measurement of aging. In: Strehler B, ed. Biology of aging. Washington, DC: American Institute of Biological Sciences 1960.

42. Bortz W. Disuse and aging. JAMA 1982;248:1203–1210.

43. Mooradian AD. Biomarkers of aging: do we know what to look for? J Gerontol Biol Sci 1990;48:183–186.

44. Kerlan R. Health and fitness through physical activity. NY: Wiley, 1978:22.

45. Kasch FW, Boyer JL, Van Camp SP, et al. The effect of physical activity and inactivity on aerobic power in older men—a longitudinal study. J Phys Sports Med 1990;8:73–83.

46. Rogers MA, Hagberg J, Martin SH, et al. Declines in VO$_2$max with aging in Master's athletes and sedentary men. J Appl Physiol 1990;68:2195–2199.

47. Henriksson J. Cellular metabolism and endurance. In: Shepard RJ, Astrand PO, eds. Endurance and sport. Oxford: Blackwell Science, 1992:46–60.

48. Bortz W. The physics of frailty. J Am Geriatr Soc 1993; 41:1004–1008.

49. Thompson, D'Arcy. On growth and form. 2nd ed. London: Cambridge University Press, 1942.

50. Braam J, Davis R. Rain, wind and touch induced expression of calmodulin and calmodulin related genes in arabidopsis. Cell 1990;60:357–364.

51. Carles DR, Won M, Orr T. Musculoskeletal anatomy, phylogeny and functional adaptation. J Biomech 1991;24: 3–16.

52. Diamond M. Extensive cortical depth measurement and neuron size increase in the cortex of environmentally enriched rats. J Comp Neurol 1967;131:357–364.

53. Bortz W. The disuse syndrome. West J Med 1984;141:89–98.

54. Kraus H, Raab W. Hypokinetic disease: disease produced by the lack of exercise. Springfield, IL: Thomas, 1961.

55. Saltin B. Cardiovascular and pulmonary adaptation to physi-

cal activity. In: Bouchard C, et al, eds. Exercise, fitness and health. Champaign, IL: Human Kinetics Books, 1990.

56. Haskell W, Sims C, Myll J, et al. Coronary artery size and dilating capacity in ultradistance runners. Circulation 1993;87:1076–1082.

57. Wood PD, Haskell W, Stern M, et al. Plasma lipoprotein distribution in male and female runners. Ann NY Acad Sci 1977;301;748–763.

58. Stratton JR, Chandler W, Schwook R, et al. Effect of physical conditioning on fibrinolytic variables and fibrinogen in young and old healthy adults. Circulation 1991;53:1692–1697.

59. Fiatarone M, Marks E, Ryan N, Evans W. Strength training in nonagenarians. JAMA 1992;63:3029–3034.

60. Mayer J. Overweight: causes, cost and control. Englewood Heights, NJ: Prentice-Hall, 1968.

61. Wood P, Stefanich M, Williams P, Haskell W. The effect on plasma lipoprotein of a prudent weight-reducing diet, with and without exercise in overweight men and woman. N Engl J Med 1991;325:461–466.

62. Litwak L, Whedon G. The effect of physical conditioning on glucose tolerance. Clin Res 1959;7:143–144.

63. Christ D, McKinnon L, Thompson R, et al. Physical exercise increases natural cellular mediated tumor cytotoxicity in elderly women. Gerontology 1989;35:66–71.

64. Bartram H, Wynder E. Physical activity and colon cancer risk? Physiologic considerations. Am J Gastroenterol 1989; 84:109–112.

65. Bernstein L, Parr R, Lobo R, et al. The effect of moderate physical activity on menstrual cycle pattern in adolescence — implications for breast cancer prevention. Br J Cancer 1987;55:681–686.

66. Lee J, Paffenbarger R, Hsieh OC. Physical activity and risk of prostate cancer among college alumni. Am J Epidemiol 1992;135:169–172.

67. Richerson H, Seebohm P. Nasal airway response to exercise. J Allergy 1968;41:269–279.

68. Johnsgaard.

69. Corrodi H, Fuxe K, Hokfelt K. The effect of immobilization stress on the activity of the central monamine neuron. Life Sci 1968;7:107–112.

70. Stewart A, King A, Preston S, et al. Functioning and well being associated with older adults' participation in exercise. Gerontologist 1991;31:9–16.

71. Blair S, Kohl H, Paffenbarger R, et al. Physical fitness and all cause mortality: a prospective study of healthy men and women. JAMA 1989;262:2395–2401.

72. Fry PS. Major social theories of aging and their implications for counseling concept and practice: a critical review. Couns Psychol 1992;20:246–329.

73. Carstensen L, Fredricksen B. Aging, illness and social preferences. Poster Presentation, Brussels: International Congress of Psychology, July 1992.

74. Carstensen L. The emerging field of behavioral gerontology. Behav Ther 1988;19:259–281.

75. Bandura A. The social foundation of thought and action: a social cognitive theory. Englewood Cliffs, NJ: Prentice-Hall, 1986.

76. Langer E, Rodin J. The effects of enhanced personal responsibility for the aged. J Pers Soc Psychol 1976;34:191–198.

77. Seligman M. Helplessness: on depression, development and death. San Francisco: Freeman, 1975.

78. Csikszentmihaly M. Flow. NY: Harper & Row, 1990.

79. Garibaldi M. *In re* Farrell. Superior Court of New Jersey 108 NJ 1987:341.

Chapter 2
Demography and Health Status

Andrew M. Kramer

There is a fountain of youth: it is your mind, your talents, the creativity you bring to your life and the lives of people you love. When you learn to tap this source, you will truly have defeated age.

Sophia Loren

Who Is Elderly?

We commonly define *elderly* as 65 years of age or older—the usual age of eligibility for retirement benefits such as Social Security and Medicare health benefits. Yet, age 65 does not necessarily reflect a time of significant change in health. Moreover, individuals over age 65 vary tremendously in terms of physiologic, cognitive, and functional capacity. As a result of this variation, it is common to distinguish subgroups of the elderly, such as the "young old" (aged 65 to 74), the "frail elderly" or the "old old" (aged 75 and older), and the "oldest old" (aged 85 and older) (1–4). Dissimilarities among these subgroups are often so pronounced that it is misleading, for most purposes, to consider individuals 65 years of age and older as a single group. For example, about 4.5 percent of elderly reside in nursing homes, but this includes only about 1 percent of those 65 to 74 years of age, close to 6 percent of those 75 to 84 years of age, and 22 percent of those 85 years of age or older (5).

Over 32 million people, or 12.6 percent of the total population, were 65 years of age or older in 1993 (6). About 57 percent of this group were 65 to 74 years of age, 33 percent were aged 75 to 84, and 10 percent were 85 years of age or older (Table 2.1). There were 50 percent more women in the over-65 age group as a whole and more than twice as many women in the over-85 age group.

Most elderly people perceive their health to be excellent, very good, or good (Figure 2.1). This finding, based on a national health interview survey, is true in all age

subgroups (5). Individuals aged 75 and older are more likely to perceive their health as fair or poor than do those 65 to 74 years of age (35% vs 28%); a smaller proportion perceive their health to be excellent or very good. Although these self-assessments of health are simple measures of health status, they tend to be strongly associated with objective measures such as physical examinations and survival rates (7,8). Thus, most elderly persons believe themselves to be healthy, and they are healthy.

Physical Functioning

Functional ability is perhaps the most important measure of health status among elderly persons because it is strongly associated with institutionalization, mortality, and need for community services (9–13). Physical functioning is generally measured in terms of ability to perform personal care activities, or activities of daily living (ADLs), including bathing, dressing, toileting, transferring, and eating. Other basic ADLs that are sometimes included are continence, grooming, walking, and getting outside. A second set of functions often measured in noninstitutionalized elderly, referred to as instrumental activities of daily living (IADLs), include home management activities (e.g., meal preparation, shopping, money management, telephone use, light housework, heavy housework).

Estimates of the size of the elderly population with functional disabilities vary in national surveys. Factors accounting for this variation are the items being measured, how disability or dependence in the activity is defined, and issues related to the sample, such as the age structure of the population (14). One major national survey of older adults, conducted in 1986, included seven personal care activities (eating, toileting, dressing, bathing, transferring, walking, and getting outside). Respondents were asked whether they had difficulty performing

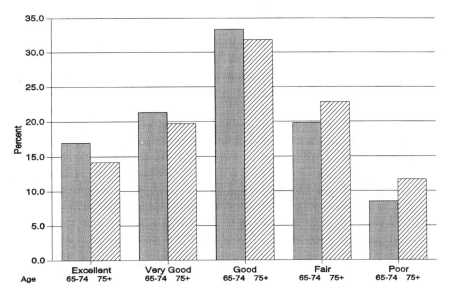

Figure 2.1. Percentage of Elderly by Age Group Rating Health as Excellent, Very Good, Good, Fair, or Poor, 1985–1987. (Reproduced by permission from National Center for Health Statistics. Data from the National Health Interview Survey. Health Data on Older Americans: United States, 1992. Series 3: Analytic and Epidemiologic Studies No. 27, DHHS Publication No. (PHS)93-1411; Hyattsville, MD, January 1993.)

Table 2.1. U.S. Elderly Population by Age and Sex, 1993.

Age (yr)	Population (×1,000,000)	Elderly (%)	Females (%)
All ages (65+)	32.6	100	60
65–74	18.7	57	56
75–84	10.6	33	62
85+	3.3	10	72

SOURCE: U.S. Bureau of the Census. Population Projections for States by Age, Sex, Race and Hispanic Origin: 1993–2020. Current Population Reports P25-111, U.S. Government Printing Office, Washington DC, 1994.

each of these specific activities, by themselves, because of a health or physical problem. On the basis of this survey, more than 75 percent of those living in the community reported no difficulty performing any of these activities. About 13 percent reported difficulty with one or two of the activities, and about 10 percent had difficulty with three or more.

As might be expected, the proportion of elderly having difficulty performing these activities increased with age (Figure 2.2). Although 83 percent of those aged 65 to 74

had no difficulty performing any of the activities, only 55 percent of those age 85 years and older were free from disability. Similarly, only 6 percent of those aged 65 to 74 had difficulty with three or more of the activities, but 14 percent of those aged 75 to 84 and 24 percent of those aged 85 or older had difficulty with three or more activities. In all age groups, more women than men reported difficulty performing these activities. White persons were less likely to have difficulty performing these activities than were persons of all other races.

Difficulty walking was the most frequent functional disability (18 percent of those 65 years of age or older) and getting outside was the second most frequent difficulty (12 percent of those 65 years of age or older). The fewest individuals had difficulty with eating and toileting (2 percent and 5 percent, respectively). This is consistent with Katz's original concept of the ADL index as hierarchical, in that functional abilities are generally lost in a sequence depending on how basic the activities are to daily life (15). Eating, continence, and toileting are more basic activities than dressing and bathing, for example, and are thus the last ones in which individuals become impaired.

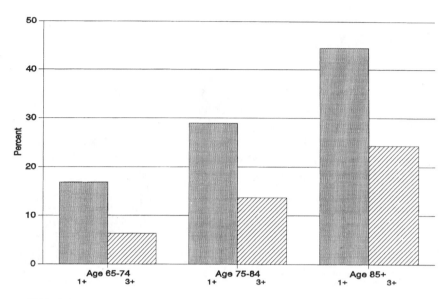

Figure 2.2. Percentage of Elderly by Age Group Having Difficulty with One or More and Three or More Activities of Daily Living (Eating, Toileting, Dressing, Bathing, Transferring, Walking, Getting Outside), 1986. (Reproduced by permission from National Center for Health Statistics. Data from the National Health Interview Survey.)

Not all persons with difficulty performing ADLs received help. Of the 23 percent of those 65 years of age or older who had difficulty with one or more activities, only 10 percent received help in performing one or more of these activities (5). However, those with difficulties in eating and toileting were far more likely to receive help with these activities than were those reporting difficulty with walking or getting outside. This probably reflects the fundamental nature of basic ADLs to human existence, in contrast to other activities in which individuals can survive without receiving help despite their disability.

Assistance with basic functional activities is one of the major reasons that elderly persons are placed in nursing homes. In their study of aging, Miller et al found that about 6 percent of those with disabilities in two or more activities were residing in nursing homes within two years of the study, in contrast to only 1 percent of those with no ADL disabilities (13). Among nursing home residents, more than 70 percent required assistance with walking and dressing, 60 percent required assistance or could not use a toilet, and about 40 percent required assistance with eating. About half had difficulty with bladder or bowel incontinence (16).

For individuals living in the community, their ability to perform social maintenance and home management activities is also critical and important to measure. The IADLs cover a range of activities that are more complex than those needed for ADLs. Some recent research suggests a hierarchical relationship between at least some of the IADL items and the ADL items, with IADL disabilities representing less severe disability (17). Of those age 65 years and older, 72 percent had no difficulty in performing the six ADLs included in the survey (18). The percentage of elderly having difficulty with one or more and three or more IADLs increased with age (Figure 2.3). Overall, there were more individuals who had difficulty in performing IADLs than in performing ADLs.

In summary, physical functioning is an important measure of health status in the elderly because of implications for institutionalization, mortality, and service needs. Maximizing functional abilities by treating specific conditions and with the use of special devices is an extremely important consideration in caring for the elderly because of the potential benefits than can accrue from enhanced functioning. Often, a small change in functional ability can have a major impact on whether an elderly person can function effectively in a relatively independent living

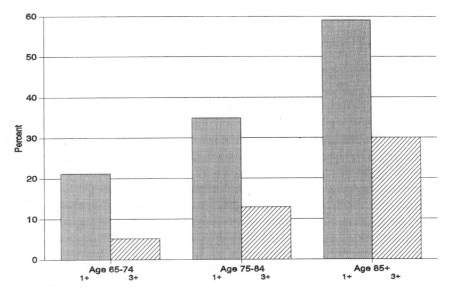

Figure 2.3. Percentage of Elderly by Age Group Having Difficulty with One or More and Three or More Instrumental Activities of Daily Living (Preparing Meals, Shopping, Managing Money, Using Telephone, Light Housework, Heavy Housework), 1986. (Reproduced by permission from National Center for Health Statistics. Data from the National Health Interview Survey.)

situation. More than three-quarters of elderly persons living in the community do not have difficulty performing basic ADLs, but these disabilities are strongly associated with age.

A wide range of functional measures are available for use in practice. Some of these measures provide fairly imprecise measures of functional disability for screening purposes (15,19), but others involve more precise functional assessments for monitoring changes in physical function (20,21). Despite ambiguities in measuring function, and some variation in results, physical functioning should be regarded as a critical measure of health status in elderly persons.

Living Arrangements and Marital Status

The likelihood that an elderly person will be living alone is related to gender and to age (Table 2.2). Elderly women are more than twice as likely to be living alone than are elderly men (5). Over half of women 75 years of age and older live by themselves. A relatively small proportion of men live alone until they reach the age of 85, at which time about one-third of men live by themselves.

The tendency for women and older persons to live alone mainly reflects declining numbers of elderly with living spouses. More than 75 percent of men 65 years of age and older are married and living with their spouse. The number of men who are widowed increases with age from 10 percent of those aged 65 to 74 to 42 percent of those aged 85 and older (22). In all age groups, many fewer women are married because over one-third of women aged 65 to 74 are widowed, and this increases to more than 80 percent of women over age 85. The substantial difference between elderly men and elderly women in terms of marital status and living arrangements reflects the greater proportion of women in the older population, a result of differences in life expectancy between men and women.

These issues are important for two reasons. First, health care providers need to be aware that large numbers of women over the age of 65 and men over the age of 85 have lost their spouse, which is a major life event. Second, most elderly persons who have lost a spouse are living alone. The numbers living with others increase with age, but it is common for elderly persons (particularly women) to live alone. Living alone is not necessarily a problem unless the person has profound functional disabilities for which

21

Table 2.2. Living Arrangements of Noninstitutionalized Elderly Persons by Age and Sex, 1985.

Living Arrangement (age, yr)	Male (%)	Female (%)
Living alone		
65+	16	43
75+	22	53
85+	34	60
Living with spouse		
65+	76	39
75+	69	24
85+	48	10
Living with others		
65+	8	18
75+	9	23
85+	18	30

SOURCE: National Center for Health Statistics. National Health Interview Survey, 1986. Functional Limitations (suppl), DHHS Publication No. (PHS)93-1411, Hyattsville, MD, 1993.

there is no assistance available, or has limited social contacts.

Surveys indicate that most elderly living at home have children or siblings with whom they visit or have telephone contact (23). In the two weeks before one survey, 73 percent of the elderly living alone had visited with relatives, 84 percent had talked with relatives on the telephone, and only 12 percent had done neither. Research suggests that living alone and having limited social supports are associated with poorer outcomes in terms of institutionalization, recovery from acute events, and mortality (24–26). Thus, both living situation and availability of social supports are important considerations in providing health care to elderly persons.

For elderly persons with disabilities in ADLs or IADLs, spouses or other relatives or individuals with whom they live often play a major role as caregivers. One must not underestimate the stress on caregivers in providing daily assistance to individuals with multiple ADL and IADL disabilities. Many caregivers, including spouses or children, are themselves elderly, which can compound the burden if the caregivers also have functional limitations. Assessment of caregiver burden is important in caring for elderly persons with functional disabilities so that, when appropriate, options for temporary assistance or relief in the form of respite care can be considered.

About twice as many women than men 65 years of age or older are placed in nursing homes (58 per 1000 population for women, in contrast to 29 per 1000 population for men) (5). This difference results not only from the differences in age distribution between women and men, but also from the fact that disabled men are more likely to live with a spouse who can provide assistance. Nevertheless, over one-quarter of 75-year-olds living alone have disabilities in one or more ADLs and more than 10 percent have disabilities in three or more activities. For these individuals, assurance that they have adequate help to function in their home is important to their health care needs.

Chronic and Acute Illness

Nearly 40 percent of individuals 65 years of age and older report activity limitation resulting from to chronic conditions (27). Chronic conditions are the major source of disability for elderly persons. Prevalence of the most common chronic conditions was obtained in a national health interview survey for all ages (Table 2.3). Prevalence is presented as the number of chronic conditions per 1000 persons.

Arthritis, hypertension, and hearing impairments were the three most common chronic conditions reported by elderly persons, and all three were reported by one-third or more of the elderly. Cataracts, chronic sinusitis, ischemic heart disease, and diabetes were reported by more than 10 percent of elderly persons. Treatment of chronic conditions, because of their high prevalence, is an important part of caring for elderly persons.

Individuals over 65 years of age experience approximately 121 acute illnesses per 100 persons per year. This is a lower rate of acute illnesses than for any other age group, with the exception of those 45 to 64 years of age. However, the rate of chronic conditions increases with age and is substantially higher for almost all conditions among those 65 years of age or older. Because of acute and chronic conditions, elderly persons experience a larger number of hospital admissions than do other age groups. In 1992, about 20 percent of those age 75 or older were hospitalized one or more times. About 15 percent of those 65 to 74 years of age were hospitalized, but less than 10 percent of those in all other age groups were hospitalized one or more times. In addition, those 75 years of age

Table 2.3. Most Common Chronic Conditions and Rate per 1000 Elderly (65 years of age or older) in 1992.

Type of Chronic Condition	No. of Chronic Conditions per 1000 Persons	Type of Chronic Condition	No. of Chronic Conditions per 1000 Persons
Skin and musculoskeletal		Genitourinary, nervous, endocrine, metabolic, blood, blood-forming	
Arthritis	481.9	Diabetes	110.4
Trouble with ingrown nails	46.5	Goiter or other disorders of the thyroid	38.7
Bursitis, unclassified	43.3	Diseases of prostate	37.2
Trouble with corns and calluses	42.1	Bladder disorders	31.3
Dermatitis	37.1	Kidney trouble	27.4
Impairments		Circulatory	
Hearing impairment	320.4	High blood pressure (hypertension)	357.6
Cataracts	166.0	Ischemic heart disease	152.7
Back impairment	99.8	Other selected diseases of heart, excluding hypertension	89.2
Tinnitus	89.4	Heart rhythm disorders	82.7
Lower extremity impairment	88.1	Cerebrovascular disease	74.4
Digestive		Respiratory	
Hernia of abdominal cavity	62.2	Chronic sinusitis	158.7
Frequent constipation	48.6	Hay fever or allergic rhinitis without asthma	82.8
Frequent indigestion	43.5	Chronic bronchitis	69.6
Diverticula of intestines	43.0	Asthma	39.8
Ulcer	33.1	Emphysema	34.6

SOURCE: National Center for Health Statistics. Number of selected reported conditions per 1000 persons, by age: United States, 1992. Table 57. Current Estimates from the National Health Interview Survey, 1992. Series 10: National Health Survey No. 189. DHHS Publication No. (PHS)94-157, Hyattsville, MD, January 1994.

and older were more likely to have been hospitalized two or more times during the year, reflecting the chronic nature of their diseases.

Life Expectancy

Life expectancy at birth is the average number of years that a group of infants born in a particular year could expect to live if they were to experience, throughout life, the age-specific death rates prevailing at the time of their birth. The life expectancy for those born in 1986 was about 75 years. Life expectancy at birth for women was seven years longer than life expectancy for men, which results in the larger proportion of women than men in later years.

For individuals who reached 65 years of age in 1986, remaining life expectancy is about 17 years—a total life span of 82 years (5). Their expected life span is greater than those born in 1986 because these individuals have already bypassed the risk of death associated with earlier ages. Those who reach age 75 can expect to live to age 86 and those who reach age 85 can expect to live to 91, with somewhat greater life expectancy for women than for men in all cases (Table 2.4).

The three leading causes of death for individuals 65 years of age or older are diseases of the heart, malignant neoplasms, and cerebrovascular disease, with the first two of these accounting for over half the deaths (5). Death rates for diseases of the heart are declining in all age groups and races. Heart disease death rates for men are consistently higher than rates for women, but the rates are declining faster in men than in women.

Between 1960 and 1986, the death rate for the population 65 years of age and older decreased by 16 percent.

Table 2.4. Life Expectancy at Selected Ages in 1986.

Age (yr)	Total (yr)	Male (yr)	Female (yr)
65	16.8	14.7	18.6
75	10.7	9.1	11.7
85	6.0	5.2	6.4

SOURCE: National Center for Health Statistics. Vital Statistics of the United States, Vol. 4. Mortality, Part A. Health Data on Older Americans: United States, 1992. Series 3: Analytic and Epidemiology Studies No. 27, DHHS Publication No. (PHS)93-1411, Hyattsville, MD, January 1993.

The decline in death rate is associated with a trend toward increased life expectancy. Life expectancy at age 65 increased approximately three years between 1960 and 1990. Although life expectancy has increased substantially during this century and is projected to continue increasing in the future, controversy exists over whether the human life span (i.e., maximum survival potential) is actually increasing. It has been suggested that the human life span is fixed and that, as morbidity is postponed until the very end of the life span, we are approaching a time at which the elderly will be living more vigorous and less dependent lives until the point of natural death (28). The evidence in recent years, however, challenges this theory. Mortality rates even among the oldest old are declining significantly, but the incidence of chronic illness and disability among the oldest ages does not appear to be declining (29,30).

We need to pay greater attention to functional or active life expectancy than to prolonging life. One study of active life expectancy found that people 65 to 69 years of age can expect to remain independent in functioning for only 10 of their expected 16 or more remaining years or life. Those independent at age 85 can expect to be dependent in functioning for about half of their estimated remaining years of life (31). Thus, maintenance of function becomes an increasingly important consideration as life expectancy increases.

Demographics in the Future

During the next 50 years, the elderly population is expected to double, whereas the total population is expected to increase by only about 35 percent (32). Thus, the elderly are expected to make up more than 20 percent of the total population by the year 2030 (Figure 2.4). Growth will be moderate until approximately 2010, at which time the "baby boom" generation will have become seniors. At this point, an increase in the proportion of young old will begin, followed by an increase in the proportion of the old old in the 2020s, and an increase in the proportion of oldest old in the 2030s.

Such projections are obviously based on assumptions about trends in fertility, immigration rates, and mortality extrapolated from historic data that may not prove to be true. All historic estimates suggest that there will be a constant increase in life expectancy for both men and women through the year 2050, and result in a greater percentage of the elderly reaching advanced ages in the future. There is considerable variation, however, in the rate at which life expectancy is projected to increase. The Social Security Administration provides three series of figures, with a wide range as an uncertainty interval (32). Past projections have generally underestimated the rate of increase in life expectancy; we may be faced with a population near the highest projections.

What are the implications of the change in demographics for the health care system and health care costs? If the age and gender mix projected for the year 2026 were imposed on the 1986 health care system, total expenditures for health care would increase about 25 percent over 1986 levels (33). Although an increasing percentage of health care dollars will be spent on the elderly, projected demographic change does not necessarily mean that the United States will spend an increasing share of the gross national product (GNP) on health. By use of different scenarios for economic growth and change in intensity of service use, demographics were found not to be the most important factor in determining health care expenditures and GNP growth was projected to offset any rise in spending. Thus, a rise in health care expenditures as a share of the GNP will be a result of other factors in addition to demographics.

As the elderly population increases, society must be prepared to meet the long-term care needs of the growing number of disabled elderly (34). Emphasis must be given to programs for minimizing disability, providing assistance in the community for those with functional disability, and treating chronic illness. This will require better

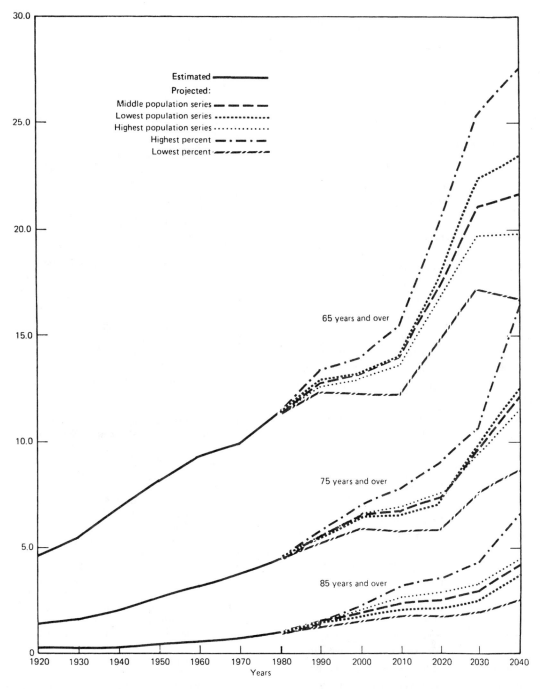

Figure 2.4. Percent of the Total Population in the Older Ages: 1920 to 2040. Estimates and projections as of July 1, except for 85 and over, 1920–1930, which relate to April 1; points are plotted for years ending in zero.

integration of traditional acute and long-term care services. Optimal care for geriatric patients, particularly those with chronic conditions and disabilities, requires the involvement of all health care providers. Physicians will have to play an active role if new approaches to old problems are to be developed.

Summary and Conclusions

• Individuals over 65 years of age vary tremendously in terms of physiologic, cognitive, and functional capacity. Thus, we often distinguish subgroups by age categories.

• Most elderly people perceive their health to be excellent, very good, or good. Only about 8 percent of those aged 65 to 74 and 12 percent of those age 75 years and older perceive their health as poor.

• Functional ability is perhaps the most important measure of health status among elderly persons because it is strongly associated with institutionalization, mortality, and need for community services. The proportion of elders having difficulty performing basic ADLs increases with age from 17 percent of those aged 65 to 74 to 45 percent of those age 85 years and older.

• Elderly women are more than twice as likely to be living alone than are elderly men; over half of women 75 years of age or older live by themselves. For those living alone, availability of social supports and assistance are critical issues in health care delivery.

• Chronic conditions are a major source of disability for elderly persons and far more prevalent than acute conditions. Thus, treatment of chronic conditions is a major focus of geriatric care.

• Life expectancy is increasing at all ages, with those 65 years of age expected to live about 17 remaining years. We must focus on minimizing disability to preserve functional or active life expectancy.

• The number of elderly persons and the proportion of the population that is over 65 years of age are expected to increase dramatically during the next 50 years. However, demographics is only one of several factors influencing health care costs and will not necessarily require health care to consume an increasing share of the gross national product. We must continue to find better approaches to treating chronic illness, minimizing functional disability,

and providing assistance in the community as the major focus of geriatric care.

References

1. Streib GF. The frail elderly: research dilemmas and research opportunities. Gerontologist 1983;23:40.
2. Suzman R, Riley MW. Introducing the "oldest old." Milbank Q 1985;63:2.
3. U.S. Bureau of the Census. American in transition: an aging society. Series P-23, no. 128. Washington, DC: U.S. Government Printing Office, 1983.
4. Rosenwaike I. A demographic portrait of the oldest old. Milbank Q 1985;63:2.
5. National Center for Health Statistics. Health data on older Americans: United States, 1992. Series 3, no. 27. (PHS)93-1411. Hyattsville, MD: Public Health Service, 1993.
6. U.S. Bureau of Census. Population projections for states by age, sex, race, and hispanic origin: 1993 to 2020. Series P-25, no. 1111. Washington, DC: U.S. Government Printing Office, 1994.
7. Kaplan G, Barell V, Lusky A. Subjective state of health and survival in elderly adults. J Gerontol 1988;43:S114–S120.
8. LaRue A, Bank B, Jarvik L, Hetland M. Health in old age: how do physicians' ratings and self-ratings compare? J Gerontol 1979;34:678–691.
9. Branch LG, Jette AM. A prospective study of long-term care institutionalization among the aged. Am J Public Health 1982;72:1373.
10. Branch L, Katz S, Kneipmann K, Papsider J. A prospective study of functional status among community elders. Am J Public Health 1984;74:266–268.
11. Harris T, Kovar MG, Suzman R, et al. Longitudinal study of physical ability in the oldest-old. Am J Public Health 1989;79:698–792.
12. Manton K. A longitudinal study of functional change and mortality in the United States. J Gerontol 1988;43:S153–S161.
13. Miller B, Prohaska T, Mermeistein R, Van Nostrand JF. Changes in functional status and risk of institutionalization and death. Vital Health Stat 1993;3:41–47.
14. Wiener JM, Hanley RJ, Clark R, Van Nostrand JF. Measuring the activities of daily living: comparisons across national surveys. J Gerontol 1990;45:S229–S237.
15. Katz S, Ford AB, Moskowitz RW. Studies of illness in the aged: the index of ADL: a standardized measure of biological and psychosocial function. JAMA 1963;184:914.
16. National Center for Health Statistics. Health United States 1992 and healthy people 2000 review. (PHS)93-1232. Hyattsville, MD: Public Health Service, August 1993.
17. Spector W, Katz S, Fulton JP. Hierarchical relationship between activities of daily living and instrumental activities of daily living. J Chronic Dis 1987;40:481–490.
18. Prohaska T, Mermelstein R, Miller B, Jack S. Functional status and living arrangements. Vital Health Stat 1993;3:23–39.

19. Stewart AL, Greenfield S, Hays RD, et al. Functional status and well-being of patients with chronic conditions. JAMA 1989;262:907–913.

20. Wade DT, Collin C. The Barthel ADL index: a standard measure of physical disability? Int Disabil Stud 1988;10:64–67.

21. Granger CV, Hamilton BB, Linacre JM, et al. Performance profiles of the functional independence measure. Am J Phys Med Rehabil 1993;72:84–89.

22. U.S. Bureau of Census. Marital status and living arrangements: March 1992. Series P-20, No 468. Washington, DC: U.S. Government Printing Office, March 1992.

23. Kovar MG, ed. Aging in the 80s, age 65 years and over, and living alone: contact with family, friends, and neighbors. National Center for Health Statistics (PHS)86-1250. Hyattsville, MD: Public Health Service, May 1986.

24. Cummings SR, Phillips SL, Wheat ME, et al. Recovery of function after hip fracture: the role of social supports. J Am Geriatr Soc 1988;36:801–806.

25. Ruberman W, Weinblatt E, Goldbert JD, Chaudary BS. Psychosocial influences on mortality after myocardial infarction. N Engl J Med 1984;311:552–559.

26. Steinbach U. Social networks, institutionalization, and mortality among elderly people in the United States. J Gerontol 1992;47:S183–S190.

27. National Center for Health Statistics. Current estimates from the national health interview survey, 1992. Series 10, no. 189. (PHS)94-1517. Hyattsville, MD: Public Health Service, 1994.

28. Fries JF. Aging, natural death, and the compression of morbidity. N Engl J Med 1980;303:130.

29. Manton KG. Changing concepts of morbidity and mortality in the elderly population. Milbank Q 1982;60:183.

30. Schneider EL, Brody JA. Aging, natural death, and the compression of morbidity: another view. N Engl J Med 1983;309:854.

31. Katz S, Branch LG, Branson MH, et al. Active life expectancy. N Engl J Med 1983;309:1218.

32. U.S. Bureau of the Census. Demographics and socioeconomic aspects of aging in the Untied States. Series P-23, no. 138. Washington DC: U.S. Government Printing Office, 1984.

33. Office of the Actuary, Health Care Financing Administration. National health expenditures, 1986–2000. Health Care Financ Rev 1987;8:1.

34. Schatzken A. How long can we live? A more optimistic view of potential gains in life expectancy. Am J Public Health 1980;70:1199.

Chapter 3
Financing, Use, and Organization of Health Care for Older Persons

Robert H. Binstock

The first wealth is health.

Ralph Waldo Emerson
The Conduct of Life

Prolonged and costly illness in later years robs too many of our elder citizens of pride, purpose and savings.

John F. Kennedy, Message to U.S. Congress
on the nation's health needs

The importance of older people in American health care is reflected by the simple facts that 1) a substantial number of health care dollars is currently spent on older persons and 2) even larger expenditures are projected for the future. Persons age 65 years and older, about 12.5 percent of the population, account for one-third of the nation's annual health care expenditures, or $300 billion of an estimated total of $900 billion in 1993 (1). Per capita expenditures for older persons are four times greater than for younger persons (2).

Government finances nearly two-thirds of health care for older Americans. The federal Medicare program, which provides a basic package of health insurance for most Americans who are age 65 years and older (as well as persons who receive federal disability insurance, and those with end-stage renal disease), accounts for 45 percent of the total expenditure. Medicaid, jointly funded by the federal and state governments, provides another 12 percent, principally for long-term care in nursing homes and residential environments. Care financed through the Department of Veterans Affairs, Department of Defense, Indian Health Services, and a variety of state and local government programs constitutes about 6 percent of the total. Only 8 percent is funded through private insurance, mainly from so-called Medigap supplemental policies; less than 1 percent comes from philanthropy (3).

Older persons pay 28 percent of the cost of their care

out-of-pocket. Much of this outlay pays for skilled nursing that along with mental health services, has only minimal Medicare coverage. Nearly two-thirds of prescription drug expenses, not covered at all by Medicare, are paid for out-of-pocket (4). Persons who can afford Medigap policies have their deductibles and co-payments covered reasonably through insurance. Poor older persons can have their deductibles and co-payments under Medicare paid for by Medicaid through a Qualified Medicare Beneficiary program enacted in 1988.

This chapter presents an overview of contemporary issues regarding the arrangements for financing older people's health care, as well as issues of health care organization and utilization. First, the chapter presents a brief overview of the patterns through which older people use health care services. Particular attention is paid to high utilization rates at advanced ages because the American older population is rapidly becoming even older. The chapter then considers the impact of population aging on national health care expenditures, contemporary pressures to curb Medicare expenditures, and related possibilities of health care for older people becoming limited informally in the contexts of managed care, as well as specific policies that might explicitly ration the care of older people. Next, the chapter examines a wide range of issues in the financing of long-term care, and describes a series of contemporary experimental demonstrations that seek to integrate acute and long-term care and financing. A brief concluding section notes some of the basic challenges that changes in the financing and organization of care will pose for physicians who practice geriatric medicine.

Health Care Utilization Patterns of Older People

Hospital costs account for 42 percent of the health care

expenditures for older people; 21 percent is spent on physician services, 20 percent on nursing homes, and the remaining 17 percent is distributed among a wide variety of other types of care, such as home health care, dental services, prescription drugs, vision and hearing aids, and medical equipment and supplies (3).

Persons 65 years of age and older currently account for 73 percent of annual deaths in the United States (5) and have higher prevalence rates of diseases and disabilities than the population at large. Consequently, older persons use most kinds of health care at much higher rates than persons under 65 years of age. At older ages within the elderly population, the rates of care utilization increase substantially.

About 35 percent of the elderly population is discharged from short-stay hospitals each year (3). Persons age 65 years and older account for 42 percent of the days of care in such hospitals and for about 31 percent of discharged patients. At ages 75 years and older and 85 years and older, each of the these dimensions of usage increases in rate. For example, the hospital discharge rate for those age 85 years and older is 90 percent higher than that for people age 65 to 74 years.

Some 1.6 million older people (5.1 percent of persons age 65 years and older) are in nursing homes (6). The rate of nursing home use increases sharply at older ages within the elderly population. About 1.4 percent of Americans age 65 to 74 years are in nursing homes, as compared with 6.1 percent of persons age 75 to 84 years and 24 percent of persons age 85 years and older.

An additional 4 million older people have limitations in activities of daily living (ADLs), instrumental activities of daily living (IADLs), or both (7), and most of them receive some form of long-term care in their own homes or some other residential facility such as a congregate living community, an adult foster home, or a board-and-care facility (8). About 80 percent to 85 percent of such community-based care to older patients is provided to them on an informal, unpaid basis by their spouses, siblings, adult children, and broader kin networks. About 74 percent of dependent, community-based older persons receive all their care from family members or other unpaid sources: roughly 21 percent receive both formal and informal services; only about 5 percent use only formal services (9). As is the case with nursing home patients, the percentage of older community residents who need help with long-term care increases dramatically at advanced old ages. For instance, the proportion needing care rises from 7.3 percent in the 65- to 74-year-old category to 14.8 percent for those in the 75- to 84- year-old category, and to 30 percent among those aged 85 and older (10).

Although older persons are about 12 percent of the population, they account for 20 percent of all contacts with physicians (11). Persons of all ages average 5.4 contacts per year, but persons age 65 to 74 years average 8.2 contacts and persons age 75 years and older average 9.9 contacts per year. Similarly, the probability of seeing a physician increases by advancing age categories. Among persons 45 to 64 years of age, 76.5 percent see a physician within a 12-month period; 85.1 percent of persons 65 to 74 years of age and 89.1 percent of people age 75 years and older have such a contact in the same time interval.

Population Aging and National Health Care Spending

Because the U.S. older population is growing absolutely and proportionally—from about 32 million persons today to an estimated 68 million in the year 2040 (12), health care costs for older persons have frequently been depicted as an unsustainable burden, or as one observer put it, "a great fiscal black hole" that will absorb an unlimited amount of national resources (13). When expected increases in the older population are combined with projections that the population conventionally termed "old" is becoming markedly older, on average, within itself, dramatic estimates can be made of staggering health care costs for older people in the future. In 1980, for example, persons 85 years of age and older were only 8.8 percent of the population age 65 years and older; in the year 2040 they will be 18 percent of the population age 65 years and older (12). As implied by comparatively higher rates of health care utilization among persons in their late seventies and eighties, described above, morbidity rates are much greater among persons in this age range than are rates for the total group age 65 years and older. Accordingly, sensational cost implications have been predicted, such as an estimate that, during the next 50 years, the national cost of nursing homes will rise from about $48 billion (today's cost) to as much as $139 billion, as projected in constant, inflation-adjusted dollars (14).

Up to now, neither increases in the number and proportions of older persons nor the aging of the older population have been major factors in the growth of health care expenditures. Demographic factors have been negligible contributors to spiraling health care costs compared with increases in per capita utilization of services, intensity of services per day or per visit, health-sector specific price inflation, and general inflation (15).

A recent study by Mendelson and Schwartz (16), for instance, indicated that although population aging accounted for about one-fifth of the annualized rise in real expenditures for long-term care from 1987 through 1990, it was a relatively negligible factor in the rise of spending for hospitals, physicians, and other forms of health care. Moreover, this analysis found a steady reduction in the contribution of population aging to health care costs between 1975 and 1990, and projected little impact of aging on costs through 2005. Earlier analyses (15,17) yielded similar findings regarding the minimal impact of aging and other demographic changes on increases in health care expenditures through the end of this century. If population aging has a major impact on U.S. health care costs, it will not be felt strongly until after 2015 when the "baby boom" population cohort joins the ranks of persons aged 65 and older; even this is not at all certain.

In fact, cross-national comparisons of health care expenditures and population aging provide no evidence that substantial or rapid population aging, or both, cause high levels of national economic burden from expenditures on health care (18). Health care costs are far from "out of control" or even "high" in many nations that have comparatively large proportions of older persons or that have experienced rapid rates of population aging. The public and private structural features of health care systems (e.g., relatively fixed or open-ended health care budgets)—and behavioral responses to them by citizens and health care providers—appear to be far more important determinants of a nation's level of health care expenditures than do population aging and other demographic trends.

Pressures to Limit Medicare Expenditures

Precisely because the U.S. health care system is undergoing structural changes, however, there are distinct possibilities that limitations on expenditures for older patients and the care they receive may increase in the years immediately ahead. Most of the specific policy actions and proposals to contain health care costs in recent years have focused on Medicare.

There are a number of fundamental reasons for this focus. First, Medicare is the biggest single source of payment for health care in America. Its large, aggregate national costs, and its rapid inflation are easily determined and highly visible. In 1993, Medicare paid about $153 billion for personal health care services. Medicare expenditures are projected to nearly triple during this decade, from $111 billion in 1990 to $328 billion in the year 2000 (1). Second, as implied by such projections, Medicare expenditures will contribute substantially to the federal deficit for many years unless drastic changes are made in the program. Third, since the federal government pays the bills for Medicare patients, Medicare costs are more directly responsive to government action than are those costs paid for through private insurance and out-of-pocket. The most far-reaching cost-containment measures undertaken to date have been changes in reimbursement procedures under Medicare, such as prospective payment on the basis of diagnosis-related groups (DRGs) to control expenditures on hospitals (19), the introduction of a "resource based relative-value scale" (RBRVS) for reimbursing physicians, and the introduction of Medicare Health Maintenance Organizations (HMOs) (20). Finally, changes in Medicare approaches to paying for care are a plausible strategy for implementing the more general goal of cost-containment because this nationwide governmental program affects the financial incentives of most American hospitals, nursing homes, physicians, and other health care providers and suppliers.

The issue of how to pay for Medicare is rather immediate. Recent annual reports of the Trustees of the Social Security Trust Funds have consistently estimated that Medicare's Part A Hospital Insurance (HI) costs will substantially exceed revenues in the latter half of the 1990s, and that by early in the next century, the HI trust fund reserves will be exhausted. The financing of Medicare's Part B (nonhospital) Supplementary Medical Insurance (SMI) has moved from being principally financed by premiums from Medicare enrollees, in the early years of the program, to being, today, 75 percent financed from general revenues.

Legislation in 1993 partially responded to these issues by enacting Medicare spending reductions and revenue increases that are estimated to total $85 billion over the five-year period from 1994 to 1998 (21). A 1994 report by a federal commission clearly indicated that further major measures to curb Medicare expenditures (22) would be put forth. And, as 1995 came to a close, President Clinton was proposing to reduce projected Medicare spending by $124 billion over seven years, while Congress was proposing $270 billion in reductions over the same time period. Whether such cutbacks in Medicare have a demonstrable impact in reducing the quantity and quality of care provided to older persons has yet to be documented.

Reduced Care in the Context of Managed Care?

The broad trend toward managed care and away from fee-for-service medicine in the U.S. may extend to older Americans and possibly affect the care that they receive. President Clinton's 1993 plan for health care reform, for example, would have enabled states to fold Medicare insurees into the purchasing alliances that were expected to arrange for health care of their members through HMOs and other managed care organizations with fixed, limited budgets (23). Older people, grouped with younger people in these budgeted plans, could have become subject to a covert, informal system of old-age-based rationing.

As doctors attempt to provide adequate care within the context of limited budgets, they tend to be pressured by administrators and colleagues *not to make available* to their older patients expensive tests and medical specialists that they do make available to their younger patients. As Robert and Rosalie Kane (24) observed, "[T]he basic incentive in any capitated system is toward under-service"; and "When care for older persons is combined with care for all others, older persons could be at a competitive disadvantage if rationing schemes were applied."

Nothing in the decade-long experience of the Medicare HMO program launched by the Health Care Financing Administration is reassuring in this area (20,25). Indeed, the likelihood of covert rationing in the context of budgeted care is indicated by the experience of the British National Health Service in which the pressures of fixed resources have resulted in older patients being routinely, though unofficially, denied tests and care made available to younger patients with the same clinical conditions (26).

Legislation proposed by Congress in 1995 included measures to expand the number of Medicare-financed managed care plans available and to encourage Medicare patients to abandon traditional fee-for-service health care by joining managed care plans. If substantial numbers of older persons opt for managed care, physicians will be challenged considerably to provide appropriate care for older patients under capitated arrangements—especially when one considers, as noted above, that present per capita expenditures are four times greater for persons age 65 years and older, than they are for the younger population.

Curbing Costs Through Old-Age-Based Rationing

Proposals to curb the costs of health care for older people have extended well beyond the scope of the Medicare program to more general propositions for limiting the care of elderly people. These proposals, which vary in specific content and in the age ranges they use to define "older persons," have been made with increasing frequency since the early 1980s. They appear to be an expression of a larger backlash against an artificially homogenized group labeled "the aged," which has become a scapegoat for a variety of societal problems that have been rhetorically unified as issues of intergenerational conflict and equity.

As expenditures for benefits to the aging have climbed to more than 30 percent of the annual federal budget (27), older people have become increasingly stereotyped in the media as prosperous, hedonistic, selfish, and politically controlling "greedy geezers." They have been blamed for problems of children, the declining strength of the U.S. economy, and the nation's general inability to free up resources for use in a variety of worthy causes (28). Especially prominent among the problems for which elderly people have been made scapegoat is health care costs. A number of academicians and public figures—including politicians—have urged vigorously that American society set limits to health care for older people. In 1984, Richard Lamm, then Governor of Colorado, was widely quoted as stating that older persons "have a duty to die and get out of the way" (29). Although Lamm subsequently stated that he had been misquoted on this specific statement, since leaving office, he has delivered the same message repeatedly in a somewhat more delicately worded fashion (30,31).

During the past decade, discussion of this notion has spread to a number of forums. Ethicists and philosophers have generated principles of equity to undergird "justice between age groups" in the provision of health care, rather than, for instance, justice between rich and poor, or justice among ethnic and racial subgroups (32,33). Conferences and books have explicitly addressed the issue with titles such as "Should Medical Care Be Rationed by Age?" (34).

Late in 1987, this theme received substantial popular attention with the publication of a book, *Setting Limits: Medical Goals in an Aging Society*, by ethicist Daniel Callahan (13). Callahan depicted the elderly population as "a new social threat" and a "demographic, economic, and medical avalanche . . . one that could ultimately (and perhaps already) do [*sic*] great harm." Callahan's remedy for this threat was to use "age as a specific criterion for the allocation and limitation of health care" by denying life-extending health care—as a matter of public policy—to persons who are in their "late 70s or early 80s" or who have "lived out a natural life span." Although Callahan described the natural life span as a matter of biography rather than biology, he used chronological age as an arbitrary marker to designate when, from a biographical standpoint, the individual should have reached the end of a natural life and should be viewing life retrospectively, not prospectively. *Setting Limits* provoked widespread and continuing discussion in the media and public forums throughout the country and directly inspired other books (35–37) and scores of journal articles dealing with the topic of old age and rationing health care. Today, the notion of limiting the health care of older people in one way or another is surfacing with increasing frequency in national magazines and newspapers (38).

Putting aside the issues of the moral implications and political feasibility of such proposals, which are considerable (36), what sorts of financial "savings" might be achieved through rationing measures such as categorically denying life-saving care to older persons? Would these savings be of economic significance?

Proponents of old-age-based rationing have not identified the magnitude of savings that their proposals might achieve. But, for illustrative purposes, one can construct an example. For a number of years, about 28 percent of annual Medicare expenditures has been for Medicare insurees who die within a year (39). On the surface, this sounds extraordinarily wasteful. But the vast majority of the 4500 Americans aged 65 and older who die every day (5) are relatively low-cost cases.

Suppose, however, care were to be denied to prospective *high-cost* Medicare decedents (although, clinically, it is rarely possible to make highly reliable prospective distinctions between high-cost survivors and decedents). Even if it were ethically and morally palatable to implement a policy that denied treatment to such high-cost patients, and thereby to eliminate "wasteful" health care, the dollars saved would be insignificant in the larger context of national health care costs.

High-cost Medicare decedents, as reasonably defined, annually account for 3.5 percent of Medicare expenditures (40–43). In 1993, when Medicare expenditures were estimated to be $153 billion, a policy that denied high-cost Medicare patients treatment would have saved $5.3 billion. Viewed in isolation, this is a substantial amount of money. But in the larger context, saving such an amount would have produced a negligible effect on the overall situation; it would have reduced national health care costs from $900 billion to just under $895 billion, a saving of about 0.006 percent, six-tenths of 1 percent.

In another approach, Emanuel and Emanuel (44) have estimated the savings that could be achieved if advance directives, hospice care, and the elimination of aggressive care could be effectively implemented for all persons aged 65 and older who will die within the year. They calculate that such methods to reduce the use of aggressive life-sustaining interventions would save, hypothetically, 6.1 percent of annual Medicare expenditures. In

1993, this would have yielded $9.3 billion, or 1 percent of total national health care expenditures.

In short, the impact on national health care costs is likely to be negligible from trying to save money by limiting aggressive, high-cost care for older patients who are going to die within a year. Even if one considered such amounts significant to save in a given year, such savings would not restrain the rate of growth in health care spending over time. As noted above, increases in service intensity, utilization rates, health-sector specific price inflation, and general inflation are vastly more significant factors in annual health care cost increases.

Such facts about the economic insignificance of futile care are not widely known and appreciated. Yet, even if they are understood, it seems very likely that issues of high-cost acute care for those older persons who *survive*, as well as for those who die, will continue to be debated. A substantial agenda of research needs to be implemented to inform such debates about specific types of aggressive care—coronary artery bypass operations, kidney and liver transplants, and so on—for patients of advanced age. At the moment, for instance, the conventional wisdom is that extraordinary amounts of money are expended on acute care for persons age 80 years and older. Yet, data suggest that this is far from true (45).

Financing Long-Term Care

More than eighty federal programs and a plethora of state and local public and private agencies are sources of funding for long-term care services (46). Each source regulates the availability of funds with rules as to eligibility and breadth of service coverage and rules change frequently; patients are often designated ineligible for funding through Medicare, Medicaid, the Veterans Administration, and other programs. Thus, despite the many sources of funding, specific patients and caregivers may find themselves ineligible for financial help and unable to pay out-of-pocket for needed services. In one study, about 75 percent of the informal caregivers for dementia patients reported that they did not use formal services because they were unable to pay for them (47).

Paying out-of-pocket for long-term care can be a catastrophic financial experience for patients and their families. The annual cost of a year's care in a nursing home

averages $37,000 (48) and can range higher than $100,000. Although the use of a limited number of services in a home or in other community-based settings is less expensive, non-institutional care for patients who would otherwise be appropriately placed in a nursing home is not cheaper (49). Patients and their families paid more than $33.5 billion out-of-pocket for long-term care services in 1993 (50). The total national expenditure for long-term care was $75.5 billion. Payments from all sources for nursing homes added up to $54.7 billion, and for home care the sum was $20.8 billion. Out-of-pocket payments accounted for 51 percent of nursing home costs and 26 percent of home care expenditures.

Private Insurance

Although Medicare pays for short-term, subacute nursing care, it does not reimburse patients for long-term care, either in nursing homes or at home. Private long-term care insurance, a relatively new product, is very expensive for most older persons, and its benefits are limited in scope and duration. The best quality policies providing substantial benefits over a long period of time charged annual premiums in 1991 averaging $2,525 for persons age 65 year and $7,675 for those age 79 years (48). About 4 percent to 5 percent of older persons have private long-term care insurance, and only about 1 percent of nursing home costs are paid for by private insurance (50). A number of analyses have suggested that even when private long-term insurance becomes more refined, no more than 20 percent of older Americans will be able to afford it (50–53). Although some studies suggest a potential for a higher percentage of customers, these studies assume limited packages of benefit coverage (54).

A variation on the use of private insurance to finance long-term care is the use of continuing-care retirement communities (CCRCs) that promise comprehensive health care services, including long-term care, to all members (55). CCRC customers tend to be middle- and upper-income persons who are relatively healthy when they become residents and who pay a substantial entrance charge and monthly fee in return for a promise of "care for life." It has been estimated that about 10 percent of older people could afford to join such communities (56). Most of the 1000 CCRCs in the US, however, do not provide complete benefit coverage in their contracts, and those that do have faced financial difficulties (57). Because most older people prefer to remain in their own homes rather than join age-segregated communities, an alternative product termed "life care at home" (LCAH) was developed in the late 1980s and marketed to middle-income customers. LCAH offered lower entry and monthly fees than those of CCRCs (58). There are, however, only about 500 LCAH policies in effect (57).

A relatively new approach for providing long-term care in residential settings is the "assisted living" facility created for moderately disabled persons who are not ready for a nursing home. An assisted living facility provides limited forms of personal care, supervision of medications and other daily routines, and congregate meal and housekeeping services (59). Assisted living has yet to be combined with an insurance component.

The Role of Medicaid

For those who cannot pay out-of-pocket for long-term care or pay through various insurance arrangements, and who are not eligible for care through programs of the Department of Veterans Affairs, the available sources of payment are Medicaid and other means-tested government programs funded by the Older Americans Act, Social Service Block Grants (Title XX of the Social Security Act), and state and local governments. The bulk of such financing is through Medicaid, which paid an estimated 52 percent of total national nursing home expenditures in 1993, accounting for one-quarter of all Medicaid spending (1).

Medicaid finances the care, at least in part, of about 60 percent of nursing home patients (48). Medicaid does not pay for the full range of home care services that are needed for most clients who are functionally dependent. Most state Medicaid programs provide reimbursement only for the most "medicalized" services that are necessary to maintain a long-term care patient in a home environment; rarely reimbursed are essential supports such as chore services, assistance with food shopping and meal preparation, transportation, companionship, periodic monitoring, and respite programs for family and other unpaid caregivers.

Medicaid does include a special waiver program that allows states to offer a wider range of nonmedical home care services if these services are limited to patients who otherwise would require Medicaid-financed nursing home care. But the volume of services in these waiver programs, which, in some states, combine Medicaid with funds from the Older Americans Act, the Social Services Block Grant program, and other state and local government sources, is small in relation to the overall need (60).

Although many patients are poor enough to qualify for Medicaid when they enter a nursing home, a substantial number become poor after they are institutionalized (61). Persons in the latter group deplete their assets to meet their bills and eventually "spend down" and become poor enough to qualify for Medicaid. Others become eligible for Medicaid by sheltering their assets—illegally or legally with the assistance of attorneys who specialize in so-called Medicaid estate planning. Because sheltered assets are not counted in Medicaid eligibility determinations, such persons, without being poor, are able to take advantage of a program designed for the poor. An analysis in Virginia estimated that the aggregate of assets sheltered through the use of legal loopholes in 1991 was equal to more than 10 percent of what the state spent on nursing home care through Medicaid in that year (62). Asset sheltering has become a source of considerable concern to the federal and state governments as Medicaid expenditures on nursing homes are increasing rapidly and are projected to triple from 1990 to 2000 (1).

Private Insurance/Medicaid Partnerships

The Robert Wood Johnson Foundation has undertaken an experimental program in four states. The program is intended to enable middle- and upper-income older persons to protect their assets from being spent down and have Medicaid pay for their long-term care (63). Through the Partnership for Long-Term Care Program, state governments agree to exempt spending of assets by Medicaid clients if these clients have previously had their long-term care paid for by a state-certified private insurance policy. In California, Connecticut, and Indiana, the Medicaid agencies allow a dollar of asset protection for each dollar that has been paid by insurance. In New York, after three years of nursing home coverage or six months of home health coverage, protection is granted for all assets; however, the individual's income must be devoted to the cost of care along with Medicaid. This experiment is in its early stages and cannot yet be evaluated.

Public Long-Term Care Insurance: An Issue on the Agenda

In response to lobbying efforts (64,65) U.S. Representative Claude Pepper introduced a bill in 1989 to provide federal long-term home care insurance coverage for persons of any age who were dependent in at least two ADLs. Since then, a number of long-term care bills have been introduced to provide coverage for nursing home and home care, with projected expenditures ranging from $10 billion to $60 billion, depending on provisions regarding the specific populations to be eligible and details regarding the timing, nature, and extent of insurance coverage. The home and community-based long-term care component in President Clinton's 1993 health reform package (23) carried forward the principle of age-irrelevance in determining eligibility for benefits. It also introduced the element of cost-sharing by clients, with the poorest having their care fully reimbursed and wealthier clients having to pay for some of their care.

Mainly because of anticipated costs, no federal long-term care program has yet been enacted. Nonetheless, the principle now seems firmly established that any long-term care policy that may emerge will rely on criteria involving need for services, not on an age-categorical approach.

Whether the principle of age-irrelevance will prove to be politically viable remains to be seen. Even if the fiscal costs of such a program become perceived as manageable, it is far from certain that older people and younger disabled people—the latter including persons with spinal cord injury, cerebral palsy, mental retardation, acquired immunodeficiency syndrome (AIDS), and other disabling conditions—will emerge as a powerful, unified, constituent coalition backing such legislation. Unity will require substantial resolution of divergent outlooks and needs among the constituencies to be served.

Traditionally, advocates for the aged and for younger disabled populations have not been united in supporting long-term care initiatives and have sometimes engaged in sharp conflict (66). From the perspective of older persons, long-term care has been seen as a problem besetting elderly people, categorically, to be dealt with through a "medical model" of health and social services. And a major, though not exclusive, element of interest in public insurance has been generated by the possibility of becoming poor through spending down and thereby becoming dependent on a welfare program, Medicaid, to pay long-term care bills. There is a distinct middle-class fear, both economic and psychological, of using savings and selling a home to finance one's own health care. This anxiety reflects a desire to preserve estates for inheritance, as well as the psychological intertwining of personal self-esteem with one's lifetime accumulation of material worth and sense of financial independence. This kind of concern has little political appeal beyond segments of the old-age constituency, of course, in the contemporary political environment structured by a generational equity paradigm (67).

In contrast to older persons, younger disabled persons and their advocates do not perceive long-term care insurance as primarily an issue of whether the government, or the individual client, or the family pays for the care. At least as important to disabled younger people are autonomy and independence. Their prime issue is basic access to services, technologies, and environments that will make feasible a "normalization" of daily life—that is, make it possible for them to do much of what they would be able to do if they were not disabled.

The Americans with Disabilities Act of 1991 helps to eliminate discriminatory and physical barriers to the participation of people with disabilities in employment, public services, public accommodations and transportation, and telecommunications. But it does not provide for disabled younger adults the elements of long-term care such as paid assistance in the home and for getting in and out of the home, peer counseling, semi-independent modes of transportation, and client control or management of services.

Although the younger disabled have advocated long-term care services, they have rejected a medical model that emphasizes long-term care as an essential component of health services. By the same token, disabled people have tended to eschew symbolic and political identification with elderly people because of traditional stereotypes of older people as frail, chronically ill, declining, and "marginal" to society.

Beyond issues of disparate philosophy lie specific divergences in service needs. For example, persons disabled through spinal cord injuries tend to remain in stable medical and functional condition for many years. Persons with AIDS have a trajectory of decline, punctuated by intermittent and continual episodes of acute illness. Although the trajectory for many elderly persons in long-term care is gradual decline, on average their need for acute care is not as frequent as that of persons with AIDS (68).

Despite their traditional differences, advocates for the aged and the disabled did work together temporarily in the planning process for President Clinton's 1993 initiative on long-term care. This was reflected in the fact that the President's proposal incorporated many specific concerns that have been put forward by advocates for the younger disabled population over the years; for example, the principle that clients should be able at their own discretion to hire and fire service providers. But unity eroded shortly thereafter in the context of considerable reservations that the respective constituencies had regarding the overall Clinton plan for health care reform (69).

Integrating Acute and Long-Term Health Care

A long-recognized problem in the financing and organization of health care for older people is the fragmentation of the delivery system. Few units of organization integrate acute and long-term care in ways that are optimal either for patient care or for cost-efficiency. Separate sources of financing for acute and long-term care—especially the separate streams of funding through Medicare and Medicaid and the incentives associated with them—tend to engender fragmentation and, often, inappropriate care. Even when acute and long-term care services are part of the same organization, as is the case for hospitals that have their own nursing home beds, financial incentives can be perverse. As Meiners notes (63):

> [T]he fact is that Medicare and Medicaid policy have contributed to our fragmented system of care. Unnecessary hospitalizations of those in nursing homes are encouraged by low Medicaid reimbursements, bed hold day payments, and DRG related payment incentives for short stay hospital admissions. Physician payments are biased toward hospital care instead of care in the office, home, or nursing home. More emergency room visits, medical transportation, and readmissions result.

Experimental models for integrating financing and care for older patients have been developed and are being refined through field demonstrations. Each involves the mechanism of managed care. But their differences illustrate some of the issues and challenges generated by various sources of funding and different types of older patient populations.

During the last decade, projects such as the National Channeling project; the Triage project in Connecticut; the ACCESS project in Rochester, New York; and the South Carolina long-term care project have used case management as a means of integrating services on a cost-effective basis. On the whole they have not proved to be cost-effective because in most case the sources of funding were not integrated (70).

A financially integrated model, initially tested at several sites in the 1980s, is the Social Health Maintenance Organization (S/HMO), financed experimentally with waivers from the federal Health Care Financing Administration (HCFA). The S/HMO offers customers a limited package of home and community-based long-term care benefits on a capitated basis as a supplement to Medicare HMO benefits, and attempts to enroll primarily healthy older customers (71). The S/HMO seeks to demonstrate what is financially feasible for such a population. Results from the early experiments were equivocal with respect to the viability of financing arrangements and target populations (72). Consequently, Congress called for a second round of S/HMO demonstrations to test refinements such as heavy involvement of geriatricians and geriatric nurse practitioners; standard protocols for obtaining adequate medical and social histories and for diagnosing and managing conditions frequently found in older patients; increased attention to the effects of prescription drugs on patients; and outpatient alternatives to hospitalization and nursing home placement.

Another approach, the On Lok model developed at a San Francisco neighborhood center in the 1970s and early 1980s, is targeted to community-based older persons who are already sufficiently dependent in ADLs and IADLs to be appropriately placed in a nursing home. Most patients are eligible for both Medicare and Medicaid. Services are organized around an adult day care program that not only serves as a social program and as a respite for caregivers, but also functions much like a geriatric outpatient clinic with substantial medical observation and supervision (73). The On Lok model, now being replicated at 10 demonstration sites as a Program for All-Inclusive Care for the Elderly (PACE), appears to have integrated acute and long-term care fairly well under its managed care approach. Whether it can be extended beyond the very frail population it has served to date—patients who are already functionally dependent, and dually eligible for Medicare and Medicaid—remains to be seen. (To some extent, this is what is being explored in the second round of the S/HMO demonstrations.) Early evaluations of the PACE demonstrations indicate that they are experiencing problems with financial viability, high staff turnover among physicians and adult day health center directors, and the right patient mix in terms of both acuity and dementia (74).

Yet another model attempting to integrate the financing and delivery of acute and long-term care for older persons is the Minnesota Long-Term Care Options Project (LTCOP). Still in the planning stage, LTCOP is incorporating elements of both the S/HMO and the On Lok models. In contrast to the S/HMO, however, LTCOP targets Medicaid-eligible enrollees and accordingly offers a benefit package that includes nursing home care as well as home and community-based care. LTCOP includes a less functionally dependent population than the On Lok model. Hence, it provides an opportunity to test broader approaches to integrating acute and long-term care than any that have been tried to date.

Conclusion

Major changes in the financing and organization of health care for older people are sure to continue taking place in the years immediately ahead. In late 1995, for instance, the 104th Congresss was attempting to eliminate the open-ended federal "entitlement" feature of Medicaid that guarantees coverage for every poor citizen, and to turn Medicaid into a block grant program that provides a fixed amount of Medicaid coverage and what benefits that coverage provides. Political conflict would ensue at the state level among competing constituencies of the poor—elderly people, children, and others. Many analysts have speculated that Medicaid-financed home- and community-based care would be eliminated in most

states. It is also likely that Medicaid reimbursement rates to nursing homes would become increasingly inadequate for maintaining quality of care.

The financing and organizational changes that have taken place and will take place are emerging in an arena of geriatric medicine that has already undergone substantial changes in recent years. Geriatric emergency medicine is developing as a specialty as a result of the complex challenges frequently involved in treating older patients beset by multiple clinical disorders (75). Multidisciplinary geriatric assessment teams have been established in the belief that they will improve the choice of treatment goals as well as discharge objectives (76). Special acute care geriatric wards are being developed as environments to facilitate functional recuperation and independence of older patients (77). Diagnostic and therapeutic interventions traditionally undertaken on an inpatient basis, such as cataract surgery, herniorrhaphy, bronchoscopy, colonoscopy, and coronary angiography, are now being done as outpatient procedures (78).

The adoption of prospective payments for reimbursing hospitals has not only shortened the average length of hospital stays (79), but also has had the salutary effect of heightening the importance of responsible discharge planning. Nearly one-fifth of elderly patients discharged from hospitals require nursing home placement for either short-term or long-term care, and in one study over 50 percent of patients age 75 years and older needed home health care (80).

Among these new developments, however, perhaps the most important challenges are those that will shape the core elements of medical practice. As finances have become a central concern, and as many more physicians function in the context of managed care structures instead of the traditional fee-for-service context, the role of the physician is becoming increasingly ambiguous. Changes in financing and organization are posing issues that will sharply affect geriatric medicine in the years immediately ahead—What or who determines the appropriate course of treatment? The third-party payers, Medicare, Medicaid, and insurance companies? Hospital administrators? How authentic is the patient's right to decide in this context? Will the physician's traditional role in determining "good care" become tenuous? What impact will ambiguity in the locus of responsibilities for medical decision making have on doctor-patient relationships, and, most important, on the quality of care provided to geriatric patients? The resolution of issues such as these, generated by the swiftly changing arena of financing and organization, will markedly shape the future of geriatric medicine and care for older people.

References

1. Burner ST, Waldo DR, McKusick DR. National health expenditures projections through 2030. Health Care Financ Rev 1992;14:1–29.
2. Waldo DR, Sonnefeld ST, McKusick DR, Arnett RH III. Health expenditures by age group, 1977 and 1987. Health Care Financ Rev 1989;10:111–120.
3. U.S. Senate, Special Committee on Aging. Aging America: trends and projections. Washington, DC: U.S. Government Printing Office, 1991.
4. U.S. Senate, Special Committee on Aging. Developments in aging: 1993. vol. 1. Washington, DC: U.S. Government Printing Office, 1994.
5. National Center for Health Statistics. Annual summary of births, marriages, divorces and death: United States, 1993. vol. 42, no. 13. Hyattsville, MD: Public Health Service, 1994.
6. U.S. Bureau of the Census. Nursing home population: 1990. CPH-L-137. Washington, DC: U.S. Government Printing Office, 1993.
7. U.S. Department of Education, National Institute on Disability and Rehabilitation Research. Disability statistics abstract. Washington, DC: U.S. Government Printing Office, 1992.
8. Leon J, Lair T. Functional status of the noninstitutionalized elderly: estimates of ADL and IADL difficulties. National Medical Expenditure Survey Research Findings 4. DHHS Pub. No. (PHS)90-3462. Rockville, MD: Agency for Health Care Policy and Research, Public Health Service, 1990.
9. Liu K, Manton KM, Liu BM. Home care expenses for the disabled elderly. Health Care Financ Rev 1985;7:52.
10. National Association for Home Care. Basic statistics about home care. Washington, DC: National Association for Home Care, 1992.
11. National Center for Health Statistics. Current estimates from the National Health Interview Survey, 1989. Vital and health statistics. ser. 10, no. 176. Hyattsville, MD: Public Health Service, 1990.
12. Taeuber CM. Sixty-five plus in America. Current populations reports, special studies, P23-178. Washington, DC: U.S. Government Printing Office, 1992.
13. Callahan D. Setting limits: Medical goals in an aging society. New York: Simon & Schuster, 1987.
14. Schneider EL, Guralnik JM. The aging of America: impact on health care costs. JAMA 1990;263:2335–2340.
15. Sonnenfeld ST, Waldo DR, Lemieux J, McKusick DR. Projec-
tions of national health expenditures through the year 2000. Health Care Financ Rev 1991;13;1–27.
16. Mendelson DN, Schwartz WB. The effects of aging and population growth on health care costs. Health Aff 1993;12:119–125.
17. Arnett RH III, McKusick DR, Sonnefeld ST, Cowell CS. Projections of health care spending to 1990. Health Care Financ Rev 1986;7:1–36.
18. Binstock RH. Health care costs around the world: is aging a fiscal "black hole?" Generations 1993;XVII:37–42.
19. Coulam RF, Gaumer GL. Medicare's prospective payment system: a critical appraisal. Health Care Financ Rev 1991; (annual suppl):45–77.
20. Brown RS, Bergeron JW, Clement DG, et al. Does managed care work for Medicare? An evaluation of the Medicare risk program for HMOs. Princeton: Mathematica Policy Research, 1993.
21. Congressional Budget Office, Congress of the United States. The economic and budget outlook: an update. Washington, DC: U.S. Government Printing Office, 1993.
22. Bipartisan Commission on Entitlement and Tax Reform. Commission findings. Washington, DC: Bipartisan Commission on Entitlement and Tax Reform, 1994.
23. White House Domestic Policy Council. The President's health security plan. New York: Random House, 1993.
24. Kane RL, Kane RA. Effects of the Clinton health reform on older persons and their families: a health care systems perspective. Gerontologist 1994;34:598–605.
25. Kasper JD, Riley GF, McCombs JS. Capitation and Medicare: Past, present, and future. In: Pauly M, Kissick WL, eds. Lessons from the first twenty years of Medicare: research implications for public and private sector policy. Philadelphia: University of Pennsylvania, 1988:239–272.
26. Aaron HJ, Schwartz WB. The painful prescription: rationing hospital care. Washington, DC: The Brookings Institution, 1984.
27. Congressional Budget Office, Congress of the United States. The economic and budget outlook: fiscal years 1995–1999. Washington, DC: U.S. Government Printing Office, 1994.
28. Binstock RH. The oldest old and "intergenerational equity." In: Suzman R, Willis D, Manton K, eds. The oldest old. New York: Oxford University, 1992:394–417.
29. Slater W. Latest Lamm remark angers the elderly. Arizona Daily Star March 29, 1984:1.
30. Lamm RD. A debate: Medicare in 2020. Medicare reform and the baby boom generation. Proceedings of the Second Annual Conference of Americans for Generational Equity. Washington, DC: Americans for Generational Equity, 1987:77–88.
31. Lamm RD. Columbus and Copernicus: new wine in old wineskins. Mt Sinai J Med 1989;56:1–10.
32. Daniels N. Am I my parents' keeper? An essay on justice between the young and the old. New York: Oxford University, 1988.
33. Menzel PT. Strong medicine: the ethical rationing of health care. New York: Oxford University, 1990.

34. Smeeding TM, Battin MP, Francis LP, Landesman BM, eds. Should medical care be rationed by age? Totowa, NJ: Rowman & Littlefield, 1987.

35. Homer P, Holstein M, eds. A good age: the paradox of setting limits. New York: Simon & Schuster, 1990.

36. Binstock RH, Post SG, eds. Too old for health care? Controversies in medicine, law, economics, and ethics. Baltimore: The Johns Hopkins University, 1991.

37. Barry RL, Bradley GV, eds. Set no limits: a rebuttal to Daniel Callahan's proposal to limit health care for the elderly. Urbana: University of Illinois, 1987.

38. Castro J. Condition critical. Time November 25, 1991:35–42.

39. Lubitz JD, Riley GF. Trends in Medicare payments in the last year of life. N Engl J Med 1993;328:1092–1096.

40. Lubitz JD, Prihoda R. The use and costs of Medicare services in the last two years of life. Health Care Financ Rev 1984;5:117–131.

41. Scitovsky AA. The high cost of dying: what do the data show? Milbank Q 1984;62:591–608.

42. Scitovsky AA. Medical care in the last twelve months of life: the relation between age, functional status, and medical care expenditures. Milbank Mem Q 1988;66:640–660.

43. Congressional Research Service, Library of Congress, Congress of the United States. Health care costs at the end of life. Washington, DC: U.S. Government Printing Office, 1990.

44. Emanuel EJ, Emanuel LL. The economics of dying: the illusion of cost savings at the end of life. N Engl J Med 1994;330:540–544.

45. Fortinsky RH, Binstock RH, Sivinski L, Rimm A. An empirical look at Medicare costs in the context of age-based rationing. Paper presented at the Annual Meeting of the American Public Health Association, Washingtion, DC, November 1, 1994.

46. Congressional Research Service, Library of Congress, Congress of the United States. Financing and delivery of long-term care services for the elderly. Washington, DC: U.S. Government Printing Office, 1988.

47. Eckert SK, Smyth K. A case study of methods of locating and arranging health and long-term care for persons with dementia. Washington, DC: Office of Technology Assessment, Congress of the United States, 1988.

48. Wiener JM, Illston LH. Health care financing and organization for the elderly. In: Binstock RH, George LK, eds. Handbook of aging and the social sciences, 4th ed. San Diego: Academic Press, 1996;427–445.

49. Weissert WG. Strategies for reducing home care expenditures. Generations 1990;XIV:42–44.

50 Wiener JM, Illston LH, Hanley RJ. Sharing the burden: strategies for public and private long-term care insurance. Washington, DC: The Brookings Institution, 1994.

51. Crown WH, Capitman J, Leutz WN. Economic rationality, the affordability of private long-term care insurance, and the role for public policy. Gerontologist 1992;32:478–485.

52. Friedland R. Facing the costs of long-term care: an EBRI-ERF policy study. Washington, DC: Employee Benefits Research Institute, 1990.

53. Rivlin AM, Wiener JM. Caring for the disabled elderly: who will pay? Washington, DC: The Brookings Institution, 1988.

54. Cohen MA, Tell E, Greenberg J, Wallack SS. The financial capacity of the elderly to insure for long-term care. Gerontologist 1987;27:494–502.

55. Chellis RD, Grayson PJ. Life care: a long-term solution? Lexingtion, MA: Lexington Books, 1990.

56. Cohen M. Life care: new options for financing and delivering long-term care. Health Care Financ Rev 1988; (annual suppl):139–143.

57. Williams TF, Temkin-Greener H. Older people, dependency, and trends in supportive care. In: Binstock RH, Cluff LE, von Mering O, eds. The future of long-term care: social and policy issues. Baltimore: Johns Hopkins University (in press:1996).

58. Tell EJ, Cohen MA, Wallack SS. New directions in lifecare: an industry in transition. Milbank Q 1987;65:551–574.

59. Kane RA, Wilson KB. Assisted living in the United States: a new paradigm for residential care for older people? Washington, DC: American Association for Retired Persons, 1993.

60. Miller NA. Medicaid 2176 home and community-based care waivers: the first ten years. Health Aff 1992;11:162–171.

61. Adams EK, Meiners MR, Burwell BO. Asset spend-down in nursing homes: methods and insights. Med Care 1993;31:1–23.

62. Burwell B. State responses to Medicaid estate planning. Cambridge, MA: SysteMetrics, 1993.

63. Meiners MR. The financing and organization of long-term care. In: Binstock RH, Cluff LE, von Mering O, eds. The future of long-term care: social and policy issues. Baltimore: Johns Hopkins University (in press:1996).

64. Fox P. From senility to Alzheimer's disease: the rise of the Alzheimer's disease movement. Milbank Q 1989;67:58–102.

65. McConnell S. Who cares about long-term care? Generations 1990;XIV:15–18.

66. Torress-Gil FM, Pynoos J. Long-term care policy and interest group struggles. Gerontologist 1986;26:488–495.

67. Binstock RH. Transcending "intergenerational equity." In: Marmor TR, Smeeding TM, Greene VL, eds. Economic security, intergenerational justice: a look at North America. Washingtion, DC: Urban Institute, 1994:155–185.

68. Benjamin AE. Trends among younger persons with disabilities and chronic diseases. In: Binstock RH, Cluff LE, von Mering O, eds. The future of long-term care: social and policy issues. Baltimore: Johns Hopkins University (in press:1996).

69. Binstock RH. Older Americans and health care reform in the 1990s. In: Rosenau PV, ed. Health care reform in the nineties. Thousand Oaks, CA: Sage, 1994:213–235.

70. Weissert WG, Hedrick S. Lessons learned from research on effects of community-based long-term care. J Am Geriatr Soc 1994;42:348–353.

71. Leutz W, Greenberg JN, Abrahams R, et al. Changing health care for an aging society: planning for the social/health maintenance organization. Lexington, MA: Lexington Books, 1985.

72. Newcomer RJ, Harrington C, Friedlob A. Social health main-

tenance organizations: assessing their initial experience. Health Serv Res 1990;25:425–454.

73. Zawadski RT, Eng C. Case management in capitated long-term care. Health Care Financ Rev 1988; (annual suppl):75–81.

74. Kane RA, Illston LH, Miller NA. Qualitative analysis of the program of all-inclusive care for the elderly (PACE). Gerontologist 1992;32:771–780.

75. Bosker G, Schwartz GR, Jones JS, Sequeira M. Geriatric emergency medicine. St. Louis: Mosby, 1990.

76. Gallo JJ, Reichel W, Andersen L. Handbook of geriatric assessment. Rockville, MD: Aspen, 1988.

77. Rubenstein LZ, Stuck AE, Sui AL, Wieland GD. Impacts of geriatric evaluation and management programs on defined outcomes: overview of the evidence. J Am Geriatr Soc 1991;39(suppl):8S–16S.

78. Macaluso J, Thomas R. Extracorporeal shock wave lithotripsy: an outpatient procedure. J Urol 1991;146:714–717.

79. Russell LB. Medicare's new hospital payment system: is it working? Washington, DC: The Brookings Institution, 1989.

80. Rubin C, Sizemore M, Loftis P, et al. The effect of geriatric evaluation and management on Medicare reimbursement in a large public hospital: a randomized clinical trial. J Am Geriatr Soc 1992;40:989–995.

Chapter 4
Geriatric Neuropsychology

Deborah C. Koltai and Gordon J. Chelune

The crucial task of old age is balance: keeping just well enough, just brave enough, just gay and interested and starkly honest enough to remain a sentient human being.

Florida Scott-Maxwell
The Measure of My Days

Clinical neuropsychology is an applied science that involves the evaluation of simple and complex brain-behavior relationships. Central to its practice is the use of standardized instruments. The use of standardized, objective tests to measure neurocognitive abilities is based on systematic theories of the structure of human abilities. Test data are then interpreted within the context of demographic, medical, and psychosocial data to yield information about the neuropsychological status of the individual. Traditional uses of these evaluations have included the identification and delineation of cognitive and behavioral manifestations of central nervous system impairment, differential diagnosis, and the development and application of behavioral plans based on the patient's functional abilities.

In contrast to evaluations based on clinical impression, the use of standardized instruments to measure cognitive abilities avoids many sources of bias or error. Domains screened during a typical mental status examination, such as judgment and insight, are among those subject to the most bias (1). Evaluations based on clinical impressions can be unreliable and imprecise, and are not quantitative (2). The lack of quantitative data precludes reliable test-retest assessments to follow changes in the patient that may be caused by illness or intervention. To address the referral question and the needs of the patient, the neuropsychologist tailors the assessment approach by using varying combinations of standardized, validated instruments, administered in the same systematic fashion to all patients (3).

The use of neuropsychological evaluations in the workup of geriatric patients has grown as primary care physicians and therapists have recognized the frequency and impact of cognitive changes in the elderly. It is well known that the size of the elderly population is growing (4), and there is some recent evidence suggesting that the incidence of dementing illness among the elderly may also be increasing (5).

In this chapter, cognitive change associated with normal aging and illnesses is briefly discussed. In addition, the role of the neuropsychologist is addressed, followed by a discussion of questions addressed by neuropsychological evaluations. Finally, commonly used tests are presented to familiarize the reader with some of the instruments used in neuropsychological batteries.

Normal Aging

Cognitive changes associated with normal aging can be most precisely measured by neuropsychological tests, which at times provide the only possible confirmation of suspected decline (6). Age-related decline is generally observed after the age of 50, with little or no nonpathological decline occurring before this age (7).

The constructs of fluid and crystallized abilities (8) can be used to address which cognitive functions tend to decline with age. Fluid abilities are skills associated with problem solving and the performance of novel tasks, sometimes under time pressure; these tend to decline with normal aging. In contrast, crystallized abilities involve overlearned knowledge and tend to be less susceptible to decline. Thus, tasks measuring verbal, rehearsed knowledge, such as the verbal subtests of the Wechsler Adult Intelligence Scale–Revised (9), tend to be more resistant to decline, whereas perceptual-organizational subtests tend to show normal, age-related decline.

Normal, age-related decline has been the subject of many investigations that have shown decrements in various skills, but particularly in memory and in abilities related to executive functions (10). Measures that use distraction and delayed free recall have been shown to be particularly sensitive to the effects of aging (11). Other investigators have reported that aging effects are noted more frequently on visual-perceptual and constructional tasks than on memory tasks (12).

Van Gorp et al (13) found that speed of processing also declines with age. Benton and Sivan (14) stated that in addition to tasks that make demands on short-term memory, tasks in which speed of response is related to perceptual-organizational scores show a greater rate of decline with age. However, there is some evidence that age-related decrements are demonstrated on performance-based tasks even when these tests are administered in an untimed manner (15), which suggests that speed of processing alone does not account for these changes.

Table 4.1 summarizes the neuropsychological domains associated with normal, age-related decline. Differences in what various investigators have reported to be the domains most affected by aging are partially a result of the different instruments used (14) and differences in methodology, such as the screening criteria for "normal, healthy elderly" adults (16). Many early studies of aging did not thoroughly screen subjects for illnesses affecting the central nervous system, resulting in conclusions that may be confounded by medical factors (4). Interindividual variability in performance also shows a tendency to increase with age (17), and this may represent another confounding variable in research on normal aging. The determinants of this variability remain only vaguely understood. It appears that some individuals carry more cognitive reserve against age-related decline than do others; this can be accounted for only partially by differences in education and medical status.

Education has been found to covary with performance

Table 4.1. Neuropsychological Domains Associated with Normal Age-Related Declines.

Learning and memory
Executive functions
Speed of information processing
Performance on timed tasks
Visual-perceptual and visual-constructional skills

on neuropsychological tests (18,19), but as is shown with age, the literature demonstrates that education does not equally influence the performance of individuals in all cognitive domains. Although an age-education interaction has been demonstrated, at the oldest age level there is no evidence that education makes any difference in age-related decline on perceptual-organizational subtests (19).

When assessing the cognitive abilities of a geriatric patient, the clinician must consider many variables that have the potential to alter test results. The effects of age and education, and their interaction, are among the variables that must be integrated with test data to make interpretations about the neurocognitive status of the geriatric patient.

Illnesses Associated with Cognitive Change

In addition to the cognitive changes encountered as a result of normal aging, some frequently encountered age-related illnesses can lead to disturbances in cognitive function. In spite of common myth, only 15 percent of individuals older than age 65 have dementia (20). Of those who do develop dementia, approximately 50 percent develop dementia of the Alzheimer's type (DAT) (6,21). Vascular dementias are the second most common organic cause of cognitive decline in the elderly (22). Approximately 5 percent of individuals older than 65 years have had at least one stroke (23), and multi-infarct dementia (MID) accounts for approximately 10 percent to 15 percent of patients with dementia (21,24). Estimates of patients with Parkinson's disease who develop substantial cognitive impairments range from 10 percent to 40 percent (24,25). Other primary neurodegenerative dementias, such as Pick's disease, are less common (6). Infections of the central nervous system, metabolic or endocrine system dysfunction, and electrolyte disturbances also have the potential to cause substantial changes in mental status.

These disease processes have multiple implications regarding the geriatric patient's functioning; some of these processes are inextricably linked to the individual's absolute and relative cognitive strengths and weaknesses. The patient's functional abilities and his or her management are greatly contingent on the integrity of the central nervous system. Neuropsychological evaluations can be used to delineate these capacities, to stage and follow cognitive decline, and to plan for treatment and management. They also can be used to monitor interventions and recovery of function through serial assessments in individuals whose cognitive decline is associated with a treatable etiology.

Neuropsychology and the Geriatric Team

Neuropsychologists traditionally provide a consultative service, but many may also be core members on specific treatment teams. The role of the neuropsychologist on a geriatric assessment and treatment team is to address the cognitive, behavioral, and affective aspects of the patient's functioning.

The use of neuropsychological input on geriatric teams has increased in the past 10 years as multidimensional geriatric assessment has grown. Some research supporting inter- and multidisciplinary approaches to geriatric assessment and treatment has demonstrated an improvement in diagnostic accuracy as well as more thorough and more cost-effective treatment and placement (26). One survey of interdisciplinary inpatient geriatric teams addressed the various goals, compositions, approaches, and usefulness of these teams (27). The investigators concluded that geriatric patients typically have medical and functional issues that require treatment by different disciplines, but that there are also concerns regarding the quality, efficiency, and cost of teams. Katz et al stated that, although the ideal way to respond to geriatric consultations is with an interdisciplinary approach, this is often too costly and that a single-physician comprehensive assessment can yield comparable results (28). However, these investigators also found that recommendations based on single-physician assessments were implemented in less than one-third of the cases, perhaps because the consultant "may have been looked upon by the ward staff as lacking credibility in the socioeconomic, psychologic, and functional rehabilitative domains." Katz et al also stated that many of the patients would have benefitted from formal psychological evaluation because mental health problems and cognitive dysfunction were numerous and a more comprehensive workup was warranted.

Clinicians serving geriatric patients have increasingly recognized the need to include functional measures in their assessments, particularly since the U.S. Commission on Chronic Illness emphasized the importance of "function" in illness (2). Ideally, the interdisciplinary evaluation of geriatric patients uses validated, quantitative instruments to assess a number of areas, such as activities of daily living (ADLs), cognitive and affective functioning, and medical and social systems. The aim of these evaluations is to yield information about the patient's functional abilities in addition to the patient's overall medical well-being. A change in the social, behavioral, psychiatric, or medical well-being of a patient impacts other domains; thus, a comprehensive evaluation must address all these aspects (29). Rubenstein's review of inter- and multidisciplinary teams revealed that, in addition to yielding improved diagnostic accuracy and more appropriate treatment and placements, improvement was also shown in functional status, affect or cognition, use of home health services, and prolonged survival. Concurrently, decreases have been shown in the number of prescribed medications, use of acute hospitals and nursing homes, and in medical costs (30).

Referral Questions

Neuropsychological instruments are designed and standardized in a way that allows the clinician to answer a number of questions relevant to the medical, psychological, and psychosocial functioning of patients. The following section discusses three areas in which neuropsychological evaluations are frequently used: differential diagnosis, functional assessments, and research.

Differential Diagnosis
Neuropsychological evaluations are frequently used to aid in diagnosis. With the advent of technologically advanced neuroimaging, such as computerized tomography (CT) and magnetic resonance imaging (MRI), the use of neuropsychological testing for localization of brain lesions has substantially decreased. CT and MRI procedures are useful in detecting gross anatomical lesions, although subtle neurological disease processes are not always detected by these methods. In addition, results from neuroimaging techniques can be misleading in terms of neurobehavioral correlates. The relationship between various levels of structural integrity and behavioral

impairments is still only vaguely understood. For instance, Johansson (31) found that among subjects in his sample, gray-matter atrophy was documented by CT in all cases demonstrating dementia, but also in 96 percent of nondemented subjects. Areas of decreased attenuation in the periventricular white matter were noted in 70 percent of the demented subjects, but also in 34 percent of the nondemented subjects. Neuroimaging techniques do not reflect compensatory behaviors or recovery of function. However, these factors can affect performance on neuropsychological tests, and thus can be considered and incorporated into interpretations about cognitive status and functional ability.

Unlike neuroimaging techniques, neuropsychological evaluation provides direct assessment of neurobehavioral functions. Various disease processes often produce relatively distinct constellations of neurocognitive change. Thus, the neuropsychologist can frequently use assessment data to characterize the nature and scope of an individual's impairment and determine its etiology. For instance, MID can be differentiated from DAT by examining the pattern of decline and relative areas of spared functioning. Structural damage to subcortical areas and their various pathways often leads to retrieval deficits despite adequate storage of information, whereas cortical damage tends to result in difficulties with the encoding and storage of information (32). Investigations have repeatedly shown that patients with DAT have impaired initial acquisition of verbal and nonverbal material, and that the information that is acquired is subject to rapid decay (33,34). Pick's disease is often characterized by marked deficits in executive functions and behavioral disinhibition, along with a relatively moderate impairment of memory (25).

Essential in the diagnostic process is the identification of treatable causes of cognitive decline. Clarfield (35) reviewed studies that provided follow-up and found that 8 percent of dementias resolved partially and 3 percent resolved fully. However, methodological flaws and inconsistencies have impeded a thorough understanding of dementias resulting from treatable causes (36). The most common sources of treatable intellectual impairment are reported as being depression, drug intoxication, and metabolic or infectious disorders (21,35). Some of these conditions have cognitive

hallmarks that aid in their identification, as in the case of depression.

Reports of clinical depression in the elderly general population have been as high as 13 percent (37). Reports of elderly individuals with medical illnesses reveal an even higher rate of depression, ranging from 20 percent to 35 percent (38). Kaszniak (39) stated that the largest source of misdiagnosis among elderly patients results from difficulty in distinguishing depression from dementia. The frequency of subjective memory complaints also increases with age and may or may not coexist with actual depression, making the distinction more difficult. Patients with dementia also may have a concurrent depression. However, a significant amount of research has investigated both the quantitative and qualitative types of errors in performance that these different subgroups make on neuropsychological tests (39–41). Results of affective screening, in combination with the pattern of deficits revealed during neuropsychological evaluation, helps the geriatric neuropsychologist to differentiate between dementias resulting from central nervous system compromise and the dementia of depression.

Functional Ability

Because many geriatricians have adopted a functional assessment model in the evaluation and treatment of the elderly, requests for neuropsychological evaluations with referral questions related to functional abilities have increased. A growing literature examining the relationship between performance on neuropsychological tests and everyday functioning has emerged (42–46). Some neuropsychological tests are now being developed with the specific goal of providing direct assessment and information about everyday tasks and activities (e.g., the Rivermead Behavioural Memory Test (47)).

Although, ideally, all neuropsychological evaluations sample all the major domains of cognitive ability, an evaluation that is designed to address functional abilities may sample specific behaviors relevant to everyday functioning in further detail. The primary difference in these assessments, however, lies not so much in the tests used as in the interpretation of the test results. Impressions will include information about what the patient can or cannot do in addition to the delineation of neurocognitive impairment and integrity. For instance, test results may reveal that a patient with specific difficulties with verbal memory may be able to learn and recall information that is presented visually. Patients can often recall information or comprehend instructions that are presented simply and sequentially, but they become overwhelmed when the information is too lengthy or complex. Assessments emphasizing the functional approach attempt to identify cognitive strengths and weaknesses and to determine what these mean relative to the everyday functioning of the patient. This information can then be applied to other essential areas, such as competency, behavioral planning, and discharge planning.

Issues of competence are among the most frequent questions addressed by the geriatric neuropsychologist (48). Although no clear standards exist at present for the evaluation of competence, some support for the use of neuropsychological data in these evaluations has emerged. Tymchuk et al (49) found that decision-making ability is related to tests of comprehension, and Stanley et al (50) demonstrated that cognitively impaired patients have difficulty comprehending important aspects of consent information. Others (51) have found that competency relates to tests of conceptualization.

Competency is defined in a variety of ways within the general context of abilities. Because there is no standard criteria to measure competence, the issue is typically approached by examining the patient's ability to understand treatment procedures, their side effects, and their alternatives. While information processing and judgment need to be relatively intact to answer these types of questions, adequate decision-making often involves more than these specific abilities alone. In addition, competency decisions may also be based on diagnoses such as dementia. These decisions provide little information about the functional capabilities of the patient (52) because he or she may function quite well in some areas but not in others.

The patient frequently benefits when assessment and decisions about the capacity of the patient are viewed in a framework that distinguishes between personal (psychosocial), financial, and medical competency. Because competence is directly linked to functional abilities, individuals may rank at different levels on a continuum of decision-making capacity (53). To appropriately maximize independence and promote the patient's autonomy,

a thorough evaluation of these different areas of competency is important. An individual may be competent for some matters but not for others (54). Neuropsychological test batteries can be tailored to address various aspects of an individual's decision-making capacity to identify areas of decline versus spared abilities. Again, the use of standardized tests to assess competency also aids in counteracting bias resulting from decisions being formed solely on the basis of clinical impression (55).

Functional assessments are also frequently applied to behavioral planning. The geriatric neuropsychologist is often consulted to design behavioral plans for individuals with significant cognitive limitations, particularly when behaviors become difficult for staff or family members to manage. An aspect of this includes education, as misunderstandings can often be minimized or avoided by understanding the sequelae of central nervous system impairment. For instance, without this understanding, a disruption of executive functions leading to disinhibition and impulsivity can be mistaken for oppositional behavior.

One survey (56) revealed that caregivers found agitation, hallucinations, and dangerous or embarrassing behaviors to be of more concern than disorientation or deficits in self-care. When designing plans to maximize behavioral compliance and independence, the neuropsychologist considers and integrates information regarding the patient's cognitive limitations, as well as the patient's behavioral and affective status. These plans can also be incorporated into plans for individual or group psychotherapy treatment for geriatric patients.

Planning for the long-term care of the geriatric patient is another area in which functional cognitive assessments are useful. Having detailed insight into a person's relative strengths and weaknesses and his or her ability to manage various levels of cognitive challenge is necessary to recommend the type of care the individual should receive. Thus, neuropsychological data can also be used to address this area of patient care.

Research

Neuropsychological assessments are also employed in empirical investigations designed to demonstrate the effects of different variables. The efficacy of pharmacological treatments or the impact of medical interventions on cognitive symptoms can be monitored by using performances on standardized neuropsychological instruments as outcome measures. Neuropsychological measures have also been used to document the course and specific pattern of cognitive decline in various diseases. Mechanisms of preservation versus decline have been investigated. For instance, investigations of various mnestic abilities have shown that procedural memory is often spared in patients with Huntington's disease, but episodic or declarative memory is not (57).

Evaluation of the Geriatric Patient

Rapport is a variable that often requires clinical sensitivity (58). Many geriatric patients have never had contact with a professional psychologist, and extra time may need to be taken to address the clinician's role and the purpose of the evaluation. Also, the geriatric patient often has visual or auditory deficits that can substantially affect test performance, and they need to be considered. These variables should be addressed before the evaluation to avoid attributing deficits in test performance to comprehension, visual-spatial, or mnestic impairment (48).

When designing the test battery, the neuropsychologist should consider the patient's stamina and overall level of ability in addition to the referral question. Because geriatric patients often fatigue easily, and patients with substantial cognitive deficits can become overwhelmed by the length of an evaluation or the level of information processing necessary to complete some tests, batteries may have to be modified to be shorter and to include less taxing instruments. Cunningham et al (59) studied the effects of fatigue and found its effects become a concern when batteries are longer than approximately 2.5 hours. Qualitative neurobehavioral approaches are also sometimes used to sample abilities when patients cannot complete comprehensive neuropsychological protocols. Although these levels of assessment do not yield the same amount or type of information, data concerning the patient's cognitive, behavioral, and affective status can still be obtained given these limitations.

The patient's history often provides information about the etiology of cognitive decline. Information about acute medical factors, remote central nervous system insults, the rate of decline, or presence of affective or behavioral changes can be essential to making a differential diagnosis (60). For instance, a change in personality involving inappropriate behavior is frequently an early symptom of Pick's disease. Stepwise deterioration is often suggestive of cerebrovascular disorders, whereas a gradual decline is frequently suggestive of primary neurodegenerative diseases.

Several cognitive domains should be measured. Typically evaluated are global intellectual functioning, attention and concentration, memory, executive functions, language and communication, visual-spatial functions, sensory-motor abilities, and mood and personality. As mentioned previously, it is essential to assess these domains because the constellation of deficits and spared areas of functioning is the cornerstone of neuropsychological interpretation.

Neuropsychological Instruments

Comprehensive test batteries, such as the Halstead-Reitan Battery (61,62) and the Luria-Nebraska Neuropsychological Battery (63) provide global measures of cognitive functioning. However, they are generally not used for elderly patients because the tests can be quite lengthy. Flexible batteries, made up of tests sampling each neurocognitive domain to measure specific abilities, are more commonly used with the geriatric population.

Screening Tests

Some tests are designed to be global screening or staging measures. Table 4.2 lists some frequently used measures, the abilities they assess, scores generated, and administration time. Most of these tests do not necessarily evaluate neurocognitive domains in depth, but instead identify the patient's overall level of cognitive functioning. However, some are designed to yield information about relative strengths and weaknesses and can be useful to evaluate patients who cannot tolerate lengthy test batteries. Caution must be exercised, however, because such tests may underestimate decline in individuals who had premorbidly superior abilities or higher levels of education, and may overestimate impairment in patients with less education (64).

The Mini-Mental Status Exam (MMSE) (65) is perhaps the most widely recognized bedside screening measure

Table 4.2. Screening Tests.

Abilities Assessed	Scores	Time
Mini-Mental Status Exam Orientation, verbal free recall, attention, calculation, repetition, comprehension, writing, visual constructional praxis	Single score	10–15 min
Neurobehavioral Cognitive Status Exam Orientation, digit span forward, verbal free recall, verbal recognition memory, psychomotor problem solving, calculation, judgment, verbal reasoning, naming, comprehension, repetition	Specific scores by subtests	20–40 min
Dementia Rating Scale Attention, digit span forward and backward, concentration, comprehension, verbal fluency, bimanual alternating motor movements, visual constructional praxis, verbal and visual reasoning, orientation, verbal free recall, verbal and visual recognition memory	Single score; specific scores for attention/concentration, memory, initiation/perseveration, construction, conceptualization	30–60 min
MicroCog Digit span forward and backward, vigilance, signal detection, incidental learning, verbal and visual recognition memory, verbal and visual reasoning, calculation, visual-spatial perception, reaction time	Specific scores by subtests; scores for information processing speed and accuracy; scores of general cognitive functioning and proficiency	30–60 min
Clock-Drawing Tasks Visual Constructional Praxis, planning	General score	1–3 min

for global cognitive functioning. This 30-item instrument requires minimal testing materials. Orientation is the most thoroughly addressed area, accounting for one-third of the MMSE items; all other areas are assessed with fewer items.

The original standardization sample for the MMSE consisted of 63 normal, elderly subjects, and early research suggested 87 percent sensitivity and 82 percent specificity for the test. However, later studies showed that age and years of education significantly affect performance and levels of sensitivity and specificity (64,66). The MMSE tends to overestimate impairment among individuals with less than nine years of education and those who are older than 60 years of age. The MMSE can also underestimate deficits in well-educated individuals who may find the items easy even in the presence of cerebral dysfunction. Factor analytic studies of the MMSE have suggested that as much as 66 percent of the variance can be accounted for by a two-factor structure consisting of an educational factor that comprises the reading and writing items and serial-sevens task, and a recent memory factor that includes the recall and orientation items (67). The

educational factor may exert a significant degree of influence on test outcome, which is consistent with other findings that level of education significantly affects MMSE scores.

Other variables also affect the overall level of performance on the MMSE. Principal lifetime occupations have been shown to relate significantly with MMSE scores, independent of age and education effects (68). Also, the MMSE has been reported to be less sensitive among patients with right hemisphere dysfunction or mild forms of cerebral dysfunction, regardless of origin (69).

The Neurobehavioral Cognitive Status Examination (NCSE) (70) is a brief, standardized screening measure of cognition that consists of 10 sections, each containing four to eight items. The NCSE utilizes a step-down procedure in which each area begins with the most difficult item, followed by easier items. If the patient is able to complete the most difficult item accurately, the easier items are not administered and the patient is given credit for them as if they had been passed.

The NCSE was standardized on 119 healthy adults between the ages of 20 years and 92 years, and normative data is presented for three age ranges (20 to 29; 40 to 66; and 70 to 92). The NCSE has been shown to be sensitive to the effects of brain dysfunction among neurosurgical patients with documented brain lesions (70). In another study (71), the sensitivity of the NCSE, MMSE, and the Cognitive Capacity Screening Examination (CCSE) (72) was examined in a group of patients with documented brain lesions. The false-negative rate for the CCSE was 53 percent, for the MMSE, 43 percent, but for the NCSE only 7 percent. The authors attributed the higher sensitivity of the NCSE to the use of independent subtests that assessed skills within the major domains of cognition, and the use of graded tasks within each of the domains.

The Mattis Dementia Rating Scale (DRS) (73) is a 144-item instrument that was specifically designed to stage the severity of dementia and to monitor the progression of cognitive decline. Although sensitive to various levels of cognitive ability among low-functioning individuals, the test is less sensitive among higher-functioning patients. Thus, the DRS is less sensitive to deficits among premorbidly high-functioning individuals who show a mild decline in cognitive ability, but who continue to function in the average range. Like the NCSE, the DRS uses a step-down procedure.

A number of investigations have been conducted to examine the psychometric properties of the DRS (74–76). Overall, the DRS has been shown to be effective in differentiating between various clinical groups with different levels of dementia. The DRS has also been shown to be sensitive to the differences between control subjects and patients with mild and moderately severe DAT (77). Another study showed that the DRS can distinguish among stages of dementia better than ratings on an Instrumental Activities of Daily Living scale (78), although the authors concluded that the use of the two measures in conjunction may improve prediction further (79).

In contrast to these studies, a recent investigation found that the attention and construction subscales of the DRS are not consistently reliable or valid, and that the initiation/perseveration subscale is not internally consistent. However, the DRS total score was found to be reliable and had good convergent and predictive validity (80). Another major drawback of the DRS is that it does not assess language functioning thoroughly and the memory items

are relatively simple (21). Because memory deficits and dysnomia are frequently observed in patients with DAT (22), the examiner may need to supplement the DRS with other measures to assess these functions.

The MicroCog: Assessment of Cognitive Functioning (81) represents a new generation of cognitive screening instrument. It is a computer administered and scored battery of tasks that is specifically designed to assess neurocognitive domains that are especially relevant to normal and pathological aging. Both a standard form and a short-form version are available. Both versions yield age- and education-corrected index scores based on a nationally representative standardization sample of 810 subjects that are grouped into three age ranges. Nine index scores are generated and are stratified into three levels, reflecting different levels of content.

Clinical studies with the MicroCog have yielded impressive sensitivity (65% to 94%) and specificity (65% to 94%) data. Green et al (82) were able to distinguish with 91.8 percent accuracy and 94 percent specificity a sample of 52 medically evaluated patients with mild cognitive impairment from a demographically matched control group of 50 individuals. Comparisons between groups with mild dementia or depression resulted in a sensitivity rate of 94.4 percent and a specificity rate of 78.9 percent.

Unfortunately, because of computer presentation of stimuli, the patient's expressive language skills and recall memory abilities cannot be evaluated. As mentioned previously, the assessment of these particular domains can be critical to the diagnosis of DAT (22). Nevertheless, although further validity studies are still forthcoming, the MicroCog can be clinically interpreted in terms of index and subtest patterns of performance that characterize the patient's cognitive strengths and limitations with respect to an appropriate age- and education-matched cohort.

Clock drawings are frequently used as a quick screening task for visual-constructional difficulties and general neurocognitive decline (83). Although many versions exist, the patient is typically asked to draw a clock, put in all the numbers, and set the hands to a predetermined time. Clock drawing has been studied in a number of investigations and there have been attempts at devising scoring criteria to examine the usefulness of the task to differentiate between groups. Libbon et al (84) found that scores based on a 10-point scoring system correlated with measures of executive functions and visual-spatial functioning. The investigators could differentiate between demented and nondemented groups, but not between patients with DAT and patients with cerebrovascular dementia. However, patients with cerebrovascular dementia performed significantly worse than patients with DAT when they were asked to copy a model of a predrawn clock. Kozora and Cullum (85) found a significant difference in the performance of healthy adults aged 50 to 70 and adults aged 70 to 95 by using three scoring systems, thus demonstrating the effects of normal aging. These investigators also found that the three scoring systems effectively differentiated between patients with DAT and matched controls.

In addition to the objective scores that can be generated, clock drawings also frequently offer qualitative information about cognitive deficits in planning, and problems with micrographia, hemi-spatial neglect, the tendency to be stimulus bound, and visual-spatial difficulties. Kozora and Cullum (85) found that patients with DAT showed deficits primarily in numerical position, time setting, proportions, spatial accuracy, and omission of details.

Intelligence Tests

Measures of intelligence are frequently included in neuropsychological evaluations to estimate the individual's premorbid and current overall levels of ability. Knowing these levels allows the examiner to estimate the expected level of functioning for the patient, to identify dissociations, and to avoid over- or underestimating impairment. Table 4.3 summarizes some frequently used intelligence measures.

The Wechsler Adult Intelligence Scale–Revised (WAIS-R) (86) is perhaps the most widely used measure of general intelligence. It consists of 11 subtests and yields verbal IQ, performance IQ, and full scale IQ scores. Norms are based on 1880 people ranging from 16 to 74 years old and are presented for nine age ranges. Because of the increasing attention to the evaluation of older individuals, various investigators have provided supplementary normative data for individuals up to age 96 (87,88).

Because intelligence is an important variable to evaluate, a number of attempts have been made to develop short forms of these tests to shorten administration time while retaining reliability and validity. A frequently used abbreviated form of the WAIS-R, the Satz-Mogel Short Form (89), substantially shortens administration time to approximately 25 minutes to 40 minutes. In this abbreviated form, some subtests are given in whole; in others, every other item or every third item is given. Formulas are then applied to estimate what the original subtest scores would be had all items been administered. This form has been shown to maintain its validity when applied to certain clinical populations, but not in others. A study by Dolske et al indicated that the use of the form is valid with elderly dementia patients (90).

The Kaufman Brief Intelligence Test (K-BIT) (91) is a relatively new instrument that is a motor-free screening measure of intelligence and yields a verbal IQ, a nonverbal IQ, and a composite IQ. It was normed on 2022 subjects from 4 to 90 years old. The manual reports

Table 4.3. Intelligence Tests.

Abilities Assessed	Scores	Time
Wechsler Adult Intelligence Scale–Revised 　General fund of information, digit span forward and backward, vocabulary, calculation, comprehension, verbal reasoning, scanning and attention to detail, nonverbal social reasoning, object assembly, psychomotor problem solving, digit symbol substitution	Specific scores by subtests; verbal, performance, full scale IQ scores	60–90 min
Kaufman Brief Intelligence Test 　Visual naming, verbal definitions, visual-spatial analogies	Verbal, nonverbal, composite IQ scores	25–40 min
Raven's Coloured Progressive Matrices 　Visual-spatial analogies	General IQ score	15–30 min

correlations between K-BIT indexes and WAIS-R IQ scores from .52 to .75 in a group of 64 normal individuals aged 16 to 47. In a mixed clinical group, correlations with the IQ scores from the WAIS-R were .83, .77, and .88 (92). However, a disadvantage of the K-BIT is that verbal IQs may be negatively biased when individuals are dysnomic, and nonverbal IQs may be negatively biased for individuals with declines in executive function.

Raven's Coloured Progressive Matrices (93) is a nonverbal test of intelligence that was designed for use with young children and elderly people. Similar to the visual-spatial analogies in the K-BIT, this test requires individuals to visually analyze stimuli and involves pattern recognition and matching. Older subject norms are presented based on the performances of 271 healthy people aged 60 to 89. As with the K-BIT, individuals with relatively circumscribed impairments in executive function may do poorly with matrices, which results in lower IQ estimates.

Learning and Memory Tests

Table 4.4 lists some frequently used memory instruments and their features. A patient with impaired attention is likely to perform poorly on many cognitive tasks, but particularly on memory tests, because of a failure to note relevant stimuli. Patients with severe attentional deficits may have a delirium (94) and cannot be evaluated reliably for dementia because the diagnosis necessitates the presence of a memory impairment within the context of adequate attentional control.

One commonly used method of evaluating attention and concentration quickly is to ask patients to repeat series of digits forward and backward. Alternatively, serial calculation tasks can be employed, such as the serial-sevens items on the MMSE, although this method of assessing attention can be confounded by calculation difficulties. Another screening procedure for attention and vigilance asks the patient to indicate when he or she has heard a certain target letter while the examiner presents letters at the rate of one per second. Errors of omission and commission can be suggestive of inattention, impulsivity, perseveration, or all these factors.

The Wechsler Memory Scale–Revised (WMS-R) (95) is a frequently used memory test that consists of several tasks. Age-corrected normative data are presented for five summary index scores derived from 316 normal individuals ranging from 16 to 74 years of age. Supplemental norms that can be applied to individuals up to 94 years old have been published to aid in the evaluation of older elderly individuals (96).

The WMS-R has been used in a large number of investigations, including many with elderly subjects. In one study, older, healthy individuals between the ages of 75 and 95 demonstrated more rapid rates of forgetting on the visual reproduction, verbal paired associates, and visual paired associates subtests than did their 50- to 70-year-old counterparts (97). A factor analytic study (98) found that when only the immediate recall subtests were analyzed, a two-factor structure consisting of a general memory factor and an attentional factor emerged. When the delayed recall subtests were added to the analysis, a verbal, nonverbal, and weaker attentional factor emerged. Although the WMS-R is a relatively comprehensive memory test with impressive research supporting its reliability and validity, it does not measure recognition memory abilities, indepth which are particularly useful in differential diagnosis.

The Rey Auditory Verbal Learning Test (RAVLT) (99) is a widely used, verbal-list-learning measure of memory. It consists of a list of 15 unrelated words presented over five trials, which allows the examiner to evaluate the patients initial recall and subsequent learning curve. Following the fifth presentation of the target list, a distractor list of another 15 unrelated words is presented, followed by a recall trial of the original list (short-term recall). A 20-minute delayed recall trial may be presented, as well as a recognition memory trial. Interference effects, confabulations, false-positive errors, and perseverations can be noted.

Rey (99) presented norms based on social class and age. Recently, normative data for RAVLT performances based on a sample consisting of 530 cognitively normal individuals aged 56 to 97 have been published (100). The RAVLT has also been used in numerous clinical investigations, including one that examined the differential affects of age on various aspects of memory in healthy, elderly patients (101).

The California Verbal Learning Test (CVLT) (102) is another verbal-list-learning measure consisting of 16 words. Again, the patient's initial recall, learning curve

Table 4.4. Memory Tests.

Abilities Assessed	Scores	Time
Wechsler Memory Scale–Revised Orientation, sequencing, visual recognition memory, short-term and long-term visual and verbal free recall, digit span forward and backward, span of visual memory forward and backward	Specific scores by subtests; specific summary index scores for attention/concentration, general and delayed memory; modality-specific scores for verbal and visual short-term memory	45–60 min
Rey Auditory Verbal Learning Test Short-term and long-term verbal free recall, recognition memory	Specific scores for verbal free recall, learning across trials, delayed recall, recognition memory	15–45 min
California Verbal Learning Test Short-term and long-term verbal free recall and cued recall, recognition memory	Specific scores for verbal free and cued recall, recognition memory, learning characteristics, recall errors, contrast measures	30–60 min
Rivermead Behavioural Memory Test Free and cued recall, and recognition of stimuli during tasks related to everyday memory (e.g., remembering a name, appointment, route)	General score; screening score	30 min
Recognition Memory Test Verbal and facial recognition memory	Specific scores for recognition of words and faces	20–30 min
Fuld Object-Memory Test Short-term and long-term free recall, verbal recognition memory, right-left discrimination, verbal fluency, tactile object recognition	Specific scores for free recall, recognition memory, storage, retrieval, repeated retrieval, ineffective reminders, verbal fluency	20–30 min
Shopping List Test Short-term and long-term verbal free recall, recognition memory	Specific scores for free recall, recognition memory	15 min

over trials, performance on a distractor list, short-term and delayed recall, and recognition memory are assessed. However, unlike the RAVLT, the target words fall into four semantic categories, which allows the examiner to evaluate learning strategies and clustering techniques. The semantic categories are also used as cues to evaluate the patient's cued recall capabilities. False-positive errors, confabulations, perseverations, and interference tendencies can also be noted. Scoring can be done manually or by computer. Normative data are presented based on a nonclinical reference group of 273 neurologically normal individuals grouped into seven age ranges from 17 years to 80 years. The main indexes of the CVLT have been shown to correlate with the original Wechsler Memory Scale (102,103). CVLT and WMS-R scores also correlated highly with one another in a mixed group of patients and controls, which provides further evidence for the construct validity of the CVLT (104). Because the CVLT meas-

ures different aspects of memory, it allows differential patterns of memory dysfunction to emerge, which can be useful in differentiating different neurological groups (102).

The Rivermead Behavioural Memory Test (RBMT) (47) uses memory tasks closely related to those involved in everyday life (e.g., keeping an appointment, learning a stranger's first name and surname, and recalling the location of a hidden belonging). The test has 12 tasks that cumulatively yield both a screening score and a more detailed profile score.

The RBMT validation study (105) demonstrated good interrater reliability and test-retest reliability coefficients. Validity was established by examining the intercorrelations between the RBMT and subjective ratings of the patients' memory and scores on other objective tests of memory. The RBMT correlated significantly with other objective memory tests and had the highest relationship among the objective memory tests with the subjective memory ratings completed by the patient, relative, and health caregivers. However, in one investigation (106), the RBMT was not found to be any better than the WMS-R in predicting subjective ratings of memory difficulty. Wilson (107) demonstrated that the RBMT was better than the WMS-R in predicting independence in a clinical group, which suggests that the RBMT may prove to be an ecologically valid alternative when measuring memory. However, more research needs to be conducted to examine further the usefulness of this instrument.

The Warrington Recognition Memory Test (RMT) (108) evaluates a patient's recognition memory for words and faces. In the word condition, 50 target words are presented to the patient, each for three seconds. To ensure attention to each item, the patient is required to respond "yes" or "no" according to whether the item is perceived as "pleasant" or "not pleasant." The patient is then shown 50 pairs of words, with one of each pair being the original target word. The patient must choose which of the two words was originally presented. The same procedure is repeated with 50 photographs of unfamiliar faces, followed by the recognition phase in which the person must identify the target face when presented with a foil. The RMT was normed on 310 volunteer subjects without a history of cerebral disease, and who ranged in age from 18 to 70 years. The RMT can provide valuable information regarding retrieval memory abilities.

The Fuld Object-Memory Evaluation (109) assesses several aspects of learning and memory and also provides information about verbal fluency, tactile object recognition, and right-left discrimination. This test consists of the patient first identifying by touch 10 common objects that are in a bag by using either the right or left hand as requested by the examiner. The patient is then given a verbal fluency trial that acts as a distractor task before the first recall-of-objects trial. After recalling as many items as possible, the patient is told the items that he or she omitted (selective reminding). The recall, reminding, and fluency tasks are repeated four more times. Recall is then assessed after a 15-minute delay, and those items not retrieved are then presented in a yes-no, forced-choice, recognition format.

The test yields information about a patient's capacity for free recall, ability to benefit from repeated presenta-

tions through selective reminding, delayed recall, and recognition abilities. Normative data were collected on 54 subjects ranging in age from 68 years to 93 years. The ability of the test to differentiate between clinical and nonclinical groups has been demonstrated (109). The performance of different groups has been shown to affect various parts of the test. For example, nonimpaired subjects benefit from repeated trials, but the recall of impaired subjects tends to level off after the second trial (109). The Fuld Object-Memory Test has recently been shown to be useful in prospectively identifying individuals who subsequently develop dementia (110).

The Shopping List Task (111) is an alternative memory test for patients who cannot be evaluated with lengthier, more demanding tests. It requires the patient to recall 10 items from a shopping list over repeated trials and uses the selective reminding procedure for omitted words. Initial recall, learning over repeated trials, delayed recall, and recognition memory are evaluated. McCarthy et al (111) demonstrated the differential sensitivity of the test by using it to differentiate between young normals and elderly normals, reflecting age-related differences. In addition, these investigators showed the usefulness of this test in differentiating between elderly normals and elderly patients with dementia.

Executive Function Tests

Performance on tests of executive function have been associated with the integrity of the frontal lobes, and frontodiencephalic connections (112). Executive functions are skills such as the ability to plan complex motor activities and initiate behavior and also are involved in mental and motor sequencing, cognitive flexibility, problem solving, abstract reasoning, judgment, response inhibition, and general information-processing abilities. Perseveration, problems with initiation, and the tendency to be stimulus bound are also signs of executive function disruption. Cerebrovascular and neurodegenerative disorders often affect these structures and their associated pathways. For instance, Pick's disease causes marked atrophy of the frontal lobes and is primarily characterized by impairments in executive functions (25). Because patients with affective and psychotic disorders can also manifest deficits in executive functions, attention must be drawn to the entire constellation of neuropsychological findings to differentiate between affective, psychotic, cerebrovascular, and neurodegenerative disorders. Table 4.5 lists some of the measures that assess executive functions.

The Executive Interview (EXIT) developed by Royall, et al (113) is an examination that can be used with patients who are moderately to severely demented, or with those who cannot tolerate lengthy traditional measures. The EXIT consists of a series of neurobehavioral tasks, such as assessing frontal release signs and mental and motor sequencing. The pilot validation study demonstrated that the EXIT could effectively differentiate between different levels of functional independence with 40 individuals (113). The EXIT correlated .73 and .64 with the Trail Making Test Part A and Part B (see discussion below), respectively, but .85 negatively with the MMSE. Currently, further validation studies are being conducted to evaluate the sensitivity and specificity of the EXIT as a measure of frontal lobe dysfunction.

The Trail Making Test (114) has two parts. Trails A is a test of visual scanning and sequencing that consists of 25 circles numbered 1 to 25. The patient is asked to connect the circles in numerical sequence as quickly as possible. Part B also consists of 25 circles, but they are numbered from 1 to 13 and lettered from A to L. The patient is asked to alternate cognitive sets during sequencing by alternating between consecutive numbers and letters while connecting the circles. Both parts are timed. Heaton et al (115) presented age- and education-corrected norms based on 486 subjects ranging from 20 to 80 years old. An impairment on the Trail Making Test, particularly Trails B, often indicates difficulties with executive functions.

The Controlled Oral Word Association (COWA) (116) consists of three word-generation trials, in which the patient is given a specific letter (e.g., "C") and is asked to name as many words that begin with that letter as he or she can within 60 seconds. Norms correcting for age, education, and gender are available for converting the raw number of words generated to percentile scores. Although this is a test of language function, many studies have demonstrated that patients with frontal lesions, particularly in the left hemisphere, generate significantly fewer words than do healthy subjects (117,118). Functional MRI studies have demonstrated activation of the frontal cortex during related tasks of word generation (119). Patients with DAT also generate significantly fewer words than do healthy controls (120).

Table 4.5. Tests of Executive Function.

Abilities Assessed	Scores	Time
Geriatric Executive Interview Mental and motor sequencing, verbal and design fluency, inhibition of various responses (e.g., anomalous sentence repetition, automatic behavior), grasp and snout reflex, motor impersistence, thematic perception, echopraxia, serial order reversal task, grip task	Single score	10–15 min
Trail Making Visual scanning, sequencing, cognitive flexibility	Specific scores for time and errors	4–12 min
Controlled Oral Word Association Verbal fluency	Single score for verbal fluency	5 min
Ruff Figural Fluency Figural fluency	Specific scores for nonverbal fluency and preseveration	7 min
Wisconsin Card Sorting Test Ability to develop and maintain appropriate problem-solving strategies across changing stimulus conditions (e.g., organized searching, utilization of environmental feedback to shift cognitive sets, modulating impulsive responding)	Specific scores for categories achieved and characteristics related to acquiring and shifting cognitive sets	20–30 min

The Ruff Figural Fluency Test (121) is a related measure that requires the patient to generate as many different novel designs as possible in five 60-second trials by using standard templates. Ruff et al (122) presented normative data for 358 subjects ranging from 16 to 70 years old. When analyzing the factor structure of the Figural Fluency Test within the context of other neuropsychological measures, Baser and Ruff (123) found that the unique designs score loaded on an "arousal or initiation" factor and a "complex intelligence" factor, and the ratio of perseverative errors to unique designs score loaded on a "planning" factor. Problems with design fluency can often be suggestive of dysfunction in the nonlanguage dominant hemisphere.

The Wisconsin Card Sorting Test (WCST) (124,125) is a standardized test of complex problem-solving abilities. The WCST evaluates the patient's ability to acquire and maintain problem-solving strategies and to benefit from feedback while doing so. This test also measures the frequency of perseverative responses. Administration can be done manually or with a computer. Norms are presented for 899 subjects ranging from 6 to 89 years old (126). Extensive validity research has been conducted on the WCST to examine its relationship to executive functions and structural lesions; Heaton et al (126) have recently presented a review of this literature.

Language and Communication Tests

Table 4.6 lists some frequently used language measures, the abilities they assess, scores generated, and time of administration. Comprehensive language test batteries are available, but many examiners choose to give selected subtests from them to assess specific abilities. A discussion of three comprehensive batteries, along with an example of the use of a single subtest follows.

The Multilingual Aphasia Exam (MAE) (116) consists of eight subtests that screen a number of receptive and expressive skills. Percentile scores corrected for age and education are provided for each subtest (127). The Boston Diagnostic Aphasia Examination (BDAE) (83) is a battery of tasks that aids in the diagnosis and treatment of aphasia. Because the complete test battery takes from one to four hours to administer, many examiners choose to give only selected subtests. Although profile scores are available, the authors do not link these to specific subtypes of aphasia. Borod et al (128) published norms and provided cutoff scores in addition to means, standard deviations, and ranges. The Western Aphasia Battery (129) was derived from the BDAE, in part as an effort to provide an instrument that would also provide diagnostic classifications (130). The patient's performances on this battery can be compared with pattern descriptions for eight aphasia

Table 4.6. Language Tests.

Abilities Assessed	Scores	Time
Multilingual Aphasia Examination		
Visual naming, written and oral spelling, controlled oral word association, sentence repetition, aural and reading comprehension, comprehension of complex syntactical instructions	Specific scores by subtests	30–40 min
Boston Diagnostic Aphasia Examination		
Conversational and expository speech, auditory comprehension (e.g., word discrimination), oral expression (e.g., repetition, naming), writing (e.g., dictation, written symbols, written formulation)	Specific scores by subtests; aphasia severity rating scale, speech characteristics rating scale	1–4 hr
Western Aphasia Battery		
Spontaneous speech, auditory verbal comprehension, repetition, naming, reading (e.g., reading commands, stimulus-object choice matching, spelled word recognition), writing (e.g., to dictation, copying), apraxia, construction, visuospatial, calculation	Specific scores by subtests; aphasia quotient, cortical quotient	30–60 min
Boston Naming Test		
Confrontation naming	Specific scores for spontaneously correct responses, number and types of cues given, and number correct with cues	15–20 min

subtypes. However, the classification system does not account for patients who have an aphasia that has components of more than one of these subtypes of aphasia. Thus, the diagnostic usefulness of the Western Aphasia Battery has been questioned (131).

The Boston Naming Test (BNT) (132) is a subtest of the BDAE that is frequently used by itself because of its usefulness as a measure of confrontation naming and semantic retrieval. Because dysnomia is a common symptom of DAT (21,22), the evaluation of the geriatric patient's naming ability can be critical. Spreen and Strauss (133) demonstrated that the BNT is sensitive to differential performances of normal, elderly subjects, patients with DAT, and patients with other dementing disorders. The BNT consists of asking the patient to identify 60 line drawings of objects that range from commonly used or seen objects (e.g., bed, tree) to uncommon or infrequently seen objects (e.g., sphinx, abacus). If the individual misidentifies the stimulus as something outside the object class (e.g., "snake" for "pretzel"), a semantic cue is given (e.g., "something to eat"). If the individual misidentifies the stimulus as something within its semantic category (e.g., "bird" for "pelican"), or if the individual cannot spontaneously name the stimulus but indicates that he or she knows the object class, a phonemic cue is given (e.g., "pel" for pelican). Through an analysis of a patient's use of these cues, the examiner can rule out visual-spatial difficulties that may have contributed to poor performance. The original norms were based on 30 normal children, 84 normal adults aged 18 to 59, and 82 aphasics. Van Gorp et al (134) published normative data on 78 individuals ranging in age from 59 years to 80 years and older in five age groups.

Visual-Spatial and Visual-Motor Tests

The Hooper Visual Organization Test (VOT) (135) assesses a patient's ability to perceive, integrate, and visual-perceptually organize information. It requires the patient to identify 30 objects that have been cut up and randomly arranged on stimulus cards. Full credit is given for the correct identification of the object, and partial credit is given for responses that are partially correct or too general to receive full credit. Age- and education-corrected norms are presented based on 231 subjects ranging in age from 25 years to 69 years. The test does require naming, and patients with dysnomia may perform poorly for reasons other than diminished visual-spatial functioning.

The Judgment of Line Orientation Test (136) is a 30-item test that evaluates a patient's ability to judge angular relationships. The patient is shown a stimulus card with two angled lines and is asked to match the lines to two of eleven angled lines forming a semicircle on a template. Benton et al (136) presented normative data and demonstrated that patients with posterior right hemisphere lesions perform poorly on this test, but patients with anterior right or left hemisphere lesions perform adequately.

Table 4.7 describes some frequently used measures of visual-spatial and visual-motor ability. The tests discussed above address the perception and processing of visual stimuli, independent of motor skill. However, visual-spatial processing tasks that require motor output also tap a number of other functions, such as planning. The clock-drawing task may reflect difficulties in planning and visual-spatial abilities, the presence of hemineglect, tremors, perseveration, and tendencies to be

Table 4.7. Visual-Spatial and Visual-Motor Tests.

Abilities Assessed	Scores	Time
Hooper Visual Organization Test		
Perception, integration, organization of perceptual information	Single score	10–20 min
Judgment of Line Orientation		
Visual-perceptual discrimination	Single score	10–20 min
Rey-Osterreith Complex Figure		
Perceptual integration and visual constructional praxis, short-term and long-term recall (optional)	Specific scores for copy, immediate and delayed recall trials	3–5 min

stimulus bound. Some examiners also use other drawings of various complexity to yield similar information.

The Rey-Osterrieth Complex Figure is derived from the work of Rey (137), who developed a complex figure in 1941 to examine perceptual and visual memory functions in patients. This test has no single, universally accepted, scoring system, but a number of administration and scoring procedures were subsequently developed. The first emerged in 1944 when Osterrieth (138) developed a scoring procedure for Rey's Figure and obtained normative data for a group of 230 children and a group of 60 adults. The adults ranged from 16 to 60 years of age. Osterrieth also collected data on a smaller group of "brain damaged" patients. The test is typically given by asking the subject first to copy the figure, which is complex and heavily detailed. While the subject copies, the examiner, at intervals, switches the color of the pencil the patient is using so that the approach to drawing the figure can be analyzed. Other examiners opt to make notes about the patient's approach to the stimuli rather than disrupt the process of drawing the figure. This task is timed, and is usually followed by one or more recall trials that yield information about visual memory. In addition to obtaining objective scores, the examiner can track the patient's approach to drawing the figure. Thus, difficulties with planning, initiation, recall, or a hemi-neglect may be revealed.

Sensory-Motor Tests

The patient's gait and motoric symptoms, such as tremor or cogwheeling, can provide useful behavioral information about underlying disease processes. The frequency, type, and severity of motoric dysfunction can aid in differential diagnosis and localization and is also helpful in judging functional adaptivity. Table 4.8 describes some of the measures commonly used by neuropsychologists.

The Finger Oscillation Test (62) uses a specially adapted manual tapper to measure fine-motor speed. The tapping speed of the index finger of the subject's dominant hand is assessed by giving 10-second trials until five consecutive trials that are within five taps of each other are obtained. The trials are then averaged to obtain the fine-motor speed for that hand. The nondominant hand is evaluated in the same way, and the examiner may alternate between dominant and nondominant hands after a specified number of trials. Various administration and scoring guidelines have been presented (139,140) to obtain the average scores of fine-motor ability. Because tapping speed declines with age, age- and education-corrected norms are available (115).

The Grooved Pegboard (141) is a measure of fine-motor coordination and dexterity. The test consists of 25 notched pegs that are placed into slotted holes angled in various directions on a small board. Time to complete the task and number of pegs dropped are evaluated for both the dominant and the nondominant hand. Norms based on various clinical and nonclinical groups are available for assessing the functional capacity of each side of the body (115,142).

The Hand Dynamometer (62) is an apparatus that assesses grip strength. The instrument fits in the palm of the patient's hand, and he or she is required to pull against a

Table 4.8. Sensory-Motor Tests.

Abilities Assessed	Scores	Time
Finger Oscillation Test Fine-motor speed	Scores for each hand	10 min
Grooved Pegboard Fine-motor coordination and dexterity	Scores for each hand	5–10 min
Hand Dynamometer Grip strength	Scores for each hand	5 min

Sensory-Perceptual Examination
  Tactile, auditory, and visual extinction to double simultaneous stimulation, graphesthesia,
  finger localization, visual fields to gross confrontation
	Specific scores by subtests	15–20 min

grip, which provides a quantitative assessment of strength in kilograms. This test of hand-grip strength has both diagnostic and functional implications. Norms based on 475 subjects are available for this measure (115).

The Reitan-Klove Sensory-Perceptual Examination (62) is a series of tasks designed to assess tactile, auditory, and visual extinction to double simultaneous stimulation in a systematic manner. Tasks of finger agnosia, graphesthesia, and visual fields on gross confrontation are also administered. Selected subtests are frequently given to reduce administration time. Normative data are available (115).

Emotional Functions and Personality Tests

Psychiatric disorders such as depression are relatively common among the elderly and may have an adverse affect on cognition. The effect of these disorders on cognition can be severe enough to cause a dementia of depression, and may also overlap with a dementia resulting from a neurologic origin. Therefore, it is essential to include measures of emotional and personality functioning in the neuropsychological evaluation. In addition, when a patient is assessed from a functional point of view, an evaluation of affective and personality factors and their impact on the patient's life is necessary. The following measures are frequently used to screen for affective and personality dysfunction in elderly populations.

The Geriatric Depression Scale (GDS) (143) is a commonly used screening questionnaire for depression in the elderly. The test takes approximately 10 minutes to administer. It consists of 30 yes/no questions selected specifically to screen for depressive symptoms in the elderly population (144). Yesavage et al (143) found that the GDS was significantly correlated (.82) with Research Diagnostic Criteria (RDC) (145) for major affective disorder (depressed) in their groups of control and depressed individuals. The GDS was also found to have 92 percent sensitivity and 89 percent specificity in an investigation involving hospitalized elderly patients (146).

The Beck Depression Inventory (BDI) (147) is also a frequently used brief questionnaire of depression. The BDI was designed for use with the general adult population. Administration time varies from about 10 minutes to 25 minutes. The inventory consists of 21 items, each rated on a 4-point scale. The BDI yields information about the intensity of depressive symptoms, not their frequency or breadth. Good correlations between the diagnosis of major depressive disorder and the BDI have been observed (148). Gallagher et al (149) found that the BDI misclassified only 17 percent of their subjects in relation to RDC.

The Hamilton Rating Scale for Depression (HRS-D) (150) yields a score about a patient's emotional functioning and is based on a structured interview with the patient and information about general functioning. The HRS-D was developed to assess the severity of depression, not as a diagnostic instrument (151). Time to complete the scale varies considerably depending on the availability of information needed to rate the individual. The HRS-D is intended to be administered by a trained rater, and validity is heavily dependent on the skill of the examiner (150).

The Minnesota Multiphasic Personality Inventory-2 (MMPI-2) (152) is a multidimensional measure of personality functioning consisting of 567 true-false statements. The test can be scored by hand or computer. Because of its length, the MMPI-2 is often not a feasible test for elderly patients. The MMPI-2 was normed on 2600 community subjects. The test yields information about both emotional and personality functioning with 10 clinical scales and seven validity scales. The configuration of the overall profile is used to make inferences about emotional and personality factors, and the information gathered typically represents stable personality characteristics rather than the immediate affective experience of the individual. Various researchers have also developed subscales, for example, Harris-Lingoes Subscales (153) and supplementary scales (154), based on item analysis, factor analysis, and clinical judgment. These scales can also be used during profile interpretation.

Conclusion

The inclusion of neuropsychological assessment in the evaluation of the geriatric patient provides objective and meaningful information about the individual's neurocognitive and emotional functioning. This information is frequently used by the clinician to evaluate functional ability, as well as to aid in differential diagnosis and competency decisions. In addition, behavioral, treatment, and discharge planning may be facilitated by implications of the neuropsychological evaluation. Standardized data obtained through neuropsychological evaluations are frequently used in research to document treatment efficacy and to enhance the understanding of disease processes as they relate to brain-behavior relationships.

In addition to discussing the role of neuropsychology in the evaluation of the geriatric patient, this chapter has presented a description of a number of commonly used neuropsychological tests. These procedures are not used in isolation, but are selected to sample various neurocognitive domains. The test data that result yields a constellation, or profile, of neurocognitive strengths and limitations. The interpretation of this constellation is used to answer questions about differential diagnosis and functional ability in the evaluation of the geriatric patient.

References

1. Tancredi LR. The mental status examination. Generations 1987;11:24–31.
2. Katz S, Stroud MW. Functional assessment in geriatrics: a review of progress and directions. J Am Geriatr Soc 1989;37:267–271.
3. Davison LA. Introduction. In: Reitan RM, Davison LA, eds. Clinical neuropsychology: current status and applications. Washington, DC: Winston, 1974:1–18.
4. Albert MS. General issues in geriatric neuropsychology. In: Albert MS, Moss MB, eds. Geriatric neuropsychology. New York: Guilford, 1988:3–10.
5. Kokmen E, Beard CM, O'Brien PC, et al. Is the incidence of dementing illness changing? Neurology 1993;43:1887–1892.
6. Heston LL, White JA. Dementia: a practical guide to Alzheimer's disease and related illnesses. New York: WH Freeman, 1983.
7. Albert MS, Heaton RK. Intelligence testing. In: Albert MS, Moss MB, eds. Geriatric neuropsychology. New York: Guilford, 1988:13–32.
8. Horn JL. The theory of fluid and crystallized intelligence in relation to concepts of cognitive psychology and aging in adulthood. In: Craik FIM, Trehub S, eds. Aging and cognitive processes. New York: Plenum, 1982:237–278.
9. Wechsler D. Wechsler Adult Intelligence Scale–Revised. New York: Harcourt Brace Jovanovich, 1981.
10. Erkinjuntii T, Laaksonen R, Sulkava R, et al. Neuropsychological differentiation between normal aging, Alzheimer's disease and vascular dementia. Acta Neurol Scand 1986;74:393–403.
11. Craik FIM. Age differences in remembering. In: Squire LR, Butters N, eds. Neuropsychology of memory. New York: Guilford, 1984:3–12.
12. Howieson DB, Holm LA, Kaye JA, et al. Neurologic function in the optimally healthy oldest old: neuropsychological evaluation. Neurology 1993;43:1882–1886.
13. Van Gorp WG, Satz P, Matrushina M. Neuropsychological processes associated with normal aging. Dev Neuropsychol 1990;6:279–290.
14. Benton AL, Sivan AB. Problems and conceptual issues in neuropsychological research in aging and dementia. J Clin Neuropsychol 1984;6:57–63.
15. Klodin VM. Verbal facilitation of perceptual-integrative performance in relation to age. Doctoral dissertation. St. Louis: Washington University, 1975.
16. Naugle RI, Cullum CM, Bigler ED. Evaluation of intellectual and memory function among dementia patients who were intellectually superior. Clin Neuropsychol 1990;4:355–374.
17. Levin HS, Benton AL. Age and susceptibility to tactile masking effects. Gerontology 1973;15:1–9.
18. Ardila A, Rosselli M. Neuropsychological characteristic of normal aging. Dev Neuropsychol 1989;5:307–320.
19. Heaton RK, Grant I, Matthews CG. Differences in neuropsychological test performance associated with age, education, and sex. In: Grant I, Adams K, eds. Neuropsychological assessment of neuropsychiatric disorders. New York: Oxford, 1986:100–120.
20. Mortimer JA, Schuman LM, French LR. Epidemiology of dementing illness. In: Mortimer JA, Schuman LM, eds. The epidemiology of dementia. New York: Oxford, 1981:3–23.
21. Albert MS. Geriatric neuropsychology. J Consult Clin Psychol 1981;49:835–850.
22. Barr A, Benedict R, Tune L, Brandt J. Neuropsychological differentiation of Alzheimer's disease from vascular dementia. Int J Geriatr Psychiatry 1992;7:621–627.
23. Funkenstein HH. Cerebrovascular disorders. In: Albert MS, Moss MB, eds. Geriatric neuropsychology. New York: Guilford, 1988:179–207.
24. Friedland RP. Alzheimer's disease: clinical features and differential diagnosis. Neurology 1993;43:45–51.
25. Moss MB, Albert MS. Alzheimer's disease and other dementing disorders. In: Albert MS, Moss MB, eds. Geriatric neuropsychology. New York: Guilford, 1988:145–178.
26. Rubenstein L. The clinical effectiveness of multidimensional geriatric assessment. J Am Geriatr Soc 1983;31:758–762.
27. Miller RL, Winograd C, Frengley D, et al. Inpatient geriatric consultive teams. Gerontol Geriatr Educ 1988;8:35–52.
28. Katz PR, Dube DH, Calkins EC. Use of a structured functional assessment format in a geriatric consultative service. J Am Geriatr Soc 1984;33:681–686.
29. Becker PM, Cohen HJ. The functional approach to the care of the elderly: a conceptual framework. J Am Geriatr Soc 1984;32:923–929.
30. Rubenstein LZ. Geriatric assessment: an overview of its impacts. Clin Geriatr Med 1987;3:1–15.

31. Johansson B. Neuropsychological assessment in the oldest-old. Int Psychogeriatr 1991;3:51–60.

32. Cummings JL, Benson DF. Subcortical dementia: review of an emerging concept. Arch Neurol 1984;41:874–879.

33. Butters N, Salmon DP, Cullum CM, et al. Differentiation of amnesic and demented patients with the Wechsler Memory Scale–Revised. Clin Neuropsychol 1988;2:133–148.

34. Moss MB, Albert MS, Butters N, Payne M. Differential patterns of memory loss among patients with Alzheimer's disease, Huntington's disease, and alcoholic Korsakoff's syndrome. Arch Neurol 1986;43:239–246.

35. Clarfield AM. The reversible dementias: do they reverse? Ann Intern Med 1988;109:476–486.

36. Barry PP, Moskowitz MA. The diagnosis of reversible dementia in the elderly: a critical review. Arch Intern Med 1988;148:1914–1918.

37. Gurland BJ. The comparative frequency of depression in various adult age groups. J Gerontol 1976;31:283–292.

38. Moffie HS, Paykel ES. Depression in medical inpatients. Br J Psychiatry 1975;126:346–353.

39. Kaszniak AW. Neuropsychological consultation to geriatricians: issues in the assessment of memory complaints. Clin Neuropsychol 1987;1:35–46.

40. Jones RD, Tranel D, Benton A, Paulsen J. Differentiating dementia from "pseudodementia" early in the clinical course: utility of neuropsychological tests. Neuropsychology 1992;6:13–21.

41. Silberman EK, Weingartner H, Laraia M, et al. Processing of emotional properties of stimuli by depressed and normal subjects. J Neurol Ment Disord 1983;171:10–14.

42. Acker M. Relationships between test scores and everyday life functioning. In: Uzzell B, Gross Y, eds. Clinical neuropsychology of intervention. Boston: Martinus Nijhoff, 1986:85–117.

43. Chelune GJ, Moehle KA. Neuropsychological assessment and everyday functioning. In: Wedding D, Horton AM, Webster J. The neuropsychology handbook: behavioral and clinical perspectives. New York: Springer, 1986:489–525.

44. Hart T, Hayden M. The ecological validity of neuropsychological assessment and remediation. In: Uzzell B, Gross Y, eds. Clinical neuropsychology of intervention. Boston: Martinus Nijhoff, 1986:21–50.

45. Sunderland A. Clinical memory assessment: matching the method to the aim. In: Tupper D, Cicerone K, eds. The neuropsychology of everyday life: assessment and basic competencies. 1990:169–183.

46. McCue M, Rogers JC, Goldstein G. Relationships between neuropsychological and functional assessment in elderly neuropsychiatric patients. Rehab Psychol 1990;35:91–99.

47. Wilson B, Cockburn J, Baddeley A. The Rivermead Behavioural Memory Test. Cambridge, UK: Thames Valley Test, 1985.

48. Mattis S. Neuropsychological assessment of competency in the elderly. Forensic Rep 1990;3:107–114.

49. Tymchule AJ, Ouslander JG, Rabbar B, Fitten J. Medical decision-making among elderly people in long term care. Gerontologist 1988;28:59–63.

50. Stanley B, Stanley M, Guido J, Garvin L. The functional competency of elderly at risk. Gerontologist 1988;28:53–58.

51. Marson D, Ingram K, Harrell L. Neuropsychological correlates of competency loss in dementia using a specific legal standard. Program and Abstracts of the International Neuropsychological Society, 1994:104.

52. Scogin F, Perry J. Guardianship proceedings with older adults: the role of functional assessment and gerontologists. Law Psychol Rev 1986;10:123–128.

53. Kloezen S, Fitten LJ, Steinberg A. Assessment of treatment decision-making capacity in a medically ill patient. J Am Geriatr Soc 1988;36:1055–1058.

54. Baker FM. Competent for what? J Natl Med Assoc 1987;79:715–720.

55. Steinberg A, Fitten LJ, Kachuck N. Patient participation in treatment decision-making in the nursing home: the issue of competence. Gerontologist 1986;26:362–366.

56. Haley WE, Brown SL, Levine EG. Family caregiver appraisals of patient behavioral disturbance in senile dementia. Clin Gerontol 1987;6:25–34.

57. Butters N, Wolfe J, Martone M, et al. Memory disorders associated with Huntington's disease: verbal recall, verbal recognition and procedural memory. Neuropsychologia 1985;23:729–743.

58. Lawton MP, Storandt M. Clinical and functional approaches to the assessment of older people. In: McReynolds P, Chelune GJ. Advances in psychological assessment. vol 6. San Francisco: Jossey-Bass, 1984:236–276.

59. Cunningham WR, Sepkoski CN, Opel MR. Fatigue effects on intelligence test performance in the elderly. J Gerontol 1978;33:541–545.

60. Albert M. Assessment of cognitive dysfunction. In: Albert MS, Moss MB, eds. Geriatric neuropsychology. New York: Guilford, 1988:57–81.

61. Halstead WC. Brain and intelligence. Chicago: University of Chicago, 1947.

62. Reitan RM, Davison LA. Clinical neuropsychology: current status and applications. New York: Hemisphere, 1974.

63. Golden CJ, Hammeke TA, Purisch AD. Manual for the Luria-Nebraska Neuropsychological Battery. Los Angeles: Western Psychological Services, 1980.

64. Anthony JC, LeResche L, Niaz U, et al. Limits of the Mini-Mental State as a screening test for dementia and delirium among hospital patients. Psychol Med 1982;12:397–408.

65. Folstein MF, Folstein SE, McHugh PR. Mini-Mental State: a practical method for grading the cognitive state of patients for the clinician. J Psychiatr Res 1975;12:189–198.

66. Launer LJ, Dinkgreve MAHM, Jonker C, et al. Are age and education independent correlates of the Mini-Mental State Exam performance of community-dwelling elderly? J Gerontol 1993;48:271–277.

67. Fillenbaum GG, Heyman A, Wilkinson WE, Haynes CS. Comparison of two screening tests in Alzheimer's disease:

the correlation and reliability of the Mini-Mental State Examination and the Modified Blessed Test. Arch Neurol 1987;44:924–927.

68. Frisoni FB, Rozzini R, Bianchetti A, Trabucchi M. Principal lifetime occupation and MMSE score in elderly persons. J Gerontol 1993;48:310–314.

69. Naugle RI, Kawczak K. Limitations of the Mini-Mental State Examination. Cleve Clin J Med 1989;56:277–281.

70. Kiernan, RJ, Mueller J, Langston JW, Van Dyke C. The Neurobehavioral Cognitive Status Examination: a brief but differentiated approach to cognitive assessment. Ann Intern Med 1987;107:481–485.

71. Schwamm LH, Van Dyke C, Kiernan RJ, et al. The Neurobehavioral Cognitive Status Examination: comparison with the Cognitive Capacity Screening Examination and the Mini-Mental State Examination in a neurosurgical population. Ann Intern Med 1987;107:486–491.

72. Jacobs JW, Bernhard MR, Delgado A, Strain JJ. Screening for organic mental syndromes in the medically ill. Ann Intern Med 1977;86:40–46.

73. Mattis S. DRS: Dementia Rating Scale: professional manual. Odessa, FL: Psychological Assessment Resources, 1988.

74. Chase TN, Foster NL, Gedio P, et al. Regional cortical dysfunction in Alzheimer's disease as determined by positron emission tomography. Ann Neurol 1984;15:170–174.

75. Coblentz JM, Mattis S, Zingesser L, et al. Presenile dementia: clinical aspects and evaluation of cerebrospinal fluid dynamics. Arch Neurol 1973;29:299–308.

76. Gardner R, Oliver-Munoz S, Fisher L, Empting L. Mattis Dementia Rating Scale: internal reliability study using a diffusely impaired population. J Clin Neuropsychol 1981;3:271–275.

77. Vitaliano PP, Breen AR, Russo J, et al. The clinical utility of the Dementia Rating Scale for assessing Alzheimer patients. J Chronic Dis 1984;37:743–753.

78. Lawton MP. Assessing the competence of older people. In: Kent D, Katenbaum R, Sherwood S, eds. Research planning and action for the elderly. New York: Behavioral, 1972:122–143.

79. Shay KA, Duke LW, Conboy T, et al. The clinical validity of the Mattis Dementia Rating Scale in staging Alzheimer's dementia. J Geriatr Psychiatry Neurol 1991;4:18–25.

80. Smith GE, Ivnik RJ, Malec JF, et al. Psychometric properties of the Mattis Dementia Rating Scale. Assessment 1994;1:123–131.

81. Powell DH, Kaplan EF, Whitla D, et al. MicroCog: Assessment of Cognitive Function: manual. San Antonio: Psychological Corporation, 1993.

82. Green RC, Green J, Harrison JM, Kutner MH. Screening for cognitive impairment in older individuals: validation study of a computer-based test. Arch Neurol 1994;51:779–786.

83. Goodglass H, Kaplan E. The assessment of aphasia and related disorders. Philadelphia: Lea & Febiger, 1983.

84. Libbon DJ, Swenson, RA, Barnoski, EJ, Sands LP. Clock drawing as an assessment tool for dementia. Arch Clin Neuropsychol 1993;8:405–415.

85. Kozora E, Cullum CM. Qualitative features of clock drawings in normal aging and Alzheimer's disease. Psychol Assess 1994;1:179–187.

86. Wechsler D. Wechsler Adult Intelligence Scale–Revised. San Antonio: Psychological Corporation, 1981.

87. Ryan JJ, Paolo AM, Brungardt TM. Standardization of the Wechsler Adult Intelligence Scale–Revised for persons 75 years and older. Psychol Assess 1990;2:404–411.

88. Malec JF, Ivnik RJ, Smith GE, et al. Mayo's older Americans normative studies: utility of corrections for age and education for the WAIS-R. Clin Neuropsychol 1992;6:31–47.

89. Adams RL, Smigielski J, Jenkins RL. Development of a Satz-Mogel short form of the WAIS-R. J Consult Clin Psychol 1984;52:908.

90. Dolske MC, Law RT, Yeoh L, et al. Utility of the Satz-Mogel WAIS-R across clincial populations. Clin Neuropsychol 1993;7:345.

91. Kaufman AS, Kaufman NL. Kaufman Brief Intelligence Test: manual. Circle Pines, MN: American Guidance Service, 1990.

92. Naugle RI, Chelune GJ, Tucker GT. Validity of the Kaufman Brief Intelligence Test. Psychol Assess 1993;5:182–186.

93. Raven JC. Guide to using the Coloured Progressive Matrices. London: HK Lewis, 1965.

94. Mesulam M, Geschwind N. Disordered mental status in the postoperative period. Urol Clin North Am 1976;3:199–215.

95. Wechsler D. Wechsler Memory Scale–Revised. New York: Psychological Corporation, 1987.

96. Ivnik RJ, Malec JF, Tangalos EG, et al. Mayo's older American normative studies: WMS-R norms for ages 56 to 94. Clin Neuropsychol 1992;6:49–82.

97. Cullum CM, Butters N, Troster AI, Salmon DP. Normal aging and forgetting rates on the Wechsler Memory Scale–Revised. Arch Clin Neuropsychol 1990;5:23–30.

98. Bornstein R, Chelune GJ. Factor structure of the Wechsler Memory Scale–Revised. Clin Neuropsychol 1988;2:107–115.

99. Rey A. L'examen clinique en psychologie. Paris: Universitaires de France, 1964.

100. Ivnik RJ, Malec JF, Smith GE, et al. Mayo's older American normative studies: updated AVLT norms for ages 56 to 97. Clin Neuropsychol 1992;6:83–104.

101. Mitrushina M, Satz P, Chervinsky A, D'Elia L. Performance of four age groups of normal elderly on the Rey Auditory Verbal Learning Test. J Clin Psychol 1991;47:351–357.

102. Delis DC, Kramer JH, Kaplan E, Ober BA. California Verbal Learning Test: research edition: manual. New York: Psychological Corporation, 1987.

103. Wechsler D. A standardized memory scale for clinical use. J Psychol 1945;19:87–95.

104. Delis Dc, Cullum CM, Butters N, Cairns P. Wechsler Memory Scale–Revised and California Verbal Learning Test: convergence and divergence. Clin Neuropsychol 1988;2:188–196.

105. Wilson B, Cockburn J, Baddeley A, Hiorns R. The development and validation of a test battery for detecting and moni-

toring everyday memory problems. J Clin Exp Neuropsychol 1989;11:855–870.

106. Koltai D. The Rivermead Behavioural Memory Test and the Wechsler Memory Scale–Revised: an analysis of convergence and divergence. Ann Arbor: University of Michigan, 1993.

107. Wilson B. Long-term prognosis of patients with severe memory disorders. Neuropsychol Rehab 1991;1:117–134.

108. Warrington EK. Recognition Memory Test: manual. Windsor, UK: Nfer-Nelson, 1984.

109. Fuld PA. Fuld Object-Memory Evaluation. Chicago: Stoelting, 1977.

110. Masur DM, Sliwinski M, Lipton RB, et al. Neuropsychological prediction of dementia and the absence of dementia in healthy elderly persons. Neurology 1994;44:1427–1432.

111. McCarthy M, Ferris SH, Clark E, Crook T. Acquisition and retention of categorized material in normal aging and senile dementia. Exp Aging Res 1981;7:127–135.

112. Luria AR. The working brain: an introduction to neuropsychology. New York: Basic Books, 1973.

113. Royall DR, Mahurin RK, Gray KF. Bedside assessment of executive cognitive impairment: the Executive Interview. J Am Geriatr Soc 1992;40:1221–1226.

114. Reitan RM: Validity of the Trail Making Test as an indication of organic brain damage. Percept Mot Skills 1958;8:271–276.

115. Heaton RK, Grant I, Matthews CG. Comprehensive norms for an expanded Halstead-Reitan Battery: demographic corrections, research findings, and clinical applications. Odessa, FL: Psychological Assessment Resources, 1991.

116. Benton AL, Hamsher K. Multilingual aphasia examination: manual of instructions. Iowa City: University of Iowa, 1976.

117. Miceli F, Caltagirone C, Gainotti G, et al. Neuropsychological correlates of localized cerebral lesions in nonaphasic brain-damaged patients. J Clin Neuropsychol 1981;3:53–63.

118. Perret E. The left frontal lobe of man and the suppression of habitual responses in verbal categorical behavior. Neuropsychologia 1974;12:323–330.

119. McCarthy G, Blamire AM, Rothman DL, et al. Echo-planar magnetic resonance imaging studies of frontal cortex activation during word generation in humans. Neurobiology 1993;90:4952–4956.

120. Miller E, Hague F. Some characteristics of verbal behavior in presenile dementia. Psychol Med 1975;5:255–259.

121. Ruff RM. Ruff Figural Fluency Test administration manual. San Diego: Neuropsychological Resources, 1988.

122. Ruff RM, Light RH, Evans R. The Ruff Figural Fluency Test: a normative study with adults. Dev Neuropsychol 1987;3:37–51.

123. Baser C, Ruff RM. Construct validity of the San Diego Neuropsychological Test Battery. Arch Clin Neuropsychol 1987;2:13–32.

124. Berg EA. A simple objective test for measuring flexibility in thinking. J Gen Psychol 1948;39:15–22.

125. Grant DA, Berg EA. A behavioral analysis of degree of reinforcement and ease of shifting to new responses in a Weigl-type card sorting problem. J Exp Psychol 1948;34:404–411.

126. Heaton RK, Chelune GJ, Talley JL, et al. Wisconsin Card Sorting Test manual: revised and expanded. Odessa, FL: Psychological Assessment Resources, 1993.

127. Benton AL, Hamsher K. Multilingual Aphasia Examination: manual of instructions. Iowa City: AJA Associates, 1983.

128. Borod JC, Goodglass H, Kaplan E. Normative data on the Boston Diagnostic Aphasia Examination, Parietal Lobe Battery, and the Boston Naming Test. J Clin Neuropsychol 1980;2:209–216.

129. Kertesz A. Aphasia and associated disorders. New York: Grune & Stratton, 1979.

130. Kertesz A, Poole E. The aphasia quotient: the taxonomic approach to measurement of aphasic disability. Can J Neurosci 1974;1:7–16.

131. Lezak MD. Neuropsychological assessment. New York: Oxford University, 1983.

132. Kaplan E, Goodglass H, Weintraub S. The Boston Naming Test. Philadelphia: Lea & Febiger, 1983.

133. Spreen O, Strauss E. A compendium of neuropsychological tests: administration, norms, and commentary. New York: Oxford, 1991.

134. Van Gorp WG, Satz P, Kiersch ME, Henry R. Normative data on the Boston Naming Test for a group of normal older adults. J Clin Exp Neuropsychol 1986;8:702–705.

135. Hooper HE. The Hooper Visual Organization Test: manual. Los Angeles: Western Psychological Servies, 1958.

136. Benton AL, Varney NR, Hamsher K. Visuospatial judgment: a clinical test. Arch Neurol 1978;35:364–367.

137. Rey A. L'examen psychologique dans les cas d'encephalopathie traumatique. Arch Psychol 1941;28:286–340.

138. Osterrieth PA. Le test de copie d'une figure complexe. Arch Psychol 1944:30:206–356.

139. Boll TJ. The Halstead-Reitan Neuropsychology Battery. In: Filskov SB, Boll TJ. Handbook of clinical neuropsychology. New York: Wiley, 1981:577–607.

140. Reitan RM, Wolfson D. The Halstead-Reitan Neuropsychological Test Battery: theory and clinical interpretation. South Tucson, AZ: Neuropsychology, 1985.

141. Klove H. Clinical neuropsychology. In: Forster FM. The medical clinics of North America. New York: Saunders, 1963.

142. Matthews CG, Haaland KY. The effect of symptom duration on cognitive and motor performance in parkinsonism. Neurology 1979;29:951–956.

143. Yesavage JA, Brink TL, Rose TL, et al. Development and validation of a geriatric depression screening scale: a preliminary report. J Psychiatr Res 1983;17:37–49.

144. Brink TA, Yesavage JA, Lum O, et al. Screening tests for geriatric depression. Clin Gerontol 1982;1:37–44.

145. Spitzer R, Endicott J, Robins E. Research Diagnostic Criteria: rationale and reliability. Arch Gen Psychiatry 1978;35:773–782.

146. Koenig HG, Meador KG, Cohen HJ, Blazer DG. Self-rated depression scales and screening for major depression in the older hospitalized patient with medical illness. J Am Geriatr Soc 1988;36:699–706.

147. Beck AT, Ward C, Mendelson M, et al. An inventory for measuring depression. Arch Gen Psychiatry 1961;4;561–571.

148. Gallagher D. Assessment of depression by interview methods and psychiatric rating scales. In: Poon LW, ed. Clinical memory assessment of older adults. Washington DC: American Psychological Association, 1986:202–212.

149. Gallagher D, Breckenridge J, Steinmetz J, Thompson LW. The Beck Depression Inventory and Research Diagnostic Criteria: congruence in an older population. J Consult Clin Psychol 1983;51:945–946.

150. Hamilton M. A rating scale for depression. J Neurol Neurosurg Psychiatry 1960;23:56–62.

151. Hamilton M. Development of a rating scale for primary depressive illness. Br J Soc Clin Psychol 1967;6:278–296.

152. Butcher JN, Dahlstrom WG, Graham JR, et al. Minnesota Multiphasic Personality Inventory (MMPI-2): manual for administration and scoring. Minneapolis: University of Minnesota, 1989.

153. Harris R, Lingoes J. Subscales for the Minnesota Multiphasic Personality Inventory. Mimeographed materials. Langley Porter Clinic, 1968.

154. Dahlstrom WG, Welsh GS, Dahlstrom LE. An MMPI handbook: clinical interpretation. vol 1. Minneapolis: University of Minnesota, 1972.

Part II General Care of the Geriatric Patient

Chapter 5
Approach to the Patient

Dennis W. Jahnigen and Robert W. Schrier

I am not afraid of tomorrow, for I have seen yesterday and I love today.

William Allen White
In Lois L. Kaufman, Old Age Is Not for Sissies

The relationship of the physician with an elderly patient involves more than simple application of the most current diagnostic and therapeutic information. This knowledge by the physician is necessary but not sufficient to ensure an optimal outcome. The relationship requires recognition of the differences and the similarities between the patient and the physician. It requires sensitivity to age-related changes that may increase the anxiety associated with illness for the patient and that may increase the difficulty of obtaining accurate historic and physical information for the physician. The relationship also involves appreciation of differences in the values among elderly patients and a willingness to negotiate what may be medically indicated or medically possible with what is most desirable from the patient's frame of reference. The goals of therapy in an elderly person may lie in relief of symptoms rather than a cure, in preservation of independent living rather than returning to employment, in easing suffering at the end of life rather than fighting death.

The relationship an elderly person has with a primary care physician can be extremely important to the older person's overall health. The relationship provides opportunity for preventive services, accurate assessment and treatment of existing conditions, and planning for the eventual need of end-of-life medical treatment. The primary care physician has the opportunity to come to know the elderly patient as an individual, as a part of his or her family and community, and to learn something about the patient's past and about the patient's hopes for the future. This type of information can be invaluable in making the decisions commonly required of the physician.

Elderly persons have high use of health services in virtually all care settings. Although the use of long-term care services, such as home care and nursing homes, is usually recognized as common among elderly populations, these persons also require acute services, including emergency care, hospital care, and intensive care services. The Emergency Department (ED) is a common point of entry into the hospital for elderly patients. Although elderly patients rarely use the ED as a source for primary care, when they do come to the ED, they are usually more seriously ill than younger patients. In a multicenter study, patients over 65 years of age were 4.4 times more likely to arrive at the ED by ambulance, 5.6 times more likely to be admitted to the hospital, and 5.5 times more likely to require intensive care on admission compared with younger patients (1,2,3) (see also Chapter 9).

Diagnosis

The identification of disease and disability in an elderly patient can be difficult. Many common geriatric conditions do not fit as discrete diseases but are better thought of as syndromes (Table 5.1). The presentation of disease can be atypical. As much as one-third of elderly patients with a myocardial infarction have no chest pain; shortness of breath is one of the most common presenting symptoms. Pneumonia without fever, peritonitis without abdominal pain, and hyperthyroidism without tachycardia are but a few atypical presentations (Table 5.2). Many of the symptoms of elderly patients are nonspecific, such as weakness, weight loss, incontinence, tiredness, dizziness, or falling (Table 5.3). A sudden change in mental function is an important clue to underlying acute illness. Likewise, a sudden decrease in functional status, such as the loss of competence at carrying out tasks associated with a given level of independence, is often the only sign

Table 5.1. Common Geriatric Problems.

Loss of autonomy
Inactivity
Gait instability
Decreased functional level
Cognitive impairment
Malnutrition
Polypharmacy
Incontinence
Infections
Decreased hearing/vision
Depression
Inadequate social support
Iatrogenesis
Substance abuse

Table 5.2. Clinical Conditions with Atypical Presentations in the Elderly.

Condition	Atypical Presentation
Myocardial infarct	No chest pain
Pulmonary embolism	No shortness of breath
Acute abdomen	No abdominal pain
Hyperthyroidism	No tremor or tachycardia
Cancer	Depression
	Mass without symptoms
Hypothyroidism	Cognitive impairment
Depression	Masked, no sadness
Alcohol abuse	Falls, weight loss
Drug reaction	Confusion
Endocarditis	Confusion
Congestive heart failure	Confusion
Pneumonia	No fever

Table 5.3. Nonspecific Symptoms of Illness in Elderly Persons.

Confusion
Weight loss
Weakness
Incontinence
Dizziness
Falling
Self-neglect
Functional decline
Apathy
Anorexia

Table 5.4. Diseases Causing Difficulty with Physical Tasks.

	Men (%)	Women (%)	Total (%)
Arthritis	39	55	49
Old age	13	11	12
Heart disease	16	13	14
Injury	10	13	12
Lung disease	7	5	6
Stroke	5	2	3

SOURCE: Modified from Ettinger W, Fried L, Harris T, et al. Self-reported causes of physical disability in older people. J Am Geriatr Soc 1994;42:1035–1044.

Table 5.5. Screens of Functional Abilities.

Activities of Daily Living (ADLs)
   Feeding
   Ambulation
   Bathing
   Continence
   Communication
   Dressing
   Toileting
   Transferring
   Grooming
Instrumental Activities of Daily Living (IADLs)
   Writing
   Cooking
   Shopping
   Climbing stairs
   Managing medication
   Ability to do outside work
   Reading
   Cleaning
   Doing laundry
   Using telephone
   Managing money
   Ability to use public transportation

of a serious underlying event. Parsimony of diagnosis, which attempts to use a single disease process to explain all symptoms, often fails with elderly patients because of the presence of multiple comorbidities that interact with each other. For example, depression can lead to anorexia and malnutrition. Tachycardia associated with sepsis can unmask coronary artery disease.

The concept of functional status is often more important than the presence of a specific disease. Functional ability is the combined effect of disease and disability on the person's ability to carry out a task associated with everyday living (Table 5.4). Functional ability can be evaluated in a number of ways. Two simple screens are the activities of daily living (ADLs) and the instrumental activities of daily living (IADLs) (Table 5.5). These are arranged in a hierarchical order from basic skills to complex skills. These skills of daily living tend to be lost sequentially. Each function is rated on degree of independence to develop an overall score. This information can help determine the type of assistance needed, appropriate living arrangements, and changes over time.

The Role of The Primary Care Physician

In the office, the role of the primary care physician is obvious, but it is equally important in the hospital (4). Even though the patient may become the primary responsibility of a surgeon, medical specialist, or intensivist, the primary care physician can provide reassurance to the patient, participate in difficult decisions, and offer continuity of medical care later in the hospital stay and after discharge. The hospital environment poses unique threats to the health of elderly patients, such as adverse outcomes from diagnosis and therapy, medication side effects, malnutrition, infections, falls, pressure ulcers, and functional decline, all of which are potentially preventable by careful medical and nursing oversight (see Chapter 10).

The first encounter a patient has with the physician is especially important (5). In addition to establishing confidence in the physician's concern and competence, the first meeting conveys the degree of respect and style of communication that will characterize future interactions. The extent to which the physician succeeds in the initial interview will have a major effect on patient trust and willingness to consider and follow future recommendations (6–9). Although, initially, geriatric patients typically take for granted physician competence they are able to judge physician concern themselves. Elderly patients usually wish to be fully included in the medical decision-making process (10,11). They want to be fully informed in terms they can understand, but they are reliant on physician authority in making medical decisions and are less likely to challenge the physician's recommendations than younger patients. Contrary to popular belief, older patients are actually less inclined to report symptoms than younger patients (12). This may be because a symptom such as incontinence is embarrassing, or because older

persons believe a symptom such as joint pain or memory loss are normal with old age. Frequently, older patients will have a friend or family member accompany them to the office or hospital to help understand and remember discussions. The setting in which this initial meeting occurs clearly influences both the manner and urgency with which information is obtained. If the first meeting is in the context of an acute or life-threatening event, a very focused, rapid assessment is needed. On most other occasions, there is sufficient time for the physician to interview and examine the patient deliberately, checking frequently to make sure the patient understands and is comfortable with what is occurring. Several practical "pointers" can assist in this process.

1. As a sign of respect, an older patient should be addressed formally (Mr., Mrs., Ms.). Avoid using the patient's first name unless invited to do so. Many elderly persons resent being treated in an overly familiar fashion, especially by a person much younger than themselves. Speak facing the person, with a slow cadence and medium voice volume. If the person has hearing problems, do not shout. A very loud voice rarely improves understanding and can actually be painful because of sudden transmission of a loud noise. An inexpensive headset amplifier can be obtained easily at electronic stores and can be available in any office or hospital setting to assist in communication. If the patient uses a hearing aid, make sure it is turned on and functioning. Examine the patient in a well-lit area that is free of extraneous noises, if possible. Check to verify that the patient is able to understand what you say by asking the patient to reiterate an understanding of what was said. The choice of words used is important because the educational range of elderly patients can be from elementary school through graduate school. The physician should attempt to use appropriate language and avoid complex medical terminology unless the patient is familiar with medical terms.

Elderly patients are usually most comfortable with ambient temperatures of 75 to 78°F. They are less efficient at maintaining comfortable body temperatures and should be provided a blanket if they must wear a hospital gown for any length of time. Few geriatric patients are able to lie flat on a standard office examination table because nearly all have kyphosis and cervical osteoarthritis, which limits neck extension. A pillow is almost always required for comfort. For frail patients, electric tables are safer and easier than standard tables. Electric tables can be lowered to approximately 20 inches; thus, they can permit a short patient to sit down without undue assistance.

2. In an ambulatory setting, the patient should initially be allowed to wear personal clothing rather than a gown, which most people find embarrassing and undignified (13). Examine the person in a position of equality; that is, address the person at the same level. Sit facing the patient rather than looking down to the person.

In a hospital setting, elevate the patient's head and sit down to communicate. Hospitals are unsettling to most people because of uncertainty about the illness that requires them to be there. Explaining each step of the examination can be reassuring. Do not sit on a patient's bed or remove the bedclothes without asking the patient's permission. The inpatient environment can be particularly frightening to elderly patients because of the rapid pace, numerous encounters with hospital personnel at all hours of the day, and loss of privacy and personal control. Small gestures, such as drawing the curtain to offer a degree of privacy, are appreciated. Although a medical team in a teaching institution often includes several physicians in training, the senior physician should ask the patient's permission for others to watch or participate in the examination. In teaching hospitals, during rounds in which a team of several individuals may participate, only one person at a time should ask questions and examine the patient.

Be aware that great differences in age, race, sex, or cultural background may influence interpretation of symptoms, expectations from medical care, communication, and the attitude of the patient toward the physician. Some of these factors can be significant barriers. For example, a youthful-appearing physician may seem "too young to know anything." An elderly male may be reticent with a female physician, or a similar disparity may occur between a doctor and a patient of a different race or cultural background. Although there is no single way to overcome these issues, clearly conveying interest in the person, as well as acknowledging and respecting differences, usually leads to satisfactory communication. The few minutes the physician spends in socializing with the patient can help accomplish rapport, can help put the patient at ease, and can enable the physician to learn

about the patient's level of comfort, method of expression, affect, and mental status.

3. Treat family members as important allies, but focus on the patient (14). Speak directly to the patient, not to adult children who may be present. With good intentions, competent adult children with a frail parent may speak as though the patient is not present. Further, they may have their own agenda for the physician, such as having the doctor "insist" the patient relocate to a "safer" environment, or prohibiting the physician from telling the patient about the medical condition. Family members usually have important information for the physician and should be included in all discussions (15), but the patient should remain the primary decision maker. When a patient is of questionable competence, courtesy is still essential, although medical history information is suspect and questioning can often be abbreviated.

4. Be culturally sensitive. Patients from Middle Eastern cultures may be extremely modest and may need to be examined while partially or completely clothed. A Native American may insist on having a room in a nursing home "smudged" before agreeing to move in. Smudging involves the use of burning sweetgrass to bless the area. (When this occurred in one nursing home, the staff initially refused, for fear of setting off the fire alarm. Eventually, the alarm was turned off so the ceremony could be performed.) Allow for variations in patient beliefs and expectations of the physician. Family members may be able to provide translation, when needed, for interpretation of symptoms and reinforcement of medical cooperation.

5. Pace the examination according to the time available and the tolerance level of the patient. Rarely is it necessary or feasible to obtain a complete history and physical examination from an elderly, frail person during a single setting. The lifelong volume of information, large number of past or current problems, and a sometimes endless series of complaints in the "review of systems" can be draining on both the patient and the physician and calls for a different method to gather information. The urgency of the apparent problem and the time allocated are the first determinants of the depth and extent of questioning. For complex patients, a complete examination can be performed over the course of two or three visits, as long as the physician has a good medical record of what needs to be done. For patients with stable chronic diseases, part of a complete examination can be performed at each regularly scheduled, three- or four-month visit, a practice known as a *rolling physical* (16). Limit to three or four the number of problems dealt with during one visit. It is difficult for patients to keep track of multiple plans. Schedule more visits as needed to deal with multiple problems. For each patient, write down instructions, changes in medications, and follow-up visits.

6. Use a team approach. Frail, elderly persons typically need professional assistance beyond medical care. If available, an interdisciplinary team can benefit the patient by offering a more thorough evaluation and access to a wider range of services, such as social services, community-based nursing, physical and occupational therapy, and psychological, nutritional, dental, and other types of support (see also Chapter 6). In a hospital setting, most of these services are available, but in an office setting, arrangement for community referral may be necessary.

7. Support the caregiver. Providing physical and emotional support for a frail, dependent person is stressful. Caregivers of persons with Alzheimer's disease have greater physical and mental illness than age-matched controls, and immunologic function is diminished under the stress of caregiving. Caregivers may delay or ignore their own health needs. The physician should monitor the vigor of the patient's support system and the apparent health needs of any primary caregivers. Respite programs can be advised to allow caregivers a period of rest.

Competence

All persons are assumed to be competent unless demonstrated to be otherwise. Although the legal determination of incompetence is made by a court (see Chapter 21), the clinical definition of competence is the ability to understand the implications of medical decisions and a willingness to participate in one's own care. A patient known to have dementia may still be medically competent. Many patients with moderate or severe dementia are unable to participate in their own care; in these situations, other persons to assist in decision making must be sought. States vary in their laws regarding surrogate decision makers. A call to the State Medical Society can lead to accurate regional information in this circumstance. Most

states accept a family member as a surrogate spokesperson for the incompetent patient, but some require a court-appointed guardian. The use of advanced directives, such as the Durable Power of Attorney for Health Care Matters may be useful. Primary care physicians should become familiar with the guidelines in the states in which they practice.

If the competence of the patient is questionable, detailed testing of mental status may be necessary (see Chapter 22). Such testing must be approached gently because it can be a great source of anxiety and frustration to an elderly person. After testing, if competency is still uncertain, a detailed evaluation by a psychiatrist or psychologist may be needed.

Truth Telling

A widely held value in Western medicine is the right of the patient to know the truth about personal medical conditions and options for treatment. Adult family members wishing to spare their elderly relative anxiety may request that the physician not inform the patient of the facts of the illness. If the patient is competent, he or she should have the option of knowing as much as they wish about the condition. This situation can be handled by discussing the findings of the examination with the patient and the family, asking the patient, first, "What do you wish to know about your illness?" and, second, "If this is a serious or life-threatening illness, would you want to know about it?" The response to the first question allows the patient to specify the type of information and level of detail desired. Most patients will answer in the affirmative to the second question, and in so doing, can help the physician speak honestly to the patient but still respect the family's concern. For patients with Alzheimer's disease or other dementing illnesses, arguments both for and against telling the patient the diagnosis have been made (17). For patients with early disease who have insight into their cognitive deficits, the offer of information should be made because some patients may wish to organize their activities and future plans accordingly. For patients with more severe cognitive impairment, the ability to retain new information may be lost, and the individual may forget each time the diagnosis is mentioned. In such circumstances, constantly reinforcing that the person has a progressive cognitive illness would seem to have little value.

The Office Visit

The office visit with an elderly person is a time-limited encounter, and few physicians in the context of a busy office can devote hours to a medical assessment. Initial data collection can be obtained during 2 or 3 visits, rather than during a single one. Typically, one or more family members may wish to participate in the interview. Their presence may be important because the patient may forget or mitigate needed information. The patient should be the clear center of attention, faced by the physician, with family members in the background. Shaking of heads in opposite directions by the patient and family in response to a question can be an early clue that memory loss is the reason for the evaluation.

After allowing the patient to describe the reason for the visit and to answer focused questions, the physician can encourage the patient who has multiple complaints to name the most troublesome problems. This list can be limited by the physician to those that can be addressed during the first visit, with others to be pursued at a future time. This approach can be very useful for the patient with 10 or more complaints.

Next, the physician can suggest that the patient change into a gown while the physician and family members step out of the room. At this juncture, the family can be asked for additional information, which may elicit essential details that the patient was unwilling or unable to reveal, such as functional deficits, self-neglect, depression, recent physical decline, or alcohol abuse. This brief encounter allows the family to participate but preserves the patient as the focal point. If there are serious family stresses underway at the time of the first visit, and social services are available on site, the family can be immediately interviewed by a social worker, psychologist, or nurse practitioner while the patient is examined. During the family interview, urgent needs such as safety, legal guardianship, meals, living arrangements, and supportive home services, can be identified and addressed.

During this first visit, the physician can examine the patient, performing as much of a complete examination as is practical in the time available. A complete examination is rarely practical or essential. Major components omitted should be documented with a plan for completing them at subsequent visits. The physician can develop a problem list and planned actions during the examination. During the examination, the physician can ask additional questions to verify or elaborate the patient's earlier responses. The patient's affect and responses to questions may be very different when he or she is alone than when a caregiver is in the room. Touching the patient during every visit is important because it makes a physical bond with the patient and can be reassuring.

After the examination, the patient can dress while the physician finishes notes, visits the family, or sees another patient. The physician can then briefly reconvene with the patient and family to discuss findings and recommendations. For a complex patient with complex problems, plans for diagnostic testing, initial therapy, referral for additional evaluations (audiology, opthalmology, physical therapy, dental, social services, and others) can be made, and arrangements for follow-up visits established. The initial evaluation can be done in one hour or less with use of a minimum data set and collection of non-duplicative information (see Chapter 6).

Subsequent Visits

Follow-up visits can be used to monitor therapy, discuss the results of tests, and pursue new or additional problems. The patient should be weighed at each visit because a decline may be a marker for underlying illness that might otherwise go unnoticed. Patients should be requested to bring all medications to each visit. Verification of the medication, dosage, and how the patient is taking the medication should be done at each visit to help improve compliance and reduce error. Unnecessary or ineffective medications can be discontinued. The patient and family can indicate whether the therapy has been effective. In addition to active problems, at least one other preventive issue should be covered at each visit (Table 5.6; see also Chapter 8). This type of follow-up visit should require only 20 to 30 minutes, even for the very old patient. Another member of the health care team can visit with the patient, assist with dressing as needed, reinforce information to the patient, and help bring the visit to a close.

Table 5.6. Planning for Follow-up Visits.

Immunization status
Counseling about: exercise, accident risks
Counseling about: diet, alcohol use
Mental status screening
Mammogram
Pelvic/pap smear
Rectal examination
Screen of gait, vision, hearing
Advance directive discussion

Patients with multiple problems or with extensive frailty should be seen as often as their condition dictates but usually at intervals no longer than 3 to 4 months. This permits the physician to do a rolling physical and to monitor for functional decline. For example, if a patient is normally seen four times yearly, the following sequence of evaluation could be used:

Visit 1   Establish rapport
           Determine primary three complaints or issues
           Review medication
           Determine urgency of evaluation
           Assess social situation
           Focus physical examination
           Give initial immunization (pneumococcal, tetanus-diphtheria)
           Examine mental status
           Assess safety issues

Visit 2   Build rapport
           Repeat weight, blood pressure, medication review
           Assess management of current problems
           Screen nutrition
           Screen vision
           Examine skin
           Screen hearing
           Finish omitted parts of initial examination
           Make specialty referrals as needed

Visit 3   Review weight, blood pressure, medication
           Continue management of ongoing problems
           Give pelvic examination
           Give rectal examination
           Schedule mammogram

           Oral evaluation
           Discuss advance directives
           Arrange community services
           Schedule laboratory procedures as indicated

Visit 4   Review weight, blood pressure, medication
           Continue management of current problems
           Evaluate gait
           Give influenza immunization
           Assess caregiver status
           Schedule laboratory procedures as indicated
           Review completeness of physical evaluation

There is little evidence that an asymptomatic elderly person needs an annual physical. Specific information about home visits and nursing home visits are discussed in detail in Chapters 13 and 14, respectively.

Medical Decision Making

Medical decision making with elderly patients can be perplexing, especially to the physician in training. The volume of complaints, the nonspecificity of symptoms, and the large number of potential diseases that a typical review of symptoms may identify can be challenging to approach in a systematic fashion. Deciding which conditions to focus on, how aggressive to be, and when to shift from attempting cure to palliation can challenge the physician. The five-step process described below can be used to rank disabilities or complaints in a way that appreciates individual wishes and values, but uses medical diagnostic and therapeutic techniques selectively. The process offers one way to avoid unwanted care and offers beneficial interventions judged to be appropriate by both patient and physician. In this way, a "best" answer can emerge in which the patient's objectives define the desired outcome, and the physician uses the best available technology to achieve this, rather than the symptom or the disease defining the "best" treatment. This process can be incorporated into a primary care relationship and accomplished over a series of visits. If necessary, this process can be used in a single visit to plan strategies. Generally, it is preferable for the process to occur in an ambulatory environment, with the patient free from the stress of acute illness, to allow issues to be raised and considered by patient and family in a deliberative fashion. The goals for the patient can be dynamic and change over time to reflect response to therapy or a change in the patient's desires.

A Geriatric-Sensitive Model of Medical Decision Making

1. Learn about the patient's values. Older persons differ from one another in what is important in their lives and differ as a group from younger populations. Younger persons typically fear death more than any other event, but elderly persons fear loss of independence and autonomy, long-term disability, being a financial burden on others, and loss of mental faculties, more than death (18). Few very old persons have not considered death, and many approach it with calm resignation or even welcome it as an end to suffering. Some older persons are "fighters" and are willing to undergo great discomfort and risk for the possible extension of any amount of life.

The current quality of life as perceived by the person is important for the physician to determine. Health professionals who project their own perceptions on the quality of life of a patient may undervalue the current quality of life as perceived by the patient. How does the patient feel about present life? Has the patient thought about circumstances under which he or she would not want to live? Does religion provide comfort or guidance as the patient approaches the end of life? Has the patient talked to others about wishes or made an advance directive or durable power of attorney? What does the patient enjoy in life—running a marathon? Caring for a beloved pet? This type of information helps set the stage on which medical decisions will be made and enforces rapport with a patient.

2. Determine the person's objectives from the medical encounter. The response from the patient to the question "Why are you here today?" may range from "Because my daughter made me come" to "I just don't feel good." The person may be seeking one or more outcomes from the medical encounter. Failure to recognize what the person is seeking can lead to major miscommunication and dissatisfaction to the patient, physician, and family. Possible patient objectives are listed in Table 5.7.

3. Determine the medical facts. Using the patient's values and objectives as guides, the physician becomes diagnostician, determining the most likely disease(s), conditions,

Table 5.7. Possible Patient Objectives.

Patient Objective	Example
a. Cure of the condition	"Please fix my painful hip."
b. Relief of symptoms	"Help me tolerate the pain of my arthritis."
c. Reassurance	"Do I have cancer?" "Do I have Alzheimer's disease?"
d. Preservation of function	"Help me control my falling so I can stay in my own home."
e. Explanation	"What's happening to me?" "What can I expect in the future?"
f. Sympathy	"I want someone to listen to me."
g. Validation	"I am important because you treat me with respect, and take my concern seriously."
h. Secondary gain	"I want my family to care more about me."

disabilities present, and an assessment of prognosis, therapeutic options, and risk-benefit estimates. The physician needs to have the most current information on the usefulness of potential interventions because elderly persons overestimate the usefulness of many interventions. Many elderly patients (and their families) have greatly inflated expectations of the success of medical interventions. For example, in one study, community elderly persons believed that in-hospital cardiopulmonary resuscitation results in a rate of discharge alive that was more than 60 percent higher than the actual rate of 13 percent (19) (Table 5.8). Overestimation occurs in part because the primary source of health information for elderly persons is television (Table 5.9). Such misconceptions emphasize the need for education on accurate prognosis and usefulness of interventions. Elderly persons are discerning about interventions on the basis of perceived usefulness; they may adjust their preferences when presented with accurate information (20). In judging the relative usefulness of many interventions for elderly persons, one should consider cohort and, more important, estimates of life expectancy (Table 5.10). Interventions near the end of a person's life may have minimal or no impact on either quantity of life or relief of symptoms. In some circumstances, the use of artifical feedings or antibiotics may be of no benefit to the patient (21,22). A recent study of hospice patients demonstrated that the symptoms associated with thirst and hunger could be well managed by

Table 5.8. Elderly Persons' Estimations vs Actual Survival Rates After In-hospital CPR*.

	Actual Survival Rate (%)	Estimated Survival Rate (%)
All patients	13	62
Healthy 80-year-olds	No Data	51
Patients from nursing homes	1	41
Patients with severe infections	1	40
Patients with widespread cancer	1	28

*CPR = cardiopulmonary resuscitation.
SOURCE: From Miller D, Jahnigen D, Gorbien M, Simbartl L. Cardiopulmonary resuscitation: how useful? Attitudes and knowledge of an elderly population. Arch Intern Med 1992:152;578–582.

Table 5.9. Elderly Persons' Source of Knowledge about CPR*.

Source	(%)
Television	66
Books and magazines	53
First aid or CPR class	35
Family and friends	35
Other health professionals	23
Never heard of CPR	9
Family physician	6
Religious teachings	2

*CPR = cardiopulmonary resuscitation.
SOURCE: Reproduced by permission from Miller D, Jahnigen D, Gorbien M, Simbartl L. Cardiopulmonary resuscitation: how useful? Attitudes and knowledge of an elderly population. Arch Intern Med 1992:152;578–582.

Table 5.10. Life Expectancy for Elderly Persons.

Current Age (yr)	Men (yr)	Women (yr)
Age 65	14.7	18.6
Age 75	9.1	11.7
Age 85	5.2	6.4

SOURCE: National Center for Health Statistics. Vital Statistics of the United States. vol. II. Mortality, Part A. Washington, DC: Public Health Service, 1986.

offering small amounts of water (21,23). The physician needs to provide judgment about the likely benefit of any proposed interventions (24). Part of what patients expect from their doctors is a recommendation. Every option

possible need not be presented. Interventions that, in the physician's opinion, are futile need not be presented. The physician can offer several courses of action that seem to be reasonable.

4. Recommend and negotiate. In this step, the physician recommends a course of diagnosis or therapy to the patient and family and "tests" it for acceptance to check how well the physician understands the patient's values and wishes. Negotiation should occur. If the patient wants something other than what the physician recommends, the reasons should be explored. If the family wants something other than what the patient wants or what the physician recommends, these issues must be discussed and reconciled.

5. Agree on a strategy and measure of success. The final step is to agree on an overall strategy for medical care and the expected outcome. In this way, patient, physician, and family can understand the expected outcome, and the measure of success. This is a dynamic process, and the outcome may change depending on response to therapy or other factors. Some examples of explicit strategies are listed in Table 5.11.

Agreement ahead of time on the goals of medical care for a specific patient helps everyone to understand what is occurring and to judge the success of the care plan. The physician needs to keep in mind that the success of his care is best judged in the patient's own terms regarding achieving the most with what life offers. The physician who knowingly accepts this challenge will be rewarded with the satisfaction of using the best skills "to cure when possible, to comfort often, to care always."

Table 5.11. Strategies for Medical Care.

Strategy	Expected Outcome
Cure	Total resolution of the problem
Rehabilitation	Recovery of lost function
Prevention	Avoidance of disease
Diagnostic	Obtain needed information for subsequent decision
Experimental	High risk/low likelihood of benefits
Acute care	Aggressive treatment of illness/stabilization
Symptom-based	Relief of discomfort without cure
Palliation	Preservation of patient control; comfort during death

References

1. Strange GR, Chen EH, Sanders AB. Use of emergency departments by elderly patients: projections from a multicenter data base. Ann Emerg Med 1992;21:819–824.
2. Singal BM, Hedges JR, Rousseau EW, et al. Geriatric patient visits. Part I: comparison of visits by geriatric and younger patients. Ann Emerg Med 1992;21:802–807.
3. Sanders A, Morley J. The older person in the emergency department. J Am Geriatr Soc 1993;41:880–882.
4. Fahs M. Primary medical care for elderly patients. II. J Community Health 1989;14:89–99.
5. Gastel B. Working with your older patient: a clinician's handbook. Bethesda, MD: National Institute on Aging, National Institutes of Health, 1994.
6. Adelman R, Green M, Charon R. Issues in physician-elderly patient interaction. Ageing and Society 1991;2:127–148.
7. Anderson L, Zimmerman M. Patient and physician perceptions of their relationship and patient satisfaction. A study of chronic disease management. Patient Educ Couns 1993;20:27–36.
8. Beisecker A, Beisecker T. Patient information-seeking behaviors when communicating with doctors. Med Care 1990;28:19–28.
9. Green M, Adelman R, Charon R, Friedman E. Concordance between physicians and their older and younger patients in the primary care medical encounter. Gerontologist 1989;29:808–813.
10. Haug MR, ed. Elderly patients and their doctors. New York: Springer, 1981.
11. Beisecker AE. Aging and the desire for information and input in medical decisions. Patient consumerism in medical encounters. Gerontologist 1988;28:330–335.
12. Branch L, Nemeth K. When elders fail to visit physicians. Med Care 1990;23:11.
13. Carlson M, Jahnigen D. The hospital gown. J Am Geriatr Soc 1991;38:A30.
14. Glasser M, Prohaska T, Roska J. The role of the family in medical case-seeking decisions of older adults. Fam Community Health 1992;15:59–70.
15. Haley W, Clair J, Saulsberry K. Family caregiver satisfaction with medical care of their demented relatives. Gerontologist 1992;32:219–226.
16. Jahnigen DW, Schrier RW. The doctor/patient relationship in geriatric care. In: Jahnigen D, Schrier RW, eds. Issues in the care of the elderly. New York: WB Saunders, 1986:457–464.
17. Drickamer MA, Lachs MS. Should patients with alzheimer's disease be told their diagnosis? N Engl J Med 1992;326:947–951.
18. Americans view aging. Alliance for Aging Research, 1991.
19. Miller D, Jahnigen D, Gorbien M, Simbartl L. Cardiopulmonary resuscitation: how useful? Attitudes and knowledge of an elderly population. Arch Intern Med 1992;152:578–582.
20. Murphy D, Burrows P, Santilli S, et al. The influence of the probability of survival on patients' preferences regarding cardiopulmonary resuscitation. N Engl J Med 1994;330:545–549.
21. Fabiszewski K, Volicer B, Volicer L. Effect of antibiotic treatment on outcome of fevers in institutionalized alzheimer's patients. JAMA 1990;263:3168–3172.
22. Quill T. Utilization of nasogastric feeding tubes in group of chronically ill, elderly patients in a community hospital. Arch Intern Med 1989;149:1937–1941.
23. McCann R, Hall W, Groth-Juncker A. Comfort care for terminally ill patients. The appropriate use of nutrition and hydration. JAMA 1994;274:1263–1268.
24. Miller D, Gorbien M, Simbartl L, et al. Factors influencing physicians in recommending in-hospital cardiopulmonary resuscitation. Arch Intern Med 1993;153:1999–2003.

Suggested Readings

Adelman R, Green M, Charon R. The physician-elderly patient-companion triad in the medical encounter. The development of a conceptual framework and research agenda. Gerontologist 1987;27:729–734.

Barsky AJ, Hochstrasser B, Coles NA, et al. Silent myocardial ischemia. Is the person or the event silent? JAMA 1990;264:1132–1135.

Ettinger W, Fried L, Harris T, et al. Self-reported causes of physical disability in older people. J Am Geriatr Soc 1994;42:1035–1044.

Fried LP, Storer PJ, King DE, et al. Diagnosis of illness presentation in the elderly. J Am Geriatr Soc 1991;39:117–123.

Nordyke RA, Gilbert FI, Harada ASM. Graves' disease. Influence of age on clinical findings. Arch Intern Med 1988;184:626–631.

Rost K, Frankel R. The introduction of older patient's problems in the medical visit. J Health Aging 1993;8(5):387–401.

Rowe JW. Health care of the elderly. N Engl J Med 1985;312:1159–1165.

Singa LB, Hedges J, Rousseau E, et al. Geriatric patient emergency visits, Part J: comparison of visits by geriatric and younger patients. Ann Emerg Med 1992;21:802–807.

Chapter 6
Geriatric Assessment

Alison A. Moore and David B. Reuben

Have you a moist eye? a dry hand? a yellow cheek? a white beard? a decreasing leg? an increasing belly? is not your voice broken? your wind short? your chin double? your wit single? and every part about you blasted with antiquity?

Chief Justice
William Shakespeare, King Henry IV, Part 2

The concept of geriatric assessment has developed in recognition of the complex medical, mental health, social problems, and attendant functional disabilities of many frail, elderly persons. By implementing the principles of geriatric assessment, health care professionals prioritize these problems and develop prevention, treatment, and rehabilitation strategies that emphasize improving or maintaining patient function. Geriatric assessment includes evaluation of older persons' physical and mental health, and their functional and social status. Other domains frequently included in the assessment are the patient's economic status, characteristics of the home environment, and a discussion of patient preferences regarding advanced directives.

Assessment of older persons may be accomplished through a variety of approaches ranging from assessment of the patient by an individual practitioner to evaluation of the patient by a multidisciplinary team of health care professionals (comprehensive geriatric assessment). This chapter focuses on the two ends of the spectrum of assessment, beginning with geriatric assessment by the individual practitioner and extending these concepts to multidisciplinary geriatric assessment.

Geriatric Assessment by the Individual Practitioner

Most older persons do not need an extensive multidimensional evaluation; this process should be reserved for those who are frail or at high risk for functional decline.

An appropriate strategy is to supplement the traditional medical assessment by briefly screening for common geriatric conditions and then performing a more comprehensive evaluation only on those patients who have potential problems identified by the screening.

Careful screening is particularly indicated for common geriatric conditions that are frequently missed during the traditional history-taking and physical examination. In addition to seeking common geriatric conditions, physicians should discuss issues that are of particular relevance to the health of older persons (e.g., advanced directives, adequacy of social support, economic status, environmental risks). Each domain should be systematically, if briefly, evaluated to determine whether a more in-depth assessment is necessary.

Theoretically, assessment instruments are not needed in clinical practice. All necessary information can be obtained by asking the right questions and performing the appropriate maneuvers in the course of gathering the medical history and physically examining the patient. However, the traditional evaluation of the patient has been limited to the medical domain and often fails to address some of the most important geriatric issues. As a result, some clinicians have turned to assessment instruments and standardized questions, which can insure comprehensiveness, increase accuracy, and save time. Standardized questions can be included as part of a questionnaire that patients (or their families) can complete before the visit or in the waiting room. Many instruments can be administered by trained office staff who do not have professional degrees.

The following sections review domains that comprise an individual physician's office-based geriatric assessment for community-dwelling older persons. In each section, brief methods of screening and longer methods for further evaluation of each problem are presented. When available, standardized validated questions or performance-based measures are provided both to screen and to further assess each domain. However, the clinician may choose to rely on less formal questions to probe potential problems.

Medical Assessment

In addition to a complete medical history and physical examination, common geriatric conditions warrant particular investigation. Problems with vision, hearing, leg mobility, malnutrition, urinary incontinence, and polypharmacy may all contribute to functional decline among older persons. These problems may be missed because older patients may not recognize that they are indicative of medical problems (e.g., falls), because they are embarrassed to mention them (e.g., incontinence), or because they believe that these symptoms are normal aspects of aging that cannot be helped (e.g., hearing loss). This section reviews the rationale and methods for assessing each of these problems.

Visual Impairment

More than 90 percent of older persons require eyeglasses, and over 20 percent of those persons over age 85 have difficulty seeing even when they wear glasses. Vision problems can increase the risk of injury (e.g., falls with resulting fractures, motor vehicle accidents) and contribute to deficits in physical and psychosocial functioning.

The two measures used commonly in practice to screen for visual impairment are the Snellen Eye Chart and the Jaeger Card (Table 6.1). The most commonly used Snellen Eye Chart requires that the patient stand 20 feet from the chart. The Jaeger Card is a handheld chart that is read at a distance of 14 inches. For both tests, patients fail the screen if they are unable to read all the letters on the 20/40 line while they are wearing corrective lenses.

A longer screen for visual problems, developed to assess visual functional status among persons with cataracts, is the Activities of Daily Vision Scale (1). This is an interviewer-administered questionnaire that assesses difficulty in performing 20 activities. The scale is both reliable and valid but has not yet been tested as a screening instrument.

Hearing Impairment

Hearing impairment is reported by 23 percent, 33 percent,

and 48 percent of those aged 65 to 74 years, 75 to 85 years, and 85 years and older, respectively. Hearing impairment is associated with reduced cognitive, emotional, social, and physical function in older adults. Hearing amplification devices have improved functional status and quality of life of older persons (2).

Among the best screens for hearing loss are the Welch Allyn Audioscope (Welch Allyn, Inc., Skaneateles Falls, NY), the whispered voice test, and the Hearing Handicap Inventory for the Elderly–Screening Version (HHIE-S) (3). The audioscope is a handheld otoscope with a built-in audiometer. It should be set at 40 decibels (dB) to evaluate hearing in the elderly. Patients fail the screen if they are unable to hear either the 1000- or 2000-hertz (Hz) frequency in both ears or both the 1000- and 2000-Hz frequencies in one ear (4).

The whispered voice test is administered by whispering 3 to 6 random words (numbers, words, or letters) at a set distance (6, 8, 12, or 24 inches) from the person's ear and then asking him or her to repeat the words. The examiner should be behind the person to prevent lipreading. The untested ear should be covered or occluded during the testing. A patient is considered to have failed the test if he or she is unable to repeat correctly 50 percent of the whispered words. The Hearing Handicap Inventory for the Elderly–Screening Version is a 10-item self-administered questionnaire that asks patients about emotional and social problems associated with impaired hearing (3) (see Appendix).

Malnutrition and Weight Loss

Prevalence estimates of malnutrition in the community-based older population vary widely because of differences in the definition and in the evaluation of malnutrition and the population studied. Malnutrition may place older people at risk for subsequent dysfunction, disability, and sometimes premature or increased morbidity and risk of death.

Low body weight and unintentional weight loss are highly predictive of mortality and morbidity in elderly patients. One question for detecting weight loss asks: "Without trying to, have you lost or gained 10 pounds in the last six months?" (5). Persons who answer "yes" to this question are at an increased risk of death during the next four years.

Table 6.1. Geriatric Screening and Assessment Instruments.

Problem	Instrument	Estimated Administration Time (min)
Vision	Snellen Eye Chart	1–2
	Jaeger Card	1
	Activities of Daily Vision Scale	10–15
Hearing	Welch Allyn Audioscope	1–2
	Whispered voice test	1
	Hearing Handicap Inventory for the Elderly	2
Malnutrition	"Without trying to, have you lost 10 lbs in the last six months?"	<1
	Body mass index	1
	Nutritional Health Checklist	1–2
Urinary incontinence	"In the last year, have you ever lost your urine and gotten wet?"	<1
	"Have you lost urine at least six separate days?"	
Mobility	"During the past 12 months, have you fallen all the way to the ground or fallen and hit something like a chair or a stair?"	<1
	Up & Go test	1–2
	Gait and balance test	1–2
	Functional reach	<1
Dementia	Recall of 3 items	2
	Clock-drawing test	1–2
	Serial-sevens test	1–3
	Mini-Mental State	5–10
Depression	"Do you often feel sad or depressed?"	<1
	"How much of the time, during the last month, have you felt downhearted and blue?"	<1
	"In the past year, have you had two weeks or more during which you felt sad, blue, or depressed, or when you lost all interest and pleasure in things that you usually cared about or enjoyed?"	≤1
	"Have you had 2 years or more in you life when you felt depressed or sad most days even if you felt OK sometimes?"	
	"Have you felt depressed or sad much of the time in the past year?"	
	Geriatric Depression Scale (short form)	5
Function	Katz Index of Independence in ADL Scale	1–5
	OARS Multidimensional Function Assessment Questionnaire	1–5
	COOP Chart	5–10
	Functional Status Questionnaire	15

Another way to screen for problems with nutrition is to measure the patient's height and weight and determine body mass index (BMI) using the formula: weight in kilograms divided by height in meters squared. Persons who have a low BMI also have an increased risk of death (6). Potential problems with nutrition may also be detected by a 10-item checklist developed by the Nutrition Screening Initiative for determining nutritional health among older persons (7) (see Appendix).

Urinary Incontinence

Urinary incontinence affects 10 percent to 30 percent of community-dwelling elderly adults. The prevalence of weekly or more frequent urine loss is 3 percent to 11 percent. From a medical standpoint, incontinent individuals are predisposed to perineal rashes, pressure ulcers, lower extremity cellulitis, urinary tract infections, urosepsis, falls, and fractures. Affected persons frequently feel embarrassed, isolated, stigmatized, and depressed. Frail persons with incontinence also place great strain on caregivers, and frail, elderly persons with many impairments are often placed in a nursing home when they become incontinent (8).

A validated screen for incontinence consists of two questions: 1) "In the last year, have you ever lost your urine and gotten wet?" and, if the respondent answers "yes" to the first question, 2) "Have you lost urine on at least six separate days?" (9). Positive answers to both questions indicate a potential problem with urinary incontinence (10).

Problems with Mobility

Gait disorders affect 15 percent to 20 percent of elderly persons. Approximately 20 percent of persons who are 75 years of age or older require help from a person or device to transfer out of a chair; over 30 percent have difficulty with stairs. Each year, one-third of community-dwelling persons who are age 75 years and older fall; of these, one-half suffer multiple episodes of falling. Three to 5 percent of falls by both community-dwelling and institutionalized older persons result in fracture. An additional 5 percent to 10 percent of falls result in restricted activity for more than a few days or in serious nonfracture injuries that require medical care. A history of falls may be obtained by asking a standardized question: "During the past twelve months have you fallen all the way to the ground or fallen and hit something like a chair or stair?" (11).

The timed "Up & Go" is a test of functional mobility for the frail elderly (12). During this test, the patient is observed and timed while rising from an arm chair, walking 3 meters (10 feet), turning, walking back, and sitting down again. Patients who cannot perform the test within 20 seconds should be evaluated further to identify specific problems with gait or balance.

A more extensive screen for gait and balance abnormalities is the Performance-Oriented Assessment of Mobility instrument (13) (see Appendix). This test takes five minutes to administer and grades different aspects of patients' balance and gait. Maximal score is 28 points. If the score is less than 19, the relative risk of falling over a three-month period is 5.7.

Functional reach is a measure of balance that also can identify persons who are likely to fall (14). Functional reach is the maximal distance one can reach forward from a standing position without stepping and is measured using a leveled yardstick secured to the wall at shoulder height. The test takes less than five minutes. Patients who cannot reach more than 10 inches are at an increased risk of falling during the next six months (15).

Polypharmacy

Older persons in the U.S. use four to five prescription drugs at any one time, and two-thirds of those over age 65 also use at least one nonprescription drug. Polypharmacy may occur because older persons often see more than one physician and may get medication from each one. They also may not either understand or be given adequate instructions to discontinue medications or change dosages.

Potential problems with polypharmacy can be assessed by having patients bring in all their medication bottles, both prescription and nonprescription. Drug regimens should be investigated for possible interactions, drug dosages should be adjusted to provide the smallest dose that achieves therapeutic effect, and certain drugs like amitriptyline and long-acting benzodiazepines should be avoided.

Cognitive Assessment

The incidence of dementia increases with age, such that approximately 5 percent to 10 percent of those older than 65 years and 15 percent to 47 percent over age 85 have some degree of dementia. In nursing homes, 50 percent to 80 percent of those older than 65 years have some degree of cognitive impairment.

Three very brief screens have good predictive values for cognitive impairment (16). These are recall of three items, the clock-drawing test, and the serial-sevens test. In the recall of three items test, the examiner asks the patient to repeat the names of three items and then remember them (17). After one minute, the examiner asks the patient to recall the three items. Patients who cannot remember at least two items are more likely to be cognitively impaired. In the clock-drawing test, the examiner draws a circle and instructs the patient to draw a clock in the circle (18). Patients who are unable to complete a normal clock are at increased risk for dementia. In the serial-sevens test, the examiner asks the patient to subtract seven from 100 five times (19). Normal results on these tests vastly reduce the probability of dementia, but abnormal results increase the odds of dementia.

A longer, commonly used instrument to screen for cognitive impairment is the Mini-Mental State (17) (see Appendix), particularly useful in screening for moderate impairment in cognitive function. The Mini-Mental State examination has a maximum score of 30, usually takes 5 to 10 minutes to administer and assesses several areas of cognition, including orientation, registration, attention and calculation, recall, and language. A score of 20 or less greatly increases the likelihood of cognitive impairment and a score of 26 or more greatly decreases the chances of impairment. Intermediate values of 21 to 25 are less helpful in making the diagnosis. Interpretation of this score must include assessment of possible factors that may affect the patient's performance, such as level of consciousness, formal education, and English language comprehension (20).

Affective Assessment

At any time, from 1 percent to 3 percent of community-dwelling elderly have major depression, but more than 10 percent of older persons in the community have important symptoms of depression that cause them to have difficulty performing their daily routines. Depressive symptoms are associated with increased morbidity and mortality. Because many depressed patients respond to pharmacotherapy, psychotherapy, or both, it is important to identify depressed elders and prescribe adequate treatment.

"Do you often feel sad or depressed?" is one validated screening question for depression among the elderly (21). A second validated question used for screening for depression is an item from the Mental Health Inventory: "How much of the time, during the last month, have you felt downhearted and blue?" Persons who answered "a good bit of the time," "most of the time," or "all of the time" when given five response choices were at increased risk for major depression (22). A third validated method for screening for depression consists of two questions. The first is: "In the past year, have you had two weeks or more during which you felt sad, blue, or depressed, or when you lost all interest and pleasure in things that you usually cared about or enjoyed?" The second question has

two parts: "Have you had two years or more in your life when you felt depressed or sad most days, even if you felt okay sometimes?" If the respondent answers "yes" to this question, he is asked: "Have you felt depressed or sad much of the time in the past year?" (23)

A longer screen is the short form Geriatric Depression Scale (24,25) (see Appendix). This is a self-administered series of 15 questions that takes five minutes to complete. Persons who score more than 5 are at risk for major depression.

Assessment of Function

Assessing functional limitations in the elderly can be useful for detecting disease and dysfunction, selecting appropriate treatments or other interventions, and evaluating the effects of these interventions. Three levels of function are commonly evaluated in older persons: basic activities of daily living (BADLs), instrumental or intermediate activities of daily living (IADLs), and advanced activities of daily living (AADLs).

National community-based surveys report 2 percent to 8 percent of the elderly population have impairments in BADLs. These include abilities the patient needs to provide basic self-care (e.g., bathing, dressing, toileting, continence, feeding, and transferring) (26).

As many as 25 percent of community-dwelling elderly have at least one disability of IADLs. These include abilities the patient needs to live independently (e.g., shopping for groceries, driving or using public transportation, using the telephone, preparing meals, doing housework, doing handyman work, doing laundry, taking medications, and handling finances) (27).

AADLs include physical and social activities that tend to be voluntary and whose loss may indicate early functional decline (28). Social AADLs include participation in social activites, traveling, being employed, or going to a movie. Physical AADLs include recreational exercise and gardening. Because AADLs are usually voluntary, they are more specific to the individual than are BADLs and IADLs (e.g., one older person prefers golf, another prefers tennis). In addition, the significance of a change in AADLs may be very different from a change in lower levels of functioning. Rarely does a change in AADL function precipitate a change in living situation. Nevertheless, asking about AADL functions may be an excellent way to monitor the function of healthy older persons. Depending on the specific activity measured, from 10 percent to 70 percent of community-dwelling elderly persons have difficulty participating in the advanced social and physical activities.

Brief scales have been developed to assess persons' functional capabilities. Ability to perform self-care activities may be assessed by the Katz Index of Independence in Activities of Daily Living (29) (see Appendix). Using this scale, an examiner rates an individual's ability to perform the six Katz ADLs either independently, or with assistance. In a similar fashion, using the Older Americans Resource and Services (OARS) Multidimensional Function Assessment Questionnaire, an examiner can rate an individual's ability to perform five instrumental activities of daily living, such as getting to places out of walking distance, shopping, preparing meals, doing housework, and handling money (30) (see Appendix).

Function can be more comprehensively evaluated by the Functional Status Questionnaire, a self-administered questionnaire that comprehensively evaluates physical, psychological, social, and role function (31). Another instrument is the COOP Chart method, a set of cartoon-like drawings of persons depicting different levels of physical, emotional, social, and other dimensions of functioning (32). Both these measures have been used in clinical settings to provide physicians with reports of their patients' functioning.

Assessment of Social Support

When older persons become progressively frail, the need for social support becomes more important. The availability of assistance from family and friends is frequently the determining factor for whether a functionally dependent older person remains at home or is institutionalized. Even with healthy older persons, it is often valuable to raise the question of who would be available to help if the patient became ill; early identification of problems with social support may prompt planning to develop resources should the necessity arise.

Economic Assessment

Economic assessment also becomes more important for functionally impaired persons who may qualify for state or local benefits, depending on income, or may need to plan to draw upon their financial reserves in a strategic manner.

Environmental Assessment

Physicians rarely personally conduct environmental assessments; however, community agencies such as visiting nurses are available to inspect homes for safety and can recommend installation of adaptive devices (e.g., shower bars, raised toilet seats). Persons who are at risk for becoming dependent in IADLs should be evaluated for the geographic proximity of necessary services (e.g., grocery shopping, banking), their need for use of such services, and their ability to use these services in their current living situations.

Advance Directives

Finally, a key component of geriatric assessment is the evaluation of the patient's wishes for care. These preferences are essential in determining a management plan. Specific advance directives are invaluable in guiding therapy if a patient is unable to speak for him or herself at a future time. The Durable Power of Attorney for Health Care, which asks the patient to designate a surrogate to make medical decisions if the patient loses decision-making capacity, is often less emotionally laden than specifying treatments that the patient may or may not want. Nevertheless, particularly for patients with early dementia, it is valuable to begin discussions about preferences for specific treatments while the patient still has the cognitive capacity to make these decisions.

Effectiveness of Geriatric Assessment by the Individual Practitioner

Many medical organizations advocate screening and assessing common geriatric conditions by primary care clinicians (33–35). Yet, the effectiveness of geriatric assessment provided by an individual physician in improving or maintaining older persons' function has not been studied. Future research should clarify whether systematic screening for problems in the multiple domains of geriatric assessment leads to identification of more treatable problems, changes patient management, and improves health outcomes. In addition, standard, brief, multidimensional screens that are useful in busy clinical settings are likely to be developed and validated.

Comprehensive Geriatric Assessment

The 1987 National Institutes of Health Consensus Development Conference defined comprehensive geriatric assessment (CGA) as being "a multidisciplinary evaluation in which the multiple problems of older persons are uncovered, described, and explained, if possible, and in which the resources and strengths of the person are catalogued, need for services assessed, and a coordinated care plan developed to focus interventions on the person's problems."

Conceptually, comprehensive geriatric assessment is a three-step process: 1) screening or targeting of appropriate patients, 2) assessment and development of recommendations, and 3) implementation of recommendations, including physician and patient adherence with recommendations. Each of these steps is essential if the process is to be successful in achieving health and functional benefits.

Within this broad conceptualization, CGA has been implemented using many different models. Some of the earliest and most successful CGA programs have used hospital-based units. However, because of changes in length of hospital stays, an increasing number of CGA programs are relying on postdischarge and community-based assessment. Furthermore, most of the early programs focused on restorative or rehabilitiative goals (tertiary prevention), whereas many newer programs are aimed at primary and secondary prevention. Therefore, making each step of the CGA operational differs according to the population being assessed, the setting for the intervention, and the goals of the assessment. For example, community-based assessment programs that are geared toward primary and secondary prevention may have very broad targeting criteria, but entry into a geriatric rehabilitation unit may require very strict criteria to restrict the use of expensive resources to those who are most likely to benefit from the intervention.

Comprehensive geriatric assessment programs have been established in acute care and rehabilitation hospitals, nursing homes, adult day hospitals, and in community-based ambulatory settings. Even within settings, different types of assessment programs have been developed. For example, acute care hospitals may offer CGA as a consultative service, as a consultative service with limited order-writing capabilities (e.g., for diagnostic tests or rehabilitative services), or as a geographically distinct geriatric evaluation and management unit that has a separate nursing staff.

To identify older persons who are most appropriate for CGA, programs have used various targeting strategies, such as chronological age, functional impairment, physical illness, geriatric conditions, and psychosocial conditions. Of these, the best supported by clinical trials have been functional impairment and geriatric conditions. However, definitions of functional impairment and the types of geriatric conditions used to target patients have varied from study to study. To date, no easily administered targeting criteria have been demonstrated to reliably identify patients who are likely to benefit from CGA in a variety of settings and institutions.

Similarly, the assessment process itself has yet to be defined in a standardized, generalizable form. The types of health care professionals comprising the assessment team, the content of information collected, and the types and intensity of services provided have differed among studies of the effectiveness of CGA. For example, ambulatory geriatric assessment teams are most commonly staffed by a physician, a nurse or social worker, and one additional member. In contrast, in hospital settings the teams are generally larger (36). In many settings, the CGA process relies on a core team consisting of a physician, nurse, and social worker and, when appropriate, draws upon an extended team of physical and occupational therapists, a nutritionist, pharmacist, psychiatrist, psychologist, dentist, audiologist, podiatrist, and optician. Although these professionals are usually on staff in hospital settings and are available in the community, access to and reimbursement for these services have limited the effectiveness of the CGA process. Frequently, the composition of the team is determined on the basis of local expertise and availability of resources rather than on programmatic needs.

In CGA, the various components of the evaluation are completed by different members of the team. For example, medical assessment of older persons may be done solely by a physician, nurse practitioner, or physician's assistant. However, additional professionals may be needed to provide more in-depth evaluations of specific aspects of the medical evaluation. For example, a dietitian may be needed to assess dietary intake and provide recommendations; an audiologist may need to conduct a more extensive assessment of hearing loss and fit an older person for a hearing aid. The input of these health professionals is particularly important when additional therapy (e.g., physical, occupational, speech) is needed in addition to a detailed diagnostic evaluation.

Effectiveness of Comprehensive Geriatric Assessment

Research is only beginning to look inside the "black box" of the intervention provided by CGA. Several studies have demonstrated that merely identifying geriatric problems is insufficient to change primary care physician behavior and improve major patient outcomes. The issue may be particularly important in ambulatory-based CGA programs in which patient adherence with recommendations is particularly important. If CGA is to be conducted on a consultative basis rather than by the team assuming primary care of the patient, successful implementation of CGA recommendations requires adherence at two levels, that of the primary care physician and that of the patient.

Studies of CGA have demonstrated significant benefits of the process, including improvements in diagnostic accuracy, placement, functional status, affect and cognition, use of home health care services, and survival. Reductions in medications, use of hospital services, nursing home days, and medical care costs have also been documented. However, each of these benefits has not been demonstrated in every study.

A recent meta-analysis has summarized data from 28 controlled trials of five models of comprehensive geriatric assessment: 1) geriatric evaluation and management units (GEMU), 2) inpatient geriatric consultation services, 3) home assessment services, 4) hospital home assessment services (i.e., in-home CGA for patients recently discharged from the hospital), and 5) outpatient assessment services (37). Although mortality was reduced overall, this benefit was not significantly demonstrated for outpatient geriatric assessment services or hospital home assessment services. Similarly, in this meta-analysis, other

benefits varied depending on the model used. Only the geriatric evaluation and management unit model demonstrated improvement in functional status, although several individual trials of outpatient and hospital home assessment have demonstrated benefit in IADL function. The GEMU model and the hospital home assessment service models were associated with increased likelihood of living at home at one year. When examining the process of care, CGA programs that had medical control over CGA recommendations or those that provided ambulatory follow-up were associated with reduced mortality. In summary, the most persuasive evidence for CGA, to date, comes from intensive and expensive versions of the process such as specialized geriatric assessment and rehabilitation units that have assumed direct control of patient care.

Conclusion

Geriatric assessment is a comprehensive approach to diagnosing and managing the complex medical and psychosocial problems of frail, elderly persons. The key underlying principles of this approach are the multidimensionality of the assessment and the goals of improving functional capabilities and overall health status. Although assessment by individual practitioners and by multidisciplinary teams are conceptually identical, they differ markedly in the resources needed to provide the assessment, in linkages to therapy on the basis of recommendations from the assessment process, and possibly with respect to benefits. The clinical usefulness of geriatric assessment depends on well-trained health care professionals, effective screening and assessment instruments, targeting appropriate patients for CGA, synthesis of information derived from the assessment to develop a suitable management strategy, and implementation of the plan. As advances are made in these areas, the effectiveness of geriatric assessment should also improve and is likely to enhance the well-being of older persons.

References

1. Mangione CM, Phillips RS, Seddon JM, et al. Development of the "Activities of Daily Vision Scale": a measure of visual functional status. Med Care 1992;30:1111–1126.

2. Mulrow CD, Aguilar C, Endicott JE, et al. Association between hearing impairment and the quality of life of elderly individuals. J Am Geriatr Soc 1990;38:45–50.

3. Ventry IM, Weinstein BE. Identification of elderly people with hearing problems. ASHA 1983;25:37–42.

4. Lichtenstein MJ, Bess FH, Logan SA. Validation of screening tools for identifying hearing-impaired elderly in primary care. JAMA 1988;259:2875–2878.

5. National Center for Health Statistics. National Health and Nutrition Examination Survey I Epidemiologic Followup Study, 1982–1984. Vital and Health Statistics, Series 1, No. 22. Hyattsville, MD: National Center for Health Statistics, 1987. DHHS publication no. (PHS) 87–1324.

6. Andres R, Elahi D, Tobin JD, et al. Impact of age on weight goals. Ann Intern Med 1985;103:1030–1033.

7. Lipschitz DA, Ham RJ, White JV. An approach to nutrition screening for older Americans. Am Fam Physician 1992;45:601–608.

8. Smallegan M. There was nothing else to do: needs for care before nursing home admission. Gerontologist 1985;25:364–369.

9. Diokno AC, Brock BM, Brown MR, Herzog AR. Prevalence of urinary incontinence and other urological symptoms in the noninstitutionalized elderly. J Urol 1986;136:1022–1025.

10. Diokno AC, Brown MR, Brock BM, et al. Clinical and cystometric characteristics of continent and incontinent noninstitutionalized elderly. J Urol 1988;140:567–571.

11. Cummings SR, Nevitt MC, Kidd S. Forgetting falls: the limited accuracy of recall of falls in the elderly. J Am Geriatr Soc 1988;36:613–616.

12. Podsiadlo D, Richardson S. The timed "Up & Go": a test of basic functional mobility for frail elderly persons. J Am Geriatr Soc 1991;39:142–148.

13. Tinetti ME. Performance-oriented assessment of mobility problems in elderly patients. J Am Geriatr Soc 1986;34:119–126.

14. Duncan PW, Weiner DK, Chandler, et al. Functional reach: a new clinical measure of balance. J Gerontol 1990;45:M192–M197.

15. Duncan PW, Studenski S, Chandler J, Prescott B. Functional reach: predictive validity in sample of elderly male veterans. J Gerontol 1992;47:M93–M98.

16. Siu AL. Screening for dementia and investigating its causes. Ann Intern Med 1991;115:122–132.

17. Folstein MF, Folstein SE, McHugh PR. "Mini-Mental State": a practical method for grading the cognitive state of patients for the clinician. J Psychiatr Res 1975;12:189–198.

18. Wolf-Klein GP, Silverstone FA, Levy AP, et al. Screening for Alzheimer's disease by clock drawing. J Am Geriatr Soc 1989;37:730–734.

19. Klein LE, Roca RP, McArthur J, et al. Diagnosing dementia. J Am Geriatr Soc 1985;33:483–488.

20. Tombaugh TN, McIntyre NJ. The Mini-Mental State Examination: a comprehensive review. J Am Geriatr Soc 1992;40:922–935.

21. Abler R, Drinka T, Mahoney J, et al. Depression in patients of a geriatric medicine clinic: comparison of two screening instruments. Gerontologist 1991;31:325.

22. Berwick DM, Murphy JM, Goldman PA, et al. Performance of a five-item mental health screening test. Med Care 1991;29:169–176.

23. Rost K, Burnam MA, Smith GR. Development of screeners for depressive disorders and substance disorder history. Med Care 1993;31:189–200.

24. Yesavage JA, Brink TL, Rose TL, et al. Development and validation of a geriatric depression rating scale: a preliminary report. J Psych Res 1983;17:27.

25. Sheikh JI, Yesavage JA. Geriatric Depression Scale: recent evidence and development of a shorter version. Clin Gerontol 1986;5:165–172.

26. Katz S, Ford AB, Moskowitz RW, et al. Studies of illness in the aged. The index of ADL: a standardized measure of biological and psychosocial function. JAMA 1963;185:914–919.

27. Lawton MP, Brody EM. Assessment of older people: self-maintaining and instrumental activities of daily living. Gerontologist 1969;9:179–185.

28. Reuben DB, Solomon DH. Assessment in geriatrics, of caveats and names. J Am Geriatr Soc 1989;37:570–572.

29. Katz S, Downs TD, Cash HR, et al. Progress in the development of the index of ADL. J Gerontol 1970;10:20–30.

30. Fillenbaum GG. Screening the elderly: a brief instrumental activities of daily living measure. J Am Geriatr Soc 1985;33:698–706.

31. Jette AM, Davies AR, Cleary PD, et al. The Functional Status Questionnaire: reliability and validity when used in primary care. J Gen Intern Med 1986;1:143–149.

32. Nelson EC, Landgraf JM, Hays RD, et al. The functional status of patients. How can it be measured in physicians' offices? Med Care 1990;28:1111–1126.

33. Lachs MS, Feinstein AR, Cooney LM, et al. A simple procedure for general screening for functional disability in elderly patients. Ann Intern Med 1990;112:699–706.

34. Almy TP. Comprehensive functional assessment for elderly patients. Ann Intern Med 1988;109:70–72.

35. Rubenstein LV, Calkins DR, Greenfield S, et al. Health status assessment for elderly persons. Report of the Society of General Internal Medicine Task Force on Health Assessment. J Am Geriatr Soc 1989;37:562–569.

36. Epstein AM, Hall JA, Besdine R, et al. The emergence of geriatric assessment units. Ann Intern Med 1987;106:299–303.

37. Stuck AE, Siu AL, Wieland GD, et al. Comprehensive Geriatric Assessment: a meta-analysis of controlled trials. Lancet 1993;342:1032–1036.

Chapter 7
Drug Use in the Elderly

John G. Gerber and Alan S. Hollister

One of the first duties of the physician is to educate the masses not to take medicine.

William Osler

Elderly persons use more drugs—both prescription and over-the-counter medications—per capita than do younger patients. Certainly, part of this greater drug use is related to the increased comorbidity of the elderly with both chronic and acute illnesses. In part because of increased drug use, aged patients have three to seven times as many adverse drug reactions as patients in the 20- to 29-year-old age group (1). In addition, because aging is associated with declining physiologic processes, once adverse drug reactions occur, the elderly patient's ability to compensate and recover from them may be also impaired (2). For these reasons, the practitioner must be aware of how to use drugs safely and efficaciously and, equally important, when to use drugs in the elderly. Because of altered physiological functions that occur with aging, elderly patients respond differently to certain groups of drugs than do younger patients. This chapter reviews the effect of aging on absorption, distribution, excretion and end-organ responsiveness of drugs. In addition to understanding of the effect of aging on pharmacokinetic parameters, one must realize that disease processes themselves may alter the way the body handles drugs. Overall, there is a large variability across a population group in the way a drug is processed by the body. Therefore, individualization of drug therapy remains the ideal method of approach.

Drug Absorption and Bioavailability in the Elderly

By far, most drugs in clinical use are administered orally. Before these drugs reach the systemic circulation, they are in contact with the stomach, the small intestine (in which most of the absorption takes place), and the liver, by way of portal circulation. Drugs that are rapidly and extensively metabolized by the liver are extracted to a large extent during their first pass through the liver via the portal vein, which thereby reduces the drug's systemic bioavailability. Once the drug reaches the systemic circulation, it can interact with key cellular components to exert a pharmacologic effect.

With aging, the gastrointestinal tract undergoes both physiologic and anatomic changes that potentially affect drug absorption. Nonetheless, studies have not demonstrated that these gastrointestinal changes affect drug absorption for the majority of the drugs used by the elderly (3). However, not all drugs have been evaluated in this regard. Gastric acid production decreases with aging, but gastric motility does not. With aging, there is about a 30 percent decrease in mucosal absorptive surface in the small bowel, as well as a decrease in gastrointestinal motility. In addition, there is about a 40 percent reduction in small intestinal blood flow. Evidence suggests diminished absorption through the active transport systems involved with galactose, calcium, thiamine, and iron absorption in the elderly, but most drugs are passively absorbed; for these drugs, the aging gut is not an obstacle (4). Rather, diseases associated with aging or the concomitant administration of several drugs may contribute to abnormal drug absorption in the elderly patient. Antacids can decrease the absorption of chlorpromazine, tetracycline, cimetidine, isoniazid, D-penicillamine, and some of the azole antifungals; cholestyramine can bind and decrease the absorption of phenobarbital, warfarin, thiazides, thyroxine, digitalis glycosides, aspirin, acetaminophen, and penicillin. Drugs with anticholinergic effects can decrease motility and delay the absorption of many drugs (5). Although these drug interactions can occur in patients of all ages, the likelihood of the use of multiple drugs is greater in the elderly.

The liver stands between drugs in the portal blood and the systemic circulation. Drugs that have high hepatic clearance (i.e., the extraction ratio in each pass through the liver is greater than 30 to 40 percent) are extensively metabolized by the liver during their first pass after absorption, thus reducing the drugs' systemic bioavailability. Aging has been reported to decrease the metabolic capacity of the liver. For orally administered, high-hepatic-clearance drugs, the first-pass elimination is therefore reduced in the elderly, and consequently, the amount of drug reaching the systemic circulation is expected to increase. Increased bioavailability has been described in the elderly for the β-adrenoceptor blocker, propranolol, and for the active enantiomer of verapamil (6). However, the variability in the hepatic extraction ratio for both drugs across a population group was of such magnitude that both the elderly and young patients had overlapping values. These observations again stress the importance of individualization of drug therapy because the genetic and environmental influences on hepatic metabolism of drugs produce a greater variation across a population than does the effect of aging itself.

Drug Distribution in the Elderly

Once a drug reaches the systemic circulation, it is distributed throughout body fluids and tissues. Drug distribution is determined mainly by body composition and plasma protein binding. The body composition is altered by aging so that the total body water both in absolute terms and in percent of body weight is reduced by as much as 15 percent between the ages of 20 years and 80 years. Lean body mass is decreased, but there is a marked increase in total body fat with age. The increase in total body fat is relatively greater in men than it is in women (7).

In addition to alterations in body composition, plasma protein binding of drugs may be different in the young compared with the elderly. Because the free drug concentration in the blood determines the ability of the drug to reach its site of action, alterations in protein binding can significantly affect drug action for a given total drug concentration. Plasma concentration of albumin tends to decrease with aging, which is probably secondary to a decrease in albumin production by the liver (8). Decrease in albumin concentration may be responsible for the decrease in the plasma protein-binding capacity of acidic drugs like phenytoin, phenylbutazone, and warfarin. However, many basic drugs such as lidocaine and propranolol bind mainly to α_1 acid glycoproteins, the concentration of which may increase with aging and with acute or chronic inflammatory diseases (9). Drugs such as meperidine can also bind to erythrocytes with very high affinity. Aging appears to reduce the binding capacity to red blood cells, and meperidine binding has been demonstrated to decrease in aged patients.

With known alterations in body composition and in protein binding with aging, how the volume of distribution of drugs will be altered in the elderly can be predicted. The volume of distribution is simply the ratio of the mass of the drug in the body divided by its concentration in the blood. Thus, the higher the volume of distribution of the drug, the lower the proportion of the drug found in the intravascular compartment. The volume of distribution of any drug is determined by the relative affinity of the drug for the tissues versus its affinity for the blood. If a drug has a very high affinity for blood components but a low affinity for tissue components, the volume of distribution is small. Alternatively, if the drug has a very high affinity for tissue components but a poor affinity for blood components, the volume of distribution is greater because the drug preferentially partitions into tissue spaces. This knowledge enables certain predictions about the volume of distribution when the body composition is altered, as in the aged.

Since total tissue water content is decreased in the aged, one would predict that the volume of distribution of drugs that distribute mainly into body water would be smaller in the elderly, if plasma protein binding is not altered. Antipyrine is a model drug that distributes into water spaces and remains essentially unbound in the plasma. Indeed, the volume of distribution of antipyrine has been reported to be reduced in the elderly (10). Ethanol also distributes into water spaces, and the volume of distribution of ethanol is reduced in the elderly. For a drug such as diazepam, which is very lipophilic, the volume of distribution is increased in the elderly, presumably because of the increased total body fat content, because diazepam plasma protein binding is unaltered (11).

For a drug such as digoxin, in which the large volume of distribution is secondary to the extensive tissue binding of the drug (primarily to muscle Na^+/K^+ ATPases), the decreased muscle mass in the elderly is associated with a decreased volume of distribution of digoxin.

How do changes in volume of distribution affect therapeutic use of drugs? Volume of distribution is one of the two determinants of the half-life of a drug. An increase in the volume of distribution produces a longer half-life, and a decrease in the volume of distribution produces a shorter half-life. This relationship is given quantitatively as (Vd = volume of distribution; $t_{\frac{1}{2}}$ = drug half-life)

$$t_{\frac{1}{2}} = \frac{0.693 \times Vd}{\text{plasma clearance}}$$

Thus, alterations in the volume of distribution influence the dosage intervals of drugs used in chronic therapy. The larger the volume of distribution, the less frequently the drug has to be administered because the plasma concentration of the drug decays more slowly. However, because both the clearance and the effects of drugs are usually related to the free drug concentration, the steady-state effects of a maintenance dosage regimen should not be altered by the volume of distribution alone. Steady-state is present when the amount of drug reaching the systemic circulation per unit of time equals the amount of drug eliminated per unit of time. At steady-state, only two variables determine the plasma level of the drug achieved: the amount of drug reaching the systemic circulation and the blood clearance of the drug. The volume of distribution, therefore, can be considered as a reservoir for drugs in the body. The blood concentration of the drug is in equilibrium with the tissue concentration of the drug. If the tissue reservoir for the drug is very large (large Vd), the rate of fall of the blood concentration of the drug will be slow, even if the clearance of the drug is high. In the absence of a loading dose, it may take a considerable length of time to reach a steady-state blood concentration if the drug's Vd is large, because a large reservoir for drug has to be filled. The partitioning of drug into this reservoir delays the time to reach steady-state. Because the drug that is partitioned into tissues and extravascular fluid spaces is not available for metabolism or excretion, the drug does not play a role in determining the blood concentration at steady-state, but it does determine the length of time necessary to reach steady-state concentration.

This principle is very important to understanding of pharmacokinetics in the elderly, in disease states, or in simple drug interactions. If the steady-state blood concentration of one drug at a fixed dosage is altered by a disease state or by another drug, the alteration must have occurred because of a change in either the bioavailability or the plasma clearance of the drug. For example, warfarin's effect on clotting factor synthesis is enhanced by the concurrent administration of the nonsteroidal anti-inflammatory drug, phenylbutazone. Phenylbutazone was found to interfere with warfarin metabolism, which caused a decrease in the clearance of warfarin (12).

Alterations in drug binding to plasma proteins alter the drug's volume of distribution and the amount of free (unbound) drug in the plasma at any total plasma drug concentration. By decreasing the fractional protein binding (that is, drug bound as a percentage of total drug in plasma) of a drug, the amount of free drug available to interact with its receptor is increased at an equivalent total drug concentration. Thus, interpretation of a total drug level under conditions of altered protein binding has to be reappraised. This concept is well understood in interpreting plasma phenytoin levels in uremia. Although the decrease in protein binding in the elderly for phenytoin is not as dramatic as it is in uremia, the decrease could potentially result in excessive drug response at an apparent therapeutic total drug concentration (13).

Because the free drug interacts with a receptor, and the free drug is available for metabolism, alterations in protein binding itself does not change the drug dosage in the elderly, unless free drug clearance is also affected. Thus, an important pharmacokinetic impact that changes in protein binding may have is the interpretation of total plasma concentrations during therapeutic drug monitoring. A total plasma phenytoin level of 20μg/ml does not have the same implication when only 80 percent of the drug is bound to albumin instead of the normal binding of 90 percent.

The Effect of Aging on Renal Elimination of Drugs

There are numerous drugs in which the major mode of elimination is through the kidneys. Some of the more important ones that are used frequently in the elderly population are digoxin, procainamide, the amino-glycoside antibiotics, penicillin, thiazide diuretics, clonidine, and the beta-adrenergic blockers, atenolol and nadolol. Renal function deteriorates with age; the glomerular filtration rate at age 70 is about 60 percent of that at age 20. In addition, renal blood flow is decreased by 40 percent in the elderly, and maximal sodium and water conservation is also impaired (14). Because aging is associated with a decrease in muscle mass (the source of creatinine), using plasma creatinine alone as a measure of renal function can be very deceptive. A plasma creatinine of 1 mg per 100 ml in a 70-year-old person does not indicate the same glomerular filtration rate as does a plasma creatinine of 1 mg per 100 ml in a 20-year-old person. Thus, one should never base the dosage of a renally excreted drug on plasma creatinine alone. Whenever possible, an endogenous creatinine clearance should be determined to estimate the glomerular filtration rate. If that is not practical, the practitioner should assume that, in the elderly, there is a 40 percent reduction in renal function if the serum creatinine concentration is normal, and thefore start a medication eliminated by renal excretion at a reduced dosage.

For drugs such as digoxin, procainamide, and the aminoglycosides, blood concentrations can be followed to assess the appropriateness of the dosing regimen. For the thiazide diuretics and clonidine, evaluating clinical response is the best way to follow the efficacy of these drugs. Interestingly, since the tubular transport system in the kidneys is diminished with aging, drugs such as furosemide that reach the active tubular site by way of the organic acid transport mechanism in the kidneys require higher dosage in the elderly to achieve the same intratubular concentration and, therefore, an equivalent diuresis to that in younger patients.

A number of dosage guidelines and nomograms have been developed on the basis of endogenous creatinine clearance (15). Because the variability of normal renal function independent of age is small and the effect of aging on this function is predictable, rational guidelines for therapy can be established for renally excreted drugs.

The Effect of Age on Hepatic Clearance of Drugs

Unfortunately, the variability of hepatic metabolism of drugs within a population is so large that simple predictions about alterations in dosage requirements with aging are impossible to make. Hepatic clearance of drugs is determined by both the intrinsic ability of the liver to metabolize a drug and the blood flow to the liver. The relative contributions of these two physiologic variables to the hepatic clearance of the drug is specific for each drug. For drugs that are avidly metabolized by the liver (i.e., the liver has a large capacity to metabolize the drugs), the hepatic blood flow is the main determinant of the liver clearance. Propranolol, lidocaine, and many of the tricyclic antidepressant drugs belong to this class. These drugs have high hepatic clearance and high hepatic extraction, and the extent of their metabolism is perfusion limited. In the case of drugs for which the liver has a limited metabolizing capacity, the intrinsic enzymatic activity within the liver determines the hepatic clearance. Warfarin, theophylline, some benzodiazepines, and the barbiturates belong to this class. These drugs have low hepatic clearance, and the extent of their metabolism is perfusion independent. Most other drugs belong somewhere between these two extremes, in which both the enzymatic activity and hepatic blood flow contribute to the determination of their hepatic clearance (Table 7.1).

Hepatic drug metabolism occurs primarily by way of two enzyme systems. Phase I reactions carried out by the microsomal mixed function oxidase systems result in a polar molecule from the parent compound that is frequently pharmacologically still active. Phase II metabolism results in conjugation of the molecule by glucuronidation, sulfation, or acetylation. Conjugated molecules are usually pharmacologically inactive and are eliminated by the kidneys or by the biliary system. It has been suggested that aging decreases phase I reactions. However, this effect is probably unrelated to any decrease in the enzymatic activity in the hepatocytes but, more likely, is secondary to the decrease in liver size associated

Table 7.1. Major Mode of Excretion of Commonly Used Drugs.

Hepatic Excretion			Renal Excretion	
High Clearance (>500 ml/min/70 kg)	Intermediate (100–500 ml/min/70 kg)	Low Clearance (<100 ml/min/70 kg)		
Amitriptyline	Acetaminophen	Carbamazepine	Acecainide	Hydrochlorothiazide
Chlorpromazine	Chloramphenicol	Chlordiazepoxide	Acyclovir	Imipenem
Diltiazem	Erythromycin	Diazepam	Aminoglycosides	Lithium
Doxepin	Prazosin	Digitoxin	Amoxicillin	Methicillin
Hydralazine	Quinidine	Ibuprofen	Ampicillin	Methotrexate
Imipramine		Indomethacin	Atenolol	Nadolol
Lidocaine		Itraconazole	Captopril	Penicillin
Meperidine		Phenobarbital	Cefazolin	Piperacillin
Metoprolol		Phenylbutazone	Cephalexin	Procainamide
Nifedipine		Salicylic acid	Chlorothiazide	Vancomycin
Nortriptyline		(concentration-dependent)	Cimetidine	
Propranolol		Theophylline	Clonidine	
Triazolam		Tolbutamide	Digoxin	
Verapamil		Valproic acid	Disopyramide	
		Warfarin	Fluconazole	
			Fluoroquinolones	
			Foscarnet	
			Furosemide	

with aging and, therefore, to a decrease in the total numbers of hepatocytes (16). Phase II conjugation reactions have not been demonstrated to be affected by aging. However, in practical terms, the liver metabolism of a low clearance prototype drug, antipyrine (which is metabolized by the phase I reaction), was not different in the young or the old population. Although the mean hepatic clearance was lower in the elderly, such overlap existed between the two population groups that meaningful population differences could not be demonstrated (17).

As noted earlier the liver blood flow plays a critical role determining the rate of metabolism of drugs with very high clearances. Liver blood flow is significantly reduced in the elderly as compared with that of the younger population. This suggests that the hepatic clearance of high-clearance drugs is reduced in the elderly; this difference has been demonstrated for intravenously administered propranolol (18). In addition, the disposition of orally administered high-clearance drugs is complex. Because these drugs undergo significant first-pass liver metabolism, alterations in liver blood flow affect the amount of drug reaching the systemic circulation. Thus, even though the systemic metabolism of these drugs is expected to be

lower in the elderly because of diminished hepatic blood flow, the systemic drug load is also expected to be lower. In addition, there is a large variability caused by genetic and environmental factors in the hepatic extraction of drugs by way of the first pass; thus, age is a relatively small component of any pharmacokinetic differences observed across a study population.

In summary, for drugs undergoing hepatic metabolism, individualization of drug therapy is of utmost importance. For drugs such as β-adrenergic blocking agents that have high therapeutic indexes, close clinical monitoring is not as important as it is for drugs such as lidocaine or warfarin, in which therapeutic monitoring is essential to avoid untoward side effects.

The Effect of Aging on End-Organ Responsiveness to Drugs

Excessive drug response in the elderly can be a result of pharmacokinetic alterations resulting in excessive blood levels of the drug or of increased sensitivity of the body to the drug. A change in end-organ responsiveness can result from alterations in receptor number or affinity, changes in the enzymes that eventually translate the effect of the drug, or structural changes in the end organ so that the organ cannot respond fully. Actual changes in end-organ responses in the elderly have been described for only a few drugs. Elderly subjects have a quantitatively lower increase in heart rate to intravenous boluses of isoproterenol (19). This effect does not seem to be secondary to alterations in the β-adrenergic receptor numbers or affinity in the elderly, but is likely caused by postreceptor mechanism. Elderly persons also have an enhanced orthostatic response to antihypertensive agents. Aging is associated with a reduced baroreceptor response to hypotension as well as a reduction in peripheral venous tone. The enhanced orthostatic hypotension to sympatholytic drugs in the elderly is an example of excessive effect as a consequence of changes in tissue responsiveness associated with aging. Elderly patients have been described to have a reduced rate of synthesis of clotting factors compared to that of a young population at an equivalent plasma concentration of free warfarin. Whether this increased sensitivity was secondary to altered vitamin K availability in the elderly or to a depressed ability to synthesize clotting factors was not elucidated. Nonetheless, investigators have reported that, in general, elderly patients require much less warfarin to achieve anticoagulation than does the younger population (20).

Elderly patients also seem to respond excessively to psychotropic drugs. One report examined psychomotor performance in elderly and younger subjects after they received 10 mg of the benzodiazepine, nitrazepam. There were no pharmacokinetic differences between the two groups, but the elderly had significantly greater impairment of psychomotor performance as compared with that of the younger volunteers (21). Elderly patients also frequently have paradoxical agitation to barbiturates. The etiology of this unusual response is unknown, but routine use of barbiturates and sedative hypnotic agents is discouraged in the elderly. These are some important examples of altered end-organ responsiveness in the elderly. This is a fertile, but still unexplored, territory in gerontology, and urgently needs more work.

Effect of Aging on the Use of Specific Drugs

The large number of drugs currently available for use and the explosion of interest in geriatric clinical pharmacology in recent years makes an exhaustive review of all drugs used in the elderly far beyond the scope of this chapter. The following discussion attempts to illustrate briefly the aforementioned principles and to note the effects of some commonly used agents in elderly patients. The pharmacokinetic and pharmacodynamic changes observed during the use of these agents in the elderly are summarized in Tables 7.2 and 7.3.

Anticoagulants
Coumarin anticoagulants such as warfarin are strongly protein bound and metabolized by the liver. The dosage of anticoagulant must be individualized with use of the prothrombin time or international normalized ratio (INR) to avoid complications from overanticoagulation or underanticoagulation. Most data suggest that the coumarin dose required for proper anticoagulation is lower in an elderly population as compared with that for young patients (20), apparently because of an increased sensitivity of the liver to inhibition of clotting factor synthesis at any plasma total warfarin concentration in elderly patients. No dramatic pharmacokinetic changes with aging have been described for warfarin.

Drug interactions with warfarin are common and may have catastrophic effects (12). Interactions may result from changes in warfarin absorption, protein binding, or metabolism. Pharmacodynamic interactions may result from administration of other drugs that alter hemostasis or by dietary changes in vitamin K availability. In the geriatric patient population, frequent changes in medications (with or without notification of the physician) and the use of treatments such as influenza vaccine that may alter warfarin action or kinetics mandate great caution and frequent reassessment of the patient during the administration of warfarin.

Antihypertensive Drugs
Aging is associated with an abnormal baroreceptor response to hypotension as well as a reduction in peripheral venous tone (22,23). Thus, it is not unusual to observe some asymptomatic orthostatic hypotension in elderly persons who take no medication (see Chapter 36). The use of drugs such as clonidine and methyldopa, that further interfere with sympathetic function may result in severe orthostatic hypotension in this population.

Table 7.2. Alterations with Aging in the Pharmacokinetics of Drugs.

Drug	Vd*	t½*	Cl*	Mechanism	Recommendation
Acetaminophen	D	U	D	Unknown	No dose adjustment
Amantadine	D	I	D	Reduced renal function	Reduce dose
Aminoglycosides	U	I	D	Reduced renal function	Reduce dose or increase dosing interval
Amitriptyline, Nortriptyline, Imipramine	?	I	D		
Atenolol	U	I	D	Reduced renal function	Assess efficacy clinically
Ceftazidime	D	I	D	Less tissue penetration	
Chlordiazepoxide	I	I	D	Unknown	
Cimetidine	?	I	D	Reduced renal function	Reduce dose
Diazepam	I	I	U	Unknown	Assess efficacy clinically
Digoxin	D	I	D	Reduced renal function	Reduce dose
Disopyramide	U	I	D	Reduced renal function	Reduce dose
Furosemide	I	I	D	Reduced renal function, decreased albumin	Not major factor in clinical use
Ibuprofen	?	?	D	Unknown	
Lidocaine	I	I	D	Decreased hepatic blood flow	Reduce dose
Lithium	?	I	D	Reduced renal function	Reduce dose
Naproxen	?	?	D	Unknown	Effect is small
Phenobarbital	?	I	?	Unknown	Monitor levels
Phenylbutazone	I	U	?	Decreased albumin	
Phenytoin	I	?	I	Reduced albumin	Monitor levels, adjust dose with caution due to saturation kinetics
Prazosin	I	I	U		
Procainamide	U	I	D	Reduced renal function	Reduce dose
Propranolol	U	I	D	Decreased hepatic blood flow	Assess efficacy clinically
Quinidine	U	I	D	Decreased metabolism	Reduce dose
Ranitidine	?	I	?	Reduced renal function, increased peak	Reduced dose may be needed
Salicylate	I	I	D	Reduced renal function, decreased albumin	
Theophylline	U	I	D	Unknown	Measure drug levels
Tocainide	U	I	D	Reduced renal function	Reduce dose
Trazodone	?	I	D	Unknown	
Valproic acid	U	U	U	Decreased free drug clearance decreased protein binding	

?* = unknown; U = unchanged; I = increased; D = decreased; Vd = volume of distribution; t½ = half-life; Cl = clearance.

Table 7.3. Alterations with Aging in Pharmacodynamics of Drugs.

Drug	Alteration	Recommendation
Antihypertensive agents	Increased risk of orthostatic hypotension	Use agents cautiously
Benzodiazepines	Increased sensitivity	Use lower maintenance dose initially
β-adrenergic blockers	Decreased β-adrenergic responsiveness	Monitor efficacy/action clinically
Coumarin anticoagulants	Increased sensitivity	Use lower maintenance dose initially
Diuretics	Decreased intratubular concentration, increased sensitivity to complications	Monitor electrolytes and orthostatic blood pressure

Prazosin, guanethidine, guanadrel, and labetalol may also cause significant orthostatic hypotension.

Aging is associated with decreased renin and aldosterone levels and reduced responsiveness of these systems to physiological stimuli (24). The implications of this change on antihypertensive drug use in the elderly has not been completely defined. Although elderly patients respond to angiotensin-converting enzyme inhibitors with a decrease in blood pressure, the use of agents that work independent of the renin-angiotensin system has been recommended for treatment of hypertension in the elderly (25) (see also Chapter 36).

Studies on pharmacokinetic alterations with aging in the handling of antihypertensive medications have been limited. Studies have suggested that the bioavailability of prazosin may be decreased in elderly patients. Also, the volume of distribution of prazosin is increased with aging, but the clearance is unchanged. The increased volume of distribution results in an increased half-life for prazosin in elderly patients (26). As discussed below, the use of diuretics and β-adrenergic antagonists is complicated by both pharmacodynamic and pharmacokinetic changes with aging (27). The safest way to treat elderly, hypertensive patients is to use drugs conservatively, and to routinely measure both lying and standing blood pressure. The incidence of cerebral and coronary arteriosclerosis is high in the elderly; thus, excessive hypotension can result in serious sequelae. The value of treating hypertension and isolated systolic hypertension in the elderly has been established (25), but it is prudent to apply the knowledge of the pharmacokinetic and pharmacodynamic alterations associated with aging in choosing which antihypertensive drugs and the frequency of monitoring necessary in therapeutics.

Antibiotics and Antiviral Drugs

Several antibiotics, including the penicillins, most cephalosporins, vancomycin, and the aminoglycosides are cleared primarily by the kidney; hence, their clearance decreases with aging. This is particularly important with respect to the aminoglycosides because their use is associated with a 5 percent to 10 percent incidence of nephrotoxicity (28). Serum creatinine concentration may not be a reliable indicator of creatinine clearance in the elderly because creatinine production is also decreased as a result of the lower muscle mass in this population. Serum concentrations of the aminoglycosides can be measured to adjust the dosing regimen to minimize the cumulative aminoglycoside exposure, and which may reduce the risk of toxicity. Fortunately, most of the commonly used antibiotics have a high therapeutic-toxic ratio and any pharmacokinetic alterations with aging are not associated with clinically significant changes. However, there are a few drugs in which pharmacokinetic alterations could have significant toxic ramifications. Erythromycin clearance has been described to be decreased in the elderly (29). At the same dosage schedule, elderly volunteers had a twofold higher serum concentration of this drug as compared with that in young subjects. Because the ototoxicity of erythromycin is concentration dependent, one should prescribe high-dose erythromycin with caution in the elderly population. The fluoroquinolones are mainly renally excreted; aging is associated with a decreased clearance for most of these drugs. In addition, the elderly have an increased absorption of ciprofloxacin as compared with that for young volunteers (30). Thus, without adjustments in dosages, one may expect that the side effects of fluoroquinolones will be exaggerated in the elderly.

Limited information is available on the pharmacokinetic changes of antiviral drugs in the elderly. Amantadine exhibits reductions in the volume of distribution and in clearance in the elderly, but the effect on clearance is greater, which causes a prolongation of serum half-life (31). Its analog, rimantadine, does not share these characteristics. Both acyclovir and foscarnet are eliminated by way of the kidneys; thus, declining renal function in the elderly will decrease clearance and increase plasma levels of these compounds. These changes are probably more critical for foscarnet because of its greater intrinsic toxicity and lack of cellular metabolism to achieve activity. At present, there are no data available on the effects of aging for zidovudine, didanosine, or dideoxycytidine. These drugs have to be taken up by cells and phosphorylated, which suggests that both pharmacokinetic and pharmacodynamic changes with aging should be examined.

Antiepileptic Drugs

Phenytoin elimination is characterized by saturable kinetics. The drug is also extensively protein bound, and only the free drug is available for metabolism and pharmacologic action. Age-related changes in kinetics have been examined for phenytoin (32). Protein binding of phenytoin decreases with aging because of the decrease in plasma albumin concentration. The total plasma clearance of phenytoin is increased in the elderly as compared with clearance in the younger population, but the free drug clearance may not be different in the two groups, which may reflect the alteration in protein binding. The saturation kinetics of phenytoin limit the clinical use of a detailed analysis of phenytoin clearance because elimination kinetics will change in an individual patient as the dose is changed, regardless of the patient's age (33). The plasma concentration at which phenytoin metabolism becomes saturated varies widely; genetic factors probably overshadow any age-dependent alterations in phenytoin metabolism.

When treating a patient with phenytoin, the practitioner must understand that phenytoin metabolism may become saturated at plasma concentrations at or below therapeutic levels. Measurement of phenytoin levels may be useful in avoiding toxicity while maximizing efficacy, but alterations in protein binding may complicate the interpretation of total phenytoin levels in the elderly. If alterations in protein binding are suspected, a specific measurement of the free phenytoin concentration is available to clarify this clinical situation.

Phenobarbital is cleared primarily by hepatic metabolism. The data available suggest that the plasma half-life of phenobarbital is increased with aging. Either a change in plasma clearance or in the volume of distribution could be responsible for this change in half-life, and its clinical significance has not been defined. Limited data indicate that the pharmacokinetics of carbamazepine are not affected by aging (34). Valproic acid's half-life, volume of distribution, and total drug clearance have not been reported to be different in young and elderly subjects (35). However, valproic acid protein binding was shown to be decreased in the elderly subjects and the free drug clearance reduced.

Antiarrhythmic Drugs

A large number of antiarrhythmic agents are now in clinical use, including drugs eliminated by hepatic metabolism, such as quinidine and lidocaine. Others are excreted to varying degrees by the kidneys (procainamide, disopyramide, tocainide) (27). As would be expected, the decrease in creatinine clearance associated with aging results in decreased clearance of procainamide, tocainide, and, presumably, disopyramide.

Lidocaine elimination by the liver is flow limited. Thus, decreased hepatic flow rates in the elderly result in decreases in lidocaine clearance with aging; this has been confirmed in some studies. In addition, the volume of distribution of lidocaine increases with age. The result of both of these changes is a prolonged half-life of lidocaine in elderly patients. The clearance of quinidine is approximately 35 percent lower in the elderly as compared with that in a younger population. Neither the volume of distribution nor the protein binding of quinidine is significantly affected by aging.

Antineoplastic Agents

Antineoplastic agents are frequently employed in elderly patients, and result in increased risk of myelosuppression, peripheral neuropathy, severe mucositis, and impairment in renal function. Most antineoplastic agents are highly metabolized, and altered hepatic function with aging, disease, or concurrent drug therapy may influence the efficacy and safety of these agents. Etoposide and methotrexate are primarily eliminated by the kidneys and both exhibit reduced clearance as renal function declines with aging. Altered organ responsiveness with aging may explain the acute dementia following high-dose interferon-α therapy in patients more than 65 years of age, although altered pharmacokinetics may also be present (36). The tolerability of antineoplastic agents may be improved by modification of the size, frequency of dosing, or both, and by the recognition that the creatinine clearance is the best estimate of residual renal function in the elderly.

Digoxin

Digoxin is commonly used in the elderly population, and its use is associated with a high incidence of adverse reactions. Plasma digoxin levels are not uniformly predictive of toxicity, and may be particularly misleading in patients older than 65 years of age (37). Digoxin is eliminated primarily through renal excretion. The decrease in creatinine clearance with aging correlates well with a decrease in digoxin clearance. Some investigators have reported a decrease in the volume of distribution of digoxin with aging, but the decrease in clearance is the dominant change with aging. Thus, the half-life of digoxin increases with aging, and the initial maintenance dose should be reduced in elderly patients. If further work confirms the reduction in the volume of distribution, the loading dose of digoxin used would also need to be reduced for the geriatric population.

β-Adrenergic Blockers

A large number of β-adrenergic blockers are now in clinical use, and complex pharmaco-kinetic and pharmacodynamic differences have been demonstrated for their use in elderly persons compared with use in young patients. Propranolol has been the most studied in this respect. Propranolol is cleared by the liver in a flow-dependent manner. With aging, the clearance of propranolol is decreased, but its volume of distribution, protein binding, and bioavailability are unchanged. The half-life of propranolol is thus increased with aging (18). However, there are also physiological changes in the β-adrenergic system that occur with aging, which may alter the action of β-adrenergic blockers. Some studies have demonstrated a decreased number of β-adrenergic receptors with aging, and a decrease in the maximal cardiac response to isoproterenol, a β-adrenergic receptor agonist (27). How these changes in adrenergic function translate to the pharmacologic use of β-adrenergic blockers is complex and the subject of ongoing investigation, but these changes may make the elderly patient more or less susceptible to β-blockade with use of drugs such as propranolol. Thus, clinical assessment is critical for balancing the varied pharmacokinetic and pharmacodynamic changes.

In general, the other β-adrenergic blockers available can be characterized as lipophilic compounds, such as propranolol, which are metabolized by the liver, or hydrophilic drugs, such as atenolol, which are eliminated by the kidneys. Aging is associated with alterations in both hepatic blood flow and creatinine clearance; thus, the clearance of both lipophilic and hydrophilic drugs is decreased in the elderly. No significant changes in the volume of distribution of these agents have been described. Decrease in clearance leads to a pro-

longation of the half-life of these agents in the geriatric population.

Diuretics

As many as 45 percent of patients older than 65 years of age admitted to an inpatient medical service will be taking diuretics. Furosemide is commonly used in elderly patients. Its volume of distribution may increase slightly with age, but the dominant pharmacokinetic alteration is a decrease in clearance which leads to a prolonged half-life (38,39). However, elderly patients are also relatively resistant to the diuretic action of furosemide. Furosemide needs to reach the intraluminal surface of the renal tubule to influence sodium chloride transport. Thus, the same decrease in renal function that results in lower furosemide clearance also decreases furosemide delivery to its site of action. These changes in the kinetics and action of furosemide need to be viewed in the context of frequent adverse reactions to diuretic therapy in geriatric populations.

Dehydration, prerenal azotemia, and hypotension are frequently associated with diuretic use in the elderly, but these complications are rarely observed in the younger population. The use of thiazide diuretics causes a greater potassium loss in the elderly as compared with that in younger patients (40). There are no clear-cut explanations for these enhanced responses in the elderly, but altered dietary intake, less effective thirst recognition, and abnormal autonomic response to hypotension may contribute to the adverse effects. A practitioner, therefore, needs to be cautious when using a diuretic in an elderly patient. Serum electrolyte determinations and measurement of orthostatic blood pressures are helpful in avoiding serious complications. The combination of a diuretic and digoxin may be dangerous because hypokalemia and hypomagnesemia from diuretic use can potentiate the cardiotoxicity of digoxin. Also, a decrease in renal function secondary to diuretic-induced dehydration can result in accumulation of digoxin to toxic levels.

Inhaled Anesthetics

The inhaled anesthetics are highly fat-soluble agents whose removal from the body is dependent on pulmonary gas exchange, hepatic metabolism, or both. The change in body composition with aging—increased percentage of body fat—and decreased cardiac output, pulmonary gas exchange, and hepatic function may all act to decrease the clearance of inhaled anesthetics. These theoretical principles were recently demonstrated for isoflurane, enflurane, halothane, and methoxyflurane, in which decreased clearances and significantly increased volumes of distribution occurred in elderly patients compared with young patients (41). Since elderly patients represent a growing segment of the surgical population, knowledge of these changes in inhaled anesthetic clearance may avoid complications in surgical and postsurgical management of the elderly.

Nonsteroidal Anti-inflammatory Drugs

Most nonsteroidal anti-inflammatory drugs (NSAIDs) are strongly protein bound and are metabolized by the liver (42). Aspirin is the mostly commonly used NSAID. Aspirin is rapidly converted to salicylate after absorption, and this conversion is unaffected by age. The volume of distribution for salicylate increases with age, but its clearance decreases. These changes result in a prolonged half-life for salicylate in the elderly. Pharmacokinetic studies have also been performed using some of the other NSAIDs. The clearances of ibuprofen and naproxen have been shown to decrease with age, but for unclear reasons the changes in ibuprofen clearance were seen in elderly men but not in elderly women. The pharmacokinetics of piroxicam and indomethacin have not been shown to change with age.

Ten to 15 percent of the population more than 65 years old take prescription NSAIDs that are associated with significant morbidity (42,43). Bleeding from peptic ulcers in patients older than 60 years has been shown to be associated with NSAID use. Many of the recent reports of severe hepatic and renal toxicity secondary to NSAID use have occurred in elderly patients. As always, the clinician needs to assess carefully the risks and benefits of treatment with these agents in geriatric patients and review periodically the need for their continued use.

Sedative, Antipsychotic, and Antidepressant Drugs

The consequences of aging on the proper use of psychoactive drugs are complex. Pharmacokinetic studies have been performed for only a few drugs. Many studies examining central nervous system (CNS) sensitivity to

these drugs in the elderly do not take into account the possibility of altered clearances or protein binding. Aging may be associated with a decrease in mental agility, a decline in intellectual responsiveness and perception, and impaired learning ability and memory. Thus, it would not be surprising that the use of sedative hypnotic drugs would lead to adverse CNS reactions more commonly in the elderly. Unfortunately, this important interaction has not been explored in adequate detail. It has been recognized for a long time that elderly patients frequently have paradoxical agitation when given barbiturates. The exact etiology of this reaction is unknown, but the routine use of barbiturates and sedative hypnotic agents should be minimized for this population.

The half-life of diazepam is increased approximately fourfold in the elderly as compared with that in a young population (11). This change in half-life is the result of an increased volume of distribution, without a change in clearance or protein binding. These kinetic changes would suggest, on the basis of pharmacokinetics, that at steady-state the total dose of diazepam should be unchanged for the elderly, but that the dosing interval could be lengthened. The half-life of chlordiazepoxide is increased with aging as a result of an increase in the volume of distribution and a decrease in the clearance. Data also suggest that the elderly are more sensitive to the central depressant effect of benzodiazepines. Adverse CNS effects during flurazepam therapy are more common in the elderly than in younger patients (44). Impairment of psychomotor performance after the administration of 10 mg of nitrazepam was greater in elderly subjects as compared with impairment in younger individuals, but no change in nitrazepam pharmacokinetics were observed (21). Thus, it is prudent to begin elderly patients on a lower benzodiazepine dose than the dose that would be used in younger patients.

Limited data are available on changes with aging in the pharmacokinetics and pharmacodynamics of the antidepressants. The clearances of amitriptyline, nortriptyline, and imipramine have been reported to be decreased in the elderly. The plasma half-life of trazodone is increased in the elderly, secondary to a decrease in clearance.

Analgesics

Early studies examining the effect of morphine sulfate

and pentazocine hydrochloride on postoperative pain concluded that elderly patients were more sensitive to the analgesic effects of these narcotics (45). Data indicate that neither the volume of distribution nor the elimination of morphine sulfate is different in young compared with elderly subjects (46). However, the rate of distribution of morphine is faster in younger patients, which results in higher plasma levels of the drug soon after administration in the elderly patients. Higher meperidine levels have also been reported after administration of the drug to elderly patients as compared with levels in young individuals. A detailed and complete analysis of pharmacodynamic and pharmacokinetic changes in narcotic analgesic handling for the elderly is not yet available.

Alterations with aging for acetaminophen pharmacokinetics are small. The volume of distribution for acetaminophen decreases, and there is also a trend towards decreased acetaminophen clearance. The combination of these changes results in little or no change with aging for acetaminophen half-life (47).

Other Drugs

Lithium is excreted by the kidneys, and its clearance is decreased in the elderly. Cimetidine is eliminated by both renal and hepatic mechanisms, and its clearance is decreased with aging. Ranitidine, a histamine-2 antagonist similar to cimetidine, is also eliminated by both renal and hepatic mechanisms. The half-life of ranitidine is increased by approximately 40 percent in elderly patients as compared with the half-life in a young population. In addition, the peak ranitidine concentration after oral administration is higher in elderly patients, which suggests a decrease with age in the first-pass elimination of the drug. Theophylline is cleared primarily by way of hepatic metabolism, and clearance has been reported to be decreased in elderly patients. For both lithium and theophylline, laboratory measurement of drug levels can be helpful in optimizing dosage regimens. Calcium channel blockers are being used with increasing frequency in elderly patients, and the clearance of verapamil and diltiazem is reduced in the elderly (48). Theoretically, the reduced hepatic blood flow and phase I metabolizing enzymes associated with aging will increase the bioavailability and prolong the half-life of all calcium channel blockers in use today.

Summary of Drug Use in the Geriatric Population

The proper use of therapeutic agents in the elderly is important for optimal functioning (Table 7.4). Yet, data have repeatedly demonstrated that the incidence of adverse drug reactions in a geriatric population is two to three times that seen in young patients, and reaches an incidence rate of above 20 percent in patients more than 80 years old (49,50). The physician must be aware of this risk and its contributing factors as well as of techniques to minimize risk.

Physiological changes that occur with aging result in

Table 7.4. Guidelines for Prescribing Drugs for the Elderly.

Diagnostic considerations
    Establish diagnosis; set realistic therapeutic endpoints.
    Take careful drug history, including all over-the-counter agents and alcohol use.
    Scrutinize medication list for potential toxicities and/or drug interactions when new symptoms arise.
    Inquire regularly about known drug side effects, especially those affecting autonomic nervous system.
Drug choice
    Employ drug therapy only after nonpharmacologic therapy has been considered and benefit clearly outweighs risk.
    Select effective drugs on basis of tolerability and ease of administration.
    Start with low doses; titrate slowly.
    Simplify drug regimens; carefully educate patient and caregiver regarding dose size, frequency, drug actions, potential side effects.
    Limit duration of drug therapy to minimum time necessary by prescribing appropriate number of doses.
Drug monitoring
    Monitor drug level frequently because of altered pharmacokinetics, pharmacodynamics, narrowed therapeutic index.
    Monitor and reinforce drug compliance.
    Reassess frequently risk vs benefit of drug therapy; consider dose reductions, drug "holidays," substitution of nondrug therapy.

predictable changes in drug distribution and elimination, and an understanding of these alterations permits the clinician to use drugs in elderly patients rationally and safely. For drugs eliminated by renal excretion, the fall in glomerular filtration in the elderly decreases drug clearance by as much as 50 percent. Hepatic drug metabolism is altered much less with aging, except for those drugs in which clearance is limited by the reduced hepatic blood flow in elderly patients. The use of measured drug levels to assist in clinical decision making (therapeutic drug monitoring) is one way to assess objectively whether the optimal dosing regimen has been chosen. Elderly patients often take a large number of medications (5 to 10 different drugs in most studies), which increases the risk of adverse drug interactions (51,52). Nonprescription medications should not be neglected in this regard. Elderly patients may also be more sensitive to drug effects, both therapeutic and toxic, at any given drug concentration. The adverse effects of many drugs may be subtle, particularly when superimposed on the changes that occur with aging and the effects of underlying diseases. Thus, it is critical that the physician specifically question and examine the patient, and keep in mind the potential for adverse drug effects.

Optimal prescribing practices by the physician will not be sufficient if the patient does not take the medications properly. Several techniques can be employed to improve patient compliance (52,53). The obvious steps are to minimize the number of medications and to caution the patient about changing drug dosages. For some patients, it may be necessary to involve family members or visiting nurses in these discussions. Patients should also be informed of the potential hazards of over-the-counter drugs. The pharmacist can also work with the patient to reinforce the instructions of the physician, to provide special packaging that includes memory aids, and to keep accurate drug lists. Obviously, to completely eliminate adverse drug reactions in the elderly is impossible; however, with care, the problems can be minimized and their consequences recognized and managed.

References

1. Schmucker DL. Age-related changes in drug disposition. Pharmacol Rev 1978;30:445–456.

2. Lamy PP. Physiological changes due to age. Pharmacodynamic changes of drug action and implications for therapy. Drugs Aging 1991;1:385–404.

3. Plein JB, Plein EM. Aging and drug therapy. Ann Rev Gerontol Geriatr 1981;2:211–254.

4. Montgomery RD, Haeney MR, Ross IN, et al. The ageing gut: a study of intestinal absorption in relation to nutrition in the elderly. Q J Med 1978;47:197–211.

5. Weiling PG. Interactions affecting drug absorption. Clin Pharmacokinet 1984;9:404–434.

6. Schwartz JB, Troconiz IF, Verotta D, et al. Aging effects on stereoselective pharmacokinetics and pharmacodynamics of verapamil. J Pharmacol Exp Ther 1993;265:690–698.

7. Novak LP. Aging, total body potassium, fat-free mass, and cell mass in males and females between ages 18 and 85 years. J Gerontol 1972;27:438–443.

8. Wallace S, Whiting B, Runcie J. Factors affecting drug binding in plasma of elderly patients. Br J Clin Pharmacol 1976;3:327–330.

9. Sjoqvist F, Alvan G. Aging and drug disposition–metabolism. J Chronic Dis 1983;36:31–37.

10. Vestal RE, Wood AJJ. Influence of age and smoking on drug kinetics in man. Studies using model compounds. Clin Pharmacokinet 1980;5:309–319.

11. Klotz U, Avant GR, Hoyumpa A, et al. The effects of age and liver disease in the disposition and elimination of diazepam in adult man. J Clin Invest 1975;55:347–359.

12. Serlin MJ, Breckenridge AM. Drug interactions with warfarin. Drugs 1983;25:610–620.

13. Hayes MJ, Langmann MJS, Short AH. Changes in drug metabolism with age. 1. Warfarin binding and plasma proteins. Br J Clin Pharmacol 1975;2:69–72.

14. Davies DF, Shock NW. Age changes in glomerular filtration rate, effective renal plasma flow, and tubular excretory capacity in adult males. J Clin Invest 1950;29:496–507.

15. Bennett WM, Aronoff GR, Golper TA, et al. Drug prescribing in renal failure. Dosing guidelines for adults. Philadelphia: American College of Physicians, 1987.

16. James OFW. Gastrointestinal and liver function in old age. Clin Gastroenterol 1983;12:671–691.

17. Wood AJJ, Vestal RE, Wilkinson GR, et al. Effect of aging and cigarette smoking on antipyrine and indocyanine green elimination. Clin Pharmacol Ther 1979;26:16–20.

18. Vestal RE, Wood AJJ, Branch RA, et al. Effect of age and cigarette smoking on propranolol disposition. Clin Pharmacokinet 1976;1:135–155.

19. Vestal RE, Wood AJJ, Shand DG. Reduced beta-adrenoceptor sensitivity in the elderly. Clin Pharmacol Ther 1979;26:181–186.

20. O'Malley K, Stevenson IH, Ward CA, et al. Determinants of anticoagulant control in patients receiving warfarin. Br J Clin Pharmacol 1977;4:309–314.

21. Castelden CM, George CF, Marcer D, et al. Increased sensitivity to nitrazepam in old age. BMJ 1977;1:10–12.

22. Caird FI, Andrew GR, Kennedy RD. Effect of posture on blood pressure in the elderly. Br Heart J 1973;35:527–530.

23. Gribbon B, Pickering TG, Sleight P, et al. Effect of age and high blood pressure on baroreflex sensitivity in man. Circ Res 1971;29:424–431.
24. Bauer JH. Age-related changes in the renin-aldosterone system. Physiological effects and clinical implications. Drugs Aging 1993;3:238–245.
25. The fifth report of the Joint National Committee on Detection, Evaluation and Treatment of High Blood Pressure (JNC V). Arch Intern Med 1993;153:154–183.
26. McNeil JJ, Drummer OH, Conway EL, et al. Effect of age on pharmacokinetics of and blood pressure responses to prazosin and terazosin. J Cardiovasc Pharmacol 1987;10:168–175.
27. Rocci ML Jr, Vlasses PH, Abrams WB. Geriatric clinical pharmacology. Cardiol Clin 1986;4:213–225.
28. Moore RD, Smith CR, Lipsky JJ, et al. Risk factors for nephrotoxicity in patients treated with aminoglycosides. Ann Intern Med 1984;100:352–357.
29. Miglioli PA, Pivetta P, Strazzabosco M, et al. Effect of age on single- and multiple-dose pharmacokinetics of erythromycin. Eur J Clin Pharmacol 1990;39:161–164.
30. Nilsson-Ehle I, Ljungberg B. Influence of age on the pharmacokinetics of ciprofloxacin. Scand J Infect Dis 1989;60(suppl):23–27.
31. Hayden FG, Minocha A, Spyker DA, Hoffman HE. Comparative single-dose pharmacokinetics of amantadine hydrochloride and rimantadine hydrochloride in young and elderly adults. Antimicrob Agents Chemother 1985;28:216.
32. Hayes MJ, Langmann MJS, Short AH. Changes in drug metabolism with increasing age. 2. Phenytoin clearance and protein binding. Br J Clin Pharmacol 1975;2:73–79.
33. Richens A. Clinical pharmacokinetics of phenytoin. Clin Pharmacokinet 1979;4:153–169.
34. Hockings N, Pall A, Moody J, et al. The effect of age on carbamazepine pharmacokinetics and adverse effects. Br J Clin Pharmacol 1986;22:725–728.
35. Perucca E, Grimaldi R, Gatti G, et al. Pharmacokinetics of valproic acid in the elderly. Br J Clin Pharmacol 1984;17:665–669.
36. Balducci L, Mowry K. Pharmacology and organ toxicity of chemotherapy in older patients. Oncology (Huntingt) 1992;6(suppl 2):62–68.
37. Boman K. Digitalis intoxication in geriatric in-patients. Acta Med Scand 1983;214:345–351.
38. Andreasen F, Hansen U, Husted JE, et al. The pharmacokinetics of furosemide are influenced by age. Br J Clin Pharmacol 1983;16:391–397.
39. Kerremans ALM, Tan Y, van Baars H, et al. Furosemide kinetics and dynamics in aged patients. Clin Pharmacol Ther 1983;34:181–189.
40. Friend DG. Drug therapy and the geriatric patient. Clin Pharmacol Ther 1961;2:832–836.
41. Strum DP, Eger EI II, Unadkat JD, et al. Age affects the pharmacokinetics of inhaled anesthetics in humans. Anesth Analg 1991;73:310–318.
42. Woodhouse KW, Wynne H. The pharmacokinetics of nonsteroidal anti-inflammatory drugs in the elderly. Clin Pharmacokinet 1987;12:111–122.
43. Griffin MR, Piper JM, Daugherty JR, et al. Nonsteroidal anti-inflammatory drug use and increased risk for peptic ulcer disease in elderly persons. Ann Intern Med 1991;114:257–263.
44. Greenblatt DJ, Allen MD, Shader RI. Toxicity of high-dose flurazepam in the elderly. Clin Pharmacol Ther 1977;21:355–361.
45. Belville JW, Forrest WH, Miller E, et al. Influence of age on pain relief from analgesics. A study of postoperative patients. JAMA 1971;217:1835–1841.
46. Owen JA, Sitar DS, Berger L, et al. Age-related morphine kinetics. Clin Pharmacol Ther 1983;34:364–368.
47. Divoll M, Abernethy DR, Ameer B, et al. Acetaminophen kinetics in the elderly. Clin Pharmacol Ther 1982;31:151–156.
48. Kates RE. Calcium antagonists. Pharmacokinetic properties. Drugs 1983;25:113–124.
49. Caird FI. Towards rational drug therapy in old age. J R Coll Phys 1985;19:235–239.
50. Leach S, Roy SS. Adverse drug reactions: an investigation on an acute geriatric ward. Age Ageing 1986;15:241–246.
51. Gosney M, Tallis R. Prescription of contraindicated and interacting drugs in elderly patients admitted to hospital. Lancet 1984;2:564–567.
52. Royal College of Physicians. Medication for the elderly. J R Coll Phys 1984;18:7–17.
53. Gryfe CI and Gryfe BM. Drug therapy of the aged: the problem of compliance and the roles of physicians and pharmacists. J Am Geriatr Soc 1984;32:301–307.

Suggested Reading

Bair FE, ed. Cancer Sourcebook. vol. 1. Detroit: Omnigraphics, 1990:818.
Jernigan JA. Update on drugs and the elderly. Am Fam Physician 1984;29:238–247.

Chapter 8
Preventive Medicine

John F. Steiner

Let me advise thee not to talk of thyself as being old. There is something in Mind Cure, after all, and, if thee continually talks of thyself as being old, thee may perhaps bring on some of the infirmities of age. At least I would not risk it if I were thee.

Hannah Whitall Smith
Logan Pearsall Smith, Philadelphia Quaker

An individual aged 65 has a life expectancy of 16.5 years, of which he or she can expect to live independently for 10.0 years, or 61 percent of that time span (1). The primary goal of preventive medicine for the elderly is to prolong the period of functional independence; prolongation of life, though important, is a secondary objective (2). Breslow and Somers defined a set of general goals for preventive care of the elderly, based on a division into the "young old" (65 to 74 years of age), and the "old old" (75 years and older) (3). The goals are described in Table 8.1. Many of these goals also apply to younger age groups, but others, such as preparation for retirement and avoidance of institutionalization, are specific to the elderly. Ideally, preventive care for older persons should begin when the individuals are young, through counseling to maintain a healthy lifestyle and age-appropriate screening to identify preventable disease. Nevertheless, many preventive measures that should be instituted earlier in life, such as smoking cessation, breast cancer detection, and hypertension treatment, are of benefit even if begun after the age of 65 (4). In addition to carryover of prevention efforts from earlier stages in the life cycle, preventive medicine for the elderly also requires identification and modification of functional problems unique to the elderly, such as age-related visual and hearing loss or environmental hazards that may cause falls. This chapter introduces some general principles of preventive care, summarizes the areas in which preventive care is most commonly recommended for the elderly, and reviews the evidence on which preventive care recommendations are based.

General Principles of Preventive Medicine

Preventive care interventions have traditionally been divided into three classes: primary prevention—activities that reduce the likelihood that disease or functional impairment will develop (e.g., immunization); secondary prevention—the early detection and treatment of disease, usually through screening of asymptomatic individuals, to forestall consequences (e.g., treatment of hypertension); and tertiary prevention—the attempt to slow the progression of established disease or reduce resulting disability (e.g., geriatric assessment) (5). All three types of preventive interventions are important for the elderly, though tertiary prevention gains significance because of the increased burden of illness and dysfunction in many older persons.

Preventive interventions for the elderly commonly involve screening, defined as "the presumptive identification of unrecognized disease or defect by the application of tests, examinations, or other procedures, which can be applied rapidly" (6). The goal of screening is to use an accurate but safe and inexpensive test to separate an asymptomatic population into groups at higher and lower risk, thereby restricting the use of expensive or potentially hazardous diagnostic evaluations to the subgroup of individuals most likely to derive benefit. The use of mammography to detect breast cancer in women without a palpable breast mass is an example of screening; any abnormality detected on mammography does not prove the diagnosis of breast cancer, but does identify patients at higher risk for the disease, and who therefore require further evaluation by biopsy.

Not all health problems are amenable to screening. Attributes of the burden of illness imposed by the health

Table 8.1. Goals for Preventive Care of the Elderly.

Age (yr)	Goals
65–74	Prolong the period of optimal physical, mental, and social activity
	Minimize handicapping and discomfort from onset of chronic conditions
	Help to prepare for retirement
75 and over	Prolong the period of effective activity and ability to live independently and to avoid institutionalization, if possible
	Minimize inactivity and discomfort from chronic conditions
	Ensure minimal physical and mental distress and provide emotional support to patient and family in the event of terminal illness

SOURCE: From Breslow L, Somers AR. The lifetime health-monitoring program. N Engl J Med 1985;312:827–835.

Table 8.2. Criteria for Evaluation of Preventive Measures.

Characteristics of the disability or disease

  Prevalence of condition in population

  Impact on individual (e.g., disability, pain, social disruption, years of life lost)

  Impact on society (mortality, morbidity, cost of care)

  Sufficiently long subclinical phase to allow effective screening

Characteristics of the test for screening or assessment

  Validity of test (likelihood that test is positive in individuals with the condition and negative in those without it)

  Acceptability to patient and health care provider

  Risk of harm from the test

    Risk, discomfort, and cost of evaluating a positive test

    Personal and social disadvantages of being labeled as diseased by the test

  Likelihood of compliance with the testing procedure by provider and patient

Characteristics of the treatment regimen

  Efficacy (does suitable treatment exist)

  Effectiveness (is treatment actually rendered)

    Availability of treatment in community

    Adherence of patients to treatment

    Acceptability of costs of treatment

    Evidence of benefit when applied in the general population

SOURCE: Adapted from U.S. Preventive Services Task Force. Guide to preventive services. Baltimore: Williams & Wilkins, 1989; Canadian Task Force on the Periodic Health Examination. The periodic health examination. Can Med Assoc J 1979;121:1193–1254; Fletcher RM, Fletcher SW, Wagner EH. Clinical epidemiology—the essentials. Baltimore: Williams & Wilkins, 1982.

problem, characteristics of the screening test, and the effectiveness of treatment for individuals found to have the disease must be considered in identifying appropriate targets for preventive screening. For example, lung cancer is a common and devastating disease, but screening for lung cancer has not proven effective (4). Even when lung cancer is detected early, existing treatments have been too ineffective to justify the effort and expense to screen all individuals at risk. Table 8.2 lists a number of general characteristics of diseases and functional impairments that must be considered in assessing suitable conditions for preventive care for any age group.

Special Considerations in Preventive Care for the Elderly

In the elderly, preventive care takes place in a context of interrelated medical, functional, and social considerations. Ultimately, the appropriateness of any preventive intervention depends on the overall goals of health care, as defined by the individual in collaboration with the health care provider. Several special considerations should guide decision making about prevention for elderly individuals.

Because the preservation of function is the main goal of preventive care, increasing emphasis should be placed on the detection of impairments such as sensory loss, muscle weakness, or gait disturbances that might predispose to falls, since such impairments might lead to a loss of abilities to maintain activities of daily living. For example, a patient with numerous medical problems, who is cared for by family or other caregivers, may be able to live at home until she or he develops cataracts that prevent social activities, make self-care more difficult, and ultimately overwhelm the caregivers' ability to cope, prompting them to seek nursing home care. Such vulnerable individuals require particular attention to functional deficits to avoid loss of their independence.

Decisions about screening should not be based on age alone; old age does not justify diagnostic or therapeutic nihilism. It may be appropriate, for example, to recommend mammography for a healthy 80-year-old, yet inappropriate to do so for a 60-year-old patient with end-stage congestive heart failure. Decisions should be based on the patient's current and anticipated level of function, as well as on an appraisal of the risks of the screening test itself, and of any further tests required if the screening test is abnormal. Although an increasing body of evidence has identified conditions for which preventive care should be started in older persons, few studies define an age at which prevention is of no further value.

Screening tests may have different diagnostic characteristics in elderly patients than they do in younger individuals. In tuberculosis screening programs, for example, the probability of a positive response to a standard intradermal (5 TU) skin test rises with age into the sixth decade but declines thereafter. One screening program for patients in long-term care facilities found that the rate of positive responses fell from 43 percent in patients aged 65 to 74 years to 19 percent in those aged 85 to 94 years, perhaps as a result of factors such as immunologic senescence, local changes in aging skin, or a decrease in reactivity as the initial infection becomes more remote (7). Since a single tuberculin skin test is less effective for screening, other strategies, such as use of a booster dose of tuberculin one week after the screening, are necessary to diagnosis tuberculosis in the elderly. In contrast, the accuracy of mammography improves with age because of changes in the aging breast that improve the ability of the procedure to distinguish cancer from normal tissue.

The effectiveness of preventive treatments may also vary with age. The usefulness of pneumococcal vaccine was first demonstrated in young men at high risk of pneumococcal pneumonia, but the efficacy of pneumococcal vaccine has been difficult to demonstrate in elderly individuals with chronic diseases because of these individuals' inability to produce or sustain antibodies to the antigens in the vaccine (8). In some cases, the effectiveness of treatment may be greater in the elderly. For example, treatment of hypertension in the elderly was long thought unnecessary and potentially hazardous. Recent randomized trials have demonstrated that individuals up to age 84 benefit from hypertension treatment through substantial reductions in the risk of stroke, and that the benefit of treating hypertension, as measured by the absolute reduction in stroke rate per 1000 patients treated, is greater in older than in middle-aged individuals (9).

In younger adults, screening is often performed during routine visits to health providers. For the elderly, as for pregnant women and for children, special visits may be necessary for comprehensive preventive care. Such encounters may occur in the provider's office, in the home, or in an institutional care setting. Because of the variety of preventive care needs in the elderly, any single health professional may lack the range of skills or the time necessary to provide comprehensive preventive care. An interdisciplinary health care team, typically including a physician, nurse, physical therapist, pharmacist, and social worker, is often needed for comprehensive preventive care, particularly for tertiary prevention through geriatric assessment (10). Many preventive activities can also be performed effectively by such interdisciplinary teams or their members, such as nurse practitioners (11).

Primary Prevention in the Elderly

Efforts at primary prevention for the elderly have focused on a number of categories, such as immunizations, accident prevention, chemoprevention, and counseling to stop smoking, improve nutrition, or promote exercise. A summary of recommended measures for primary prevention is provided in Table 8.3.

Influenza Immunization

Fifteen times between 1957 and 1982, influenza epidemics in the United States were associated with 10,000 or more excessive deaths. Most deaths occurred in the elderly (12). In epidemic and nonepidemic years, influenza leads to an increase in hospitalizations of elderly individuals for pneumonia, other acute and chronic respiratory illnesses, and congestive heart failure (13). Although patients with chronic cardiorespiratory diseases and residents of long-term and chronic care facilities are particularly vulnerable to the consequences of influenza, healthy elderly individuals are also at risk.

Influenza vaccine is less efficacious in the elderly than it is in younger individuals, though overall vaccine has an efficacy of 60 percent to 70 percent (12). Despite continued public concern about vaccine side effects, a randomized trial has shown no excess of systemic symptoms in individuals given active influenza vaccine compared with those given placebo (14). No randomized trials to assess the effectiveness of influenza vaccination in the elderly have been conducted, but cohort studies in nursing

Table 8.3. Recommendations for Primary Prevention in the Elderly.

Condition	Preventive Measure	Frequency	Comments
Influenza	Immunization	Yearly	Also amantadine during outbreaks
Tetanus	Immunization	Every 10 yr	Women less likely to have primary immunization
Cigarette use	Counseling	Ongoing	Use of multiple strategies is most effective
Poor nutrition	Counseling, dietary supplements	Ongoing	Hospitalized, chronically ill, functionally impaired individuals at high risk.
Sedentary life style	Exercise counseling and prescription	Ongoing	In both community-living and institutionalized persons

homes and among community-living seniors have shown substantial reductions in the incidence of influenza, hospitalizations for cardiorespiratory disease, and mortality among individuals receiving the vaccine (15,16). Population-based analyses suggest that influenza immunization is also economically advantageous because the reduction in hospitalization costs as a result of immunization of the elderly more than outweighs the costs of a vaccination program (17). On the basis of such information, annual immunization against influenza is recommended for all individuals aged 65 and older.

Pneumococcal Immunization

Although most national guidelines advise immunization with a 23-valent pneumococcal vaccine at age 65 years to prevent pneumococcal infections, evidence for this recommendation is inconclusive. Pneumococcal disease can affect healthy seniors, but individuals who are immunosuppressed or have chronic cardiorespiratory, hepatic, renal disease, or diabetes are at higher risk. Randomized trials in high-risk groups have found that pneumococcal vaccine was not effective in preventing pneumococcal infections, primarily because many individuals failed to produce or sustain protective antibodies (8,18). In contrast, numerous case-control studies have

suggested that pneumococcal vaccine substantially reduces the incidence of extrapulmonary pneumococcal infection, with estimated vaccine efficacy of 50 percent to 60 percent. Much of this benefit is hypothesized to occur in healthy elderly individuals (19,20). In an attempt to synthesize these findings, some authorities have suggested that pneumococcal vaccine should be administered to healthy persons between the ages of 55 to 65 to obtain an immune response before chronic diseases that would reduce immunocompetence develop (21). Others have argued that the lack of effectiveness in randomized trials, along with the relatively low attack rates in healthy individuals and the population costs of mass vaccination, preclude pneumococcal immunization for any group (18). Given this controversy, no evidence-based recommendations can be made about the role of pneumococcal vaccination in the elderly. However, many authorities continue to recommend vaccination at age 65 on the basis of the low cost per vaccination and the minimal side effects of the vaccine (22).

Tetanus Immunization

In the U.S., tetanus is primarily a disease of the elderly: 70 percent of cases in recent years have occurred in individuals aged 50 years and older (23). Serologic surveys have suggested that 50 percent or more of elderly individuals lack protective titers of tetanus antitoxin. Elderly men are more likely than elderly women to have been immunized, often during military service. After a primary immunization series, most authorities recommend booster immunization every 10 years throughout the life span (4). However, given the 15- to 25-year persistence of protective tetanus antitoxin levels, the rarity of tetanus cases in the population, and the expense of mass immunization, some authorities suggest that a single tetanus booster at age 60 or 65 may be a more cost-effective immunization strategy (24).

Prevention of Falls

Falls are common in the elderly, occurring in about one-third of community-living seniors each year and in a higher proportion of individuals in hospitals and long-term care. In community-living elderly, serious injury results from about 5 percent of falls; injury rates from falls in institutions range from 10 percent to 25 percent (25). Risk factors for falls include muscle weakness, disturbances in gait or balance, visual impairment, cognitive dysfunction, orthostatic hypotension, and drugs, especially psychotropic and cardiovascular medications (25).

Strategies for primary prevention of falls, or of injuries resulting from falls, have been tested in two randomized trials. In an attempt to modify risk factors for falling, half a group of almost 3200 community-dwelling seniors received a series of educational presentations concerning environmental safety, modification of risky behaviors in the home (such as unsafe use of chairs to reach high places), and demonstration of an exercise program to improve strength, range of motion, and proprioception in the legs (26). This intervention resulted in a 7 percent reduction in falls (after adjustment for other fall-risk factors) and a 4 percent reduction in falls leading to injury; neither of these declines was statistically significant, however. Thus, this community-based educational intervention may not have been of sufficient intensity or duration to protect community-dwelling older persons from subsequent falls or injuries, and it did not target individuals at highest risk. In another study, residents of a nursing home in Denmark were randomly assigned to wear external trochanteric hip protectors, which were fixed in special underwear and were designed to direct impact away from the greater trochanter during falls. Hip protectors reduced subsequent hip fractures by 56 percent, but, not surprisingly, had no effect on the incidence of falls or on nonhip fractures resulting from falls (27). The use of such protectors is a promising strategy for primary prevention of serious injuries in at-risk individuals. At present, however, no proven strategies exist for primary prevention of falls in the general population of elderly persons.

Prevention of Other Accidental Injuries

A variety of other strategies for primary prevention of injuries have been proposed, such as interventions to increase use of safety belts in automobiles, improve driving safety, reduce pedestrian accidents, and prevent burns (through use of smoke detectors and reduction of water-heater settings to 120° to 125°F), but randomized trials to evaluate the effectiveness of these measures are lacking (28).

Primary Chemoprophylaxis with Aspirin

Some authorities, such as the United States Preventive Services Task Force (USPSTF), recommend the use of 325 mg of aspirin every other day as primary prevention for cardiovascular disease in elderly men who have other cardiovascular risk factors (29). Two randomized trials that have assessed the role of aspirin in primary prevention reached somewhat conflicting conclusions, however. The British aspirin trial found no decrease in myocardial infarction, no difference in cardiovascular or all-cause mortality, and a slight but nonsignificant increase in stroke among male physicians randomized to take 500 mg of aspirin daily compared with those receiving placebo (30). The U.S. Physicians Health Study found a 69 percent decrease in fatal myocardial infarction among men randomized to 325 mg of aspirin every other day, no difference in cardiovascular or all-cause mortality, and an increase in stroke rate (especially hemorrhagic strokes) among men randomized to aspirin (31). When the results of these studies were pooled, the decline in myocardial infarction rate remained statistically significant, and the rise in stroke rate became statistically significant (32). On the basis of these data, the Canadian Task Force on the Periodic Health Examination recently concluded that routine use of aspirin as primary prevention for cardiovascular disease in the elderly could not be justified, and that the decision to use aspirin must be individualized (32). The effects of aspirin for primary prevention in women have not been assessed with a randomized trial, but observational studies suggest some benefit (33). Although many studies have demonstrated the benefit of aspirin in preventing further cardiovascular events in patients with known cardiac or cerebrovascular disease (a form of tertiary prevention), current evidence appears too inconclusive to recommend widespread use of aspirin for primary prevention.

Smoking Cessation

The prevalence of smoking among older adults remains distressingly high, 17.2 percent in men and 13.7 percent in women aged 65 and older in 1987 (34). A young person's decision to quit smoking cigarettes may be richly rewarded by better health and longer life. Substantial evidence suggests that an elderly, lifelong smoker also benefits from quitting. Prospective cohort studies have found that relative risks of all-cause mortality and coronary artery disease were two- to threefold higher among elderly male smokers, and twofold higher among women (34). A number of studies have also demonstrated that smoking cessation after age 65 results in a decline in mortality rate within one to five years. The decline in risk after quitting was slower among male smokers, probably because of earlier onset and higher lifetime consumption of cigarettes. In patients with known coronary artery disease, smoking cessation produces an immediate decline in cardiovascular mortality, evident within the first year after smoking cessation (35,36). Other research has suggested that physical function, as measured by improved ability to walk and climb stairs, was also better among nonsmokers or former smokers compared with that of current smokers (34).

Smoking cessation is most successful if multiple modalities are used (such as face-to-face counseling by physicians or nonphysicians, nicotine replacement with gum or patches, and written materials), if individualized advice is provided in both individual and group sessions, and if reinforcing sessions are continued after the initial treatment effort (37). Thus, smoking cessation in older individuals remains a major focus for primary prevention.

Nutritional Counseling

Estimates of the prevalence of malnutrition in the elderly vary widely, depending on the population studied and on the nutritional indexes measured. Malnutrition has been reported in as much as 61 percent of individuals admitted to hospitals or residing in long-term care facilities, and specific nutritional deficits have been found in 5 percent to 10 percent of community-living individuals, especially those chronically ill or socially isolated (38,39). Risk factors for poor nutrition include depression, cognitive impairment, poverty, and problems with eating-related functional abilities, such as difficulties in feeding oneself, shopping, or preparing food (40). Markers of poor nutritional status include low serum cholesterol (<160 mg/dl), low serum albumin, and involuntary weight loss (40). Dietary supplementation has been shown to reduce the rate of postoperative complications, and the duration of hospitalization and inpatient rehabilitation stays among patients with hip fracture (41), to improve immune responsiveness and reduce morbidity from infections in elderly individuals (42), and to reduce overall mortality in a population of long-term care patients (43). Thus, physicians should attempt to identify undernourished individuals through inquiry about activities of daily living relating to eating, ongoing monitoring of weight, and scrutiny of laboratory markers indicative of poor nutrition.

Exercise Counseling

Most elderly individuals are physically inactive. Population surveys suggest that 40 percent to 60 percent of older adults are completely sedentary, and only 5 percent to 10 percent are sufficiently active to maintain or improve cardiorespiratory fitness (44). The benefits of exercise at all ages include reductions in the incidence of coronary artery disease, hypertension, noninsulin-dependent diabetes mellitus, and depression. Increased physical activity also increases bone mineral content, reduces the risk of osteoporotic fractures, and increases overall longevity (45). In long-term prospective studies, ongoing physical activity in men aged 60 to 84 was associated with half the risk of mortality over a follow-up period of more than 10 years (46).

Numerous studies have demonstrated that conditioning programs for elderly individuals can enhance aerobic exercise capacity, but fewer have demonstrated benefits of exercise on the functional outcomes crucial to the overall goals of health promotion for seniors. However, statistically significant improvements in gait and balance with physical conditioning have been shown (47), and a recent study of nursing home residents demonstrated improvement in strength, mobility, activities of daily living, and reduction in depression with regular exercise (48). Although additional research is necessary to define programs that maximize the functional benefits of exercise conditioning in the elderly, existing interventions support the usefulness of physician counseling to encourage exercise throughout the life span.

Secondary Prevention in the Elderly

In addition to attempts to prevent disease through primary prevention, secondary prevention for early disease may be beneficial in a number of conditions that afflict elderly persons, such as functional impairments (vision,

Table 8.4. Recommendations for Secondary Prevention in the Elderly.

Condition	Screening Test	Frequency	Definitive "Gold Standard" Test	Comments
Visual impairment	Visual acuity	1–5 yr	Ophthalmologic examination	—
Hearing impairment	Portable audioscopy or questionnaire	1–2 yr	Audiometry	—
Hypertension	Blood pressure measurement	1–2 yr	Blood pressure measurement	Up to age 80–84
Cervical cancer	Pap smear	1–3 yr	Biopsy	In women not screened earlier in life
Breast cancer	Clinician breast examination	Yearly	Biopsy	—
	Mammography	Every 2 yr		Up to age 75
Colorectal cancer	Fecal occult blood testing	Yearly	Colonoscopy/biopsy	—
	Flexible sigmoidoscopy	3–5 yr		
Alcohol abuse	CAGE questionnaire	As needed	Detailed clinical history	—
Hypothyroidism	T_4 or TSH*	1–2 yr	TSH, clinical findings	Elderly women only
Osteoporosis	None	—	None	Perimenopausal estrogen for at least 7 yr
				Calcium and vitamin D supplementation
Tuberculosis	PPD	Yearly	Chest radiograph to identify active disease, mycobacterial culture	In nursing home residents

*T_4 = thyroxine; TSH = thyrotropin.

hearing, dementia), cardiovascular disease (hypertension, cholesterol), cancer (cervix, breast, colorectal, and prostate), and other health conditions (alcohol abuse, hypothyroidism, osteoporosis, and tuberculosis). A summary of recommended measures for secondary prevention is provided in Table 8.4.

Visual Impairment

Visual impairment in the elderly can result from a variety of treatable conditions such as cataracts, diabetic retinopathy, and glaucoma. Whatever the cause, diminished vision restricts functional independence directly and contributes to other health hazards such as motor vehicle accidents and falls. Several studies have demonstrated that poor vision, usually identified through testing of static visual acuity, is associated with decrease in ability to perform activities of daily living, depression, less satisfying social relationships, and decreased frequency of driving (49,50). Randomized trials to demonstrate the benefits of correction of visual impairment on function in the elderly have not been performed. A nonexperimental evaluation of elderly persons before and after cataract surgery found that the procedure not only enhanced visual acuity, but increased functional abilities

such as driving and reading a newspaper. After cataract surgery, individuals also demonstrated improvements in measures of mental status and manual performance (51). Another common sense intervention to compensate for diminished visual acuity is home evaluation to improve lighting and reduce hazards for falls. To prevent the functional losses that result from decreased vision, regular screening for visual acuity is prudent for elderly persons.

Hearing Impairment

Audiologic evidence of hearing loss is present in over one-third of persons over the age of 65, but only about 25 percent of elderly individuals report problems with hearing (52). Impaired hearing, whether alone or combined with other sensory deficits such as visual impairment, results in substantial loss of functional independence among the elderly. Numerous studies have shown associations between hearing impairment and communication problems, cognitive loss, depression, and social isolation (53). A 10-item screening questionnaire, the Hearing Handicap Inventory for the Elderly–Screening version (HHIE-S), was developed to identify functional consequences of hearing impairment (54). This questionnaire had an overall accuracy of about 75 percent, in comparison with the "gold standard" of pure-tone audiometry (53). A portable Audioscope (Welch Allyn, Inc., Skaneateles Falls, NY) has also been evaluated and shows a sensitivity of roughly 90 percent and a specificity of approximately 80 percent for detecting hearing loss (53,54). The best evidence to justify screening for hearing impairment in the elderly derives from a recent randomized trial that evaluated improvement in functional abilities after provision of hearing aids (52). In this study, over 80 percent of the 194 patients who enrolled reported adverse effects on functional status because of hearing impairment at baseline. In comparison with individuals randomized to a waiting list for hearing aids, those who received the hearing aid immediately demonstrated significant improvements in social and emotional function, communication, cognition, and depression. Periodic screening for hearing loss by questionnaire or audioscopy should be performed regularly in the elderly.

Screening for Dementia

Early detection of cognitive impairment in the elderly has been advocated to identify potentially reversible causes, such as depression or adverse drug reactions, to modify the home environment and provide guidance to caregivers, and to prompt discussion of advance directives. Severe dementia occurs in 2.5 percent to 5.0 percent of community-dwelling seniors; mild dementia occurs in 4.3 percent to 12.7 percent. The prevalence of dementia is substantially higher among the oldest old, with rates as high as 47 percent among nonagenarians (55). Of the screening tests advocated for dementia, the Folstein Mini-Mental State Examination (MMSE) has been used most widely because of its brevity and ease of administration. Although the test has age-, race-, and education-dependent norms, the customary cutoff defines mild dementia as a score of 23 or less of the 30 points possible, and severe dementia as a score of 17 or less. At a cutoff of 23, the MMSE has a sensitivity of 84 percent and a specificity of 90 percent among Caucasians, and an overall accuracy of 94 percent in distinguishing cognitively normal seniors from those with dementia (56,57).

Despite the substantial burden of illness imposed by dementia and the existence of an accurate screening test,

the role of screening for cognitive impairment in community-dwelling seniors remains controversial. No randomized trials have demonstrated that early detection of cognitive impairment improves health, and some authorities raise concerns that individuals identified with dementia may be stigmatized by their social network or by health professionals (55). The lack of clear benefit for screening combined with the possibility of negative "labeling" led the Canadian Task Force on the Periodic Health Examination to conclude that existing evidence is insufficient either to include or exclude screening for cognitive impairment in the package of preventive services for the elderly (55). Although concurring with this conclusion, the USPSTF suggests that clinicians inquire into the functional status of elderly patients at home to identify any functional decline that might signal the onset of cognitive impairment, and thereby prompt comprehensive geriatric assessment to maintain functional independence (58).

Hypertension Screening

Blood pressure in elderly patients should be checked at every office visit and at least every two years. Hypertension can be diagnosed after several readings, ideally obtained both in and outside the office setting, show diastolic blood pressure consistently greater than 90 mm Hg or systolic blood pressure greater than 160 mm Hg. In the last 10 years, several studies have demonstrated that treatment of diastolic hypertension or isolated systolic hypertension (systolic blood pressure greater than 160 mm Hg without concurrent elevation of diastolic blood pressure) reduces strokes and cardiac events in elderly individuals (9,59–61). From a public health perspective, the number of elderly hypertensives who must be treated to prevent a stroke is substantially lower than that for younger hypertensives. The benefits of treating hypertension persist at least to the age of 84; existing studies have enrolled too few patients of ages older than 84 years to demonstrate the continuing efficacy of treatment.

Cholesterol Screening

In contrast to the clear benefits of treating hypertension, the role of cholesterol screening and treatment of hyperlipidemia in the elderly is highly controversial. The prevalence of hypercholesterolemia is very high in the elderly; nearly 50 percent of women and one-third of men have serum cholesterol levels of 240 mg/dL (6.2 mmol/liter) or greater (62). However, the association between elevated cholesterol and cardiovascular disease is weaker in the elderly than it is in younger individuals. Elevated serum cholesterol remains a risk factor for coronary artery disease, with a relative risk of 1.5 to 1.7 in the highest quartile of serum cholesterol (63), but little relationship has been shown between serum cholesterol and all-case mortality in elderly individuals (64). In younger individuals, randomized trials of lipid-lowering medications have demonstrated a small absolute reduction in coronary artery disease in hyperlipidemic men, but no reduction in all-cause mortality (65,66). No comparable studies exist for the elderly. In contrast to individuals without known coronary artery disease, substantial evidence exists showing that tertiary prevention through lipid-lowering is appropriate for persons with known coronary artery disease (67). Thus, existing evidence does not conclusively demonstrate the benefit of screening and treatment for elevated serum cholesterol in the elderly. Dietary modification, which can reduce low-density lipoprotein (LDL) levels by 5 percent to 15 percent, seems prudent for all individuals aged 65 and older (62). If serum cholesterol remains elevated despite dietary changes, medication may be warranted in individuals with known coronary artery disease. Given the high cost and uncertain effectiveness of lipid-lowering medications in asymptomatic elderly individuals, however, the use of lipid-lowering drugs for primary prevention cannot yet be recommended.

Cervical Cancer Screening

Cervical cancer is often viewed as a problem of young women, but the incidence of the disease is as much as four times higher in women more than age 65; 25 percent of new cervical cancers and 40 percent of total cervical cancer deaths occur in the elderly (68,69). In one survey, 38 percent of women older than age 75 and 14 percent of women aged 65 to 75 reported *never* having had a Pap smear; an additional 28 percent reported that they had not had regular screening (70). Since widespread cervical cancer screening was not instituted until the 1950s, after

many now-elderly women had completed their reproductive years, the proportion of elderly women who have received no screening for cervical cancer is likely to decline over time. In women who have had normal Pap smears every 1 to 3 years since early adulthood, cervical cancer very rarely develops after age 65. Continued screening for these women is not necessary. For women who were not screened early in life, and particularly for disadvantaged elderly women at high risk of inadequate screening, Pap smears should be continued every 1 to 3 years after the women reach age 65. A study of a single screening Pap smear in elderly women in an inner-city clinic identified a high prevalence of cervical neoplasia (13.5 per 1,000 examinations) (68). In this same population, cervical cancer screening was cost saving, with a reduction of health care costs of about $6,000 per 100 Pap smears performed (69). Thus, screening for cervical cancer appears to be justified on both clinical and economic grounds for elderly women who have had few or no previous Pap smears and who have not had hysterectomies.

Breast Cancer Screening

Two methods have been proposed for breast cancer screening: manual breast examination by clinician and mammography though controlled trials have compared breast examination by clinician without mammography to no screening at all, annual breast examinations are recommended by all preventive care guidelines (4). The role of mammography has been defined in a series of randomized trials during the last 30 years. The relative risk of dying of breast cancer for women aged 60 to 69 who received screening mammograms every 18 months to 33 months was 0.69, that is, a 31 percent risk reduction (71). Too few women over age 70 have been entered into existing trials to estimate the effectiveness of breast cancer screening for older women. Despite this lack of information, the consensus of advisory groups is that mammographic screening and clinician breast examinations should be continued until about age 75 (72). The optimal screening interval (i.e., yearly or longer) is unknown; currently, Medicare reimburses for screening mammography performed every two years.

Colorectal Cancer Screening

About 75 percent of the 145,000 new cases of colorectal cancer each year occur in persons 65 or older (73). Two screening strategies, fecal occult blood testing (FOBT) and sigmoidoscopic examination of the rectum and distal colon, have long been advocated for colorectal cancer screening. Several recent studies have substantially bolstered evidence for the effectiveness of colorectal cancer screening of the elderly. FOBT has been advocated to detect bleeding, colonic, premalignant adenomas or carcinomas. The sensitivity of FOBT, with either of two common reagents, was approximately 26 percent; in other words, only one-fourth of malignant colorectal neoplasms were detected by this means (74). Although the specificity of FOBT was about 95 percent to 98 percent, most positive tests were not a result of colon cancer, with a positive predictive value of only 5 percent to 9 percent. Despite the low sensitivity and positive predictive value, a program of yearly FOBT was recently shown, in a randomized controlled trial, to reduce colon cancer mortality by 33 percent (75). No reduction in colorectal cancer mortality was observed in this study when screening occurred every other year. Since most of the positive FOBTs were false positives, further diagnostic evaluation (usually including colonoscopy) was performed in about 20 percent of the more than 46,000 enrollees in the study. As a result, some of the reduction in mortality observed in this study may have been caused by coincidental discovery of nonbleeding neoplasms during a colonoscopy prompted by a false-positive FOBT (76).

The sensitivity and specificity of sigmoidoscopy, whether performed with a rigid or flexible instrument, are presumed to be in excess of 90 percent. Recent case-control studies have suggested that a strategy of sigmoidoscopic screening every three to five years resulted in a 70 percent reduction in colorectal cancers occurring within the reach of the sigmoidoscope, but mortality for colorectal cancers beyond the reach of the sigmoidoscope was not affected (77). No randomized trials have confirmed this observation. However, a program of periodic flexible sigmoidoscopy may be a reasonable preventive strategy for colorectal cancer in the elderly because fewer flexible sigmoidoscopic screening examinations are necessary to prevent one colorectal cancer death in individuals aged 60 to 69 years, compared with screening in younger persons (78).

Several unresolved issues remain before a coordinated screening strategy can be recommended for colorectal cancer. First, the optimal combination of FOBT and sigmoidoscopic screening is unknown. Screening sigmoidoscopy as infrequently as every 10 years may prevent some deaths from colorectal cancer (77). Second, the effort and expense of a mass screening program for colorectal cancer in the elderly need to be assessed in the context of other health care needs. Promising approaches include selective screening of individuals at highest risk of colorectal cancer, on the basis of age or genetic markers for colorectal cancer.

Prostate Cancer Screening

In 1993, an estimated 165,000 new cases of prostate cancer were diagnosed, with 35,000 deaths. Currently, a 50-year-old American man has about a 40 percent chance of developing microscopic prostate cancer, a 10 percent chance of being diagnosed with prostate cancer, and a 2 percent to 3 percent chance of dying of the disease (79). Despite this substantial burden of illness, evidence for the effectiveness of prostate cancer screening is not compelling. Assessment of serum prostate-specific antigen (PSA), the most intensively studied screening test, is limited by the lack of studies defining the true sensitivity and specificity of the test in a screened population. In most studies, the "gold standard" test of prostate biopsy has been reserved for individuals with an abnormally high PSA, which prevents calculation of the false negative rate, and thereby the sensitivity, of the PSA (80). Further, no conclusive evidence from randomized controlled trials indicates that early diagnosis of prostate cancer reduces mortality from the disease. Some observational studies have demonstrated that the survival of individuals with early-stage prostate cancer who defer treatment until symptoms develop is comparable to that of patients treated with radiotherapy or radical prostatectomy (81). Thus, neither the performance of the most widely recommended diagnostic test nor the effectiveness of early treatment for prostate cancer are sufficiently well defined to justify a recommendation for mass screening with PSA in elderly men.

Screening for Alcohol Abuse

Alcoholism affects up to 10 percent of the elderly, and contributes to 15 percent to 20 percent of nursing home admissions, yet the problem is commonly overlooked or misdiagnosed among older adults (83). Few clinical characteristics distinguish elderly patients with alcoholism from non alcoholic seniors admitted to the hospital (84). Even when alcohol abuse was identified, physicians less often recommended specific treatment for alcoholism in elderly persons than they did for younger individuals (84).

In recent years, screening questionnaires have been used to establish the diagnosis of alcoholism in the elderly. Of these, the CAGE is the shortest and most readily adaptable for clinical use. The questionnaire consists of four questions: 1) Have you ever felt you should Cut down on your drinking? 2) Have people ever Annoyed you by criticizing your drinking? 3) Have you ever felt Guilty about your drinking? 4) Have you ever had a drink first thing in the morning (Eye opener) to steady your nerves or to get rid of a hangover? (85). Using a cutoff of two or more positive responses of four, the sensitivity of the CAGE questionnaire has been reported as 48 percent to 70 percent, with a specificity of 91 percent to 99 percent (85,86). The sensitivity of the CAGE may be lower in elderly alcohol abusers than in younger individuals.

Rigorous studies of treatment strategies in elderly individuals with alcoholism are lacking, but randomized trials in younger individuals have demonstrated the effectiveness of alcoholism detection and counseling in primary care (87). Thus, screening for alcohol abuse with instruments such as the CAGE seems justified in the elderly.

Screening for Hypothyroidism

Thyroid deficiency is common in the elderly. Estimates of the prevalence of hypothyroidism depend on whether abnormal biochemical tests alone or a combination of biochemical findings and clinical symptoms are used to define the condition. The estimated prevalence of overt hypothyroidism ranges from 0.3 percent to 1.8 percent, and the prevalence of biochemical hypothyroidism (serum thyrotropin (TSH) levels greater than $10\,\mu U/liter$) is 5.9 percent for elderly women and 2.3 percent for men (88,89). Overt hypothyroidism is more common in admis-

sions to geriatric hospitals or long-term care settings, with a prevalence of 2 percent to 4 percent (89). Both the total thyroxine (T_4) and the sensitive TSH have been advocated as screening tests for thyroid deficiency. Using a cutoff of $7\,\mu g/dL$, T_4 was reported to have a sensitivity of roughly 93 percent and a specificity ranging from 68 percent to 81 percent, and TSH had a sensitivity of 99 percent and a specificity ranging from 80 percent to 99 percent, using a cutoff greater than $5\,\mu U/liter$ (89,90). The choice of screening tests (T_4 or TSH) may depend in part on the comparative cost of the two tests.

Most authorities concur that mass screening for hypothyroidism is not justified in men of any age or in young women because of the low prevalence of the disease. However, there is greater justification for screening in older women because of the higher prevalence of overt or biochemical hypothyroidism in the context of symptoms that might be attributable to thyroid disease. On the basis of the prevalence of the disease, the ease and inexpensiveness of screening, and the efficacy of thyroxine replacement for individuals with overt hypothyroidism, the USPSTF has suggested that screening for thyroid dysfunction in elderly women may be "clinically prudent" (4), but this recommendation is not supported by evidence from randomized trials.

Osteoporosis Prevention

Although bone loss in women usually accelerates at the time of menopause, the health consequences of osteoporosis are most prominent in the elderly. Twenty-five percent of women more than 70 years of age have had vertebral fractures, which are often asymptomatic. Over 90 percent of hip fractures occur in women older than age 70 (91). Until recently, most studies of osteoporosis prevention focused on therapy during the perimenopausal years and excluded elderly women. Recent studies concerning the role of screening for osteoporosis, the use of estrogens, and the importance of dietary supplementation with calcium and vitamin D have clarified an approach to prevention of bone loss and fractures in older women.

Although methods of screening for osteoporosis using bone densitometry have been developed, no studies demonstrate that the long-term outcomes of asymptomatic women are improved by osteoporosis screening. Thus, universal screening is not currently recommended, and emphasis in osteoporosis prevention has been placed on pharmacologic measures (92).

Randomized trials beginning in the perimenopausal period have demonstrated the effectiveness of estrogens (typically, conjugated estrogens at doses of 0.625 mg/day) in preventing bone loss and vertebral fractures; epidemiologic studies have suggested that estrogen use also reduces hip and wrist fractures (92). Among older women in the Framingham study, bone density measured at a mean age of 76 years was significantly higher in women who had used estrogen for seven years or more than it was in women who had used estrogen replacement for shorter periods of time or not at all (93). Benefit was limited to women less than 75 years of age, which led many authorities to conclude estrogen is of little benefit to women older than age 75 (94).

In women 70 years and older, ongoing bone loss is often caused by increased parathyroid hormone secretion stimulated by inadequate dietary intake of vitamin D and calcium. A recent randomized trial demonstrated that dietary supplementation with 1.2 gm/day of elemental calcium and 800 IU of vitamin D_3 preserved bone density and reduced the rate of hip fractures and total nonvertebral fractures in a large group of women whose mean age was 84 years (95). Thus, a lifelong strategy for osteoporosis prevention should include institution of estrogen therapy for at least seven years after menopause, with ongoing supplementation with calcium and vitamin D if dietary intake is insufficient.

Observational studies have suggested that estrogen replacement reduced the risk of coronary artery disease by 50 percent (96). The impact of concurrent progestin use on the protective effect of estrogen is unclear. As yet, however, no randomized trials have confirmed that estrogen replacement prevents coronary artery disease; a large study to address this question is ongoing. Thus, although the role of estrogen in primary or secondary prevention of osteoporosis and its complications is well defined in the elderly, the use of estrogen as primary prevention for cardiovascular disease requires further study.

Tuberculosis Prevention

Tuberculosis continues to be a problem in the elderly, particularly in residents of nursing homes. In 1987, the 6150 cases of tuberculosis that occurred in persons aged 65 or older represented 27 percent of the total U.S. cases, although this age group comprised only 12 percent of the population (97). The incidence of endemic or nosocomial tuberculosis among nursing home residents is approximately twice that of elderly persons living in the community (97,98). Health care workers in nursing homes are also at high risk. As noted earlier, the proportion of individuals with a positive tuberculin skin test declines with age, for a variety of reasons that may include immunologic or cutaneous changes and the increasing remoteness of the primary tuberculosis infection (7). Tuberculosis screening in the elderly should consist of first-step testing with purified protein derivative tuberculin (PPD-T) (5 TU), followed by a second PPD-T of the same strength one week later in individuals whose initial test is negative (97). A positive response is defined by 10 mm of induration on either test. Individuals with a positive skin test should receive a chest radiograph to identify current or past disease. Most positive tuberculosis skin tests in the elderly are caused by remote primary infection and should not be treated with isoniazid prophylaxis. However, active tuberculosis should be considered in these individuals if the person develops signs or symptoms such as a prolonged cough, weight loss, or unexplained fever. PPD skin testing should be repeated yearly in all nursing home residents to identify recent converters who may require isoniazid treatment (99).

Summary

Over the past 10 years, substantial research has accrued to define appropriate primary and secondary prevention strategies for the elderly. Although some authorities advocate additional preventive measures in the elderly (Table 8.5), clinicians should insist on a high standard of evidence before incorporating preventive maneuvers into clinical practice. Preventive care, in which the physician makes a recommendation to an individual without symptoms, differs in important ways from most health care encounters, in which the patient seeks the guidance of the physician to remedy a specific complaint (80). This crucial difference imposes a special obligation on the physician to ensure that preventive care recommendations are based on high-quality evidence for effectiveness and (if possi-

Table 8.5. Health Conditions for Which Preventive Measures Have Been Advocated, But Proof of Benefit Is Lacking.

Primary Prevention
    Pneumococcal immunization
    Injuries due to falls
    Other accidental injuries
    Aspirin chemoprevention
    Adverse drug reactions
Secondary Prevention
    Dementia
    Hyperlipidemia
    Prostate cancer
    Skin cancer
    Oral cancer
    Depression
    Urinary tract infection
    Urinary incontinence
    Elder abuse

---

ble) cost-effectiveness, because preventive efforts not justified by improved outcomes may cause anxiety or expense without improvement of function or longevity.

References

1. Katz S, Branch LG, Branson MH, et al. Active life expectancy. N Engl J Med 1983;309:1218–1225.
2. Rowe JW. Health care of the elderly. N Engl J Med 1985;312:827–835.
3. Breslow L, Somers AR. The lifetime health-monitoring program. N Engl J Med 1977;296:601–608.
4. U.S. Preventive Services Task Force. Guide to clinical preventive services. Baltimore: Williams & Wilkins, 1989.
5. Canadian Task Force on the Periodic Health Examination. The periodic health examination. Can Med Assoc J 1979; 121:1193–1254.
6. Fletcher RM, Fletcher SW, Wagner EH. Clinical epidemiology–the essentials. Baltimore, Williams & Wilkins, 1982:67.
7. Dorken E, Grzybowski S, Allen EA. Significance of the tuberculin test in the elderly. Chest 1987;92:237–240.
8. Simberkoff MS, Cross AP, Al-Ibrahim M, et al. Efficacy of pneumococcal vaccine in high-risk patients. N Engl J Med 1986;315:1318–1327.
9. SHEP Cooperative Research Group. Prevention of stroke by antihypertensive drug treatment in older persons with isolated systolic hypertension. JAMA 1991;265:3255–3264.
10. Applegate W, Deyo R, Kramer A. Meehan S. Geriatric evaluation and management: current status and future research directions. J Am Geriatr Soc 1991;39(suppl):2S–7S.
11. Beers MH, Fink A, Beck JC. Screening recommendations for the elderly. Am J Public Health 1991;81:1131–1140.
12. LaForce FM. Adult immunizations: are they worth the trou-
ble? J Gen Intern Med 1990;5(suppl):S57–S61.
13. McBean AM, Babish JD, Warren JL. The impact and cost of influenza in the elderly. Arch Intern Med 1993;153:2105–2111.
14. Margolis KL, Nichol KL, Poland GA, Pluhar RE. Frequency of adverse reactions to influenza vaccine in the elderly. JAMA 1990;264:1139–1141.
15. Gross PA, Quinnan GV, Rodstein M, et al. Association of influenza immunization with reduction in mortality in an elderly population. Arch Intern Med 1988;148:562–565.
16. Nichol KL, Margolis KL, Wuorenma J, Von Sternberg T. Efficacy and cost savings of influenza vaccination among community living seniors. J Gen Intern Med 1994;9(suppl 2):89. Abstract.
17. Nichol KL, Margolis KL, Wuorenma J, Von Sternberg T. The efficacy and cost effectiveness of vaccination against influenza among elderly persons living in the community. N Engl J Med 1994;331:778–784.
18. Hirschmann JV, Lipsky BA. The pneumococcal vaccine after 15 years of use. Arch Intern Med 1994;154:373–377.
19. Shapiro ED, Berg AT, Austrian R, et al. The protective efficacy of polyvalent pneumococcal polysaccharide vaccine. N Engl J Med 1991;325:1453–1460.
20. Butler JC, Breiman RF, Campbell JF, et al. Pneumococcal polysaccharide vaccine efficacy. JAMA 1993;270:1826–1831.
21. LaForce FM, Eickhoff TC. Pneumococcal vaccine: an emerging consensus. Ann Intern Med 1988;108:757–759. Editorial.
22. Recommendations of the Immunization Practices Advisory Committee: pneumococcal polysaccharide vaccine. MMWR Morb Mortal Wkly Rep 1989;38:64–76.
23. Richardson JP, Knight AL. The prevention of tetanus in the elderly. Arch Intern Med 1991;151:1712–1717.
24. LaForce FM. Routine tetanus immunizations for adults: once is enough. J Gen Intern Med 1993;8:459–460.
25. Josephson KR, Fabacher DA, Rubenstein LZ. Home safety and fall prevention. Clin Geriatr Med 1991;7:707–731.
26. Hornbrook MC, Stevens VJ, Wingfield DJ, et al. Preventing falls among community-dwelling older persons: results from a randomized trial. Gerontologist 1994;34:16–23.
27. Lauritzen JB, Petersen MM, Lund B. Effect of external hip protectors on hip fractures. Lancet 1993;341:11–13.
28. Wolf ME, Rivara FP. Nonfall injuries in older adults. Annu Rev Public Health 1992;13:509–528.
29. Woolf SH, Kamerow DB, Lawrence RS, Medalie JH, Estes EH. The periodic health examination of older adults: the recommendations of the U.S. Preventive Services Task Force. Part 1. Counseling, immunizations, and chemoprophylaxis. J Am Geriatr Soc 1990;38:817–823.
30. Peto R, Gray R, Collins R, et al. Randomized trial of prophylactic daily aspirin in British male doctors. BMJ 1988;296:313–316.
31. Steering Committee of the Physicians' Health Study Research Group. Final report of the aspirin component of the ongoing Physicians' Health Study. N Engl J Med 1989; 321:129–135.

32. Canadian Task Force on the Periodic Health Examination. Periodic health examination, 1991 update: 6. Acetylsalicylic acid and the primary prevention of cardiovascular disease. Can Med Assoc J 1991;145:1091–1095.

33. Manson JE, Stampfer MJ, Colditz GA, et al. A prospective study of aspirin use and primary prevention of cardiovascular disease in women. JAMA 1991;266:521–527.

34. LaCroix AZ, Omenn GS. Older adults and smoking. Clin Geriatr Med 1992;8:69–87.

35. Jajich CL, Ostfeld AM, Freeman DH. Smoking and coronary heart disease mortality in the elderly. JAMA 1984;252:2831–2834.

36. Hermanson B, Omenn GS, Kronmal RA, Gersh BJ. Beneficial six-year outcome of smoking cessation in older men and women with coronary artery disease. N Engl J Med 1988;319:1365–1369.

37. Kottke TE, Battista RN, DeFriese GH, Brekke ML. Attributes of successful smoking cessation interventions in medical practice: a meta-analysis of 39 controlled trials. JAMA 1988;259:2882–2889.

38. Bienia R, Ratcliff S, Barbour GL, Kummer M. Malnutrition in the hospitalized geriatric patient. J Am Geriatr Soc 1982; 30:433–436.

39. Goodwin JS, Goodwin JM, Garry PJ. Association between nutritional status and cognitive functioning in a healthy elderly population. JAMA 1983;249:2917–2921.

40. Morley JE. Why do physicians fail to recognize and treat malnutrition in older persons? J Am Geriatr Soc 1991; 39:1139–1140.

41. Delmi M, Rapin CH, Bengoa JM, et al. Dietary supplementation in elderly patients with fractured neck of the femur. Lancet 1990;335:1013–1016.

42. Chandra RK. Effect of vitamin and trace-element supplementation on immune responses and infection in elderly subjects. Lancet 1992;340:1124–1127.

43. Larsson J, Unosson M, Ek AC, et al. Effect of dietary supplement on nutritional status and clinical outcome in 501 geriatric patients—a randomized study. Clin Nutr 1990;9:179–184.

44. Wagner EH, LaCroix AZ, Buchner DM, Larson EB. Effects of physical activity on health status in older adults. I. Observational studies. Annu Rev Public Health 1992;13:451–468.

45. Surgeon General's Workshop on Health Promotion and Aging. Summary recommendations of physical fitness and exercise working group. MMWR Morb Mortal Wkly Rep 1989;38:700–707.

46. Paffenbarger RS, Hyde RT, Wing AL, Hsieh CC. Physical activity, all-cause mortality, and longevity of college alumni. N Engl J Med 1986;314:605–613.

47. Buchner DM, Beresford SAA, Larson EB, et al. Effects of physical activity on health status in older adults. II. Intervention studies. Annu Rev Public Health 1992;13:469–488.

48. McMurdo ME, Rennie L. A controlled trial of exercise by residents of old people's homes. Age Ageing 1993;22:11–15.

49. Marx MS, Werner P, Cohen-Mansfield J, Feldman R. The relationship between low vision and performance of activities of daily living in nursing home residents. J Am Geriatr Soc 1992;40:1018–1020.

50. Carabellese C, Appollonio I, Rozzini R, et al. Sensory impairment and quality of life in a community elderly population. J Am Geriatr Soc 1993;41:401–407.

51. Applegate WB, Miller ST, Elam JT, et al. Impact of cataract surgery with lens implantation on vision and physical function in elderly patients. JAMA 1987;257:1064–1066.

52. Mulrow CD, Aguilar C, Endicott JE, et al. Quality of life changes and hearing impairment. A randomized trial. Ann Intern Med 1990;113:188–194.

53. Mulrow CD, Lichtenstein MJ. Screening for hearing impairment in the elderly: rationale and strategy. J Gen Intern Med 1991;6:249–258.

54. Lichtenstein MJ, Bess FH, Logan SA. Validation of screening tools for identifying hearing-impaired elderly in primary care. JAMA 1988;259:2875–2878.

55. Canadian Task Force on the Periodic Health Examination. Periodic health examination, 1991 update: 1. Screening for cognitive impairment in the elderly. Can Med Assoc J 1991;144:425–431.

56. Fillenbaum G, Heyman A, Williams K, et al. Sensitivity and specificity of standardized screens of cognitive impairment and dementia among elderly black and white community residents. J Clin Epidemiol 1990;43:651–660.

57. Ritchie K, Fuhrer R. A comparative study of the performance of screening tests for senile dementia using receiver operating characteristics-analysis. J Clin Epidemiol 1992;45:627–637.

58. Woolf SH, Kamerow DB, Lawrence RS, et al. The periodic health examination of older adults: The recommendations of the U.S. Preventive Services Task Force. Part II. Screening tests. J Am Geriatr Soc 1990;38:933–942.

59. Amery A, Birkenhager W, Brixko P, et al. Mortality and morbidity results from the European Working Party on High Blood Pressure in the Elderly trial. Lancet 1985;2:1349–1354.

60. Dahlof B, Lindholm LH, Hansson L, et al. Morbidity and mortality in the Swedish Trial in Old Patients with Hypertension (STOP–Hypertension). Lancet 1991;338:1281–1285.

61. Beard K, Bulpitt C, Mascie-Taylor H, et al. Management of elderly patients with sustained hypertension. BMJ 1992;304:412–416.

62. Garber AM, Littenberg B, Sox HC, et al. Costs and health consequences of cholesterol screening for asymptomatic older Americans. Arch Intern Med 1991;151:1089–1095.

63. Rubin SM, Sidney S, Black DM, et al. High blood cholesterol in elderly men and the excess risk for coronary heart disease. Ann Intern Med 1990;113:916–920.

64. Kronmal RA, Cain KC, Ye Z, Omenn GS. Total serum cholesterol levels and mortality risk as a function of age. Arch Intern Med 1993;153:1065–1073.

65. Lipid Research Clinics Program. The Lipid Research Clinics Coronary Primary Prevention Trial results: I. Reduction in incidence of coronary heart disease. JAMA 1984;251:351–364.

66. Frick MH, Elo O, Haapa K, Heinonen OP. Helsinki Heart

Study: primary prevention trial with gemfibrozil in middle-aged men with dyslipidemia. N Engl J Med 1987;317:1237–1245.

67. Blankenhorn DH, Nessim SA, Johnson RI, et al. Beneficial effects of combined colestipol-niacin therapy on coronary atherosclerosis and coronary venous grafts. JAMA 1987; 257:3233–3240.

68. Mandelblatt J, Gopaul I, Wistreich M. Gynecological care of elderly women: another look at Papanicolaou smear testing. JAMA 1986;256:367–371.

69. Mandelblatt JS, Fahs MC. The cost-effectiveness of cervical cancer screening for low-income elderly women. JAMA 1988;259:2409–2413.

70. Celentano DD, Shapiro S, Weisman CS. Cancer preventive screening among elderly women. Prev Med 1982;11:454–463.

71. Nystrom L, Rutqvist LE, Wall S, et al. Breast cancer screening with mammography: overview of Swedish randomized trials. Lancet 1993;341:973–978.

72. Nattinger AB, Goodwin JS, Screening mammography for older women. Arch Intern Med 1992;152:922–925.

73. Wagner JL, Herdman RC, Wadwha S. Cost effectiveness of colorectal cancer screening in the elderly. Ann Intern Med 1991;115:807–817.

74. Ahlquist DA, Wieand HS, Moertel CG, et al. Accuracy of fecal occult blood screening for colorectal neoplasia. JAMA 1993;269:1262–1267.

75. Mandel JS, Bond JH, Church TR, et al. Reducing mortality from colorectal cancer by screening for fecal occult blood. N Engl J Med 1993;328:1365–1371.

76. Lang CA, Ransohoff DF. Fecal occult blood screening for colorectal cancer. Is mortality reduced by chance selection for screening colonoscopy? JAMA 1994;271:1011–1013.

77. Selby JV, Friedman GD, Quesenberry CP, Weiss NS. A case-control study of screening sigmoidoscopy and mortality from colorectal cancer. N Engl J Med 1992;326:653–657.

78. Ransohoff DF, Lang CA. Sigmoidoscopic screening in the 1990s. JAMA 1993;269:1278–1281.

79. Garnick MD. Prostate cancer: screening, diagnosis and management. Ann Intern Med 1993;118:804–818.

80. Sox HC. Preventive health services in adults. N Engl J Med 1994;330:1589–1595.

81. Johansson JE, Adami HO, Andersson SO, et al. High 10-year survival rate in patients with early, untreated prostatic cancer. JAMA 1992;267:2191–2196.

82. Dorr VJ, Williamson SK, Stephens RL. An evaluation of prostate-specific antigen as a screening test for prostate cancer. Arch Intern Med 1993;153:2529–2537.

83. Solomon DH. Alcoholism and aging. In: West LJ. Alcohol-ism. Ann Intern Med 1984;100:411–412.

84. Curtis JR, Geller G, Stokes EJ, Levine DM, Moore RD. Characteristics, diagnosis, and treatment of alcoholism in elderly patients. J Am Geriatr Soc 1989;37:310–316.

85. Jones TV, Lindsey BA, Yount P, et al. Alcoholism screening questionnaires: are they valid in elderly medical outpatients? J Gen Intern Med 1993;8:674–678.

86. Buchsbaum DG, Buchanan RG, Welsh J, et al. Screening for drinking disorders in the elderly using the CAGE questionnaire. J Am Geriatr Soc 1992;40:662–665.

87. Wallace P, Cutler S, Haines A. Randomized controlled trial of general practitioner intervention in patients with excessive alcohol consumption. BMJ 1988;297:663–667.

88. Sawin CT, Castelli WP, Hershman JM, et al. The aging thyroid: thyroid deficiency in the Framingham study. Arch Intern Med 1985;145:1386–1388.

89. Helfand M, Crapo LM. Screening for thyroid disease. Ann Intern Med 1990;112:840–849.

90. Schectman JM, Pawlson LG. The cost-effectiveness of three thyroid function testing strategies for suspicion of hypothyroidism in a primary care setting. J Gen Intern Med 1990;5:9–15.

91. Resnick NM, Greenspan SL. "Senile" osteoporosis reconsidered. JAMA 1989;261:1025–1029.

92. Melton LJ, Eddy DM, Johnston CC. Screening for osteoporosis. Ann Intern Med 1990;112:516–528.

93. Felson DT, Zhang Y, Hannan MT, et al. The effect of postmenopausal estrogen therapy on bone density in elderly women. N Engl J Med 1993;329:1141–1146.

94. Riggs BL, Melton LJ. The prevention and treatment of osteoporosis. N Engl J Med 1992;327:620–627.

95. Chapuy MC, Arlot ME, Duboeuf F, et al. Vitamin D_3 and calcium to prevent hip fractures in elderly women. N Engl J Med 1992;327:1637–1642.

96. Psaty BM, Heckbert SR, Atkins D, et al. A review of the association of estrogens and progestins with cardiovascular disease in postmenopausal women. Arch Intern Med 1993;153:1421–1427.

97. Advisory Committee for Elimination of Tuberculosis. Prevention and control of tuberculosis in facilities providing long-term care to the elderly. MMWR Morb Mortal Wkly Rep 1990;39 RR-10:7–20.

98. Stead WW, Lofgren JP, Warren E, Thomas C. Tuberculosis as an endemic and nosocomial infection among the elderly in nursing homes. N Engl J Med 1985:1483–1487.

99. Stead WW, To T, Harrison RW, Abraham JH. Benefit-risk considerations in preventive treatment for tuberculosis in elderly persons. Ann Intern Med 1987;107:843–845.

Chapter 9
Emergency Care of the Older Person

Arthur B. Sanders

Being over seventy is like being engaged in a war. All our friends are going or gone and we survive amongst the dead and the dying as on a battlefield.

Muriel Spark
Memento Mori

Most older persons need emergency care sometime in their lives. Data from the National Center For Health Statistics (NCHS) indicates that emergency medical services (EMS) are a major point of care for older patients. In a 1992 NCHS survey of hospital ambulatory care services, persons aged 65 to 74 years had an estimated 31.4 emergency department (ED) visits per 100 persons per year. Persons age 75 years and older had 55.8 visits per 100 persons per year (1). The need for emergency medical care increases with age. Persons 75 years and older are more than twice as likely to use EMS than are younger persons aged 45 to 64 years (1).

Two studies over the past several years have demonstrated the importance of the emergency medical care system to older persons. An analysis of 1.2 million emergency department visits in 1992 found that 15 percent of all ED visits were by persons 65 years of age or older (2). This data projects to a total of 13.7 million ED visits by older persons in 1990. The breakdown of this group by age was as follows: 6.3 million ED visits for patients age 65 to 74 years, 5 million visits by patients age 75 to 84 years, and 2.3 million visits by patients 85 or older (2). A more recent study by the NCHS reviewed ED visits in 1992 and estimated that 12.6 million patients aged 65 or older visited EDs. These data included 5.8 million patients age 65 to 74 years and 6.8 million age 75 years or older (1).

Most elderly patients come to the ED because they feel they are "too sick to wait for an office visit" (3). About one-third of older patients are referred to the ED by their primary care provider (3). Evidence from multicenter studies indicates that elderly persons who visit EDs represent an ill population. On admission to the ED, 78 percent of elderly were classified as either high or intermediate urgency (4).

The level of emergency medical resources used by older persons appears to be quite high. To get to emergency departments, 30 percent of older patients use ambulance transport compared with 9 percent ambulance use for the nonelderly population (2). In fact, 36 percent of all ambulance transports to EDs were for patients 65 years or older. Similarly, 46 percent of elderly patients received comprehensive ED services (2). Approximately one-third to one-half of elderly patients seen in EDs are admitted to the hospital; 7 percent go to intensive care units (2,4), compared with 8 percent of nonelderly patients admitted to the hospital and 1.3 percent of nonelderly admitted to intensive care units. In addition, 78 percent of elderly persons cared for in EDs receive laboratory tests, and 77 percent receive radiographs (4). The elderly spend about 30 minutes longer in the ED than do the nonelderly (4). Additional time is needed for the higher level of service and diagnostic tests.

Elderly patients discharged from the ED are more likely than nonelderly patients to have problems in caring for themselves as a result of their acute illness. Twenty-one percent of older persons discharged from EDs reported a change in their ability to care for themselves as a result of their injury or illness (4). Despite noting problems with waiting time and expense of ED care, 96 percent of older patients were satisfied with their emergency medical care (4,5). These data reinforce the concept that emergency medical care is a major element in the overall management of older persons. The EMS system needs to be integrated into the care plan for older patients.

Emergency Medicine Model of Care

Emergency medicine was recognized in 1979 by the American Board of Medical Specialties as the twenty-third medical specialty and certification board examinations began in 1980. In 1994, there were more than 100 residency training programs in emergency medicine and approximately 23,000 emergency physicians. Because these disciplines are so new, many primary care physicians may not be familiar with the model of care used in EDs and the principles and elements of the emergency medical care system. Because older persons use EMS so frequently, primary care physicians and geriatricians need to understand the emergency medical care system in their community—both the prehospital EMS system and care in the ED.

Prehospital Care

The EMS system begins in the prehospital phase with response to a medical call for help. In many communities, public service agencies such as the fire departments provide prehospital services and interface with ambulance companies. In other communities, a mix of private sector and public EMS services is available.

The extension of medical services into the community is a major change that has evolved over the last 20 years in our health care system. In the 1960s ambulances were regarded as horizontal taxis. Many ambulance services were run by funeral homes. There were no standards or medical control for emergency attendants. Experience with well-trained paramedics in the military in Vietnam and Korea proved that nonphysicians can provide life-saving treatment in the field for seriously ill victims of multisystem trauma (6).

At the same time, cardiologists noted that the large investments that hospitals made in developing cardiac care units for patients with acute myocardial infarction made little impact on overall mortality. Most patients died of ventricular fibrillation in the first few hours after their infarct before they ever reached the cardiac care unit. Pioneering efforts in several cities demonstrated that quality emergency medical care can be extended outside the hospital into the community (7–10). Paramedics can be taught to provide sophisticated medical care, including defibrillation, endotracheal intubation, and adminis-

tration of cardiac drugs at the scene for a patient with a myocardial infarction or cardiac arrest. This effort has made a major impact in survival from cardiac arrest (11–13). For example, data from Seattle show that if cardiopulmonary resuscitation (CPR) is provided within four minutes and defibrillation within eight minutes of cardiac arrest, 43 percent of patients with ventricular fibrillation survive to hospital discharge (12). Twenty years ago, these patients would have died before arriving at the hospital.

To be successful, EMS must be a coordinated system of care involving communications, triage, transportation, documentation, medical control, training, and continuing education. Each state has a lead EMS agency that sets standards and provides resources for communities (cities or counties) to implement. Each community's EMS system is unique; therefore, geriatricians and primary care providers need to be familiar with the system of EMS in their community. Table 9.1 lists a summary of the training and capabilities of prehospital care providers in the United States (6).

Table 9.1. Prehospital Care Providers.

Level	Training (hr)	Capabilities
Dispatch	25	Prioritize calls, dispatch appropriate level of care
First responders	50	CPR, first aid
EMT-A*	120–150	CPR, extrication, splinting, spinal immobilization, airway bagging, oxygen support, transport
EMT-D*	40	Duties of EMT-A plus defibrillation
EMT-P*	500–1500	Endotracheal intubation, defibrillation, medications, intravenous support, chest decompression, cricothyrotomy

Modified from Kromer JR, Hunt R. Emergency medical services and prehospital personnel in emergency medicine. In: Hamilton GC, Sanders AB, Trott AT, Strange CR, eds. Emergency medicine: an approach to clinical problem solving. Philadelphia: WB Saunders, 1991:1119.
*EMT-A = emergency medical technicians; EMT-D = emergency medical technicians with training for defibrillation; EMT-P = paramedics; CPR = cardiopulmonary resuscitation.

First responders are generally police or fire department personnel and are used in some communities to render first aid or give CPR until more sophisticated care arrives. Basic emergency medical technicians (EMT-A) receive 120 to 150 hours of training. They can perform CPR, patient extrication, splinting and immobilization, administer oxygen, and communicate with other EMS providers. EMTs generally work on defined community protocols under the direction of an emergency physician (6). Some EMTs have also received additional training in the use of a defibrillator (EMT-D) and can defibrillate patients in ventricular fibrillation in the field by use of defined medical protocols (14–16).

Paramedics (EMT-P) receive about 1000 hours of training and must pass certifying examinations mandated by each state's EMS agency. They are capable of delivering sophisticated emergency medical care such as endotracheal intubation, intravenous fluid and drug administration, defibrillation, needle thoracostomy, and cricothyrotomy. Paramedics usually operate under the direction of their base station emergency physicians, but some communities use standardized protocols for certain conditions (6).

Since EMS providers frequently respond to older patients in their homes, they are often able to assess the living environment of the patient. In one study, paramedics in Akron, Ohio were taught to evaluate the home environment of elderly patients with regard to risks for health or safety (Figure 9.1) (17). Over a nine-month period, 6000 elderly patients were screened. Problems involving 197 people were identified to the Area Agency on Aging. Assessments were completed on 124 people, with problems confirmed in 121; useful interventions were implemented for 94 of 121 people with identified problems (17).

Once the patient enters the EMS system, transport to the hospital may be dictated by the medical condition of the patient. Primary care providers need to understand their local EMS system with regard to specialized care. For example, many communities have designated trauma centers capable of providing immediate surgical care to trauma victims. Other hospitals may have burn centers, pediatric centers, or hyperbaric oxygen chambers that provide specialized care for specific injuries or illnesses. Some patients may be regarded as too "unstable" to transport across town and must be brought to the nearest hospital capable of caring for the patient. Thus, occasionally, patients may not be brought to the hospital that the primary care physician is affiliated with; this policy can create inconvenience but is ultimately in the best interest of the patient. The paramedics are taught to do what they feel is best for the patient during a crisis situation. Once the patient is evaluated and stabilized in an ED, transfer to another hospital for admission can be arranged. Close communication between primary care providers and emergency physicians is the key for the optimal management of older patients.

FOLLOW-UP REPORT

Name	Priority	Hospital	Run No. ☐ ☐ ☐ ☐ ☐ ☐ ☐
Street No. City State Zip			No Problem Noted ☐ Could Not Evaluate ☐ Date ☐☐ ☐☐ ☐☐

Age	Race	Sex	Contact / Telephone	Home	Lives Alone	Original Patient	More Than 1 Patient
	W B O	M F		Y N	Y N	Y N	Y N

Names of Additional Persons: ____________

Environmental
- Temperature ____________
- Order ____________
- Sanitation ____________
- Hazards ____________

Social
- Support ____________
- Trauma ____________
- Food ____________

Activities of
- Daily Living ____________

Medical
- Hygiene ____________
- Senses ____________
- Medicines ____________
- Conditions ____________

Mental
- Confusion ____________
- Affect ____________
- ETOH ____________

____
Paramedic

Figure 9.1. Paramedic Report Form. Reproduced by permission from Gerson LW, Schelble DT, Wilson JE. Using paramedics to identify at-risk elderly. Ann Emerg Med 1992;21:6.

Emergency Department Care

In the ED, patients are often initially triaged by a nurse.

Almost 80 percent of older patients are classified as high or intermediate urgency (4). A patient with higher urgency classifications is evaluated sooner by the emergency physicians, regardless of the time of the patient's arrival. The emergency physician is usually seeing multiple patients and is constantly making priority decisions about time and ED resources. The ED must always be ready to shift gears to devote its resources to a critical patient arriving by ambulance. When the patient arrives, a focused history and physical is done on the basis of two underlying questions: 1) Is a life-threatening process causing this patient's complaint? 2) Is there an urgent disease process or injury that needs prompt diagnosis? Anticipation of urgent of emergent conditions is the underlying theme or emergency medicine. Emergency medicine tries to anticipate the worst conditions until they can be reasonably ruled out.

Often decisions are made on the basis of limited data. For example, an older patient coming to the ED complaining of chest pain, shortness of breath, dizziness, or syncope would immediately be placed on an electrocardiographic monitor, have intravenous fluids started, and have a 12-lead electrocardiograph (ECG) taken. These events would occur before, or simultaneously while the basic history and physical examination were completed. Anticipatory monitoring takes precedence over the usual orderly process of history-taking, physical examination, differential diagnosis, diagnostic tests, and so forth. The patient's final diagnosis may be bronchitis or costochondritis; this is irrelevant in the ED, however, because one of the principles of emergency care would be violated if a high-risk patient were not monitored and were not given appropriate tests to rule out life-threatening problems. The patient with a *potential* myocardial infarct can suffer cardiac arrest from ventricular fibrillation at any moment and must be treated with anticipation of this life-threatening complication. The ED workup focuses on reasonably ruling out such life- or limb-threatening processes.

Older patients are difficult to evaluate because important diseases or events such as acute myocardial infarction may present with atypical symptoms. Therefore, a more complete evaluation of older persons is often necessary during their ED visit. Also, older persons may not give a single complaint; they may reiterate a complex

of symptoms. Further, most older patients have comorbid diseases. In one multicenter ED study, 94 percent of older patients had one or more comorbid diseases (4). The ED complaint may represent a new disease process, manifestation of a chronic disease, or complication of treatment. Arriving at the correct diagnosis is frequently not possible or practical in the ED. If one can reasonably rule out immediate life-threatening processes, a full diagnostic workup can be done by primary care providers in a controlled office or clinic setting.

An understanding of these principles helps explain the data on ED resource use for older patients. Older persons are more likely to have life-threatening diseases or events such as myocardial infarction, subdural hematoma, or infarcted bowel. Since older persons present with atypical symptoms for such life-threatening conditions, more extensive ED workups such as ECGs, head computed tomography (CT) scans, or laboratory tests must be done. For example, less than half of patients over 75 years of age present with chest pain while having a myocardial infarction (18). Older persons frequently present with vague, nonspecific complaints such as "not feeling well," "weak" or "dizzy," which may necessitate a comprehensive ED assessment to rule out emergent conditions. Table 9.2 reviews some of the distinguishing factors about the emergency medical model of care.

It is only by understanding the EMS system and the model used to care for patients that one can appropriately advise and educate older patients. The EMS system works best for sick patients who are injured or acutely ill. It is not so appropriate for patients with manifestations of chronic problems or patients in whom acute and serious illness is not an important concern. In the last few years, another level of care in our health care system has developed, the "urgent care" center. These clinics or offices are equipped like a doctor's office. The medical model used is analogous to an unscheduled appointment in a doctor's office rather than to emergency medical care model. Urgent care centers may be appropriate for patients with less serious illnesses or injuries.

Perception of Older Patients of the Emergency Department Environment

The ED environment does not easily accommodate the needs of older persons. Many EDs have a high volume of

Table 9.2. Principles of Emergency Care.

The emergency medical system focuses on caring for acutely ill or injured patients.

Emergency medicine focuses on the patient's chief complaint.

Emergency health care providers try to anticipate and monitor patients for life- or limb-threatening illness or injury.

Beyond life-threatening processes, emergency health care professionals focus on acute disease processes that need prompt attention and on common diseases.

Making a diagnosis is not as important as ruling out life- or limb-threatening processes.

The emergency department must always be ready to divert its staff and resources to new patients with acute injuries or illnesses.

Emergency health care professionals are constantly making priority decisions regarding multiple patients and ED resource availability because of the constantly changing emergency department clientele.

Emergency health care professionals often must make immediate decisions on the basis of limited data.

Time pressures and limited resources are important elements in the care of emergency department patients.

patients with rapid turnover. The ED is a stressful environment for both patients and emergency health care providers. Privacy may not be available in every room. Occasionally, patients must be seen and treated in hallways. Patients, especially older patients, are often anxious about their condition (5). The EMS model, with its emphasis on anticipating complications and ruling out life-threatening conditions, can be very stressful for older people who do not understand the system. For example, if an older patient with a cough and vague chest tightness is treated as if he is having a heart attack, he thinks he is having a heart attack. This increases the patient's anxiety.

A report of interviews in a multicenter focus group regarding the perceptions of emergency care by the elderly documented their concerns (5). Although older patients were generally satisfied with the medical care they received in EDs, the long waits were uncomfortable for the patients and for their families. They were very anxious and frightened by their injury and illness. Most patients said that they went to the ED because they thought they had a serious or life-threatening problem. Their anxiety was not relieved until the final disposition was made (5). The ED environment was thought to be cold and noisy; patients had trouble hearing and understanding

health care professionals. Amenities such as pillows or blankets were not always available. Patients were not always informed of what was happening to them and why (5). Patients were unfamiliar with the emergency care system; they did not know when to call "911." They did not understand the concept of trauma centers, or why they may be taken to hospitals that they may not choose. Those released from the ED expressed problems with transportation and safety in getting home (5).

Primary care providers usually have the luxury of time in getting to know their patients, their values, and their family and support system before a crisis occurs. They have built an important trust relationship with the patient. The emergency care provider is unable to develop such a relationship in the short period of time while the patient is in crisis. Time pressures and ED priorities limit the amount of time the emergency physicians can spend with each patient.

Many EDs are taking steps to improve the physical environment for the patients by measures such as incorporating better lighting, making private rooms available, and adding more comfortable beds. A critical factor, however, is staff time and the ability to take the time to talk and reassure older patients. Over the past 30 years, EDs have experienced a steady growth in the number of patients seen. It is estimated that in 1992 92 million patients visited EDs (19). Resources available to EDs have not expanded proportionately. Many hospitals and EDs, especially in the inner cities, are experiencing crisis in health care reflecting overall problems in the health care system. Overcrowding, budget cuts, and lack of resources exacerbate the problem.

Optimizing Emergency Care

To optimize the care of older patients, primary care physicians must integrate emergency medicine into the health care network for their patients. This can most readily be done through patient education and the transfer of information to emergency health care providers.

Patient Education

It is very important that older patients and their caretakers understand how the EMS system works and how and when to access it. In some communities, there are systems in which frail patients can be provided with a personal emergency alarm and response device to activate the EMS system. These systems can provide a level of security and independence for some older people (20).

There is evidence in the literature that for some problems older patients wait too long before accessing EMS and coming to an ED (21–24). For example, Weaver et al found that only 5 percent of patients age 75 years or older with acute myocardial infarction had been treated with thrombolytics (21). The reason for this is multifactorial, but includes some issues that can be addressed by patient education. Older patients with acute myocardial infarction often delay seeking medical care and present with atypical symptoms such as shortness of breath or syncope (21). Ironically, the older patient can benefit most from thrombolytic treatment for acute myocardial infarction. Because of their higher mortality from myocardial infarction, older patients have the most to gain from aggressive treatment with thrombolytics (Figure 9.2) (22). Treatment, however, is only effective if given within a limited time from the onset of symptoms.

Older patients must thus be taught the signs and symptoms of acute myocardial infarction and be instructed to call "911" (if available) for immediate transport to an ED. CPR training classes can be encouraged, especially for spouses of high-risk patients. The American Heart Association "chain of survival" stresses the importance of each link in the EMS system—from patient education, bystander CPR, EMT, and paramedics to ED and critical care treatment for patients with acute vascular disease (25). When the EMS system is appropriately implemented, older persons have similar outcomes for cardiac arrest compared with those for younger persons (26,27). Therefore, aggressive treatment for cardiac arrest should be provided to all persons, regardless of age, unless advance directives indicate that the patient does not want to be resuscitated (11). An important part of geriatric practice is to work with the emergency physicians and EMS providers to educate older patients and their caretakers on the appropriate use of ambulances, EDs, urgent care centers, trauma centers, and the EMS system.

Information Transfer
One of the major problems that emergency health care professionals have in caring for older persons is acquiring

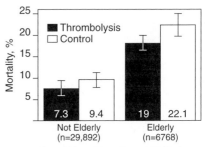

Figure 9.2. Acute myocardial infarction mortality rates in subgroups after treatment with thrombolytic therapy (with 95% confidence intervals). Although the percentage of mortality reduction is similar in the elderly (19%) and nonelderly (22%), the absolute mortality difference in lives saved per 100 patients treated is greater in the elderly group (4.2) ($P < 0.0001$) than in the nonelderly group (2.1) ($P < 0.0001$). It must be noted that the number of elderly and nonelderly patients reflects the number of patients in the compiled data, not the proportion of elderly acute myocardial infarction patients potentially eligible for thrombolytic therapy. Many of these studies specifically excluded elderly patients. Reproduced by permission from Doorey AJ, Michelson EL, Topol EJ. Thrombolytic therapy of acute myocardial infarction. JAMA 1992;268:3109.

information about the patient's baseline functional and cognitive status and their medical history. In the ED setting, with the patient in an acute medical crisis, it is often difficult for emergency care professionals to get a concise, accurate history. A survey of 433 emergency physicians regarding ED management of elderly patients revealed communication issues to be a major problem (28). Ninety-one percent of physicians reported moderate or frequent problems obtaining information from older patients, and 77 percent reported moderate or frequent problems obtaining information from a nursing home transferring the patient to the ED. In addition, 44 percent reported moderate or frequent problems obtaining information from the patient's primary care physician (28). In the same survey, information about ethical issues, such as advance directives specifying limitation of care for patients, was something that emergency physicians needed but frequently could not ascertain in the ED (28).

Primary care providers and geriatricians can work with emergency health care professionals to develop systems

Table 9.3. Emergency Medicine Information Transfer

Patient Name _____
Primary Care Physician _____
   Contact Telephone # _____
Caretaker _____
Next-of-Kin _____
ADL (list deficits) _____
IADL (list deficits) _____
Baseline Cognitive Status _____
Advance Directives _____
Chronic Diseases _____
Medications _____
Allergies _____
EKG (copy if possible)
Comments To Emergency Physician:

_____
_____
_____

Form Updated: _____

for information transfer. One simple method is for the primary care physician to provide the patient with a summary of his or her medical information. The physicians can ask the patient or caretaker to provide this information if emergency care is needed. Copies can be kept in wallets, automobiles, or other convenient places. In some systems, the information can be provided on laminated, wallet-sized cards. An example of types of information needed in EDs is provided in Table 9.3.

Advance directives are a crucial part of the medical information needed by emergency health care providers. The more detailed and more specific the information is, the more useful it will be. Many states and communities recognize portable advance directives through the EMS system (29,30). Figure 9.3 is an example of such a prehospital form endorsed by the American College of Emergency Physicians (30). If the patient does not want to have CPR performed, a standardized form acceptable to the local EMS providers can be presented to the EMTs when help is needed and the form will be respected (29,30). Similarly, some advance directives may include limitation of some aspects of care but make provision for others; these wishes must be transmitted to emergency physicians. For example, one patient may want to be treated with antibiotics for an acute infection but not want treatment for progression of a chronic disease such as

metastatic cancer. The emergency physician can use the information to guide the diagnostic tests and treatment.

The second area of information transfer involves the baseline functional and cognitive status of older persons. Many older persons have cognitive or functional deficits. The crucial question for the emergency physician is whether these deficits are new or old. Has there been a change in the patient's status? For example, a patient who comes to the ED and who has a change in functional status and no orders for limitation of care will be extensively examined for systemic problems that may be manifest as the functional change. These may include problems such as occult infections, myocardial infarction, metabolic abnormality, or stroke. If, however, the functional deficit is old and has not recently changed, exten-

---

REGIONAL EMS AUTHORITY

'DO NOT RESUSCITATE' ORDER

I, (patients full legal name), have been diagnosed as having a terminal medical illness. I have discussed both the prognosis of this illness and the treatment options with my physician, (patient's attending physician). Based on this information, I have requested that in the event of a cardiac arrest, no CPR be undertaken.

_____   _____
Patient's Signature   Attending Physician's Signature

_____   _____
Elective Date   Seal of Authorizing Agency
                                     (Optional)

_____
Expiration Date

_____
Signature of Patient Surrogate

_____
Signature of Witness

Figure 9.3. Sample authorization form by a competent patient to initiate a "do not resuscitate" order. Reproduced by permission from Emergency Medical Services Committee of the American College of Emergency Physicians. Guidelines for "Do Not Resuscitate" Orders in the Prehospital Setting. Ann Emerg Med 1988;17:1107.

sive workup may not be necessary. Similarly, baseline cognitive deficits are important to document. The use of a standardized cognitive instrument such as the Mini-Mental Status Examination can be repeated in the ED to determine changes and the extent of workup.

Summary

Older patients frequently need emergency medical care. Their experience with the EMS system can be greatly enhanced with attention to their needs by interdisciplinary programs between emergency medicine, geriatrics, and primary care physicians. Education programs that teach patients about CPR and early warning signs of acute medical conditions can also inform them of the process of EMS care. Information transfer, especially with regard to baseline function and advance directives, can help emergency care professionals provide the level of care desired by the patient.

References

1. McCraig LF. National hospital ambulatory medical care survey: 1992 emergency department summary. National Center for Health Statistics, Centers for Disease Control and Prevention, US Department of Health and Human Services, 1994.
2. Strange GR, Chen EH, Sanders AB. Use of emergency departments by elderly patients: projections from a multicenter data base. Ann Emerg Med 1992;21:819–824.
3. Hedges JR, Singal BM, Rousseau EW, et al. Geriatric patient emergency visits Part II: Perceptions of visits by geriatric and younger patients. Ann Emerg Med 1992;21:808–813.
4. Singal BM, Hedges JR, Rousseau EW, et al. Geriatric patient emergency visits Part I: Comparison of geriatric and younger patients. Ann Emerg Med 1992;21:902–807.
5. Baraff LJ, Bernstein E, Bradley K, et al. Perceptions of emergency care by the elderly: results of multicenter focus group interviews. Ann Emerg Med 1992;21:814–818.
6. Krohmer JR, Hunt R. Emergency medical services and perhospital personnel. In: Hamilton GC, Sanders AB, Trott AT, Strange GR, eds. Emergency medicine: an approach to clinical problem solving. Philadelphia: WB Saunders, 1991:1117–1130.
7. Hackett TP, Cassem NH. Factors contributing to delay in responding to the signs and symptoms of acute myocardial infarction. Am J Cardiol 1969;24:651–658.
8. Pantridge JF, Geddes JS. Cardiac arrest after myocardial infarction. Lancet 1966;1:807–808.
9. Grace WJ, Chadborun JA. The mobile coronary care unit. Dis Chest 1969;55:452–455.
10. Pantridge JD, Geddes JS. A mobile intensive care unit in the management of myocardial infarction. Lancet 1967;2:271–273.
11. Guidelines for cardiopulmonary resuscitation and emergency cardiac care. JAMA 1992;268:2171–2302.
12. Eisenberg MS, Bergner L, Hallstrom A. Cardiac resuscitation in the community. Importance of rapid provision and implications for program planning. JAMA 1979;241:1905–1907.
13. Eisenberg MS, Copass MK, Halstrom AP, et al. Treatment of out-of-hospital cardiac arrests with rapid defibrillation by emergency medical technicians. N Engl J Med 1980;302:1379–1383.
14. Stults KR, Brown DD, Schug VL, Bean JA. Prehospital defibrillation performed by emergency medical technicians in rural communities. N Engl J Med 1984;310:219–223.
15. Stults KR, Brown DD, Kerber RE. Efficacy of an automated external defibrillator in the management of out-of-hospital cardiac arrest: validation of the diagnostic algorithm and initial clinical experience in a rural environment. Circulation 1986;73:701–709.
16. Weaver WE, Hill D, Fahrenbruch CE, et al. Use of the automatic external defibrillator in the management of out-of-hospital cardiac arrest. N Engl J Med 1988;319:661–666.
17. Gerson LW, Schelble DT, Wilson JE. Using paramedics to identify at-risk elderly. Ann Emerg Med 1992;21:688–691.
18. Bayer AJ, Chadha JS, Farag RR, et al. Changing presentation of myocardial infarction with increasing old age. J Am Geriatr Soc 1986;34:166–263.
19. American Hospital Association. Hospital Statistics, 1989–1990, Chicago, American Hospital Association, 1990.
20. Ruchlin HS, Morris JN. Cost-benefit analysis of an emergency alarm and response system: a case study of a long-term care program. Health Serv Res 1981;16:65–80.
21. Weaver WD, Litwin PE, Martin JS, et al. Effect of age on use of thrombolytic therapy and mortality in acute myocardial infarction. J Am Coll Cardiol 1991;18:657–662.
22. Doorey AJ, Michelson EL, Topol EJ. Thrombolytic therapy of acute myocardial infarction: keeping the unfulfilled promises. JAMA 1992;268:3108–3114.
23. Topol EJ, Califf RM. Thrombolytic therapy for elderly patients. N Engl J Med 1992;327:45–47.
24. Krumholz HM, Pasternak RC, Weinstein MC, et al. Cost effectiveness of thrombolytic therapy with streptokinase in elderly patients with suspected acute myocardial infarction. N Engl J Med 1992;327:7–13.
25. Cummins RO, Ornato JP, Thies WH, Pepe PE. Improving survival from sudden cardiac arrest: the "chain of survival" concept: a statement for health professionals from the Advanced Cardiac Life Support Subcommittee and the Emergency Cardiac Care Committee, American Heart Association. Circulation 1991;83:1832–1847.
26. Van Hoeyweghen RJ, Bossaert LL, Mullie A, et al. Survival after out-of-hospital cardiac arrest in elderly patients. Ann Emerg Med 1992;21:1179–1184.
27. Longstreth WT, Cobb LA, Fahrenbruch CE, Copass MK.

Does age affect outcomes of out-of-hospital cardio-pulmonary resuscitation? JAMA 1990;264:2109–2110.

28. McNamara RM, Rousseau EW, Sanders AB. Geriatric emergency medicine: a survey of practicing emergency physicians. Ann Emerg Med 1992;21:796–801.

29. Miles SH, Crimmins TJ. Orders to limit emergency treatment for an ambulance service. JAMA 1985;254:525–527.

30. American College of Emergency Physicians: Guidelines for "do not resuscitate orders" in the prehospital setting. Ann Emerg Med 1988;17:1106–1108.

Chapter 10
Acute Hospital Care

Robert M. Palmer

It may seem a strange principle to enunciate as the very first requirement in a hospital is that it should do the sick no harm.

Florence Nightingale
Notes on Hospitals

Older patients account for 30 percent of all hospital discharges and 41 percent of all inpatient days in the United States (1). The rate of hospitalization is nearly twice as high in the age group 85 years and older compared with that in the age group 65 to 74 years (2). These trends persist despite the decline in hospitalization rates and the average length of hospital stay that occurred after the introduction of Medicare's Prospective Payment System (PPS) (3). In addition, the practice of geriatric medicine is being influenced by the evolution of managed health care, home care, other long-term care services, and the increasing prevalence of chronic diseases that often require hospitalization for acute exacerbations (4,5). Even with a shift in care from hospital to community-based settings, older patients, because of their physical frailty and severity of illness, often require admission to a hospital where they may experience an adverse event. Indeed, the hospital experience is often stressful for the older patient, who faces the risks of iatrogenic illness, functional decline, institutionalization, and a diminished quality of life. The patient's admission to a hospital may be stressful to family members as well, generating fear, anxiety, and negative expectations of the patient's outcome. Although adverse effects of the hospital experience may not always be preventable, an understanding of their causes and consequences may enable physicians to identify opportunities to optimize patient care and improve the outcomes of hospitalization.

The Hospital Experience

Adverse Effects of Hospitalization

The risks of hospitalization for elderly patients are well described (Figure 10.1) (6). Acutely ill older patients are vulnerable to the adverse effects of the hospital for several reasons. First, they often have multiple comorbid conditions that increase the severity of acute illness. Second, their homeostatic reserves may be exceeded and lead to multiorgan system failure. For example, muscle mass, muscle strength, and aerobic capacity are diminished with aging, and may be further compromised by the deconditioning effects of sustained bed rest. Postural instability, which may manifest as orthostatic hypotension or falls, is associated with impaired baroreceptor reflexes and is also exacerbated by prolonged bed rest. Third, the older patient's independent performance of the physical, mental, and social activities of daily living may be limited by elements of hospitalization and the fast-paced and technology-intensive environment of the hospital (6). Patients with cognitive impairment, arthritis and joint diseases, and chronic heart and respiratory disease are at particular risk for functional decline (a loss of independent physical functioning) during hospitalization (6).

Indeed, 25 to 60 percent of older patients experience functional decline during the course of an acute illness requiring hospitalization (7–10). The loss of independent functioning is associated with serious sequelae such as prolonged hospital stay, nursing home placement, and mortality (11). In one study of elderly veterans, the patient's level of activities of daily living (ADL) in hospital was the strongest independent predictor of six-month mortality (11). Functional decline is more likely to occur in patients with a pressure sore, cognitive impairment, functional dependency, and low social activity level (10). Delirium (acute confusional state), which occurs in about

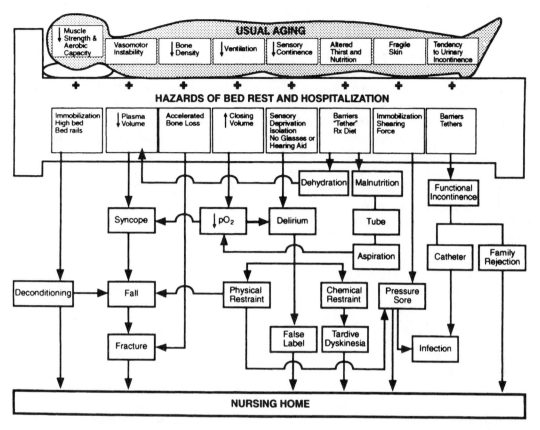

Figure 10.1. The risks of hospitalization and bed rest. Reproduced with permission from Creditor MC. Hazards of hospitalization of the elderly. Ann Intern Med 1993;118:219–223.

25 percent of medically ill elderly patients during hospitalization, is perhaps the most important predictor of functional decline in medically ill patients (12) and is most likely to occur in patients with severe systemic illness, dementia (chronic cognitive impairment), dehydration, and sensory impairments (13). Cognitive impairment and level of psychosocial functioning are also important predictors of surgical outcomes. In a prospective study of functional recovery one year after hospital discharge for hip fracture, recovery was poorer among elderly patients who had chronic or acute cognitive impairments and depressive symptomatology while hospitalized; patient contact with the social network after hospital discharge was associated with greater recovery (14). In another study, good pre-fracture physical functioning and cognitive status were associated with satisfac-

tory recovery and physical function after hip fracture. Postsurgical depression was associated with poorer recovery in both functional and psychosocial status (15). These studies serve to underscore the important effects of physical, cognitive and social dysfunction on clinical and functional outcomes of hospitalization and suggest the potential to prevent or ameliorate adverse outcomes through early detection and treatment of functional impairments.

The extent of functional decline in elderly patients hospitalized for acute medical illness may exceed the decline attributable to the acute illness itself. Of the many factors potentially contributing to the patient's loss of independent functioning, four are of particular importance: iatrogenic illness, bed rest and immobility, undernutrition, and the physical environment.

Iatrogenic Illness

Iatrogenic illness, defined as any illness that results from a diagnostic procedure, from any form of therapy, or any harmful occurrences that are not natural consequences of the patient's disease (16), occurs most commonly in older patients (17). Complications of drug therapy and of diagnostic and therapeutic procedures (18), nosocomial infections (19,20), fluid and electrolyte disturbances (21), and trauma (e.g., falls) are common examples of iatrogenic illnesses. Other examples include pressure sores resulting from forced immobilization by physical restraints, hematomas from venipuncture and arterial catheterization, dehydration and hypernatremia after preparation for gastrointestinal studies, and acute renal failure resulting from the administration of contrast agents. Omission of therapeutic services may contribute to the risk of iatrogenic illness. Patients may miss scheduled treatment, meals, or therapy, which result in undertreatment of the acute illness, temporary starvation, and dehydration (22).

Iatrogenic illness is common in hospitalized patients. In a study of general medical patients, the incidence of iatrogenic illness was 36 percent (16). An incidence of 45 percent was found in a study of elderly veteran males (17). The risk of an iatrogenic event is related to the level of disease severity, the presence of impaired cognitive function, and the duration of hospital stay. In one study, iatrogenic complications—over half considered preventable—occurred in 58 percent of medically ill patients hospitalized for 15 or more days (23). Advanced age and severe underlying disease increase the risk for nosocomial infections such as urinary tract infections, bacteremia, pneumonia, and wound infection (24). Iatrogenic complications occur while patients are preparing for or completing diagnostic procedures and studies. Adverse events from errors of omission and negligence also occur more often in older patients (25).

Medications, by causing adverse drug reactions (ADR), are the most common recognized cause of iatrogenic illness (see Chapter 8). The most important risk factor for ADR is the number of medications received by the patient, but the class of medication is also important (26). Becase they have multiple illnesses and take more medications (polypharmacy), elderly patients are more likely to experience ADR than are younger patients. Examples of ADR in hospitalized older patients are delirium from psychotropic medications (26), falls associated with the use of benzodiazepines that have long elimination half-lives (e.g., diazepam) (27), and urinary retention from medications with anticholinergic properties (28). The increased risk for ADR in elderly patients can also be attributed to alterations in drug disposition, tissue sensitivity associated with aging, and to drug interactions (29).

Although age-related changes in serum proteins and protein binding are generally inconsequential, older hospitalized patients often have reduced levels of serum albumin as a result of multiple chronic diseases or protein-calorie malnutrition. Consequently, the doses of albumin-bound drugs (e.g., phenytoin, sulfa, warfarin) need to be adjusted when a patient's albumin level is low. Doses of drugs that are metabolized by microsomal oxidation need to be adjusted when other drugs with similar metabolism are added to the patient's regimen (e.g., the dose of theophylline is reduced when cimetidine is started).

Changes in hepatic drug metabolism and renal elimination can be related to both aging and illnesses. Daily endogenous creatinine production declines with age because of decrease in lean body mass: serum creatinine may appear "normal" despite a substantial decrease in glomerular filtration rate as a result of chronic renal disease (see Chapter 49). Maintenance doses of renally excreted drugs (e.g., aminolgycosides, angiotensin-converting enzyme inhibitors) are usually lower for older patients. Changes in liver metabolism are highly variable; no useful formula exists to help guide dosage of drugs metabolized by the liver. For most drugs undergoing phase II metabolism (nonmicrosomal oxidation), changes with aging are not clinically important (29).

Age-related changes in tissue sensitivity (pharmacodynamics) are less clearly documented. Although hospitalized older patients are believed to be more sensitive to medications, the greater effects of drugs at lower doses is largely attributable to age-related changes in drug disposition. Increased sensitivity to some medications has been documented. For example, tissue sensitivity to potent analgesics, some benzodiazepines (e.g., triazolam) (30) and warfarin (31) is increased with aging. Beta-receptor sensitivity (e.g., to isoproterenol) is decreased, which may account for the lack of tachycardia with stress or adrenergic stimulation seen in some elderly patients (32).

Bed Rest and Immobility

Although bed rest during hospitalization is often desired by elderly patients, prolonged or sustained bed rest has deleterious physiologic effects (33). For example, prolonged bed rest reduces the patient's cardiac reserve and aerobic capacity and can lead to joint contractures and inability to walk. Cardiac and muscular deconditioning occur within days of sustained bed rest in older patients (33). Generalized weakness and postural lightheadedness or hypotension are common symptoms of the deconditioning that accompanies sustained bed rest; these effects often prohibit the patient's independent ability to transfer from bed or to walk (34). Bed rest also predisposes patients to pressure sores, hypoxemia, accelerated bone loss, and constipation (6). Enforced bed rest and immobility are abetted by high beds, various tethers such as intravenous lines and Foley catheters, and physical restraints (6). Patients who remain in bed or in a chair often fail to receive physical therapy or to perform exercises with the nurses, which may accelerate functional decline (35). Psychoactive drugs may be prescribed as chemical restraints to prevent patients from falling or pulling out lines and tubes. However, despite the common use of physical and chemical restraints in hospitalized patients, their effectiveness is not well established and their use is controversial.

Physical or mechanical restraints are devices used to inhibit free movement. They include vest, belt, mitten, jacket, wrist, and ankle restraints. Bed rails, geriatric chairs, and wheelchairs are sometimes classified as mechanical restraints (36). Patient factors predictive of restraint use include advanced age, cognitive impairment, risk of injury to self or others, physical frailty, presence of monitoring or treatment devices, and need to promote body alignment (36). Administrative pressure to avoid litigation, availability of restraint devices, staff attitudes, and insufficient staffing also augur restraint use (36). Restraints are most often used to control problematic behaviors, treatment interference, and falls. Nurses are more likely to initiate the application of physical restraints than are physicians (37). Physical restraints often create adverse physical and psychological effects. Falls,

injuries, and death from strangulation may occur (38). Patients may suffer a loss of autonomy and become agitated and angry when restraints are applied against their wishes (39). Furthermore, outcomes of hospitalization are worse in restrained patients: greater morbidity and mortality rates occur in restrained than unrestrained patients, although this relationship is confounded by severity of disease (37,39).

Undernutrition

Elderly patients are often malnourished at hospital admission and at high risk for incident undernutrition during hospitalization (40). Chronic disease, cognitive impairment, social isolation, poor dentition, impaired thirst perception (41), and limited access to food and fluids predispose patients to protein-calorie undernutrition and dehydration during hospitalization. Some patients with protein-calorie malnutrition are admitted to the hospital with a diagnosis of failure to thrive; these patients often have a history of functional decline, social withdrawal, and recent weight loss (42,43). These patients also often have dementia, delirium, depression, drug toxicity, or chronic diseases such as cancer and heart failure (42). Deleterious effects of malnutrition include impaired wound healing, predisposition to pressure sores, impaired immunity, prolonged hospital stay, and mortality (44,45). The impact of malnutrition on hospital outcomes was demonstrated in a subacute rehabilitation setting in which the risk of elderly patients developing at least one medical complication was correlated with both functional status and serum albumin concentration at admission, amount of weight lost in the year before admission, and the presence of renal or pulmonary diseases (46). In other studies of older patients during acute hospitalization, two measures of protein-calorie malnutrition, hypoalbuminemia and hypocholesterolemia, are associated with prolonged length of stay and inhospital mortality (45,46). Inhospital undernutrition may delay wound healing and contribute to the development of pressure sores. Short-term semistarvation induces disturbances in fluid and electrolyte balance and exacerbates generalized weakness (47).

Physical Environment

The importance of a supportive physical environment has

been demonstrated in long-term care settings but has been less appreciated in the acute care hospital (48). The typical American hospital is structured to meet the needs of physicians and caregivers, not patients. For the older patient, the physical features of the acute care hospital may render it a hostile environment: raised beds can make getting up and down difficult and risky; cold, shiny floors may look wet and make getting out of bed uncomfortable and frightening; cluttered hallway corridors may discourage independent ambulation and contribute to the risk of falls; sterile appearing walls and corridors may fail to provide the orienting clues that often permit independent way-finding; and the many disturbing, unfamiliar, and often unanticipated routines and procedures may clash with the patient's usual or desired routines (48). These environments may impede functional independence, accelerate functional decline, and exacerbate delirium (e.g., "intensive care unit psychosis").

In summary, the physical environment and the process of care in the hospital may threaten independent physical and cognitive functioning of older patients. Their limited homeostatic reserves, high severity of illness, and multiple comorbid conditions predispose these patients to functional decline, prolonged hospitalization, and greater risk of nursing home placement. By recognizing the deleterious effects of hospitalization, however, physicians working with other health professionals and hospital administrators can modify the practice of medicine and potentially attenuate the adverse effects of hospitalization.

Principles of Hospital Care

The principles of optimal care of hospitalized older patients include modification of the physical environment, efforts to prevent iatrogenic illness, early detection of functional impairments and their management, promotion of mobility and physical activity, nutritional assessment and intervention, attention to psychosocial needs and personal values, and interdisciplinary care (Table 10.1).

Physical Environment
Modifications of the physical and functional environment have been described in acute care geriatric units (48–51)

Table 10.1. Principles of Hospital Care: Key Points.

Principle	Key Points
Modify physical environment	Carpeting Clocks, calendars Visual contrasts Floor lighting Handrails Activity room
Prevent iatrogenic illness	Avoid polypharmacy Lower initial doses of medications Use of psychoactive medications judiciously Use alternatives to physical restraints Avoid unneeded studies
Detect/treat functional impairments	Conduct comprehensive assessment of basic ADL, IADL, cognition, mood, social function Link assessment to specific interventions (e.g., assistive devices, exercise, toileting schedule) Detect, evaluate, and treat delirium
Promote mobility	Do not limit physical activity Order bedside exercises to maintain muscle strength and joint flexibility
Assess/treat nutritional needs	Screen for protein-calorie malnutrition (weight loss, muscle wasting, low serum albumin and cholesterol, anemia) Prescribe dietary fluids and calorie intake (monitor daily) Use dietary supplements or calorie-dense snacks
Recognize psychosocial needs and personal values	Attend to patient's need for comfort, relief of pain, and rest Maintain continuity of nursing care Optimize sensory input (vision, hearing) Encourage social visits Review advance directives
Practice interdisciplinary care	Collaborate with health care team Formulate early discharge planning Consider home care as option to nursing home placement Discharge patients when stable (afebrile, normotensive, no new symptoms)

Reproduced by permission from Palmer RM. Acute hospital care of the older patient. Cleve Clin J Med 1995;62:117-128.

(Table 10.2) and are similar to successful modifications reported in the settings of long-term care, psychiatry, and rehabilitation. In some geriatric units, the environment is modified to foster functional independence and to allay the disorienting effects of the unfamiliar environment of the hospital (48,51). The hallway corridor and patient rooms are carpeted, and clocks and calendars are prominently placed in each room. Carpeting patterns and wall coverings with visual contrasts are chosen to aid patient orientation and way-finding. In addition, space for personal items from home are provided, special beds with floor lighting are selected, additional lighting behind each patient's bed is installed, cubical curtains are added, and visually appealing paint and wallpaper colors are chosen. Patient rooms are designed to permit privacy; a large common space (activity room) encourages dining outside rooms, socializing, and light exercise. The addition of handrails to the hallway corridors and grab bars in bathrooms promote patient safety and encourage independent mobility. Many of these environmental modifications are inexpensive and are suitable for all hospitalized patients; for example, clocks in rooms and handrails or grab bars.

Prevention of Iatrogenic Illness

The incidence of iatrogenic illness is potentially reducible through rational drug prescribing, avoidance of physical restraints and immobility, and proper selection of diagnostic procedures. Principles of drug prescribing for elderly patients are applicable to the hospital setting (52) (see Chapter 8). Physicians should know the pharmacology of the prescribed drugs and use a few drugs well; consider age-related alterations in drug disposition and tissue response; anticipate common drug interactions and consider the effects of alcohol and cigarette smoking; use lower than standard doses of most drugs; and consider adverse drug effects as the cause of new symptoms (52). Physicians should also consider consulting a pharmacist or using a computer software program for help when they prescribe new or unfamiliar medications to elderly patients (53).

Alternatives to drug therapy for behavioral symptoms should be considered before psychotropic medications are prescribed. For example, anxious or mildly confused patients can be treated with environmental changes (soft lights, quiet room, background music), behavioral approaches (soft voice, handholding, reality orientation) or the recruitment of families and sitters to the patient's bedside. Psychoactive medications should be reserved for use when the patient's health or comfort is immediately threatened. When anxiolytic therapy is indicated, benzodiazepines with short to intermediate elimination half-lives should be preferred to those with long elimination half-lives (53). The metabolism of the anxiolytic, lorazepam, and the hypnotic, temazepam, unlike diazepam or flurazepam, are not significantly affected by aging; with intermittent use, these agents may be less likely to produce ataxia, cognitive impairment, and falls (27). Although tricyclic antidepressants and antipsychotic drugs are often sedative, the high incidence of adverse effects of these agents limits their application as anxiolytics or hypnotics. These agents and the antihistamines (e.g., diphenhydramine) have prominent anticholinergic properties that predispose patients to delirium, constipation, tachyarrhythmias, and urinary retention (28). Although a role for antipsychotic agents (e.g., haloperidol) is well established for the treatment of agitated delirium in critical care units (54), their therapeutic index has not been established. Haloperidol, in low doses of 0.5 mg to 3.0 mg per 24 hours, is often effective, but extrapyramidal symptoms may prove problematic. Haloperidol is less anticholinergic and is less likely to cause hypotension than other neuroleptics. Often, a combination of low doses of haloperidol and lorazepam reduces the agitation and delusions or hallucinations of delirium more effectively than high doses of the individual drugs given alone (54).

The alternative approaches to restraint use developed in long-term care settings can be adapted for use in the hospital. One hospital, using a policy similar to one used in nursing homes, reduced the use of mechanical and chemical restraints without increasing the incidence of serious injury from falls (55). Some practical measures that reduce the need for restraining patients include relieving pain with analgesics or a change in body position, changing treatment (e.g., removing catheters), increasing sensory inputs (e.g., hearing and visual aids), improving patient orientation, and employing a family companion or sitter to stay with the patient.

Psychotropic agents and physical restraints are best

Table 10.2. Acute Care Geriatric Units*.

Study	Design	Patient Mix	Targeting Criteria	Environmental Modification	Intervention	Outcomes
Saunders et al, 1980	Descriptive	M, S, N	Age ≥65 years; "restorative nursing care"	Calendar in room; hand held shower heads; communal dining room; medications in patient's drawers; exit door alarms; satellite OT/PT room	Multidisciplinary assessment and care; nurse coordinator; discharge planning at admission	Unit patients had shorter hospital length of stay and fewer nursing home admissions than expected
Collard et al, 1985	Randomized, controlled trial (2 hospitals)	M, S	Age ≥65 years; predicted length of stay ≥48 hours; participating physician	Communal dining area	Primary nurse assessment at admission; home assessments of elective admissions; discharge planning at admission; interdisciplinary conferences; home visit by nurse	Unit patients had shorter hospital length of stay and lower total charges at 1 hospital; no differences in self-rated health or mobility
Boyer et al, 1986	Randomized, controlled trial	M, S, N	Age ≥70 years; potentially reversible disease	Communal dining room; bedside commodes and walkers	Primary nurse assessment; multidisciplinary conferences; rehabilitation emphasis	Unit patients had better functional and mobility scores; lower ancillary charges
Meissner et al, 1989	Controlled study	M	Age ≥70 years; potential for functional recovery; specific medical conditions	Congregate area for meals and PT/OT; group rooms	Nurse assessment at admission; nurse coordinator; multidisciplinary team and conference	Unit patients had greater improvement in ADL scores; longer length of stay and total charges; fewer hospital readmissions over 1-year period; no differences in discharge destinations
Fretwell et al, 1990	Randomized, controlled trial	M	Age ≥75 years; attending physician consent; direct admissions and ICU transfers	None reported	Consultation team on an acute care unit; functional assessment by primary nurse; interdisciplinary team meetings; nurse coordinator; follow-up telephone calls	Unit patients with depression at admission had improved mood at follow-up; no difference in ADL, length of stay, discharge destination
Huber and Kennard, 1991	Controlled study	M, S	Age ≥55 years; potential for functional recovery	Calendars and clocks in each room; handrails in corridors; home-like atmosphere	Multidisciplinary assessment and conference; specially selected nursing staff	Unit patients with high disease acuity improved functioning; trend toward shorter length of stay and lower hospital costs

*ADL = activities of daily living; ICU = intensive care unit; M = medical; N = neurologic; OT = occupational therapy; PT = physical therapy; S = surgical.
SOURCE: Palmer RM, Landefeld CS, Kresevic D, Kowal J. A medical unit for the acute care of the elderly. J Am Geriatr Soc 1994;42:545–552.

avoided unless alternatives are ineffective and the patient's safety requires immediate intervention (e.g., to prevent accidental removal of a central line) (56). When restraints are considered necessary, the reasons should be documented in the patient's chart and discussed with the patient, nurse, and family, when applicable, at the first opportunity. Restraints should be used for the shortest time necessary and their indications should be reevaluated at each nursing shift. Every two hours, restraints should be removed to check the patient's skin and to reposition the patient to prevent pressure sores. If patients become more agitated after restraints are applied, physicians should consider removing the restraints and trying alternative strategies.

Detection and Management of Functional Impairments

A comprehensive functional assessment identifies physical and cognitive impairments and leads to improved clinical outcomes of hospitalization: prolonged survival, reduced medical care costs, reduced use of acute care hospitals and nursing homes, and improved mood and cognition (57). In one clinical trial that compared usual care with a geriatric evaluation unit, patients assigned to the geriatric unit intervention were less often discharged to a nursing home and less likely to spend any time in a nursing home following discharge; hospital readmissions and mortality over the subsequent one year were more common in the control group (58). In a clinical trial that compared usual care to a geriatric assessment and rehabilitation unit, patients assigned to the geriatric unit intervention were discharged less often to nursing homes and had significantly more functional improvement in several basic self-care activites; in addition, more were residing in the community six months after admission to the study (59).

Comprehensive functional assessment is performed by an interdisciplinary team, usually beginning with the primary nurse's evaluation (Table 10.3). In some settings, geriatric clinical nurse specialists or geriatric resource nurses are specially trained to detect and manage functional impairments (48,60). These nurses or the patient's primary nurse perform an initial functional assessment and initiate interventions according to guidelines. For ex-

Table 10.3. Interdisciplinary Geriatric Assessment: Team Members and Roles*.

Team Member	Role
Primary nurse/ Nurse specialist	Assessment of functional status (basic ADL, IADL, falls risk, cognition, mood, special senses, nutrition; skin condition); implement guidelines to prevent functional decline; conduct daily interdisciplinary rounds; teach patient self-care.
Social worker	Assess patient's social support network, health insurance coverage, caregiving needs; review advance directives (living will, durable power of attorney for health care); evaluate family dynamics (potential caregiver stress or elder abuse); arrange referrals to community agencies (e.g., home care); arrange transfer to nursing home or rehabilitation hospital.
Physical therapist	Evaluate gait and mobility; maintain or improve strength, flexibility, and endurance of muscles and range of motion of joints; recommend assistive devices for ambulation; administer treatment modalities.
Occupational therapist	Evaluate and improve ability to perform ADL; fit splints for upper extremities; perform environmental assessment (home visit) and recommendations; teach use of assistive and safety devices.
Dietitian	Assess nutritional status; recommend nutritional interventions (e.g., special diets and food supplements); monitor enteral and parenteral alimentation.
Speech pathologist	Evaluate patients with aphasia or dysphagia; recommend swallowing techniques to prevent aspiration.
Home care coordinator	Participate in comprehensive discharge planning; assure smooth transition of care from the hospital to home; coordinate posthospital care with patient's physician and other providers.

*ADL = activities of daily living, IADL = instrumental activities of daily living.
Reproduced by permission from Palmer RM. Acute hospital care of the older patient. Cleve Clin J Med 1995;62:117–128.

ample, the nurse dispenses bedside commodes or urinals to patients who are having difficulty toileting themselves independently. A detailed functional assessment is time-consuming, but the use of standardized screening instruments may simplify the process of assessment and allow detection of mild degrees of functional impairment (61). Validated instruments that have good sensitivity and specificity are available for the bedside detection of delirium (62), cognitive impairment (63), and depression (64). These instruments can be administered to patients by nonphysicians. Repeated reassessment of the patient by nurses throughout the day improves detection of functional impairments. For example, nurses have an excellent opportunity to observe the fluctuation in level of attention that is characteristic of patients with delirium. Nurses are also likely to first observe changes in the patient's level of independence in performing basic ADLs.

The early detection of delirium is important in the prevention of functional decline (see Chapter 23). Detection of delirium in hospitalized patients is achievable through observation of the patient and application of brief bedside tests of attention and cognition (e.g., serial sevens, days of week backwards, digit span, sentence writing), interviewing family members and caregivers to ascertain whether cognitive changes have occurred, and talking to nurses or reading their notes to determine whether the patient is disoriented, inappropriate in communication or behaviors, or has delusions or hallucinations (65). The accuracy of the bedside diagnosis of delirium is remarkably good with simplified diagnostic criteria that are observable at the bedside such as an acute onset and fluctuating course, and disorganized thinking, altered level of consciousness, or both (62). Once delirium is detected, a search for the etiology is pursued. Infections, systemic diseases, adverse drug effects, and neurologic events are common etiologies of delirium (see Chapter 23). Treatment of the underlying etiology is of foremost importance. In some instances, this may require stopping or reducing doses of medications. In postoperative delirium, the use of supplemental oxygen; pressor agents or volume expanders; or the treatment of an underlying infection such as pneumonia, urinary tract infection, or wound infection is often helpful (66). Continuity of nursing care, correction of sensory deficits, orientation stimuli (reality orientation), and social visits from family members should also be considered.

Mobility and Physical Activity

Physical therapy or graded exercises to maintain joint flexibility and muscle strength and to prevent pressure sores, should be prescribed as activity orders on the first hospital day (Table 10.4). Helpful measures include changing the patient's position from supine to standing several times a day, aerobic exercises such as assisted ambulation, and resistive exercises of the lower extremities performed in bed or in a chair (34). To prevent dependence in gait or transfers, patients can be taught to ambulate or stand at least three times daily and to walk to the activity room for group exercises and meals daily. They can also be taught active or passive range of motion

Table 10.4. Graded Bedside Exercises: Activity Orders.

Exercises focus on the lower extremities and trunk, in which muscle strength and flexibility are most important to postural stability and gait.

Patient Capability	Description
Level 1—Requires bed rest	For bed-confined patients, passive or active range-of-motion exercises for hips, knees, ankles, and trunk.
Level 2—Sits in Chair	Conducted in bed or in a chair; Level 1 exercises plus exercises for trunk flexibility and strengthening of the plantar and dorsal flexors of the ankle.
Level 3—Has bathroom privileges	Done with the patient standing; includes full range-of-motion exercises for the trunk and lower extremities and for weight-bearing
Level 4—Walks at will	Includes Level 3 exercises and walking in room or hallway.

exercises, weight-bearing exercises, and resistive and aerobic exercises. Independent patient mobility is promoted by avoiding physical and chemical restraints and dispensing assistive devices (walkers, quad canes and grab bars) and bedside appliances such as trapeze bars, wheelchairs, and Hoyer lifts. Patients who need assistance with transfers and mobility can be referred to a physical or occupational therapist for further evaluation and treatment. Patients can exercise in the activity room or in the physical therapy department. Patients can be taught by nurses or therapists to perform bedside range-of-motion exercises and low-impact resistive exercises. Patients with impaired ability to transfer or walk independently may benefit from the dispensing of assistive devices such as canes and walkers. Physical activity should not be limited unless there are explicit contraindications (6). Physicians should coordinate their interventions with nurses, therapists, and other health professionals.

Mobility is further enhanced by the avoidance of physical and chemical restraints. As the patients convalesce from acute illnesses, they can spend increasing lengths of time in the activity room, where they may exercise and socialize with other patients, or in the physical therapy department. Occupational therapy can be helpful in restoring the patient's performance of personal ADLs. An occupational therapy evaluation can also suggest modifications in the patient's home that will promote independent and safe functioning.

Nutritional Assessment and Intervention

The patient's medical history, physical examination, and laboratory evaluation are all critical components of the assessment of malnutrition. A history of weight loss is an important and sensitive antecedent of malnutrition and is predictive of posthospitalization mortality (40). The diagnosis of protein-calorie malnutrition is often based on physical features such as loss of lean body mass, temporal muscle wasting, generalized weakness, and glossitis as well as objective assessments of serum albumin, serum cholesterol, hemoglobin, and other biochemical markers (67). These physical and biochemical features, however, may be insensitive to early or mild presentations of malnutrition. Prevalent malnutrition at admission is suspected in patients with recent unintentional weight loss,

generalized weakness, muscle atrophy, a serum albumin less than 3.0 gm/dl, a serum cholesterol less than 150 mg/dl, or an unexplained normocytic anemia (44,67). Diagnostic evaluation of these patients may reveal evidence of underlying chronic diseases, dysphagia, dementia, or depression (42,43). Therapeutic interventions often include high-calorie and high-protein diets with nutritional supplements or snacks, and, less commonly, enteral or parenteral alimentation (68,69). Social visits and meals with family members can be helpful in restoring the patient's appetite. Elderly patients may have defects in thirst perception or their access to sufficient fluids and calories might be limited (41). Fluid and caloric requirements, therefore, should be prescribed and monitored daily to prevent undernutrition during hospitalization. The value of nutritional intervention was shown when oral nutrition supplements given to elderly patients with femoral neck fractures resulted in fewer hospital complications and a shorter length of hospital stay (70).

Psychosocial Needs and Personal Values

Anxiety, fear, and distress are common symptoms during hospitalization and may be exacerbated by negative expectations of hospital outcomes harbored by the patients or their family members. Symptoms of depression may interfere with recovery of physical functioning. Family caregivers may wonder how they will provide care at home for a physically and functionally impaired older person. The stress of caregiving may affect their health or lead them to make hurried and poorly planned decisions. To lessen the adverse effect of these psychosocial factors, the personal values and needs of patients and their families should be addressed by physicians and nurses early in the patient's hospital stay. Family and patient conferences may serve to allay fear and clarify confusing aspects of the patient's personal needs during and after hospitalization. Periodic updates and consultation with the patient and family keep them aware of the patient's progress and engaged in the process of decision making. The patient's perceptions of the hospital experience and personal preferences should be elicited. Advance directives and the patient's wishes for treatment should be discussed early in the hospitalization. The importance of these discussions was shown in one study in which patients' self-reported wishes and physician judgment of medical utility influenced physician recommendations about resuscitation (71). Ideally, discussion of advance directives should take place before the patient's hospitalization. Total hospital and professional charges are lower when patients are admitted with an established nonresuscitation order than they are when the order is made during hospitalization (72). Thus, early effort to determine patient expectations of hospitalization, attitudes regarding cardiopulmonary resuscitation, and advance directives may serve to improve clinical outcomes.

Comfort measures, including adequate control of pain with analgesic medications, should be provided. Patient fear can be alleviated through nursing interventions, correction of sensory deficits, and reality orientation; increasing social visits from family members; and a quiet environment that promotes periods of relaxation and sleep at night.

Interdisciplinary Care

The expertise required to coordinate the assessment and treatment of older patients demands an interdisciplinary team approach to hospital care. Physicians work with a wide range of health professionals who collaborate in the care of patients (Table 10.3). The evolution of interdisciplinary collaboration reflects the importance of a multidimensional evaluation and intervention to address the complex physical and psychosocial needs of elderly hospitalized patients. However, since not every patient needs the services of every team member it is most important for physicians to initiate the interdisciplinary process with the primary nurse. After the physician and nurse evaluation, other team members can be recruited as needed into the process of patient care.

A major focus of the interdisciplinary team is discharge planning, which, ideally, begins early in the patient's hospitalization (73). Models for interdisciplinary discharge planning have been designed to identify high-risk patients, evaluate and optimize their functional status, develop a comprehensive plan that is reassessed throughout hospitalization, and assure continuity of care during the transition from hospital to home (74). In one hospital unit that emphasized discharge planning, mean hospital lengths of stay and total hospital charges were significantly reduced (49). In another setting, discharge planning coordinated by a gerontological nurse specialist

helped to reduce the incidence of rehospitalization 12 weeks after patient discharge from the hospital (75).

Early discharge planning by an interdisciplinary team achieves several objectives. First, the team can identify patients at risk of nursing home placement related to nonmedical predictors such as inadequate social support network, patient functional dependency, and cognitive impairment. Second, the team can estimate the patient's hospital length of stay and need for functional assistance or formal supports at home (76). Third, the team can educate patients and their families about diagnosis, prognosis, medications, home safety, and appropriate self-care at home (e.g., diet, exercise). Finally, the team can coordinate home care with physicians and, when warranted, with home nursing services. A coordinated process of transitional care should reinforce the advice given the patient by the team during hospitalization and reduce the risks of functional deterioration, medication noncompliance, and early unplanned hospital readmission.

Decisions about the timing of hospital discharge and of patient disposition present great challenges to physicians and team members. Nonterminal patients should not be discharged from the hospital if there is the following evidence of clinical instability on the day of planned discharge: 1) a new finding of incontinence, chest pain, dyspnea, delirium, tachycardia, or hypotension; 2) a temperature more than 38.3°C; or 3) a diastolic blood pressure of 105 mm Hg or higher (77). Elderly patients who are sent home in an unstable condition are twice as likely to die within 30 days after hospitalization compared with those whose condition is stable (77). Patients who need assistance in ADLs or who have inadequate social supports in the community are more likely to require nursing home placement compared with functionally independent patients (76). However, some carefully selected elderly patients may improve their independent functioning with a structured home care intervention after short-stay hospital treatment (78). These patients are often independent in ADLs before their acute illness and have good social support networks. Short-term rehabilitative services enable older patients to regain their independence in ADLs. Patients receiving early, systematic discharge planning experience an increased likelihood of successful return to home after hospital admission and a decreased chance of unscheduled readmission (78). However, home health care is used more often by patients with low educational levels, inaccessible social supports, and impairments in one or more instrumental ADLs (79).

In summary, modifications of the physical environment and the other principles of hospital care, can attenuate the adverse effects of hospitalization. Despite today's fast-paced and technology-oriented acute care hospital, the personal, physical, and functional needs of older patients need not be ignored. Through a comprehensive assessment and interdisciplinary collaboration those needs can be addressed and patient outcomes potentially improved (80).

References

1. Vital and Health Statistics. Health data on older Americans, 1992. Hyattsville, MD: U.S. Department of Health and Human Services, 1993.

2. Edwards WO, Gibson DA. Geographic variations in Medicare utilization of short-stay hospital services, 1981–1988. Health Care Financ Rev 1990;11:107.

3. Libson CL, Naessens JM, Campion ME, et al. Trends in elderly hospitalization and readmission rates for a geographically defined population: pre- and post-prospective payment. J Am Geriatr Soc 1991;39:895–904.

4. Kosecoff J, Kahn KL, Rogers WH, et al. Prospective payment system and impairment at discharge. The "Quicker and Sicker" story revisited. JAMA 1990;264:1980–1983.

5. Kahn KL, Keeler EB, Sherwood MJ, et al. Comparing outcomes of care before and after implementation of the DRG-based prospective payment system. JAMA 1990;264:1984–1988.

6. Creditor MC. Hazards of hospitalization of the elderly. Ann Intern Med 1993;118:219–223.

7. Gillick MR, Serrell NA, Gillick LF. Adverse consequences of hospitalization and the elderly. Soc Sci Med 1982;16:1033–1038.

8. Warshaw GA, Moore JT, Friedman SW, et al. Functional disability in the hospitalized elderly. JAMA 1982;248:847–850.

9. Hirsch C, Sommers L, Olsen A, et al. The natural history of functional morbidity in hospitalized older patients. J Am Geriatr Soc 1990;38:1296–1303.

10. Inouye SK, Wagner DR, Acampora D, et al. A predictive index for functional decline in hospitalized elderly medical patients. J Gen Intern Med 1993;8:645–652.

11. Narain P, Rubenstein LZ, Wieland GD, et al. Predictors of immediate and 6-month outcomes in hospitalized elderly patients: the importance of functional status. J Am Geriatr Soc 1988;36:775–783.

12. Murray AM, Levkoff SP, Wetle TT, et al. Acute delirium and functional decline in the hospitalized elderly patient. J Gerontol Med Sci 1993;48:M181–M186.

13. Inouye SK, Viscoli CM, Horwitz RI, et al. A predictive model for delirium in hospitalized elderly medical patients based on admission characteristics. Ann Intern Med, 1993;119:474–481.

14. Magaziner J, Simonsick EM, Kashner TM, et al. Predictors of functional recovery one year following hospital discharge for hip fracture; a prospective study. J Gerontol 1990;45:M101–M107.

15. Mossey JM, Mutran E, Knott K, et al. Determinants of recovery twelve months after hip fracture: The importance of psychosocial factors. Am J Public Health 1989;79:279–286.

16. Steel K, Gertman PM, Crescenzi C, Anderson J. Iatrogenic illness on a general medical service at a university hospital. N Engl J Med 1981;304:638–642.

17. Jahnigen D, Hannon C, Laxson L, LaForce FM. Iatrogenic disease in hospitalized elderly veterans. J Am Geriatr Soc 1982;30:387–390.

18. Schroeder SA, Marton KI, Strom BL. Frequency and morbidity of invasive procedures: report of a pilot study from two teaching hospitals. Arch Intern Med 1978;138:1809–1811.

19. Haley RW, Houton TM, Culver DH, et al. Nosocomial infections in U.S. hospitals 1975–1976. Estimated frequency by selected characteristics of patients. Am J Med 1981;70:947–959.

20. Hanson LC, Weber DJ, Rutala WA, Samsa GP. Risk factors for nosocomial pneumonia in the elderly. Am J Med 1992;92:161–166.

21. Snyder NA, Feigal DW, Arieff AI. Hypernatremia in elderly patients: a heterogeneous, morbid, and iatrogenic entity. Ann Intern Med 1987;107:309–319.

22. Patterson C. Iatrogenic illness. Clin Geriatr Med 1986;2:121–136.

23. Lefevere F, Feinglass J, Potts S, et al. Iatrogenic complications in high-risk, elderly patients. Arch Intern Med 1992;152:2074–2080.

24. Gorbien MJ, Bishop J, Beers MH, et al. Iatrogenic illness in hospitalized elderly people. J Am Geriatr Soc 1992;40:1031–1042.

25. Leape LL, Brennan TA, Laird N, et al. The nature of adverse events in hospitalized patients. Results of the Harvard medical practice study II. N Engl J Med, 1991;324:377–384.

26. Lamy PP. Adverse drug effects. Clin Geriatr Med 1990;6:293–307.

27. Ray WA, Griffin MR, Schaffner W, et al. Psychotropic drug use and the risk of hip fracture. N Engl J Med, 1987;316:363–369.

28. Peters NL. Snipping the thread of life. Antimuscarinic side effects of medications in the elderly. Arch Intern Med 1989;149:2414–2420.

29. Montamat SC, Cusack BJ, Vestal RE. Management of drug therapy in the elderly. N Engl J Med 1989;321:303–309.

30. Greenblatt DJ, Harmatz JS, Shapiro L, et al. Sensitivity to triazolam in the elderly. N Engl J Med 1991;324:1691–1698.

31. Gurwitz JH, Avorn J, Ross-Degnan D, et al. Aging and the anticoagulant response to warfarin therapy. Ann Intern Med 1992;116:901–904.

32. Abernethy DR. Altered pharmacodynamics of cardiovascular drugs and their relation to altered pharmacokinetics in elderly patients. Clin Geriatr Med 1990;6:285–292.

33. Harper CM, Lyles YM. Physiology and complications of bed rest. J Am Geriatr Soc 1988;36:1047–1054.

34. Hoenig HM, Rubenstein LZ. Hospital-associated deconditioning and dysfunction. J Am Geriatr Soc 1991;39:220–222.

35. Lazarus BA, Murphy JB, Coletta EM, et al. The provision of physical activity to hospitalized elderly patients. Arch Intern Med 1991;151:2452–2456.

36. Evans LK, Strumpf NE. Tying down the elderly. A review of the literature on physical restraint. J Am Geriatr Soc 1989;37:65–74.

37. Mion LC, Frengley JD, Jakovcic CA, Marino JA. A further exploration of the use of physical restraints in hospitalized patients. J Am Geriatr Soc 1989;37:949–956.

38. Miles SH, Irvine P. Death caused by physical restraints. Gerontologist 1992;32:762–766.

39. Robbins LJ, Boyko E, Lane J, Cooper D, Jahnigen DW. Binding the elderly: a prospective study of the use of mechanical restraints in an acute care hospital. J Am Geriatr Soc 1987;35:290–296.

40. Sullivan D, Patch JA, Walls RC, Lipschitz DA. Impact of nutrition status on morbidity and mortality in a select population of geriatric rehabilitation patients. Am J Clin Nutr 1990;51:749–758.

41. Phillips PA, Rolls BJ, Ledingham JGG, et al. Reduced thirst after water deprivation in healthy elderly men. New Engl J Med 1984;311:753–759.

42. Palmer RM. "Failure to thrive" in the elderly: diagnosis and management. Geriatrics 1990;45:47–55.

43. Berkman B, Foster LWS, Campion E. Failure to thrive: paradigm for the frail elderly. Gerontologist 1989;29:654–659.

44. Rudman D, Feller AG. Protein-calorie undernutrition in the nursing home. J Am Geriatr Soc 1989;37:173–183.

45. Constans T, Bacq Y, Brechet JF, et al. Protein-energy malnutrition in elderly medical patients. J Am Geriatr Soc 1992;40:263–268.

46. Noel MA, Smith TK, Ettinger WH. Characteristics and outcomes of hospitalized older patients who develop hypocholesterolemia. J Am Geriatr Soc 1991;39:455–461.

47. DeHaven J, Sherwin R, Hendler R, Felig P. Nitrogen and sodium balance and sympathetic-nervous-system activity in obese subjects treated with a low-calorie protein or mixed subject. New Engl J Med 1980;302:477–482.

48. Palmer RM, Landefeld CS, Kresevic D. A medical unit for acute care of the elderly. J Am Geriatr Soc 1994;42:545–552.

49. Meissner P, Andolsek K, Mears PA, et al. Maximizing the functional status of geriatric patients in an acute community hospital setting. Gerontologist 1989;29:524–528.

50. Collard AF, Bachman SS, Beatrice DF. Acute care delivery for the geriatric patient: An innovative approach. Q Rev Bull 1985;6:180–185.

51. Boyer N, Chuang JC, Gipner D. An acute care geriatric unit. Nurs Manage 1986;17:22–25.

52. Vestal RF. Pharmacology and aging. J Am Geriatr Soc 1982;30:191–200.

53. Schader RI, Greenblatt DJ. Use of benzodiazepines in anxiety disorders. N Engl J Med 1993;328:1398–1405.

54. Fish DN. Treatment of delirium in the critically ill patient. Clin Pharm 1991;10:456–462.

55. Powell C, Mitchell-Pedersen, Fingerote E, Edmund L. Freedom from restraint: consequences of reducing physical restraints in the management of the elderly. Can Med Assoc J 1989;141:561–564.

56. Robbins LJ. Restraining the elderly patient. Clin Geriatr Med 1986;2:591–599.

57. National Institutes of Health Consensus Development Conference Statement: geriatric assessment methods for clinical decision making. J Am Geriatr Soc 1988;36:342–347.

58. Rubenstein LZ, Josephson KR, Wieland GD, et al. Effectiveness of a geriatric evaluation unit: A randomized clinical trial. N Engl J Med 1984;311:1664–1670.

59. Applegate WB, Miller ST, Graney MJ, et al. A randomized, controlled trial of a geriatric assessment unit in a community rehabilitation hospital. N Engl J Med 1990;322:1572–1578.

60. Inouye SK, Acampora D, Miller RL, et al. The Yale geriatric care program: a model of care to prevent functional decline in hospitalized elderly patients. J Am Geriatr Soc 1993;41:1345–1352.

61. Applegate WB, Blass JP, Williams TF. Instruments for the functional assessment of older patients. N Engl J Med 1990;322:1207–1214.

62. Inouye SK, VanDyck CH, Alessi CA, et al. Clarifying confusion: the confusion assessment method. Ann Intern Med 1990;113:941–948.

63. Folstein MF, Folstein SE, McHugh PR. "Mini-Mental State." A practical method for grading the cognitive state of patients for the clinician. J Psychiatr Res 1975;12:189–198.

64. Yesavage JA, Brink TL, Rose TL, et al. Development of a geriatric depression screening scale: a preliminary report. J Psychiatr Res 1983;17:37–49.

65. Francis J. Delirium in older patients. J Am Geriatr Soc 1992;40:829–838.

66. Gustafson Y, Brannstrom B, Berggren D, et al. Geriatric-anesthesiologic program to reduce acute confusional states in elderly patients treated for femoral neck fractures. J Am Geriatr Soc 1991;39:655–662.

67. Mitchell CO, Lipschitz DA. Detection of protein-calorie malnutrition in the elderly. Am J Clin Nutr 1982;35:398–406.

68. Drickamer MA, Cooney LM. Geriatrician's guide to enteral feeding. J Am Geriatr Soc 1993;41:672–679.

69. McMahon MM, Farnell MB, Murray MJ. Nutritional support of critically ill patients. Mayo Clin Proc 1993;68:911–920.

70. Delmi M, Rapin CH, Bengoa JM, et al. Dietary supplementation in elderly patients with fractured neck of the femur. Lancet 1990;335:1013–1016.

71. Miller DL, Gorbien MJ, Simbartl LA, Jahnigen DW. Factors

influencing physicians in recommending in-hospital cardiopulmonary resuscitation. Arch Intern Med 1993; 153:1999–2003.

72. Maksoud A, Jahnigen DW, Skivinski CI. Do not resuscitate orders and the cost of death. Arch Intern Med 1993;153:1249–1253.

73. Evans RL, Hendricks RD. Evaluating hospital discharge planning: a randomized clinical trial. Med Care 1993;31:358–370.

74. Wertheimer DS, Kleinman LS. A model for interdisciplinary discharge planning in a university hospital. Gerontologist 1990;30:837–840.

75. Naylor MD. Comprehensive discharge planning for hospitalized elderly: a pilot study. Nurs Res 1990;39:156–161.

76. Wachtel TJ, Fulton JP, Goldfarb J. Early prediction of dis-

charge disposition after hospitalization. Gerontologist 1987;27:98–103.

77. Brook RH, Kahn KL, Kosecoff J. Assessing clinical instability at discharge. The clinicians responsibility. JAMA 1992;268:1321–1322.

78. Melin AL, Bygren LO. Efficacy of the rehabilitation of elderly primary health care patients after short-stay hospital treatment. Med Care 1992;30:1004–1015.

79. Solomon DH, Wagner DR, Marenberg ME, et al. Predictors of formal home health care use in elderly patients after hospitalization. J Am Geriatr Soc 1993;41:961–966.

80. Inouye SK, Wagner DR, Acampora D, et al. A controlled trial of a nursing-centered intervention in hospitalized elderly medical patients: the Yale geriatric care program. J Am Geriatr Soc 1993;41:1353–1360.

Chapter 11
Surgery in the Geriatric Patient

Dennis W. Jahnigen

The most important thing we have learned about the aged is the necessity to give them the shortest possible period "down," the longest period "up." When a patient is "up," he is a citizen, an individual. When he is "down," he and his doctor are in trouble . . . "Down" is bad, "up" is life.

Dr. Martin R. Steinberg
Saturday Evening Post, 1967

This chapter reviews some of the physiologic effects of surgery on the elderly patient, common complications, general and specific risk assessments, and management of common comorbidities during the perioperative period.

Surgery for the elderly patient requires the best abilities of the primary care physician, the operating room team, the recovery room personnel, and the hospital ward staff to achieve optimal outcomes. Because of better understanding of the stress of surgery and improvements in anesthetic and operative techniques over the past 20 years, it is now possible to perform extensive surgical procedures on patients 90 or even 100 years of age (1). Although mortality rates for elderly persons are higher than those for younger patients, age alone should not be the criterion to exclude consideration of surgery (Table 11.1). The primary care physician has important roles in helping decide whether to refer a patient for consideration for surgery, in providing an assessment of preoperative status, in alerting others to likely problems, in monitoring postoperatively, in acting as the patient's advocate throughout the process, and in reassuming primary responsibility at some point during the patient's convalescence. In some instances, the primary care physician may know the patient well and may raise the initial consideration of surgery with the patient. In other instances, the first encounter the physician has with the patient may be in the emergency or hospital ward, as a consultant asked to help evaluate the patient for an emer-

gency surgical procedure. As a consultant, the physician should focus on identifying and optimizing medical conditions that may affect the success of the surgical procedure. Avoid recommendations as to the type of anesthesia or obvious suggestions such as "avoid hypoxemia" or "watch electrolytes" as these are not helpful to a surgeon or anesthesiologist. The choice of anesthetic agent and method, likewise, is the prerogative of the anesthesiologist. While spinal anesthesia has lower pulmonary complications than general anesthesia, they both have significant potential for cardiac complications.

Stress of Surgery

Major surgery places great stress on many organ systems. Oxygen consumption increases 30 percent to 70 percent during the postoperative period compared with that at baseline. Cardiac output and myocardial oxygen demands also increase proportionally. The hypothalamic-pituitary-adrenal axis is activated with an increase in plasma cortisol levels and catecholamine concentrations (2,3). Nutritional needs increase dramatically in the postoperative period. If the patient is malnourished before surgery, the likelihood of a postoperative complication increases (4). In the elderly patient, homeostatic reserve may be diminished by known illness, subclinical disease, or normal aging. The demands of surgery may exceed reserves or unmask subclinical disease, either of which can lead to a poor or undesired outcome.

Decision Making About Surgery

The primary care physician or surgeon should ask a number of questions as part of the preoperative assessment: 1) Given the patient's current functional status and life expectancy, is the proposed surgery reasonable? 2) Is the proposed procedure understood by the patient and

Table 11.1. Mortality for Selected Surgical Procedures in the Elderly.

Operation	Mortality (%)	
	Adult Patients	Patients age 65+
All procedures	0.9	5–10
Amputation	2–4	3–17
Cataract	0.01–0.05	0.01–0.2
Hernia (elective)	0.01	3.
Mastectomy	0.1	0.6
Transurethral prostate resection	0.4	0.2–2.0
Total hip replacement		5
Appendectomy (no perforation)	0.01	0.6
Appendectomy (perforation)	0.1	6
Cholecystectomy	0.3–7.0	3–7
Colon resection	5	10
Pneumonectomy	3–6	10–20
Coronary artery bypass	2	3–5
Aortic aneurysm	5	5–10

SOURCE: Kammerer WS, Gross RJ, eds. Medical consultation. Baltimore: Williams & Wilkins, 1990.

consistent with his or her wishes? 3) Are postoperative nursing and rehabilitative services available, and are they experienced in caring for geriatric patients? Older patients have more surgical complications than do younger patients, mainly because of the presence of comorbid disease, although homeostatic reserve in most organ systems diminishes with advanced age. The baseline prevalences of some comorbid conditions for geriatric patients are cardiovascular disease, 50 percent; respiratory disease, 30 percent; neurological disease, 30 percent; nutritional problems, 30 percent; and diabetes, 20 percent. An awareness of common morbid events in the postoperative period can help target areas for close monitoring (5,6,7) (Table 11.2).

Risk Assessment

A careful assessment of the elderly patient should be done long enough before surgery to permit identification of potential problems and plan optimal management. The Dripps Scale of the American Society of Anesthesiologists (ASA) provides a general estimate of risk (8) (Table 11.3). Mortality rates from the ASA may also be useful in evaluating overall risk (9) (Table 11.4).

Table 11.2. Postoperative Causes of Mortality in Elderly Patients.

Heart disease
　Myocardial infarction
　Congestive heart failure
Pulmonary emboli
Chronic obstructive pulmonary disease
Infection
　Pneumonia
　Sepsis
Gastrointestinal problems
　Liver disease
　Bleeding
Renal failure
Stroke

Table 11.3. Dripps Scale.

Level	Patient Characteristics
Class 1	Healthy, localized pathology, patient age <80 yr
Class 2	Mild to moderate systemic disturbance, patient age >80 yr
Class 3	Severe systemic pathology
Class 4	Severe systemic disorder and life-threatening disease, may not be correctable with surgery
Class 5	Moribund patient, little chance of survival for 24 hr without surgery

SOURCE: Dripps DR, Lamont A, Eckenhoff JE. The role of anesthesia in surgical mortality. JAMA 1961;178:261–266.

Table 11.4. Mortality Rates By Age and Physical Status.

Dripps Level	Mortality (%)			
	Age 0–34 yr	Age 35–64 yr	Age 65+ yr	All Ages
1, 2	0.1	0.3	1.0	0.3
3	5.0	3.9	5.2	4.6
4	27.5	21.4	31.0	25.9
5	70.2	71.3	75.8	72.4
All Levels	1.0	2.6	5.8	2.6

SOURCE: Hirsh R, et al (eds). Health care delivery in anesthesia. Philadelphia: G.F. Stickley 1979:100.

Table 11.5. Goldman Multifactorial Index.

Item	Points
History	
Myocardial infarction within 6 mo	10
Age >70 yr	5
Physical exam	
S$_3$ gallop or jugular venous distension	11
Aortic stenosis	3
Electrocardiogram	
Rhythm other than sinus	7
>5 premature ventricular contractions/min	7
Poor general medical status	3
Intraperitoneal, intrathoracic, or aortic surgery	3
Emergency surgery	4
Total possible points	53

SOURCE: Goldman L, Caldera DL, Nussbaum SR, et al. Multifactorial index of cardiac risk in noncardiac surgical procedures. N Engl J Med 1977;297:845–850. Permission Requested.

Table 11.6. Risk of Complications after Noncardiac Surgery.

Class	Points	Life-threatening Complication (%)	Cardiac Death (%)
I	0–5	0.7	0.2
II	6–12	5	2.0
III	13–25	11	2.0
IV	26	22	56.0

SOURCE: Goldman L, Caldera DL, Nussbaum SR, et al. Multifactorial index of cardiac risk in noncardiac surgical procedures. N Eng J Med 1977;297:845–850. Permission Requested.

Table 11.7 Risk of Cardiac Events for Vascular Surgery Patients.

Predictor	Odds Ratio
Angina	2.6
Q waves on electrocardiogram	4.2
History of ventricular ectopy	3.5
Diabetes	2.6
Positive Thallium scan	9.8
Age >70 yr	2.0

SOURCE: Eagle KA, Coley CM, Newell JB, et al. Combining clinical and thallium data optimizes preoperative assessment of cardiac risk before major vascular surgery. Ann Intern Med 1989;110:859–866.

A careful history and physical examination of the patient should be done if major surgery is contemplated. The patient's use of over-the-counter medications, smoking, and alcohol use should be evaluated. Patients should discontinue aspirin 7 to 10 days before surgery. The overall level of the patient's physical fitness can be assessed and "prehabilitation," a program to improve flexibility, strength, and aerobic fitness before elective surgery, can begin. At minimum, the patient's resting electrocardiogram (ECG), chest radiograph, complete blood count, plasma electrolytes, glucose, and creatinine should be obtained, with additional evaluations as indicated below (10,11).

Cardiac Risk Screens

General risk screens are useful in stratifying patients into high, moderate, or low risk for postoperative cardiac complications. Depending on the type of surgery contemplated, more specific tests of cardiac function may be indicated. The Goldman Index was developed in the 1970s to predict cardiac risk in noncardiac surgery (12,13) (Table 11.5). This index has been validated in several subsequent studies, although its sensitivity has been questioned. The presence of clinical heart failure is the single most important predictor of cardiac death, followed closely by myocardial infarction (MI) within the past 6 months. The total score can be used to predict minor or life-threatening cardiac complications (Table 11.6). For patients undergoing vascular surgery, Eagle criteria have been used to evaluate risk for cardiac events (14,15). This scale uses clinical evidence of coronary artery disease (CAD) applied among patients undergoing vascular study and has been shown to be 83 percent sensitive in predicting postoperative ischemic events (Table 11.7).

Patient-Specific Cardiac Evaluations

The extent of the cardiac evaluation needed is determined by the patient's history of significant CAD and the type of procedure planned. If the patient has had MI, a delay of 6 months before surgery, if possible, should be made. If more urgent surgery is needed, a 4- to 6-week period after MI will allow scar formation, and a successful operation can then be performed. Patients who have undergone coronary artery bypass (CABG) and are currently asymptomatic have a lower risk of perioperative MI; the risk is reduced from 9 percent to 2.4 percent. Patients with known, stable CAD and who are to undergo elective surgery may need a stress test of some type because evidence of severe CAD may influence the decision whether to perform surgery. For the patient who has stable angina and a reasonable functional status, such as the ability to climb two flights of stairs or exercise vigorously without exacerbating symptoms, no further functional testing may be needed. For patients with symptomatic CAD and who are undergoing urgent surgery, an echocardiogram can provide useful information on contractility, valve function, and wall motion abnormalities.

Patients undergoing peripheral vascular surgery have more than 50 percent risk of having significant CAD (16,17). If such persons have hypertension, diabetes, angina, or previous MI, coronary angiography and revascularization before the vascular surgery should be considered. For surgical patients with vascular disease, identified predictors of cardiac events include age older than 70 years, diabetes, angina, and previous MI. For elderly patients with no risk factors, 5 percent will have a cardiac event; with one or two risk factors, 15 percent will have a cardiac event; and with three or more factors, 50 percent will have a cardiac event. Postoperative ischemia on ECG with 1 mm depression confers a relative risk of cardiac event of 16. In one study of vascular surgery patients, 14 of 16 patients who had a postoperative cardiac event showed postoperative ischemia on ECG (18).

Patients at high risk should be considered for cardiac catheterization; those with intermediate risk require a functional test (19). Evaluation of myocardial function can include one or more of the following tests:

1. For patients who can exercise, use of a treadmill or bicycle ergometer is the desired functional test. This can be combined with thallium perfusion scanning to detect abnormal perfusion.

2. Dipyridamole stress thallium imaging identifies very low cardiac risk. The predictive value of positive tests to indicate subsequent cardiac events is not good, and another test may be needed (20).

3. Stress echocardiography can be performed with patients using a treadmill, or by use of intravenous dobutamine. A negative test has high predictive value for no CAD. The predictive value of a positive test is lower,

60 percent to 90 percent, depending on the specific agents used (21). If target heart rate is not reached, atropine can be used to improve predictive value (22).

4. If a major procedure is contemplated, the presence of symptoms of angina along with a positive functional test may suggest cardiac catheterization. Angioplasty can be done with a short recuperation period before surgery, if necessary (23,24).

In a population with a known 88 percent prevalence of CAD, the sensitivity of exercise, dobutamine, and dipyridamole stress echocardiography was 88 percent, 82 percent and 74 percent, respectively. Specificity was 82 percent, 77 percent and 94 percent, respectively (20). Another recent study investigated dipyridamole-thallium scanning and single photon-emission computerized tomography (SPECT). This combination did not accurately predict postoperative cardiac complications (25). The best predictor of postoperative coronary events was clinical evidence of CAD (known MI, angina, ECG evidence of MI), which had an odds ratio of 2.6, and age older than 65 years, which had an odds ratio of 2.3 for adverse cardiac events. Perioperative myocardial ischemia on ECG is a potent risk factor for a postoperative myocardial event (26). Preoperative nitroglycerine paste is often used until 24 to 48 hours after surgery, but data to support this practice are lacking.

The presence of an asymptomatic carotid bruit is not a predictor of postoperative stroke. Unless the patient has a history of stroke or symptoms to suggest transient ischemic attacks (TIA), further studies of the carotid arteries are not needed. There is no evidence that prophylactic endarterectomy is indicated in the asymptomatic patient. Because carotid bruits are associated with atherosclerosis in other areas, the presence of CAD and other vascular pathology should be carefully considered. For patients with recent stroke or TIA, surgery should be postponed, if possible, until the patient is neurologically stable, the etiology of the event has been determined, and appropriate measures to prevent recurrence have been undertaken.

Dementia

Although only 5 percent of individuals over 60 years of age have cognitive impairment, nearly 40 percent of those older than 80 years do. As much as 50 percent of elderly patients undergoing hip surgery may develop delirium postoperatively (27). A baseline measure of cognition is important. A screening test such as the Folstein Mini-Mental Status Examination can be administered in only a few minutes and often will reveal unsuspected impairment (28). If dementia is detected, the anesthesiologist and nursing staff should be alerted. With some medications that affect mental function, lower doses can be used, and others can be avoided entirely. Liberal visiting by the patient's family before and after the surgery may help reduce the patient's confusion. Close nursing attention with orientation and careful explanations can be reassuring. Some patients may require an anxiolytic or neuroleptic medication (see Chapter 22).

Congestive Heart Failure

Preoperative pulmonary edema, an S_{-3} gallop, or jugular venous distention are associated with as much as 40 percent risk of postoperative congestive heart failure (CHF) (12). The patient's volume status must be carefully managed throughout the perioperative period. Patients who have a borderline overloaded volume status or in whom large volume shifts are anticipated may need preoperative invasive monitoring. Current indications for invasive monitoring include major cardiovascular procedures, the presence of significant aortic stenosis, shock, difficult-to-manage heart failure, cardiac or vascular surgery, adult respiratory distress syndrome (ARDS), or complex hemodynamics (29).

Hypertension

Mild to moderate hypertension (diastolic pressure <110 mm Hg) does not increase operative risk, but higher pressures should be controlled preoperatively. Patients already taking antihypertensive medications should continue medication until the morning of surgery and may take medication with a sip of water. Patients on routine diuretics may have unsuspected hypokalemia, which must be corrected before surgery. Special care must be taken to avoid abrupt cessation of beta blockers or clonidine because rebound hypertension can occur. Intravenous labetalol, propranolol, or a clonidine patch can be used to control blood pressure if the patient can have nothing orally. Diuretics should be withheld on the day of surgery because volume status can be managed with intravenous fluids. The anesthesiologist must be informed of all medications the patient may be taking.

Dysrhythmias

Preoperative dysrhythmias are present in 6 percent to 15 percent of elderly patients, with the higher rates seen among those with known CAD. A significant increase in cardiac mortality seems to exist for patients with dysrhythmia, particularly for those with atrial fibrillation (12). Preoperative management consists of correcting blood pressure and electrolyte and acid-base disorders. A Holter monitor or long rhythm strip can help to quantitate and estimate the significance of the dysrhythmia. Cardiac event monitors that can be used for several weeks, if needed, are now available to document and quantitate suspected dysrhythmias. For ventricular tachycardia, multiform, premature ventricular contractions, or atrial fibrillation with rapid ventricular response, specific antiarrhythmic treatment is indicated. Prophylactic digoxin should not be used because it can potentiate serious dysrhythmias. If rate control is needed, intravenous preparations can be used.

Pacemakers

Chronic bifascicular block is present in 4.5 percent of preoperative patients over 40 years of age (12). Of these, 2.3 percent have right bundle branch block (RBBB) with left anterior hemiblock, 2 percent have left bundle branch block alone, and 0.2 percent have RBBB and left posterior hemiblock. There is very little risk of any of these conditions progressing to complete heart block (CHB). Among 145 patients with partial block who underwent 68 procedures, only one progressed to CHB (30–32). There is no reason for such patients to have a prophylactic pacemaker. Similarly, first degree atrioventricular (AV) block does not increase operative risk.

Patients who should have a preoperative pacemaker are those with CHB, high grade AV block, Mobitz type II AV block, symptomatic sinus node dysfunction, and symptomatic bradyarrhythmia.

For patients who already have a pacemaker, the anesthesiologist needs to know the type, pacing mode, and rate. A cardiologist should determine the function of the patient's pacemaker and evaluate possible surgical risks.

Chronic Pulmonary Disease

Surgery on the thorax or upper abdomen causes noticeable decreases in certain aspects of respiratory function, which can lead to hypoxemia, atelectasis, and pulmonary infection. With upper abdominal surgery, forced expiratory volume in one second (FEV_1) decreases 40 percent to 60 percent in the postoperative period. Forced residual capacity can drop 50 percent with an increase in tidal volume and respiratory rates that normally maintain minute ventilation. Forced vital capacity (FVC) declines as much as 40 percent of baseline values. These values usually return to preoperative values in 7 to 14 days. For patients with known lung disease, FEV_1 greater than 0.5 liter and FVC greater than 1 liter are usually accepted as minimum for thoracic or abdominal operations. Factors that increase risk of postoperative pulmonary infections include thoracic and upper abdominal surgery, surgery lasting over 4 hours, advanced age, obesity, known obstructive lung disease, general anesthesia (33), abnormal pulmonary function tests, and absence of respiratory therapy. Elderly patients should have pulse oximetry before major surgery and an arterial blood gas determination if abnormal lung function is suspected. These tests can provide important baseline measurements if the patient shows a clinical change postoperatively.

Efforts to optimize the patient's pulmonary status should be undertaken. These can include respiratory therapy, bronchodilators, and smoking cessation. Although there are immediate benefits from smoking cessation (lowering carboxyhemoglobin levels, enhanced oxygen carrying capacity, alveolar macrophage adherence), the effect on mucociliary clearance and airflow obstruction is delayed, with no change seen for at least 2 months. Thus, 2 months is the current recommendation for optimal time for smoking cessation before surgery (34). Cessation less than two weeks before surgery has been associated with an increase in pulmonary complications (34). For patients with reversible airway disease, bronchodilator therapy with inhaled agents or low dose corticosteroids is favored over aminophylline, which can have a toxic interaction with halothane.

Diabetes

Diabetes is common among geriatric patients. Diabetes also is a predictor of atherosclerotic vascular disease. Diabetics have increased platelet aggregation, decreased tissue oxygenation, impaired resistance to infection, pressure ulcer development, and greater likelihood of subclinical coronary, vascular, or renal disease (35). Special care is necessary to maintain normal blood glucose levels because this facilitates wound healing; care is also needed to prevent complications from these conditions. Glucose management for patients undergoing major surgery is as follows:

1. Diet-controlled diabetics—check blood glucose every 6 hours.

2. Oral hypoglycemic-treated patients—administer usual agent on the day of surgery with an infusion of 5% dextrose and glucose determinations every six hours.

3. Insulin-dependent diabetics—give 1/2 the usual total daily dose as an intermediate-acting insulin the morning of surgery, begin a 5% dextrose infusion, check glucose every 2 hours through recovery room stay, then every 6 hours with additional regular insulin, as needed, to keep serum glucose at approximately 150 mg/dL. It is most important to prevent symptomatic hypo- or hyperglycemia.

4. For patients who have total parenteral nutrition, check serum glucose hourly through surgery and until the patient is stable.

Steroid Dependence

If the patient has been taking systemic steroids 2 weeks or longer during the previous 6 months, parenteral steroids (intravenous hydrocortisone, 100 mg/6 hr) should be begun the night before surgery and tapered to the patient's usual dose when oral corticosteroids can be resumed.

Nutrition

Before surgery the patient should have carefully controlled nutrition. Poor nutrition increases surgical risk, delays wound healing, lowers the threshold for infections, and potentiates development of pressure ulcers (4). A simple screen for adequacy of nutrition includes the following:

1. Serum albumin at or more than 3.5 mg/dL

2. Total lymphocyte count over 1800/ml

3. Weight more than 80 percent of ideal or body mass index (BMI) at or more than 21 kg/m²

4. Total cholesterol more than 160 mg/dL

5. Patient taking adequate calories

If these parameters are not met, the patient should receive nutritional intervention before surgery, if possible, with use of oral supplements, multivitamins, and 1 to 2 gm/day of ascorbic acid. Total calories of 30 to 35 cal/kg/day and 1.50 gm/kg/day of protein should be provided. If the patient's gastrointestinal tract is functioning, oral supplements may be adequate. More seriously ill patients may need peripheral or central hyperalimentation. For patients who are wasted, have not been eating before surgery, and for whom gastrointestinal function will not be normal promptly after surgery, prompt hyperalimentation should be considered.

Nurses should give special attention to elderly patients who are able to tolerate oral food. Simply placing a tray at the patient's bedside may be inadequate because elderly patients may be confused or otherwise unable to feed themselves. Monitoring self-feeding, encouragement, or hand-feeding the patient may be needed to ensure adequate intake.

Anemia

If the patient has chronic anemia (more than 9 gm/dL), transfusion is not usually required. If the patient has recently lost blood, has known underlying cardiac or pulmonary disease, or if large intraoperative blood losses are expected, transfusion may be needed. Transfusion should be done at least 24 hours before surgery, if possible, to allow equilibration of circulating blood volume. For euvolemic patients, only one unit of packed red blood cells should be given at a time to minimize the risk of volume overload.

Patients Taking Warfarin

If risk of embolization is low (atrial fibrillation without dilated atrium, porcine aortic valve) patients can discontinue medication 36 to 48 hours before surgery and 5 to 10 mg of vitamin K can be administered subcutaneously. Prothrombin times should be checked every 12 hours. One to 2 days after surgery, warfarin can be restarted. If the patient can have nothing by mouth, heparin can be used. Patients at high risk for embolization (nontissue mitral valve) can stop taking warfarin 18 to 36 hours before surgery and 10 to 15 mg of vitamin K can be given intravenously. Heparin should be given 24 to 72 hours after surgery, and warfarin resumed when the patient is stable.

Prophylaxis

Deep Vein Thrombophlebitis

Venous thrombophlebitis is a common complication of surgery (Table 11.8). Geriatric patients undergoing virtually any major surgery are at high risk. Without prophylaxis, 50 percent to 70 percent of patients undergoing knee or hip replacement surgery develop deep vein thrombophlebitis (DVT). Patients with major trauma have similarly high rates (36). Prophylaxis of DVT is intended to prevent pulmonary emboli and postphlebitic venous incompetence. A variety of measures are available (37,38) (Table 11.9). The best choice in a clinical setting depends on the patient's risk for hemorrhagic complication. New low-molecular-weight heparin preparations are effective and do not require laboratory monitoring of clotting times because they have more predictable action and bioavailability.

Talbe 11.8. Risk of Deep Vein Thrombophlebitis.

Surgery	With Prophylaxis (%)	Without Prophylaxis (%)
General surgery	5–10	20–25
Hip replacement	20	45–55
Hip fracture	20	50–70
Total knee replacement	25–35	70
Spinal surgery	4–25	50–70
Abdominal hysterectomy	12–15	35
Femoral fracture	10–40	80

Table 11.9. Methods of Prophylaxis for Deep Venous Thrombosis.

Heparin
  5000 U subcutaneously 2 hr before surgery
  5000 U subcutaneously every 8 hr until ambulatory
Warfarin
  .15 mg/kg on evening before surgery
  .075 mg/kg on evening of surgery
Adjust INR to 1.5–2.0
External pneumatic compression
  Place before surgery
  Continue until discharge
  Can be used with warfarin
Low-molecular-weight heparin
  Enoxaparin 30 mg subcutaneously twice a day after surgery until ambulatory

Table 11.10. Prophylaxis for Infective Endocarditis*.

High-Risk Conditions	Prophylaxis
Prosthetic valvular heart disease History of infective endocarditis Acquired valvular heart disease Mitral valve prolapse Hypertrophic cardiomyopathy	Ampicillin, 1–2 gm IV/IM + gentamycin, 80 mg IV before surgery + amoxicillin, 1.5 gm PO at 6 hr OR Vancomycin, 1 gm IV before 1 hr + gentamycin, 1.5 mg/kg (not to exceed 50 mg) IV hr before surgery

*IV = intravenously; IM = intramuscularly; PO = by mouth.
SOURCE: American Heart Association Antimicrobial prophylaxis for the prevention of bacterial endocarditis. JAMA 1990;264:2919.

Infection

Overall surgical infection rates are approximately 7 percent to 10 percent and include wound, urinary, respiratory, and skin infections, and bacteremia. Infections vary with the type of surgery and whether the wound is clean or dirty. Gastrointestinal surgeries have wound infection rates of 10 percent to 15 percent. The use of prophylactic antibiotics has been examined for many types of surgery. Although many early studies had design deficiencies, the reduction of febrile episodes and overt wound infections has been remarkably consistent at 50 percent compared with those for placebo for most surgical sites. Prophylactic antibiotics should be given no earlier than two hours before surgery and continued for no more than 24 hours after surgery (39). The antibiotic selected should cover the microorganisms most likely to be encountered. For patients with clean upper gastrointestinal, gall bladder, orthopedic, gynecologic, neurosurgical, or vascular surgery, a dose of cephalosporin given preoperatively and continued for 24 hours should be adequate. Patients with colon or rectal surgery should have additional coverage with metronidazole and an aminoglycoside. For patients at risk for bacterial endocarditis (prosthetic heart valves or valvular heart disease) or infection of a prosthetic joint, prophylaxis should be used according to American Heart Association guidelines (40) (Table 11.10).

Prevention and Management of Postoperative Problems

Pain Management

Adequate analgesia without causing abnormal mentation is the goal of postoperative pain management. Mild pain can be managed with nonsteroidals and local treatment (e.g., ice pack). Narcotics are needed for more severe pain. Using narcotics "as needed" (PRN) leads to peak and trough effects (41). Further, it relies on patient and nurse communicating effectively. If pain is expected to be severe and continuous, patient-controlled analgesia has been shown to be both safe and effective, even for frail, elderly persons with lung disease (42). This technique reduces the peak serum levels associated with intermittent dosing and is associated with a much lower risk of postoperative delirium. Contraindications include a baseline dementia or delirium that precludes the patient's ability to understand and remember how to operate the equipment.

Coronary Artery Disease

Postoperative MI occurs in about 1 percent of all adult surgical patients. If surgery is within 6 months of a previous MI, the rate of MI can be 25 percent to 35 percent with a high mortality. If the MI is a reinfarction, mortality is 50 percent to 80 percent; if there was no previous MI, mortality is 35 percent to 40 percent. Only 50 percent of patients with MI have chest pain; CHF or hypotension are the most common presentations. The peak enzyme evidence of MI occurs 24 to 48 hours after surgery.

Patients with known CAD should have an ECG 24 hours after major surgery, and myocardial enzymes should be obtained. These patients need careful monitoring, additional oxygen therapy, and a delay of normal postoperative physical activity until they are clearly stable (43).

Hypertension

Postoperative hypertension can occur as a result of pain, anxiety, hypoxemia, volume overload, alcohol withdrawal, urinary bladder distention, MI, previous hypertension, or shivering. CABG, aortic aneurysectomy, carotid endarterectomy, and urologic surgery are all associated with postoperative hypertension. Because pressures over 200/110 mm Hg can lead to adverse myocardial, renal or cerebral events, the patient's blood pressure should be brought slowly to preoperative levels. If the patient is unable to take oral medications, intravenous preperations of furosemide, propranolol, labetalol, nicardipine, or enalaprilat can be used. Sublingual nifedipine should be avoided because precipitious blood pressure drops can occur.

Pressure Ulcers

Elderly patients commonly have risk factors that predispose them postoperatively to pressure ulcers. Normal age changes in the skin include thinning of the stratum corneum and decreased water content. Specific risk factors are malnutrition, a decline of 1.0 gm/dL of total serum albumin while the patient is in the hospital, immobility, confusion, urinary or fecal incontinence, and fracture. Risk factors should be identified early and attended to with use of nutritional intervention, frequent position changes, and pressure-relieving devices. The physician should inspect the patient's skin daily for signs of early breakdown (see also Chapter 27).

Fever

Postoperative fever in a geriatric patient should have the same attention it would receive in a younger patient, but because of the effect of fever on metabolic demands and cardiac output, fever in elderly patients can lead to CHF. The most common sources are surgical site wound infection or abscess formation, respiratory infection including atelectasis and pneumonia, urinary infection, clostridium difficile infection, intravascular device infection, drug fever, thrombophlebitis, or pulmonary emboli. Principles of evaluation and management of fever are the same as for younger patients.

Transfusions

Postoperative anemia can be caused by intra- or postoperative blood loss, dilution from intravenous fluids, blood drawing, occult loss, and poor hematopoiesis. One study showed an average of 500 to 100 ml of whole blood removed by blood draws during a 3- to 4-week hospital stay (44). In the first few days after major surgery, the patient may have dilutional anemia. Careful attention to the patient's overall volume status is essential to prevent prema-

ture transfusion with increased interstitial fluid and CHF. If the patient's hemoglobin falls below 10 gm/dL or if the patient shows symptoms of angina or CHF, transfusion should be considered. In elderly patients, it is prudent to give only a single unit of packed cells at a time. This allows for a clinical assessment to determine whether signs of CHF are present. If the patient needs more blood, a low dose of a loop diuretic (10 to 20 mg of furosemide given intravenously) may be used to decrease the mobilization of interstitial fluid that occurs when plasma oncotic pressure rises with transfusion.

Deconditioning

Prolonged bed rest has several negative effects on the older patient (45,46), such as cardiac deconditioning, atelectasis, bone demineralization, loss of joint flexibility, reduced strength, and decreased baroreceptor response. The effects can diminish stability and may make standing or walking impossible without assistance. Loss of functional integrity can preclude the patient's return to an independent living arrangement, even though the patient's surgery achieved the desired results. Rehabilitation efforts should begin as early as possible, including having the patient out of bed on the day of surgery, when feasible. Even with optimal therapy, a slow period of functional recovery is normal for a geriatric patient. Hip fracture with surgical repair, for example, is associated with a one-year mortality rate of 25 percent and a 30 percent rate of permanent nursing home placement (47).

Discharge Planning

For a frail, elderly patient, being hospitalized can produce major declines in functional status. Plans for discharge needs should begin preoperatively. The patient who was previously independent may, on discharge, need rehabilitation, skilled nursing services, or assistance with activities of daily living. The patient may need specialized dressings or equipment. With elective surgical procedures, a discharge plan can be developed even before the patient is admitted. In other circumstances, discharge planning should begin as soon as the patient stabilizes and an appropriate living arrangement can be identified. A person skilled in discharge planning for elderly patients and knowledgeable of community service providers is an essential member of the patient's team. The nurse(s) and any therapists working with the patient in the hospital can recommend ongoing services and teach family caregivers how to follow up hospital procedures. Who will assume responsibility for the various components of the patient's subsequent care must be determined. The patient's primary care physician must be identified. If the patient goes to a nursing home, current information and planned treatments should be made available as rapidly as possible to the physician assuming the patient's care.

The discharge plan should address cognitive and behavioral factors that affect the patient's posthospital needs, the patient's functional status, postdischarge environmental barriers, nursing and other care requirements, available family and community support resources, patient goals and preferences, and options consistent with patient needs.

Summary

Age alone need not preclude major surgery if the surgery is likely to benefit the patient. Careful attention to preoperative preparation, communication with the anesthesiologist and surgeon regarding important premorbid conditions, and close postoperative monitoring with early mobilization can lead to a satisfactory outcome.

References

1. Hosking MP, Warner MA, Lobdell CM, et al. Outcomes of surgery in patients 90 years of age and older. JAMA 1989;261:1909–1915.
2. Waxman K. Hemodynamic and metabolic changes during and following operation. Crit Care Clin 1987;2:241–248.
3. Clowes GHA, Del Guercio LM. Circulatory response to trauma of surgical operations. Metabolism 1960;9:67–81.
4. Christou NV, Tellado-Rodriguez J, Chartrand L, et al. Estimating mortality risk in preoperative patients using immunologic, nutritional, and acute-phase response variables. Ann Surg 1989;210:69–77.
5. Seymour DG, Vaz FG. A prospective study of elderly general surgical patients: preoperative medical problems. Age Ageing 1989;18:309–315.
6. Seymour DG, Vaz FG. A prospective study of general surgical patients II: postoperative complications. Age Ageing 1989;18:316–326.
7. Boyd JB, Bradford B, Watne AL. Operative risk factors of colon resection in the elderly. Ann Surg 1980;192:743–746.
8. Dripps DR, Lamont A, Eckenhoff JE. The role of anesthesia in surgical mortality. JAMA 1961;178:261–266.
9. Hirsh R, et al. In: Stickley GF, ed. Health care delivery in anesthesia. Philadelphia: Saunders, 1979.
10. Daly M. The medical evaluation of the elderly preoperative patient. Prim Care 1989;16:361–376.
11. Kammerer WS, Gross RJ, eds. Medical consultation. Baltimore: Williams & Wilkins, 1990.
12. Goldman L, Caldera DI, et al. Cardiac risk factors and complications in non-cardiac surgery. Medicine 1978;57:357–370.
13. Goldman L, Caldera DL, Nussbaum SR, et al. Title. N Engl J Med 1977;297:845–850.
14. Detsky AS, Abrams HB, Forbath N, et al. Cardiac assessment for patients undergoing noncardiac surgery. Arch Intern Med 1986;146:2131–2134.
15. Eagle KA, Coley CM, Newell JB, et al. Combining clinical and thallium data optimizes preoperative assessment of cardiac risk before major vascular surgery. Ann Intern Med 1989;110:859–866.
16. Raby K, Goldman L, Creager M, et al. Correlation between preoperative ischemia and major cardiac events after peripheral vascular surgery. N Engl J Med 1989;321:1296–1300.
17. Golden MA, Whittemore AD, et al. Selective evaluation and management of coronary artery disease in patients undergoing repair of abdominal aortic aneurysms. Ann Surg 1990;212:415–420.
18. Raby K, Barry J, Creager M, et al. Detection and significance of intraoperative and postoperative myocardial ischemia in peripheral vascular surgery. JAMA 1992;268:222–227.
19. Wong T, Detsky A. Perioperative cardiac risk assessment for patients having peripheral vascular surgery. Ann Intern Med 1992;116:743–753.
20. Beleslin B, Ostojic M, Stepanovic A, et al. Stress echocardiography in the detection of myocardial ischemia. Head-to-head comparison of exercise, dobutamine, and dipyridamole tests. Circulation 1994;90:1168–1176.
21. Marwick TH, Nemec JJ, Pashkow FJ, et al. Accuracy and limitations of exercise echocardiography in a routine clinical setting. J Am Coll Cardiol 1992;19:74–81.
22. Poldermans D, Fioretti P, Boersma E, et al. Dobutamine-atropine stress echocardiography in elderly patients unable to perform an exercise test: hemodynamic characteristics, safety, and prognostic value. Arch Intern Med 1994;154:2681–2686.
23. Mahar LJ, Steen PA, Tinker JH, et al. Perioperative myocardial infarction in patients with coronary artery disease with and without aorto-coronary artery bypass grafts. J Thorac Cardiovasc Surg 1978;76:533–537.
24. Huber KC, Evans MA, Bresnahan JF, et al. Outcome of noncardiac operations in patients with severe coronary artery disease successfully treated preoperatively with angioplasty. Mayo Clin Proc 1992;67:15–21.
25. Baron J, Mundler O, Bertrand M, et al. Dipyridamole-

thallium (scintography and gated radionuclide angiography to assess cardiac risk before abdominal aortic surgery). N Engl J Med 1994;330:663–669.

26. Mangano DT, Hollenberg M, Fegert G, et al. Perioperative myocardial ischemia in patients undergoing noncardiac surgery–I: incidence and severity during the 4-day perioperative period. J Am Coll Cardiol 1991;17:843–850.

27. Gustafson Y, Brannstrom B, Berggren D, et al. A geriatric anesthesiologic program to reduce acute confusional states in elderly patients treated for femoral neck fractures. J Am Geriatr Soc 1991;39:655–662.

28. Folstein MF, Folstein S, McHuth PR. Minimental state: a practical method for grading the cognitive state of patients for the clinician. J Psychiatr Res 1975;12:189.

29. Schrader LL, McMillen MA, Watson CB, MacArthur J. Is routine hemodynamic evaluation of nonagenarians necessary? J Am Geriatr Soc 1991;39:1–5.

30. Pastore JO, et al. The risk of advanced heart block in surgical patients with right bundle branch block and left axis deviation. Circulation 1978;57:677–680.

31. Bellocci F, et al. The risk of cardiac complications in surgical patients with bifascicular block. Chest 1980;77:343–348.

32. Ventkateraman K, et al. Indications for prophylactic preoperative insertion of pacemakers in patients with right bundle branch block and left anterior hemiblock. Chest 1975;68:501–507.

33. Yeager MP. General versus regional anesthesia and cardiovascular safety. Anesthesiol Rev 1989;16:42–46.

34. Stoller J. Preoperative preparation of the patient. In: Kacmarek RM, Stoller J (eds.) Current Respiratory Care. Toronto: B.C. Decker, 1988.

35. Murray JF. Wound healing with diabetes mellitus. Surg Clin North Am 1984;64:769–777.

36. Geerts W, Code K, Jay R, et al. A prospective study of venous thromboembolism after major trauma. N Engl J Med 1994;331:1601–1606.

37. Collins R, Scrimgeour A, Yusuf S, et al. Reduction in fatal pulmonary embolism and venous thrombosis by perioperative administration of subcutaneous heparin. N Engl J Med 1988;318:1162–1173.

38. Weinman E, Saltzman E. Deep-vein thrombosis. N Engl J Med 1994;331:1630–1641.

39. Classen DC, Evans SR, Pestotnik SL, et al. The timing of prophylactic administration of antibiotics and the risk of surgical wound infection. N Engl J Med 1991;326:281–286.

40. American Heart Association. Antimicrobial prophylaxis for the prevention of bacterial endocarditis. JAMA 1990;264:2919.

41. Ferrell B. Pain management in elderly people. J Am Geriatr Soc 1991;39:64–73.

42. Egbert AM, Parks LH, Short LM, Burnett ML. Randomized trial of postoperative patient-controlled analgesia vs intramuscular narcotics in frail elderly men. Arch Intern Med 1990;150:1897–1903.

43. Boyd O, Grounds RM, Bennett DE. A randomized clinical trial of the effect of deliberate perioperative increase of oxygen delivery on mortality in high-risk surgical patients. JAMA 1993;270:2699–2707.

44. Eyster E, Berene J. Nosocomial anemia. JAMA 1973;223:73–74.

45. Creditor MC. Hazards of hospitalization of the elderly. Ann Intern Med 1993;118:219–223.

46. Hirsch C, Sommers L, Olsen A, et al. The national history of functional morbidity in hospitalized older patients. J Am Geriatr Soc 1990;38:1296–1303.

47. Lu-Yao G, Baron J, Barrett J, et al. Treatment and survival among elderly Americans with hip fractures. A population-based study. Am J Public Health 1994;84:1287–1292.

Chapter 12
Geriatric Rehabilitation

Laura Mosqueda and Kenneth Brummel-Smith

It is quite wrong to think of old age as a downward slope. On the contrary, one climbs higher and higher with the advancing years, and that, too, with surprising strides. Brain work comes as easily to the old as physical exertion to the child. One is moving, it is true, toward the end of life, but that end is now a goal, and not a reef in which the vessel may be dashed.

George Sand

One of the most important goals of geriatric care is the preservation or enhancement of the patient's functional abilities. Rehabilitation provides the mechanism for achieving this goal. Knowledge of rehabilitation is important to primary care physicians and other specialists caring for elderly patients because of the high prevalence of functional disabilities among the older population (1) and because access to the services of a specialist in physical medicine and rehabilitation may be limited for geriatric patients in some settings.

In geriatric care settings, rehabilitation is often conducted by a team of providers. Physicians work in concert with nurses, allied health therapists, and others to strengthen, retrain, and teach new activities to those with functional deficits. Function is viewed as an interplay between biological, psychological and social realms of life (2) (Figure 12.1). The rehabilitation team tends to each of these areas to maximize the person's performance.

Older persons may lose the ability to function independently for a variety of reasons. Classic reasons for receiving rehabilitation include such conditions as a recent stroke or amputation. However, in geriatrics, there are often many reasons, acting on one another, that create the need for rehabilitation. An episode of congestive heart failure in a person with diabetes and mild peripheral neuropathy may leave the patient so deconditioned that living alone is not possible. The latter form of functional decline is perhaps more common, and more frequently overlooked, than the classic cases.

The perception of functional loss and its treatment may be affected by personal and cultural variables. For instance, some persons may view old age as a time to be cared for, as having a "right to dependency." In those families in which only female members have functioned as homemakers, loss of some skills in instrumental activities of daily living (IADL), such as house cleaning or shopping, by males may not be seen as a deficit. Many older persons have never experienced an interdisciplinary care setting. Treatments provided by someone other than a physician or a nurse may be very upsetting.

What Is Unique About Geriatric Rehabilitation?

Several important steps are involved in rehabilitation (2) (Table 12.1). Stabilization of the primary problem is important in any rehabilitation program. Older adults, however, often have more than one primary problem or the primary problem may be difficult to define. For example, an elder who undergoes coronary artery bypass surgery and then has a stroke has at least two primary problems (coronary artery disease and hemiparesis), both of which must be addressed for a rehabilitative program to be effective. Another elder may have multiple chronic illnesses (e.g., diabetes, hypertension, history of myocardial infarction, osteoarthritis, depression), all of which contribute to a general decline or deconditioning that would improve with a rehabilitation program. For a patient to benefit fully from any rehabilitation program, the illnesses must be treated to maximize the individual's function and ability to participate.

While the health care team is identifying and treating the primary problem(s), they must also take care to prevent secondary disabilities. Older adults are particularly susceptible to secondary disabilities because they are also experiencing normal changes of aging (1). For example, bed rest is a form of treatment that carries many risks in

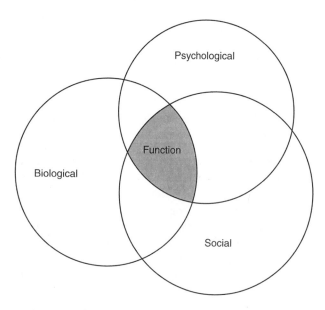

Figure 12.1. Function as a product of biological, psychological and social factors. The interplay of biological, psychological, and social realms of life creates function.

Table 12.1. Steps in Rehabilitation.

Stabilize the primary disorder
Prevent secondary disabilities
Promote functional recovery
Promote adaptation

the geriatric patient. Compared with a 35-year-old, an 85-year-old has a thinner epidermis and greater capillary fragility, which makes skin breakdown a greater threat; muscle mass is smaller and causes rapid loss of strength if the muscles are not used; intestinal motility is decreased, which makes impaction more likely. Yet, the typical geriatric patient in an acute care hospital is left to lie in bed most of the day, thereby increasing the likelihood for many secondary disabilities.

Other secondary disabilities are more specific to the underlying illness. In a patient who experiences a stroke, for example, care must be taken not to pull on the patient's affected arm and worsen a shoulder subluxation. If the physician and other health care staff are thinking about prevention from the outset, the patient is more likely to be ready for a rehabilitation program at

an earlier stage and is more likely to benefit from the program.

Functional deficits should be identified, evaluated, and treated in a timely manner. Many older adults who have an acute illness also have a history of functional problems. Therefore, obtaining information about the person's previous functional status is important to develop a realistic rehabilitation plan. The acute illness itself may have caused new functional deficits to appear. It is not uncommon for a functional deficit to be the result of a number of factors, some of which may be modifiable. For example, if the physician notices that a patient's ability to walk is severely impaired after a hysterectomy, it is important that the physician first perform a functionally-based examination to identify the problem. Next, the physician must seek the causes: Is this a result of prolonged bed rest after surgery? An exacerbation of congestive heart failure? A side effect from medications? All of these may be occurring simultaneously, and all may be modified to maximize function.

As the patient moves through the rehabilitation process, health care providers should assist with adaptation: of the person to his disability, of the environment to the person, of the family to the person, and of the person to the family (Table 12.2). All too often we try to adapt the person to the environment, rather than the other way around. Rehabilitation programs provide many strategies for altering the environment to promote maximal independence for the patient.

Disability is often accompanied by disbelief. As the patient moves through the rehabilitation process it is important to help the patient gradually understand the impact of the disability, and the physician must be vigilant in looking for evidence of depression. Encouragement is always needed, but counseling and medication are often useful adjuncts. The physician and rehabilitation team should also assist the family and patient in the transition to new roles that often occur with the onset of a new

Table 12.2. Adaptation.

Person to their disability
Environment to the person
Family to person
Person to family

disability, especially if the older adult has accompanying cognitive changes. Disability never affects just one individual; its impact is felt by all those who are a part of the patient's social network. Many losses occur as a person grows older: loss of friends, family, social roles, and function. A successful rehabilitation process must also address these factors.

Rehabilitation in Different Care Settings

Acute Rehabilitation

In acute rehabilitation, the most intensive approach to rehabilitation, the patient must be able to tolerate as much as 3 hours of combined physical and occupational therapy, speech pathology, or all three, per day. A physician knowledgeable in rehabilitation should oversee the patient's program, and an interdisciplinary team should be involved. Patients with recent stroke, spinal cord injury, multiple fractures, and traumatic brain injury are often rehabilitated in an acute rehabilitation unit. Medicare (and most third-party payors) require the patient show progress that is measurable and goal directed (3). If the expected place of discharge is a nursing home, payors will not usually reimburse.

Skilled Nursing Facility

A skilled nursing facility can offer an ideal environment for rehabilitation of the elderly patient. Therapy is provided 5 to 6 days per week but sessions are often short and held in groups. All standard therapists are available. Patients with mixed causes of decline, such as stroke with deconditioning, may particularly benefit from this approach. Patient progress toward goals and a periodic team meeting are required for reimbursement by Medicare. The Council on Accreditation of Rehabilitation Facilities (CARF) is developing accreditation standards for subacute facilities, most of which will be located in nursing homes. Meanwhile, there is wide variability in the quality of rehabilitative care offered in nursing homes.

Outpatient Clinics

Outpatient clinics that provide rehabilitation are often located in hospitals with rehabilitation departments. In some states, physical and occupational therapists func-tion as private practitioners accepting referrals. Certified Outpatient Rehabilitation Facilities (CORF) are in many communities. Transportation to the facility is often the limiting factor for older persons.

Home

Home rehabilitation is useful to those patients with good family support and less severe deficits. All therapies can be provided, but to receive reimbursement under Medicare the patient must, at minimum, receive physical therapy. Patients should have reasonable cognitive retention skills because the ability to remember past therapy strategies is important to progress. Patients can receive rehabilitation only as long as they are "house-bound."

Assessment of Rehabilitation Potential

"Rehabilitation potential" is a nebulous concept. The notion of rehabilitation potential implies that some patients will benefit from a rehabilitation program and others will not. How does one distinguish between these patients? Potential must be examined in the context of the patient's goals and those of the patient's support system. The goals should be compared with the predicted outcome to judge whether they are realistic. If so, or if the goals are modifiable to make them realistic, the patient has good rehabilitation potential (4).

Rentz states ". . . the assessment of rehabilitation potential estimates the individual's capability of cooperating with a rehabilitation program and making measured functional gains. It also appraises whether the patient's current quality of life can be improved upon despite chronic or multiple disabilities" (5). Assessment should include an evaluation of the person's physical status, psychological or cognitive status, or both, and socioeconomic status because all these factors influence the patient's and family's goals as well as the outcome.

Evaluation of Physical Status

In addition to the components of a routine physical examination, the physician should focus on a functional assessment of the patient. This encourages the examiner to search for the patient's *abilities* as well as his *disabilities*. Optimizing the patient's function is a prerequisite for conducting a fair assessment.

Cardiovascular Assessment

A careful history includes a probe for symptoms of angina, claudication, orthostatic hypotension, and congestive heart failure. The routine cardiac examination is accompanied by a careful search for evidence of peripheral vascular disease. If a patient is at high risk for ischemic heart disease, this may need to be addressed before a vigorous rehabilitation program is initiated. Echocardiography and stress testing may be needed in some cases.

Pulmonary Assessment

Normal changes of aging cause an increase in a person's functional residual capacity and residual volume, but the total lung capacity remains the same (6). These changes lead to a decrease in vital capacity and forced expiratory volume in 1 second (FEV_1), thereby reducing the older adult's pulmonary reserve. In addition to these normal changes, if the patient also has a history of lung disease (e.g., smoking, asthma), the patient's pulmonary status may limit a rigorous rehabilitation program.

Neuromuscular Assessment

The neuromuscular exam should be functionally based to assess an individual's strengths and weaknesses. There is a natural tendency to examine the affected area more thoroughly than the nonaffected area. However, nonaffected areas are often called upon for extra duty during a rehabilitation program. For example, an elderly woman with limited range of motion in her left shoulder because of an old injury may have never experienced any problems as a result. However, if she has a left-sided stroke with resultant right hemiparesis, the limitations in her left shoulder may greatly affect her rehabilitation potential.

Cognitive Assessment

A careful assessment of cognition should be the first part of the neurological examination. There are many tools available for this purpose. The Mini-Mental State questionnaire is a brief and easy-to-use example of a practical screening tool (7). To participate in an intensive rehabilitation program, patients must be able to learn. Learning involves the ability to pay attention, register, and recall information. Interestingly, patients with memory loss, such as the type that occurs in Alzheimer's disease or in multi-infarct dementia, are able to relearn overlearned tasks such as walking and feeding as long as new information (e.g., complicated instructions for using a walker) is not necessary for success. The ability to remember motor skills may be preserved even when the ability to remember verbal information has been severely impaired (5). Those who have limited attention may do better in a less intensive program that requires only short periods of concentration.

Evaluation of Psychological Factors

The importance of diagnosing and treating common psychological injuries that often accompany aging and disability cannot be overestimated. A patient who is depressed may be lethargic, withdrawn, and uninterested in getting better, and thus appear to be a poor rehabilitative candidate. However, once the depression is treated the patient may be able to participate in a program and make good progress. Many tools are available for the evaluation of depression (see Chapter 43). Health care team members, such as psychologists and social workers, may be called upon to assist with the evaluation. A study by Rosillo and Fagel demonstrated that a person's self-assessment of his potential for recovery was positively correlated with improvement in a rehabilitation program (8).

The physician should begin with the assumption that all geriatric patients have rehabilitation potential until proven otherwise. If the patient is judged to be a poor candidate for any type of rehabilitative program, there is a question to be asked: "What can I do to improve this person's rehabilitation potential?" The answer may range from removing medications to treating a depression to improving blood sugar control if the patient is diabetic.

The Physician's Role in Rehabilitation

Though much of the day-to-day effort in rehabilitation is provided by therapists and nurses, the role of the physician is paramount to a patient's success. The physician should participate in defining the causes of the patient's functional problems and review the assessment and plan of other team members. The physician should also participate in determining measurable goals or outcomes for the patient. An especially important task is to identify risks and special considerations in treatment that may effect the interventions of therapists. For instance, clarification of the patient's cardiopulmonary status is important to the physical therapist when he or she treats a stroke patient. Early diagnosis and treatment of medical and psychological conditions facilitates the patient's progress in rehabilitation and ensures good outcomes.

Rehabilitation Team Members

Rehabilitation is conducted in a team setting. Home and outpatient care is usually multidisciplinary; that is, various team members see the patient individually and communicate with one another by telephone or through the patient's chart. In more intensive care settings, such as the acute rehabilitation unit or the nursing home, an interdisciplinary team meets regularly to discuss assessment findings and plans, exchange reports of patient progress, and deal with problems.

Physical Therapist

The physical therapist assesses transfers, mobility, and conditioning and treats deficits in strength and endurance. Even simple mobility may be a problem for older persons. Physical therapists can optimize balance and mobility functions through a variety of treatment strategies.

Occupational Therapist

The occupational therapist assesses the patient's skills in Activities of Daily Living (ADL) and Instrumental Activities of Daily Living (IADL), treats deficits in self-care activities, and optimizes the patient's upper extremity function. In geriatrics, occupational therapists often participate in cognitive assessments and facilitate recovery of sensory and perceptual abilities.

Speech Pathologist

The speech and language pathologist evaluates and treats disorders of communication, speech, and swallowing and work closely with audiologists when the patient has hearing difficulties. Speech pathologists may also assess cognition.

Nurse/Restorative Aide

Especially in defined rehabilitation units, the nurse plays a crucial role in assessing the patient's ability to carry over activities learned in training. The nurse is with the patient in more normal settings than that of the therapy gymnasium and can reinforce newly learned techniques. The nurse also assists with family training, adaptation, and education.

Nutritionist

Nutritional deficits are common in rehabilitation patients. Stroke survivors are at particular risk [9]. A registered dietitian should assess nutritional status in most rehabilitation patients. The nutritionist can recommend modifications in diet to optimize the patient's functional improvements and can provide education to the patient and family.

Social Worker

In rehabilitation settings, psychosocial evaluation and assessment of mood are often the purview of the social worker. Social workers may assess family stress and coping skills and play a key role in coordination of discharge planning.

Recreation Therapist

The recreation therapist is very important to the rehabilitation of elderly persons. Some older persons may be more active in a social, recreational environment than they are in the standard therapy gymnasium. After a disabling condition develops, leisure skills and desires may determine whether the patient responds with hope or despair. The recreation therapist can provide new experiences and help the patient explore new options.

Rehabilitation of Functional Deficits

Regardless of the cause of disability, the treatment of functional deficits requires attention to many important factors. The primary functions and activities dealt with in rehabilitation include balance, transfers, gait and mobility, feeding and dressing, toileting, bathing, and grooming. Cognition and communication are other important areas addressed.

Many assistive devices can be prescribed for the patient

so that he or she can complete these activities more efficiently or independently. However, no tool should be prescribed without the patient receiving training in its use. Inadequate training may lead to the tool ending up in a closet or drawer instead of being used.

Balance

Balance involves the ability to maintain one's center of gravity over the base of support. Balance is essential for safety and independence. If balance is poor, arising from a chair may be an impossibility; walking may become a dangerous activity; independence in the performance of many common activities is jeopardized.

We use primarily visual, vestibular, and proprioceptive inputs to sense where we are in space and maintain our equilibrium. All these senses undergo some decline as a consequence of normal aging (10). The overlay on normal aging of a disability, as occurs with Parkinson's disease or osteoarthritis, for example, may cause severe difficulty with balance for the older adult.

The patient's sitting and standing balance need to be assessed. While the patient is seated, the clinician should observe whether the patient is leaning or using an upper extremity to remain upright. When the patient stands, the physician should watch for sway. If the patient keeps her feet wide apart, she requires a large base of support to maintain balance. If the patient looks stable, a gentle but firm nudge on the sternum will test the patient's ability to recover when her center of gravity is displaced (11).

Any abnormalities in balance should lead to a search for cause(s) and cure(s). The physician should consider medical conditions that may be causing pain, fatigue, or weakness and find out whether these conditions are being treated fully. The physician should also look for evidence of depression or anxiety, both of which may contribute to inattention. The patient should discontinue medications that may have side effects such as lightheadedness or sedation. The physician should examine the patient's feet and notice the type of footwear being used (slippers are slippery).

Treatment usually involves evaluation by a physical therapist who may initiate an exercise program designed to strengthen weak muscles and teach the patient compensation strategies. If the patient uses a wheelchair, the therapist should assess the appropriateness of the chair.

An adjustment in the type of chair or cushion may lead to a major improvement in sitting balance. Sitting balance involves the use of trunk muscles that can be strengthened with exercises such as catching and throwing a beach ball from the seated position. If sitting balance is adequate, the patient may work on improving standing balance.

Patients who have had prolonged bed rest may have symptomatic orthostatic hypotension even after all medications that may have contributed to the problem are removed (12). These patients may be placed on a tilt table with gradual increases in the angle and length of time at steeper angles every day (Figure 12.2). Use of parallel bars can improve balance further. With initial training, the patient holds the bars with both hands and learns to maintain balance while leaning in the lateral and anterior/posterior planes. Eventually the patient learns to keep in balance while holding the bars with one hand. As the patient moves the free hand more and more, he becomes ready to maintain balance outside the parallel bars.

Transfers

A transfer involves movement from one surface to another. Good sitting balance, along with adequate strength and flexibility are prerequisites for successful transfers. Examples of transfers are moving on and off the toilet, from bed to wheelchair, and from sitting to standing positions. A patient's inability to transfer is a major obstacle to independence.

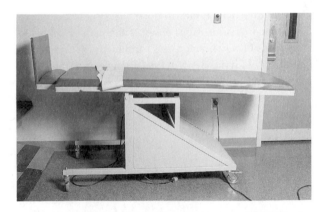

Figure 12.2. Tilt Table. Table allows gradual elevation toward vertical position and thus enables the patient with orthostatic hypotension to recover vascular homeostatic mechanisms.

An evaluation of transfer ability involves taking a history and observing the patient's movements and safety judgment. Transfers require adequate physical and cognitive status. For example, a patient who has the physical ability to arise from a wheelchair but lacks the capacity to remember to lock the brakes is at high risk of falling. One test to evaluate a patient's transfer ability is to ask the patient to get up from a chair without using his hands. Weakness of the lower extremities will make this task difficult or impossible. Some patients rock back and forth several times to gain the necessary momentum to arise. Once up, they are usually unsteady, at least for an instant. These same patients will probably "plop" into the chair when asked to sit down without using their hands. "Rockers" and "ploppers" benefit from an evaluation by a physical therapist, who may prescribe an exercise program, adaptive equipment, or both. Simple interventions such as using chairs with arm rests and high seats may be all that is needed.

Because adaptive equipment should promote independence not foster dependence, a trained specialist such as a physiatrist or rehabilitation therapist should order or recommend most devices. Raised toilet seats with a frame may permit a patient with weak or painful lower extremities to remain independent with toileting activities. A tub transfer bench can allow a patient who has difficulty getting in and out of the bathtub to do so with minimal, if any, assistance.

Stand to Sit Transfer Pattern

The patient turns his back to the chair until he feels the seat against the back of his legs. He then reaches for the arm rest with his stronger arm. While flexing forward, he places his other hand on the arm rest and then gently sits down.

Stand Pivot Transfer Pattern

This type of transfer is particularly useful for persons who use wheelchairs and have limited use of one side of the body. The patient sits on the side of the bed with the wheelchair parallel to the bed. While standing on the stronger leg, the patient reaches for the far arm rest with the stronger arm. She then pivots 90 degrees so that the wheelchair is behind her and lowers herself into the chair.

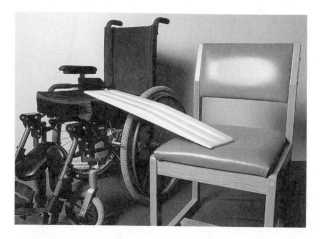

Figure 12.3. Sliding Board. A sliding board enables a person who is unable to stand to transfer from a bed to a wheelchair.

Sliding Board Transfer Pattern

This technique is useful for those who are unable to bear weight on their lower extremities, but it requires good upper extremity strength. A sliding board is placed between the two surfaces, for example, between a wheelchair and a car seat (Figure 12.3). The patient pushes downward with his arms, raises his body, and shifts to the board. He continues to move sideways until he shifts to the car seat.

Gait and Mobility

Proper treatment and prescription of assistive devices for gait and mobility begins with an accurate assessment of the patient's functional deficits. Most older persons greatly desire to walk independently. Often, this function is perceived as the most important one determining independence. However, deficits in sensory and perceptual function more accurately determine independence. The physician should measure alterations in gait patterns with use of a standardized tool such as the Tinetti gait and balance scale, or by formal pathokinesiology assessment (11).

A wide variety of canes, walkers, and wheelchairs exist for use by someone with an ambulation problem (Figure 12.4). A physical therapist should always be involved in prescribing these devices. Canes provide minimal stability and must be sized to allow the patient a slight bend at

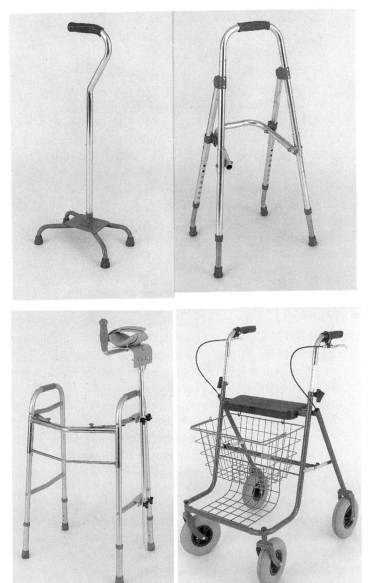

the elbow when he or she stands erect. A cane can be used to help "unweight" an affected hip, for example; thus, it should be held in the hand opposite the involved side. Four-prong canes are useful indoors but hard to manage outside. Pick-up walkers (no wheels) provide great stability and can be used when the patient is not allowed to bear weight on one side. A "hemiwalker" is useful for those who have had a stroke and who need a moderate amount of balance stability to walk. Front-wheeled walkers provide good stability and are less prone to slipping away than are four-wheeled models. Patients also like the new walkers with three or four wheels, handbrakes, and attached cargo baskets. These walkers tend to be less medical in appearance and therefore may be more readily accepted by the patient.

The choice of a wheelchair also requires the expertise of a physical therapist. The patient's size (both height and weight), locomotion and transfer needs, disability, skin integrity, stability, amputation status, and other features all affect the choice of a proper wheelchair. For the stroke patient, the seat is lowered from the normal 22 inches to 18 inches above the ground to facilitate directional control with the unaffected leg. Lightweight systems are available for patients with upper extremity weakness (Figure 12.5). Posterior tipping ("wheelies") can be prevented with casters. A special seating system can promote proper positioning and prevent skin breakdown. Arm troughs and lapboards can be attached to position flaccid upper extremities.

Many older persons benefit from a motorized wheelchair or scooter. Even those able to walk short distances may find these devices helpful in getting out into the community. The patient must have adequate sensory function of vision and hearing and adequate cognition to operate motorized devices safely.

Figure 12.4. Walking Aids. *A.* Standard straight canes do not usually provide enough support for a patient with a stroke. The platform cane provides more stability than a straight cane. *B.* A hemiwalker is used when the patient needs greater stability but a regular walker is inappropriate because the patient has unilateral upper extremity weakness. *C.* Patients with wrist arthritis, or partial control of an upper extremity, may benefit from having a trough attachment on a standard walker. *D.* If the patient has good control of both upper extremities, a four-wheeled walker may be best because it is more maneuverable and the basket allows the patient to carry objects.

Feeding and Dressing

The physician should observe the patient at first meeting: Is the patient wearing a sweater or pullover dress because he or she is unable to manipulate buttons? Is the patient wearing slippers because he or she is unable to tie shoelaces? When dressing or undressing, does the patient have the balance, strength, and flexibility to put on socks? Does a female patient have adequate range of motion in her shoulders and adequate strength in her arms to fasten

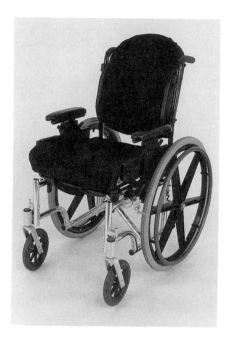

Figure 12.5. Lightweight Wheelchair. Lightweight chairs may be easier for the patient to propel and may require less energy than standard models.

her brassiere? Ask the patient to drink from a cup: Does a tremor disrupt the process? Can the patient grasp the cup firmly?

These types of observations are simple, quick, and provide valuable functional information about dressing and feeding abilities. It is important to determine whether and how a patient is able to carry out these tasks. A person who is unable to feed or dress himself, or who does so with difficulty, often benefits from a referral to an occupational therapist. In addition to teaching the patient exercises and techniques, the occupational therapist is familiar with the myriad of adaptive equipment available.

Some patients are physically able to dress themselves, but have a cognitive impairment that interferes with the process. They may be unable to choose the appropriate clothes, or may require prompting during the dressing process. Experience shows that these patients are often "dressed" by the caregiver, when all that is really needed are simple verbal instructions from the caregiver. An analogous situation sometimes exists for the cognitively impaired elder who lacks motivation to feed himself.

Many types of adaptive equipment assist with dressing and feeding (13) (Figure 12.6). Buttonhooks are appropriate for those who do not have fine-motor control but do have gross grasping ability. Long-handled shoe horns and sock aids are helpful to many who have poor range of motion at the hips, poor balance, or weak grip. Shoes with hook and loop fasteners may enable a person to put on shoes. For people who have difficulty with feeding because of weak upper extremities there are a variety of arm supports and hand splints that maximize remaining function. Many older adults have one "good" arm and one "bad" arm, which makes keeping a plate in position problematic while they eat. Nonslip mats that hold the plate in place and rimmed dishes can make one-handed eating an easier task.

Toileting, Bathing and Grooming

When a patient has weak hip extensors that cause the patient to be unable to rise from a chair without using hands, a raised toilet seat facilitates safe transfers and personal hygiene (14). Arm attachments can be mounted to any toilet and are cheaper than purchasing a new toilet (Figure 12.7). The patient may also benefit from using zipper pull loops or hook and loop clothing closures. Patients in wheelchairs need a tilt mirror to perform personal grooming. Toothbrushes with handles built-up with foam tubes are useful if the patient has hand weakness or limitation in range of motion.

If the patient can make safe transfers but does not have the balance or endurance to stand in a shower, a tub seat with suction cups on its feet is helpful. A bathtub transfer bench allows the person with transfer problems to sit, then slide into the tub area (Figure 12.8). In either case, a handheld shower hose attachment is also needed. A long-handled back brush helps those with limited range of motion in the upper extremities. Vertical grab bars are helpful in showers and above tubs.

Communication

Speech pathology evaluation usually determines what type of special adaptive equipment is required for those with communication deficits. Patients with expressive aphasia may benefit from the use of a picture communication board. Telephones with large numeric pads and automatic dialers are often helpful. An electronic alert

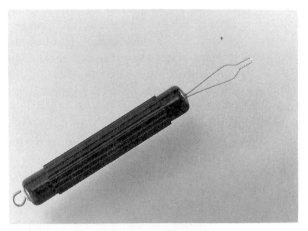

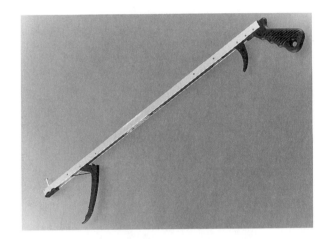

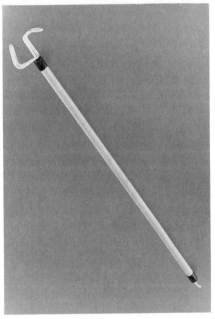

Figure 12.6. Dressing Aids. *A.* The buttonhook is useful to button clothes with one hand. *B.* A clothes hook is a simple but useful device. It can be used to pull off socks, undo hook and loop closures, or pull sweaters over the head. *C.* A reacher is used to grab objects from the floor, from over one's head, or from any place that requires a long reach.

necklace may be useful when the patient has a high risk of falling. Touch or clapping systems for turning on and off electrical equipment are easy to install and are helpful.

Maintenance Rehabilitation

Unless the patient can demonstrate improvement with rehabilitation, Medicare does not reimburse for therapy, that is, maintenance therapies are not covered. However, many older persons are on a downhill slide in terms of

functional abilities and any intervention that "maintains" their skills is useful. Such interventions are mandated by the Omnibus Budget Reconciliation Act of 1987 and may play a role in the prevention of secondary disabilities. These interventions are less intense and of longer duration than standard rehabilitation activities. In the nursing home, they are often provided by "restorative aides," nurses' aides who have special training.

All patients should be encouraged or assisted to maintain a regular program of range-of-motion (ROM) exer-

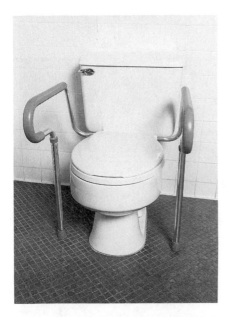

Figure 12.7. Toilet Arm Attachments. Toilet arm attachments enable a person with weak hip extensors to rise from the toilet without assistance. They also permit safer descent to the toilet. These attachments are relatively inexpensive and simple to install.

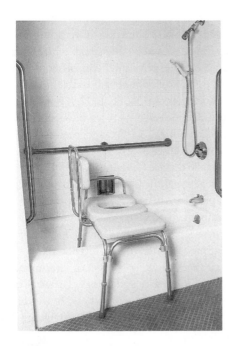

Figure 12.8. Bathtub Transfer Bench. This bench attaches to the bathtub and provides a stable base for transfers.

cises, bedside exercises, transfers, and supervised walking. The performance of simple activities of daily living (ADL) help to maintain conditioning, balance, and flexibility.

Chair-bound patients are particularly prone to complications. Contractures can be prevented by ROM exercises twice daily, with special attention to the hips and knees. Pressure sore prevention and upper extremity strengthening require a proper seating system, performing arm depressions every 30 minutes, and doing exercises using elastic bands or light weights (1 to 2 pounds).

Group exercises for maintenance rehabilitation are often well accepted by patients and stimulate mental function and socialization. For instance, a parachute game, in which a circle of patients seated in wheelchairs hold the edges of a round piece of material and attempt to block passing a ball off one edge, stimulates reaction time, upper extremity range of motion, and is fun.

Rehabilitation of Common Geriatric Conditions

Stroke

Stroke is the most common diagnosis for which older persons receive rehabilitation. Early rehabilitation interventions are important to prevent secondary disabilities and to set the stage for functional recovery (15). Proper bed positioning, turning, ROM exercises, and attention to hydration, nutrition, and maintenance of an appropriate blood pressure (>135/85) is emphasized in the acute rehabilitation hospital.

The patient and family need information about outcomes and plans. Overall, about 85 percent of persons survive stroke (90 percent survive the more common infarction and 50 percent survive hemorrhage). Functional abilities show complete recovery, 10 percent; minor disability, 40 percent; major disability, 40 percent; and dependent status, 10 percent (16).

Certain features allow further prognostication. Patients with less severe paralysis, less perceptual neglect, no (or only receptive aphasia), less sensory loss, no pseudobulbar palsy, and good cognition do better (17). Most gains in motor function will be seen during the first month, with virtually all recovery completed by 6 months. However, speech, swallowing, and sensory return may occur as late as 2 years after the stroke.

Physical therapy promotes both static and dynamic balance, first while the patient is sitting on the bed, then during transfers, and finally, while the patient is walking. The patient learns bed mobility, transfers from bed to wheelchair and from chair to toilet.

Gait training can begin when the person can maintain standing balance, support weight on the unaffected side, and advance the affected limb somewhat. Depending on the person's strength and balance, some sort of walking aid is usually needed. Straight canes are rarely used because they do not provide adequate stability. Patients who must support more of their weight with their upper extremities use hemiwalkers. A four-prong cane is used when less support is needed. Regular walkers may be very difficult for patients with stroke to use because these patients often have one weak arm. Wheelchairs are often used, even by those who can walk, to negotiate long distances. Whenever a patient has a wheelchair, it should be fitted by a physical therapist, who can make certain it is the right height and width. The patient can steer the chair with the unaffected leg to allow propulsion with one arm.

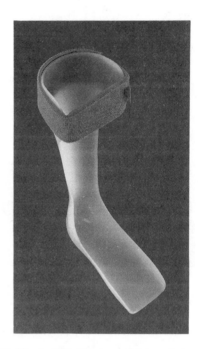

Figure 12.10. Plastic AFO. This is used for weak dorsiflexor muscles or foot drop.

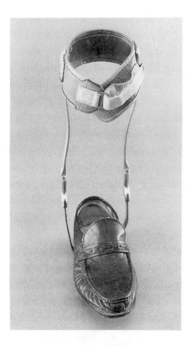

Figure 12.9. Metal Ankle-foot-orthosis (AFO). An AFO is used for stabilization of weak ankles and control of spasticity.

Therapists often use functional electrical stimulation (FES) to enhance the contraction of weak muscles, control spasticity, and provide biofeedback. Braces are commonly used and the physical therapist should help select appropriate types. A double-adjustable, upright, metal, ankle-foot-orthosis (AFO) (Figure 12.9) is heavy, unattractive, and difficult to don, but it is the brace of choice for those with spasticity. The plastic posterior AFO helps those with muscle weakness but has limited use for controlling spastic muscles (Figure 12.10).

The occupational therapist provides training in ADLs. The therapist teaches new methods of dressing, feeding, and grooming early and gives attention to sensory, perceptual and cognitive deficits. A wide variety of adaptive equipment may be offered, such as rocker knives for one-handed cutting, dressing sticks, or buttonhooks. The training in grooming includes use of special bathroom equipment such as bathtub benches, shower hoses, and raised toilet seats. Specific aids for ADLs are listed in Table 12.3.

Speech pathologists provide much more than retraining in communication for patients with stroke. Cognitive

Table 12.3. Aids for Activities of Daily Living.

Feeding—Rocker knives, cutting boards, plate retainers
Dressing—Buttonhooks, velcro-closures, tilted mirrors, reachers
Toileting—Grab bars, arm frames, raised seats
Bathing—tub bench, shower hose, grab bars, long-handled brush
Grooming—tilt mirror, built-up handles
Safety—"Lifeline" service, remote-control lights, telephone
 dialers, stair rails, removal of throw rugs

reorganization, training in the use of alternative communication techniques (such as picture boards), and evaluation and retraining for swallowing problems are all pursued.

The role of the geriatrician for patients with stroke varies with the site of care. In the inpatient setting the geriatrician is responsible for medical management and patient advocacy. The patient's blood pressure must not be allowed to drop too low. All drugs that may cause confusion or depression must be removed or reduced. Depression must be recognized early for intervention to provide optimal results. Malnutrition caused by swallowing dysfunction may require temporary tube placement, but neither nasogastric tubes nor gastrostomy tubes significantly reduce the risk of aspiration compared with that of oral feeding (18). Anticoagulation for deep venous thrombosis is controversial (19). Many authorities recommend it for patients with infarction during the immobile period of recovery. Once ambulation has begun, most physicians discontinue anticoagulation. However, all patients with atrial fibrillation should be anticoagulated after an infarction (20).

Amputation

Amputations occur primarily in older patients. Almost 75 percent of all amputees are older than age 65 (21). Peripheral vascular disease is the most common cause of amputation and that presents special problems. First, there is a high incidence of contralateral amputations later in the patient's life. Second, the patient is also likely to have underlying cardiac disease. This is important because walking with a prosthesis after below-the-knee (BK) amputation requires approximately 25 percent more energy than does bipedal ambulation. Nevertheless, more than 75 percent of geriatric amputees eventually achieve independent ambulation after a BK procedure (22). However, the energy cost of walking with an above-the-knee amputation is so great (approximately 65 percent above normal) that few older patients ever walk again. Therefore, when an amputation is being considered, the geriatrician should advocate a BK procedure whenever possible.

All patients should have optimal physical and emotional status before undergoing amputation. Preoperative education and training are essential. Patients should be encouraged to practice ROM and quadriceps strengthening exercises. Having the patient lie prone for 10 to 15 minutes helps prevent hip and knee flexion contractures. Upper body strengthening is also important.

After the operation, the head of the patient's bed must not be raised higher than a few degrees and pillows must not be placed under the patient's knees. These measures help to prevent hip and knee flexion contractures. Exercises can begin the second postoperative day. Patients must learn single-limb standing and transfers. Once the patient's stump has healed, he or she must learn stump care. Massage, wrapping, and inspection for signs of skin breakdown or irritation must be done on a daily basis.

A permanent prosthesis is usually fitted about 6 to 8 weeks after surgery to allow the stump to shrink completely. Most older patients use a solid ankle, cushioned heel (SACH). In addition to a fitted socket, a waist belt is also used for attachment. Proper fitting is important; prostheses can cost more than $2500.

Wheelchair training is also important because most older patients also use a wheelchair when traveling long distances. Although for some patients a prosthesis is inappropriate (e.g., those with moderate cognitive deficits, severe contralateral vascular disease or weakness, or joint disease), the patient may desire a cosmetic prosthesis.

Patients frequently have phantom limb sensation, but pain, fortunately, is uncommon. Pain is best treated with a combination of analgesic drugs, massage, and sometimes, local anesthetic injections. Skin breakdown is usually caused by poor stump care and an improperly fitting prosthesis.

Hip Fractures

Many geriatric patients benefit from rehabilitation after a hip fracture. Unfortunately, since the advent of diagnosis-related groups, fewer patients are receiving therapy and functional outcomes have declined (23). Patients in special need are those with underlying arthritis, cardiopulmonary disease, or conditions in which unsupervised exercise may be contraindicated. Generally, the earlier the patient can begin walking, the better the long-term prognosis. Some surgical procedures, such as percutaneous pinning, require the patient to only use "partial weight bearing" for as long as 8 weeks post-operatively. Most older people have difficulty with partial weight bearing and choose not to walk at all. With a compression screw or a prosthetic replacement, the patient can begin walking after 2 to 3 days.

All patients should be medically stabilized before surgery. The uninvolved limb can be ranged and exercised while the patient is waiting for surgery. The day after surgery, the patient can sit up and can start quadriceps exercises. The hip should not be flexed more than 90 degrees or excessively adducted.

Supervised walking can begin with the patient using a walker or cane to "unweight" the affected leg. The walker should be fitted so the patient's arms are bent at 20 to 30 degrees when they are at the side, resting on the grips. The patient should advance the walker 20 to 30 cm, then move the weak leg forward first. No more than 20 percent to 25 percent of the patient's weight should be placed on the walker or the patient is likely to fall; energy expenditure is extreme. Special walkers are needed to climb stairs. The patient should lead with the good leg when ascending stairs and lead with the affected leg when descending ("up with the good, down with the bad"). A basket or bag on the walker will allow the patient to carry things.

Other Conditions

Arthritis

Pain management is the cornerstone of treatment. Without pain, the patient can perform daily ROM exercises, lie prone for 10 to 15 minutes, and exercise. Judicious use of intra-articular injections are helpful and easy to perform. Occupational therapists can be particularly helpful in providing adaptive equipment and training in joint protection techniques.

Parkinson's Disease

Early group rehabilitation, dance classes, and singing classes all may be beneficial in promoting functional abili-

ties (24). Patients should not use canes because of the tendency to catch the cane between the legs and cause a fall. A walker is a safer choice when assistance is needed. Speech therapy may help patients with breath and voice control (25).

Deconditioning

This is commonly seen in patients who have had prolonged bed rest or hospitalization. Symptoms are an exaggerated blood pressure response to exercise, unusual dyspnea on exertion (with no evidence or other causes), and lack of endurance during ADLs. The patient should practice stretching, strengthening, and ROM exercises. Supervised ambulation training may be required. The best treatment for deconditioning is prevention. There is very little reason for an older person to be placed on "bed rest." Unless specifically contraindicated, all geriatric patients in hospitals should sit in chairs most of the time, walk or be helped to the bathroom, and eat their meals sitting up. If possible, they should walk or be helped to walk to diagnostic procedures.

Summary

Rehabilitation is a basic component of care for the geriatric patient. Efforts to detect and prevent functional losses and to restore functional abilities should proceed in all health care settings. Although the involvement of a physiatrist or other rehabilitation specialist may be necessary, primary physicians caring for older persons should be able to develop or coordinate most rehabilitation interventions for most older people with functional decline.

References

1. Gershkoff AM, Cifu DX, Means KM. Geriatric rehabilitation. 1. Social, attitudinal, and economic factors. Arch Phys Med Rehabil 1993;74:S402–S405.
2. Brummel-Smith K. Introduction. In: Kemp B, Brummel-Smith K, Ramsdell JW, eds. Geriatric rehabilitation. Boston: Little, Brown, 1990.
3. Torres-Gil FM, Wray IA. Funding and policies affecting geriatric rehabilitation. In: Brummel-Smith K, ed. Clinics in geriatric medicine 1993;9:831.
4. Mosqueda IA. Assessment of rehabilitation potential. In: Brummel-Smith K, ed. Clinics in geriatric medicine 1993; 9:831.

5. Rentz DM. The assessment of rehabilitation potential: cognitive factors. In: Hartke RJ, ed. Psychological aspects of geriatric rehabilitation. Gaithersburg, MD: Aspen, 1991.

6. Knudson R. Physiology of the aging lung. In: Crystal RG, West JG, eds. The lung: scientific foundations. New York: Raven, 1990.

7. Folstein MF, Folstein S, McHugh PR. Mini-mental state: a practical method for grading the cognitive state of patients for the clinician. J Psychiatr Res 1975;12:189.

8. Rosillo RA, Fagel ML. Correlation of psychologic variables and progress in physical therapy: degree of disability and denial of illnesses. Arch Phys Med Rehabil 1970;51:227.

9. Axelsson K. Nutritional status in patients with acute stroke. Acta Med Scand 1988;224:217.

10. Rees TS, Duckert IG. Auditory and vestibular dysfunction in aging. In: Hazzard WR, et al., eds. Principles of geriatric medicine and gerontology. San Francisco: McGraw-Hill, 1990.

11. Tinetti ME, Ginter SF. Identifying mobility dysfunctions in elderly patients. JAMA 1988;259:1190.

12. Harper C, Lyles Y. Physiology and complications of bed rest. J Am Geriatr Soc 1988;36:11.

13. Mitchell SCM. Dressing aids. BMJ 1991;302:167.

14. Arborelius UP, Wretenberg P, Lindberg F. The effects of armrests and high seat heights on lower-limb joint load and muscular activity during sitting and rising. Ergonomics 1992;35:1377.

15. Lorish TR. Stroke rehabilitation. In: Brummel-Smith K, ed. Clinics in geriatric medicine 1993;9:705.

16. Folger WN: Epidemiology of cerebrovascular disease. In: Brandstater ME, Basmajian JV, eds. Stroke rehabilitation. Baltimore: Williams & Wilkins, 1987.

17. Combovy M, Sandok B, Basford J. Rehabilitation for stroke: a review. Stroke 1986;17:363.

18. Clocon JO, Silverstone FA, Graver LM, Foley CJ. Tube feedings in elderly patients—indications, benefits and complications. Arch Intern Med 1988;148:429–433.

19. Charness ME. Controversies in the medical management of stroke—Medical Staff Conference, University of California, San Francisco. West J Med 1985;142:74–78.

20. Peterson P, Boysen G, Godtfredsen J, et al. Placebo-controlled, randomized trial of warfarin and aspirin for prevention of thromboembolic complications in chronic atrial fibrillation. Lancet 1989;175.

21. Key HW, Newman JD. Statistical comparisons of 6000 new amputations. Prosthet Orthot 1975;29:24.

22. Clark GS, Blue B, Bearer JB. Rehabilitation of the elderly amputee. J Am Geriatr Soc 1983;31:439.

23. Fitzgerald JF, Moore BS, Dittus RS. The care of elderly patients with hip fractures. N Engl J Med 1988;319:1392.

24. Formisano R, Pratesi L, Modarelli FT, et al. Rehabilitation and Parkinson's disease. Scand J Rehabil Med 1992;24:157.

25. Johnson JA, Pring TR. Speech therapy and Parkinson's disease: a review and further data. Br J Disord Communi 1990;25:183.

Chapter 13
Home Care

George Taler and Timothy Keay

In all the world there are no people so piteous and forlorn as those who are forced to eat the bitter bread of dependency in their old age, and find how steep are the stairs of another man's house.

Dorothy Dix

Long-term care in the home is the fastest growing sector of health services delivery in the United States (1), with Medicare expenditures for home health care increasing from $2.12 billion in 1988 to $10.5 billion in 1993 (2). Approximately half these national expenditures, or $5 billion, are medically oriented, and homemaker and personal care services cost an additional $6 billion to $7 billion per year (3). The 1992 National Home and Hospice Care Survey conducted by the National Center for Health Statistics found over 1 million patients receive in-home services on any given day. Growth of home care services has been stimulated by the boom in the elderly population, changes in the hospital environment, and financial implications of nursing home placement.

Efforts to reduce the costs of care to the chronically ill have led practitioners to explore increasingly more complex care in the home rather than extending hospital stays or institutionalization. Advances in technology and loosened restrictions on location of service have allowed the home care industry to respond to patients' needs with equipment previously restricted to the acute care setting. Also, most long-term care insurance policies include provisions for home care, which facilitates access to these services.

Five to 10 percent of patients in the average primary care practice receive services in their home under the direction of the physician. Contrary to popular belief, a recent survey of primary care physicians showed that 53 percent to 82 percent make house calls (4). Most patients who receive in-home services are female (67%) and older than age 65 (75%), with an average age of 70 years. The most frequent diagnoses included heart disease, diabetes, arthritides, malignant neoplasms, cerebrovascular disease, hypertension, and fractures. In addition to assistance with activities of daily living (ADL), most patients receive a variety of rehabilitative, skilled nursing services, and social services. The average length of service before discharge is 94 days, with most patients demonstrating improvement or stabilization of their underlying condition (5). Therefore, developing the skills and organization to efficiently handle these cases is advantageous to every primary care physician.

Benefits of Home Care

There are several advantages in developing home care as an important component of the spectrum of primary care service. First, medical groups that offer home care services are perceived as caring and compassionate. The improved public relations enhances the attractiveness of the practice in a competitive market. Also, the patients appropriate for house calls are usually more efficiently seen at home. When seen in the office, multiply impaired patients require additional staff time to assist with dressing, mobility, or continence; the stretcher-bound patient who occupies an examination room waiting for ambulance transport can seriously undermine office flow; and it takes extra physician time to review a complex medical treatment plan while the patient is in the office (especially if the patient is not accompanied by the primary caregiver) and to make decisions for adjustments to the patient's regimen.

The rate of hospital admission for home-bound patients is 0.5 admissions per patient per year, the highest rate among ambulatory patients, and higher than the rate for those in nursing homes (6). Familiarity with the potential of in-home services and the willingness to see the patient at home for follow-up facilitates discharge planning. Home care may reduce hospitalizations among certain populations. Hospital recidivism from respiratory, cardiac, endocrine, and mental illnesses may all respond to intensive in-home monitoring and support. The Social/ Health Maintenance Organization (S/HMO)—a Health Care Financing Administration (HCFA) demonstration project that includes patients with physical frailty among its Medicare clientele—incorporates home care to programmatic advantage and to improve patient satisfaction.

The house call presents an array of professional challenges for which the physician must be prepared, mostly through self-study. Few residency training programs incorporate home care experiences and few role models exist in the academic world. There is a natural trepidation to venture outside the familiar surroundings of the hospital or ambulatory settings, without the immediate support of the nursing staff, ancillary diagnostic facilities, or easy accessibility of colleagues and consultants.

House calls are also good for the physician because they add an important dimension to the knowledge of the patient's circumstances, sharpen primary care skills, and develop greater appreciation for the costs and invasiveness of medical interventions. A study by Ramsdell (7) showed that approximately two new problems per patient were found among patients who were initially evaluated in the office and subsequently evaluated at home. Twenty-three percent of these new problems had a potential for significant morbidity or mortality, approximately equally divided between medical, psychiatric, and safety concerns. As a result, from one to eight new recommendations were needed in the patient's plan of care.

Safety issues, compliance problems, hygiene, and extra medications the patient has obtained over-the-counter, from family or friends, or from other physicians are rarely considered when the patient is seen in the physician's office. Seeing patients in their homes uncovers situations that require skills of other health professionals, such as family counseling, financial planning, home safety, assessment for rehabilitative equipment, and linkage with community resources. As technology applicable to home care becomes more complex, primary care practitioners must learn to manage devices previously encountered only in the hospital, but mastery of this management opens the way to one of the most personally rewarding experiences in all of primary care.

Practicing in the patient's home presents a real test of the physician's skills in obtaining a history, performing a physical examination, and developing a diagnostic differential on which to base therapy. The physician's diagnostic skills must be finely honed to succeed in providing high quality care. The added costs and inconvenience of diagnostic testing and consultation promote a stepwise, algorithmic strategy that is generally more appropriate in geriatric practice. Negotiating with patients on their own "turf" reinforces the importance of patient autonomy and ethical decision making, and reaffirms the balance in the doctor-patient relationship.

Patients who are considered suitable for home care benefit from more than the convenience of the physician's visits; in-home supports have been shown to improve the patient's overall health and functional and cognitive status (8). In addition, a house call obviates the cost of specialty transport and the possible embarrassment to the patient of public exposure.

Developing an Office-Based House Call Program

A well-conceived and deliberate plan is necessary to run an efficient house call program.

Choosing the Right Patients

The best candidates for house calls are patients with mobility impairments or disruptive behaviors. Wheelchair-bound persons who have difficulty transferring to the examination table and patients who are quadriplegic require extra staff and time to have an adequate physical evaluation. Patients who suffer dementia, retardation, or severe psychiatric disorders may decompensate in a public waiting room and cause discomfort for all involved. Others who may be suitable for house calls are patients with complex, chronic, medical and psychiatric problems, especially patients with multiple medications or a plethora of issues that need to be addressed at each visit. Patients to whom the physician is committed through personal relationships or familial obligations but who are chronic "no-shows," disruptive to office scheduling, and not managable by telephone are also candidates for house calls.

For some patients, house calls need to be scheduled only for a short period of time. For patients recently discharged from the hospital and whose course was either prolonged or complicated, a home visit highlights the appliances and services needed for support during convalescence. Terminally ill patients who find it a hardship to come to the office and who have become homebound are more effectively seen at home to address their physical and emotional needs. Patients not responding to what should be adequate therapy, or whose response is inconsistent, may benefit from a diagnostic home visit. In these perplexing situations, a house call often elucidates nutritional problems (or indiscretions), allows verification of the purchase of prescribed medications, or reveals the presence of extra medications that are interfering with the expected response. Situations of suspected caregiver burnout or elder abuse are also better assessed by a diagnostic house call. In short, much more information comes from a house call than from an office visit.

Subacute problems arising between visits often may be managed very effectively by initiating a nursing visit and an in-home laboratory or radiologic assessment. The nurse can usually see the patient within 24 hours and provide an assessment. Diagnostic tests are also usually available within this time frame, allowing a reasonably accurate basis for diagnosis and therapy. However, house calls are generally not appropriate for patients with an acute, serious illness. An Emergency Department is better suited to efficiently evaluate a patient with unstable vital signs, acute delirium, or significant trauma. An exception is in the case of the imminently terminal patient who has elected to forgo hospitalization. Because the medical care plan will require careful consideration and negotiation with the family, an intercurrent house call will often result in more humane care.

Establishing an Office Organizational Structure

Two components are necessary for a successful house call program based in a private office setting. The first is to organize the information flow; the second, to establish a house call team from community resources. The objective is to manage the house call aspect of the service spectrum with maximum efficiency and least disruption to the physician's ambulatory practice.

House Call Coordinator

A house call coordinator is the pivotal component in a successful house call practice. All calls, including those from patients, nurses, and vendors, are channeled through the coordinator. For the patients, emergency triage is managed through simple algorithms. Special beeper codes convey the relative importance of messages to the physician. The role of a care coordinator for the patients and their caregivers provides a vital link to the office and saves much physician time on the telephone. Other providers become comfortable working through the coordinator, which saves time both for them and for the office. Home care nurses who leave messages and updates have assurance that a written note will document their report and that true emergencies will be conveyed promptly. The physician can aggregate return calls on the basis of verification that the parties will be available at the designated time and that the patients' chart information is accessible for an efficient interchange. The coordinator also organizes correspondence, charting, and scheduling arrangements for special clinic appointments or for office visits to consultants.

House Call Team

The house call team comprises the physician who makes house calls, the house call coordinator, representatives from the home care agency, and other vendors with whom the program has an informal working arrangement. It is best to align with one home care agency. The choice of agency should be made on the basis of several factors, such as the service area, affiliation with major hospital(s) at which the physician has privileges, adequate size to provide timely services, and a solid reputation. Coordinating services with a limited number of nursing agencies ensures a more cohesive health care team. If an agency is willing to assign nurses, social workers, and therapists who can participate in team meetings to the patients in the practice, the physician can get to know their capabilities, and the agencies can become more comfortable with the style of the physician and the office.

Other members of the house call team who should attend team meetings are a pharmacist and a durable medical equipment vendor. A community pharmacist can work in consultation with the physician in reviewing drug profiles and alerting the team to new medications and formulations. By delivering to the home, the pharmacist is more likely to increase the number of initial referrals; by assuming responsibility for oversight of patient compliance, repeat business is assured. Affiliation with the house call program can also have a beneficial effect through increased referrals from the practice and from improved public relations with the community. Similarly, a durable medical equipment vendor benefits by receiving referrals and by the built-in forum for marketing new products. The patient also benefits by having access to the most current services and devices with a minimum of bureaucratic hassles.

House call team meetings are important for communication, for interdisciplinary consultation, and also for the timely completion of all the required documentation. A regular agenda facilitates the flow of information. While the physician reports, others can complete paperwork associated with house call patients and listen for information that may be pertinent for cross-covering. The principal nurse reports on the patients requiring skilled services; the home care liaison supervisor conveys information from the physical therapists, occupational therapists, or other nurses who have seen patients under the practice's care. The pharmacist should supply printed profiles for active patients, report on compliance issues, and review any intercurrent changes in a patient's medical regimen for cross-checking by a drug interaction program and discuss interaction findings with the physician. New orders for nursing, equipment, or medications issued during the presentations, can be written and signed immediately. Weekly team meetings for programs that cover 100 patients generally last about 1 hour.

Financial Considerations

Financial considerations are essential to the success of the house call program. The first issue is to determine the size of the home care practice to ensure an adequate number of calls will be made to warrant the time commitment. The second issue is to determine appropriate remuneration for the services rendered.

Determining Practice Size

Time management and preparation are also essential components for a successful house call practice. The physician should set aside a specific time period to make house calls, preferably during the day. Generally, one-half day per week is sufficient to manage 50 to 60 patients seen quarterly for routine visits and as needed if they are less stable. There are no restrictions on remuneration for number of visits as long as the progress notes show sufficient justification for the visits. However, patients who need to be seen by a physician more than once a week should be considered for hospitalization or hospice services. Patients who need only additional supervision may have home care nurses visit as often as twice daily, for a short time.

The physician should define a reasonable geographic area for house calls. The area can be divided into quadrants, each visited once monthly, or visits can be clustered along a specified route to reduce travel time. Generally, five to seven patients can be seen in their homes during a half-day session; 10 to 12 patients can be seen when visits can be clustered in a few locations. The physician may refer patients outside the catchment area to other doctors willing to make house calls. The physician should also keep a calendar and plan return visits at the conclusion of each house call. This allows the flexibility to see patients as appropriate to their conditions, coordinate visits with other house calls in the neighborhood, and to fit into the patient's family schedule. Keeping a calendar also establishes a timetable and prevents overscheduling.

Optimizing Remuneration

The key to ensuring justification for remuneration is documentation. Records of telephone contacts with patients, family, home care staff, and team meetings are advisable, in addition to the patients' progress notes. Documentation of patient encounters should include history-taking data, physical examination findings, a therapeutic reassessment reflective of all active diagnoses, and an evaluation of the patient's functioning, caregiver issues, and evidence of a medical care plan for the ensuing period.

A hindrance for the involvement of physicians in home care is lack of reimbursement for case management services. Current procedural terminology (CPT) codes have been established for team conferences and prolonged telephone consultations.

As of 1995, Medicare has agreed to pay on a monthly basis for Care Plan Oversight (CPO) at a rate comparable to a high-level, established-patient home visit. Criteria defining eligibility for remuneration under the CPO code are different than for any other evaluation and management service; early experience suggests that approximately one quarter of the home care case load may be eligible. The patient must be under the active care of the physician as demonstrated by a face-to-face encounter within the six months prior to the initiation of CPO billing, and must be under the care of a Medicare-certified home care agency for a Medicare covered service (for example, home infusion therapy is excluded under Medicare, and so, excluded under CPO). There is a minimum requirement for 30 minutes per calender month of documented time devoted exclusively to the coordination, monitoring and adjusting of the medical care plan, beyond that needed for routine care. Billable time includes only interactions with other health professionals through meetings, telephone calls or in review of correspondence and medical records. Services usually provided as part of the follow-up of office or home visits may not contribute to CPO time. Therefore, telephone calls with the patients or their family, contacts with other office staff and routine matters, such as prescription renewals or signing home care agency orders, may not be counted. CPO may not be billed for care covered under a global fee arrangement, such as for follow-up of a surgical procedure, or services provided by the Medical Director or an employee of a Medicare Hospice. Finally, certain professional relationships may exclude physicians from billing under the CPO code. Physicians who hold a 5% or greater ownership share in the home care agency providing services, or receive greater than $25,000 in compensation from the agency are ineligible for billing for CPO provided through that agency. Since CPO is a new code with a novel set of criteria, the Medicare intermediaries are likely to be scrutinizing the documentation supporting the charges, underscoring the importance of comprehensive medical record keeping.

A medical director contract with a home care agency can also enhance revenue to the practice. Such contracts require approximately 4 to 8 hours a week for chart reviews for quality assurance purposes, inservice training for the agency staff, liaison with other physicians, and policy review and development. Criteria must be met to ensure compliance with certain "self-referral" statutes enacted in many states. It is prudent not to own stock in the home care agency, or any other entity that is financially aligned with the practice. No more than 25 percent of the home care agency's revenues may derive from affiliation with the practice, and the services rendered must not be types that would normally be given without compensation or types reimbursable through patient care. Under no circumstances can the physician accept remuneration for referrals on a patient-by-patient basis or through an exclusivity contract.

Conducting a Home Visit

Appointments should be scheduled to allow adequate time for assessment and to ensure that responsible family members will be present. For a first appointment, at least one hour is needed. Observation begins with the neighborhood: its cleanliness, its proximity to convenience stores, pharmacy, and the like, and the condition of the other houses in relation to the patient's home. Disparities between the patient's house and those surrounding it may offer clues to the level of functioning of the patient, the patient's financial status, and the possible availability of friendly neighbors for assistance to the patient.

For patients new to the practice who will be managed under the house call program, the physician should provide as much information before the first visit as is practicable. An advance packet of information about the services available through the program, selected history questionnaires, and requests for copies of recent medical records, including hospitalizations, will streamline the first visit (Table 13.1). Questionnaires should be completed by the patient and family in preparation for the visit. Listing the patient's chief complaints can help focus the encounter and ensure that all issues are addressed. Including an advance directive form in the packet encourages the patient and family to discuss these matters, and opens discussion concerning the nature and extent of care the patient desires and expects. After reviewing the advance packet materials, the initial visit priorities for new patients are to obtain a working history based on the patient's chief complaints and current problems, a targeted physical examination, an assessment

Table 13.1. The Advance Packet.

Letter of introduction to the house call program
  Names and telephone numbers of personnel in the physician's
    office with whom patients can expect to interact
  House call visit policies for regular, subacute, and acute visits
  Physician's affiliations with hospitals, home care agencies, and
    other vendors
  Physician's availability by telephone
  Charges for services
Questionnaires and forms
  Medical, family, and social histories of the patient
  Review of systems and preventive medicine
  List of prescription and over-the-counter medications that the
    patient takes regularly and as needed
  Medical allergies of the patient
  Nutritional review
  Functional assessment of the patient
  Advance directive form

Table 13.2. House Call Bag Equipment.

Blood pressure cuffs with interchangeable bulb and gauge
  Regular
  Obese
  Pediatric
Gloves with lubricant and hemoccult slides
Otoscope/ophthalmoscope kit
Glucometer
Peak flow meter
Digital thermometer
Goniometer
Tape measure
Hammer/reflex tuning fork
Bandage scissors
Toenail clippers
Portable bathroom scale
Optional equipment
  Sterile scissors, forceps, disposable scalpel
  Sterile 4 × 4 gauze and tape
  Hand-held EKG
  Hand-held otoscope/audiometer

Table 13.3. House Call Bag Stationery.

Prescription blanks
Appointment cards
Progress note paper, history forms, drug flow sheets
Advance directive forms
Release of information forms
Informed consent forms
  Tetanus, pneumovax, influenza vaccinations
  Debridement
  Other procedures
Assessment forms
  Mini-Mental State Examination
  elder abuse checklist
  home safety assessment checklist
Information and referral phone numbers

of mental function and the patient's capabilities with ADLs and instrumental activities of daily living (IADLs) function.

The physician should have a house call bag, a lightweight case capable of carrying 10 to 15 pounds. A durable soft attaché case with multiple pockets works well. Having compact equipment purchased specifically for the bag avoids removing instruments from the office (Table 13.2). Having a folder with supplemental stationery and forms is also helpful (Table 13.3). It is better not to carry any medications, needles or syringes, except as needed for vaccinations. All "sharps" should be returned to the office for proper disposal. If local pharmacies permit telephone prescriptions, it is safer and easier to call in medications so that only a limited number of prescription blanks need to be taken from the office.

A home safety check, an assessment of the need for any appliances within the living areas of the patient, and an evaluation of the capabilities of the caregiver and caregiver supports is other data the physician should gather (see below). Documentation on the patient should also include a problem list, a medication list, and (for new patients or established patients without them) decisions concerning advance directives. This information helps to develop the management goals (e.g., maintenance care or terminal care) and the necessity for further laboratory tests and consultations. A scheduled follow-up appointment completes the visit.

On subsequent visits, a review should encompass ongoing problems—a check of problem and medication lists and monitoring parameters—any intercurrent problems, functional status, and health maintenance such as vaccinations. Some time should be set aside with the caregiver to answer questions, clarify monitoring parameters, and give emotional support.

Special Considerations

Care in the home presents many issues that are outside the usual practice of medicine in the hospital, office, or nursing home. The knowledge gained from house call experiences broadens the scope of concerns that are included in the primary care considerations of patients with multiple impairments. Including home medical care in the spectrum of available options leads to referral to the most appropriate care in the least restrictive environment.

Nursing Home Care Versus Home Care

Three basic questions must be addressed when the possibility of nursing home care, instead of home care, arises. First, are the patient's needs able to be met by the caregiver(s) at home? This consideration rests primarily on the balance between the patient's dependencies and the caregiver's abilities and willingness to supplement or assume responsibilities. Dependencies are best defined through a functional status testing and an assessment for specialized treatments. If the patient's needs cannot be addressed by streamlining the medical regimen or through rehabilitation, they fall to the caregiver. The caregiver's abilities to fill these gaps can be evaluated, and if needed, enhanced through training. If the caregiver is either unable or unwilling to assume responsibility, other caregivers may be recruited from informal or formal supportive networks. Informal caregivers include other family members, friends, or members of a church or fraternal organization willing to fill the breach. Formal service providers are those whose care is usually purchased, either privately or through insurance coverage (e.g., Medicare, Medicaid, or the state Department of Social Services).

Second, can the home environment support the needs of the patient? Are there barriers to mobility that will lead to undue confinement and social isolation within the home, or which may be unsafe? Is there adequate room for appliances and can appropriate rails and other supports be installed? If there is a requirement for a special bed, commode, or other durable medical equipment, are there provisions for privacy and maintenance of personal dignity? Is the level of hygiene appropriate to the management of wounds, enteral feedings, parenteral therapies, or a ventilator?

Third, can the patient or family afford home care? Home care is not always the less expensive alternative. Out-of-pocket costs may prove beyond the means of the patient or family when care is provided in an outpatient setting, but may be covered in the nursing home. Examples include incontinence aids, supplemental feedings, dressings, and medications. Custodial care is included in the nursing home fee, but is most often not covered in the home unless a skilled service is provided concomitantly.

Ultimately, the decision must be made by the patient and the family, but the physician has an obligation to ensure that all factors are fully weighed. Most patients and many families are inclined toward home care but give weight to the opinions of the physician. In instances in which the choices seem contrary to reason, referral to a social worker or to an adult protective services agency may be indicated.

Safety

Safety in the home is an often overlooked concern while evaluating patients in the office. A house call quickly focuses attention on these concerns. The physician should encourage the patient to remove scatter rugs, electric cords, and furniture that may cause an accident. Safety features such as nightlights in the hallway, at the top and bottom of stairways, or a bright colored tape at the top and bottom steps will also help to prevent falls. Rubber mats in the bathroom and in the shower are also important. Families may wish to install remote-control light fixtures or "touch lamps" so the patient can avoid excessive reaching or bending. A home safety checklist can help to organize and focus the review (9) (Table 13.4).

Other aspects of the patient's environment can help to elucidate the overall care provided. The general hygiene of the home is important, especially if the patient is immunocompromised or if wound dressings are required. Glancing into the cupboards and refrigerator gives a sense of the adequacy of nutrition. Barriers to free passage within the home may give clues to whether additional appliances needed by the patient could be accommodated and to the problems that may occur if the patient is left alone for an extended length of time.

Family Dynamics

Family caregivers provide at least 80 percent of the care received by individuals in the community (10). Nearly two-thirds of the caregivers are women, either spouses or

Table 13.4. American Geriatric Society Home Safety Checklist.

This checklist is used to identify fall hazards in the home. After identification, hazards should be eliminated or reduced. One point is allowed for every NO answer. A score of 1 to 7 is excellent, 8 to 14 is good, 15 or higher is hazardous.

	YES	NO
Housekeeping		
1. Do you clean up spills as soon as they occur?		
2. Do you keep floors and stairways clean and free of clutter?	___	___
3. Do you put away books, magazines, sewing supplies, and other objects as soon as you're through with them and never leave them on floors or stairways?	___	___
4. Do you store frequently used items on shelves that are within easy reach?	___	___
Floors		
5. Do you keep everyone from walking on freshly washed floors before they're dry?	___	___
6. If you wax floors, do you apply 2 thin coats and buff each thoroughly or else use self-polishing, nonskid wax?	___	___
7. Do all small rugs have nonskid backings?	___	___
8. Have you eliminated small rugs at the tops and bottoms of stairways?	___	___
9. Are all carpet edges tacked down?	___	___
10. Are rugs and carpets free of curled edges, worn spots, and rips?	___	___
11. Have you chosen rugs and carpets with short, dense pile?	___	___
12. Are rugs and carpets installed over good-quality, medium-thick pads?	___	___
Bathroom		
13. Do you use a rubber mat or nonslip decals in the tub or shower?	___	___
14. Do you have a grab bar securely anchored over the tub or on the shower wall?	___	___
15. Do you have a nonskid rug on the bathroom floor?	___	___
16. Do you keep soap in an easy-to-reach receptacle?	___	___
Traffic Lanes		
17. Can you walk across every room in your home, and from one room to another, without detouring around furniture?	___	___
18. Is the traffic lane from your bedroom to the bathroom free of obstacles?	___	___
19. Are telephone and appliance cords kept away from areas where people walk?	___	___
Lighting		
20. Do you have light switches near every doorway?	___	___
21. Do you have enough good lighting to eliminate shadowy areas?	___	___
22. Do you have a lamp or light switch within easy reach from your bed?	___	___
23. Do you have night lights in your bathroom and in the hallway leading from your bedroom to the bathroom?	___	___
24. Are all stairways well lighted?	___	___
25. Do you have light switches at both the tops and bottoms of stairways?	___	___
Stairways		
26. Do securely fastened handrails extend the full length of the stairs on each side of stairways?	___	___
27. Do rails stand out from the walls so you can get a good grip?	___	___
28. Are rails distinctly shaped so you're alerted when you reach the end of a stairway?	___	___
29. Are all stairways in good condition, with no broken, sagging, or sloping steps?	___	___
30. Are all stairway carpeting and metal edges securely fastened and in good condition?	___	___
31. Have you replaced any single-level steps with gradually rising ramps or made sure such steps are well lighted?	___	___
Ladders and Step Stools		
32. Do you have a sturdy step stool that you use to reach high cupboard and closet shelves?	___	___
33. Are all ladders and step stools in good condition?	___	___
34. Do you always use a step stool or ladder that's tall enough for the job?	___	___
35. Do you always set up your ladder or step stool on a firm, level base that's free of clutter?	___	___
36. Before you climb a ladder or step stool, do you always make sure it's fully open and that the stepladder spreaders are locked?	___	___
37. When you use a ladder or step stool, do you face the steps and keep your body between the side rails?	___	___
38. Do you avoid standing on top of a step stool or climbing beyond the second step from the top on a stepladder?	___	___
Outdoor Areas		
39. Are walks and driveways in your yard and other areas free of breaks?	___	___
40. Are lawns and gardens free of holes?	___	___

Table 13.4. *Continued.*

	YES	NO
41. Do you put away garden tools and hoses when they're not in use?	——	——
42. Are outdoor areas kept free of rocks, loose boards, and other tripping hazards?	——	——
43. Do you keep outdoor walkways, steps, and porches free of wet leaves and snow?	——	——
44. Do you sprinkle icy outdoor areas with deicers as soon as possible after a snowfall or freeze?	——	——
45. Do you have mats at doorways for people to wipe their feet on?	——	——
46. Do you know the safest way of walking when you can't avoid walking on a slippery surface?	——	——
Footwear		
47. Do your shoes have soles and heels that provide good traction?	——	——
48. Do you wear house slippers that fit well and don't fall off?	——	——
49. Do you avoid walking in stocking feet?	——	——
50. Do you wear low-heeled oxfords, loafers, or good-quality sneakers when you work in your house or yard?	——	——
51. Do you replace boots or galoshes when their soles or heels are worn too smooth to keep you from slipping on wet or icy surfaces?	——	——
Personal Precautions		
52. Are you always alert for unexpected hazards, such as out-of-place furniture?	——	——
53. If young grandchildren visit, are you alert for children playing on the floor and toys left in your path?	——	——
54. If you have pets, are you alert for sudden movements across your path and pets getting underfoot?	——	——
55. When you carry bulky packages, do you make sure they don't obstruct your vision?	——	——
56. Do you divide large loads into smaller loads whenever possible?	——	——
57. When you reach or bend, do you hold onto a firm support and avoid throwing your head back or turning it too far?	——	——
58. Do you always use a ladder or step stool to reach high places and never stand on a chair?	——	——
59. Do you always move deliberately and avoid rushing to answer the phone or doorbell?	——	——
60. Do you take time to get your balance when you change position from lying down to sitting and from sitting to standing?	——	——
61. Do you hold onto grab bars when you change position in the tub or shower?	——	——
62. Do you keep yourself in good condition with moderate exercise, good diet, adequate rest, and regular medical checkups?	——	——
63. If you wear glasses, is your prescription up-to-date?	——	——
64. Do you know how to reduce injury in a fall?	——	——
65. If you live alone, do you have daily contact with a friend or neighbor?	——	——
	SCORE:	——

SOURCE: Developed by the National Safety Council in cooperation with the National Retired Teachers Association and the American Association of Retired Persons. *Falling — the Unexpected Trip. A Safety Program for Older Adults. Program Leader's Guide*; 1982. Reprinted with permission from Beck JC. Geriatrics review syllabus. ●●: American Geriatrics Society, 1991:491–493.

daughters, and nearly three-fourths of the frail elderly are cared for by family members who live in the same household. Caregiving requires from 4 to 8 hours per day and may last from 1 to 4 years or more (11).

As might be expected, the stress of caregiving can prove burdensome. Approximately half of caregivers experience symptoms of depression and stress and suffer an increased susceptibility to their own health problems. The sense of burden stems from a complex interaction of factors. Patient-specific factors include behavioral problems, the skills required in providing the treatment and maintenance regimens, and the ability or willingness of the pa-

tient to assist in care. The caregiver's health, perceived competence, and commitment are all important factors in the caregiving role. The nature of the relationship and the ability of both parties to compromise and adjust to the needs of one another are essential in this relationship.

The physician's role in support of the caregivers is multifactorial (12).

1. The patient and caregiver must be perceived as a single unit. The dependencies of the patient must be matched by the capabilities and the willingness of the caregiver to provide assistance and support.

2. A comprehensive home-based approach to care can

provide the full range of treatment and service resources necessary to support the patient-caregiver unit. Formal supports through public and private agencies may complement those skills and abilities that the caregiver cannot provide.

3. Caregivers and patients must be frequently reassessed to identify behavioral, functional, and physiologic problems that may threaten the patient-caregiver unit.

4. Training the caregiver to meet the needs of the patient ensures the caregiver's competence and the safety and well-being of the patient. Most families are highly motivated and can be successfully trained in a wide variety of therapeutic, diagnostic, and behavioral management skills. Educating the family to the specific signs and symptoms of illness as pertains to their loved one greatly facilitates clinical management and avoids untoward developments.

5. Behavioral problems must be managed expeditiously. Aberrant behaviors of the patient lead to a high level of concern in the caregiver. Often, these behaviors are the first manifestations of an acute delirium requiring prompt diagnostic and therapeutic intervention. If the behaviors are not based on a physiologic change in the patient, the physician should make specific recommendations involving either behavioral management or psychopharmacologic therapies. Recognition of the caregiver's frustration is an important element in preventing abuse or premature institutionalization of the patient.

6. The physician should validate the caregiving role by affirming the work of caregiving and acknowledging its stress and burden. A home visit provides as much emotional support to the caregiver as it provides a means for continuing medical management of the patient. Caregivers often feel a sense of isolation and are very dependent on their relationship with the primary care physician.

7. The primary care physician is the case manager and provides appropriate connections with health, social service agencies, and specialty referrals to assist in clinical management.

Detection and Treatment of Elder Abuse

Mistreatment of the elderly often manifests as unintentional neglect, usually caused by ignorance, inexperience, or lack of ability or desire of the caregiver to provide adequate care (13). Less frequent are intentional neglect, physical abuse, and financial exploitation. Verbal or emotional abuse and abrogation of civil rights are generally not included in reports on elder abuse, but clearly play a role in the mistreatment of older individuals. A 1991 Congressional report suggested that between 1.5 and 2 million older adults are abused annually in the United States. A community-based, cross-sectional survey reported incidence rates of approximately 26 new cases per 1000 persons aged 65 and older (14).

Although victims of elder abuse in the home are similar in demographics and clinical profile to the patients found in other long-term care settings, the problems of elder abuse in the home focus mainly on the caregivers. Family violence may be a learned behavior, passing from generation to generation as a means of dealing with frustration or coercion. The caregiver may have been victimized in the past and may resort to abuse when dependency roles are reversed. Not infrequently, psychopathology in the caregiver, such as alcoholism, drug addiction, or severe emotional problems, may predispose to abusive behavior. In other cases, frustration, stress, and burden in the role of caregiver, while financially dependent on the older person, may lead to resentment and contribute to mistreatment. Given these factors, it is not unlikely that abuse is repetitive in a given patient-caregiver unit and that more than one type of abuse is occurring in this setting.

The recognition of elder mistreatment often depends on a sensitivity to the circumstances that may precipitate abuse, and diagnosis is greatly aided by evaluation in the home. In situations in which an acute, unexpected change in the patient's mental or physical status has significantly increased the burdens on the caregiver, stresses are more likely to emerge as some form of abuse. Caregivers who suffer their own physical problems, are fragile emotionally, or who have poor coping and caregiving skills are more likely to resort to abusive behaviors. This is also true when the caregiver is isolated and without family or community supports. Recognition of warning signs should prompt interventions on behalf of the caregiver to prevent a situation that may result in abuse (15).

Evidence of elder abuse is most easily obtained during a home visit. Neglect is sometimes manifest as poor hygiene, inadequate nutrition, or noncompliance with

171

medications. Nevertheless, the physician should not over-interpret these findings because some patients do refuse to eat, take their medications, or resist treatments or personal attention. Verbal and emotional abuse may be suspected, however, if a patient demonstrates fear or hostility in the presence of the caregiver. Another sign may be prescriptions from several physicians for multiple medications, especially for tranquilizers. Conversely, the absence of prescribed medications may suggest intentional neglect or problems with finances. Physical abuse may result in bruises or welts on the patient's trunk, rope burns around the patient's wrists or ankles, hemorrhages in the patient's scalp, or fractures of the patient's long bones or ribs. Recurrent cancellations of previously scheduled house call appointments should also alert the physician to the potential for abuse.

A planned strategy for intervention is most likely to result in a resolution accepted by all involved. The most successful approach includes counseling for both the victim and the caregiver. If the patient is able to give a consistent history, a private discussion of care and well-being may help to elucidate the problems. Documentation of physical abuse should include drawings, and when available, photographs, x-rays, and other laboratory studies. However, many competent individuals are unwilling to accept services, and their wishes should be respected. In these instances, it is important to educate the patient about the likelihood of repetition and increased frequency of future abuse and to provide the patient with written information for emergencies and referral resources. The patient should have a safety plan that includes a mechanism for notifying the physician that he or she wishes intervention in the future. Incompetent patients should be assessed for the need for a financial or personal guardian. Confronting the caregiver in a supportive, nonjudgmental manner is more likely to result in help-seeking behavior. In counseling the caregiver, it is important to stress the positives of intervention. Recognizing the caregiver's needs and identifying stressors helps to focus skills training and coping strategies.

The degree of further risk dictates whether the patient should be immediately hospitalized or whether care can continue at home with added supports. With the strong encouragement of the primary care physician, other family members may be willing to assume caregiving responsibilities on an alternating or rotating basis. Sometimes, the best course of action is a planned nursing home admission for respite care, if all parties agree.

Mandatory reporting laws have been enacted in most states and provide protection for both the physician, the patient, and the caregiver. Notification of an adult protective services agency may facilitate access to respite services or alternative placements. During the period in which additional resources are being mobilized, such notification may also obviate an effort to pursue criminal prosecution of the caregiver if the patient requires an emergency room evaluation or hospitalization. If criminal prosecution is appropriate, the adult protective services agency can facilitate the collection of evidence and pursuit of legal action.

Hospice

Hospice is a Medicare program designed to provide care to a specific group of individuals who are expected to live at least 2 weeks but less than 6 months. Hospice programs generally are very selective because of financial risk imposed by Medicare, and they usually accept cancer patients with a well-defined course of disease.

Home care is much more versatile, can take care of a wide variety of functionally impaired individuals, including terminally ill patients. In our experience, home care patients are often quite debilitated—frequently equivalent to nursing home patients—and usually die from underlying illness within 2 years of entering a house call program, although there is considerable variability.

Knowledge of hospice care by home care physicians is vital. Especially important is knowledge of modalities of pain relief, methods to reduce dyspnea and other symptoms of dying, as well as attention to hygiene and psychosocial support (16) (see also Chapter 15).

Functional Supports/Durable Medical Equipment

Because functional dependence is the primary reason for considering home care, home modifications should be considered as part of a maintenance or rehabilitiation plan. Many patients have difficulty getting on or off the toilet, or in and out of the bathtub. Toilet seat attachments that raise the seat or provide arm rests may facilitate sitting and standing. Grab bars near the toilet and near the tub can facilitate transfers. A shower seat promotes safety in the bathtub and allows the patients to move safely over the side of the tub. A bedside commode should be considered for those capable of transferring, but unable to walk to a nearby bathroom.

The patient may also need other home modifications to allow full access within the home and to the outside. For patients who require a walker or wheelchair, removal of the doorsills addresses both access and safety issues. Chair lifts on a straight stairway may facilitate access to more than one level in the home. Portable ramps may be used for access to the outside, however the recommended grade of one foot ramp for each inch of height should be considered in designing these modifications. Shorter ramps of a steeper grade may be considered for individuals with good upper arm strength, or for patients with electric wheelchairs. An occupational therapy consultation can be very helpful in identifying other personal care and assistive devices that might be helpful for dressing, grooming, meal preparation, and housekeeping (17).

High-Tech Options

Although the home is usually considered the setting most consistent with a high-touch, low-tech approach to care, advances in technology have led to miniaturization, improved safety, and have facilitated management of complex equipment. Enteral therapies can be easily administered through a pump by a gastrostomy tube. Caregivers can learn clean techniques for filling the reservoir with feeding solutions, how to add medications and skills in site care. Intravenous therapies require more sophisticated skills but experience has shown that at least half the families who assume home care responsibilties can master the necessary skills to provide long-term antibiotics, parenteral nutrition, and some chemotherapies. Many communities now have infusion therapy vendors who provide excellent support and the close supervision needed to ensure success.

Specialized durable medical equipment includes ventilators and machines for peritoneal dialysis and hemodialysis. These appliances require extensive training, but the management of these devices can also be learned by a family willing to put in the effort. Both home care and medical support are necessary, with ready access to in-home laboratory testing, for this to be a viable option. Nevertheless, physicians who develop a sizable home care practice can expect to encounter these circumstances more frequently under the imperatives of health care reform. Less demanding appliances include support surfaces such as low-air-loss and air-fluidized beds for patients with pressure ulcers. The primary restrictions for these devices are weight and an electrical supply requirements. Ironically, all these therapies may be available for home use, but may not be available in nursing homes in many communities.

Computerization of the environment is most appropriate for individuals with long-term disabilities but who are expected to remain cognitively intact. Patients with quadriplegia, amyotrophic lateral sclerosis, or muscular dystrophies may retain control over their living area and continue to communicate with the outside world through specially designed computer interfaces. There are even dedicated bulletin boards on the Internet for patients with disabilities, providing both companionship and a means to stay abreast of medical and technological advances.

Conclusions

Home care is a useful option for medical management of a particular group of functionally impaired people. Patients are often very ill with progressive, debilitating diseases that frequently lead to their deaths, yet receive great benefit from care in their home. The physician doing home visits needs to acquire the knowledge and skills that aid in providing effective care in the home, and work within an organized and supportive system that maximizes team efficiency. Especially important is the awareness of the interprofessional nature of delivering home care. Further information is available through the American Medical Association and the American Academy of Home Care Physicians (17).

References

1. Kavesh WN. Home care: process, outcome, cost. Annu Rev Gerontol Geriatr 1986;6:135–195.
2. Health Standards and Quality Bureau. Online survey, certification and reporting system. Washington, DC: Health Care Finance Administration, 1993.
3. Letsch SW, Lazenby HC, Levit KR, Cowan CA. National

health expenditures, 1991. Health Care Financ Rev 1992;14:1–30.

4. Siwek J. Housecalls: current status and rationale. Am Fam Physician 1985;31:169–174.

5. MMWR 1993;42:820–824.

6. Master RJ, Feltin M, Jainchill J, et al. A continuum of care in the inner city: assessment of its benefits for Boston's elderly and high-risk populations. N Engl J Med 1980;302:1434–1440.

7. Ramsdell JW, Swart JA, Jackson JE, Renvall M. The yield of a home visit in the assessment of geriatric patients. J Amer Geriatr Soc 1989;37:17–24.

8. Council on Scientific Affairs. Home Care in the 1990s. JAMA 1990;263:1241–1244.

9. Beck JC. Geriatrics review syllabus. New York, New York: American Geriatrics Society, 1991:491–493.

10. Shanas E. Social myth as a hypothesis: the case of the family relations of old people. Gerontologist 1979;19:3–9.

11. Stone R, Cafferata GL, Sangl J. Caregivers of the frail elderly: a national profile. Gerontologist 1987;27:616–626.

12. Diagnostic and treatment guidelines on elder abuse and neglect. American Medical Association, 1992.

13. Pillemer K, Finkelhor D. The prevalence of elder abuse: a random sample survey. Gerontologist 1988;28:51–57.

14. Taler G, Ansello EF. Elder abuse. Am Fam Physician 1985;32:107–114.

15. Enyck, RE. The medical care of terminally ill patients. Baltimore: Johns Hopkins, 1994.

16. Axtell LA, Yasuda YL. Assistive devices in home modifications in geriatric rehabilitation. Clin Geriatr Med 1993;9:803–821.

17. Department of Geriatric Health, American Medical Association. Guidelines for the medical management of the home care patient. Chicago: American Medical Association, 1992.

Chapter 14
Nursing Home Care

Paul R. Katz

Loneliness and the feeling of being unwanted is the most terrible poverty.

Mother Teresa

Few phrases in medicine conjure up as picturesque and frightening images as do the words "nursing home." Much of the negative imagery, equally prevalent among physicians and the public, is rooted in the history of nursing homes. As recently as the early 1990s, nursing homes functioned as havens for the indigent and mentally disturbed of all ages. The care delivered in these settings was unregulated and, not surprisingly, often substandard. It was not until 1935, with passage of the Social Security Act, that the nursing home industry began evolving into its present-day form (1). Although the Social Security Act stimulated financial support for institutional long-term care services, oversight of care remained rudimentary. Indeed, it was not until 1965, with passage of Titles 19 and 20 of the Social Security Act (Medicare and Medicaid), that federal standards for nursing homes were established. Before these developments, the oversight of care in nursing homes was mainly the responsibility of individual states that were generally considered to be ineffectual.

Despite seemingly intense scrutiny, a consensus developed in the 1970s and early 1980s that quality of care in nursing homes was seriously lacking. In response to these concerns and the Health Care Financing Administration's (HCFA) failure to affect, in any substantive way, the care in nursing homes, the Institute of Medicine (IOM) in 1983, under the auspices of the National Academy of Sciences, undertook an extensive review of nursing home practice (2). The final IOM report highlighted an array of deficiencies concerning nursing home care and offered a series of recommendations designed to improve the delivery of health care in nursing homes. Central to these recommen-

dations were efforts to further professionalize the nursing staff in nursing homes, enhance residents' rights, and shift from process-based criteria in the assessment of quality to outcome-based criteria. The majority of the IOM's recommendations were incorporated into law with passage of the nursing home reform amendments contained within the Omnibus Budget Reconciliation Act (OBRA) of 1987. The following year, HCFA revised Medicare and Medicaid requirements for long-term facilities, the first such revision since 1974.

The impact of OBRA 87 on medical practice in the nursing home is outlined in Table 14.1 (3). Of note is a requirement that all nursing home residents receive a comprehensive, standardized assessment within 14 days of admission and periodically thereafter if there is a noticeable change in condition. This multidisciplinary assessment, which emphasizes functional capacity, is embodied in the minimum data set (MDS). The responsibility for completing the MDS generally falls on the nursing service, although input from a variety of disciplines, including medicine, is solicited. A number of clinical issues are highlighted in the MDS (Table 14.2), many of which fall directly under the purview of the physician. If and when problems that relate to any of the 18 highlighted issues are identified, the health care team must review accompanying resident assessment protocols (RAPs) that outline standard diagnostic and therapeutic approaches to the specific problem in question. Although each RAP is, in essence, a practice guideline, RAPs are not necessarily based on expert consensus. Although physicians are likely to be apprised of the RAP guidelines, they are under no obligation to follow them, if a clear rationale is presented in the medical record on the basis of a comprehensive medical assessment. Adherence to RAPs by nursing home practitioners and the response of state surveyors to issues regarding medical practice have yet to be determined.

Table 14.1. OBRA 87 Mandates Relating to Medical Practice in the Nursing Home*.

1. Nursing facilities must conduct, initially and periodically, a comprehensive, accurate, standardized, reproducible assessment of each resident's functional capacity.
2. Residents have the right to be free from any physical restraints imposed for the purposes of discipline or convenience, and not required to treat a resident's medical symptoms.
3. Residents have the right to be free from any psychoactive drug administered for the purpose of discipline or convenience and not required to treat a resident's medical symptoms.
4. Residents must be free from unnecessary drugs.
5. Residents have the right to a dignified existence, self-determination, and communication with and access to persons and services inside and outside the facility.
   5a. Residents have the right to choose a personal attending physician.
   5b. Residents have the right to refuse treatment.
   5c. Residents have the right to personal privacy, which includes privacy during medical treatment.
6. Residents must receive in the facility and the facility must provide the necessary care and services to attain or maintain the highest practicable physical, mental, and psycho-social well-being in accordance with the resident's comprehensive assessment and plan of care.

*OBRA = Omnibus Budget Reconciliation Act, 1987.
SOURCE: Elon R, Pawlson LG. The impact of OBRA on medical practice within nursing facilities. J Am Geriatr Soc 1992;40: 958–963.

In addition to comprehensive assessments, the physician must also clearly document the need for all medications, particularly psychoactive agents (3). Unnecessary drugs are defined as those that are given in excessive doses, for excessive periods of time, without adequate monitoring, without adequate indications for use, or in the presence of adverse consequences that indicate that the dose should be reduced or discontinued.

The mandates stemming from OBRA, particularly those requiring a standardized, comprehensive assessment for every nursing home resident, have in many ways revolutionized nursing home practice. Unfortunately, no empiric evidence exists that documents improved outcomes or enhanced quality of care for nursing home residents as a result of the changes prescribed by the 1987 Nursing Home Reform Act. Whether the time nurses spend completing each assessment might be better spent at the resident's bedside remains conjecture. Never-

theless, practice patterns in the nursing home have been changing for the better. The unwarranted use of neuroleptics, for example, appears to be declining despite the fact that one-third to one-half of all medications prescribed in nursing homes may be unnecessary (4).

Another important piece of legislation affecting nursing homes, the Patient's Self-Determination Act (PSDA), was passed in 1990 as part of the Omnibus Reconciliation Act of that year. The PSDA, fully implemented in 1992, required each state to establish policies regarding life-sustaining medical treatments. Although state statues vary considerably in definitions of surrogate decision makers and the conditions under which certain treatments might be "withheld or withdrawn," all patients admitted to Medicare- or Medicaid-certified facilities must now be apprised of their options regarding medical care (5). The impact of this legislation on nursing homes has been notable; the rate of having a living will increased from 4.5 percent in 1990 to 13.3 percent in 1993; do-not-resuscitate (DNR) orders increased from 30.1 percent to 51.4 percent during the same time period. Orders to forgo hospitalization or artificial nutrition (5 percent of residents), however, did not change appreciably between

Table 14.2. Clinical Issues Highlighted in Minimum Data Set.

Delirium
Cognitive loss/dementia
Visual function
Communication
ADL functional/rehabilitative potential*
Urinary incontinence and indwelling catheter
Psychosocial well-being
Mood state
Behavior problem
Activities
Falls
Nutritional status
Feeding tubes
Dehydration/fluid maintenance
Dental care
Pressure ulcer
Antipsychotic drug use
Physical restraints

*ADL = activities of daily living.
SOURCE: Elon R, Pawlson LG. The impact of OBRA on medical practice within nursing facilities. J Am Geriatr Soc 1992;40: 958–963.

1990 and 1993 (6). Physician sensitivity to and knowledge of advance directive precepts remains critical not only in the implementation of such directives but also in their restrictiveness (7).

Medical practice in the nursing home is guided by mandates set forth in federal legislation and by the manner in which oversight of medical care is accomplished. Because the regulatory model in the United States remains predicated on an adversarial relationship between government and health care provider, the opportunity to enhance care by means of education is often lost. The ever-present threat of government sanctions further complicates a decision-making process for nursing home residents already replete with a host of medical, social, and ethical issues. Unfortunately, many providers believe that the guidelines established by HCFA to help direct local survey teams in applying regulations, known as interpretive guidelines, remain arbitrary and at times "go beyond the intent of the law" (3). Physicians who remain sensitive to the potential rift between regulator and provider enhance their chances of avoiding conflict and optimizing patient care.

Demographics

By age 65, a person's risk of nursing home admission before death is estimated at 43 percent (8). Although only 5 percent of the elderly are institutionalized at any given time, nursing home use increases from 6 percent for persons age 75 to 84 years to 22 percent in the population aged 85 and older (9). Paralleling an increase in the population 85 years and older, the number of nursing home residents is expected to exceed 2 million by the turn of the century and 4 million by the year 2040 (10). Although some recent trends (11) point to improvements in disability rates associated with aging, any dramatic change is unlikely. The need for services will probably increase proportionate to the growth of the elderly population. Although disability rates for black, Hispanic, Asian and Native American older persons exceed those of similarly aged whites, these minorities tend to be underrepresented in nursing homes. Cost, discrimination, personal choice, and social or cultural differences are among the reasons most often cited to explain this paradox (12).

Table 14.3. Selected Characteristics of Nursing Home Residents.

Subject	Living in Nursing Homes 1985 (%)	Living in Community 1984 (%)
Age (yr)		
65–74	16.1	61.7
75–84	38.6	30.7
85+	45.3	7.6
Sex		
Men	25.4	40.8
Women	74.6	59.2
Race		
White	93.1	90.4
Black	6.2	8.3
Other	0.7	1.3
Marital status		
Widowed	67.8	34.1
Married	12.8	54.7
Never married	13.5	4.4
Divorced or separated	5.9	6.3
With living children	63.1	81.3
Requires assistance in		
Bathing	91.0	6.0
Dressing	77.6	4.3
Using toilet room	63.2	2.2
Transferring	62.6	2.8
Eating	40.3	1.1
Difficulty with bowel and/or bladder control	54.5	—
Total Age 65+yr		
No. (thousands)	1,318	26,343
Percent	100.0	100.0

SOURCE: Aging America. Trends and Projections. Washington, DC: U.S. Senate Special Committee on Aging and the American Association of Retired Person. USDHHS Pub. No. (FCOA)91-28001, 1991.

The average nursing home resident is characterized by important impairments in all physical activities of daily living (ADL), including bowel and bladder incontinence. Selected characteristics of nursing home residents compared with community-residing elderly are presented in Table 14.3 (13). Of note is a very high prevalence of psychiatric-related illness in nursing homes. A variety of studies suggest that dementia, mood and anxiety disorders, psychosis, sleep disorders, and nonspecific disturbances such as restlessness or aggression are notable sources of morbidity in long-term care facilities (14). Indeed, 70 percent of nursing home residents may meet diagnostic criteria for dementia (15), and 90 percent of nursing home residents have at least one form of behavioral disturbance (16). Although behavioral problems are very prevalent, specific psychiatric diagnoses are applied in only a small minority of cases. Zimmer et al observed that serious behavioral problems are documented by the attending physician in less than 10 percent of cases and psychiatric consultations are appropriately requested in only one of seven patients (17).

Although the prevalence of psychiatric behavioral problems in the nursing home is, in part, a consequence of the growth of the elderly population, additional factors may be implicated. Specifically, deinstitutionalization of large numbers of mentally ill individuals over the past quarter-century has forced nursing homes to fill many of the functions previously addressed by state mental hospitals.

Of the approximately 16,000 nursing facilities in the United States, 68 percent are proprietary; occupancy rates approach 92 percent, and 90 percent of homes have 25 to 199 beds (18,19). Surprisingly, the number of total nursing home beds per 1000 persons 65 years and older declined 2 percent from 1970 to 1989 despite a 24 percent increase in bed supply during the same period (20). The decline in the bed-to-person ratio for individuals 85 years and older was even more dramatic, 13 percent. The impact of continued bed restrictions in many states on quality of care and availability of community-based, long-term care services remains to be seen.

The financing of nursing home care is, in contrast to acute care, borne to a large extent by the care recipient. Government or other third-party insurers pay for the bulk of acute care services, but the primary source of payment for nursing home patients is self-pay (48 percent at time of admission), with Medicaid accounting for 41 percent of nursing home revenues at admission. Medicare contributes very little to nursing home finances (1 percent overall, 5 percent at time of admission) similar to private long-term care insurance. Unfortunately, 20 percent of persons admitted to nursing homes as self-payors spend down to qualify for Medicaid within 1 year (21). This is sobering in view of estimates that, of individuals turning age 65 in 1990, 9 percent will spend 5 or more years in a nursing home and will account for 64 percent of nursing home costs (22).

Since implementation of the prospective payment system (PPS), nursing homes have accommodated to an increasingly sick population as evidenced by a 22 percent increase in the number of patients discharged from acute care in an "unstable condition" (e.g., new incontinence, shortness of breath, confusion, chest pain, and heart rate or blood pressure abnormality, or both). Of patients discharged to nursing homes, approximately one-fourth have one or more instabilities, half have one or more measures of sickness (fever, new incontinence, new decubiti), and one-third have abnormalities in their most recent laboratory studies (23). Fitzgerald et al (24), in comparing outcomes among elderly hip fracture patients, reported decreases in the number of physical therapy sessions, maximal distance walked in the hospital, and percentage discharged back to the community after the advent of PPS. Similarly, Tresch et al (25) described 100 consecutive admissions to a hospital-based nursing home care unit, after PPS, wherein 27 percent required readmission to the acute care hospital within 30 days. This percentage was almost triple the incidence for readmission before prospective payment. Reflecting a "sicker" population, the number of nursing home deaths increased from 18.9 percent in 1982 to 21.5 percent in 1985 (26).

Although the nursing home population is generally sicker than previous cohorts, it remains heterogenous. Length of stay remains less than 3 months for 45 percent of older nursing home residents (27), which reflects admissions for terminal illness and acute orthopedic-neurologic diseases such as strokes and hip fractures. Stroke and hip fracture are generally amenable to rehabilitation but require longer recovery times than acute-based rehabilitation units typically allow. Short-stayers are also more likely to be male, married, and to be discharged back to the community. Nonetheless, short-stayers account for only 5 percent of all nursing home days; the average length of stay for all residents is approximately 19 months (27).

Of all discharges from nursing homes, two-thirds are accounted for by death. Although approximately 25 percent of patients discharged from the nursing home return home, only 7 percent remain alive at home after 2 years (28). The reasons underlying nursing home deaths typically remain unproven, as evidenced by a nursing home autopsy rate of less than 1 percent (29). Infection and cardiac decompensation figure prominently in nursing home-related morbidity and mortality.

Risks for Nursing Home Placement

Predicting nursing home placement for a given individual remains difficult. Although several variables have been useful as predictors of institutionalization (e.g., age, gender, cognitive impairment, incontinence, poor socioeconomic support, and nursing home bed supply), quantifying risk has been problematic (30). Variability in the availability and accessibility of community-based, long-term care services figure prominently in this equation. In a recent 9-year longitudinal study of 1600 older persons residing in a large metropolitan area (31), four factors among a host of demographic, physical, psychological, and functional variables stood out as notably favoring community care. These included young age, male gender, higher income, and living with children. Notably, measures of impairment or disability alone were found to be relatively insensitive predictors of site of care. Combinations of factors, however, such as age, cognitive and functional impairments (ADL and instrumental ADL [IADL]) have been found to predict *permanent* nursing home placement (32,33). Inoye et al (34) recently noted a 67 percent rate of nursing home admission in hospitalized patients with at least three of the following four risk factors—decubitus ulcer, low social activity level, self-reported need for help with basic skills, and cognitive impairment. In contrast, only 4 percent of patients were admitted to nursing homes when none of these risk factors were present. Although nurses, physicians, and social workers tend to agree in their estimates of the probability of nursing home placement, mental and functional impairments are commonly underestimated and impede the discharge process (35).

Although nursing home admissions are not inappropriate to the extent that they were 20 to 30 years ago, a bias towards institutionalization persists. Often health care providers, particularly physicians, are reluctant to take risks; as a result, they may forgo community-based services for those that are institution-based. Although nurses are onsite in nursing homes and are able to monitor complex medical conditions more closely than nurses can in many home care settings, individual patients may deteriorate under the more rigid living situation typical of nursing homes. The risk for functional deterioration in nursing homes can be great, in part a result of learned dependency. However, home care is not preferred to nursing home care in all instances. Indeed, it remains unclear whether home care notably reduces the need for hospitalization or use of nursing home services. Overall cost effectiveness of home care has also been debated. Home health care programs have, however, been shown to have positive effects on patient survival, functional level, and patient and caregiver satisfaction (36).

Acute-Long-Term Care Interface

Greater than half of all nursing home admissions originate from short-stay hospitals. Indeed, approximately one-third of women age 85 years and older who are discharged from hospitals are transferred to long-term care facilities (37). Conversely, nursing home residents have rates of hospitalization that range from 212 to 549 per 1000 nursing home beds per year (38). In view of the numbers of patients transferring between hospitals and nursing homes, health care providers must be knowledgeable of and sensitive to issues affecting medical care in each of these settings. The failure of hospital-based physicians to fully appreciate the limits and benefits of nursing home care has resulted in the often hasty discharge of patients to nursing homes, resulting in iatrogenic complications, untimely readmissions to the hospital, or both. Tresch et al, for example, demonstrated that 30 percent of patients transferred from the nursing home to the hospital returned to the nursing home with new pressure sores (39).

Information that is transferred in an expedient and complete way is one important means to ensure continuity and reduce risk for iatrogenesis. Such information generally includes a review of active problems and medications as well as a rationale for the patient's care plan. Information about the patient's level of functioning before the onset of acute illnesses is especially valuable when patients are transferred to the care of physicians who are unfamiliar with the patients. Equally important is substantiation of advance directives. Cognitively intact nursing home residents generally have concise views regarding life-sustaining treatments but may not offer them unless specifically solicited (40). For cognitively impaired residents, documenting previous wishes, facilitating the selection of a health care proxy, or both, often make a noticeable difference in the overall approach to a given patient.

Transfer of nursing home residents to short-stay hospitals generally occurs on the basis of a patient's acute illness in the context of extensive comorbidity. In such instances, lack of support services (x-ray, laboratory), and lack of adequate numbers of nursing staff who are comfortable with treating acute disease, figure prominently in the transfer decision. Unfortunately, financial incentives that favor hospitalization and accrue to both nursing homes and physicians remain in place. Innovative programs have been described, however (41), that allow for the treatment of acutely ill nursing home residents in long-term care settings treatment at substantial savings to the health care system, and with enhanced quality of care.

Staffing Patterns

Staffing patterns in nursing homes greatly affect overall quality of care. Although caring for a "sicker" population, professional nurses account for just over 10 percent of all nursing home employees. On average, nursing homes have only one registered nurse (RN) per 49 patients compared with a 1:5 ratio in acute care hospitals (42). Further, although the federal government has mandated minimum nursing staff requirements, one-third of nursing homes have been unable to comply. Since RNs are required to be present in nursing homes only 8 hours per day, it is not surprising that 40 percent of nursing facilities report 6 minutes or less of RN time per patient per day (42). The fact that both total nursing hours and the ratio of professional to nonprofessional nursing staff have been used as reliable markers of quality care has important implications for the future.

Understandably, much of the hands-on care in nursing homes is provided by nursing assistants. Retention of such staff remains problematic as evidenced in turnover rates averaging 70 percent to 100 percent per year. Professional nurses and nursing assistants often earn from 35 percent to 60 percent less than their counterparts in acute care facilities, despite similar responsibilities and training.

Staffing problems, of course, are not limited to nursing. Limited physician involvement in nursing homes remains problematic partly because of perceived burdensome amounts of paperwork, reimbursement and regulatory inequities, and, importantly, a lack of role modeling during formative training years (43,44,45,46). Currently, only about one-fifth of primary care physicians spend more than 2 hours per week in a nursing facility. Although internists comprise 60 percent of all nursing home care providers, they remain less likely to spend as much time in nursing homes as their family practice counterparts (Katz et al, personal communication). Even for those physicians practicing in nursing homes, a notable proportion may be leaving such practice. In a recent American Medical Directors Association survey, 51 percent of the medical director respondents noted a 10 percent decrease in the number of attending physicians in the nursing home, and 21 percent cited a 20 percent or greater decline (43).

Medical Care Issues in the Nursing Home

The care of nursing home residents has become increasingly complex over the past several years. Not surprisingly, much of the illness manifest in the nursing home presents in a subtle or atypical fashion consistent with the physical and psychological frailty of the patient population. Furthermore, limited access to biotechnology, frequent dependence on nonphysicians such as nurses and nursing assistants for patient evaluation, and the high prevalence of cognitive impairment in a setting of intense regulatory oversight and cost constraints particularly complicate the medical decision-making process. The heterogeneity among nursing home residents is another factor that affects overall care and precludes a uniform approach for each resident. Success in such a setting demands diligence on the part of each physician and a thoughtful, reasoned approach to the medical and ethical problems frequently encountered. Problems in nursing facilities that often require unique diagnostic and treatment strategies include incontinence, falls, syncope, infection, depression, dysthymia, confusion, malnutrition, and pressure sores (Table 14.4) (47–53).

Table 14.4. Medical Problems Frequently Encountered in the Nursing Home.

Condition	Estimated Prevalence (%)	Potential Causes	Examples of Treatment Options
Incontinence	50	Urethral obstruction Vaginal atrophy Poor mobility Confusion Diabetes Urinary tract infection Fecal impaction Diuretics	Prompted voiding Transurethral prostatectomy Limit medications Laxatives Insulin Estrogen Conditioning exercises
Malnutrition	35	Limited socialization Poor appetite Dental/swallowing Disorders Malabsorption Catabolic state (hyperthyroid; neoplasm) Increased protein excretion (nephrotic syndrome; exudative skin ulcer)	Appetite stimulants Antidepressants Dental/speech evaluation Antithyroid medications Enteral/parenteral nutrition Cancer treatment
Falls	30 (0.6–3.6 falls per bed)	Sensory impairment Hypertensive/sedative Medication Postprandial effects Poor Lighting/obstacles Musculoskeletal disorders Deconditioning Arrhythmia/valvular Disease	Improved lighting Glasses Lower extremity strengthening Limits on medication use Pacemaker Avoidance of standing after meals
Infection	10	Immunologic disorders Malnutrition Trauma Indwelling catheter Pressure ulcer Limited vaccination Undetected tuberculosis	Skin emollients Vitamins Nutritional supports Antibotics Discontinue/decrease catheter use Routine vaccinations/yearly tuberculin test Prophylaxis (e.g., Amantadine)
Depression/dysthymia	9	After cerebrovascular accident Cyclic Loss of social supports Medications Lack of intellectual stimulation Learned dependency	Enhanced recreational activity Increased visitation from family volunteer Encouragement of independence Antidepressants Electroconvulsive therapy Counseling
Pressure sores	9	Reduced mobility Poor nutrition Incontinence Confusion Fracture	Urinary catheter Occlusive dressing Vitamin supplements Nutritional support Low-pressure mattress Antibiotics Surgery Frequent turning

SOURCE: (48–53).

Health Maintenance

Health maintenance issues in the nursing home also offer unique challenges. As in other settings, decisions regarding health maintenance and disease prevention must be made on the basis of individual patient wishes, the impact of interventions on quality of life, and the cost effectiveness of treatment. Periodic screening tests for cancer such as fecal occult blood test, mammograms and Pap smears may be warranted for a sizable proportion of nursing home residents. An annual review of immunizations and tuberculin skin test reactivity is also applicable to most nursing home residents. Although not proven, yearly examinations directed specifically to podiatric, opthalmalogic, and dental problems also seem warranted for most nursing home residents. Routine laboratory screening, however, should be individualized and based on underlying illness and associated treatment regimens (54). Additional health maintenance issues can be addressed throughout the year during the mandated visits every 30 or 60 days. Review of patients medications, nutritional status, need for restraint's or urinary catheters, and changes in physical status, psychologic status, or both, can be addressed during these encounters. The role of exercise in restoring and optimizing function should not be underestimated, even for the very frail nursing home resident (55).

Physician Practice in the Nursing Home

Unfortunately, nursing home practitioners have traditionally not taken the time and effort needed to ensure consistently high standards of care (56). Although some practices have changed for the better over the past several years, as evidenced by a reduction in use of physical restraints, other therapies require similar scrutiny. In a study of 52 randomly selected nursing homes in Maryland and involving 3899 residents followed for 1 year, only 11 percent of patients with four common types of infection received an evaluation "judged by a consensus panel to be minimally appropriate to establish the diagnosis, severity and treatment of a particular infection" (57). In this study, a patient was examined by a physician in only 49 percent of cases before an antibiotic was initiated; specimens for bacterial culture were obtained in 46 per-

cent of infectious episodes in patients, and confirmatory chest x-rays were taken in only 37 percent of cases of presumed lower respiratory tract infection. Failure to respond appropriately to culture reports or to document underlying diagnoses in nursing home residents treated with antibiotics has also been reported (58,59). Kayser-Jones et al (60), in analyzing all episodes of acute illness resulting in patient transfer to a hospital in three California nursing homes, noted that in 48 percent of cases, the nursing home resident did not warrant the level of care provided in the acute care setting.

Fortunately, physicians can improve their practice in nursing homes in several ways. One very helpful approach is to become an active member of the "care team." Nowhere in geriatrics is the team more important than in the nursing home, because the interplay between acute and chronic disease in the context of extreme frailty provides constant diagnostic and therapeutic challenges. Success in such an environment depends very much on the physician's willingness to seek out and listen to the opinion of others, whatever their professional standing. Linkage with other health care providers in the nursing home, such as the administrator, director of nursing, and pharmacist-consultant, can also be forged if the physician makes an effort to understand the specific role of each nursing home practitioner and, importantly, the constraints on individual practices engendered by state and federal regulations.

In the context of the team and through interaction with staff, residents, and family, physicians often serve as role models in the nursing home. Skill at communication, clear and concise documentation in the medical record, and an overriding respect for individual rights and dignity are cornerstones of medical practice in this setting. Additional responsibilities of the attending physicians are outlined in Table 14.5 (61). Procedures to facilitate the attending physician's role in the nursing home are presented in Table 14.6 (61). The reader is also directed to several comprehensive reviews that detail policy and procedures germane to medical practice in the nursing home and offer a number of relevant protocols and guidelines (54,62).

Examination of the quality of care and the intensity of services delivered in nursing homes shows that factors other than individual physician characteristics may be

Table 14.5. Role of the Attending Physician in the Nursing Home.

1. Comprehensively assess each resident and coordinate all aspects of medical care. Implement specific treatments/services to enhance and/or maintain physical and psychosocial function.
2. Participate in the development of individual care plans and review and revise such plans periodically in conjunction with the health care team.
3. Review progress of each resident relating to individualized therapy (e.g., speech, OT, PT)* and, in concert with appropriate therapists, approve continued use.
4. Evaluate the need for rehabilitative services. Order appropriate measures and assistive devices to reduce the risk of accidents.
5. Evaluate the need for physical and/or chemical restraints, minimizing their use whenever possible.
6. Periodically review all medications and monitor for both continued need and adverse drug reactions. Respond appropriately to periodic review and recommendations of the consultant pharmacist.
7. Physically attend to each resident in a timely fashion consistent with established state and federal guidelines.
8. Respond in a timely fashion to medical emergencies.
9. Facilitate information transfer when possible and appropriate between acute and long-term care facilities.
10. Inform residents of their health status and, whenever possible, optimize each resident's decision-making capacity while assisting in establishing advance directives.

*OT = occupational therapy; PT = physical therapy.
SOURCE: Calkins E, Ford AB, Katz PR. Practice of geriatrics. 2nd ed. Philadelphia: WB Saunders, 1992.

important. The manner in which the medical staff is organized, for example, has been shown to affect some care issues. Karuza and Katz (63) recently demonstrated that facilities with closed medical staffs (i.e., restricted to a limited group of physicians responsible for all care delivery) are more likely to have physicians onsite daily, provide cross-coverage for acute patients, and have quicker physician emergency response times. Although, theoretically, closed staffs may constrain a nursing home resident's freedom of choice for physicians, they offer several advantages including cross-coverage, consistency and regularity of visits, greater medical accountability, enhanced staff communication, and improved cost monitoring and cost containment.

Physician practice in the nursing home can be further optimized with an understanding of the role of the medi-

cal director. Physicians should attempt to work cooperatively with the individual to shape medical care standards and, in the process, help to ensure quality and further staff education. The various roles of the medical director are outlined in Table 14.7. Formal certification as a nursing home medical director is now offered through the American Medical Directors Association in recognition of the medical director's critical leadership role in helping to define the goals and mission of the nursing home.

A detailed overview of issues relating to medical direction in long-term care, notably the impact on quality of care by the interplay of laws, regulations, and the organization of medical care in nursing homes can be found in Levenson's revised text (64).

Education in the Nursing Home

A variety of health care providers have found that the nursing home is a valuable educational site. The heterogeneity of the nursing home population, the manner in which care is organized, and the complex medical, legal, and ethical issues typifying nursing home care combine to provide a substrate on which clinical skills can be ad-

Table 14.6. Activities to Facilitate the Role of Attending Physician in the Nursing Home.

Schedule routine visitations with nursing staff every 30 or 60 days

Chart and/or bedside rounds with nurses, during routine visits; schedule several resident evaluations per visit to optimize efficiency

Provide nurses with protocols defining routine emergent and urgent medical situations

Collaborate with the medical director on a structured format for patients' bimonthly and annual reviews*; a structured transfer form to be used by referring acute care facilities

Arrange routine meetings with medical director to keep apprised of relevant administrative issues

*Bimonthly patient reviews should emphasize intercurrent illness, medication review, changes in function, nutrition, and rationale for use of catheters, restraints, or psychotropic agents. Annual patient reviews should include note of patient's advance directives, appraisal of patient's life satisfaction, and update of patient's health maintenance and prevention issues such as screening tests and immunizations.

Table 14.7. Role of the Medical Director.

1. Participate in administrative decision making and recommend and approve policies and procedures.
2. Participate in the development and conduct of education programs.
3. Organize and coordinate physician services and services of other professionals as they relate to resident care.
4. Participate in the process to ensure the appropriateness and quality of medical and medically related care.
5. Help articulate the facility's mission to the community and represent the facility in the community.
6. Participate in the surveillance and promotion of the health, welfare, and safety of employees.
7. Acquire, maintain, and apply knowledge of social, regulatory, political, and economic factors that relate to resident care services.
8. Provide medical leadership for research and development activities in geriatrics and long-term care.
9. Participate in establishing policies and procedures to ensure that the rights of individuals are respected.

SOURCE: Calkins E, Ford AB, Katz PR. Practice of geriatrics. 2nd ed. Philadelphia: WB Saunders, 1992.

vanced. Although many nursing home residents are frail and suffer from a variety of chronic ailments, the potential to enhance their physical and psychological function remains great, as does the provider's ability to affect the patients' overall quality of life.

Unfortunately, physicians have been slow to take advantage of the educational opportunities inherent in the nursing home. Although several accrediting bodies have supported the idea of including nursing homes in the spectrum of training sites, much work remains. Few internal medicine training programs offer a nursing home experience to their residents. When such rotations are offered, they are likely to be optional and not involve a longitudinal care component. In contrast, almost 9 of 10 family practice training programs offer nursing home training; it is usually required and longitudinal (45). Involvement of medical residents in the care of nursing home patients may translate into improved care and patient outcomes (65), as well as stimulate interest in primary care for the chronically infirm and promote clinical research in this area.

Research in nursing homes remains challenging because of the frail nature of the population being studied,

difficulties in obtaining informed consent, and a reluctance among some staff to participate in such inquiry. Thoughtful approaches to research in the nursing home have been described and may prompt needed clinical trials (66,67).

Conclusions

The ever-changing nursing home environment creates a complex but extremely challenging place in which to practice medicine. Opportunities to enhance quality of care and learn from the geriatric population abound; these opportunities will hopefully attract the best and brightest physicians in the profession.

References

1. Johnson CL, Grant LA. The nursing home in American society. Baltimore: Johns Hopkins, 1985.
2. Hawes C. The institute of medicine study: improving the quality of nursing home care. In: Katz PR, Kane RL, Mezey MD, eds. Advances in long-term care. vol. I. New York: Springer, 1991.
3. Elon R, Pawlson LG. The impact of OBRA on medical practice within nursing facilities. J Am Geriatr Soc 1992;40:958–963.
4. Avorn J, Soumerai SB, Everitt DE, et al. A randomized trial of a program to reduce the use of psychoactive drugs in nursing homes. N Engl J Med 1992;327:168–173.
5. Kapp, M. State statutes limiting advanced directives: death warrants or life sentences? J Am Geriatr Soc 1992;40:772–776.
6. Teno J, More V, Branco K. Impact of the Patient's Self-Determination Act in long-term care facilities. Presented at the Annual Meeting of the American Geriatrics Society, Los Angeles, May 1994.
7. Batchelor AJ, Winsemius D, O'Connor PJ, Wetler T. Predictors of advanced directives, restrictiveness, and compliance with institutional policy in a long-term care facility. J Am Geriatr Soc 1992;40:679–684.
8. Kemper P, Murtaugh CN. Lifetime use of nursing home care. N Engl J Med 1991;324:595–600.
9. Hing E. Use of nursing homes by the elderly: preliminary data from the 1985 National Nursing Home Survey. Vital and Health Statistics, No. 135. Hyattsville, MD: National Center for Health Statistics, 1987.
10. Schneider EL, Guralnik JM. The aging of america: impact on health care costs. JAMA 1990;263:2335.
11. Manton KG, Corder LS, Stallard E. Estimates of change in chronic disability and institutional incidents and prevalence rates in the U.S. elderly population from the 1982, 1984, and 1989 National Long-Term Care Survey. J Gerontol 1993;48:S153–S166.

12. Minority elders: longevity, economics and health. Building a public policy base. Washington, DC: Gerontological Society of America, 1991.

13. Aging America. Trends and Projections. Washington, DC: U.S. Senate Special Committee on Aging and the American Association of Retired Persons. USDHHS Pub. No. (FCOA) 91-28001, 1991.

14. Borson S, Liptzin B, Nininger J, et al. Psychiatry and the nursing home. Am J Psych 1987;144:1412–1418.

15. Rovner BW, German PS, Broadhead J, et al. The prevalence and management of dementia and other psychiatric disorders in nursing homes. Int Psychogeriatr 1990;2:13–24.

16. Tariot PN, Podgorski CA, Blazina L, Leibovici A. Mental disorders in the nursing home: another perspective. Am J Psych 1993;150:1063.

17. Zimmer JG, Watson N, Treat A. Behavioral problems among patients in skilled nursing facilities. Am J Public Health 1984;74:1118–1121.

18. Hing E, Sekscenski E, Strahan G. The National Nursing Home Survey: 1985 summary for the United States. National Center for Health Statistics. Vital and Health Statistics. Series 12, No. 97. Public Health Service. Washington, DC: U.S. Government Printing Office, 1986.

19. Sirrocco A. Nursing homes and board and care homes. Vital and Health Statistics, No. 244. Hyattsville, MD: National Center for Health Statistics, 1994.

20. Harrinton C, Preston S, Grant L, Swan JH. Revised trends in states' nursing home capacity. Health Aff 1992;11:170–180.

21. Mor V, Instrator O, Liberte L. Factors affecting conversion rates to Medicaid among new admissions to nursing homes. Health Serv Res 1993;28:1–25.

22. Kemper P, Spillman BC, Murtaugh CM. A lifetime perspective on proposals for financing nursing home care. Inquiry 1991;28:333–344.

23. Koescoff J, Kahn KL, Rogers WH, et al. Prospective payment system and impairment at discharge. The "quicker-and-sicker" story revisited. JAMA 1990;264:1980–1983.

24. Fitzgerald JF, Moore PS, Dittus RS. The care of elderly patients with hip fracture. Changes since implementation of the prospective payment system. N Engl J Med 1988;319:1392.

25. Tresch DD, Duthie EH, Newton M, Bodin B. Coping with diagnosis-related groups: the changing role of the nursing home. Arch Intern Med 1988;148:1393.

26. Sager MA, Easterling DV, Kindig DA, Anderson OW. Changes in the location of death after passage of Medicare's prospective payment system. N Engl J Med 1989;320:433.

27. Spence DA, Wiener JM. Nursing home length of stay patterns: results from the 1985 National Nursing Home Survey. Gerontologist 1990;30:16.

28. Lewis MA, Kane RL, Cretin S, Clark V. The immediate and subsequent outcomes of nursing home care. Am J Public Health 1985;75:758.

29. Katz PR, Seidel G. Nursing home autopsies: survey of physician attitudes and practice patterns. Arch Pathol Lab Med 1990;114:145.

30. Kane RA, Kane RL. Evidence about the need for long-term care. In: Long-term care—principles, programs and policies. New York: Springer, 1987.

31. Ford AB. Impaired and disabled elderly in the community. Am J Public Health 1991;81:1207–1209.

32. Jette AM, Branch LG, Sleeper LA, et al. High-risk profiles for nursing home admission. Gerontologist 1992;32:634–640.

33. Coughlin TA, McBride TD, Liu K. Determinants of transitory and permanent nursing home admissions. Med Care 1990;28:616–631.

34. Inoye SK, Wagner R, Acampora D, et al. A predictive index for functional decline in hospitalized elderly medical patients. J Gen Intern Med 1993;8:645–652.

35. Hickman DH, Hedrick SC, Gorton A. Clinician's predictions of nursing home placement for hospitalized patients. J Am Geriatr Soc 1991;39:176–180.

36. Cummings JE, Weaver FM. Cost-effectiveness of home care. Clin Geriatr Med 1991;7:865–874.

37. Chart book on health data on older Americans: United States, 1992. Vital and Health Statistics. Washington, DC: USDHHS Series 3, No. 29, 1993.

38. Rubenstein LZ, Ouslander JG, Wieland D. Dynamics and clinical implications of the nursing home—hospital interface. Clin Geriatr Med 1988;4:471–491.

39. Tresch DD, Simpson WW, Burton JR. Relationship of long-term care and acute care facilities. The problem of patient transfer and continuity of care. J Am Geriatr Soc 1985;33:819.

40. Cohen-Mansfield J, Rabinovich BA, Lipson SL. The decision to execute a Durable Power of Attorney for Health Care and preferences regarding the utilization of life sustaining treatments in nursing home residents. Arch Intern Med 1991;151:289–294.

41. Zimmer JG, Eggert GM, Treat A, et al. Nursing homes as acute care providers: a pilot study of incentives to reduce hospitalizations. J Am Geriatr Soc 1988;36:124–129.

42. Mezey M, Knapp M. Nurse staffing nursing facilities: implications for achieving quality of care. In: Katz PR, Kane RL, Mezey M, eds. Advances in long-term care. Vol. II. New York: Springer, 1993.

43. Katz PR, Karuza J, Parker M, Tarnove L. A national survey of medical directors. J Med Direct 1992;2:81–94.

44. Katz PR, Williams TF. Medical resident education in the nursing home. A new imperative for internal medicine. J Gen Intern Med 1993;8:691–693.

45. Katz PR, Karuza J, Hall N. Residency education in the nursing home: a national survey of internal medicine and family practice programs. J Gen Intern Med 1992;7:52–56.

46. Lawhorne LW, Walker G, Zweig SC, Snyder J. Who cares for Missouri's Medicaid nursing home residents? Characteristics of attending physicians. J Am Geriatr Soc 1993;41:454–458.

47. Rudman D, Arora VD, Feller AG, et al. Epidemiology of Malnutrition in Nursing Homes. In Book Geriatric Nutrition. A Comprehensive Review. Morlew J, Glick Z, Rubenstein LZ (editors). Raven Press, New York, 1990.

48. Kayser-Jones JS. Influence of the Environment on Falls in

Nursing Homes. A Conceptual Model. In Advances in LTC. Katz, Kane and Mezey (editors). Advances in LTC, vol. 2. Springer Publishing Co., New York, 1993.

49. Rubenstein LZ, Robbins AS, Josephson KR. Falls in the Nursing Home Setting: Causes and Preventive Approaches. In Advances in LTC, vol. 1. Katz, Kane, Mezey (editors). Springer Publishing Co., New York, 1991.

50. Katz PR. Antibiotics for Nursing Home Residents. Postgraduate Medicine 1993;93:173–189.

51. Tariot PN, Podgorski CA, Blazina L, Liebovici A. Mental Disorders in the Nursing Home. Another Perspective. Am J Psychiatry 1993;150:1063–1069.

52. Barndeis GH, Morris JN, Nash DJ, Lipsitz LA. The Epidemiology and Natural History of Pressure Ulcers in Elderly Nursing Home Residents. JAMA 1990;264:2905–2909.

53. Ouslander JG, Osterweil D. Physician evaluation in management of nursing home residents. Ann Intern Med 1994;121:584–592.

54. Fiatrone M, Marks EC, Ryan ND, et al. High-intensity strength training in nonagenarians. JAMA 1990;263:3029–3034.

55. Siu AL. The quality of medical care received by older persons. J Am Geriatr Soc 1987;35:1084–1091.

56. Warren JW, Palumbo FB, Fitterman L, et al. Incidence and characteristics of antibiotic use in aged nursing home patients. J Am Geriatr Soc 1991;39:963–972.

57. Katz PR, Beam TR, Brand F, et al. Antibiotic use in the nursing home. Physician practice patterns. Arch Intern Med 1990;150:1465–1468.

58. Zimmer JG, Bentley DW, Valenti WM, et al. Systemic antibiotic use at nursing homes. A quality assessment. J Am Geriatr Soc 1986;34:703–710.

59. Kayser-Jones JS, Wiener CL, Barbaccia JC. Factors contributing to the hospitalization of nursing home residents. Gerontologist 1989;29:502–510.

60. Calkins E, Ford AB, Katz PR. Practice of geriatrics. 2nd edition. Philadelphia: WB Saunders, 1992.

61. Ouslander JG, Osterweil D, Morlew J, eds. Medical care in the nursing home. New York: McGraw-Hill, 1991.

62. Karuza J, Katz PR. Physician staffing patterns correlates of nursing home care: an initial inquiry and consideration of policy implications. J Am Geriatr Soc 1994;42:1–7.

63. Levenson SA, ed. Medical direction in long-term care. A guidebook for the future. Durham: Carolina, 1993.

64. Wieland D, Rubenstein LZ, Ouslander JG, Martin S. Organizing at an academic nursing home. JAMA 1986;255:2622–2627.

65. Ouslander JG, Schnelle JF. Research in nursing homes: practical aspects. J Am Geriatr Soc 1993;41:182–187.

66. Sachs GA, Rhymes J, Cassel CK. Biomedical and behavioral research in nursing homes. Guidelines for ethical investigations. J Am Geriatr Soc 1993;41:771–777.

Chapter 15
Geriatric Hospice Care

Karyn P. Prochoda and Paul A. Seligman

Lord save us all from old age and broken health and a hope tree that has lost the faculty of putting out blossoms.

Mark Twain

Hospice is derived from the Latin words, hospes (guest), and hospitum (hospitality). A hospice was a place of rest and entertainment for traveling pilgrims (1). This changed in the eleventh century when the Knights of Hospitallers of the Order of St. John established hospices along the routes of the crusades for the ill and dying. Believing that death brought one more rapidly to God, the knights wanted to make the way comfortable.

During the reign of Henry VIII in the sixteenth century, a hospice was a shelter for the sick, poor, and blind (2). In the 1800s, the Sisters of Charity, in Dublin, established a home for the incurably ill. The idea traveled to England, where St. Joseph's Hospice was started in 1905. It was here that Dame Cicely Saunders worked as a nurse in the early days of her career. Dame Saunders later became a physician and was instrumental in promoting hospice as a philosophy of care for the terminally ill. She opened St. Christopher's Hospice in London, England, in the 1960s. St. Christopher's became the model hospice and training center for the American hospice movement.

Components of Hospice Care

As a concept, hospice continues to evolve. Presently, *hospice* is defined as a program of palliative and supportive services for dying persons and their families. These services include psychological, social, spiritual, and physical care (3,4). The services can be provided in any of the following settings: a freestanding hospice in which patients are discharged from the hospital and admitted to a professionally staffed self-contained unit; a hospital-based, free-standing hospice affiliated with a hospital but physically in a separate building; a community-based, nonprofessional agency offering home care; a program sponsored by a home health agency such as the visiting nurse service; or a program within a general hospital (5). Whatever the setting, care is provided by a physician-led, multidiscipinary team (3,4).

Hospice Philosophy

The philosophy of hospice is to recognize death as a natural process. Hospice seeks to improve the quality of life to those with a limited quantity of life. The purpose is not to hasten or postpone death, but to prepare the dying individuals and their families in a psychological and spiritual way that is comfortable for them (3). The general principles are outlined in Table 15.1.

Care becomes the focus of any hospice program. Once a patient arrives at the decision to come to hospice, the patient, family, and physician have accepted that the disease is no longer curable or controllable. There is a shift in care toward meeting basic needs of daily comfort. For physicians this is a difficult transition. Palliative care is not well taught in medical education; the emphasis is on cure and prolongation of life. Dame Saunders states "Palliative and terminal care should not only be facets of oncology but of geriatric medicine, neurology, general practice and throughout medicine" (6).

Physicians may withdraw from patients they can no longer cure, which isolates the geriatric patient and family. The patient experiences abandonment in addition to the anticipation of death. It was from the belief that the experiences of isolation, abandonment, and poor symptom control were widespread that the hospice movement began in the United States. In 1974, the first American hospice opened in Connecticut under the direction of Dr. Silvia Lack, a trainee of Dame Saunders, and then many other hospice programs opened; by 1983 there were

Table 15.1. General Principles of Hospice.

1. A program of palliative and supportive care in a variety of settings with an emphasis on home care.
2. A program of palliative care that neither hastens nor postpones death.
3. Hospice care is available 24 hours a day, 7 days a week, on an on-call basis.
4. The patient plus family, or an identified caregiver, is the unit of care, not the patient in isolation.
5. An interdisciplinary team of trained hospice professionals and volunteers work together to meet the physiologic, psychologic, social, spiritual, and economic needs of hospice patient-family-caregiver unit facing terminal illness and bereavement.
6. Management of physical and psychological symptoms is the focus of an interdisciplinary, patient-directed plan of care. This includes palliation of pain and other physical symptoms and support for psychological stresses and concerns.

SOURCE: National Hospice Organization. Standards of a hospice program of care. Arlington, VA: National Hospice Organization, 1993:1–5.

518, and by 1991, 1700. The National Hospice Organization formed in 1978 to provide guidelines and standards for the newly formed movement (7). In 1981, the Joint Commission for Accreditation of Hospitals (JCAH) developed a set of guidelines for monitoring the growth of hospices.

Medicare Reimbursement

The early hospices were volunteer run with variable sources of funding, mostly private. Because the elderly had the greatest utilization of acute care facilities at the end of life, the feasibility of lowering Medicare costs by including hospice as a Medicare benefit was considered (8). In 1980, the National Hospice Study (9,10) was started to evaluate objectively the effect of hospice payment on the Medicare program. The study included 1754 patients in 40 hospice programs. Before the study was completed, Congress, believing Medicare expenditures could be lessened by millions of dollars per year, added hospice coverage (11). However, data collected from the study were invaluable for evaluating aspects of hospice care other than financing. These areas included pain control, symptom management, analgesic use, and satisfaction with care (9,10,12–15).

The addition of hospice benefits to Medicare was passed by Congress in 1982 with the Tax Equalization and Fiscal Responsibility Act (TEFRA). To qualify for Medicare hospice benefits, an individual needs to meet the following criteria: terminally ill with a life span of 6 months or less; unable to benefit from further aggressive or curative therapy; able to receive most care in the home; and have a willing primary caregiver available in the home (16). The recipient waives rights for treatment of terminal illness-related conditions under Medicare A, but conditions not related to the terminal illness will be reimbursed. Hospice reimbursement is divided into four benefit periods; two 90-day periods, one 30-day period, and a fourth indefinite period. The fourth period was added to the benefit in 1990 in the Omnibus Budget Reconciliation Act (OBRA). Before this legislation, hospice reimbursement was not available for individuals who remained in a hospice longer than 210 days, but the hospice was required to continue to provide care for those individuals. At the beginning of each benefit period the recipient must be recertified as having a terminal illness. A hospice-benefit recipient may decide to reject the hospice benefit and return to full Medicare A coverage, forfeiting the remainder of that hospice benefit period. The entire benefit is not lost, however, and the individual may elect to return to hospice care at a later time. There is an allowance of three revocations per recipient.

The Health Care Financing Administration (HCFA), which oversees the Medicare program, specifies four levels of reimbursement for hospice care: 1) routine home care, including a health aide and some skilled nursing services; 2) continuous home care, with skilled nursing in the home for a brief period of intensive care during a crisis; 3) general inpatient care for short periods in an acute care setting to facilitate treatment of an acute problem or worsening of a chronic one; 4) inpatient respite care, to minimize caregiver fatigue.

Data from the National Hospice Study (1980) showed that 90 percent of patients in hospice had a diagnosis of cancer (10). However, in 1992, the Centers for Disease Control and Prevention (CDC) conducted a survey of hospices and their patients and found cancer as the primary diagnosis in only 65 percent of the patients. Cardiovascular disease was listed as the primary diagnosis in 10 percent of those surveyed (17). The remaining diagnoses were not specified. Other terminal illnesses present in the geriatric population for which hospice care is sought include neuromuscular disease such as amyotrophic lateral sclerosis (ALS), chronic obstructive pulmonary disease, renal disease, cerebrovascular disease and dementia.

Each disease presents unique problems when a physician is asked to accurately predict a patient's time until death. In particular, severe dementia is the prime example of a disease state that is difficult to predict. Recent studies have evaluated family and caregiver preferences in caring for the demented elder. Most of the individuals surveyed favored nonaggressive palliative care (18,19). Patients benefit from a nonaggressive approach to care when they are allowed to stay in their home environment during acute illnesses. Symptoms can be contolled with a combination of pharmacologic and nonpharmacologic methods minimizing the stress, discomfort, and disorientation of an acute hospitalization. Families benefit when Medicare hospice services are available, especially the benefits of health aides, respite care, and bereavement counseling (19). The difficulty with hospice care for these individuals is primarily the length of stay within a hospice program. The duration of stay in one study was found to be 17 to 60 months (18). This time period is well outside of the Medicare reimbursement period of 6 months.

Symptom Control

Symptom control is a key principle of hospice care. Pain affects more than 80 percent of terminally ill cancer patients with an increased prevalence toward the very end of life (20). At most, 17 percent of this pain is not related to the terminal illness (20). Assessing a pain complaint should include the type of pain, the location, and any exacerbating or alleviating factors. For patients with a diagnosis of cancer, there are several mechanisms of pain to consider. Solid tumors most commonly cause pain through organ and tissue infiltration; tumor infiltration of nervous tissue; and compression of organs, vasculature, and nerves (21). Other sources of pain related to a cancer diagnosis include pathologic fractures; and disease modifying treatments (surgery, chemotherapy, radiation therapy) (22). Nonmalignant etiologies are frequent among elderly hospice patients and are caused by exacerbations of comorbid illness. Most illnesses common

in the elderly—osteoporosis, osteoarthritis, chronic constipation, diabetes mellitus, angina, congestive heart failure, venous and arterial insufficiency, chronic pain, and cognitive impairment—are worsened when immobility, deconditioning, and additional medications occur as a result of treating pain and other symptoms caused by the terminal illness (23).

Pain occurs in three forms. Visceral pain, described as vague and nonlocalizing, is related to stretching and inflammation of tissues. Usually this form of pain is very responsive to opioids. Somatic pain is well localized, constant, and aching (21). A common type of pain in cancer patients with bone invasion, somatic pain is less sensitive to opioids alone, but responds best to a combination of nonsteroidal anti-inflammatory drugs (NSAIDS) and opioids. Neuropathic pain, deafferentation, is described as constant, dull, squeezing, burning, or aching. This type of pain is difficult to treat with opioids, but anticonvulsants and antidepressants have some efficacy for this problem.

Assessing the type of pain is important in determining the type of treatment. The cognitively impaired elder who is unable to express pain complaints needs to be observed for indicators of discomfort through behaviors. Discussions with caregivers can facilitate assessment in these individuals. Frequently, this group is difficult to treat because of the presence of comorbid illnesses in addition to cognitive impairment and terminal illness.

Although nonpharmacologic methods of pain control have some usefulness, drugs are the mainstay in pain control (20). The World Health Organization (WHO) advocates the following analgesic ladder (24). For mild pain, NSAIDs, aspirin, or acetominophen are recommended. These drugs are given on a scheduled basis. There is a ceiling at which no further efficacy is obtained by increasing the dose. Therapeutic effects take 24 to 48 hours to be noticed. Moderate pain is controlled with a combination of those drugs and a mild opioid such as codeine or oxycodone. Medication side effects, predominately consisting of nausea and constipation, become more problematic in the elderly with this step. Close monitoring and early interventions can minimize these effects. Stronger opioids are used for severe pain. The drug most commonly used by the principles outlined in Table 15.2 is morphine sulfate.

Table 15.2. Principles of Pain Control.

1. Schedule narcotic dosages around the clock.
2. Use long-acting narcotics when able, with immediate-release analgesic for breakthrough pain as needed.
3. Reassess pain complaint if narcotic needs are changing. Determine whether an adjuvant is needed.
4. Use oral route of administration, if possible, instead of parenteral and rectal routes.
5. Assess and control side effects from narcotic administration.

Initiating morphine therapy requires following the principles listed. A long-acting preparation of sustained release morphine is given every 8 to 12 hours. The initiating dose varies with the level of narcotic exposure the elder has had because of the development of tolerance and cross-tolerance to narcotics. A usual starting dosage in an individual with minimal exposure is 15 mg to 30 mg of sustained-release morphine preparation every 12 hours. An immediate-release morphine preparation is made available for breakthrough pain in dosages of 5 mg to 10 mg every 2 to 4 hours. Every 48 hours an assessment is made to determine the amount of breakthrough medication being used. Converting one-to-one, an adjustment is made in the sustained-release preparation to minimize the requirement for breakthrough medication. For example, if a geriatric patient is receiving 30 mg of sustained-release morphine every 12 hours, but is using an average of 60 mg of immediate-release morphine over a 24-hour period, the sustained-release dose can be safely increased to 90 mg every 12 hours.

Oral morphine is preferable to parenteral. About 60 percent of patients can take oral medications until within 48 hours of death (25). Individuals unable to tolerate oral medications can be given sublingual and rectal preparations of morphine (25).

A small percentage of patients are unable to tolerate morphine because of allergic reactions or side effects, especially delirium in elderly individuals. Hydromorphone is the next drug of choice. It has a short half-life of 2 to 3 hours and requires frequent administration, although a long-acting preparation is available. A rectal suppository can be used for the geriatric patient unable to tolerate oral medications.

Fentanyl citrate transdermal therapeutic system (TTS) is a time-released transdermal patch that offers controlled release of fentanyl over a 72-hour period. Its efficacy in the terminally ill elder is variable. Medication delivery depends on stable skin factors such as temperature, moisture, and absence of skin irritation. Titration of medication dosage is more difficult in the elderly individual who is close to death because of the alterations in tissue perfusion that occur before death. One author outlined four guidelines for the use of the TTS fentanyl citrate patch (24).

1. The patient should have adequate pain control by a stable dose of narcotics before the patch is placed on the patient.

2. During periods of dose adjustments or when use of the patch is begun, the patient should have liberal doses of immediate-acting analgesia available.

3. Long-acting opioids should not be used in conjunction with the patch because of the increased risk of side effects.

4. Skin sites need to be rotated to avoid accumulated narcotic in subcutaneous tissue.

The use of strong opioids in the elderly is limited by the side effects of respiratory and central nervous system depression. Therefore, beginning a geriatric patient on strong narcotics, requires starting at lower doses and increasing the dose as needed for pain control. Other side effects, such as nausea, anorexia, and delirium are common among the elderly; if these effects are unable to be controlled, symptoms may improve with a change in narcotic. Because the patient may develop tolerance and cross tolerance, changing narcotics requires calculation of the equianalgesic dose of the substituted medication. The patient should start at 50 percent to 70 percent of that dose with a rapid escalation as needed. Equianalgesia of commonly used narcotics is presented in Tables 15.3 and 15.4.

Table 15.3. Equianalgesia of Commonly Used Drugs in the Terminal Elder.

Pain Level	Drug	Parenteral Route (mg)	Oral/Sublinqual Route (mg)
mild to moderate pain	Ibuprofen		600
	Acetominophen		1000
	Codeine		30
moderate to severe pain	Morphine sulfate	10	30
	Codeine	130	200
	Hydromorphone	1.5	7.5

Table 15.4. Equianalgesia of Morphine to Fentanyl.

Total 24-hour Oral Morphine (mg)	Transdermal Fentanyl Patch (µg/hr)
50–125	25
125–225	50
225–300	75
300–400	100
400–500	125

Many elderly patients have more than one type of pain. In one survey, more than 81 percent had more than two types of pain and more than 35 percent had more than three types (30). Control of pain frequently requires the use of adjuvant medications. For example, NSAIDS are helpful in the management of bone pain, and these can be used in lower doses in the elderly, thus augmenting the effect of opioids. Indomethacin should be avoided in the geriatric population because of increased incidence of confusion.

Antidepressants are efficacious in the treatment of neuropathic pain in addition to their antidepressant effects. The tricyclics, primarily amitriptyline, are the most extensively studied. Given in lower doses than that used for antidepressant effect, they enhance the action of opioid analgesia. Among the serotonin reuptake inhibitors, paroxetine is the first to be shown effective in the treatment of neuropathic pain (26). Pain relief with the use of antidepressants occurs in 40 percent to 70 percent of patients. The onset of pain relief can occur within 48 hours because of improved sleep and lessened anxiety (26). The choice of antidepressant, in the elderly, is related to the side effect profile. A drug with minimum anticholinergic effects is desired, and should begin with low dose that is gradually escalated.

Lancinating pain, a form of neuropathic pain, is particularly difficult to control. Occasionally antidepressants give relief but anticonvulsants, specifically carbamazepine, phenytoin, and clonazepam, are most effective (20). Steroids, such as dexamethasone and prednisone, have also been successful (20).

Anxiolytics and neuroleptics have a role in augmenting pain control. Although anxiolytics have no direct analgesic effects, they decrease the anxiety associated with pain. There is evidence that neuroleptics, such as phenothiazines and haloperidol, have direct analgesic effects in addition to sedating effects (20,26–28). Low doses, adjusted upwards as needed, minimize confusion and delerium in the terminally ill elder.

Effective analgesia in the elderly is associated with an increased prevalence of side effects such as constipation, nausea, itching, and delirium. Constipation is the most frequent side effect and can evolve into an uncomfortable, painful ileus. Any narcotic regemin is incomplete unless a laxative is ordered concomittently. Ducosate sodium with a senna derivative is most commonly used. Lactulose is also used but may cause nausea, abdominal bloating, and flatulence in elders with lactose intolerance. Nausea occurs during the initiation of most narcotics, but as tolerance develops, becomes less problematic. A patient beginning a narcotic regimen should have an antiemetic as a routine medication for the first 5 to 7 days, but continue the antiemetic only as needed. Itching, a result of histamine release with the use of some narcotics, is controlled with antihistamines. Occasionally, a change in narcotic is required. Among terminal elders, especially those with cognitive impairment, delirium frequently occurs. Causes of delirium are multifactorial. General principles for managing delirium are indicated and are primarily directed at determining the underlying cause. If the narcotic is implicated, naloxone should not be used because the analgesic effects will be blocked in addition to the central nervous system effects. A change in the narcotic should be made as outlined above. In this situation, adequate control of pain is essential, for its presence increases agitation and delirium. If other measures fail to control symptomatic delirium, a low dose neuroleptic, Most such as haloperidol in dosages of 0.5 mg to 2 mg every 6 hours is often recommended (24,27,29).

Sometimes there is a geriatric patient whose pain symptoms cannot be controlled with an adequate trial of systemic narcotics or whose pain is controlled but the narcotic side effects are intolerable. For these elderly individuals, several invasive nerve blocking or ablative procedures, anesthetic and neurosurgical, can be considered. Anesthetic techniques are either destructive (e.g., chemoneurolysis with phenol or alcohol) or nondestructive (e.g., local intermittent or continuous infusions of narcotic through a sterilely placed catheter into the epidural or subarachnoid space). Narcotic side effects are less of a problem with epidural or intrathecal infusions. One author cited five conditions in which an anesthetic procedure would be ideal: 1) chemotherapy is no longer effective and pain continues to be a problem; 2) pain is poorly controlled with systemic opioid analgesics; 3) the patient and family understand and accept the risks and benefits of the planned procedure; 4) the patient has localized pain and no contraindications to the procedure; 5) bodily functions important to the patient are not compromised (i.e., sexual function, bowel and bladder control) (31). Contraindications for an invasive procedure are coagulopathy, septicemia, local infection at site of catheter insertion, poorly controlled diabetes mellitus, and lack of caregiving supports for catheter management after insertion (33).

Anesthetic ablative procedures, chemoneurolysis, are done through percutaneous injection of either phenol or alcohol. Depending on the location and quality of the pain these can be placed centrally with an epidural or intrathecal block, peripherally with a somatic or sympathetic nerve blockade, or viscerally with a celiac plexus block. The most effective ablative procedure is a celiac plexus block for control of visceral abdominal pain resulting from pancreatic, gastric, or colon cancer, as well as metastatic disease. The success rate is reported to be 57 percent to 95 percent (31). Success rates for intrathecal or epidural blockades are less impressive, 46 percent to 63 percent and 33 percent to 90 percent, respectively (31).

Neurosurgical procedures are ablative. A trial of anesthetic blockade is done before the procedure to determine patient tolerance to the numbing sensation. Some patients prefer pain to the presence of numbness. Anesthetic blocks with local anesthetic help to localize areas to be altered permanently. The two most common neurosurgical procedures performed percutaneously on the debilitated elder are dorsal rhizotomy and cordotomy. A dorsal rhizotomy, the severing of sensory nerve root fibers, is most useful for thoracic or abdominal wall pain but not effective for visceral pain. Cordotomy, commonly performed before the availability of intraspinal opioids, is effective in patients with unilateral lower extremity pain resulting from sacral plexus invasion by rectal or gynecologic cancers (32). Although these invasive techniques of pain control exist, the risk-to-benefit ratio for each individual needs to be evaluated. In general, a noninvasive approach to symptom control is advocated in the geriatric hospice patient.

Dyspnea, an unpleasant awareness of the action of breathing, occurs in over 70 percent of terminally ill patients (34). It is most common in patients with lung cancer and in those who have received chemotherapy with agents known to have pulmonary toxicity. Radiation therapy to more than 25 percent of lung tissue also predisposes an individual to develop dyspnea. Noncancer causes related to comorbid conditions also occur. Treatment depends on the underlying cause. For symptomatic relief, invasive procedures such as placement of a chest tube for a pneumothorax or a thoracentesis for a new pleural effusion can be done. For most elders, comfort is best achieved with pharmacologic interventions. Given in doses that do not suppress respiratory drive, morphine sulfate is effective for relieving the sensation of dyspnea by reducing ventilatory responses to carbon dioxide and hypoxia. Morphine can be given parenterally, orally, or via nebulizer. Nebulized morphine has the least negative effects on ventilatory drive (35). Anxiety contributes to the sensation of inadequate ventilation and can be relieved with a combination of morphine and anxiolytic agents.

Anorexia is multifactorial and commonly found in elderly hospice patients. It may result from persistent nausea, medication side effects, cancer effects, or depression. Culturally, food and drink are considered nurturing and life sustaining, therefore anorexia is most difficult for family members to accept. Physiologically, anorexia has been described as an adaptive, protective mechanism that will lead to a gentler death because death from dehydration and starvation is not painful (36). In contrast, overhydration may cause a more uncomfortable death because of the increase in pulmonary and oral secretions. Although treating anorexia is difficult, a trial of methylphenidate or dextroamphetamine may stimulate appetite and a sense of well-being, hence improving oral intake of nourishment (27). Force-feeding is not recommended, including enteral and parenteral nutrition. Family members will need support, education, and reassurance that force-feeding a dying elder may aggravate some symptoms and increase anxiety, and thus cause a worsened quality of life (37). Use of artificial sustenance requires discussion with the patient and family. The presence of advance directives is helpful for decision making if the patient is incompetent.

Multidisciplinary Team

Controlling symptoms, and providing comfort, palliation, and support for the geriatric hospice patient requires the skills of a multidisciplinary team. Medicare requires that this team be led by a physician. Ideally, the patient's primary care physician assists with developing a patient-focused plan of care for the patient. When the primary physician is unable to continue to care for the geriatric patient in hospice, the hospice's attending physician assumes care. The attending physician is employed by the hospice as an individual with an interest and expertise in palliative care to act as a consultant or to assume care on agreement with the primary physician. A hospice medical director oversees the patient's medical care to ensure quality and compliance with the hospice's standards of care.

Essential to the team are its nonphysician members. Nursing provides day-to-day care of the geriatric hospice patient and family. Nurses are responsible for ongoing assessments of symptoms and the quality of control provided by therapeutic interventions. Most important, nursing acts as the liaison between the patient-family unit and the rest of the team.

Evaluation of medication regimes and offering alternatives is a valuable service provided by the hospice-employed, consulting pharmacist. Periodic reviews of medications assist in eliminating unnecessary drugs and their potential side effects. Immobility predisposes the geriatric patient to further discomfort from loss of function and the development of contractures. Physical and occupational therapists have a role in assisting the team to maintain patient functional status and thus minimizing these discomforts. Social service workers can assist the family in several ways. They can provide counseling for both patient and family dealing with the dying process, as well as assist the family with finding emotional and financial supports within the community. Pastoral counselors assist the patient and family with spiritual issues, which frequently arise as death nears. Volunteers are the backbone of any hospice. They function in any capacity on the team, as their training allows, and provide emotional support to patients and their families. Earlier hospices were begun and run by volunteers; they remain an important and necessary part of any hospice program.

Summary and Conclusions

Hospice care is an attractive alternative for the dying individual. Earlier comparison studies have shown greater satisfaction with end of life care among individuals and their families in hospice programs (13,38,39). Since the beginning of the U.S. hospice movement in 1974, research in pain and symptom control in oncology patients has helped to improve both pharmacologic and nonpharmacologic methods of symptom control in hospice patients. Education of the medical community is progressing slowly, but more training programs are recognizing the need to teach hospice care. Previously palliative care was not well taught. An inability to cure a patient has been perceived as a failure limiting a physician's ability to focus on the alternative of providing comfort only. In the future, training in hospice care should dispel this myth.

The expansion of hospice programs in the U.S. testifies to the increased recognition of hospice as an alternative to conventional care. Further education of the medical and nonmedical community is required, especially in an environment in which physician-assisted suicide and euthanasia are being debated; hospice care provides a reasonable alternative.

Hospice care is an important component of geriatrics. The average age of the hospice patient is 71 years (17). Cancer remains the principal diagnosis of hospice patients, but the advanced age of these individuals has brought more chronic diseases and symptoms to palliative care. Symptom control is more challenging in this age group and requires the skills of an individual with training in geriatrics as well as palliative care. An awareness of disease processes, other than cancer, that can benefit from hospice care is needed to further improve the quality of an elderly individual's life when improving quantity is no longer reasonable. A period of 6 months from diagnosis to death has been legislated by Congress as the period of hospice benefits, but physicians determine when an elder patient would benefit more from a palliative approach to disease than from a curative approach. Further research and education in the area of geriatric hospice is required to continue to provide quality care through the end of life.

References

1. Stoddard S. The hospice movement: a better way of caring for the dying. New York: Vintage, 1978.
2. Mathew LM, Scully JH. Hospice Care. Clin Geriatr Med Care 1986;2:617–633.
3. National Hospice Organization. Standards of a Hospice Program of Care. Arlington, VA: National Hospice Organization, 1981.
4. National Hospice Organization. Standards of a Hospice Program of Care. Arlington, VA: National Hospice Organization, 1993.
5. Torrens PR. Hospice programs and public policy. Chicago: American Hospital, 1985.
6. Saunders C. Principles of symptom control in terminal care. Med Clin North Am 1982;66:1169–1183.
7. Plumb JD, Ogle KS. Hospice Care. Prim Care 1992;19:807–820.
8. Emanuel E, Emanuel L. The economics of dying. N Engl J Med 1994;330:540–544.
9. Aiken LH. Evaluation research and public policy: lessons from the National Hospice Study. J Chronic Dis 1986;39:1–4.
10. Greer DS, Mor V. An overview of National Hospice Study findings. J Chronic Dis 1986;39:5–7.
11. Levy MH. Living with cancer: hospice/palliative care. J Natl Cancer Inst 1993;85:1283–1287.
12. Goldberg RJ, Mor V, Wiemann M, et al. Analgesic use in terminal cancer patients: report from the National Hospice Study. J Chronic Dis 1986;39:37–45.
13. Greer DS, Mor V, Morris JN, et al. An alternative in terminal care: results of the National Hospice Study. J Chronic Dis 1986;39:9–26.
14. Morris JN, Mor V, Goldberg R, et al. The effect of treatment setting and patient characteristics on pain in terminal cancer patients: a report from the National Hospice Study. J Chronic Dis 1986;39:27–35.
15. Morris JN, Suissa S, Sherwood S, et al. Last days: a study of the quality of life of terminally ill cancer patients. J Chronic Dis 1986;39:47–86.
16. Balkin W, Lukashok H. Rx for dying: the case for hospice. N Engl J Med 1988;318:376–378.
17. Centers for Disease Control. Home health and hospice care—United States, 1992. MMWR 1993;42:820–823.
18. Volicer L. Need for hospice approach to treatment of patients with advanced progressive dementia. J Am Geriatr Soc 1986;34:655–658.
19. Luchins DJ, Hanrahan P. What is appropriate care for end-stage dementia? J Am Geriatr Soc 1993;41:27–30.
20. Walsh TD, ed. Symptom control. Boston: Blackwell Science, 1989.
21. Payne R. Cancer pain: anatomy, physiology, and pharmacology. Cancer 1989;63(suppl):2266–2273.
22. Amlot P. Cancer therapy: side effects of radiotherapy and chemotherapy. In: Walsh TD, ed. Symptom control. Boston: Blackwell Science, 1989.
23. Besdine RW. Geriatric medicine: an overview. Annu Rev Gerontol Geriatr 1980;1:135–160.
24. Enck RE. The medical care of the terminally ill patients. Baltimore: Johns Hopkins, 1994.
25. Hanks GW. Psychotropic drugs. Clin Oncol 1984;3:135–151.
26. Breitbart W, Passick R. Psychological and psychiatric interventions in pain control. In: Doyle D, Hanks G, MacDonald N, eds. Oxford textbook of palliative care. Oxford: Oxford Medical, 1993.
27. Breitbart W. Psychiatric managment of cancer pain. Cancer 1989;63(suppl):2336–2342.
28. Corr CA, Corr DM. Hospice care: principles and practice. New York: Springer, 1983.
29. Breivik H, Rennemo F. Clinical evaluation of combined treatment with methadone and psychotropic drugs in cancer patients. Acta Anaesthesiol Scand 1982;74(suppl):135–140.
30. Portenoy RK. Cancer pain: epidemiology and syndromes. Cancer 1989;63(suppl):2298–2307.
31. Ferrer-Brechner T. Anesthetic Techniques for the Management of Cancer Pain. Cancer 1989;63(suppl):2343–2347.
32. Sundaresan N, Digiacinto G, Hughes J. Neurosurgery in the treatment of cancer pain. Cancer 1989;63(suppl):2365–2377.
33. Swarm R, Cousins M. Anesthetic techniques for pain control. In: Doyle D, Hanks GW, MacDonald N, eds. Oxford Text of Palliative Care. Oxford: Oxford Medical, 1993.
34. Cooke N. Dyspnea. In: Walsh TD, ed. Symptom control. Boston: Blackwell Science, 1989.
35. Kaye P. Notes on symptom control in hospice and palliative care. Essex, CT: Hospice Education Institute, 1989.
36. Miller RJ. Force feeding the dying: an act of kindness or cruelty. Am J Hospice Care 1989;Nov/Dec:13–14.
37. Miles S. The terminally ill elderly: dealing with the ethics of feeding. Geriatrics 1985;40:112–120.
38. Kane R, Bernstein L, Wales J, et al. A randomized controlled trial of hospice care. Lancet 1984;1:890–894.
39. Kane R, Klein S, Bernstein L, et al. Hospice role in alleviating the emotional stress of terminal patients and their families. Med Care 1985;23:189–197.

Suggested Readings

Abel EK. The hospice movement: Institutionalizing innovation. Int J Health Serv 1986;16(1):71–85.
Berry ZS, Lynn J. Hospice medicine. JAMA 1993;270(2):221–222.
Brody H, Lynn J. The physicians' responsibility under the new medicare reimbursement for hospice care. N Engl J Med 1984;310(14):920–921.
Carney K, Burns N. Economics of Hospice Care. Oncol Nurs Forum 1991;18(4):761–768.
Doyle D, Hanks GW, MacDonald N, ed. Oxford Textbook of Palliative Medicine. Oxford: Oxford Medical, 1993.

Foley K. Controversies in Cancer Pain: Medical Perspectives. Cancer 1989;63(suppl):2257–2265.

Friel PB. Death and Dying. Ann Intern Med 1982;97(5):767–771.

Handy R. The elderly. In: Walsh TD, ed. Symptom Control. Boston: Blackwell Scientific, 1989.

Inturrisi C. Management of Cancer Pain: Pharmacology and Principles of Management. Cancer 1989;63(suppl):2308–2320.

Kidder D. The effects of hospice on medicare expenditures. Health Serv Research 1992;27(2):195–217.

Kissick PD. Hospice: Medicare's best kept secret. Philadelphia Med 1989;84:328–330.

Loeser J. Neurosurgical Approaches in Palliative Care. In Doyle D, Hanks G, MacDonald N, eds. Oxford Text of Palliative Care. Oxford: Oxford Publications, 1993.

Lubitz JD, Riley GF. Trends in medicare payments in the last year of life. N Engl J Med 1993;328(15):1092–1096.

Lukashok H. Hospice care under medicare—an early look. Prev Med 1990;19:730–736.

Lynn J. Dying and dementia. JAMA 1986;256(16):2244–2245.

Magni G. The use of antidepressants in the treatment of chronic pain. Drugs 1991;42(5):730–748.

Mathew LM, Jahnigen DW, Scully JH, Rempel P, Myer TJ, LaForce FM. Attitudes of House Officers Toward a Hospice on a Medical Service. J Med Educ, 1983;58:772–777.

McCracken AL, Gerdsen L. Hospice care principles for terminally ill elders. J Gerontological Nursing 1991;17(2).

Miller RJ, Albright PG. What is the role of nutritional support and hydration in terminal cancer patients? Am J Hospice Care 1989;Nov/Dec:33–38

Monfardini S, Yancik R. Cancer in the elderly: Meeting the challenge of an aging population. J National Cancer Institute, 1993;85(7):532–538.

Mor V, Birnbaum H. Medicare legislation for hospice care: Implications of national hospice study data. Health Aff 1983;2(2):80–90.

Ogle K, Warren D, Plumb J. Pain management in advanced cancer. Primary Care 1992;19(4):793–805.

Paradis LF. Hospice Handbook: A Guide for Managers and Planners. Rockville, MD: Aspen Publications, 1985.

Patt R. Nonpharmacologic measures for controlling oncologic pain. Am J Hospice Palliative Care 41–47 Nov/Dec, 1992.

Rhymes J. Hospice care in America. JAMA 1990;264(3):369–372.

Rhymes J. Home hospice care. Clin Geriatri Med 1991;7(4):803–817.

Rhymes J. Clinical management of the terminally ill. Geriatrics 1991;46(2):57–62.

Sager MA, Easterling DV, Kundig DA, Anderson OW. Changes in the location of death after passage of medicare's prospective payment system. N Engl J Med 1989;320(7):433–439.

Saunders C, Baines M. Living with Dying (2nd ed.) Oxford: Oxford Medical Publications, 1989.

Smith JF. Pain Treatment in a Palliative Unit or Team of a University Hospital. Acta Anaesthesiol Scand 1982;74(suppl):119–123.

Streim JE, Marshall JR. The dying elderly patient. Am Fam Physician 1988;38(5):175–183.

Volicer L, Rheame Y, Brown J, Fabigzewki K, Brady R. Hospice approach to the treatment of patients with advanced dementia of the Alzheimer type. JAMA 1986;256(16):2210–2213.

Zimmerman JM. Hospice: Complete Care for the Terminally Ill (2nd ed.) Baltimore: Urban and Schwartzenberg, 1986.

Chapter 16
Nutrition

Ronni Chernoff

If we could give every individual the right amount of nourishment and exercise, not too little and not too much, we would have found the safest way to health.

Hippocrates

Nutrition is a vital factor in all phases of the life cycle, in health and disease, and in the prevention of and recuperation from illness. Each phase of life has unique demands that contribute to the individual's need for nutrients. Growth, development, maturity, and acute chronic illnesses all have inherent nutrient demands that must be met to best meet dynamic metabolic states. Nutritional requirements and interventions vary because of changing physiologic conditions. Nutritional requirements necessary to maintain health and prevent disease may be different from those required in the treatment of chronic medic conditions or the recovery of health after an acute medical episode. Nutritional needs of elderly individuals who require rehabilitation are unique and may change as physical condition changes.

Normal aging is associated with physiologic changes that contribute to modifications in nutrient requirements. The major physiologic changes that occur are a reduction in total body protein, a decrease in total body water, a loss in bone density, and an increase in total body fat with a redistribution of fat stores. Although these changes occur in all aging people, they occur at different rates among individuals and may be affected by the existence of chronic diseases.

Aging is a uniquely individual process that may be affected by a person's nutritional intake throughout earlier stages (1). Some changes in the nutritional requirements of older individuals can be accommodated if clinicians are alert to their presentations and etiologies. Distinguishing between physiologic, age-induced changes and nutritional deficiencies may be difficult. Observing nutritional intake, physical strength, functional status, and physiologic alterations that occur over time yields important clues to potential nutritional problems in elderly people. The basal requirements to maintain homeostasis, the demands of chronic disease, and the extraordinary needs of acute illness make the provision of nutritional care to elderly patients a challenge for their caregivers.

Nutritional Needs of the Elderly

Energy Needs

To avoid nutritional problems, to maintain health, and to provide adequate nutrition to elderly people requires an understanding of the impact of age on nutritional requirements. The most well-documented change that occurs with advancing age is decrease in energy metabolism (2). Reduction in energy requirements is related to the decrease in protein mass that occurs with age rather than to the metabolic activity of aging tissue. Basal energy requirements reflect the total energy needed for all metabolic processes involved in maintaining cell function; reduction of active metabolic mass results in lowered energy needs.

Energy requirements are markedly affected by a reduction in time spent on a physical activity or in intensity of physical activity (3,4). Results of experiments conducted as part of the Baltimore Longitudinal Study on Aging indicated that there is an age-related decline in physical activity for both men (5) and women (6). Decreases in physical activity may be related to the onset of bone and joint diseases, the progression of chronic diseases of the heart and lungs, neurological disorders, failing vision, or fractures related to poor balance or osteoporosis. It is noteworthy that the lowered energy requirements are more closely associated with the decrease in energy expenditure than they are to a decrease in basal energy rate (5).

There is increasing evidence that frail, older adults can benefit from strength training exercises. Muscle strength can be rehabilitated by regular training and greater independence can be fostered by increased confidence in functional ability (7). Regular exercise stimulates protein turnover, maintains muscle mass, and burns more calories (8,9).

One method that may be used to ensure slower declines in energy and nutrient intake is the development of an exercise program. Data indicate that exercise training is associated with higher levels of energy and nutrient intake in older adults (6,7). Thus, there is a reconditioning of physical fitness, even through the very late years, even though there may not be an improvement in dietary quality (8). Exercise may contribute to a retention of lean body mass over time, or at least to a slower decline than occurs in nonexercising, aging people (9). Fat distribution patterns can change with exercise (10), although exercise may or may not have a noticeable impact on bone density or muscle loss in elderly individuals (11,12). Exercise may have many positive benefits beyond changes in body composition: improvement of cardiorespiratory endurance, reduction of cardiovascular risk, control of blood pressure, prevention of obesity or osteoporosis, and elevation of basal metabolic rate (13,14). Instituting an exercise program in aging individuals is controversial, and often older women are reluctant to engage in exercise programs (15), but physical activity that starts at an early age and continues throughout life has only positive effects as long as exercise regimens are not overdone to the point of injury (16). A third cause for a reduction in energy requirements with advancing age is alteration in hormone production, particularly growth hormone and testosterone, both of which promote anabolism or lean tissue growth (17).

Usually, energy requirements are extrapolated from studies conducted on younger adults, but this is not a very reliable process. Metabolic studies show that several factors alter estimation of energy expenditure or demands in older versus middle-aged or younger individuals (4,18–20). Actually measuring the metabolic rate of older people, if the resting metabolic rate (RMR) is an important factor, is crucial in planning therapeutic interventions for them; there is too much variability among individuals to rely on extrapolated or generalized data.

Protein Requirements

Protein requirements of elderly individuals might be expected to decrease to accommodate a lower total lean body mass. However, research indicates that protein requirements may be slightly higher in older subjects (21). One explanation is that lower energy intake leads to decreased retention of dietary nitrogen, therefore more dietary protein is needed to achieve nitrogen balance.

As people age and experience a decrease in skeletal tissue mass (22), the protein store represented by skeletal muscle may be inadequate to meet the demands for protein synthesis, and therefore dietary protein intake becomes more important to meet essential needs (23,24). Protein needs are also affected by immobility (25), which contributes to negative nitrogen balance. Elderly people who are bed-bound, wheelchair-bound, or otherwise immobilized require higher levels of dietary protein to achieve nitrogen equilibrium.

For healthy, free-living elderly, protein requirements have not been shown to increase or decrease significantly. Protein requirements for adults have been determined on the basis of needs for younger adults and do not compensate for age-related changes in physiology or in the body's responses to stress, trauma, infection, injury, or chronic disease. Surgery, sepsis, long-bone fractures and unusual losses, such as those that occur with burns or gastrointestinal disease, increase the need for dietary protein. In studies conducted with elderly subjects, protein requirements per kilogram of body weight were demonstrated not to decline with age (26) and the recommended dietary allowance of 0.8 grams protein per kilogram body weight as determined for younger adults was not adequate to maintain nitrogen equilibrium for elderly adults (21).

Failure to maintain nitrogen balance with dietary protein intake that meets the recommended dietary allowance may be more significant for older adults than seems apparent. Protein calorie malnutrition has been noted in many different populations of elderly people (27–31) and the slow, continuous decline of protein stores may certainly be a contributing factor in the etiology of this condition. Chronic protein inadequacy may also be a determinant in depressed immune function, loss of muscle strength, poor wound healing, and pressure ulcer development in elderly individuals. New tissue cannot be made, ulcers cannot heal, and immune responses cannot be mounted without adequate dietary protein substrate.

Some clinicians have been reluctant to provide high levels of dietary protein for fear of exacerbating renal problems in elderly individuals. Research has shown no evidence that dietary protein induces deterioration of renal function for individuals who have no evidence of renal disease (32,33). For older adults who have a measurable decline in renal function, appropriate therapeutic regimens should be followed.

Fasting plasma amino acids may be good indicators of dietary protein adequacy. Plasma amino acids may reflect changes caused by protein-energy malnutrition, by protein malnutrition, by a deficient intake of essential amino acids, or by an imbalance in dietary protein intake (34,35). Protein is a very important dietary component because it is essential in the production of a vast array of physiologic compounds, including, for example, blood components such as erythrocytes, leukocytes, and platelets; hormones such as epinephrine, insulin, and estrogen; enzymes such as proteases, disaccharidases, and lipases; smooth and striated muscle cells, epithelial tissue, and organ tissues.

Evaluating plasma proteins is a valuable tool in the nutritional assessment of older women. In general, women have smaller protein stores than men do; thus, a decrease in protein stores may contribute to increased frailty, muscle weakness, diminished ambulatory ability, and lower reserve capacity. The most valuable laboratory measure is serum albumin. Although serum albumin may be affected by various disease processes (cancer, renal failure, liver disease), it is generally not affected by age. Normal serum values ranges from 3.5 to 5gm/dL, although there may be variation in this range, depending on the methodology used in different laboratories. Serum albumin is the most reliable indicator of protein nutriture; other serum proteins often used in nutrition assessment (transferrin, urea nitrogen, total protein) are less reliable (36). Gross estimates of body composition, such as skinfold measures, have not been derived from older adult populations and, therefore, are not valid indicators of body protein or fat stores and do not account for the vast variability among elderly subjects.

Dietary protein intake is an important factor to assess. Protein-rich foods are often expensive, difficult to chew,

and perceived to be high in fat or cholesterol. As a result, these foods (meat, fish, poultry, legumes, eggs, dairy products) are often voluntarily excluded from the diets of many older adults. However, these foods contain many essential nutrients, and should be encouraged in the diets of elderly people.

Fat Requirements

Fat is essential in the diet for energy, essential fatty acids, and fat-soluble vitamins. Only small amounts of fat are needed to provide essential fatty acids, and fat-soluble vitamins are available from other dietary sources; therefore, the primary contribution from dietary fat is the provision of calories. At least 10 percent of total energy intake should be from dietary fats to provide an adequate amount of fat-soluble vitamins and essential fatty acids (23,37). The American diet contains approximately 40 percent energy from fat; altering dietary intake of fat to 30 percent or less of total energy has been recommended to reduce risk for heart disease (38). For older people, restricting dietary fat, and thereby reducing calorie intake, is a reasonable strategy to maintain calorie balance without restricting intake of other nutrients; however, for some individuals, too rigid restrictions of dietary fat may contribute to dietary energy deficits.

Modifying the type and amount of dietary fat for older adults has been controversial. There are many differences of opinion regarding the need for dietary fat modification in adults over age 65 as a means to control the incidence of heart disease (39–41). A direct correlation seems to exist between decreases in dietary fat intake, including total fat and cholesterol, and decreases in plasma cholesterol (42–44). Data also indicate that there may not be any age-related differences in effect, although this, too, is controversial (45–47). Many cardiologists believe in the benefits derived from dietary alteration of fat regardless of the age of the individual. Geriatricians tend to be somewhat more focused on health maintenance and quality of life issues and to be more conservative than others in prescribing modified diets that may lead to limited dietary intake. There is evidence that risk factors for heart disease change with advancing age and that management of systolic hypertension may be more important than lowering serum cholesterol unless cholesterol levels are far greater than 250 mg/dL.

Dietary fat has also been associated with the possible etiology of breast, colon, and endometrial cancer (48–50). Limiting dietary fat intake has been suggested to decrease the risk for cancer development; however, the value of this recommendation to prevent cancer in elderly individuals must be carefully examined. Cancer often takes many years to develop, and no evidence shows that dietary fat reduction has an impact on cancer risk in elderly persons. Fat does add texture and flavor to foods; reducing dietary fat may decrease the appeal of certain foods, which may have a detrimental effect on overall nutrient intake. Altering the diets of older adults requires compelling health promotion or reasons for disease prevention because compliance is poor and many elderly people consume diets that are low in essential nutrients before other restrictions are imposed.

Carbohydrate Needs

Carbohydrate intake in diets of elderly people should be approximately 55 percent to 60 percent of total caloric intake, with an emphasis on complex carbohydrates because the ability to metabolize carbohydrates seems to decline with advancing age (51). Fasting blood glucose levels tend to increase slowly over time; 140 mg/dL is the mean for individuals over age 65. Therefore, it has been suggested that glucose tolerance tests be compared to age-cohorts with use of age-adjusted glucose tolerance tables (52).

Elderly people should be encouraged to eat foods high in complex carbohydrates because they provide fiber. The many reported effects of fiber include improving glucose tolerance (53), reducing incidence of constipation and formation of colonic diverticuli (54–56), and lowering serum lipids (54). The potential benefits of fiber in the diets of older people support the efforts of health educators to increase the amount of dietary fiber in the American diet. As people age, the amount of dietary fiber they consume tends to decrease, often because of the difficulty with chewing foods high in fiber or to a perceived problem with digestion of foods high in fiber (57). Fresh fruits and vegetables are difficult to chew if oral health status is not optimal or dentures do not fit properly, and these foods are expensive when they are out of season. Cereal fibers should be encouraged as an alternative, but obtaining adequate fiber from cereal foods alone is difficult. Encour-

aging the incorporation of foods high in fiber, rather than recommending fiber additives, will increase nutrient density of the complete diet (58,59).

Fluid Requirements

Water is an important nutrient for older people. The problems associated with inadequate fluid intake in elderly people may be profound because dehydration is difficult to diagnose and often more difficult to prevent. Inadequate fluid intake may lead to rapid dehydration and precipitate hypotension, elevated body temperature, constipation, nausea, vomiting, mucosal dryness, decreased urine output, and mental confusion. What is particularly noteworthy is that these problems are rarely attributed to fluid imbalances that are easily corrected.

Fluid intake should be adequate to compensate for normal losses (through kidneys, bowel, lungs, and skin) and for unusual losses associated with increased body temperature, vomiting, diarrhea, or hemorrhage. A reasonable estimate of fluid needs is approximately 1 mL of fluid per kilocalorie ingested or 30 mL/kg of actual body weight. The minimum intake for all older adults, regardless of their size or caloric intake, should be approximately 1500 mL/day.

Elderly persons are at risk for dehydration for a variety of reasons. First, as protein stores become reduced so does total body water; therefore, it is easier to become depleted rapidly (60,61). Second, adaptation to water deprivation is inefficient because aging kidneys no longer concentrate urine as rapidly (62). Third, renal antidiuretic hormone receptors may lose efficiency with advanced age, and therefore contribute to difficulty in maintaining fluid volume (63,64). Fourth, elderly people have a diminished thirst sensation and osmoreceptors decrease with advancing age. These factors make the elderly individual less sensitive to fluid needs (65–67). Fifth, many older adults voluntarily do not drink adequate amounts of fluid because of minor but chronic problems with incontinence (68). Fever, infection, and excess climatic heat also contribute to increased fluid needs that may not be met with voluntary fluid intake, and institutionalized, immobile, demented, arthritic, or comatose individuals do not have ready access to dietary fluid. Patients dependent on nutrition support may be underhydrated simply because they are receiving inadequate volumes of nutrient solutions and adequate, solute-free water is not provided as part of their nutrition regimen (68).

Identification of dehydration may be difficult because the presenting symptoms are often assumed to be associated with normal aging or assumed to be signs that are expected in elderly people. If dehydration is identified, intervention may be simple, but achieving compliance with rehydration regimens may be difficult because subjects have reduced thirst sensitivity and are reluctant to consume large volumes of fluid because of their problems with incontinence. Ironically, the treatment plan to manage incontinence includes consuming large volumes of fluid so that regularly scheduled voiding is reinforced when there is urine in the bladder to be evacuated.

Fluid may be taken as water, juices, carbonated beverages or ades, tea or coffee, or gelatin or frozen desserts that are liquid at room temperature. For patients dependent on tube feeding, it is important to know that tube-feeding formulas contain approximately 750 mL water per liter of solution and that adding 25 percent of the volume of the tube feeding as additional solute-free water will compensate for the solid displacement of solids.

Vitamins

Vitamin requirements for people over age 65 are mostly speculative at present, but there is much ongoing research. The Recommended Dietary Allowances (RDA) (69) offer suggested intake levels for individuals over age 51, but these amounts allow much variability in requirements for people in middle age through old age; since more people are living longer, the range in which intake and requirement levels may vary is becoming wider (70).

Subclinical vitamin deficiencies may exist in older adults, particularly for some water-soluble vitamins. When the stress of an illness or an injury occurs, depleted stores may not be able to compensate for rapid tissue depletion and the individual may become overtly deficient. Subclinical deficiencies may exist in people who have adequate but no excess dietary intake, because the absorption and utilization of vitamins may be compromised by unusual metabolic demands, the use of multiple medications, or abuse of single-nutrient supplements. A drug profile, including both prescription and over-the-counter medications, should be part of every history taken for an elderly person (36).

Water-Soluble Vitamins

The water-soluble vitamins that require some attention in the diets of elderly people include vitamins C, B_6, and B_{12}. Vitamin C has been a nutrient of controversy for many years. Although there is no evidence that vitamin C absorption or use is impaired in elderly persons, vitamin C has been claimed to be associated with a reduced risk for cancer, cataracts, and coronary heart disease, and with an increase in life expectancy (70). Deficiency of vitamin C has been associated with poor wound healing, easy bruisability, inflammation of mucosal tissue, capillary fragility, and the deficiency disease, scurvy. Vitamin C has been identified as the most potent antioxidant in the blood and may, therefore, be effective in protecting against stress-related and degenerative diseases (70,71). Although the recommended dietary allowance is 60 mg/day, some investigators have suggested that 140 mg/day is necessary to saturate tissues with ascorbic acid (vitamin C), and they have recommended that maintaining tissues at full saturation is desirable (71).

In epidemiologic studies, vitamin assessments in elderly people, particularly those who are sedentary, homebound, institutionalized, and chronically ill, have shown significant vitamin C deficiency, with use of plasma ascorbic acid levels as the marker. In the Dutch Nutrition Surveillance System, vitamin C status was examined in both free-living and institutionalized elderly women. The investigators found that vitamin C status is most closely associated with daily dietary intake and that food preparation practices were a significant factor in the losses of vitamin C in food (72).

In one study of healthy, noninstitutionalized elderly women (73), acceptable vitamin C status was associated with plasma levels of vitamin E and folate. Supplemental vitamin C has been shown to spare vitamin E and to augment its antioxidant activity (74). Smokers have lower plasma ascorbic acid levels than do nonsmokers and longitudinal studies indicate that plasma ascorbic acid levels tend to decline with advancing age.

Supplementation with very large doses (greater than 1 gm/day) may contribute to some serious side effects such as the formation of oxalate kidney stones or chronic diarrhea in sensitive individuals. There is little evidence that massive doses of vitamin C aid in wound healing, ward off the common cold, or cure cancer (75).

In many countries, the elderly population has been found to be deficient in vitamin B_6. For example, in one study conducted on older adults in Holland, 10 percent to 45 percent of the population, depending on the indicator used (aspartate aminotransferase activity coefficient or plasma pyridoxal phosphate level), were identified as deficient in vitamin B_6 (70). The RDA for vitamin B_6 is the same for adults, regardless of age; the amount is based on a ratio of 0.16mg of vitamin B_6 per gram of dietary protein, and, therefore, there is a different allowance for males and females (2.0mg and 1.6mg, respectively). However, a depletion-repletion study demonstrated that once depleted, elderly subjects required several periods of repletion to bring their urinary xanthurenic acid excretion back to baseline levels after a load of tryptophan (76). The conclusion was that the RDA for vitamin B_6 for adults may be too low for elderly people and should be re-examined for this population.

Vitamin B_6 may be more important in older subjects because vitamin B_6 deficiency has been demonstrated to impair specific measures of cell-mediated immunity. Both lymphocyte proliferation and interleukin-2 production are depressed with vitamin B_6 deficiency in elderly persons (77). Avoiding this vitamin deficiency should be a goal of dietary modification in elderly people. The primary source of vitamin B_6 in free-living elderly seems to be fruits and vegetables, which suggests that these foods should be encouraged to provide this nutrient in addition to the many other nutrients contained in these foods (78).

Vitamin B_{12} is a vitamin for which many older adults may be at risk for deficiency. On the basis of low serum levels, elderly people have a relatively high prevalence of vitamin B_{12} deficiency (70,79). The major dietary source for vitamin B_{12} is red meat and organ meats, which many elderly people eliminate from their diets because of the fat and cholesterol content and difficulties they may have with chewing. Some of the findings of vitamin B_{12} deficiency may be the result of undetected pernicious anemia, but they also may be more associated with gastric atrophy, a condition of gastric acid hyposecretion. Gastric atrophy may interfere with vitamin B_{12} bioavailability because there is less gastric secretion of acid and pepsin, which leads to impaired digestion of cobalamin (vitamin B_{12}) from food sources and to the binding of cobalamin to bacteria that are usually killed in the more acid environ-ment of normal stomach. Although the person may have a normal output of intrinsic factor, not enough vitamin B_{12} is released from its food carriers to be absorbed in adequate amounts.

For patients who have atrophic gastritis, providing supplemental intrinsic factor does not correct the malabsorption, but, giving acid or acid plus pepsin with supplemental vitamin B_{12} can reverse the malabsorption (80). Another study demonstrated that a course of tetracycline therapy aimed at eradicating the bacteria that bind vitamin B_{12} corrects abnormal absorption of the vitamin (81).

Vitamin B_{12} deficiency is a concern with elderly people because it has been associated with impaired cognitive function, dementia, and neuropsychiatric disorders. These symptoms are associated with normal serum vitamin B_{12} levels, normal Schilling tests, and the absence of anemia or macrocytosis, but with elevated serum homocysteine or methylmalonate levels (82). Vitamin B_{12} deficiency frequently manifests itself in nonspecific symptoms; one case report describes oral epithelial dysplasia associated with vitamin B_{12} deficiency that responded to vitamin therapy (83). It is important to be aware that this vitamin deficiency is a possible etiology for vague complaints of lethargy, malaise, and forgetfulness.

Fat-Soluble Vitamins

Elderly people are less likely to be deficient in fat-soluble vitamins (vitamins A, D, E, K) because of the body's ability to store these vitamins in liver tissue. For example, the risk of vitamin A toxicity is greater than the risk of vitamin A deficiency (84). This is especially true of older people who are taking over-the-counter vitamin supplements, many of which have very high levels of vitamin A. In older people, greater vitamin A storage pools have been observed, as well as an age-related delay in clearance of retinyl esters and elevated levels of unbound circulating plasma vitamin A. These factors suggest that elderly people have a lower margin of safety in intake requirements for vitamin A (79). Although population surveys often indicate an inadequate dietary intake of vitamin A, liver levels of vitamin A do not drop with age (70). This finding may be attributed to the decreased clearance of blood vitamin A levels, particularly retinyl esters, which are indicators of toxicity (85). Vitamin A requirements may actually be lower in older adults, but more extensive longitudinal studies are needed to substantiate this claim.

Vitamin A has been associated with the possible prevention of some types of cancer. Studies on the roles of retinol, preformed vitamin A, and beta carotene are somewhat controversial (86,87). The long-term effects of high doses of beta carotene have not been adequately explored, and since most cancers take 20 years or more to develop, the long-range benefits for older people will be difficult to assess. Thus far, no toxic side effects have been observed from ingestion of high levels of carotenoids in young subjects or in old subjects; thus, no recommendations regarding this nutrient are available (70).

The greatest risk of deficiency is for vitamin D, particularly for home-bound or institutionalized elderly. Older adults maintain lower levels of active vitamin D (1,25-dihydroxyvitamin D) than do younger adults because they have lower dietary consumption, a decrease in sunlight exposure, and overuse of sunscreens (70). Vitamin D is unique in that the body has the ability to synthesize its biologically active form, but advancing age is associated with a decreased capacity to produce 7-dehydrocholesterol (provitamin D_3) in the skin and to convert 25-hydroxyvitamin D to the active 1,25-dihydroxyvitamin D in the kidney (70).

The various roles of vitamin D in body make it a very important nutrient. The best-known function for vitamin D is to retain bone and to facilitate calcium absorption and use (88). A recently elucidated role of vitamin D is that it acts as a modulator of mononuclear phagocyte and lymphocyte biology; it has a potential clinical relevance in regulating host immune defenses (89). Curiously, depressed immune function has been noted in elderly people; this observation raises questions regarding the relationship between dietary vitamin D intake and immune responsiveness in the elderly.

The RDA for vitamin D for older adults is 200 IU. Despite one study in which the average vitamin D intake was approximately 380 IU/day, many elderly people apparently require supplementation to maintain serum calcitriol levels (90). Dietary vitamin D intake is often inadequate (91–93) and, therefore, contributes to the risk of vitamin deficiency which, in turn, contributes to re-

duced bone mass in elderly women (91). Offering vitamin D supplementation to elderly individuals has a beneficial effect on maintaining bone density (94,95) and should be considered for at-risk populations.

Vitamin K deficiencies may occur, usually associated with the use of sulfa drugs, antibiotics, or vitamin K antagonists as anticoagulation therapy.

Minerals

Except for iron, which has a decreased requirement because of the body's tendency to increase tissue iron stores with advancing age and a cessation of menstrual blood loss in women, requirements do not change for most minerals as a result of age. Calcium requirements have attracted much attrention in recent years. Investigators have suggested that dietary calcium intake recommendations increase from 800 mg/day to 1200 or 1500 mg/day to reduce the risk of osteoporosis. The controversy surrounding calcium requirements for older people has not yet been settled (96).

For most other major minerals, such as sodium and potassium, requirements are not changed by the aging process but are affected by the presence of acute or chronic diseases and their treatments. Serum levels of minerals or electrolytes should be maintained within normal limits or controlled as part of disease management. In elderly people, drastic shifts in electrolyte levels and hydration status can be very debilitating because to adapt or compensate takes longer for them than it does younger people. There does not appear to be any significant change in requirements for other minerals, such as zinc, chromium, copper, manganese or selenium, in normal, healthy, elderly people. However, various disease states along with inadequate diet, such as occurs with alcoholism, drug-nutrient interactions, severe chronic malabsorption, or chronic undernutrition, may lead to deficiencies in all micronutrients.

Assessment of Nutritional Status

One of the more difficult determinations in elderly people is the accurate assessment of their nutritional status; because of the physiologic changes that occur with normal aging, many of the commonly used assessment standards are not reliable in this population (36).

Anthropometric Measures

Anthropometric measures, including height, weight, and skinfold measures, are usually important components of a nutritional assessment. These parameters are the ones most affected by the aging process (97). The most apparent age-related change occurs in height. Height decreases as people get older as a result of changes in skeletal integrity, most noticeably those that affect the spinal column. Loss of height may be caused by thinning of the vertebrae, compression of the vertebral discs, development of kyphosis, and the effects of osteomalacia and osteoporosis (98). Loss of height occurs in both males and females, although it may happen more rapidly to elderly women with osteoporosis. Therefore, stature changes and body appearance may be altered. As older people lose their ability to stand erect, the organs in the thoracic cavity become displaced, and breathing and gastrointestinal problems may ensue (99).

Loss of height may range from 1.0 to 2.5 centimeters per decade after maturity. Also, height is difficult to measure in individuals who are unable to stand erect. Height measurements cannot be obtained from people who cannot stand unaided; who cannot stand at all because of neuromuscular disorders, paralysis, or loss of lower limbs; or who are bed-bound from muscle contractures or other problems. The best estimate of stature in these individuals is to measure their recumbent height or to choose selected anthropometric sites (i.e., bony prominences) and measure the distance between a number of selected points (100). This estimate of stature may not be very reliable, but it provides some estimate of height, or recumbent length, to use to determine whether body weight is appropriate for the individual's height.

Weight is another important anthropometric measure that is altered with advancing age. Weight tends to increase into middle age (age 40 to 50), stabilize for 15 to 20 years, and then decrease progressively (97). It is important to note that these changes occur at different rates among elderly people. Use of most standardized height and weight tables is not valid for older people because most reference tables do not include elderly people in their subject pool, and most are not age-adjusted. The most appropriate tables can be compiled from the Health and Nutrition Examination Surveys (HANES, HANES II, and HANES III). These surveys provide average weight-for-height data and rank individuals on percentiles compared with others in their age group.

A more commonly used measure is body mass index (BMI), which evaluates relative weight-for-height with a mathematical ratio of weight (in kilograms) divided by height (in square meters) $-$ $Wt(Kg)/Ht(M)^2$. This formula yields a whole number that should be greater than 21 and less than approximately 35 (101). However, nomograms and tables are available that minimize the need for calculation. There is some controversy among experts regarding the range of acceptable BMI measures for elderly people (102).

Skinfold measurements (triceps, biceps, subscapular, suprailiac, thigh) are often included in a thorough nutritional assessment. Loss of muscle mass, shifts in body fat compartments, changes in skin compressibility and elasticity, and lack of age-adjusted references decrease the reliability of skinfold measures in the assessment of nutritional status in elderly people. The reference populations used in the derivation of skinfold standards do not include older people and do not adjust for age-related changes. Skinfold measures provide only gross estimates of body composition under the best conditions; with elderly subjects, these measures can provide baseline information against which changes can be assessed over time (51).

Biochemical Measures

Biochemical assessment parameters are also affected by advancing age, although not as dramatically as anthropometric indexes (36). Laboratory measures may be affected by an age-related decline in renal function, by fluid imbalances or hydration status, by the effects of long-term chronic illnesses, and by drug-drug or drug-nutrient interactions. Among the commonly used biochemical markers, serum transferrin is one that is markedly affected by advancing age. Because tissue iron stores increase with age, circulating serum transferrin levels are reduced. Iron stores and transferrin are related in an inverse relationship. Therefore, a lower than normal serum transferrin should be evaluated in relation to other biochemical measures and to serum iron levels, if obtainable (103,104).

The most reliable predictor of nutritional status in elderly people is serum albumin. It is uncommon to find a serum albumin below 4.0 g/dL in a healthy, elderly person unless the subject is overhydrated; has cancer, renal, or hepatic disease; or is taking medications that may interfere with hepatic function. Recent evidence suggests that serum albumin is a prognostic indicator of potential infectious complications and other nosocomial problems in hospitalized, frail, or dependent elderly individuals (105,106). Serum albumin is also a primary prognostic indicator of rehospitalization, extended lengths of stay, and other complications associated with protein energy malnutrition in elderly people (30). Unless there is drug interference or the person has existing chronic disease processes, most biochemical measures should remain within normal limits.

Immunologic Assessment

Tests for immunocompetence are often included as part of a nutritional assessment because malnutrition results in compromised host-defense mechanisms. However, the incidence of anergy is reported to increase with advanced age and the response to skin test antigens appears to peak after longer intervals in older people (107). Distinguishing between alterations related to protein energy malnutrition and those related to a depressed immune response from other causes is difficult (108). The value of these tests is therefore limited for elderly people.

Evaluation of Socioeconomic Status

Accurate nutrition assessment of an elderly person who is suspected of being malnourished requires a comprehensive evaluation. Social history, economic status, drug history, oral health condition, family and living situations, and alcohol use should be evaluated along with the physical and physiologic measures usually assessed (36). Although the parameters commonly used to assess nutritional status are unreliable because of the lack of age-adjusted standards, they can contribute information to develop a comprehensive picture of an individual's health and nutrition status and can be used to effectively track changes that occur in people over time.

It is also useful to assess elderly individuals with use of instruments that evaluate how well elderly people perform the activities of daily living. Available tools assess the capability of an individual in managing the activities

necessary for independence; these tools add another valuable dimension to the assessment of elderly people (109,110).

Protein Energy Malnutrition in the Elderly

Protein energy malnutrition in the hospitalized elderly individual is usually associated with a primary disease, either chronic or acute, including cancer, chronic cardiac failure, chronic pulmonary disease, renal failure, hepatic failure, and gastrointestinal problems (111). As many as 40 percent of institutionalized and hospitalized elderly are below the fifteenth percentile of their weight for height. One of the most serious consequences of undetected protein energy malnutrition in elderly people is impairment of the immune system. Already affected by advanced age, immune responses may be even more compromised by protein energy malnutrition (108). Complications associated with this problem are an increased risk of infection and a decreased ability to mobilize host defenses, which may lead to increased morbidity and mortality.

The most frequent symptom of protein energy malnutrition is confusion or a recent history of alterations in mental status. This symptom may be present on the patient's admission or may develop during the patient's hospitalization and can usually be linked to a history of chronic weight loss. The probable mechanism for confusion is dehydration, which is often present and is usually related to inadequate fluid intake (112).

Primary protein energy malnutrition is most effectively diagnosed by taking a reliable history that indicates a recent and significant weight loss associated with a serum albumin less than 3.0 gm/dL that is not related to hepatic or renal disease or to overhydration causing serum dilution. The presence of anemia, lymphocytopenia, and anergy provides confirmation of the diagnosis of protein energy malnutrition.

Once protein energy malnutrition has been identified, clinical judgment is important in setting therapeutic priorities and appropriate initiation of nutritional intervention. Once the acute phase has subsided and recuperation is underway, daily calorie counts should be instituted and the patient encouraged to consume an adequate diet.

Smaller, frequent meals may be accepted more readily by elderly patients with smaller appetites and early satiety. Oral liquid supplements can be added to solid food consumption if fluid overload is not contraindicated. The goal of refeeding should be to provide 35 kcal/kg of the patient's actual weight and at least 1 gm of protein per kilogram. Investigators have demonstrated that only 10 percent of elderly people who have protein energy malnutrition can consume adequate calories to correct their nutritional deficiencies; most subjects require more aggressive nutritional intervention (113). Others have shown that protein energy malnutrition that is not corrected contributes to medical complications and an increased rate of morbidity and mortality in this group of individuals (114,115).

Unfortunately, in recent years, nursing home placement for recovering elderly is occurring earlier in their convalescence as a result of the economic conditions of hospital reimbursement systems. Because of this, nursing home patients are often sicker and require more skilled care. Nutritional requirements for sicker residents are increased by nature of recovering illness. Nursing home diets need adjustment to provide higher density nutritional foods to accommodate patients who are still in the recovery phase of their illness. If their nutritional requirements are not met, patients are at greater risk of becoming malignantly malnourished. One of the common outcomes of this problem is frequent readmission to the hospital of nursing home patients with urinary tract, upper respiratory, and other infections, and the development of pressure ulcers (116,117).

Nutrition Support Options

Enteral Feeding
Aggressive nutritional interventions that should be considered if the malnourished patient cannot consume adequate calories orally are enteral or parenteral feeding. Except for patients who have nonfunctioning gastrointestinal tracts, enteral feeding by tube is the intervention of choice. Feeding can be accomplished with use of pliable, small-bore (8 Fr to 12 Fr) feeding tubes placed nasogastrically or nasoenterically (into the duodenum or proximal jejunum) through a gastrostomy or jejun-

ostomy. For long-term feeding, indwelling tubes should be considered because they reduce the possibility of aspiration and are less likely to be pulled out by a confused or combative patient.

Enteral nutrition support provides a reasonably safe, cost-effective method of providing adequate protein, calories, vitamins, and minerals and in meeting fluid requirements for a patient who is not able to meet his own needs by eating. Ensuring appropriate nutrient intake contributes to the individual's recovery from acute illnesses, improves the prognosis for chronic conditions that may hamper rehabilitation, and corrects subclinical or overt nutrient deficiencies (118,119). Most standard tube feeding formulas require 1500 to 2000 ml to provide 100 percent of the RDA for most nutrients.

Parenteral Nutrition
For severely debilitated, malnourished individuals who have dysfunctional gastrointestinal tracts, parenteral feeding may be the only option. Intravenous feeding in elderly, sick patients requires very careful, diligent monitoring, particularly to maintain fluid and electrolyte equilibrium. The patient's blood glucose levels must be checked regularly to avoid hyperglycemia, and, if fat emulsions are included as part of the regimen, serum lipid levels must also be carefully monitored (120). Parenteral nutrition should be provided only if there is an experienced health care professional available; the safest place for provision of parenteral feeding is the acute care hospital. Extended care facilities often lack professional staff with knowledge of or experience with parenteral feeding.

Other Chronic Conditions

Other chronic conditions in which nutrition plays an important role in rehabilitation are chronic anemias, alcoholism, and pressure ulcers. These, among others, are linked to nutritional intake and status and require nutritional intervention to facilitate recovery and rehabilitation.

Anemias
Elderly people may have chronic anemias that are related to aging, chronic illness such as chronic renal conditions,

or may be nutritional in their etiology. An unexplained anemia that occurs in some elderly people is not precipitated by the most common etiologic factors, such as chronic diseases and their processes and treatments. Epidemiologic evidence indicates that nutrition may be an important etiologic factor; anemias are more prevalent in elderly people with low socioeconomic status because they have greater risk of malnutrition (121).

A remarkable similarity between the hematopoietic and immunologic changes that occur with aging and those that occur with protein deprivation has been demonstrated. Nutritional deficiencies respond to nutritional rehabilitation (refeeding with a diet rich in nutrients); the anemia of senescence is not noticeably affected by refeeding the individual. Correcting other serum parameters affected by undernutrition may not correct immune or hematopoietic function, but reserve capacity will improve and the patient may develop a sense of well-being, feel stronger, and respond more positively to therapy (121).

Alcoholism

Alcoholism is a serious problem that severely compromises nutritional intake. Alcoholism affects dietary intake because alcohol, a rich source of calories, replaces nutrient-dense foods. However, alcohol contributes no other nutrients and precludes the alcoholic from eating other foods. Alcoholics are often deficient in water-soluble vitamins and are protein malnourished. The chronic problems alcoholics develop are often related to chronic nutritional deficiencies (122). Certainly replacing alcohol with nutritious food corrects simple deficiencies, but some changes, such as cirrhosis, are irreversible. Nutritional rehabilitation contributes to better health in elderly alcoholics.

Pressure Ulcers

Pressure ulcers are potentially serious in frail, elderly chronically ill people (see also Chapter 20). Pressure ulcers are easier to prevent than they are to cure. The patients most susceptible are those who are among the most debilitated, those confined to bed or wheelchair (123). Pressure ulcers develop from prolonged direct pressure over bony prominences. Chronic weight loss leads to a decrease in subcutaneous fat, fragile epidermis, de-

creased blood flow in both large and superficial dermal vessels, and a depressed immune function. Once breaks in the skin occur, irritation from incontinence, exposure to bacterial contaminants, and compromised blood flow contribute to further breakdown of skin, subcutaneous fat, and muscle. There are many common treatments: turning patients frequently, use of air or fluid-filled mattresses, surgical debridement, antibiotics, dressing changes, hormones, and other agents (124). However, restoration of nutritional status is essential to healing decubitus ulcers. Achieving nitrogen balance by providing sufficient protein for the body to make new tissue, and providing with adequate levels of calories to protect the protein from being used for energy, are primary goals (117). Vitamin C (ascorbic acid) and zinc are also essential for making new tissue and closing wounds. Healing pressure ulcers is undoubtedly among the greatest challenges for a chronic care patient; avoiding ulceration involves maintaining nutritional status and preventing weight loss that reduces subcutaneous fat compartments.

Conclusion

Nutritional requirements and therapies in older adults are affected by the physiologic alterations associated with human aging, the need to maintain health status in the presence of chronic conditions, and the demands of acute medical problems. Consideration of the unique aging experience of every individual and making recommendations that meet the specific needs of that person is most important. Nutrition has a significant role in health and disease and should not be overlooked when taking a patient's history or planning a patient's care regimen.

References

1. Chernoff R, Lipschitz DA. Nutrition and aging. In: Shils ME, Young VR, eds. Modern nutrition in health and disease. 7th ed. Philadelphia: Lea & Febiger, 1988:982–1000.
2. Shock NW, Gruelich RC, Andres R, et al, eds. Normal human aging: the longitudinal study of aging. NIH Publ. No:84-2450. Washington, DC: National Institutes of Health, 1984.
3. Shepard JW. Interrelationships of exercise and nutrition in the elderly. In: Armbrecht HJ, Prendergast J, Coe R, eds. Nutritional intervention in the aging process. New York: Springer-Verlag, 1984.

4. Reilly JJ, Lord A, Bunker WW, et al. Energy balance in healthy elderly women. Br J Nutr 1993;69:21–27.

5. McGandy R, Barrows CH, Spanias A, et al. Nutrient intakes and energy expenditures in men of different ages. J Gerontol 1966;21:581.

6. La Porte RE, Black-Sandler R, Cauley JA, et al. The assessment of physical activity in older women: analysis of the interrelationships and reliability of activity monitoring, activity surveys, and caloric intake. J Gerontol 1983;38:394–397.

7. Fiatarone MA, Marks EC, Ryan ND, et al. High-intensity strength training in nonagenarians: effects on skeletal muscle. JAMA 1990;263:3029–3034.

8. Butterworth DE, Neiman DC, Perkins R, et al. Exercise training and nutrient intake in elderly women. J Am Diet Assoc 1993;93:653–657.

9. Fiatarone MA, O'Neill EF, Doyle ND, et al. The Boston FICSIT study: the effects of resistance training and nutritional supplementation on physical frailty in the oldest old. J Am Geriatr Soc 1993;41:333–337.

10. Kohrt WM, Obert KA, Holloszy JO. Exercise training improves fat distribution patterns in 60- to 70-year-old men and women. J Gerontol 1992;47:M99–M105.

11. Owens JF, Matthews KA, Wing RR, et al. Can physical activity mitigate the effects of aging in middle-aged women? Circulation 1992;85:1265–1270.

12. Rutherford OM, Jones DA. The relationship of muscle and bone loss and activity levels with age in women. Age Ageing 1992;21:286–293.

13. Ideno KT, Kubena KS. Nutrition, physical activity, and blood pressure in the elderly. J Nutr Elder 1990;9:3–15.

14. Evans WJ. Exercise, nutrition and aging. J Nutr 1992; 122:796–801.

15. Shangold MM. Exercise in the menopausal woman. Obstet Gynecol 1990;75(suppl):53S–58S, 81S–83S.

16. Lee C. Factors related to the adoption of exercise among older women. J Behav Med 1993;16:323–334.

17. Morley JE, Glick Z. Endocrine aspects of nutrition and aging. In: Chernoff R, ed. Geriatric nutrition: the health professional's handbook. Gaithersburg, MD: Aspen, 1991: 311–335.

18. Voorrips LE, Tineke M-CvA, Deurenberg P, et al. Energy expenditure at rest and during standardized activities: a comparison between elderly and middle-aged women. Am J Clin Nutr 1993;58:15–20.

19. Niskanen L, Piirainen M, Koljonen M, et al. Resting energy expenditure in relation to energy intake in patients with Alzheimer's disease, multi-infarct dementia and in control women. Age Ageing 1993;22:132–137.

20. Arciero PJ, Goran MI, Gardner AM, et al. A practical equation to predict resting metabolic rate in older females. J Am Geriatr Soc 1993;41:389–395.

21. Gersovitz M, Motil K, Munro H, et al. Human protein requirements: assessment of the adequacy of the current recommended dietary allowance for dietary protein in elderly men and women. Am J Clin Nutr 1982;35:6–14.

22. Munro HN, Young VR. Protein metabolism in the elderly. Postgrad Med 1978;63:143–152.

23. Carter WJ. Macronutrients requirements for elderly persons. In: Chernoff R, ed. Geriatric nutrition: the health professional's handbook. Gaithersburg, MD: Aspen, 1991:1–24.

24. Uauy R, Winterer JC, Bilmazes C, et al. The changing pattern of whole body protein metabolism in aging humans. J Gerontol 1978;33:663–671.

25. Fiatarone MA, O'Neill EF, Ryan ND, et al. Exercise training and nutritional supplementation for physical frailty in very elderly people. N Engl J Med 1994;330:1769–1775.

26. Crim MC, Munro HN. Proteins and amino acids. In: Shils ME, Olson JA, Shike M, eds. Modern nutrition in health and disease. 8th ed. Philadelphia: Lea & Febiger, 1994:3–35.

27. Bienia R, Ratcliff S, Barbour GS, et al. Malnutrition in the hospitalized geriatric patient. J Am Geriatr Soc 1982;30:433–436.

28. Linn BS. Outcomes of older and younger malnourished and well-nourished patients one year after hospitalization. Am J Clin Nutr 1984;39:66–73.

29. Sullivan DH, Patch GA, Walls RC, et al. Impact of nutritional status on morbidity or mortality in a select population of geriatric patients. Am J Clin Nutr 1990; 51:749–758.

30. Sullivan DH, Walls RC, Lipschitz DA. Protein-energy undernutrition and the risk of mortality within 1 year of hospital discharge in a select population of geriatric rehabilitation patients. Am J Clin Nutr 1991;53:599–605.

31. Volkert D, Kruse W, Oster P, et al. Malnutrition in geriatric patients: diagnostic and prognostic significance of nutritional parameters. Ann Nutr Metab 1992;36:97–112.

32. Tobin J, Spector D. Dietary protein has no effect on future creatinine clearance. Gerontologist 1986;26:59A.

33. Lindemann RD: The aging renal system. In: Chernoff R, ed. Geriatric nutrition: the health professional's handbook. Gaithersburg, MD: Aspen, 1991:253–269.

34. Rudman D, Mattson DE, Feller AG, et al. Fasting plasma amino acids in elderly men. Am J Clin Nutr 1989;49:559–566.

35. Caballero B, Gleason RE, Wurtman RJ. Plasma amino acid concentrations in healthy elderly men and women. Am J Clin Nutr 1991;53:1249–1252.

36. Mitchell CO, Chernoff R. Nutritional assessment of the elderly. In: Chernoff R, ed. Geriatric nutrition: the health professional's handbook. Gaithersburg, MD: Aspen, 1991: 363–396.

37. Siguel EN, Schaefer EJ. Aging and nutritional requirements of essential fatty acids. In: Beare-Rogers J, ed. Dietary fat requirements in health and disease. Champaign, IL: American Oil Chemists Society, 1988:163–189.

38. Garry PJ, Hunt WC, Koehler KM, et al. Longitudinal study of dietary intakes and plasma lipids in healthy elderly men and women. Am J Clin Nutr 1992;55:682–688.

39. Nutrition. In: Berg RL, Cassells JS, eds. The second fifty years: promoting health and preventing disability. Washington DC: National Academy, 1990:157–92.

40. Kaiser FE. Cholesterol, heart disease, and the older adult. Clin Appl Nutr 1992;2:35–43.

41. Schaefer EJ, Moussa PB, Wilson WF, et al. Plasma lipoproteins in healthy octogenarians: Lack of reduced high density lipoprotein levels. Results from the Framingham Heart Study. Metabolism 1989;38:293–296.

42. American Heart Association. Dietary guidelines for healthy American adults: a statement for physicians and health professionals by the nutrition committee. Dallas: American Heart Association, 1986.

43. Garry PJ, Hunt WC, Koehler KM, et al. Longitudinal study of dietary intakes and plasma lipids in healthy elderly men and women. Am J Clin Nutr 1992;55:682–688.

44. Löwik MRH, Wedel M, Kok FJ, et al. Nutrition and serum cholesterol levels among elderly men and women (Dutch Nutrition Surveillance System). J Gerontol 1991;46:M23–M28.

45. Kaiser FE. Cholesterol, heart disease, and the older adult. Clin Appl Nutr 1992;2:35–43.

46. Harris T, Cook EF, Kannel WB, et al. Proportional hazards analysis of risk factors for coronary heart disease in individuals aged 65 or older. J Am Geriatr Soc 1988;36:1023–1028.

47. Benfante R, Reed D. Is elevated serum cholesterol level a risk factor for coronary heart disease in the elderly? JAMA 1990;263:393–396.

48. Pariza MW. Diet, cancer, and food safety. In: Shils ME, Olson JA, Shike M, eds. Modern nutrition in health and disease. 8th ed. Philadelphia: Lea & Febiger, 1994:1545–1558.

49. Crighton IL, Dowsett M, Hunter M, et al. The effect of a low-fat diet on hormone levels in healthy pre- and post-menopausal women: relevance for breast cancer. Eur J Cancer 1992;28A:2024–2027.

50. Lissner L, Kroon U-B, Bjürntrop P, et al. Adipose tissue fatty acids and dietary fat sources in relation to endometrial cancer: a retrospective study of cases in remission, and population-based controls. Acta Obstet Gynecol Scand 1993;72:481–487.

51. Chernoff R, Mitchell CO, Lipschitz DA. Assessment of the nutritional status of the geriatric patient. Ger Med Today 1984;3:129–141.

52. Andres R. Aging and diabetes. Med Clin North Am 1971;55:293–296.

53. Vinik AI, Jenkins DJA. Dietary fiber in the management of diabetes. Diabetes Care 1988;11:160–173.

54. Schneeman BO, Tietyen J. Dietary fiber. In: Shils ME, Olson JA, Shike M, eds. Modern nutrition in health and disease. 8th ed. Philadelphia: Lea & Febiger, 1994:89–100.

55. Snustad D, Lee V, Abraham I, et al. Dietary fiber in hospitalized geriatric patients: too soft a solution for too hard a problem? J Nutr Elder 1991;10:49–63.

56. Wolfsen CR, Barker JC, Mitteness LS. Constipation in the daily lives of frail elderly people. Arch Fam Med 1993;2:853–858.

57. Cashman MD. The aging gut. In: Chernoff R, ed. Geriatric nutrition: the health professional's handbook. Gaithersburg, MD: Aspen, 1991:183–227.

58. Hermann JR, Hanson CF, Kopel BH. Fiber intake of older adults: relationship to mineral intakes. J Nutr Elder 1992;11:21–32.

59. Timmons KH, DuFord S. Quick and easy steps to a high fiber diet for the elderly. J Nutr Educ 1991;23:250G.

60. Schoeller DA. Changes in total body water with age. Am J Clin Nutr 1989;50:1176–1181.

61. Reiff TR. Water loss in aging and its clinical significance. Geriatrics 1987;42:53–62.

62. Rowe J, Shack N, Defronzo R. The influence of age on the renal response to water deprivation in man. Nephron 1976;17:270–278.

63. Rolls B, Wood R, Rolls E, et al. Thirst following water deprivation in humans. Am J Physiol 1980;239:R476–R482.

64. Phillips P, Rolls BJ, Ladingham DM, et al. N Engl J Med 1984;311:753–759.

65. Leaf A. Dehydration in the elderly. N Engl J Med 1984;311:753–759.

66. Rolls BJ, Phillips PA. Aging and disturbances in thirst and fluid balance. Nutr Rev 1990;48:137–143.

67. Thirst and osmoregulation in the elderly. Lancet 1984;2:1017–1018.

68. Chernoff R. Thirst and fluid requirements in the elderly. Nutr Rev 1994;52(8):132–136.

69. Food and Nutrition Board. National Research Council. Recommended dietary allowances. 10th ed. Washington, DC: National Academy, 1989.

70. Blumberg JB. Changing nutrient requirements in older adults. Nutr Today 27(5):15–20, 1992.

71. Jacob RA, Skala JH, Omaye ST. Biochemical indices of human vitamin C status. Am J Clin Nutr 1987;46:818–826.

72. Löwik MRH, Hulshof KFAM, Schneijder P, et al. Vitamin C status in elderly women: a comparison between women living in a nursing home and women living independently. J Am Diet Assoc 1993;93:167–172.

73. Jacob RA, Otradovec CL, Russell RM, et al. Vitamin C status and nutrient interactions in a healthy elderly population. Am J Clin Nutr 1988;48:1436–1442.

74. Niki, E. Interaction of ascorbate and alpha-tocopherol. Ann NY Acad Sci 1987;498:186–199.

75. Jacob RA. Vitamin C. In: Shils ME, Olson JA, Shike M, eds. Modern nutrition in health and disease. 8th ed. Philadelphia: Lea & Febiger, 1994.

76. Ribaya-Mercado JD, Russell RM, Sahyoun N, et al. Vitamin B_6 requirements of elderly men and women. J Nutr 1991;121:1062–1074.

77. Meydani S, Ribaya-Mercado JD, Russell RM, et al. Vitamin B_6 deficiency impairs interleukin-2 production and lymphocyte proliferation in elderly adults. Am J Clin Nutr 1991;53:1275–1280.

78. Manore MM, Vaughan LA, Lehman WR. Contribution of various food groups to dietary vitamin B_6 intake in free-living, low-income elderly persons. J Am Diet Assoc 1990;90:830–834.

79. Russell RM. Micronutrient requirements of the elderly. Nutr Rev 1992;50:463–466.

80. King CE, Leibach J, Toskes PP. Clinically significant vitamin B_{12} deficiency secondary to malabsorption of protein-bound vitamin B_{12}. Dig Dis Sci 1979;24:397–402.

81. Suter PM, Golner BB, Goldin BR. Reversal of protein-bound vitamin B_{12} malabsorption with antibiotics in atrophic gastritis. Gastroenterology 1991;101:1039–1045.

82. Lindenbaum J, Healton EB, Savage DG, et al. Neuropsychiatric disorders caused by cobalamin deficiency in the absence of anemia or macrocytosis. N Engl J Med 1988; 318:1720–1728.

83. Theaker JM, Porter SR, Fleming KA. Oral epithelial dysplasia in vitamin B_{12} deficiency. Oral Surg Oral Med Oral Pathol 1989;67:81–83.

84. Krasinski SD, Russell RM, Otradovec CL, et al. Relationship of vitamin A and vitamin E to fasting plasma retinol, retinol-binding protein, retinyl esters, carotene, α-tocopherol, and cholesterol among elderly people and young adults: increased plasma retinyl esters among the vitamin A supplement users. Am J Clin Nutr 1989;49:112–120.

85. Krasinski SD, Cohn JS, Schaefer EJ, et al. Postprandial plasma retinyl ester response is greater in older subjects compared with younger subjects. J Clin Invest 1990;85:883–892.

86. Slater TF, Block G, eds. Antioxidant vitamins and beta carotene in disease prevention. Am J Clin Nutr 1991;53:189S–396S.

87. The Alpha: Tocopherol, Beta Carotene Cancer Prevention Study Group. The effect of vitamin E and beta carotene on the incidence of lung cancer and other changes in male smokers. N Engl J Med 1994;330:1029–1035.

88. Anderson, JJB. The role of nutrition in the functioning of skeletal tissue. Nutr Rev 1992;50:388–394.

89. Yoder MC, Manolagas SC. Vitamin D and its role in immune function. Clin Appl Nutr 1991;1:35–44.

90. O'Dowd KJ, Clemens TL, Kelsey JL, et al. Exogenous calciferol (vitamin D) and vitamin D endocrine status among elderly nursing home residents in the New York City area. J Am Geriatr Soc 1993;41:414–421.

91. Villareal DT, Civitelli R, Chines A, et al. Subclinical vitamin D deficiency in postmenopausal women with low vertebral bone mass. J Clin Endocrinol Metab 1991;72:628–634.

92. Webb AR, Pilbeam C, Hanafin N, et al. An evaluation of the relative contributions of exposure to sunlight and of diet to the circulating concentrations of 25-hydroxyvitamin D in an elderly nursing home population in Boston. Am J Clin Nutr 1990;51:1075–1081.

93. Gloth FM, Tobin JD, Sherman SS, et al. Is the recommended daily allowance for vitamin D too low for the homebound elderly? J Am Geriatr Soc 1991;39:137–141.

94. Dawson-Hughes B, Dallal GE, Krall EA, et al. Effect of vitamin D supplementation on wintertime and overall bone loss in healthy postmenopausal women. Ann Intern Med 1991;115:505–512.

95. Chapuy MC, Arlot ME, Duboeuf F, et al. Vitamin D_3 and calcium to prevent hip fractures in elderly women. N Engl J Med 1992;327:1637–1642.

96. Heaney RP. Calcium intake and bone health in the adult: a critical review of recent investigations. Clin Appl Nutr 1992;2:10–29.

97. Mitchell CO, Lipschitz DA. Detection of protein-calorie malnutrition in the elderly. Am J Clin Nutr 1982;35:398–406.

98. Chumlea WC, Garry PJ, Hunt WC, et al. Serial changes in stature and weight in a healthy elderly population. Hum Biol 1988;60:918–925.

99. Silverberg SJ, Lindsay R. Postmenopausal osteoporosis. Med Clin North Am 1987;71:41–57.

100. Martin AD, Carter JEL, Hendy KC, et al. Segment lengths. In: Lohman TG, Roche AF, Martorell R, eds. Anthropometric standardization reference manual. Champaign IL: Human Kinetics, 1988.

101. Dwyer JT. Screening older American's nutritional health: current practices and future possibilities. Washington DC: Nutrition Screening Initiative, 1991.

102. Potter JF, Schafer DF, Bohi RL. In-hospital mortality as a function of body mass index: an age-dependent variable. J Gerontol 1988;43:M59–M63.

103. Lipschitz DA, Cook JD, Finch CA. The clinical evaluation of serum ferritin as an index of iron stores. N Engl J Med 1974;290:1213–1216.

104. Bothwell TH, Charlton R, Cook JD, et al. Iron metabolism in man. Oxford: Blackwell Science, 1979:295–297.

105. Morrow FD. Assessment of nutritional status in the elderly: application and interpretation of nutritional biochemistries. Clin Nutr 1986;5:112–120.

106. Finucane P, Rudra T, Hsu R, et al. Markers of the nutritional status in acutely ill elderly patients. Gerontologist 1988; 34:304–309.

107. Cohn JR, Buckley CE, Hohl CA, et al. Persistent cutaneous cellular immune responsiveness in a nursing home population. J Am Geriatr Soc 1983;31:261–264.

108. Goodwin JS, Burns EL. Aging, nutrition and immune function. Clin Appl Nutr 1991;1:85–94.

109. Katz S. Assessing self-maintenance: activities of daily living, mobility, and instrumental activities of daily living. J Am Geriatr Soc 1983;31:721–727.

110. Spector WD. Functional disability scales. In: Spilker B, ed. Quality life assessments in clinical trials. New York: Raven, 1990.

111. Lipschitz DA. Protein calorie malnutrition in the hospitalized elderly. Prim Care 1982;9:531–543.

112. Hoffman NB. Dehydration in the elderly: insidious and manageable. Geriatrics 1991;46:35–38.

113. Lipschitz DA, Mitchell CO. The correctability of the nutritional, immune, and hematopoietic manifestations of protein calorie malnutrition in the elderly. J Am Coll Nutr 1982;1:17–25.

114. Morley JE. Nutritional status of the elderly. Am J Med 1986;81:679–695.

115. Shaver JH, Loper JA, Lutes R. Nutritional status of nursing

home patients. J Parenter Enter Nutr 1980;4:367–370.

116. Sullivan DH, Chernoff R, Lipschitz DA. Nutritional support in long-term care patients. Nutr Clin Pract 1987; 2:6–13.

117. Breslow RA, Hallfrisch J, Guy DG, et al. The importance of dietary protein in healing pressure ulcers. J Am Geriatr Soc 1993;41:357–362.

118. Chernoff R, Lipschitz DA. Enteral feeding and the geriatric patient. In: Rombeau JL, Caldwell MD, eds. Clinical nutrition. Vol. 1. Enteral and tube feeding. 2nd ed. Philadelphia: WB Saunders, 1990.

119. Ouslander JG, Tymchuk AJ, Krynski MD. Decisions about enteral tube feeding among the elderly. J Am Geriatr Soc 1993;41:70–77.

120. Chernoff R, Lipschitz DA. Total parenteral nutrition: considerations in the elderly. In: Rombeau JL, Caldwell MD, eds. Clinical nutrition. Vol. II. Parenteral nutrition. Philadelphia: WB Saunders, 1986.

121. Lipschitz DA, Mitchell CO, Thompson C. The anemia of senescence. Am J Hematol 1981;11:47–54.

122. Barboriak JJ, Rooney CB. Alcohol and its effects on the nutrition of the elderly. In: Watson RR, ed. Handbook of nutrition in the aged. Boca Raton: CRC, 1985.

123. Pinchofsky-Devin GD, Kaminski MV. Correlation of pressure sores and nutritional status. J Am Geriatr Soc 1986;34:435–440.

124. Gilchrest BA. Skin. In: Rowe JW, Besdine RW, eds. Health and disease in old age. Boston: Little, Brown, 1982.

Chapter 17
Exercise

Joel Posner and Kevin McCully

Exercise and temperance can preserve something of our early strength even in old age.

Cicero, 106 BC–45 BC
On Old Age X

The major goals of geriatric medicine are 1) the prevention of preventable disease, 2) the prevention of premature death, 3) and the maintenance of independent function for as long as possible. Exercise can play an important role in achieving these goals. Unfortunately, medical education and health care reimbursement have left the exercise of middle aged and elderly clients an orphan activity. Nevertheless, it has become clear that a comprehensive program of vigorous endurance and strength training can prevent disease and prolong independent function. To provide such a program, it is important to understand the basics of exercise physiology, the changes in exercise capacity seen with age, and the benefits of specific exercises for older people.

Determination of Exercise Capacity

The gold standard for measuring exercise capacity in anyone, including the elderly, is the maximal oxygen consumption during exercise (VO_2max). Since early in this century, the performance of physical work by human beings has been known to require oxygen (1). The earliest studies quantifying the amounts of oxygen that had to be consumed to do specific amounts of work were by Lindhard in Copenhagen (2), Liljestrand and Stenstrom in Stockholm (3), and Herbst in Berlin (4). They measured oxygen consumption in runners and swimmers. They showed that swimmers used larger amounts of oxygen as they increased their swimming speed and that runners used more oxygen as they ran faster. Herbst found there was a limit to the amount of oxygen used: oxygen con-

sumption by an athlete running in place at 280 steps per minute was the same as consumption when the athlete ran at 320 steps per minute.

Later, English physiologist and Nobel Laureate AV Hill measured the amount of oxygen used by himself and other subjects as they ran around a small grass track at different speeds (1). He seemed to demonstrate that for each person there was a running speed above which oxygen consumption did not increase. This and later work led to the idea that each individual possesses, at a given time in his or her life, the ability to take in, distribute, and use a certain maximum amount of oxygen, VO_2max. Taylor, at the University of Minnesota, and others, while developing measures of functional ability during and after the World War II, standardized the technique of measuring VO_2max and suggested it as the best objective measure of cardiorespiratory performance (5). These and later workers believed that the maximal amount of oxygen a person can consume reflects the maximal amount of work he or she can perform. VO_2max has become generally accepted as the standard measure of exercise capacity for young and old people.

To measure VO_2max, the subject is exercised on a treadmill, bicycle, or arm ergometer. During the test, the subject is required to do increasing work until he or she can do no more. Work is increased by continuously increasing either the speed and elevation of the treadmill or the resistance of the bicycle pedals or ergometry handles. During exercise, the person's electrocardiogram is measured continuously, blood pressure is monitored minute by minute, and the subject's expired gas is collected and measured for volume, carbon dioxide, and oxygen content. Inspired gas volume is assumed to be the same as expired gas volume. If the oxygen and carbon dioxide content of the inspired air is known, and the volume, oxygen, and carbon dioxide content of each expired breath is known, both oxygen consumption and carbon dioxide production can be determined during the whole exercise period.

Figure 17.1 shows a continuous plot of work intensity, oxygen consumption, and carbon dioxide production by breath-by-breath sampling of expired gas during an exercise test. There is a point at which work increases but oxygen consumption levels off. The presence of this plateau with increases of work has been accepted as necessary for a test to have been "maximal." The level of oxygen consumption attained at this plateau is VO_2max.

This plateau rarely occurs in older people (6). The highest level of oxygen consumption attained during the exercise test is called VO_2peak. If VO_2peak is measured repeatedly, there is consistency. Because older persons lack a plateau, a number of investigators have suggested alternative criteria for determining maximal effort, such as attainment of at least 85 percent of predicted maximal heart rate, respiratory exchange ratios ($RQ = CO_2$ production/O_2 consumption) of at least 1.15, and blood lactate levels greater than 8 mM.

Much research has been aimed at understanding the factors that make up an individual's VO_2peak (7–11): 1) the ability of the lungs to take in oxygen and diffuse it across alveolar surfaces into the bloodstream reflected by measures such as maximum minute ventilation (MVV) and lung diffusing capacity, 2) the ability of blood to carry and deliver oxygen (determined by factors such as hemoglobin concentration and 2,3 diphosphoglycerate (DPG) levels), 3) the ability of the heart to circulate oxygenated blood toward working muscles (maximum cardiac output), 4) the ability of vessels to shunt blood to working muscles, 5) the ability of working muscles to transport oxygen from hemoglobin to mitochondria, and 6) the ability of mitochondria to use oxygen (Figure 17.2).

The importance of understanding the various factors that can limit VO_2peak is that the limiting factor may be different in different individuals and may be different in older persons compared with younger people. Furthermore, the limiting factor may change for an individual as a result of an exercise training program or the onset of disease.

Many clinical laboratories perform only electrocardiographic monitoring during a cycle ergometer or treadmill exercise test. Often these tests are not performed to a

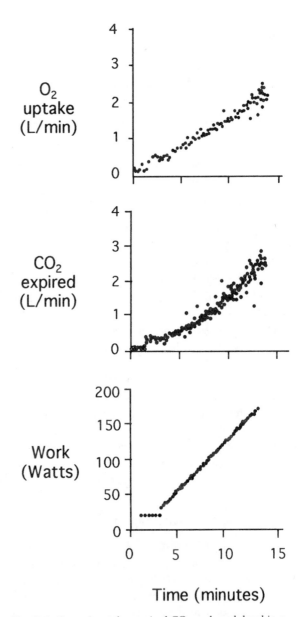

Fig. 17.1. Oxygen uptake, expired CO_2, and work level in a normal female subject during a cycle ergometer stress test. After collection of resting data, the subject performed 2 minutes of unloaded cycling (zero work) before the work level was gradually increased. Note that this subject did not show a plateau in O_2 uptake at the end of the test.

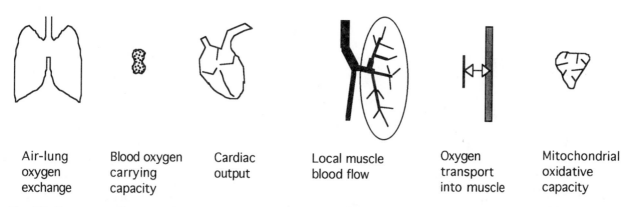

| Air-lung oxygen exchange | Blood oxygen carrying capacity | Cardiac output | Local muscle blood flow | Oxygen transport into muscle | Mitochondrial oxidative capacity |

Fig. 17.2. Factors controlling O_2 consumption during whole body exercise. Aging and disease can have differential effects on these factors. (Adapted from Wagner PD. Gas exchange and peripheral diffusion limitation. Med Sci Sports Exerc 1992;24:54–58.)

maximal work level, but to a heart rate that is approximately 85 percent of maximal predicted heart rate. This approach provides information concerning potential cardiovascular abnormalities, which is an important reason for conducting the exercise test. However, performing an exercise test with only electrocardiographic monitoring and without measures of oxygen consumption often misses important pathology. Furthermore, not performing the exercise test to maximum work levels can also miss potential cardiac abnormalities (Shaw CE, personal communication, 1995).

Exercise Capacity and Age

Exercise capacity and specifically VO_2peak declines with age (12–14). Because the above six factors have been postulated to be those that limit VO_2peak, a decline in one or more of them is apparently responsible for the age-related decrease in exercise capacity. Most researchers believe that, although the decline is multifactorial, a decline in maximum cardiac output is probably the major cause, but some researchers feel that working muscle's ability to diffuse oxygen from hemoglobin to mitochondria is, in general, the major factor limiting VO_2peak (11).

Whatever the exact mechanism, the decline can be striking. In a classic paper summarizing the changes in VO_2peak seen in trained and untrained men and women, Heath et al (15) listed the average decline with age as approximately 1 percent per year (Figure 17.3). The implications of this decline were enormous. People were be-

lieved to be able to operate over long periods of time at about 50 percent of their VO_2peak (16). Figure 17.3 shows that VO_2peak declines from about 50 ml/kg/min in healthy, untrained 20-year-old males to about 20 ml/kg/min in healthy, untrained 80-year-old males. This means that 20-year-olds can readily perform work that requires about 25 ml of oxygen/kg of body weight/minute, but healthy 80-year-olds must limit themselves to work that requires only about 10 ml/kg/min.

The oxygen costs of various activities have been measured. For example, an individual sitting quietly in a chair expends 3.5 mL of oxygen per kg of body weight each minute. For this reason, 3.5 ml/kg/min has been designated as one metabolic unit (one MET). Making a bed uses 7 ml/kg/min, slow dancing uses 10 to 12 ml/kg/min, shoveling 10 to 15 lbs of earth per minute uses approximately 25 ml/kg/min, and running 8-minute miles uses 45 ml/kg/min (17).

If Jones et al. (16) were correct, and a person could operate at only about half his or her VO_2peak, healthy 80-year-old males would need to limit their activities to quiet bed making and very slow dancing. This is simply not so.

Looking only at oxygen extraction and oxidative work misses important facts about exercise, particularly in the elderly. Even the earliest investigators in this century recognized that once a muscle worked above a certain level, it produced lactic acid. In fact, muscles can produce energy for work in two ways: they can use oxygen and produce carbon dioxide working essentially oxidatively,

213

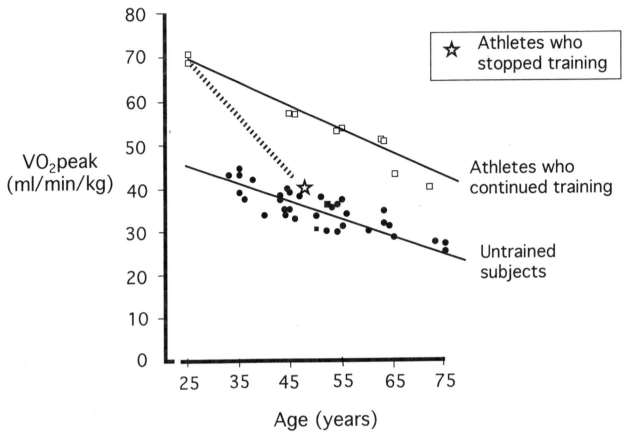

Fig. 17.3. Peak oxygen consumption during treadmill exercise in men of various ages. Each symbol represents the average results from a different study. (Adapted from Heath GW, Hagberg JM, Ali A, et al. A physiological comparison of young and older endurance athletes. J Appl Physiol 1981;51:634–640.)

or they can produce energy by glycolysis of sugars, fats, and proteins without the use of oxygen and with the production of lactic acid and, eventually, of carbon dioxide. It is likely that at most exercise intensities, both glycolytic and oxidative metabolism occurs. Lactate is used as a fuel source by muscle and accumulation of lactate in the blood occurs only when lactate production exceeds lactate uptake (18).

The significance of the point at which increasing levels of lactate occur is that this indicates a transition between steady-state work and nonsteady-state work. Below this level, people can maintain work intensity for almost indefinite times, but above this point, people fatigue and have to stop exercising (19). The higher above this point, the quicker the fatigue occurs. One of the reasons for this

is that increasing lactate causes an increase in pH concentration. Lactic acidiosis is a major cause of muscle fatigue. By measuring blood lactic acid levels continuously during exercise, one can detect the point at which this happens. This point has been named the *anaerobic threshold* (19). Subsequent studies have shown that the onset of significant glycolysis is not a result of a lack of oxygen (18). Thus the term *glycolytic threshold* is currently used in place of the term *anaerobic threshold* to indicate the point at which significant glycolysis occurs.

Work below the glycolytic threshold is almost exclusively oxidative and clearly depends on the six factors listed above. Work performed above the glycolytic threshold is mixed oxidative and glycolytic work and also depends on the capacity of glycolytic muscle fibers. When the glycolytic threshold is reached, the amount of work being performed is more than can be done purely oxidatively. Working muscles then begin glycolyzing sugars, fats, and protein, and lactic acid accumulates. This acid is buffered into water and carbon dioxide.

Glycolytic threshold can be measured simply in two ways. Blood can be continuously sampled during exercise and the concentration of lactic acid measured. The level of work at which the concentration of lactic acid rises is termed the *lactic acid threshold* (LaT). There are minor but definite practical problems using this method. A second easier method, devised by Beaver et al (20), depends on changes in expired gas concentrations during exercise. During increasing levels of exercise, but before the onset of glycolysis, the amount of carbon dioxide produced is predictably related to the amount of oxygen being used. As work increases, CO_2 production and O_2 consumption increase proportionately. At glycolytic threshold, because of the increase in lactate, then buffered into water and carbon dioxide, there is a sudden increase in carbon dioxide production without a similar increase in oxygen consumption. This change is easily detected when oxygen consumption is plotted against carbon dioxide production (Figure 17.4). Glycolytic threshold measured this way is termed the *ventilatory threshold* (VeT).

It is easy to study VeT in large numbers of subjects at all ages, including older ones. We did this in the early 1980s, measuring VO_2peak and VeT with the use of bicycle ergometry and breath-by-breath gas analysis in large numbers of older and younger subjects. We found a decline in VO_2peak that was as sharp as those found by previous investigators, but we also found that VeT declined little with age (Figure 17.5) (21). The major change as people age seems to be that the VeT is closer to the VO_2peak, which suggests that people can operate closer and closer to their VO_2peak as they get older. This is in keeping with the findings of Allen et al (22) among older and younger distance runners. The older athletes had lower VO_2peak than the younger ones, but their lactic acid thresholds were the same as those of the younger ones. Most significantly, the older athletes had running performances as good as the younger athletes (18). In short, we believe a reason why healthy older men and women can do more than one would have predicted from the earlier studies of VO_2peak and age is that glycolytic

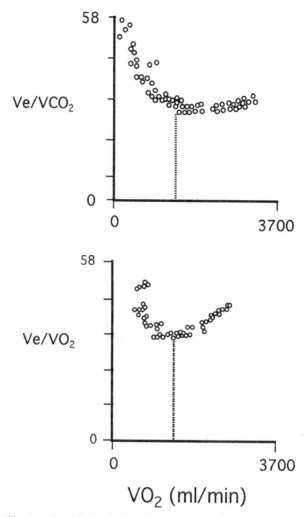

Fig. 17.4. Ventilation (Ve) to CO_2 production and O_2 consumption versus O_2 consumption during cycle ergometer exercise in a normal subject. The vertical dotted lines indicate the ventilatory threshold (VeT).

threshold declines little with age and glycolytic threshold is the predictor of ability to perform prolonged work.

Careful examination of our early data also suggested a different way to look at the age-related decline in exercise capacity. Any major decline in purely oxidative mechanisms (lungs, heart, hemoglobin, blood shunting, oxygen diffusion into muscle, mitochondria) should seemingly have resulted in a sharper decline in the measure of ability to perform predominantly oxidative work: glycolytic

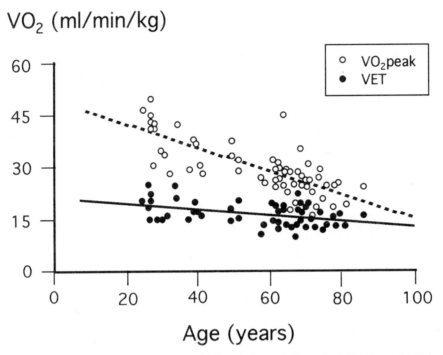

Fig. 17.5. VO₂peak and VeT in male subjects of various ages. The lines indicate the linear best fit of the data. (Adapted from Posner J, Gorman K, Windsor-Landsberg L, et al. Low to moderate intensity endurance training in healthy older adults: physiological responses after 4 months. J Am Geriatr Soc 1992;40:1–7.)

threshold. However, what actually declines with age is the ability to perform work between the onset of significant glycolysis and the maximal level of work that can be done (Figure 17.6). We call this the "gly-ox reserve" (14). Since the predominantly oxidative measure declines little, a mechanism other than a purely oxidative one must be involved. Decreases in muscle strength and endurance may be contributing factors.

Strength measured in a number of different muscle groups has been shown to decline with age (23). It is clear there is a loss of muscle mass and strength. This loss appears to be predominantly glycolytic either because of changes in the relative area of glycolytic fibers or because of a drop across all fibers in the proportion of their glycolytic metabolism (24). Some studies have also suggested that there is a loss of muscle fibers (25). Decline in other performance tests has also been seen, such as a decline in age-group records in swimming and running, two sports with numerous age-group competitions. Figure 17.7 shows age-related changes in sprint and endur-

ance running performance (26). The rate of decline is similar to that seen for VO₂peak.

The effect of age on muscle metabolism and endurance performance is less clear. A number of studies found no change in muscle metabolism from muscle biopsies (27) and in endurance measurements, but other more recent studies found age-related declines in muscle metabolism (28,29). The decline in age-group endurance performance times also supports the idea that muscle endurance is reduced. However, these results do suggest that the age-related declines in muscle metabolism are less clear and perhaps less important than age-related changes in muscle strength. Further studies are needed to clarify this issue.

In addition, there are mixed results of studies examining potential changes in blood flow capacity with age (30,31). Maximum cardiac output, for example, is preserved in healthy subjects between the ages of 20 and 80 years (32). In fact, the ratio VO₂peak/muscle mass does not change at least until age 80 (32): maximum oxygen

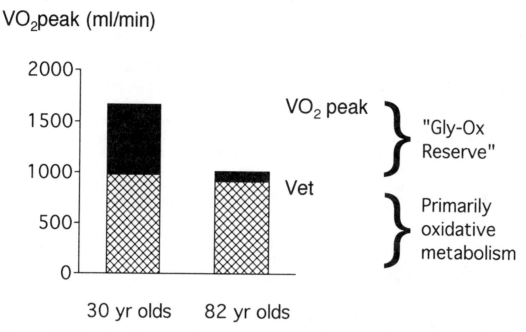

Fig. 17.6. VO₂peak and VeT showing differences in the "gly-ox reserve" in younger and older subjects.

consumption does not decline when it is normalized for muscle mass. However, some studies have reported decreased capillary densities in muscles from older subjects (28). Vasodilation as a response to exercise may be reduced, but this may be related to cardiovascular disease.

We believe the loss in muscle mass and in glycolytic capacity is a major cause of the age-related decline in exercise capacity, even as reflected by VO₂peak (14). To understand this, imagine and compare the exercise test of a healthy older subject with that of a healthy younger one. As the intensity of work is increased, both eventually reach glycolytic threshold, which occurs at about the same level of work in each subject. This suggests that for both subjects their whole oxygen delivery apparatus is working almost equally well. As work becomes both glycolytic and oxidative, lactic acid accumulates and CO_2 production increases. The older subject stops exercising before the younger one, usually because of leg fatigue. We believe this reflects the fact that limitation of exercise in older subjects is caused by multiple factors, at least one of which is the inability of older muscles to sustain glycolytic work for as long as younger muscles can. The younger subject continues working, then stops because of a feeling of shortness of breath. Older people stop exercising because their muscles give out; younger subjects can continue glycolytic work to a level at which the limiting factor seems to be a limitation in the oxidative system.

Benefits of Exercise

An exercise program for older clients should incorporate both strength and endurance training. A number of studies have reported improvements in strength in older female subjects with exercise training (33). Strength training has an important role for at least three reasons: 1) the strength of certain muscles is necessary for independent function in older women; 2) the size and strength of muscles may be important in reversing some age-related physiologic losses such as increased insulin resistance and peripheral vascular resistance; 3) global exercise capacity may depend, at least in part, on muscle strength.

To describe the physiologic profile of the functionally independent older woman, we studied 50 cognitively intact older women with different levels of functional ability (34). We measured functional ability using both self-reported indexes of ability to perform activities of daily living (ADLs) and performance tests, including standard ones and a new one that we developed—the "bag test." This test has the subject carry bags of increasing weight over a 15-meter course with three steps and a turn around in the middle. The subject continues with heavier and heavier bags until she feels she can no longer go on. The highest weight carried is her eventual score. We have found this test to be reproducible and to correlate well with other measures of ability to function independently. As expected, VO$_2$peak correlated well with the ability to

function independently (Figure 17.7); the purely oxidative glycolytic threshold did not. The strength of the leg muscles was also predictive of independent functional ability, with the strength of the calf muscles being the single best physiologic predictor of overall function (Figure 17.7). We are now exploring whether leg and calf strength are a result or a cause of independent function. In other studies, weak leg muscles have been found to predict falls in the elderly (35,36). It may be that strong hip abductors protect against hip fractures.

The relationship between independent activities and physical capacity can show a threshold response (37), as

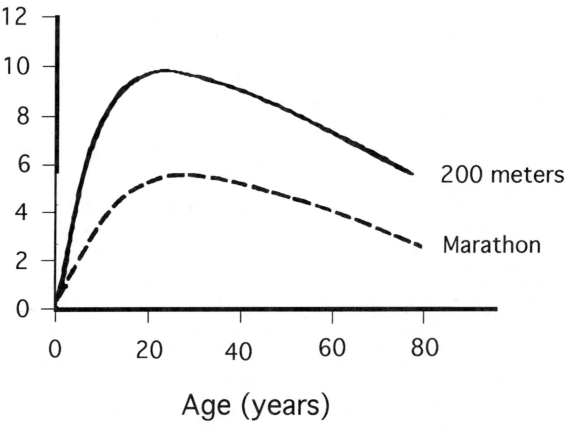

Fig. 17.7. Running speed from established age-group track records for the 200-meter dash and the marathon for men. (Adapted from Moore DH. A study of age-group track and field records to relate age and running speed. Nature 1975;253:264–265.)

shown in the case for ADL scores and VO₂peak in Figure 17.8. Below the threshold, there is a strong relationship between measures of independence and physical capacity; above the threshold, there is little relationship. The presence of a threshold depends to a large degree on the design and scoring of the test used to measure independent activities. However, the concept of a threshold is useful. In general, changes in physical capacity, both decline and improvement, have a greater impact on older and frailer people.

Increased muscle size and strength may have important metabolic and hemodynamic benefits. There is an age-related decrease in insulin sensitivity marked by increasing fasting blood glucose levels and increasing fasting blood insulin levels (38). There are many possible causes and implications for this age-related insulin resistance. One association may be with increasing peripheral vascular resistance and hypertension. It is known that younger hypertensives are almost always insulin resistant. It has been shown that insulin resistance occurs at the level of striated muscle (39). Endurance exercise decreases insulin resistance in older subjects (40). A combination of endurance exercise and resistive strength training, which increases muscle size and strength, may have even greater metabolic benefits as well as benefits for simple endurance and physical capacity. Loss of vigor with age

may be a result of loss of muscle strength and endurance in addition to any decline in lung, blood, or heart function.

This is not to suggest that endurance training is unimportant. Vigorous endurance training does have an important place in any exercise program for the elderly. This training has real and measurable benefits that may occur at many levels at once, including increases in physical capacity, prevention of cardiovascular disease, and increasing longevity in general. It has been shown that endurance training improves VO₂peak in the elderly (21,28,33) and in the young, but with interesting differences. In the young, VO₂peak increases mainly because of increases in ability to do work before glycolytic threshold; in the elderly, there is an increase mainly in the ability to do work after the onset of significant glycolysis (14). Whatever the mechanisms, there are clearly health benefits. Paffenberger showed that Harvard graduates who engaged in vigorous exercise lived longer than those who do not (41); we did a controlled study among healthy subjects over age 60, two-thirds of whom we exercised and one-third of whom we simply met with regularly. The incidence of new onset cardiovascular disease was significantly lower among the exercisers than it was among the contact group (42).

One of the important issues in terms of benefits of exer-

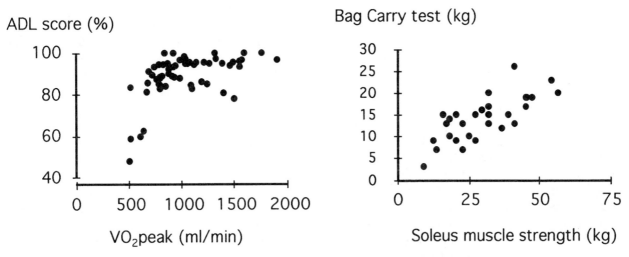

Fig. 17.8. The relationship between measures of independence activities (ADL and bag carrying test) and measures of physiological capacity (VO₂peak and soleus muscle strength) in older women (mean age, 69 years). ADL versus VO₂peak shows a threshold value around a VO₂peak of 900 mL/min, but bag carrying versus soleus strength does not.

cise in the elderly is the effect of lack of exercise. Older people show rapid declines in physical capacity when forced to undergo bed rest (43).

The Exercise Program

Considering the benefits of vigorous exercise, it is a mistake to recommend simply "keeping active" or "gardening" for most older clients; we believe that a serious program of resistive strength, endurance, and flexibility training has an important role in aiding people to age optimally. The major reason for promoting keeping active is that some exercise is better than nothing, and keeping active maybe a more realistic goal for a large part of the elderly population than is a regular, supervised exercise program. It is difficult to get people to join and maintain exercise training programs (44), and this difficulty is most likely magnified when increasing exercise intensity is part of the regimen because significant adaptations to exercise require high training intensities (45,46). More research is needed to learn how to overcome factors that tend to limit exercise compliance in the eldery.

Providing supervised exercise training programs for the elderly is also not easy. For an exercise program to be both safe and effective, clients need a careful pre-exercise evaluation and exercise prescription and some mechanism for monitoring of their progress. This is currently difficult to finance and may become even more difficult in the future. Nevertheless, exercise programs for the elderly are being set up. For example, we have been able to operate an exercise program that involves about 1000 older people in two separate centers in Philadelphia.

Pre-Exercise Evaluation

A pre-exercise evaluation has two goals: to detect disease that will make unmodified exercise dangerous, and to gather the data needed to write an efficient, safe exercise prescription. The evaluation should include a review of the client's medical records, a history, and a physical exam. Diseases or conditions that make an exercise evaluation dangerous include tight aortic stenosis, idiopathic hypertrophic subaortic stenosis, aortic aneurysm, uncontrolled congestive heart failure, unstable angina, and ventricular arrhythmias that have not been fully assessed.

If deemed safe for the client, an exercise stress test with gas exchange data should be performed. The test commonly uses a cycle ergometer or a motorized treadmill. The cycle ergometer produces fewer motion artifacts and provides less risk of injury from falling because the subject is supported by the ergometer seat. The subject can stop the test by stopping pedaling and remaining seated. For this reason, the cycle ergometer is particularly recommended for testing frail clients. The treadmill test has the advantage of involving use of larger muscle mass, and thus generally produces higher VO_2peak values. The risk of falling during the treadmill test is reduced by having the subject wear a supporting harness. Even so, treadmill exercise can be quite intimidating to many elderly people.

If there is a specific medical indication, such as chest pain of undiagnosed origin, palpitations or arrhythmias of undiagnosed origin, or unexplained shortness of breath, the test fee can be billed to the client's insurance company or to Medicare. Whether hypertension, severe hyperlipidemias, or peripheral vascular disease are acceptable indications is not clear.

Most exercise stress tests in the United States are performed by cardiologists in facilities without gas collection capabilities. However, it is preferable also to collect gas exchange data because gas collection reveals whether a test is maximal and, often, adds information on cardiac and pulmonary pathology not available from a simple stress electrocardiogram.

Even when the stress test is not done to diagnose a specific medical condition, it still has purpose:

1. In asymptomatic patients, it may detect conditions that need further workup or that make unrestricted exercise dangerous, such as exercise-induced ventricular arrhythmias; ischemic electrocardiographic response to exercise; hypertensive response to exercise (systolic blood pressure of 220 or more or diastolic pressure of 120 or more); signs of exercise-induced congestive failure, including dyspnea, the development of rales, drop in blood pressure with increased work, and early onset of glycolytic threshold. About one-fifth of all clients presenting for an exercise program with no significant medical history, symptomatology, or signs of disease have a stress test result necessitating further workup; 5 percent of patients presenting in this way have a condition that needs treatment or makes unrestricted exercise dangerous. These patients are referred to their own physicians for

further workup and treatment; many eventually need a specially modified, monitored exercise program.

2. It allows for the design of a precise endurance exercise program based on VeT, VO$_2$peak attained, and changes in the respiratory quotient (RQ) seen during exercise (see below).

Beyond the standard evaluation, exercise stress test with gas exchange data, and physical therapy evaluation, specialized evaluations can be made, depending on the individual. A physical therapy evaluation needs to be included for many older clients before they begin resistive strength training. Older people with elevated cholesterol, for example, should have lipoprotein analysis and body fat estimation. Their program should include a more emphatic low-fat diet and inclusion of longer endurance training periods to encourage more fat mobilization.

Ideally, the design of an individualized program of endurance and flexibility training includes input from a physician, nurse practitioner or physician assistant, exercise physiologist, and physical therapist. The exercise program should include an introductory period of stretching and aerobic exercise that lasts about four weeks. At this point, assuming no complications, the older exerciser should be evaluated by a physical therapist and exercise physiologists to design a resistive strength training program. This approach will result in an individualized resistive strength training program that takes into account musculoskeletal weaknesses of each older exerciser.

Endurance Exercises

There are four elements to the endurance exercise prescription: duration, frequency, type, and intensity (47). Subjects should endurance train for at least 40 minutes three times a week. The session should include a 5-minute warm up, 30 minutes of training, and 5 minutes of cool down. To combat boredom, the workout can be divided and performed on a number of different machines such as a stationary bicycle, an arm ergometer, a treadmill, and a rowing machine. Subjects warm up and spend 10 to 12 minutes each on different machines. Running, using a cross-country ski machine, a stair-climbing machine, and swimming are other good types of endurance exercises.

Each exercise offers specific benefits and poses special problems. For cardiovascular fitness, the subject must exercise at an intensity that provokes an appropriate training heart rate. This is best determined by examining the gas exchange data collected during the exercise test. After a 5-minute warm up, healthy subjects should exercise to the heart rate they attained at a VO$_2$ that was 70 percent to 85 percent of their VO$_2$peak. If gas exchange data are not available, exercise target heart rate can be determined by the Korvonen formula, which uses only the pulse rate attained during a monitored maximal exercise test. By this formula, healthy older subjects should exercise at

heart rate = (0.70 to 0.85) × [(maximum attained

heart rate − resting heart rate) + resting heart rate].

In older subjects, the simple formula maximum heart rate of 220 − age often does not apply. As people age, their heart rate response to exercise changes. Also, many older people take medication that interferes with heart rate response to exercise. The intensity of the exercise can be modified for subjects with heart or lung disease: the intensity can be cut to that needed to attain the heart rate at 60 percent or 50 percent of the VO$_2$peak.

For clients who need to lose fat, an additional 30 to 45 minutes of exercise at a lower intensity should be added. The intensity that best mobilizes fat is one that produces the heart rate corresponding to the heart rate at which the RQ was lowest after exercise was begun during the exercise test.

Resistive Strength Training

Leg muscles, and particularly calf muscles, play a key role in a person's ability to perform the activities necessary for independent living (14). A number of studies have shown that resistance training can be done safely with young and even very old people with proper evaluation and prescription (14,44,45), although the precise benefits of exercise-induced increases in the strength and size of other muscles on the health and well-being of elderly people has not been fully assessed. Fiatarone et al (45) had 90-year-old subjects perform a 6-week exercise resistance training program of some upper leg and hip muscles. The resistance training resulted in large changes in specific muscle strength, smaller changes on performance tests that rely on the muscles that were trained, and even smaller changes in muscle mass (Figure 17.9). This study and others demonstrate that large improvements in muscle strength are possible in the elderly. However, they also demonstrate that improvements in muscle strength

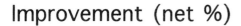

Improvement (net %)

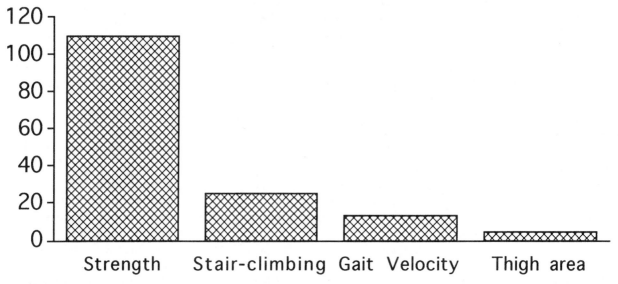

Fig. 17.9. Net improvement of leg muscle strength, stair-climbing ability, gait velocity, and thigh muscle area following an intensity resistance training program in very old subjects. The values shown are differences in adaptation seen in the exercise group compared with the control group. For gait velocity and thigh area, the control group showed slight decreases over the experimental period. (Data from Fiatarone MA, Marks EC, Ryan ND, et al. High-intensity strength training in nonagenarians: effects on skeletal muscle. JAMA 1990;263:3029–3034.)

do not necessarily translate into large changes in functional capacity. There is a need for additional studies to look at the influence of a comprehensive, long-term resistance training program on functional capacity in the elderly.

The prescription for resistance exercise includes the type of exercise and its intensity and frequency. Muscle groups can be worked with use of free weights or weight-training machines. Either can be effective, but free weights are, in general, harder to use properly and therefore more likely to cause injury. If machines are used, those that feature the ability to place limitations on the range of motion of any given exercise and the ability to add resistance in small increments are best. The biomechanics of the machines are also important. There is little agreement about the best exercise intensity. For older people, we favor low to moderate resistance with frequent repetitions, not use of heavy resistance with few repetitions (44,45). Low to moderate resistance levels may

provide less stimulus for adaptation, but they require less supervision and risk of injury. In studies that used high resistance with low repetitions, Fiatarone et al (44,45) used a subject-to-staff ratio of 1:1 or 2:1. This kind of labor-intensive training program is not practical in most settings.

In general, exercise consisting of low to moderate resistance levels requires much less staffing. Resistance is set so that subjects can perform each exercise for three sets of 10 repetitions with good form. Strict insistance on good form not only increases the training stimulus, but also reduces the risk of injury. Once the older exerciser can perform three sets of 12 to 15 repetitions with good form, the weight is increased slightly, but never enough so that 10 repetition sets cannot be done. Proper breathing technique during the exercise is also important, particularly to prevent Valsalva maneuvers during resistive portions of the exercise. Proper breathing also helps to prevent the occurrence of dangerously high blood pressure levels.

Good form and breathing can be taught by well-trained exercise physiologists.

Stretching

All clients should be instructed in a good stretching routine that includes stretching all major muscle groups. Stretching exercise should consist of slow, steady stretching without bouncing. If done properly, stretching should never be painful. Ideally, stretching exercises should be incorporated into the start and finish of each exercise session.

Implementing a Program

To implement an exercise program for the elderly requires the same expertise and support as do programs for younger people (48): good exercise facilities, knowledgeable staff, and efficient administration.

The numbers and qualifications of the exercise staff depend on the types of older subjects in the program. An exercise program for older exercisers without major clinical problems requires a staff-to-client ratio of 1:10. Cardiac rehabilitation programs require staffing ratios of 1:4 because of the extra cardiac monitoring that is required. Other disease rehabilitation programs also may need higher staffing levels. Because exercise programs for the elderly almost always include some special rehabilitation programs, the final staffing ratio is rarely as low as 1:10 (our program currently has an exerciser-to-staff-to-client ratio of 1:7).

There are two general models of staffing an exercise program for older people, an exercise physiologist model and a nursing model. In both models, physician coverage is desirable, and required if cardiac rehabilitation programs are being conducted. The exercise physiologist model uses a combination of bachelor's and master's level exercise physiologists. Certification of the exercise physiologists in cardiopulmonary resuscitation and pulmonary care is necessary; certification as an exercise trainer by a national organization such as the American College of Sports Medicine is desirable. In addition, some of the staff must be certified in cardiac rehabilitation and advanced life support. The nursing model uses nurses, nurse practitioners, and physical therapists. This model works well in a clinical setting.

Other models, such as exercise programs at community centers and YMCAs, may not allow satisfactory staffing requirements. In this case, the general health of the older exercisers must be carefully evaluated and the exercise program adjusted (such as screening out less healthy older people, reducing exercise intensities, types of equipment used) to reduce risks.

Future of Exercise Centers for the Elderly

The benefits of exercise programs for older people has been demonstrated. The major limitation to implementing exercise programs for the elderly is lack of funding. Commercial exercise programs for younger people have flourished, but they require efficient management, carry significant costs to the exerciser, and often rely on low compliance from clients who sign up for long-term memberships. Exercise centers for older people carry additional requirements and this makes them more expensive to run. To make exercise programs for older people affordable for most Americans, they will require increased government or private support. Increasing knowledge of the health benefits of exercise, coupled with increased emphasis on preventive medicine may provide the funding needed to result in more exercise centers for the elderly. Future research will determine whether additional components or modifications are needed to persuade more older people to exercise and to increase the efficiency of exercise training programs. Regular exercise is likely to be one of the tools used with hormonal therapy and aggressive vitamin and nutrition therapy to reduce the impact of aging on limiting function in people as they get older.

References

1. Hill AV, Lupton H. Muscular exercise, lactic acid, and the supply and utilization of oxygen. Q J Med 1923;16:135–171.
2. Lindhard J. Über das minutenvolum des herzens bei ruhe und bei muskelarbeit. Pflugers Arch 1915;161:233–283.
3. Liljestrad G, Stenstrom N. Studien über die physiologie des schwimmens. Skand Arch 1920;39:1–63.
4. Herbst R. Der gastroffwechsel als mab der körperlichen leistungsfähigkeit. Dtsch Arch 1928;162:33–50.
5. Taylor HL, Buskirk E, Henschel A. Maximal oxygen intake as an objective measure of cardio-respiratory performance. J Appl Physiol 1955;8:73–80.

6. Noakes TD. Implications of exercise testing for prediction of athletic performance: a contemporary perspective. Med Sci Sports Exerc 1988;20:319–330.

7. Green HJ, Patla AE. Maximal aerobic power: neuromuscular and metabolic considerations. Med Sci Sports Exerc 1992; 24:38–46.

8. Honig CR, Connett RJ, Gayeski TE. O_2 transport and its interaction with metabolism: a systems view of aerobic capacity. Med Sci Sports Exerc 1992;24:47–53.

9. Sutton JR. VO_2 max–new concepts on an old theme. Med Sci Sports Exerc 1992;24:26–29.

10. Saltin B, Strange S. Maximal oxygen uptake: "old" and "new" arguments for a cardiovascular limitation. Med Sci Sports Exerc 1992;23:30–37.

11. Wagner PD. Gas exchange and peripheral diffusion limitation. Med Sci Sports Exerc 1992;24:54–58.

12. Health GW, Hagberg JM, Ehsani AA, Holloszy JO. A physiological comparison of young and older endurance athletes. J Appl Physiol 1981;51:634–640.

13. Kohrt WM, Malley MT, Coggan AR, et al. Effects of gender, age, and fitness level on response of VO_2max to training in 60 to 71-yr-olds. J Appl Physiol 1991;71:2004–2011.

14. Posner JD, Gorman KM, Klein HS, Cline CJ. Ventilatory threshold: measurement and variation with age. J Appl Physiol 1987;63:1519–1525.

15. Heath GW, Hagberg JM, Ali A, et al. A physiological comparison of young and older endurance athletes. J Appl Physiol 1981;51:634–640.

16. Jones NL, Markrides L, Hitchcock C, et al. Normal standards for an incremental progressive cycle ergometer test. Am Rev Respir Dis 1978;131:31–39.

17. Ainsworth BE, Haskell WL, Leon AS, et al. Compendium of physical activities: classification of energy costs of human physical activities. Med Sci Sports Exerc 1993;25:71–80.

18. Brooks GA. Lactate production under fully aerobic conditions: the lactate shuttle during rest and exercise. Fed Proc 1986;45:2924–2929.

19. Wasserman K, Whipp BJ, Koyal SN, Beaver WL. Anaerobic threshold and respiratory gas exchange during exercise. J Appl Physiol 1973;35:236–243.

20. Beaver WL, Wasserman K, Whipp BJ. A new method for detecting anaerobic threshold by gas exchange. J Appl Physiol 1986;60:2020–2027.

21. Posner J, Gorman K, Windsor-Landsberg L, et al. Low to moderate intensity endurance training in healthy older adults: physiological responses after 4 months. J Am Geriatr Soc 1992;40:1–7.

22. Allen WK, Seals DR, Hurley BF, et al. Lactate threshold and distance-running performance in young and older endurance athletes. J Appl Physiol 1985;58:1281–1284.

23. Cartee GD. Aging skeletal muscle: response to exercise. Exerc Sports Sci Rev 1994;22:91–120.

24. Larsson L. Histochemical characteristics of human skeletal muscle during aging. Acta Physiol Scand 1983;117:469–471.

25. Grimby G, Saltin B. The aging muscle. Clin Physiol 1983; 3:209–218.

26. Moore DH. A study of age-group track and field records to relate age and running speed. Nature 1975;253:264–265.

27. Orlander J, Kiessling KH, Larsson L, et al. Skeletal muscle metabolism and ultrastructure in relation to age in sedentary men. Acta Physiol Scand 1978;104:249–261.

28. Coggan AR, Spina RJ, King DS, et al. Skeletal muscle adaptations to endurance training in 60- to 70-yr-old men and women. J Appl Physiol 1992;72:1780–1786.

29. McCully K, Fielding R, Evans W, et al. Correlations between in vivo and in vitro metabolism in young and old human skeletal muscles. J Appl Physiol 1993;75:813–819.

30. Brooks SV, Faulkner JA. Maximum and sustained power of extensor digitorum longus muscles from young, adult, and old mice. J Gerontol 1991;46:1328–1333.

31. Laforest S, St. Pierre DM, Cyr J, Gayton D. Effects of age and regular exercise on muscle strength and endurance. Eur J Appl Physiol 1990;60:104–111.

32. Lakatta EG. Changes in cardiovascular function with aging. Eur Heart J 1990;11(suppl C):22–29.

33. Cress ME, Thomas DP, Johnson J, et al. Effect of training on VO_2max, thigh strength and muscle morphology in septuagenarian women. Med Sci Sports Exerc 1991;23:752–758.

34. Posner PD, McCully K, Landsberg L, et al. Physical determinants of independence in older women. Gerontologist 1992; 32:190.

35. Tinetti ME. Instability and falling in elderly patients. Semin Neurol 1989;9:39–45.

36. Whipple RH, Wolfson LI, Amerman PM. The relationship of knee and ankle weakness to falls in nursing home residents: an isokinetic study. J Am Geriatr Soc 1987;35:13–20.

37. Buchner DM, de Laeur BJ. The importance of skeletal muscle strength to physical function in older adults. Behav Med 1991;13:91–97.

38. Gudat U, Berger M, Lefebvre PJ. Physical activity, fitness and non-insulin-dependent (Type II) diabetes mellitus. In: Bouchard C, Shephard RJ, Stephens T, eds. Physical activity, fitness, and health. Champaign, IL: Human Kinetics, 1994: 669–683.

39. Defronzo R, Jacot E, Jequier E, et al. The effect of insulin on the disposal of intravenous glucose: results from indirect calorimetry and hepatic and femoral venous catheterization. Diabetes 1981;30:1000–1007.

40. Reaven G, Ho H, Hoffman B. Attenuation of fructose-induced hypertension in rats by exercise training. Hypertension 1988;12:129–132.

41. Paffenbarger RS, Hyde RT, Wing AL, et al. Some interrelations of physical activity, physiological fitness, health, and longevity. In: Bouchard C, Shephard RJ, Stephens T, eds. Physical activity, fitness, and health. Champaign, IL: Human Kinetics, 1994:119–133.

42. Posner JD, Gorman KM, Gitlin LN, et al. Effects of exercise training in the elderly on the occurrence and time to onset of cardiovascular diagnoses. J Am Geriatr Soc 1990;38:205–210.

43. Clark LP, Dion DM, Barker WH. Taking to bed: Rapid func-

tional decline in an independently mobile older population living in an intermediate-care facility. J Am Geriatr Soc 1990;38:967–972.

44. Sallis JF, Hovell MF. Determinants of exercise behavior. Exerc Sports Sci Rev 1990;18:307–330.

45. Fiatarone MA, Marks EC, Ryan ND, et al. High-intensity strength training in nonagenarians: effects on skeletal muscle. JAMA 1990;263:3029–3034.

46. Fiatarone MA, O'Neill EF, Ryan ND, et al. Exercise training and nutritional supplementation for physical frailty in very elderly people. N Engl J Med 1994;330:1769–1775.

47. Haskell WL. Health consequences of physical activity: understanding and challenges regarding dose-response. Med Sci Sports Exerc 1994;26:649–660.

48. Kamen RL, Patton RW. Cost benefits of an active versus an inactive society. In: Bouchard C, Shephard RJ, Stephens T, eds. Physical activity, fitness, and health. Champaign, IL: Human Kinetics, 1994:134–144.

Chapter 18

Evaluation and Management of Common Symptoms in Geriatric Care

Martin J. Gorbien and Donna L. Miller

Years steal
Fire from the mind as vigor from the limb;
And Life's enchanged cup but sparkles near the brim.

Byron

Childe Harold's Pilgrimage

The challenge of caring for frail, elderly persons with multiple problems, unusual combinations of signs and symptoms, and important psychosocial stressors demands a pristine history and physical examination. In geriatric care, unusual presentations of common illnesses occur and subtle changes provide clues to accurate diagnosis. In this chapter, six complaints that geriatricians frequently face in office practice are presented: unintentional weight loss, constipation, pruritus, cough, weakness, and sleep disorders. They are instructive examples of the approach required in providing care for elderly patients.

Unintentional Weight Loss

Many physicians consider loss of 5 percent or more of usual body weight during a period of 6 to 12 months to be significant and to warrant further investigation (1). Unintentional weight loss in an elderly person can be the presenting symptom of a myriad of medical and psychosocial problems and may be an ominous marker of disease. The physician is first obligated to determine that weight loss has truly occurred, as approximately half of older patients cannot substantiate their complaint through serial weight charts, review of old medical records, collaboration by family members, or an obvious change in clothing size (1).

Physiologic changes of weight related to aging do oc-

cur. Maximal body weight is generally reached by men between ages 34 and 54 and by women between ages 55 and 65. Loss in lean body mass and total body water accounts for some limited decline in body weight after age 65. Fat atrophy and changes in fat distribution may cause anatomical changes that contribute to the appearance of significant weight loss. Distinguishing between natural changes and pathological weight loss is important.

A careful history and physical examination combined with limited laboratory studies has been shown to adequately identify older patients who need additional testing. In one study, 91 ambulatory patients (mean age, 59.3 ± 17.5 years) with at least 5 percent weight loss during a period of 6 months were evaluated at a Veterans Affairs hospital. Twenty-six percent had no apparent cause for the weight loss, 19 percent had malignancy, 14 percent had benign gastrointestinal problems, and 9 percent suffered from depression (2). In most cases, the initial evaluation accurately predicted patients who needed further testing. Another study showed similar findings in 154 hospitalized patients (3). In spite of extensive evaluation, 23 percent of subjects had no identifiable cause for weight loss. Psychiatric illness (10%) was more likely in patients with normal laboratory testing (Table 18.1).

Elderly patients are more likely than younger patients to have multiple problems or impairments that contribute to weight loss (1). These can be summarized by the mnemonic "WEIGHT LOSS" shown in Table 18.2.

Willingness to Eat

Morley outlined multiple psychological causes for weight loss in the elderly (4). Depression is often underrecognized and undertreated in this age group. Weight loss and apathy may be the presenting symptoms,

Table 18.1. Unintentional Weight Loss in the Elderly: Summary of Studies.

Authors	Sample and Data Base	Setting	Age (±SEM) and Sex Ratio	Etiology of Comments No. (%)	Weight Loss after Evaluation of Multiple Possible DX
Marton et al (2)	91 patients; weight loss ≥5% of usual body weight over 6 mo; prospective study	Veterans Administration clinics and hospital	59.3 (±17.5) M/F ratio: 90:1	No apparent cause 24 (26) Cancer 18 (19) GI 13 (14) Cardiovascular 8 (9) Psychiatric 8 (9) Alcohol 7 (8) Other DX 18 (19)	1. 35% with no identifiable physical cause after 1 yr of evaluation 2. Physical causes clinically apparent on initial evaluation in 55 of 59 pts 3. 25% of pts died within 1 yr of study entry
Rabinovitz et al (3)	154 inpatients; weight loss ≥5% of usual body weight over 6 mo; retrospective chart review	Internal medicine service hospital admissions	64.2 (±12.8) M/F Ratio: 1.2:1.0	Neoplasm 56 (35) Unknown 36 (23) GI disorder 26 (17) Psychiatric 16 (10) Misc 20 (13)	1. Patients with malignancy were older and had more abnormal physical findings 2. Low albumin and high alkaline phosphatase seen more often in patients with neoplasm 3. 36% had neoplasms 4. 23% no identifiable cause
Thompson and Morris (12)	45 outpatients; weight loss of ≥7.5% baseline weight in 6 mo; retrospective chart review after computer search	7 family practice centers in Southeast US	71.9 M/F ratio: 1:2	Unknown 11 (24) Depression 8 (18) Cancer 7 (16) GI 5 (11) Hyperthyroid 4 (9) Misc 6 (13)	1. 24% with no identifiable etiology after 2 yr 2. Diagnosis of depression more common than cancer 3. Only 4 deaths within 2 yr, all cancer-related 4. CT scans not helpful as screening test

CT = computed tomography; DX = diagnosis; GI = gastrointestinal; pts = patients.

although atypical presentations of pseudodementia and hypochondriasis may hamper early diagnosis and treatment. Standardized screening instruments for depression should be administered to elderly patients with weight loss. Depressed patients usually respond well to low-dose antidepressants. However, careful monitoring of therapy must occur because weight loss and anorexia may be an undesirable side effect of therapy, especially with the newer class of selective serotonin reuptake inhibitors such as fluoxetine, sergiline, and paroxetine.

Bereavement often causes anorexia, which leads to re-duced food intake and ketosis that further suppresses appetite. The problem may be compounded by poor culinary skills or social isolation, especially in men.

Some older persons may voluntarily reduce their food intake in the final months of their life because they view their life as excessively burdensome. Physicians should exclude treatable depression as a cause of this behavior.

Late-life paranoia may manifest as a refusal to eat because of the belief that the food is poisoned. After determining whether these beliefs are paranoid delusions or factual (e.g., elder abuse), physicians may prescribe a

Table 18.2. Causes of Weight Loss in the Elderly.

W	E	I	G	H	T

Willingness to eat
  Depression
  Bereavement
  Psychiatric illness
  Anorexia
  Manipulation
	End-stage chronic/
	  diseases
	  Carcinoma
	  Congestive heart
	  failure
	  COPD
	  CAD
	  Neurologic disorders
		Intoxication
		  Alcohol
		  Sedatives
		  Hypnotics
		  Gastric pathology
			Gastrointestinal
			  disorders
			  Dysphagia
			  Diarrhea
			  Parkinson's disease
			  Pancreatic cancer
				Hypermetabolic states
				  Hyperthyroidism
				  Prolonged febrile
				  states
				  Xerostomia
				  Pheochromacytomia
					Tooth problems
					  Odynophagia
					  Periodontal
					  disease

	L	O	S	S	

	Loss of memory
	  Dementia
		Olfactory changes/
		  dysgeusia
		  Impaired senses
		  Dietary restriction
			Social problems
			  Poverty
			  Isolation
				Side effects of medications
				  ACE inhibitors
				  Digoxin
				  Antidepressants
				  Antihypertensives
				  Nonsteroidals
				  Theophylline
				  Acetazolamide	

ACE = angiotensin-converting enzyme; CAD = coronary artery disease; COPD = chronic obstructive pulmonary disease.

neuroleptic such as haloperidol that often eliminates such delusions and restores normal appetite.

Manic behavior with prolonged periods of sleeplessness and frenetic activity may cause weight loss. Treatment with lithium often resolves this problem.

Food refusal may be used as a means of manipulating family or nursing home staffs, especially in situations in which elderly patients have developed dependence for activities of daily living (ADL) because of disease or disability.

Anorexia nervosa may occur in elderly patients who had classic cases of this disorder in their teens. Morley et al described a group of older patients with anorexia tardive, a syndrome that resembles anorexia nervosa (5). The patients had extremely abnormal attitudes about eating and feared becoming overweight despite profound weight loss. Some of them were following excessively restricted diets to lower cholesterol levels or to promote longevity.

End-Stage or Chronic Diseases

Cancer is always a possible cause of weight loss in the elderly because of the production of cachectin (tumor necrosis factor) and interleukin, both of which have anorectic effects (6). Some tumors produce bombesin that sends false messages of satiety to the central nervous system. Zinc deficiency associated with tumors may contribute to dysgeusia and anorexia of malignancy.

A number of chronic diseases may cause significant weight loss, especially in the later stages of illness. Cardiac cachexia occurs in patients with congestive heart failure in association with severe weight loss, protein-losing enteropathy and hypoalbuminemia (7). In addition, some patients with severe coronary artery disease may experience angina during eating or during the process of digestion, which leads to reduced oral intake to avoid pain. Anginal symptoms caused by mesenteric artery ischemia may respond to calcium channel blockers or nitrates.

Patients with chronic obstructive pulmonary disease (COPD) may lose weight as a result of higher energy requirements of accessory respiratory muscles for breathing and early satiety. Patients with COPD may become dyspneic while eating, and thus reduce their caloric intake.

Neurologic disorders such as stroke, amyotrophic lateral sclerosis (ALS), and Parkinson's disease may cause weight loss directly because of dysphagia or functional limitations that result in inability to transport food to one's mouth. In addition, depression often accompanies these disorders and exacerbates weight loss. A thorough swallowing evaluation with speech therapy is often diagnostic and may suggest strategies for eating. Treatment of depression may also stimulate appetite and improve caloric intake.

Intoxication

Alcohol abuse, like depression, is underdiagnosed in elderly patients. Depression and bereavement often trigger late-life alcoholism. Alcohol may become a food substitute and lead to malnutrition and weight loss. Any patient who presents to a medical office visit under the influence of alcohol most likely suffers from alcohol abuse. However, careful questioning of the patient and loved ones or screening with the CAGE or MAST-G questionnaire may be necessary to uncover this problem.

Gastrointestinal Disorders

Dysphagia is a relatively common problem caused by a wide range of diseases. Oropharyngeal dysphagia is manifested by difficulty in initiating swallowing, coughing, or nasal regurgitation of food during swallowing. This form of dysphagia is seen in primary neurological disorders, upper pharyngeal and esophageal obstructive processes, primary muscle disorders, and esophageal motility problems.

Esophageal dysphagia is characterized by the sensation of food sticking in the esophagus, usually retrosternally. This type of dysphagia is caused by extrinsic compression on the esophagus, intrinsic esophageal structural lesions, or motility disorders. Although treatment of the primary process is paramount, proper positioning during feeding of appropriate food textures (thickened liquids, pureed or finely chopped foods) may improve a patient's oral intake by reducing aspiration.

Diarrhea is an uncommon cause of unintentional weight loss in the elderly patient, except in disorders such as sprue or amyloidosis that result in malabsorption. When diarrhea is osmotic, a meal may precipitate the problem and lead to food aversion to control the diarrhea.

Gastric pathology such as gastritis, peptic ulcer disease, gastric outlet obstruction, and carcinoma may present as weight loss. Pancreatic carcinoma may present as unex-

plained weight loss. Esophageal candidiasis should be considered in immunocompromised patients with dysphagia, anorexia, and weight loss.

Hypermetabolic States

Hyperthyroidism causes weight loss through increased metabolic demands. However, in elderly patients, apathetic hyperthyroidism may cause an atypical presentation with atrial fibrillation, ptosis, weight loss, myopathy, or congestive heart failure. Thyroid hormone levels may be at the upper limits of normal when hyperthyroidism is accompanied by malnutrition, but thyroid-stimulating hormone (TSH) will be depressed.

Other metabolic causes of weight loss include pheochromocytoma and prolonged febrile states (e.g., infections). Parkinson's disease may be viewed as a hypermetabolic state because of the increased caloric requirements caused by constant fine tremor, which is analogous to continuous exercise.

Teeth Problems

Odynophagia (pain with eating) caused by ill-fitting dentures or other native teeth problems may cause weight loss from reduced caloric intake. Poorly cleaned dentures, gingivitis, periodontal disease, medication side effects, neuropathies, and systemic illness may adversely alter taste perception and the enjoyment of eating.

About 44 percent of the elderly may have dry mouth (xerostomia) (8). This condition may be the result of medication side effects, previous head or neck radiation treatments, salivary gland disorders, or Sjögren's syndrome. Commercial saliva substitutes are generally unsatisfactory to most patients, and efforts should be focused on preventive dental care and symptomatic relief.

Loss of Memory

Routine office weights are very important for demented patients who cannot provide a reliable history. Early in Alzheimer's disease, concomitant depression may cause weight loss. Olfactory deficits and poor dental hygiene may dull taste perception. As the disease progresses, impaired swallowing, feeding apraxia, and blunted thirst and hunger drives contribute to the problem. Assistance with mealtime is often required in the later stages. Patients may improve their caloric intake with protein supplements and finger foods that do not require utensils to enjoy.

Olfactory Changes and Dysgeusia

Physiologic decline in taste and smell perception often interfere with appetite stimulation and food enjoyment. Many older patients prefer a more seasoned diet because of these changes. Sodium-restricted diets may interfere with taste perception and may lead to reduced caloric intake. Visual impairment may decrease visual appetite cues and hinder food preparation.

Social Problems

Approximately 11.4 percent of the elderly live below the poverty level (9), and total daily caloric intake of less than 1000 calories is twice as common in this group as it is in the general population (10). Limited financial resources may cause persons to choose between paying bills, buying medicine, or purchasing food.

Social isolation or lack of family and social supports may cause a person to be unable to procure food from a store. Bereaved individuals may dislike eating alone or have limited food preparation skills. Fear of leaving home because of concerns about personal safety in high-crime areas or during inclement weather may also contribute to a patient's poor oral intake and weight loss.

Strong ethnic food preferences may make community or institutional food programs less appealing for some individuals. Stringent dietary modifications for elevated cholesterol, diabetes, or congestive heart failure should be avoided whenever feasible because bland foods are much less desirable.

Side Effects of Medications

Medications can interfere with appetite and caloric intake in several ways. Some medications, such as angiotensin-converting enzyme (ACE) inhibitors and digoxin, cause dysgeusia and suppress appetite. As much as 25 percent of patients on digoxin may develop anorexia and weight loss (11). Psychotropic drugs, antidepressants, some antihypertensives, and diuretics may cause dry mouth and exacerbate xerostomia and odynophagia. Nausea, dyspepsia, and abdominal pain may accompany use of nonsteroidals and theophylline preparations. The carbonic anhydrase inhibitor acetazolamide may cause

weight loss in patients with glaucoma. Evaluating whether medications are a cause of weight loss is an important first step in the older patient.

Management of Weight Loss

Early intervention at the first sign of weight loss is the key to successful management of this problem. A focused history and physical may provide the starting point for medical evaluation. Ask the patient if the weight loss is intentional or caused by another problem or physical symptom associated with eating. Food diaries for community-dwelling patients or formal calorie counts for institutionalized or hospitalized patients are helpful to document actual food consumption and preferences. These may serve as a guide for the physician and dietician and lead to practical ways to improve intake, such as adding snacks, adjusting food consistency, and eliminating restrictive diets. A patient's preferred meal should be maximized by adding increased calories or nontraditional foods at mealtime. Problem foods, such as those that cause excessive bloating or flatulence, should be avoided. Consumption of liquids should occur after or between meals to reduce early satiety. Regular exercise and management of constipation or diarrhea may improve appetite. Oral hygiene should be emphasized.

The history may also uncover psychosocial issues contributing to weight loss. Appropriate measures can then be undertaken, such as soliciting help from family and friends, increasing socialization for mealtimes, and arranging for community services such as Meals-on-Wheels.

All patients with dysphagia need a complete swallowing evaluation and consultation with a speech pathologist and an occupational therapist for optimal management. Other medical problems contributing to weight loss should be investigated and treated appropriately. Periodic review of all medications, both prescription and over-the-counter, is helpful.

Laboratory and diagnostic testing should be guided by the history and physical examination. Table 18.3 outlines tests that have been shown to have the highest yield in a geriatric weight loss workup (3,4,12). Computed tomography (CT) scans are not useful as initial tests for evaluating of weight loss in ambulatory geriatric patients (11) because cancer is usually not the cause of weight loss.

Table 18.3. Diagnostic Testing for Weight Loss.

Test	Value
Serum albumin	<3.5 gm/dL
Serum calcium	>10.5 mg/dL
Serum hemoglobin	<12.0 gm/dL men; <10.0 gm/dL women
Serum cholesterol	<160 mg/dL
Serum creatinine	>2.0 mg/dL
Serum glucose	>200 mg/dL
Liver function	AST or GGTP >2× normal; elevated INR, Alk phos, or bilirubin
Thyroid function	TSH > 15 μmol/ml or FTI > 5.5
Total lymphocyte count	<1500 μL
Other	
Chest x-ray	
Stool hemoccult	
Urinalysis	

AIK phos = alkaline phosphatase; AST = Aspartare aminotransferase; FTI = free thyroxine index; GGTP = γ-glutamyltranspeptidase; INR = international normalized ratio; TSH = thyroid-stimulating hormone.

SOURCE: Modified from Robbins LJ. Evaluation of weight loss in the elderly. Geriatrics 1989;44:31–35.

Nutritional Supplements and Appetite Stimulants

When oral intake is inadequate to maintain a patient's weight, despite caloric supplements and other measures, tube feedings should be considered. The risks, benefits, and goals of treatment need to be clearly understood by all involved in the decision-making process. Short-term tube feeding is reasonable, particularly for problems that are expected to be reversible. However, when the patient is incompetent, or when the underlying disease process is expected to be terminal, decisions about tube feeding are more difficult and controversial. Nutritional issues are covered in detail in Chapter 16.

Medications have a limited role in stimulation of appetite. Megestrol acetate has been shown to increase appetite and promote weight gain, especially in women with advanced breast cancer (13). This observation has also been noted in a small group of acquired immuno-deficiency syndrome (AIDS) patients (14). However, this drug has not been studied in elderly populations with weight loss.

Preliminary studies show that growth hormone increases muscle mass and contributes to more rapid weight gain in severely malnourished elderly (15). Addi-

tional research is needed before this expensive hormone can be recommended to correct weight loss.

Low-dose prednisone and tricyclic antidepressants have been used by clinicians to enhance appetite and promote weight gain in selected patients. However, none of these medications are specifically approved to control or correct weight loss.

Constipation

Although there may not be consensus on the definition of constipation, this complaint is quite familiar for elderly patients living in the community, as well as for those in hospitals or in extended care facilities. When patients describe a constipated state they may mean that the frequency of stools is inadequate, the defecation is incomplete, or the movements are difficult or painful. Physicians in office practice are often asked to address this problem. If the simple definition of constipation as "a condition in which bowel movements are infrequent or incomplete" (16) is accepted, the issue becomes quite common.

Studies of the bowel habits of elderly individuals in the community have been difficult to interpret because of wide variations in prevalence of constipation. Many of these studies rely on self-reporting, which complicates interpretation. In a study of almost 500 community-dwelling adults over age 62, approximately 70 percent of respondents had a daily bowel movement, although the use of laxatives ranged from 38 percent (men) to 50 percent (women) (17). Donald et al (18) reported that 30 (23%) of 129 outpatients (mean age, 76.3) suffered from constipation yet 96 percent of the population reported having three to five or more stools each week. Connell (19) and colleagues reported that over 90 percent of elderly participants in his study had normal bowel function with a range of three stools per day to three stools per week. In a study of 209 individuals ages 65 to 93, 30 percent of participants described themselves as constipated, but only 2 percent to 3 percent had fewer than three stools per week. The number of nonlaxative medications and chronic illnesses correlated with the complaint of constipation in women and the number of psychological symptoms correlated with perceived constipation in both men and women (20). Despite variation in the reported prevalence of constipation, the National Center for Health Statistics concurs that as individuals age, they report an increase in constipation, incomplete evacuation, and scybalous stools, as well as abdominal pain and distention.

Although a variety of physiologic changes take place in the aging colon, the changes do not provide an adequate explanation for the age-related increase in constipation. The changes include atrophy of the mucosa, abnormal changes in intestinal glands, and cell infiltration of the lamina propria and mucosa. Also noted are hypertrophy of the lamina muscularis mucosae, atrophy of the muscle layer, an increase in connective tissue, and arteriolar sclerosis.

Much attention has been paid to the topic of age-related changes in colonic transit time. Review of the collective data on colonic transit time suggests that, in general, young and old subjects appear quite similar. There is much overlap when comparing the transit time of constipated and nonconstipated elderly, with the possibility of slow transit time in the rectosigmoid region as a possible etiology of constipation (21). Many investigations looking at colonic transit time of dietary fiber fail to reveal clinically significant differences among young and old subjects. In addition, electrophysiological evaluation of sigmoid and rectal motility did not show differences among healthy young and healthy old participants when measurements were taken before, during, and after a meal (22). Nevertheless, motor abnormalities have been found in the pelvic floor and colon in patients with long-standing chronic constipation (23).

Fecal impaction is a serious complication of constipation, whether acute or chronic (24). This disorder is often overlooked in both inpatient and outpatient settings. Impaction can occur in the presence of an incomplete daily bowel movement. Fecal soiling (which may be described by the patient as diarrhea) can be an important clue to the presence of impaction. The wide-ranging signs and symptoms of fecal impaction can be confusing. Chest pain, shortness of breath, leukocytosis, low-grade fever, dysuria, or anuria represent some of the more unusual signs and symptoms of fecal impaction. Although individuals with early impaction can usually be managed as outpatients, fecal impaction is not infrequently cause for hospital admission (25). The practicing physician in geriatric practice should be aware of this common problem to prevent its development and to avoid resultant morbidity (26).

A thorough history must be taken when a patient complains of constipation. An extensive list of medical conditions can lead to constipation; these are outlined in Table 18.4 (27). The number and quality of the stools, chronicity of the problem, associated weight loss, the presence of blood in the stool, and a diet history are essential elements for review.

Medications are common culprits in causing constipation and a partial list of drugs that can cause constipation is included in Table 18.5 (27). Physical examination should focus on an abdominal examination, with atten-

Table 18.4. Causes of Constipation.

Lesions of the gut
  Aganglionosis
  Obstruction
  Idiopathic megacolon
  Colon cancer
  Ulcerative colitis
  Irritable bowel syndrome
  Solitary rectal ulcer
  Rectal fissure, stricture, or hemorrhoids
  Hirschsprung's disease
  Volvulus
Neurological disorders
  Autonomic neuropathy
  Multiple sclerosis
  Stroke
  Spinal cord tumors
  Cauda equina tumors
  Paraplegia/quadriplegia
Metabolic disorders
  Hypothyroidism
  Hyperparathyroidism
  Adrenal and pituitary hypofunction
  Uremia
  Porphyria
Psychiatric disorders
  Dementia
  Depression
  Affective disorders
Lesions of the pelvis
  Rectocele
  Cystocele
  Uterine prolapse
  Prostatic disease
  Hernia
  Pelvic tumors

Table 18.5. Drugs Associated with Constipation.

Minerals
    Albumin
    Bismuth
    Calcium
    Iron
Sympathomimetics
    Ephedrine
    Isoproterenol
    Phenylpropanolamine
Antidepressants
    Amitriptyline
    Doxepin
    Imipramine
Heavy Metals
Opiates
    Codeine
    Diphenoxylate
    Hydrocodone
    Meperidine
Antiarrhythmics and antihypertensives
    Disopyramide
    Narcoleptics
    Antiparkinsonian agents
Nonsteroidal anti-inflammatory agents

tion to the presence of a distended bladder and the character of bowel sounds, and on a digital rectal examination, looking for impaction, mass, abnormalities of sphincter tone, and the presence of occult blood. A study of the colon by sigmoidoscopy, colonoscopy, or an air-contrast barium enema may also be elected, depending on details of the patient's history and physical examination. Once it has been established that the patient is constipated and a primary lesion of the colon and as systemic medical condition have been ruled out as causes for the constipation, attention should turn to treatment.

Castle's step care approach (28) for treatment of constipation provides an ordered series of steps in the treatment of constipated patients. Bowel retraining is an important part of the care of patients, even when medications are used. Encouraging patients to respond to the periods of high-motility, the "call to stool," can be achieved by having patients try to evacuate 30 to 60 minutes after breakfast in an attempt to restore the gastrocolic reflex that may be impaired in older adults. This may be accomplished initially with the aid of glycerin suppositories. Bulk laxatives can be safe and effective. Patients must be urged to

be certain that intake of liquids is adequate to avoid creating hard, uncomfortable stools. Individuals who have had diets low in fiber should titrate doses slowly to avoid gas and bloating. Stool softeners can be helpful to patients who report having hard stool. However, older patients more commonly have soft stool that is difficult to evacuate from the rectum. Exercise is an important adjunct to any bowel regimen.

There is a wide variety of laxatives from which to choose if modification of diet, activity, and scheduled toileting has not proven successful. Stimulant laxatives should generally be avoided because they lead to dependence and can have long-term side effects. Constipated individuals with long-standing history of irritant laxative use are among the most difficult to treat. Saline (magnesium citrate) laxatives and stimulant (bisacodyl, phenolphthalein) laxatives should be reserved for use as needed for more difficult situations. Hyperosmolar laxatives such as lactulose or sorbitol can be helpful in resistant cases and can generally be titrated with great success.

Pruritus

Pruritus (itching) is a common and annoying complaint that plagues geriatric patients and their physicians. However, a careful history and physical examination often yields the proper diagnosis and obviates the need for dermatologic referral. Studies of elderly populations have suggested that from 29 percent to 50 percent of patients over age 75 suffer from pruritus (29,30). This symptom may represent a primary dermatologic disease or be the harbinger of systemic illness. In the elderly, xerosis is the most likely cause of pruritus (31–33).

A thorough history and physical examination help distinguish acute from chronic pruritus and localized from generalized pruritus. Important information includes onset and duration of the pruritus; location (general or localized); presence of a rash; new or recurrent problem; exposure to potential sensitizing agents such as chemicals, cleaning products, or cosmetics; a complete medication history; and response to therapies (over-the-counter and prescription). The entire body and scalp should be inspected for signs of scratching or skin lesions.

With few exceptions, localized pruritus is caused by regional dermatitis. However, some diffuse disorders are more likely to become manifest in susceptible body areas that have dense cutaneous innervation or in those more convenient to scratching. Examples of generalized disorders are psoriasis, urticaria, and pityriasis rosea. Table 18.6 lists the most common dermatologic causes of pruritus by body region. Extensive discussion of treatments for these conditions is available in other sources (32–36), but general treatment guidelines are outlined in Table 18.7.

If the history and physical examination do not reveal an obvious primary dermatologic disorder or systemic illness, xerosis (dry skin) is the most likely cause of the pruritus. Aging skin holds less water and is especially prone to scaling and cracking under conditions of decreased humidity and changes in ambient temperature. The patient should be instructed in a 2-week trial of therapy designed to provide symptomatic relief. These

Table 18.6. Causes of Localized Pruritus by Body Region.

Scalp	Psoriasis
	Seborrheic dermatitis
Hands	Contact dermatitis
	Eczema
	Scabies
Trunk	Contact dermatitis
	Erythrasma
	Psoriasis
	Scabies
	Seborrheic dermatitis
	Urticaria
Inguinal	Candida
	Contact dermatitis
	Erythrasma
	Pediculosis
	Scabies
	Tinea cruris
Anal	Candida
	Contact dermatitis
	Gonorrhea
	Hemorrhoids
	Psoriasis
	Tinea cruris
Legs	Atopic dermatitis
	Dermatitis herpetiformis
	Eczema
	Neurotic excoriations
	Stasis dermatitis
Feet	Contact dermatitis
	Tinea pedis

Modified from Greco PJ, Ende J. Pruritis: a practical approach. J Gen Intern Med 1992;7:340–349.

Table 18.7. Treatment Guidelines for Common Dermatologic Causes of Pruritus.

Problem	Suggested Initial Treatment
Contact dermatitis	Topical corticosteroids Eliminate offending agent
Dermatophyte (fungal) infections	1% clotrimazole or 2% miconazole nitrate cream or powder
Eczema	Topical corticosteroids
Erythrasma	Oral/topical erythromycin or imidazoles
Psoriasis	Topical corticosteroids
Scabies	1% lindane or 5% permethrin topically
Seborrheic dermatitis	Topical corticosteroids, selenium sulfide, or tar-containing shampoo

Table 18.8. Dermatologic Causes of Generalized Pruritus.

Obvious Eruptions	Nonspecific or No Eruptions
Drug reactions	Aquagenic pruritus
Folliculitis	Atopic dermatitis
Fungal infections	Bullous pemphigoid
Mycosis fungoides	Contact dermatitis
Pemphigus	Dermatitis herpetiformis
Pityriasis rosea	Insect bites
Psoriasis	Pediculosis
Sunburn	Scabies
	Urticaria
	Xerosis

Modified from Greco PJ, Ende J. Pruritis: a practical approach. J Gen Intern Med 1992;7:340–349.

measures include reduction in bathing frequency and duration, use of mild soaps, liberal application of emollients, and the use of a humidifier. When the pruritus does not significantly improve after these measures, a systemic etiology should be considered.

Careful skin inspection usually identifies dermatologic causes of generalized pruritus (Table 18.8). Systemic disorders (Table 18.9) should be considered in undiagnosed patients after 2 weeks of treatment for xerosis and after medication reactions and primary dermatological conditions have been excluded. Useful laboratory tests for evaluation of systemic etiologies are listed in Table 18.10.

Table 18.9. Systemic Causes of Generalized Pruritus.

Organ System	Etiology	Laboratory Clues
Endocrine	Carcinoid tumor	Elevated urinary 5-HIAA
	Diabetes mellitus	Elevated FBS
	Thyroid disease	Abnormal TSH
Hematologic	Iron deficiency anemia	Abnormal CBC and iron studies
	Mastocytosis	Abnormal peripheral smear
	Myeloproliferative	Abnormal CBC and smear
	Paraproteinemias	SPEP/SIEP
	Polycythemia vera	Elevated sedimentation rate; abnormal CBC
Infection	AIDS	HIV test
	Infestation	Skin scrapings
Neurologic	Brain abscess	CT scan/MRI
	Cerebral infarct	CT scan/MRI
	Multiple sclerosis	MRI/LP
	Tumor	CT scan/MRI
Obstructive biliary disease	Drug-induced cholestasis	Elevated LFTs/drug history
	Extrahepatic obstruction	Ultrasound/CT scan
	Primary biliary cirrhosis	Elevated alk phos/Antimicrosomal Ab
Psychiatric	Depression	History and physical
	Emotional stress	
	Parasitosis	
Renal	Chronic renal failure	Elevated BUN, creatinine
Other	Cancer	
	Medication reactions	Drug history
	Xerosis	Visual inspection of skin

Ab = antibody; alk phos = alkaline phosphatase; BUN = blood urea nitrogen; CBC = complete blood cell count; CT = computed tomography; FBS = fasting blood sugar; 5-HIAA = 5-hydroxyindoleacetic acid; LFT = liver function test; LP = lumbar puncture; MRI = magnetic resonance imaging; SIEP = serum isoenzyme electrophoresis; SPEP = serum protein electrophoresis; TSH = thyroid-stimulating hormone.

Table 18.10. Laboratory Evaluation for Systemic Disorders.

Initial screening	CBC with differential
	BUN, creatinine
	Liver function tests
	TSH
	Fasting glucose
	Chest x-ray
	Stool for occult blood
Additional testing	Iron studies
	SPEP, SIEP
	Skin biopsy
	Stool, for ova and parasites
	Radiologic studies
	Bone marrow biopsy

BUN = blood urea nitrogen; CBC = complete blood cell count; SIEP = serum isoenzyme electrophoresis; SPEP = serum protein electrophoresis; TSH = thyroid-stimulating hormone.

If no specific diagnosis can be determined, the patient requires periodic evaluation because the pruritus may precede a systemic illness such as primary biliary cirrhosis by months or years. Treatment of the underlying disorder is usually necessary for relief of itching in systemic illness such as thyroid disorders or myeloproliferative diseases.

Psychogenic pruritus (itching caused by anxiety, associated depression, or both) is a diagnosis made only after other dermatologic and systemic illnesses have been excluded. Often these patients have extensive excoriations of their skin because of their scratching. Antidepressants are generally successful in treating this problem.

Pruritic patients are often very uncomfortable and require aggressive symptom control. Topical or systemic corticosteroids are reserved for patients with a steroid-responsive dermatitis. Topical anesthetics and antihistamines are generally avoided because they may cause allergic sensitization of the skin. However, the topical anesthetic pramoxine has been shown to cause few allergic reactions and may be more effective than 1% hydrocortisone (37). Compounds containing phenol or menthol may be soothing and provide temporary relief.

Antihistamines are often used as adjunctive therapy but present a special problem for the geriatric patient who is particularly vulnerable to their side effects of sedation, delirium, or urinary retention.

A low dose of a sedating antihistamine at bedtime such as hydroxyzine, diphenhydramine, or cyproheptadine may be useful in carefully selected and monitored patients. The nonsedating antihistamines such as terfenadine or astemizole are better tolerated for daytime use, although their experience in the treatment of pruritus is limited to date (38). Doxepin, a tricyclic antidepressant used at low doses, increases the threshold for histamine-induced itching and may be considered for bedtime use in some patients. Histamine (H_2) blockers have been effective treatments in chronic urticaria and Hodgkin's disease. Less traditional adjunctive therapies include acupuncture, transcutaneous nerve stimulation, and oral opiate antagonists.

Cough

Cough is a very common complaint for elderly individuals in the ambulatory care setting. Despite the fact that older patients may neglect to report cough and minimize its presence, cough is abnormal at any age (39). The age-associated change in the respiratory system are legion but, nevertheless, do not provide adequate explanation for the existence of cough (40,41). However, these changes may leave the aging patient at higher risk for acute and chronic respiratory problems. Clearly, several conditions that can cause cough increase in incidence with age. These include infection (bronchitis and pneumonia), congestive heart failure, and COPD. As patients age, the co-existence of multiple medical problems and related medications can make definitive diagnosis of cough, both acute and chronic, quite challenging.

The evaluation of cough begins with the patient's his-

tory, the most important portion of the evaluation. Special attention should be paid to cardiopulmonary history and review of systems, with careful questioning in regard to smoking history and environmental issues (allergies, other exposure). Whether the patient has had a history of pulmonary infection is important to know. Details regarding the chronicity and daily pattern of the cough are very important. For example, nocturnal cough may provide a clue to the diagnosis of gastroesophageal reflux. Again, altered presentations of common diseases appear in older adults. Cough may be the sole harbinger of early congestive heart failure, cough-type asthma (42), microaspiration, or very mild forms of neurologic disease such as stroke, motor neuron disease, or Parkinson's disease. In addition, the patient's medication history should be completed to determine whether drugs such as captopril (ACE inhibitor) and related agents can be incriminated (43).

Irwin and Curley (44) cited four common causes of chronic cough: postnasal drip syndrome, asthma, chronic bronchitis, and gastroesophageal reflux. These investigators showed that, beyond the patient's history and physical examination, other studies are of very limited usefulness. Although pulmonary function surveys, methacholine inhalational challenge, chest x-ray, sinus CT, and bronchoscopy are sometimes appropriate on an individualized basis, their use should be based on the specific findings of the patient's history and physical examination.

Postnasal drip syndrome has special significance for older adults. It is a common complaint and can be a result of chronic sinusitis and rhinitis of various etiologies. Empirical treatment with antihistamines, decongestants, and inhaled nasal steroids or cromolyn sodium can often prove effective. However, the anticholinergic side effects of antihistamines and the cardioactive effects of decongestants (e.g., pseudoephedrine) often prohibit their use. Decongestants are often inappropriate for patients with hypertension, coronary artery disease, and tachyarrhythmias. They should be used short-term with caution.

Chronic bronchitis, asthma, and emphysema are increasingly important entities for elderly patients. Improved care and subsequent longevity has led to increased awareness of these conditions in old patients.

236

The prevalence rates for asthma, chronic bronchitis, and emphysema for those over age 60 are 30, 40, and 60/100,000 men, respectively (46). The mortality from these diseases more than doubles between age 65 and 75 (48). Although asthma is generally considered to be a disease of younger people, it can develop at any age. The older a person is at the time of onset, the more challenging the diagnosis. Separating cardiac from pulmonary causes for cough or wheezing can be formidable. Clearly, an individual can have more than one cause of cough, wheezing, or shortness of breath. Individualized testing by echocardiogram, methacholine challenge, and spirometry can assist in clarifying the diagnosis.

The treatments for these three conditions have much in common. Inhaled beta-agonists and steroids may be difficult for older patients to use because they may have poor coordination or trouble understanding the proper use of meter-dosed inhalers. Several adaptive devices ("spacers") exist to help increase compliance with these medications. Oral beta-agonists have significant cardiac effects and theophylline interacts with a number of other medications. The need for such substances should be carefully reviewed.

Gastroesophageal reflux may result in a variety of symptoms, such as heartburn, dysphagia, and cough. Occasionally, cough is the prominent symptom of gastroesophageal reflux and other complaints may be absent. Any medication or substance that may impair normal antireflux mechanisms of the lower esophageal sphincter (LES) can lead to this condition. Caffeine, alcohol, tobacco, nitrates, beta-adrenergic agents, calcium channel blockers, and aminophylline are common examples of agents that affect the integrity of the LES. When symptoms caused by esophagitis are not prominent, the diagnosis may be elusive. Although diagnosis is being made by endoscopy and other dynamic swallowing studies, empiric treatment with proton pump inhibitors or H_2 blockers should be initiated. Inhaled beta-agonists (e.g., albuterol) can be helpful in treating associated cough along with other common-sense advice, such as elevation of the head during sleep and diet modification. Hiatal hernias are common in older patients but play a far less prominent role in the etiology of gastroesophageal reflux than previously believed.

A variety of other conditions with accompanying swallowing disorders seen in elderly patients may have cough as a common presenting feature. Zenker's diverticulum, esophageal dysmotility, stroke, Parkinson's disease, multi-infarct dementia, late-stage Alzheimer's disease, and motor neuron disease can lead to swallowing-related problems and associated cough. Because many of these conditions are seen in elderly patients, they must be considered as potential causes of cough.

The treatment of cough is sometimes difficult despite the large selection of prescription and over-the-counter agents available to practitioners (47). Studies of efficacy are not particularly encouraging, and adverse drug reactions associated with cough and cold medications are particularly important for elderly patients (48). Antihistamines are used for cough caused by colds and allergies. Despite the recent development of newer, less sedating preparations, the anticholinergic properties are well known for causing acute confusion, gait imbalance, dry mouth, constipation, and urinary retention. Decongestants such as phenylpropanolamine and pseudoephedrine can cause cardiac side effects, including elevated arterial blood pressure, tachycardia, and angina pectoris. Guaifenesin is a safe, widely available expectorant but is only minimally effective. Cough suppressants (e.g., dextromethorphan or codeine) can be helpful when cough prevents patients from sleeping.

Regardless of its etiology (Table 18.11), cough can be quite debilitating. Chronic cough can impair one's ability to eat, to converse, to socialize, and to sleep. Musculoskeletal strain with occasional rib fractures are troubling aspects of chronic cough. In evaluating cough in elderly patients, thorough history and physical examination with properly selected studies can lead to accurate diagnosis. Only after meticulous investigation should the diagnosis of psychogenic cough be considered (49). Many patients have more than one cause for their cough. Thoughtful review of the patient's medication, diet, and sleep pattern are helpful in better understanding the etiology of the cough and may lead to effective intervention.

Weakness

The older patient's complaint of weakness presents a challenging problem for a physician, especially because weakness may have multiple interpretations. Although weakness usually refers to a decrease in or lack of muscle strength, patients may use this term to mean fatigue, pain, or lack of interest in usual activities. Weakness implies a perceived change from the patient's baseline level of function, and it is important to determine what the patient means by his complaint and to establish a previous level of activity during the history-taking. Family members may also provide pertinent information and observations that can help the physician. The complaint should not be viewed as trivial or as an expected consequence of aging, especially in previously healthy older patients, nor should weakness be attributed to progression of chronic illnesses such as diabetes or heart disease without a medical evaluation to exclude other etiologies.

Table 18.11. Frequent Causes of Cough.

Pulmonary
Chronic bronchitis
Asthma
Emphysema
Postnasal drip syndrome (vasomotor or allergic rhinitis)
Interstitial fibrosis
Pneumothorax

Cardiac
Congestive heart failure

Infection
Pneumonia
Bronchitis (bacterial or viral)
Tuberculosis
Chronic infection (e.g., empyema, bronchiectasis)

Neoplasm
Primary neoplasm of lung
Metastatic neoplasm of lung or mediastinum

Gastrointestinal
Gastroesophageal reflux
Zenker's diverticulum
Esophageal dismotility

Drugs
ACE inhibitors
Substances that impair tone of LES

Neurologic
Stroke
Parkinson's disease
Motor neuron disease
Multi-infarct dementia
Neurotic cough

Table 18.12. Common Causes of Weakness in the Older Patient.

Psychosocial
Depression
Life stressors
Alcoholism

Medications
Digoxin
Diuretics
Antiarrhythmics
Benzodiazepines
Neuroleptics

Metabolic
Electrolyte abnormalities
Renal disease
Thyroid disease
Diabetes mellitus
Parathyroid disease
Adrenal insufficiency

Neuromuscular disease
Motor neuron diseases
Peripheral neuropathy
Myopathy
Stroke
Parkinson's disease
Myasthenia gravis

Medical disease
Cardiac disease
Peripheral vascular disease
Anemia
Polymyalgia rheumatica
Infection
Malignancy

No good data exist as to the prevalence or causes of weakness in older persons. Waltman has observed that depression or other psychosocial problems seem to be the primary precipitator in his experience (50). Table 18.12 outlines five categories of disorders or problems that may be manifested as weakness in the office setting.

Psychosocial Problems

Depressive symptoms affect about 15 percent of the community population over age 65, with higher rates reported in long-term care settings (51). Older patients are more likely to develop somatic symptoms such as weight loss, insomnia, lassitude, and lack of interest in usual activities rather than report a depressed mood. This may result in the complaint of weakness. ("I'm so weak that I just can't do anything anymore.") Treatment with appropriate antidepressants should relieve depressive symptoms.

Stressors such as loss of a spouse or loved one, financial concerns, a significant decline in function of independence because of medical illness, or a change in residence may trigger a complaint of weakness as a depressive equivalent. Patients should be questioned about alcohol use, especially under these circumstances. Depression may occur following a stroke or be manifested as memory loss. The physician should elicit this information as part of the patient's history to avoid unnecessary diagnostic testing or drug therapy.

Medication Use
The risk of adverse drug reactions in older patients is two to three times greater than that for younger patients because of polypharmacy, age-related changes in pharmacokinetics and pharmacodynamics, greater severity of medical illness, and changes in body composition (52). Prescription or over-the-counter medications may cause undesirable symptoms, such as weakness, at therapeutic or toxic drug levels.

Certain medications are notorious for their potential deleterious effects in older patients. For example, digoxin may cause problems even at therapeutic serum levels (53). Simultaneous use of antiarrhythmic agents such as verapamil or quinidine increases serum digoxin levels and the risk of toxicity. Concomitant usage of diuretics may contribute to hypokalemia-induced arrhythmia. Antiarrhythmic drugs such as mexilitine, quinidine, and procainamide may cause weakness and fatigue and should be limited to use in symptomatic patients. Potassium-wasting diuretics may cause hypokalemia and weakness. Drug-induced hyponatremia and weakness may be seen with diuretics such as sulfonylurea, and fluoxetine. Hyperkalemia or renal insufficiency may occur in some older patients who are prescribed nonsteroidals, ACE-inhibitors, or potassium-sparing diuretics. Careful monitoring of medications and serum electrolytes can minimize problems with these medications.

Some drugs may cause delirium and weakness even at low doses. Psychotropic medications, benzodiazipines, and antihistamines all have this potential.

It is desirable for a patient to bring all medications to an initial office visit to establish an accurate medication history. Medicines should be reviewed and doses verified and recorded at each subsequent office visit to minimize errors and diminish the likelihood of adverse drug reactions. All unnecessary medications should be discontinued and discarded. Written instructions should accompany a detailed verbal description of the proper dosage, purpose of the drug, and possible side effects. In demented patients, a responsible caregiver should receive the instructions. These prescribing practices can reduce the incidence of adverse drug reactions in the elderly.

Metabolic Abnormalities
Disturbances in potassium, sodium, or calcium levels may cause weakness. Weakness and fatigue are frequently presenting symptoms of endocrine disorders such as thyroid disease, adrenal insufficiency, parathyroid disease, or diabetes. Azotemia and renal failure may also cause these symptoms. Anemia, a marker for a wide array of hematological and medical diseases, may be discovered during a workup for the complaint of weakness.

Neuromuscular Weakness
Complaints of weakness that are limited to a specific body region or are gradual in onset with reduced muscle strength are suggestive of a neuromuscular disorder. Questions about functional abilities (ability to rise from a chair, climb stairs, perform self-care activities) are useful in differentiating true weakness caused by neuromuscular disease from generalized fatigue, which is more consistent with a systemic illness. Muscle atrophy, fasciculations, and normal sensation usually accompany muscle weakness in patients with motor neuron diseases such as ALS.

Peripheral nerve disease is suggested by sensory abnormalities and distal muscle weakness. Common causes in the elderly include diabetes mellitus, alcohol toxicity, vitamin B_{12} deficiency, and autonomic dysfunction.

A diagnosis of myopathy is suggested in a patient with impaired proximal muscle strength, relative preservation of reflexes, normal sensation, and weakness of gradual onset. Acquired myopathies include polymyositis, thyroid disease, alcohol toxicity, and steroid-induced.

Myasthenia gravis characteristically has ocular involvement and fluctuating fatigability of muscles.

Progressive or fixed neurological deficits may occur with strokes or subdural hematoma. The patient's history and physical examination should help distinguish these clinical events from other disorders.

In early Parkinson's disease, a patient may first notice a change in energy level and functional abilities and may call this weakness. Until the hallmark features of this disorder are apparent (tremor, bradykinesia, masked facies), the diagnosis may be overlooked.

Other Medical Illnesses

Serious infections and malignancy may be a cause of weakness. Patients with polymyalgia rheumatica complain of proximal muscle weakness and generalized fatigue. An elevated sedimentation rate and anemia are laboratory clues to this diagnosis.

Myocardial infarction, cardiac ischemia, and arrhythmia need to be considered in elderly patients who complain of fatigue and weakness, especially when accompanied by dyspnea or reduced exercise capacity. Leg weakness that occurs when the patient walks may be the patient's description of intermittent claudication.

Laboratory testing is often comprehensive for a patient's complaint of weakness because of the wide range of diagnostic possibilities (Table 18.13). Testing should be supplemented with other screening procedures and x-rays depending on the patient's history and physical examination.

Treatment hinges on the diagnosis made after complete evaluation. Patients may also benefit from dietary modifications, vitamin supplements, and regular exercise. How-

Table 18.13. Initial Laboratory Evaluation of Weakness.

Blood chemistry
Chest x-ray
CBC
ECG
Erythrocyte sedimentation rate
Serum drug levels
Thyroid function tests
Urinalysis

CBC = complete blood cell count; ECG = electrocardiogram.
SOURCE: Modified from Gordon M. Differential diagnosis of weakness: a common geriatric symptom. Geriatrics 1986; 41:75.

ever, if no definite etiology can be determined, the physician should reassure the patient and avoid attributing symptoms to old age. Ongoing medical follow-up is important in these cases because other symptoms that help elucidate an underlying illness may emerge.

Sleep Disorders

Physicians caring for older adults will likely be challenged when they address sleep-related complaints (55). The high prevalence of sleep complaints from older individuals has made this problem almost accepted as a normal, age-related phenomenon. Nevertheless, the physician should give thoughtful consideration to this issue.

A review of more than twenty studies completed between 1931 and 1971 concluded that older subjects spend more time in bed despite decreased sleep time, have increased nocturnal awakenings and sleep latency, and take more daytime naps (56). A study of almost 2500 persons aged 65 to 75 years demonstrated that 15 percent of older subjects arise before 5 A.M. and sleep less than 5 hours per night. Twenty-five percent of men and 40 percent of women over age 65 describe themselves as "light sleepers" (57). Karacan (58) studied 1645 individuals over age 16 and found that 45 percent had trouble falling asleep and that this complaint increased with age. The use of sleeping pills increases with age and is more common in women. The study found that 10 percent of respondents used medication for sleep. Interestingly, mortality rates are higher for those who us sleeping pills and for those who sleep less than 7 hours per night (59).

A number of well-documented neurophysiologic changes in sleep do occur with aging, and their clinical relevance is a topic of intense research. Despite much knowledge regarding the electroencephalographic stages of sleep and associated changes with age, the aggregate significance of these changes is not yet well synthesized. Normal sleep consists of rapid eye movement (REM) sleep and non-REM sleep. The latter is categorized in stages 0 through 4. A typical night of sleep for a young adult begins with a short period of stage 1 (descending) and stage 2 (unequivocal) sleep, followed by longer periods of stage 3 (deep), and stage 4 (cerebral) sleep. In 1 to 2 hours, REM sleep begins. The cycle repeats every 90 minutes. REM periods lengthen and alternate with non-

REM stages 2 or 3. Approximately 4 to 6 REM periods occur nightly and account for 20 percent to 25 percent of all sleep.

For older adults, stages 3 and 4 sleep are significantly decreased, with some individuals having no stage 4 sleep; more time is spent in stage 1 in a typical night. REM sleep periods grow shorter as one ages, but occur with the same frequency as they do in younger adults (60).

Obtaining an accurate sleep history from the patient is essential because treatment is contingent on this information. Common terms used to describe sleep are found in Table 18.14. Since many people have difficulty in relating accurate information regarding sleep patterns, it is helpful to have information from a patient's bed partner or some other close observer of the patient.

Many medical problems have impact on the quality of sleep. Any respiratory symptom such as cough, wheezing, paroxysmal nocturnal dyspnea, orthopnea, or sleep apnea can result in insomnia. Congestive heart failure, emphysema, and asthma are a few conditions that can precipitate these symptoms. A study of healthy, elderly individuals (mean age, 73 years) revealed that 27.5 percent had more than five sleep disturbances per hour that resulted in some degree of arousal (61). Nighttime arousals seem to increase with age and their etiologies must be explored. For example, true sleep apnea (cessation of airflow for more than 10 seconds during sleep) was found in 37.5 percent of older subjects (mean age, 72.7 years) and may go unrecognized in elderly individuals (61). Although the classic image of an individual with sleep

apnea is that of an obese man who snores and has daytime somnolence, the presentations in older individuals may not be classic in nature.

Any condition that causes pain can disturb sleep. Osteoarthritis, peptic ulcer disease, or other chronic abdominal pain (e.g., reflux), and angina pectoris commonly effect the quality of sleep. Nocturnal myoclonus (restless leg syndrome) may cause frequent nocturnal awakenings. Nocturnal leg cramps caused by vascular disease may lend themselves to medical or surgical treatment, and appropriate workup should be initiated.

Nocturia is very common in older persons. More than two-thirds of healthy men and women over age 65 arise at night to urinate. The incidence rises in those who take certain medications or who have chronic diseases that lead to increased urinary output. Diuretic therapy, benign prostatic hypertrophy, congestive heart failure, poorly controlled diabetes, or loss of bladder distensibility can lead to nocturia.

A variety of sleep disorders can be caused by prescription and over-the-counter medications. Such drugs should be reviewed carefully to determine whether they play a role in a patient's sleep disturbance. Caffeine, decongestants, and certain antidepressants can cause unwanted excitation. Dosages should be reviewed at each visit.

The relationship between psychiatric disturbances and sleep disorders is both interesting and important. In recognizing that sleep disturbances of any type can be associated with depression, the physician must be vigilant in assessing this potential association. Roehrs and Lineback (62) identified that more sleep disturbances occur in age-matched subjects with psychiatric illness than with those without psychopathology. However, a short form of the Minnesota Multiphasic Personality Inventory revealed a significantly higher frequency of abnormal scores in younger subjects with sleep disorders than in older subjects (61). Adjustment disorders, generalized anxiety, bereavement, and other affective disorders can result in disturbances of sleep architecture. Treating depression with co-existing sleep disorders with a sedating tricyclic antidepressant or an agent such as trazadone is often helpful.

Quite often, improvements in sleep practices can ameliorate the patient's problem and allow the individual to

Table 18.14. Terms Relating to Sleep.

Term	Definition
Time in bed	Time spent in bed, regardless of actual sleep
Total sleep time	Total time spent asleep during nocturnal time in bed
Sleep difficulty	Ratio of total sleep time at night to total nocturnal time in bed
Sleep latency	Time from deciding to sleep and turning the lights out until actually sleeping
Wake after sleep onset	Arousal from sleep in which periods of brief or prolonged wakefulness occur between time of sleep onset and final awakening

avoid medications. Daytime napping should be limited to no more than one 30 to 60 minute nap in the afternoon. Caffeine should be avoided if the individual is sensitive to its effects. Alcoholic beverages are sometimes used as an aid to sleep, but they often result in a subtle withdrawal that can actually exacerbate the sleep problem. Quite often, people cannot sleep because, simply, they are not tired. Therefore, exercise can become an integral part of the solution and should take place early in the day.

When nonpharmacologic methods fail, the physician may elect to use a sedative-hypnotic agent (Table 18.15). Sedatives promote sleep by relaxing the patient; hypnotics induce sleep and decrease sleep latency, and therefore, improve sleep efficiency (63). Sedative-hypnotics are known to decrease REM sleep. When a benzodiazepine is chosen, the physician should select an agent with a short half-life to avoid the patient's having daytime drowsiness and problems of gait and balance. Low-dose, short-acting benzodiazepines can be used for a brief period on an as needed basis, but tolerance to these medications develops quickly. They can exacerbate sleep apnea and dull cognition and memory. Antihistamines can also cause confusion, dry mouth, constipation, and gait disturbances because of their anticholinergic properties.

Benzodiazepines are well known for their association with falls (64,65). Medications that have half-lives longer than 24 hours significantly increase the patient's risk of hip fracture related to falls. Patients with chronic illnesses and dementia who take benzodiazepines are also more likely to sustain falls and related injuries (66).

Pharmacologic therapy can be employed safely if the physician individualizes the choice of agent, and remains aware of age-related pharmacokinetics, duration of use, and potential side effects. An ongoing dialogue can be helpful in a patient's transition from drug to nondrug therapy.

References

1. Robbins LJ. Evaluation of weight loss in the elderly. Geriatrics 1989;44:31–35.
2. Marton KI, Sox HC, Krupp JR. Involuntary weight loss: diagnostic and prognostic significance. Ann Intern Med 1981; 95:568–574.
3. Rabinowitz M, Pitlik SD, Leifer M, et al. Unintentional weight loss. A retrospective analysis of 154 cases. Arch Intern Med 1986;146:186–187.
4. Morley JE. Anorexia in older patients: its meaning and management. Geriatrics 1990;45:59–66.
5. Morley JE, Silver AJ, Miller DK, Rubenstein LZ. The anorexia of the elderly. NY Acad Sci 1989;575:50–59.
6. Morley JE. Neuropeptide regulation of appetite and weight. Endocr Rev 1987;256–287.
7. Gorbien MJ. Cardiac cachexia. In: Morley JE, Glick Z, Rubenstein LZ, eds. Geriatric nutrition: a comprehensive review. New York: Raven, 1990:315–324.
8. Sullivan DH, Martin W, Flaxman N, Hagen JE. Oral health problems and involuntary weight loss in a population of frail elderly. J Am Geriatr Soc 1993;41:725–731.
9. National Center for Health Statistics. Health statistics on older persons, United States—1986. Vital and Health Statistics, Series 3, No. 25. Washington DC: US Government Printing Office, DHHS Publ. No. (PHS)87-1409, 1987.
10. Morley JE. Nutritional status of the elderly. Am J Med 1986;81:679–695.
11. Morley JE, Reese SS. Clinical implications of the aging heart. Am J Med 1989;86:77–86.
12. Thompson MP, Morris LK. Unexplained weight loss in the ambulatory elderly. J Am Geriatr Soc 1991;91:497–500.
13. Tchekmedyian NS, et al. Megestrol acetate in cancer anorexia and weight loss. Cancer 1992;69:1268–1274.
14. Von Roenn JH, Murphy RL, Weber KM, et al. Megestrol acetate for treatment of cachexia associated with human immunodeficiency virus (HIV) infection. Ann Intern Med 1988;109:840–841.
15. Kaiser FE, Silver AJ, Morley JE. The effect of recombinant human growth hormone on malnourished older individuals. J Am Geriatr Soc 1991;39:235–240.
16. Stedman's Medical Dictionary. 23rd ed. Baltimore: Williams & Wilkins, 1976:313.
17. Milne JS, Williamson J. Bowel habits in older people. Gerontol Clin 1972;14:56–60.
18. Donald IP, Smith RG, Cruikshank JG, et al. A study of consti-

Table 18.15. Medications Used to Treat Insomnia.

Drug	Half-life (hrs)	Recommended Starting Dose (mg)
Estazolam	10–24	1
Lorazepam	10–20	0.5
Oxazepam	5–20	10
Temazepam	9.5–12.4	7.5
Triazolam	1.5–5.5	0.125
Zolpidem tartrate	≈2.5	5

SOURCE: Reproduced by permission from Gorbien MJ. When your older patient won't sleep: how to put insomnia to rest. Geriatrics 1993;48:72.

pation in the elderly living at home. Gerontology 1985; 31:112–118.

19. Connell AM, Hilton C, Irvine G, et al. Variation of bowel habits in two population samples. BMJ 1965;2:1095–1099.

20. Whitehead WE, Drinkwater D, Chestkin LJ, et al. Constipation in the elderly living at home – definition, prevalence and relationship to lifestyle and health states. J Am Geriatr Soc 1989;37:423–429.

21. Melkerson M, Andersson H, Bosaeus I, Falkheden T. Intestinal transit time in constipated and non-constipated geriatric patients. Scand J Gastroenterol 1983;18:593–597.

22. Cummings JH, Jenkins DJ, Wiggins HS, et al. Measurement of mean transit time of dietary residue through the human gut. Gut 1976;17:210–218.

23. Shouler P, Keighley MRB. Changes in colorectal function in severe idiopathic chronic constipation. Gastroenterology 1986;90:414–420.

24. Wright BA, Staats DO. The geriatric implications of fecal impactions. Nurse Pract 1986;11:53–66.

25. Read NW, Abouzekry L, Read MG, et al. Anorectal function in patients with fecal impaction. Gastroenterology 1988; 89:959–966.

26. Wrenn K. Fecal impaction. N Engl J Med 1989;321:658–661.

27. Gorbien MJ. Constipation in the elderly. Ger Med Today 1988;7:53–63.

28. Castle SC. Constipation. A pressing issue. Arch Intern Med 1987;147:1702–1704.

29. Beauregard S, Gilchrest BA. A survey of skin problems and skin care regimens in the elderly. Arch Dermatol 1987; 123:1638–1643.

30. Fleischer Ab. Pruritus in the elderly: management by senior dermatologists. J Am Acad Dermatol 1993;28:603–609.

31. Greaves MW. Pathophysiology and clinical aspects of pruritus. In: Fitzpatrick TB, Eisen AZ, Wolff K, et al, eds. Dermatology in general medicine. 4th ed. New York: McGraw-Hill, 1993:313–421.

32. Greaves MW. Pruritus. In: Champion RH, Burton JL, Ebling FJG, eds. Textbook of dermatology. 5th ed. Boston: Blackwell Science, 1992:527–535.

33. Greco PJ, Ende J. An office-based approach to the patient with pruritus. Hosp Pract 1992;27:121–128.

34. Greco PJ, Ende J. Pruritus: a practical approach. J Gen Intern Med 1992;7:340–349.

35. Phillips WG. Pruritis. What to do when the itching won't stop? Postgrad Med 1992;92:34–36, 39–40, 43–46.

36. Kantor GR. Evaluation and treatment of generalized pruritus. Cleve Clin J Med 1990;57:521–526.

37. Fisher AA. Allergic reactions to topical (surface) anesthetics with reference to the safety of tronothane (pramoxine hydrochloride). Cutis 1980;25:584, 586, 589–91, 625.

38. Woodward JK. Pharmacology and toxicology of nonclassical antihistamines. Cutis 1988;42:5–9.

39. Braman SS, Correo WM. Cough: difficult diagnosis and treatment. Clin Chest Med 1987;8:177–188.

40. Donnerberg RL, Dixon GI. Pulmonary disease in the practice of geriatrics. In: Calbins E, Davis PJ, Ford AB, eds. Geriatrics Philadelphia: WB Saunders 1986:327–338.

41. Allen SC. Aging and the respiratory system. In: Brocklehurst JC, Tallis RC, Fillit HM, eds. Textbook of geriatric medicine and gerontology. 4th ed. London: Churchill-Livingstone 1992:739–767.

42. O'Connell EJ, Rojas AR, Sachs MI. Cough-type asthma: a review. Ann Allergy 1991;66:278–285.

43. Stoller JK, Mehta AC, Vidt DG. Captopril-induced cough. Chest 1988;93:659–660.

44. Irwin RS, Curley FJ. The diagnosis of chronic cough. Hosp Pract 1988;23:82–92.

45. U.S. Dept. of Health, Education, and Welfare. Prevalence of selected chronic respiratory conditions. Vital Health Statements No. 84. Washington DC: US Government Printing Office, 1970.

46. U.S. Veterans Study. Am Med News 1984.

47. Irwin RS, Curley FJ. The treatment of cough: a comprehensive review. Chest 1991;99:1477–1484.

48. Hendeles L. Efficacy and safety of antihistamines and expectorants in non-prescription cough and cold preparations. Pharmacotherapy, 1993;13:154–158.

49. Gay M, Blazer F, Bartsek K, et al. Psychogenic habit cough: review and case reports. J Clin Psychiatry, 1987;14:12:483–486.

50. Waltman RE. Weakness. In: Yoshikawa TT, Cobbs EL, Brummel-Smith K, eds. Ambulatory geriatric care. St. Louis: Mosby-Year Book, 1993; Chapt. 33.

51. National Institutes of Health. Consensus statement. The diagnosis and treatment of depression. JAMA 1992;268:1018–1024.

52. Nolan L, O'Malley K. Prescribing for the elderly. Part I. Sensitivity of the elderly to adverse drug reactions. J Am Geriatr Soc 1988;36:142–149.

53. Morley JE, Reeve SS. Clinical implications of the aging heart. Am J Med 1989;86:77–86.

54. Gordon M. Differential diagnosis of weakness: a common geriatric symptom. Geriatrics 1986;41:75.

55. Gorbien MJ. When your older patient won't sleep: how to put insomnia to rest. Geriatrics 1993;48:65–75.

56. Miles LE, Dement WE. Sleep and aging. Sleep 1980;3:119–220.

57. McGhie A, Russell S. The subjective assessment of normal sleep patterns. J Ment Sci 1962;10:238–244.

58. Karacen I, Thornby J, Anch M, et al. Prevalence of sleep disturbance in a primarily urban Florida county. Soc Sci Med 1976;10:239–244.

59. Kripke D, Simons R, Garfindel L, et al. Short and long sleep and sleeping pills. Arch Gen Psychiatry, 1979;36:103–116.

60. Dement W, Miles L, Carskadon M. "White paper" on sleep and aging. J Am Geriatr Soc 1982;30:25–50.

61. Carskadon M. Respiration during sleep in the elderly. J Am Ger Soc 1982;30:312–315.

62. Roehrs T, Lineback W, Zorick F, et al. Relationship of psycho-

pathology to insomnia in the elderly. J Am Ger Soc 1982;
30:312–315.

63. Roth T. Pharmacological and medical considerations in hypnotic use. Sleep 1982;5:546–552.

64. Ray W, Griffin M, Schaffner W. Psychotropic drug use and the risk of hip fracture. N Engl J Med 1987;316:363–406.

65. Greenblatt D, Allen M, Shader R. Toxicity of high dose flurazepam in the elderly. Clin Pharmacol Ther 1977;21:355–361.

66. Tinetti M, Williams T, Mayewski R. Fall risk index for elderly patients based on number of chronic disabilities. Am J Med 1986;80:429–434.

Chapter 19
Ethical Aspects of Geriatric Care

Stephen G. Post

The young man knows the rules but the old man knows the exceptions.

Oliver Wendell Holmes
Old Age is not for Sissies

The exponential growth of biomedical technology empowers geriatricians to do more than they ever have to rescue elderly people from death (1). Against this background, one task of geriatric ethics is to prevent overtreatment that may occur when elderly people are subject to biomedical technology (2). Continuing communication between the physician and individual patients and their families regarding their objectives in treatment and whether these objectives can be realistically achieved is the salutary and proper response. The possibility of undertreatment requires the physician to advocate optimal medical care while adhering to the principle that the competent patient has the final power of decision. But geriatric ethics is not only about making good decisions; it is also about care in the sense of solicitude or anxiety about the well-being of the patient. Quandary ethics or decisionism is no more important than virtue and character (3). Good decisions are negotiated with patients in the communicative context that solicitude and loyalty alone establish. Continuity of care with a primary physician is essential.

This chapter focuses on communicative ethics with undemented and demented patients and their families and addresses a number of pressing ethical issues that confront the contemporary geriatrician.

Communicative Ethics

No physician can practice the art of medicine as a mere technician, for moral values are inherent in the goals of restoring health or providing palliation and comfort care (4). The geriatrician must, if necessary, actively generate concern in patients that futile or nonbeneficial use of technology should be avoided; the physician should voice his or her moral conscience in relation to patients, families, and society. According to Hippocratic tradition, the practitioner of medicine can countenance only that which is beneficial to patients. The mainstays of the Hippocratic tradition are "do no harm," beneficence, confidentiality, and justice. Over the past several decades, the principles of respect for patient autonomy and the correlative of truth telling have ascended in the context of a wide cultural revolt against authority and evidence indicating that patients are, in general, benefitted by veracity (5).

Patient autonomy was most recently confirmed with the passage of the Patient Self-Determination Act (PSDA), a federal law that went into effect in December 1991. All home health care agencies, hospitals, nursing homes, hospices, and health maintenance organizations receiving Medicaid or Medicare dollars must present patients with written statements of their rights to accept or refuse treatments under state law as well as their right to prepare advance directives. Although it is arguable that the act imposes on some patient groups, many older patients will eventually face decisions of life and death, and the act should encourage clarification of values through substantial communication with physicians. Unfortunately, the act does not require the primary physician to initiate the discussion of rights and values, which would enable an admissions clerk to make papers available routinely to patients.

The morally and legally established shift away from the classic image of the healer who decides strictly in accord with his or her judgment to the current image of the healer who must consider patient values and autonomy *never* reduces the physician to a mere technician stripped of moral conscience and voice. The geriatrician makes treatment recommendations directly or indirectly by words used to present and describe options to the patient. The idea of a value-neutral physician is both impossible and wrong. Respect for patient autonomy requires the geriatrician to engage in active communication with patients, listening attentively to the patient's goals, but articulating his or her views on whether those goals are realistic and whether specific treatments are beneficial. Physician and patient are usually able to reach a consensus on the basis of good communication (6). In cases of deep-felt disagreement, the geriatrician can, for reasons of conscience, refer a patient to another competent physician who may accommodate that patient's decision (7).

Some geriatricians are raising the moral voice, arguing that certain treatments are futile or devoid of benefit and therefore ought not to be provided, although the precise definition of futility remains a matter of ongoing debate. Nevertheless, the physician must communicate to patients and families why he or she considers a treatment futile (8). Good communication is essential to conveying the meaning of futility to a particular patient or family without insensitivity or creating unnecessary despair (9). In this process, futility must not be used to mask other logically distinct moral concerns, such as quality of life, which deserves discussion on its own terms (10). For example, the geriatrician who believes that patients with severe or terminal dementia should receive only palliative and comfort care because of the quality of life should explain this view and offer families the opportunity to pursue another physician. Studies of geriatricians indicate tremendous variation in opinion on quality of life, dementia, and treatment levels (11).

The duties of the geriatrician in communicative ethics *always* go beyond merely laying out for the patient a laundry list of treatment options, either verbally or with the help of a written directive. The ethical geriatrician must personally communicate, recommend, and carefully negotiate reasonable medical decisions with autonomous patients or their families (12). That patient autonomy holds trump in decision making does not require the physician to relinquish the classic commitment to the patient's good, although that good now includes the patient's values (13). The good geriatrician is a moderate autonomist and a moderate patient welfarist.

There is danger in the overemphasis on patient autonomy if this means the loss of any concern with the patient's good and a moral abandonment in the garb of respect for patient self-determination. Whenever a patient refuses treatment that is clearly in his or her best interests or requests what is reasonably deemed futile, the geriatrician is obliged to engage in substantial conversation rather than agree with the first words a patient utters. The moral tension between respect for patient autonomy and the patient's good is both necessary and creative (14). This tension defines many moral dilemmas (15).

The example of cardiopulmonary resuscitation (CPR) further illustrates communicative ethics. Too often geriatric patients are provided with a paper form in which they merely check "yes" or "no" to CPR. But a paper form is meaningful only if it symbolizes a continual communication (16). Physicians should always inform patients of the probabilities of failure and success, of what "success" means, and of the extensive trauma sometimes associated with CPR, which may include the breaking of ribs. In a 4-year study of Milwaukee nursing homes, 196 people received CPR and were admitted to hospitals. Only 19 percent survived, and a mere 5 percent (10 patients) became well enough to return to the nursing homes (17). The responsible geriatrician must present such data in simple terms to competent elderly people for them to make realistic choices; a physician may go so far as to recommend against CPR, although the "do not resuscitate" (DNR) decision rests with patient or family. Physicians are not required to present information to patients in a value-neutral and unbiased fashion, and, in many cases, they should not (18).

Treatment Refusal and Withdrawal

Although two decades ago treatment refusal and withdrawal ("passive euthanasia") was morally and legally controversial, it is now clearly established that all competent people of age have a right to refuse or to request withdrawal of any medical technology, including artificial nutrition and hydration.

The words "active euthanasia" and "passive euthanasia" suggest two instances of a continuum of the same action. It is perhaps better to speak of "killing" and "allowing to die," which emphasizes a moral difference between aiming to end a life and removing treatment knowing that, if the patient continues to live, he or she will be cared for steadfastly. In the second instance, if the patient does die, the result is the same as killing, but what the physician *does* and *becomes* as an intentional moral agent is very different. In the withdrawal of treatment, a covenant of care and support remains, demonstrating that the intent underlying withdrawal of treatment is not death, but relief of technological bondage (19).

It is much clearer ethically to speak of refusal, withdrawal, assisted suicide, and finally euthanasia, reserving the latter term strictly for cases in which death is caused directly by one person through injection or some other impingement upon another, even if requested. Euthanasia, then, refers to "mercy killing," although because of tremendous advances in palliative care and preserving lucidity, a better term might be "control killing," a final assertion of human control over the moment of death previously left in the hands of nature or of nature's God (20).

Some physicians feel that withdrawal of treatment is ethically unacceptable but refusal of treatment is not. In other words, they will agree not to start a treatment, but once it is started, they will not withdraw it. However much standard philosophical analysis indicates that these actions are indistinguishable, the psychological fact is that withdrawing treatment makes the physician feel that he or she is more directly responsible for death. There is action in "pulling the plug." Although these feelings are understandable, they should not be morally determinative (21). Typically, the physician has the responsibility to the patient to experiment with interventions and determine their efficacy or futility so that the patient or the patient's proxies can make judgments based on greater certitude.

Some physicians are concerned that ordinary treatment should be neither refusable nor withdrawable. But what is extraordinary treatment today may be ordinary treatment tomorrow; thus, the distinction is unhelpful. However, the physician can rightfully reject any requests to refuse or withdraw palliative care, because the art of medicine includes the removal of pain as well as promotion of healing. Palliative care may have the unintended side effect of extending life.

Assisted Suicide and Euthanasia

A classic and valid objective of medicine is to remove suffering but not the sufferer. If the citizens of some states

in the U.S. passed referendums that pushed the art of medicine beyond treatment refusal and withdrawal to physician-assisted suicide or to voluntary euthanasia, many physicians would resist such requests because they consider assisted suicide and euthanasia contrary to the healing and palliative goals of medicine. This is a plausible argument emerging from consideration of the art of medicine and should not be confused with the art of killing. For this reason physicians do not participate in capital punishment by lethal injection.

In the event that assisted suicide and euthanasia referendums are passed, physicians can insist that these policies not be implemented without the development of enhanced comfort care, palliation, and long-term care. Assisted suicide and voluntary euthanasia, if legalized, must follow, not preempt, implementation of a comprehensive, nationwide care program for the dying and the dependent. This is especially relevant for frail elderly people. If good palliation, comfort care, and long-term care cannot be provided as a first option, then assisted suicide or euthanasia, while ostensibly voluntary, will in fact be matters of default rather than of genuine selection from existing alternatives. The incompatibility thesis states: in a health care system that fails to provide adequate palliative and comfort care for the dying, or long-term care for the dependent and elderly, an increased toleration for and perhaps legalization of assisted suicide and voluntary euthanasia would likely remove the social pressure for improved care. Assisted suicide and euthanasia could easily become the only options, and thus forced options.

In the event that policies permitting assisted suicide or voluntary euthanasia are implemented without a fully adequate care system being established first, it can be reasonably anticipated that these policies would diminish the political will to develop a care system. There are the risk of (1) diverting funds from hospice and long-term care; (2) undermining the training of physicians, nurses, and others for hospice and long-term care; and (3) diminishing research in palliation or in better long-term care design. These are all areas of marginal investment in our current health care system. Albert R. Jonsen, who opposes assisted suicide, asks, "If pain can be ended by the death of the patient, why persist in the careful titration of medicine and emotional support that relieves pain and, at the same time, supports life?" (22). Jonsen marshals his line of argument in a categorical criticism of assisted suicide and euthanasia.

Others are concerned with the incompatibility thesis, but in the final analysis this does not deter them from defending assisted suicide. An article by Timothy E. Quill et al defends assisted suicide, but still supports enhanced palliation and comfort care, for when properly applied such care usually results in a tolerable death (23). Physician-assisted suicide, the authors contend, should not become a substitute for comprehensive comfort care, which must "at least have been considered" and preferably tried. Thus, an important articulation of guidelines for physician-assisted suicide takes the incompatibility thesis seriously enough to urge the hospice option as a first resort. The authors do not require this as a first resort, although they recommend it.

Perhaps the availability of assisted suicide and euthanasia would spur opponents of these practices to mobilize resources and develop a state-of-the-art hospice and long-term care system. However, in hard economic times, such an effort may not garner widespread support, especially because assisted suicide and mercy killing are cost efficient.

Geriatricians, because they care for many frail people whose social worth in an age-conscious society can be marginal, have a special obligation to encourage the enhancement of old age, not its termination. Alzheimer's disease is on the cutting edge of the national and international debate over physician-assisted suicide. Although requests for suicide from the terminally ill are often shaped by untreated pain and inadequate psychosocial conditions, what should be done about requests by people with diagnoses of progressive dementia?

Reports consistently indicate that in the Netherlands, where assisted suicide and mercy killing are accepted, about 10 percent of requests come from patients with chronic, degenerative neurological disorders (24). Margaret P. Battin writes of progressive dementia: "This is the condition the Dutch call *entluistering*, the 'effacement' or complete eclipse of human personality, and for the Dutch, *entluistering* rather than pain is a primary reason for choices of [active] euthanasia" (25). Battin makes a partial defense of assisted suicide or mercy killing in cases of progressive dementia if requested by a living will or by personal directive.

In 1990, Jack Kevorkian assisted Janet Adkins in suicide. She was a 54-year-old member of the Hemlock Society, had been diagnosed with Alzheimer's disease, was happily married with three grown sons, was intellectually very active, and was horrified by the prospects of decline. One year after diagnosis, she perceived the "first symptoms" of dementia and assisted suicide soon followed. Although many would not accept such an early, preemptive suicide as morally justifiable, one surmises that many in our society would prefer to be killed rather than endure the more severe stages of dementia. People justifiably fear progressive neurodegenerative diseases that dismantle the self.

But if assisted suicide and euthanasia were legally permitted before the development of good Alzheimer's disease care programs that enable patients to better adapt to their incapacities, then the incompatibility thesis would become relevant. Why invest in research, training, and facilities for dementia care when assisted suicide or euthanasia were already available and cheaper? Because of the likelihood that impact on investment would be negative, the appropriate compromise may be firm avoidance of assisted suicide policies and the further development of supportive environments that can enhance quality of life for patients with dementia.

The incompatibility thesis can be extended beyond dementia care to the care of the aged in general. For example, Derek Humphrey of the National Hemlock Society suggests that elderly people are crying out for death. He argues that old age is "sufficient cause to give up" even without unbearable suffering. It is a preemptive alternative to growing old. He presents the case of a recently widowed Hemlock Society member who at 85 took an overdose of medication and died: "There was no terminal illness, but her horror of having a stroke and spending her final years in the hospital was unbearable now that her beloved husband was gone and her children grown and scattered" (26). The woman's neighbor had called Humphrey and remarked that just the previous day the woman had been walking happily in the garden. Humphrey reminded the caller that the woman was a "regular attender of Hemlock conferences for years and had clearly thought the matter through very thoroughly." At no point does Humphrey consider the possibility that improved social supports might provide an alternative to preemptive suicide among elderly people.

If assisted suicide and mercy killing were to become the way of death for the elderly, a practice defended in C.G. Prado's book on preemptive suicide in advanced age, it is difficult to imagine continuing social commitment to institutions that enhance the quality of life for those who grow old (27). In a society in which the traditional teaching functions of the elderly have all but disappeared, it is regretfully easy for the choice of preemptive suicide to become the expected one.

Assessing Competency

Another area in which considerable misconception exists is in judgments of competency, important because, once made, they remove self-determination from the affected person. Competency judgments are made for specific tasks, principally with respect to a patient's decisions about finances and about medical care. A person may lack competency to handle financial affairs but still have a sense of self-identity and the ability to make decisions about place of residence and medical care. It is imperative to take seriously those areas of competence that remain as dementia progresses to avoid premature judgments of global incompetency.

It is contrary to human dignity to judge people incompetent without justification, as can occur when specific competencies are not distinguished. The judgment of incompetency is morally significant because it effectively removes a human being from the sphere of moral agency, denies liberty of choice, and justifies paternalistic powers of control. Not infrequently, pressure is exerted on psychiatrists by family members who, for their own convenience, desire a judgment of incompetence, or by physicians who wish to proceed with a treatment despite patient reluctance. Such pressure must be resisted.

In almost all cases, judgments of competency for medical decision making are made in health care settings without need for legal proceedings. Only judgments of competency with respect to property, usually made while the patient is living in the community, require a legal context to establish property guardianship in the absence of a durable power of attorney. People without family generally require competency assessment in the legal con-

text to assign guardians responsible for decision making. But in the clinical context, there is rarely a need to have recourse to courts. Judgments of competency are made informally, avoiding *de jure* technocracy.

Most determinations of competency in the health care setting are made by the attending physician, sometimes with the assistance of a psychiatrist. Such determinations make it important for geriatricians, more than other primary care specialists, to understand how to judge incompetency in their patients, many of whom are enfeebled. Judgments of specific competencies are sometimes difficult, but they are often remarkably straightforward, as when an elderly patient is obviously incoherent in conversation and has no insight into the consequences of a decision or its alternatives.

Such judgments usually occur when the patient is refusing a treatment that the geriatrician deems essential, and the standards for competency are often more stringent the greater the risk of harm to the patient. Thus, judgments of competency in the clinical setting are partially understandable as a negotiation at the interface of self-determination and objective best interests. If a patient refuses a clearly beneficial surgery that promises to restore a good quality of life, one would want a high standard of competence and measure of certitude; if the consequences of a decision are minor, the standards of competence can be lowered.

Geriatricians are often better able to assess competency than psychiatrists are because, as primary caregivers, geriatricians may know their patients over a long period of time and thus have greater knowledge of the variability of the patients' cognitive state. Competency for medical decision making requires an ability to communicate choices; understanding of the relevant information disclosed regarding diagnosis, prognosis, physician recommendations, and likely outcome (requiring memory for words and ideas, comprehension of meanings, and causal relations); and rational manipulation of information (28).

In dementia, periods of incompetence may exist with periods of relative lucidity. Intermittent competence should be used to advantage. Especially in the progression of dementia, sensitive and humane discussion and negotiation are necessary as each task-specific competency is dismantled by the disease.

Although it is vital that geriatricians communicate directly with the competent, elderly patient rather than assume that simply because people are old their autonomy can be circumvented, the solicitous family should be a significant part of the process of communication. In some cultural traditions that view the self as essentially social-familial, patients will not want to distinguish their autonomy from family wishes. However, in most cases, previously indicated wishes of the patient supersede, and, ideally, were conveyed to the family members before incompetence manifested.

Family Involvement

In cases of incompetency for medical decision making, the informal family conversation is the established ritual of American health care. Only in cases of family conflict is a case likely to go to court. Withdrawal or refusal of treatment requires judicial resolution when there is active dissent among interested parties (contentious and embattled families) that is resistant to informal resolution, when previous statements of the patient indicate desire for unlimited treatment ("do everything") that is now non-beneficial, and sometimes in cases on the legal frontier (e.g., rationing limited resources and removal of nutrition and hydration in states in which these practices remain highly controversial) (29).

With good communication skills, the physician and family can resolve to everyone's satisfaction cases that would otherwise be of legal concern. Discussions with the family should be entered in the patient's records and, when a difficult decision is negotiated, it is wise to have the records countersigned by family members.

A moral task of the geriatrician is to serve as a consensus builder. If the patient has attempted to extend his or her autonomy past the point of decisional incompetence via a living will, the geriatrician must support this. Ideally, the living will is combined with a Durable Power of Attorney for Health Care, so that an individual designated by the patient is free to make decisions in the instances in which a living will is almost impossible to interpret in the specific situation. The physician must be in close communication, offering information on the burdens and consequences of specific treatments and making recommendations. In the absence of a previously designated surrogate, the physician must find a representative family proxy, usually selected as a spokesperson by the

family if not specified by patient. The rule of thumb is that for nonminors this representative will be the spouse, an adult child, siblings, or parents, in lexical priority. The goal of communication ethics is mutual, informal agreement.

Practically, the physician should ask family members not what they would like to do but rather what they think the patient would have wanted (substituted judgment). The geriatrician has the expert knowledge to focus discussion on broad outcome goals. If the patient would have accepted treatment in the hospital so as to return home, that goal should be indicated as possible or as no longer achievable. If the geriatrician knows with reasonable certainty that the patient's death is imminent, he or she can encourage familial acceptance and perhaps wait a few days to suggest treatment withdrawal once the family has adjusted emotionally. With older patients, it is important to communicate with a family member who is also old, because adult children may not share the same lifespan perspective on mortality (30). Once desired outcomes are clear, specific decisions generally fall into line.

It has been reported that about half of elderly patients with living wills would want family to make medical decisions in case of incompetency (31). Therefore, it is important for the physician to ask patients how seriously they would want their living wills to be considered, given a preference to entrust loved ones. The readiness to place decisions ultimately in the hands of family members is to be expected because of the social nexus of values shared by the family unit, and this is consistent with the general practice in medicine to rely on family members to make decisions for incompetent patients. The preferences of the elderly to rely on family to render surrogate decisions should continue to be protected as an informal institution in health care settings, even if occasionally recourse to the courts is necessary. As a general rule, the less legal involvement in intimate family decisions, the better.

Age-Based Rationing

Communicative ethics allows for individualized decision making (32) and allows patients' families, or both to work toward the best decision. Unless geriatricians give systematic attention to this form of decision making, they indirectly encourage popular support for assisted suicide (i.e., if physicians tend not to communicate and take patient values seriously, why should they not take the more reliable course) as well as support age-based cutoffs of beneficial treatments (i.e., if cost containment cannot be achieved in the physician-patient-family nexus, why should society not ration to achieve it). Age-based cutoffs for life-saving treatment have been endorsed by a number of important thinkers. Daniel Callahan is pessimistic about patients and geriatricians avoiding overtreatment (33). Critics have been more optimistic, and some have warned against "scapegoating the elderly" (34).

Briefly, there are four reasons against age-based rationing: 1) however imperfect some individual patient decision making may appear in retrospect, leaving choices about when to cease the struggle against death to personal conscience is preferable to draconian measures; 2) if society moves toward rationing experiments in health care distribution, this should presume an age-neutral framework that looks at particular conditions such as advanced dementia, advanced acquired immunodeficiency syndrome (AIDS), and neonatal intensive care rather than devaluing a demographic group, "the aged," which then must bear the entire burden; 3) age-based cutoffs disregard heterogeneity in the physical and psychological condition of elderly people; and 4) such cutoffs suggest that the wisdom and generativity of many elderly people is unimportant to society.

Assisted suicide and age-based cutoffs for life-saving treatment do succeed in challenging the geriatric community to take proactive and preemptive responsibility for the enhancement of good, individualized decision making that avoids overtreatment through the art of focused values communication.

Dementia Ethics

Because so many of the dilemmas of geriatric medical care involve patients with dementia, the remainder of this chapter is devoted to a brief overview of representative topics in dementia ethics.

Maintaining Solicitude

To maintain solicitude, the experience of people with dementia must not be interpreted against a background ideal of pure reason and self-control. What pictures shall we draw of the patient with dementia? No ethical question is more basic. If the pictures are sketched with achievement-oriented, socioeconomic, and cognitive values, harm results.

Metaphors commonly heard in discussions of patients with dementia are worthy of attention. Is the patient only a "shell" of his or her former self, a mere "husk?" Is the glass "half empty?" (35). Shall we think of dementia patients as "useless eaters," as "life unworthy of life?" Ethically, there is much at stake in the culture's metaphorical images of the experience of dementia, for these images surely shape our response to this growing moral challenge. Shall we nurture the well-being of people with dementia, shall we give them a disrespectful and insensitive pseudocare, shall we efficiently dispatch them to a prompt death?

These are not abstract and theoretical questions. The abuse of demented people is widespread. Jay Katz devoted the first chapter of *Experimentation with Human Subjects* to a case in Brooklyn's Jewish Chronic Disease Hospital (36). In July 1963, three physicians from Sloan-Kettering Memorial Hospital injected live cancer cells subcutaneously into 22 chronically ill, senile patients at the Jewish Chronic Disease Hospital. The physicians did not inform the subjects that live cancer cells were being used; they were willing to inflict potential wanton harm. Moreover, a considerable number of these subjects were demented. The purpose of the experiment was to measure immune response to see whether the cells would take hold and grow. Robert J. Levine lists this case, along with the Tuskegee syphilis study, the Willowbrook studies on hepatitis, and the San Antonio contraceptive study in which poor Mexican-American women seeking birth control were given placebos, as among examples of unethical research that directly fomented development of guidelines for research ethics in the 1970s (37).

From 1940 to 1945 an inconspicuous agency in Nazi Germany operated from offices in Berlin at Tiergartenstrasse 4. The "T-4 Project," begun in 1939 and concluded in 1941, was directed by Wurzburg Professor of Psychiatry, Werner Heyde. An estimated 94,000 psychiatric patients were killed—some in gas chambers, others in psychiatric hospitals and sanatoriums—with overdoses of sedatives. Many were demented, although the exact proportion is unknown (38). Demented people were dubbed "useless eaters" who wasted precious national resources. Such an attitude was in part grounded in the eugenic theories that shaped Nazi medical policies and granted moral consideration or standing only to the "fit," and cast aside the principle that the weak of mind and body are among us in part to strengthen our tendencies to solicitude for and tolerance of those whose lives are different.

In hard economic times, will we be solicitous? The question is pressing because Alzheimer's disease is common in older age groups who, in significant degree, are alive because of successful biomedical extension of the human lifespan. Alzheimer's disease afflicts an estimated 1 of 1000 people aged 60 to 65 years, 4 of 100 over age 65, and as many as half of those older than age 85 (39). As the population continues to age, financial burdens will increase. Will solicitude be too costly? There are currently nearly 4 million cases of Alzheimer's disease in the U.S.; 9 million cases are projected by the year 2040; recent analysis indicates that the total cost of caring for a patient with Alzheimer's disease in northern California is approximately $47,000 per year whether the patient lives at home or in a nursing home; the total U.S. national cost for Alzheimer's disease care is estimated at more than $100 billion (40).

Well-Being and Dementia

What is morally required for dementia care is a deep commitment to well-being; a commitment that sets aside bias against cognitive impairment. Tom Kitwood and Kathleen Bredin include 12 indicators of well-being in people with severe dementia: the assertion of will or desire, usually in the form of dissent despite coaxings; the ability to express a range of emotions; initiation of social contact (e.g., a person with dementia who has a small toy dog that he treasures places it before another person with dementia to attract attention); affectional warmth (e.g., a woman without much sociality who wanders back and forth in a facility but, when someone says hello to her, gives the person a kiss on the cheek and then continues her wandering); social sensitivity in the form of a smile or taking another's hand; self-respect (e.g., a woman who has defecated on the floor in the sitting room attempts to clean up after herself); acceptance of other sufferers of dementia (e.g., a fast wanderer who takes the hand of a

slow wanderer and leads the person); humor (e.g., when a person with severe dementia unexpectedly blurts out "Try putting a coin in the slot" when a technical problem with a video system develops); creativity and self-expression, often achieved through art or music therapy; showing evident pleasure through smiles and laughs in an exercise event; helpfulness, as in the case of a man who provided a cushion for a woman seated on a hard floor; and relaxation (e.g., a person with dementia who takes the hand of another who has a habit of lying on the floor tensely curled up and leads the person to a sofa where she relaxes) (41). These indicators "are virtually independent of the complex cognitive skills that most adults continuously employ," but they have tremendous importance and validity (p. 282). The goal of dementia care ethics is to enhance patient's well-being by facilitating a sense of personal worth, a sense of agency and social confidence, and a basic trust or security in the environment and in others.

Diagnostic Disclosure

In most situations, people with the probable diagnosis of Alzheimer's disease should be told their diagnosis. This disclosure can be empowering and beneficial when support groups (such as the Alzheimer's Association) are available to the person diagnosed and to the family, and when counseling and other services can be provided to facilitate emotional adjustment to the diagnosis. Even when support is limited, because many individuals already sense that something is wrong and may suspect Alzheimer's disease, a sensitive disclosure is often well received.

The diagnosis should be communicated by the physician in a meeting with the affected individual and family together, although in some cases it may be advantageous to inform family members first. The content, timing, and manner of disclosure must be appropriate for the affected person and family and be consistent with cultural variations and knowledge of family dynamics. Disclosure of diagnosis should occur with sufficient time allotted for questions from family and the person diagnosed and for recommendations from the physician or health care team. It is helpful to include an additional member of the health care team, such as a social worker or nurse, in the family meeting to follow up questions and discuss recommendations and resources. Another session to further discuss diagnosis and support systems is also beneficial (42).

With diagnostic disclosure comes the moral duty for the physician to direct the affected individual and family to available resources. A specific care plan should be discussed and agreed on, and in this nurses and social workers can be very helpful. The physician should emphasize the health care team's availability to give direct assistance or to make referrals; the physician should also stress that although the patient's dementia cannot be cured, efforts will be made to treat its effects and to assist the affected person and family in coping with the illness.

Among the advantages of telling individuals about their diagnosis are that executing advance directives (such as durable powers of attorney or living wills), obtaining consent for the patient to participate in Alzheimer's disease research, and preparing other forms of life planning and treatment planning become possible. Most important, disclosure permits active participation in psychological interventions, by the person with dementia, and thus helps to alleviate anger, self-blame, fear and depression.

Driving Privileges

Diagnosis of dementia is never itself sufficient reason for loss of driving privileges. An early and sensitive issue for people with dementia is limitation of driving privileges. Individuals with dementia are at risk of driving impairments, and if they are actually impaired, privileges must be limited for public safety (43). The obviously impaired person should not drive at all, and eventually all people with dementia must stop driving entirely. But people with mild dementia present a more complicated situation.

Individuals are often capable of driving for several years after their diagnosis, depending on the rate of disease progression (44). Often partial limits can be designed for the individual who may be able to drive safely in a familiar neighborhood, in daylight, or in good weather. Although there is an indisputable duty to prevent people from driving if they threaten community safety, the principle should not be applied prematurely or without individualized risk appraisal that demonstrates impairment of driving ability.

Duties of geriatricians to prevent dangerous driving are unclear, but mandatory reporting of people with demen-

tia has disadvantages. Mandatory reporting singles out people with dementia. Significantly, the most thorough recent study indicated that during the first 3 years after the onset of Alzheimer's disease, a person's risk of automobile crashes is well within the accepted range for other drivers, and that with unofficial restraints on driving (miles driven and familiar neighborhoods) along with informal termination of driving at a time decided by the person with dementia and his or her family, "the overall risk to society does not exceed a level well accepted for others groups of drivers." Indeed, the risk is considerably less than that for young men between the ages of 16 and 24 years. After 2 to 3 years have elapsed, most people with dementia stop driving (45).

Beyond the fact that unofficial and informal restrictions on driving suffice, mandated reporting of people with dementia raises serious questions about confidentiality. Such reporting may dissuade people with dementia from seeking help. More consistent with confidentiality, the physician can send a letter to the person with dementia and family reminding him or her of an agreement to limit driving, but implementation remains largely a matter of family responsibility.

Behavior Control

Family caregivers sometimes put tremendous pressure on the psychiatrist to do something quickly about patient behaviors that are offensive or frightening, and thus result in emotional strain. Our society has come to expect prompt control of such behaviors, often through chemical means. Caregivers may be dealing with various competing obligations, so that an aging parent in a delusional or agitated state is the straw that can break the caregiver's back. For these and other reasons, some of them economic, it is difficult to sustain the commitment to methods that are environmental and psychosocial rather than pharmacologic (46).

With specific reference to Alzheimer's disease and associated dementias, Richard J. Martin and Peter J. Whitehouse argued that "Behavioral interventions (i.e., making modifications in the environment) are generally preferable to medications for the treatment of most behavioral problems" (47). These authors point out that use of medications is important in cases of depression, psychosis, anxiety, and sleep disturbances. But they urge a cautious use of psychoactive drugs and offer two basic guidelines: 1) treatment should be purposeful, with the target symptom well defined, and 2) use of as few drugs as possible, low doses, slowly increased dosages, and careful monitoring for side effects. Polypharmacy and overmedication are particular problems in this patient population.

Nancy L. Mace suggests caution in using drugs to reduce disturbed behaviors (wandering, restlessness, irritability) "at dosages that interfere with remaining cognitive function and at which side effects occur" (48). Geriatricians must keep abreast of new research protocols that indicate control of patients' behavior at lower dosages than are customarily given. Mace also stresses the importance of first changing the patient's physical or psychosocial environment before drugs are used.

The range of moral issues in geriatric medicine is wide. In this chapter, consistent emphasis has been on communicative ethics because with this method most particular problems can be resolved successfully. The geriatrician must, in the care of each patient, deal with ethical issues and make the discussion of them a regular part of good practice. Everyday clinical ethics requires practical wisdom and experience and is the responsibility of every physician. Law can provide some framework for clinical ethics, but can never substitute for the moral duties of the physician.

References

1. Office of Technology Assessment. Life-sustaining technologies and the elderly. Washington, DC: U.S. Government Printing Office, 1987.
2. Winner L. Autonomous technology: technics out-of-control as a theme in political thought. Boston: MIT, 1977.
3. Pincoffs EL. Quandaries and virtues: against reductivism in ethics. Lawrence, Ks: University of Kansas, 1986.
4. Kass L. Toward a more natural science: biology and human affairs. New York: Free Press, 1985.
5. Beauchamp TL, Childress JF. Principles of biomedical ethics. New York: Oxford University, 1989.
6. Pellegrino ED, Thomasma DC. For the patient's good: the restoration of beneficence in health care. New York: Oxford University, 1988.
7. American Medical Association. Current opinions of the council on ethical and judicial affairs. Chicago: American Medical Association, 1993.
8. Miles SH. Informed demand for nonbeneficial medical treatment. N Engl J Med 1991;325:229–233.
9. Delvecchio MJ, Good BJ, Good CS, Lind SE. American oncology and the discourse on hope. Cult Med Psychiatry 1990; 14:59–79.
10. Birren JE, Lubben JE, Rowe CR, Deutchman DE, eds. The concept and measurement of quality of life in the frail elderly. New York: Academic Press, 1991.
11. Alemayehu E, Molloy DW, Guyatt GH, et al. Variability in physicians' decisions on caring for chronically ill elderly patients: an international study. Can Med Assoc J 1991; 144:1133–1138.
12. Katz J. The silent world of doctor and patient. New York: Free Press, 1984.
13. Moody HR. Ethics in an aging society. Baltimore: Johns Hopkins University, 1992.
14. Wicclair MR. Ethics and the elderly. New York: Oxford University, 1993.
15. Waymack MH, Taler GA. Medical ethics and the elderly: a case book. Chicago: Pluribus, 1988.
16. High DM. A new myth about families of older people? Gerontologist 1991;31:611–618.
17. Tresch AR. Outcomes of cardiopulmonary resuscitation in nursing homes: can we predict who will benefit? Am J Med 1993;95:123–130.
18. Lynn J. Conflicts of interest in medical decision making. J Am Geriatric Soc 1988;36:945–950.
19. Post SG. Inquiries in bioethics. Washington, DC: Georgetown University, 1993.
20. Kilner JF. Life on the line: ethics, aging, ending patients' lives and allocating vital resources. Grand Rapids, MI: Eerdmans, 1992.
21. President's Commission for the Study of Ethical Problems in Medicine and Biomedical and Behavioral Research. Deciding to forego life-sustaining treatment: ethical, medical, and legal issues in treatment decisions. Washington, DC: U.S. Government Printing Office, 1983.
22. Jonsen AR. Reflection. In: Hamel, eds. Active euthanasia, religion, and the public debate. Chicago: Park Ridge Center, 1991:100–105.
23. Quill TE, Cassel CK, Meier DE. Care of the hopelessly ill: proposed clinical criteria for physician-assisted suicide. N Engl J Med 1992;327:1380–1384.
24. de Wachter MAM. Euthanasia in the Netherlands. Hastings Cent Rep 1992;22:23–30.
25. Battin MP. Euthanasia in Alzheimer's disease? In: Binstock RH, Post SG, Whitehouse PJ, eds. Dementia and aging: ethics, values and policy choices. Baltimore: Johns Hopkins University, 1992:118–137.
26. Humphrey D. Rational suicide among the elderly. In: Leenaars AA, Maris RW, McIntosh JL, Richman J, eds. Suicide and the older adult. New York: Guilford, 1992:125–129.
27. Prado CG. The last choice: preemptive suicide in advanced age. New York: Greenwood, 1990.
28. Appelbaum PS, Grisso T. Assessing patients' capacities to consent to treatment. JAMA 1988;319:1635–1638.
29. Schwartz RL. Refusal of treatment: rights, reasons, responses. In: Anderson GR, Glesnes-Anderson VA, eds.

Health care ethics: a guide for decision makers. Rockville, MD: Aspen, 1987:127–137.

30. Uhlmann RF, Pearlman RA, Cain KC. Physicians' and spouses' predictions of elderly patients' resuscitation preferences. J Gerontol 1988;43:M115–M121.

31. Sehgal A, Galbraith A, Chesney M, et al. How strictly do dialysis patients want their advance directives followed? JAMA 1992;267:59–63.

32. Jahnigen DW, Binstock RH. Economic and clinical realities: health care for elderly people. In: Binstock RH, Post SG, eds. Too old for health care? Controversies in medicine, law, economics, and ethics. Baltimore: Johns Hopkins University, 1991:13–43.

33. Callahan D. Setting limits: medical goals in an aging society. New York: Simon & Schuster, 1987.

34. Binstock RH, Post SG. Old age and the rationing of health care. In: Binstock RH, Post SG, eds. Too old for health care? Controversies in medicine, law, economics, and ethics. Baltimore: Johns Hopkins University, 1991:1–12.

35. Howell M. Caretakers' views on responsibilities for the care of the demented elderly. J Am Geriatr Soc 1984;32:657–660.

36. Katz J. Experimentation with human beings. New York: Russell Sage, 1972.

37. Levine RJ. Ethics and regulation of clinical research. Baltimore: Urban & Schwarzenberg, 1986.

38. Muller-Hill B, Fraser G.R. trans. Murderous science: elimination by scientific selection of Jews, Gypsies, and others, Germany 1933–1945. New York: Oxford University, 1988.

39. Katzman R, Saitoh T. Advances in Alzheimer's disease. FASEB J 1991;5:278–286.

40. Rice DP, Fox PJ, Max W, et al. The economic burden of Alzheimer's disease care. Health Aff 1993;12:164–176.

41. Kitwood T, Bredin K. Towards a theory of dementia care: personhood and well-being. Aging Soc 1992;12:269–287.

42. Riley KP. Psychological interventions in Alzheimer's disease. In: Gilmore GC, Whitehouse PJ, Wykle ML, eds. Memory, aging and dementia. New York: Springer, 1989:199–211.

43. Gilley DW, Wilson RS, Bennett DA, et al. Cessation of driving and unsafe motor vehicle operation by dementia patients. Arch Intern Med 1991;151:941–946.

44. Hunt L, Morris JC, Edwards E, Wilson BS. Driving performance in persons with mild senile dementia of the Alzheimer type. J Am Geriatr Soc 1993;41:747–753.

45. Drachman DA, Swearer JM. Driving and Alzheimer's disease: the risk of crashes. Neurology 1993;43:2448–2456.

46. Dworkin G. Autonomy and behavior control. Hastings Cent Rep 1976;6:23–28.

47. Martin RJ, Whitehouse PJ. The clinical care of patients with dementia. In Mace NL, ed. Dementia care: patient, family, and community. Baltimore: Johns Hopkins University, 1990:22–31.

48. Mace NL. The management of problem behaviors. In: Mace NL, ed. Dementia care: patient, family, and community. Baltimore: Johns Hopkins University, 1990:74–114.

Chapter 20
Ethnic Issues in Geriatric Care

Evelyn Hutt, Terri Richardson, Spero Manson, and Lynn Mason

The fact that we are human beings is infinitely more important than all the peculiarities that distinguish human beings from one another.

Simone de Beauvoir
The Second Sex

The geriatric population of the United States, destined to nearly triple in size during the next 50 years, will become increasingly more diverse during that same time. The 1990 U.S. census estimates that about 1 of every 10 people over age 65 is a member of a racial or ethnic minority (African American, Hispanic, Asian, Pacific Islander, or Native American). By 2050 that number will be about 1 of every 3 people (1). Changes will also take place in the population older than age 80. These elders have diverse histories, life experiences, and languages. The quality of their lives will be affected by how well health care providers understand their diverse health care needs and points of view.

The purpose of this chapter is to provide a broad framework and some basic information about each of five major ethnic groups, chosen either because they are numerically large or because their recent arrival in the United States makes them particularly puzzling to health care providers. Some general issues in cross-cultural understanding and research are considered, and principles of a culturally sensitive approach to the geriatric patient are proposed. The remainder of the chapter gives information on each of five major ethnic groups: 1) basic demographic facts—the size of the population, its age, gender, income distribution, and major subgroups; 2) cohort analysis—the important unique historic events experienced by each ethnic group that shaped its world view; 3) the health status of the group and the diseases that are particularly prevalent or important; 4) the group's distinctive cultural beliefs about health and health care; and 5) prevalent and impor-

tant typical geriatric syndromes (e.g., falls) and their variation in ethnically distinct populations.

What is an ethnic group? It is easier to say what it is not: an ethnic group is not a racial group, an economically disadvantaged minority, a national group, or a religious group, although it may have some or all of those components. Instead, an ethnic group is "a group of individuals with a shared sense of peoplehood" (2) and "a sociologic construct that is highly correlated with behavior and cultural phenomena, particularly language, dress, adornment, food preference, religion, patterns of social interactions, choice of marriage partner and family composition" (3). The distinction is important because it prevents the confusion of socioeconomic status with culture as a determinant of behavior and emphasizes the divergence that may exist between cultural norms and actual practice (4). The guiding principle in this definition is that it focuses on who the individual perceives him or her *self* to be in relation to other people. It may mean that such a person will define family differently from the dominant culture, speak a different language, and have a different set of beliefs about causality, health, and the relative importance of various human activities.

From this definition arises the first principle of a culturally sensitive approach to the geriatric patient: listen to what the patient says, directly and indirectly, about him or herself and what matters most to the person. Presume that you are ignorant, but that human experience is universal enough that if you listen carefully, patients can tell you what is wrong and something about what they need.

Second, an ethnic group is as internally diverse as it is distinct from the dominant culture. For example, the Hispanic population in the United States comprises at least four major subcultures grouped by country of origin (Cuba, Mexico, Puerto Rico, and Central America). Each has its own dialects, foods, customs, and habits. Additional diversity is introduced by local variation in the interaction among majority and minority cultures, the number of generations by which an ethnic group or person is removed from cultural homogeneity or isolation, and whether English is spoken.

In the face of this diversity and our ability to present only the broadest outlines of the cultural influences on geriatric patients, making facile assumptions on the basis of inadequate data may cause serious error. Inquiring directly about specific cultural beliefs and practices and the degree to which an individual or family adheres to them is always useful, if the inquiry is made in a respectful manner.

Third, many ethnic groups have within them recent immigrants who have experienced torture. Numerical estimates are unavailable, but it is known that torture is practiced in almost 100 countries (5). Victims of torture may be extremely reluctant to discuss their experience directly. They fear disbelief, the pain of their memories, and possible retribution against family and friends left behind. They have both physical and psychological sequelae. Physical complaints commonly include skin lesions, pulmonary infections, gait disturbances from beatings on the soles of the feet, headaches, abdominal pain, dental problems, fractures, and genital tract disorders. Psychological symptoms may include depression, night-mares, irritability, difficulties with memory and concentration, persistent shame, despair, and humiliation.

Care providers can assist these patients by being aware of their possible history of torture and being open to hearing the patient's experience. Confidentiality is of utmost importance. "It is also crucial for health professionals to follow through on all promises made, with clear and concise time frames included. Alleviating symptoms with medication often can be an aid to building a level of trust and rapport" (5).

A word must must be said about language barriers. The word is interpreter. When both patient and care provider are not fluent in a common language, using an interpreter is essential, but it complicates an already difficult interaction. Problems can result from bad paraphrasing, interpreter-patient interactions, the interpreter's self-image, and ethnocentric expectations. Tips that can make using a translator easier are presented in Table 20.1 (6).

African Americans

Demography and History

The African American elderly population is growing faster than the white elderly population and is the most rapidly increasing segment of the African American population. Currently more than 2.5 million African Americans are age 65 and older (7). This figure represents 8.2 percent of the total U.S. population older than age 65. The U.S. Census Bureau estimates that by the year 2000 African American elderly will number 3 million persons. Compared with other segments of the population, larger numbers of older African Americans are poor; they are less educated; they have less adequate housing; they have more chronic, physically limiting diseases, and they have fewer years of life remaining.

A significant number of African American elders are poor. In 1991, 32.7 million (33%) African Americans lived below the poverty level compared with 11.3 percent of whites. Most African American elders rely on Social Security for more than half their income. To cover medical expenses, 54.4 percent of African American elders rely on government help—from Medicare (37.9%) or from a combination of Medicare/Medicaid (16.5%) (8). In contrast, 77.3 percent of white elders have supplemental private insurance.

Table 20.1. Tips for Using an Interpreter.

1. Avoid using family members.
2. Learn basic words and phrases in the target languages, and ask the interpreter about words or comments that have not been translated.
3. Become familiar with special terminology used by patients.
4. Meet regularly with the interpreter.
5. Address the patient directly.
6. Invite correction.
7. Use a mode of communication as conversational as possible.
8. Pursue seemingly unconnected issues that the patient raises.
9. Provide written instruction and ask the patient to feed back understanding.
10. Emphasize by repetition.
11. Reassure the patient that confidentiality will be respected.
12. Be patient.

Adapted from Putsch RW. Cross-cultural communication: the special case of interpreters in health care. JAMA 1985;254: 3344–3348.

An estimated 6 percent of African American elderly have no formal education, and only 17 percent of African American elders have a high school education; 41 percent of white elders have attended high school (8).

Most African American men are married, but the majority of African American women are widowed, and widowhood comes earlier to African Americans than to others. In 1990, 45.1 percent of African American women and 19.8 percent of men age 65 to 74 years were widowed. Relatively more African American elders than others had never married, and many African American elders lived alone. Among African American men age 65 and older, 22.2 percent lived alone and 59.6 percent lived with a spouse (9). Among African American women, 38.7 percent lived alone and 44.5 percent lived with a spouse.

In the 1980s a dramatic increase occurred in the number of grandparents serving as primary caregivers for grandchildren and great-grandchildren. Among African Americans, approximately 12 percent of children live with their grandparents compared with 3.6 percent of white grandchildren (10). Rates may be higher in some inner cities. This is felt in part to be due to the crack/cocaine epidemic.

From 1910 to 1970, approximately 6.5 million African Americans moved from the South to the North and West. In 1980, 52 percent of 26 million African Americans lived in the South, 18 percent in the Northeast, 20 percent in the Midwest, and 9 percent in the West (10). Three-fourths of all African Americans live in metropolitan areas.

Most African Americans share a common history of slavery. Table 20.2 briefly summarizes their life experiences. Although the Emancipation Proclamation of 1863 technically freed African Americans from slavery, black codes and Jim Crow laws kept African Americans separate and unequal. It was not until the 1960s, with the Voting Rights Act and the Civil Rights Act, that African Americans received basic rights that other American citi-

Table 20.2. Cohort Experiences for African Americans.

	Historic Experience			
	1900–1920	1920–1940	1940–1960	1960–Present
	Ku Klux Klan	Red summer	WWII–Segregated units and factory work in U.S. North and West.	Civil rights movement
	Lynchings	W.E.B. Dubois		Dr. Martin Luther King's nonviolent protests
	NAACP organization	Marcus Garvey's Back to Africa movement	1954–U.S. Supreme Court ruling to desegregate education	Black pride
	Participation in WWI	Harlem renaissance		Desegregation and affirmative action
		Great Depression		Vietnam War Crack epidemic HIV epidemic

Current Age of Cohort (yr)	Life Stage at Historic Experience			
	1900–1920	1920–1940	1940–1960	1960–Present
85+	Child–adolescent	Young adult	Middle-aged	Elder
75–85	Child	Adolescent–young adult	Young adult–middle-aged	Middle-aged–old
65–75		Child, adolescent	Adolescent–young-adult	Young adult–middle-aged
55–65		Child	Child–young adult	Young adult–middle-aged

SOURCE: Adapted from Yeo, G. Teaching Materials and Handouts. Stanford Geriatric Education Center, Stanford, CA 1991.

zens had. Despite their common history, African Americans are a heterogeneous group.

Health Status

Life expectancy for African Americans trails that of whites, especially for African American men (Table 20.3) (8). However, a crossover phenomenon exists—at approximately age 75, African American mortality rates are lower than white rates, and African Americans who survive to age 75 have a greater life expectancy than do white Americans (11,12). Crossover is probably a result of selective survival of healthier African Americans. African American women surviving to 85 years of age have the longest life expectancy for women and men of both races.

In the United States, a disproportionate number of African Americans become sick sooner and die earlier than do whites. Causes for excess mortality in African Americans include cancer, cardiovascular disease, diabetes, infant mortality, violence and human immunodeficiency virus (HIV) disease (13).

Decades of research have documented the high risk of

Table 20.3. Life Expectancy for births in 1992.

Race	Male (yr)	Female (yr)	Total (yr)
White	71.8	79.4	76.1
Black	64.5	73.6	69.1

Adapted from National Center for Health Statistics. Health, United States, 1992. U.S. Department of Health and Human Services, DHHS Pub. No. (PHS)93-1232. Hyattsville, MD: U.S. Public Health Service, 1993.

Table 20.4. Persons Aged 65 to 74 with Hypertension and Obesity.

Sex	Race	Hypertension (%)	Obesity (%)
Female	White	70.6	36.5
Female	Black	85.0	60.8
Male	White	65.8	25.8
Male	Black	75.1	26.4

Adapted from National Center for Health Statistics. Health, United States, 1992. U.S. Department of Health and Human Services, DHHS Pub. No. (PHS)93-1232. Hyattsville, MD: U.S. Public Health Service, 1993.

hypertension (HTN) among African Americans. The rates of HTN and obesity in the African American elderly are shown in Table 20.4 (7). African Americans tend to develop HTN earlier than whites, and at every age their HTN is more severe than it is in whites. Because HTN is a major risk factor for cardiovascular disease and stroke, African Americans have a 1.3-fold greater rate of nonfatal stroke and 1.8-fold greater rate of heart disease than do whites (14). The reason for higher rates of HTN is not entirely known. Excessive body weight, stressful lifestyle, and high salt intake have been offered as possible explanations. Recently, Grim and Wilson (15) postulated that ocean passage and other periods of entrenched slavery were characterized by excessive sodium depletion from sweating, diarrhea, and vomiting. Evolutionary pressure favored development of genetic machinery that conserved sodium beyond normal levels. This is consistent with most African American HTN being low-renin, salt sensitive. Reduction in salt intake and weight, and the use of diuretics and calcium channel blockers have been shown to be effective in treating and preventing hypertension in African Americans.

Since the turn of the century, there has been a considerable increase in the prevalence of diabetes mellitus (DM) in African Americans. African Americans over the age of 65 have nearly three times the incidence of type II diabetes as their white counterparts. Although relatively more African American than white diabetics are obese, and obesity is the most important risk factor for DM, the higher prevalence of DM among African Americans is not fully explained by differences in obesity (16). African Americans are at greater risk than whites for diabetic complications such as heart disease, stroke, kidney failure, blindness, and peripheral vascular disease. Age- and sex-adjusted incidence of diabetic end-stage renal disease is at least fourfold higher in African Americans than in whites. Death rates from DM are twice as high in African Americans than they are in whites.

Over 7 million African Americans smoke (17); 24.3 percent of African American men 65 years of age and older, compared with 14.2 percent of elderly white men, smoke, although African Americans smoke fewer cigarettes. Fewer African American women older than 65 years (9.6%) smoke than do white women over 65 years of age

(12.1%). African American smokers start smoking at a later age than white smokers, but they have higher mortality rates for smoking-related diseases. Approximately 75 percent of African American smokers consume mentholated cigarettes, which have a higher tar and nicotine content than do regular cigarettes. For several decades, the rate of lung cancer among African American males has been increasing at a faster rate than it has among white men (18), and rate increases are greatest in those 65 years of age and older.

Health Beliefs

Because elderly African Americans are a heterogeneous group, descriptions of cultural beliefs may not be equally applicable. Nevertheless, some African Americans seek formal medical help only when their condition becomes incapacitating, partly because some older African Americans remember when outpatient clinics and hospital wards for blacks were relegated to a dingy basement and the clinics were staffed by unlicensed doctors and nurses. Blacks have encountered culturally insensitive physicians, inaccessibility of medical facilities, and language barriers. Therefore, many turned to a traditional medical system that has its roots in the slave culture of the American South and stems from West Africa and the Caribbean. Although physicians are increasingly the practitioners of choice for most African Americans, many also consult specialists in folk medicine.

Traditional black folk medicine integrates a belief in magic with Protestant Christian theology (19). The universe is seen as a hostile place in which the forces of good and evil struggle for control. Illness in this system affects both the mind and body, and has either a natural or unnatural cause. Natural illness results when an individual upsets the harmony of the physical or spiritual world. Unnatural illness results from the deliberate evil acts of others. Patients may consult any of three practitioners: the "old lady" (also called "granny" or "Ms. Markus") who is well versed in herbal medicine; the spiritualist who is believed to have been "called by God," has a basis in Christianity, and is not well versed in voodoo; and the voodoo priest or priestess who casts spells, reads bones, and is well versed in voodoo rituals and procedures. The priest also has a thorough knowledge of herbs and animal habits (19). In addition to these formal folk medicine practices, many elders rely on home remedies such as cod liver oil, herbal teas, garlic, and Epsom salts.

Geriatric Syndromes

Glaucoma

Glaucoma is the leading cause of blindness among African Americans in the United States. The prevalence of blindness from glaucoma in African Americans is sevenfold that of the white population in general and becomes 15-fold for those age 45 to 64 years (20). Glaucoma is more common and more aggressive in African Americans. The reason is not known, but early screening and treatment are likely to decrease visual loss.

Primary open-angle glaucoma (POAG) accounts for 70 percent of all glaucoma cases. POAG is characterized by 1) an intraocular pressure consistently above 21 mm Hg in at least one eye, 2) an open, normal-appearing anterior chamber angle with no apparent ocular or systemic abnormality that might account for the elevated intraocular pressure, and 3) typical glaucomatous visual field, optic nerve head damage, or both. Risk factors for POAG include diabetes, extreme myopia, or family history of glaucoma. POAG has no associated symptoms or other warning signs before the development of advanced field loss.

Depression

In the past, African Americans were believed to be immune to depression as a result of underdeveloped higher brain function. This view has subsequently been dismissed. Rates of depression for African Americans are the same as they are for whites when adjustments are made for socioeconomic status. However, that clinicians have more difficulty diagnosing depression among African Americans has been suggested (21), possibly because of the increased prevalence of somatic complaints in elders or because African American elders may be stoic and reluctant to share personal troubles with careproviders. Moreover, none of the diagnostic instruments easily usable in a primary care setting have been validated in African Americans or in any low-literacy population. Studies of gender differences in rates of depression have yielded varying results, but most report more depressive symptoms in women (22).

Social support and religious participation may have a positive influence on depression among African American elders. African Americans report greater levels of religious involvement and they turn to religion more often than whites do to cope with feelings of depression. Given the role of the church in African American culture, religious identification may provide a protective function for African Americans. Without the informal networks of friends, the extended family, church, and folk practitioners, African American elders might suffer more depression. If these institutions suffer further erosion over the next half-century, depression rates in African Americans may rise.

American Indians and Alaska Natives

Demography and History

American Indians and Alaska Natives, who number approximately 2 million (0.08% of the general U.S. population), are among the fastest growing minority groups in the United States (1). There are over 300 reservation communities, 212 Alaska villages, and 505 federally recognized tribes. Many people assume that this special population lives largely in rural America; however, more than one-third make their homes in cities. Indians and Natives are culturally diverse, and may differ markedly in terms of language, kinship systems, social organization, and religious practice. Nonetheless, certain core values appear to be common among them: orientation to the present, cooperation, generosity and sharing, respect for age, harmony with nature, and humility (23,24). Other commonalities seem to be a consequence of shared histories of colonization, including dramatic military resistance, externally imposed forms of governance, forced dietary changes, mandatory boarding school education, and active missionary movements.

Compared with other minority groups, the number of Indians and Natives 65 years of age and older is significantly lower, about 100,000 persons (1). The number of elderly Native Americans is primarily a result of past fertility patterns and secondarily of improved chances of survival. Their life expectancy at birth, now 76.9 years, began to rise dramatically in the middle part of this century as preventive health measures brought many infectious diseases under control. Like Indians and Natives in general, three-fourths of all Native American elders live in the West and South. Nearly 40 percent can be found in Oklahoma, California, and Arizona, the three states with the largest Indian populations. The percentage of older Native Americans living beyond 80 years, often referred to as the "old old", is estimated to remain about the same in 2050 as it is now — slightly less than 1 percent. However, the old old will, in 2050, be a much greater proportion (increasing from 18% to 39%) of all elderly Indians. Consequently, Indian and Native families, already committed culturally to caring for their elder members, will be called on to provide increasing support for growing numbers of older, frail relatives.

Table 20.5 presents a number of prominent historic events and experiences that have affected the lives of this special population. Most of these events involve the introduction of federal policies that dramatically altered the physical, social, and economic climates of the times. For example, the Dawes Act (1887) provided the allotment of property rights to individual Indians, which in turn led to the sale of trust lands, and subsequent disenfranchisement of landless Native people. About the same time, moved by the devastating consequences of largely unchecked infectious diseases, the Bureau of Indian Affairs (BIA) launched a major health initiative that laid the groundwork for the present-day Indian Health Service. Several decades later, in 1924, Native Americans were formally granted U.S. citizenship and the right to vote. This was accompanied by a major reorganization of local government, which swept away traditional forms of leadership and instituted tribal councils and formal elections.

The Dawes Act also brought about wholesale change in diet and subsistence practices and made available free refined wheat, sugar, lard, bacon, and cheese. Also during the early twentieth century, the federal government's educational policies — which revolved around boarding schools as mechanisms of assimilation — reached their zenith, resulting in massive upheavals of Indian family structure.

World War II brought a brief respite from these pressures. Indian and Native men entered military service in large numbers. After the war, they returned to their homes as a new political force and brought an unprecedented level of knowledge and sophistication to local governance. However, assimilationist policies were re-

Table 20.5 Cohort Experiences for American Indians and Alaska Natives.

	Historic Experience			
	1890–1920	1920–1940	1940–1960	1960–Present
	Aftermath of Dawes Severalty Act	Citizenship granted to all Indians in 1924	WWII service	Economic Opportunity Act
	Medical division established in Indian Service	Indian Reorganization Act	Hoover Commission and termination of BIA urban relocation program	PL 638 Indian Self-Determination Act
		Peak BIA boarding school education		PL 437 Health Improvement Act
	Prohibition of liquor sales on reservations		PL 280 Transfer of Jurisdiction Act	Alaska Native lands claim settlement

Current Age of Cohort (yr)	Life Stage at Historic Experience			
	1900–1920	1920–1940	1940–1960	1960–Present
85+	Child–adolescent	Young adult	Middle-aged	Elder
75–85	Child	Adolescent–young Adult	Young adult–middle-aged	Middle-aged–Elder
65–75		Child–adolescent	Adolescent–young adult	Adult–young Elder
55–65		Child	Child–young adult	Young adult–middle-aged

BIA = U.S. Bureau of Indian Affairs; PL = U.S. Public Law; WWII = World War II.
SOURCE: Adapted from Yeo, G. Teaching Materials and Handouts. Stanford Geriatric Education Center, Stanford, CA 1991.

vived with even greater vigor. Economically successful reservations were encouraged to divest themselves of federal guardianship. BIA programs relocated thousands of families to cities such as Denver, Los Angeles, and Chicago to provide vocational training and employment opportunities. Many reservations saw jurisdiction over their legal matters transferred from federal to state governments.

The Johnson Administration, through its Great Frontier and War on Poverty programs, signaled a radical turnabout. Economic development began in Indian communities and focused on local employment opportunities and necessary infrastructure. Unparalleled increases in health care funding, including, for the first time, urban Indian programs, were authorized. Long-standing disputes over Alaska Native lands were settled, which established regional corporate self-governments. These events, and the experiences that they spawned, touched the lives of all Native Americans, albeit at various points in their personal histories, and thus have construed varying meanings to them. As a result, there are cohort and intergenerational differences in cultural values, social organization, and health behavior within this special population, and these differences should be anticipated.

Health Status

The major health problems of older American Indians and Alaska Natives include non-insulin-dependent diabetes mellitus (NIDDM), high blood pressure, tuberculosis, rheumatoid arthritis, heart disease, cancer, and liver and kidney disease (25). Alcohol abuse appears to contribute greatly to the risk of these and other health problems. Heart disease and cancer rank first and second, respectively, as the most frequent causes of death among Native elders, followed closely by pulmonary illnesses. More than half (59%) of all Indians and Natives 65 years of age and older experience significant limitation in activities of daily living (26). Not surprising, depressive symptomatology is quite common among older Native Americans (27). Unfortunately, providers often fail to detect depression, mainly because this population seldom volunteers such information (25).

Health Beliefs

Native elders' understanding of and narratives about illness are firmly grounded in the local dimensions of the self. Yet, they may sharply distinguish between the acute aspects of a health problem (e.g., pain, gastrointestinal distress, shortness of breath), for which help may be sought from physicians, and ultimate cause (e.g., social transgressions, spiritual imbalance, witchcraft), usually thought to be the purview of indigenous healers. Careful, supportive inquiry can elicit important clinical findings in regard to these matters (28).

Asian and Pacific Island Americans

Demography and History

The Asian/Pacific Islander group is both the most diverse and the fastest growing ethnic elderly population in the United States. This category includes more than 20 different ethnic and language groups. One may question the usefulness of grouping them together. Lui and Yu (29) explain:

> In the strictest sense, the term Asian/Pacific American is a meaningful concept only insofar as it identifies the geographic origins of a group of people who are visibly different from the majority white population.... [T]he importance of having at least some preliminary baseline information on this ethnic group seems to override the disadvantages

of lumping such diverse populations together (p. 36).

According to the 1990 U.S. census, one-half million Asians age 65 and older live in the United States, or 1 percent of all elderly in the U.S. This group doubled in size from 1980 to 1990. By 2050, Asians are projected to represent 8 percent of all elders, 6.2 million people. Their current distribution among major national groups can be seen in Figure 20.1 (1).

The Asian elderly have a higher proportion of men than do other groups in the United States. The ratio of men to women among older Asians is 100:82. In contrast, among older African Americans, the ratio is 100:62. The increased proportion of elderly males is a result of immigration patterns during the past 100 years.

Asian elders tend to be younger than the elders of other groups. Twenty-three percent of white elders are age 80 or older, but only 10 percent of Asian elders are that age. Asians also have a longer life expectancy: 82.9 years, compared with 76.6 for Anglo Americans and 70.4 for African Americans. Overall, Asians are better educated and have more evenly distributed incomes than other ethnic minorities. These figures, however, obscure important pockets of poverty and illiteracy in Asian communities. Of note, 40 percent of elderly Asians are linguistically isolated, that is, they live in a household in which no one age 14 or older speaks English (1).

Very broad outlines of the major historic events in the

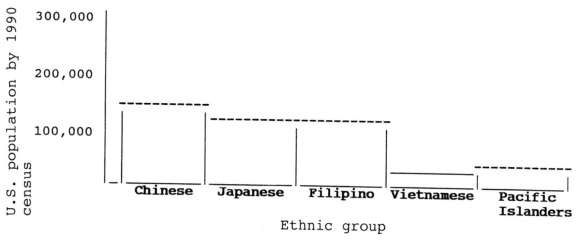

Fig. 20.1. Major national groups of Asian elders

Table 20.6. Cohort Experiences for Asian and Pacific Island Elders.

Ethnic Group	Historic Experience			
	1900–1920	1920–1940	1940–1960	1960–Present
Chinese	Immigration Exclusion Act—Residents mostly male laborers from South China	Family associations, Tongs Pearl Buck novels	Chinese in World War II Repeal of Exclusion Acts Fear of Chinese Communists Immigration to U.S. of wives	Increase in education Immigration to U.S. from Hong Kong and Taiwan
Japanese	Beginning of immigration to U.S.	Immigration Exclusion Act	Internment camps World War II	Rise of Japan in world economic order
Filipino	Filipinos lose Philippine-American War Male laborer immigration to U.S.	1934 Tydings-McDuffie Act limits immigration Labor riots	Philippine independence Filipino men in U.S. Armed Forces immigrate	1965 Immigration Act abolishes quotas Family immigration
Pacific Islander	Hawaii U.S. protectorate Guam U.S. territory Samoa U.S. Naval control		Guam under Japanese control	Hawaii statehood
Southeast Asian	French colonization	French colonization	French colonization ends Vietnam War	1975 – Vietnam War ends Boat People

Current Age of Cohort (yr)	Life Stage at Historic Experience			
	1900–1920	1920–1940	1940–1960	1960–Present
85+	Child–adolescent	Young adult	Middle-Aged	Elder
75–85	Child	Adolescent–young adult	Young adult–middle-aged	Middle-aged–Elder
65–75		Child–adolescent	Adolescent–young adult	Adult–young Elder
55–65		Child	Child–young adult	Young adult–Middle-aged

Adapted from Morioka-Douglas N, Yeo G. Aging and health: Asian and Pacific Island American elders. SGEC Working Paper, series 3. Stanford: Stanford Geriatric Education Center, 1990.

lives of Asian and Pacific Island Americans can be seen in Table 20.6. Different as these experiences are from each other, some common themes emerge to distinguish the experience of this group from others. All members of this group experienced discrimination by restrictions on immigration. Most Asians and Pacific Islanders experienced the dominant U.S. culture as colonizer or hostile combatant. The first immigrants from China, Japan, and the Philippines were groups of single men who came to the U.S. as laborers. Their social isolation is likely to be especially intense as they age. Although the years after 1960 brought

increasing social liberalization and opportunity for Asian minorities, these factors are sometimes accompanied by thinly disguised envy and resentment from members of the majority culture (29).

Health Status

Morbidity and mortality information for Asian and Pacific Island elders is limited and spotty. Some information, organized by national groups, is available from Morioka-Douglas and Yeo (29). In general, age-adjusted mortality rates seem to be lower for Asians than for other groups and the incidence of specific diseases within major disease categories is also lower. Place of birth is an important variable; death rates for foreign-born elders are at least double the rates for American-born Chinese, Japanese, and Filipinos.

Chinese

Although the prevalence and incidence of coronary artery disease and myocardial infarction are lower in the Chinese than they are in others, the incidence of cerebrovascular disease, stroke, and multi-infarct dementia (as contrasted with Alzheimer-type) is higher (30,31), possibly because of a greater prevalence of diabetes among Chinese women and smoking among Chinese men; other risk factors have not been well delineated.

Malignant neoplasms cause proportionately the same percentage of deaths in the Chinese as they do in other ethnic groups, but among the Chinese there is a higher incidence of liver, esophageal, and pancreatic cancers and a lower incidence of breast cancer. Osteoporosis rates may also be higher. Suicide rates among elderly Chinese women are at least three times those of Anglo American women in the same age group.

Japanese

The profile of major diseases and morbidity is similar for Japanese and Chinese people, but the Japanese have a relatively higher incidence of stroke and diabetes and relatively lower incidence of coronary disease. Among the malignant neoplasms, stomach and esophageal cancer are more prevalent in Japanese men. Japanese women older than 75 years of age and men older than age 85 have very high suicide rates.

Filipinos

Hypertension is particularly common in Filipinos and is comparable with rates for African Americans. Rates of vascular disease are rising. Gout is especially prevalent among Filipinos. The reason for the prevalence of gout is not known, but may reflect an inherited renal tubular defect.

Southeast Asians

Because of their very recent immigration, the Indochinese have had major health problems of malnutrition and in-fections: tuberculosis, intestinal parasites, hepatitis B, and dental abscesses. A recent study of cardiovascular risk factors in this population suggests a potential for increased incidence of atherosclerotic disease. Hypertension and cigarette smoking are particularly common (32). Several studies have also found increased rates of depression.

Pacific Islanders

Information is most scanty for this group, but of particular concern are diseases associated with obesity.

Health Beliefs

Cultural beliefs and health practices are more diverse than the number of distinct ethnic groups in this population, but some useful generalizations may be made. The health beliefs of Chinese, Japanese, and some Southeast Asians are based in the Chinese system of thought wherein health is viewed as a state of dynamic equilibrium between opposing energy forces, often termed "hot" and "cold."

> "Hot" and "cold" have no relation to temperature but represent two energy forces, Yin and Yang, that need to be in balance. Yin includes darkness, cold and emptiness, whereas Yang is light, warmth, and fullness. Old people are predisposed to the "cold."
>
> "Chi" is a form of energy that moves through human beings along pathways called meridians. Like "chi", blood circulates in the body. Where there are imbalances of "chi" or blood, illness occurs. Balance is restored by stimulating the flow of chi at various focal points on the meridians with needles, as in acupuncture or pressure as in acupressure or shiatsu. External forces that cause disease include wind or "feng" which is a noxious substance that enters the body to cause symptoms such as bloating, flatulence, depression and joint pain (29).

Practitioners of traditional Chinese medicine work in cities in which substantial populations of Asian immigrants live. Herbs and herb combinations are sold over the counter and are poorly regulated. In California, the Department of Health Services has collaborated with the Oriental Herbal Association to identify potential toxins.

For the Japanese, the Chinese system of dynamic balance exists along with Shinto beliefs that disease is caused by outside spirits who bring retribution on people who have succumbed to temptation. These spirits can be removed by various purification rites and the use of purgatives. In addition, Japanese culture places a high value on avoiding shame or embarrassment and deferring to authority. This combination of values may make it particularly difficult for Japanese elders to seek or accept nursing or social service assistance.

Among Southeast Asians, Chinese beliefs about health prevail within an older animist system. Animist notions about spirit possession are particularly prevalent among the Hmong, Mien, and the Thai Dam people of Laos. Dermabrasive practices (cupping, pinching, coin-rubbing, burning) are used to extract toxic "wind" from the body or to transfer "heat" back into the body. The marks from these procedures should not be misinterpreted as signs of abuse (33).

Filipinos also subscribe to the balance theory of health, which they call "timbang." They have a hot and cold categorization which is somewhat different from the Chinese in that it came from Mexican beliefs by way of Spanish colonial priests. Filipinos have a fatalistic attitude about disease:

> Imbalances that threaten health can be brought about by personal disorderliness and by irregularity more generally. Filipinos believe that we get pretty much what we deserve—that is, everything balances out (34).

A physician should take special care when informing Filipinos about the extent or severity of disease because stress is believed to exacerbate the imbalance that originally caused the illness.

Traditional health beliefs and practices are less common among Pacific Island Americans because of their long domination by Westerners. Further information is available in Palafox and Warren's book, *Cross-Cultural Caring* (35).

Common to all these cultures, and indeed to geriatric patients in general, is the desire to be treated with respect. This involves addressing the patient as "Mr." or "Mrs." with the surname and inquiring about traditional practices without condescension or disdain. Recognizing the surname may present a problem to the health care provider because a common Southeast Asian practice is to place the surname first. The first name may also be a clan or dynasty name. On initial contact, it is appropriate to use Mr. or Mrs. with the given name and then to ask the patient how he or she wishes to be addressed (33).

Geriatric Syndromes

Little, if any, data have been collected on the prevalence of typical geriatric syndromes in this population. However some comments about traditional Asian beliefs about family, filial piety, and the impact of cultural norms on geriatric patients may be useful. Traditional Asian family structures are highly patriarchal, with the eldest male having the most power and authority. The eldest son is expected, in return for receiving the largest inheritance, to respect and provide for his parents in their dependent years.

Like other cultural norms, however, these values and practices are changing as families acculturate and more women join the work force. "Although the pattern of inlaws living with younger children is still common, the influence of older adults has diminished over recent generations and ethnic identity and values have changed from generation to generation" (36). The gap between traditional beliefs and actual practice is likely to produce disappointment, if not bitterness, in the elder and tension, if not guilt, among their children. Moreover, because of immigration patterns, an increased proportion of the oldest Asians are men without families. There will be a growing need for bilingual, bicultural services for these elders.

Hispanic Americans

Demography and History

The term Hispanic covers numerous distinct, regional populations and local communities throughout urban and rural America. This convenient but overly broad category encompasses much historical, geographic, social, political, cultural, linguistic, and genetic diversity. Of the 20.8 million documented and undocumented individuals identified as Hispanic in the 1990 U.S. census, approximately 1 million (5%) are age 65 or older. These elders make up about 4 percent of the older population of the U.S. (37).

The largest group of U.S. Hispanic elders is Mexican American (48%), followed by Cuban immigrants (18%),

Table 20.7. Cohort Experiences for Hispanic Americans.

Ethnic Group	Historic Experience			
	1900–1920	1920–1940	1940–1960	1960–Present
Mexican American	Massive immigration to U.S. Mexican revolution	Founding families and migrant laborers Zoot suiters/riots	WWII participation U.S. Armed Forces forum Barrios	Chicano movement La Raza New poverty Bilingual education Latino arts and media
Cuban American	Spanish-American War Island dependence on U.S.	Batista era	Castro–Island communism Health/education reforms Exodus to U.S.–Wave 1	Exodus to U.S.–Waves 2 and 3 Miami colony
Puerto Rican	Spanish-American War	Colonial relationship with U.S. Severe depression Immigration to U.S.	Commonwealth status Immigration to U.S. Nationalist movement Operation Bootstrap/Reforms	Operation Bootstrap/reforms to commonwealth status

Current Age of Cohort (yr)	Life Stage at Historic Experience			
	1900–1920	1920–1940	1940–1960	1960–Present
85+	Child–adolescent	Young adult	Middle-aged	Elder
75–85	Child	Adolescent–young adult	Young adult–middle-aged	Middle-aged–Elder
65–75		Child–adolescent	Adolescent–young adult	Young adult–middle-aged
55–65		Child	Child–young adult	Young adult–middle-aged

WWII = World War II.
Adapted from Morioka-Douglas N, Yeo G. Aging and health: Asian and Pacific Island American elders. SGEC Working Paper, series 3. Stanford: Stanford Geriatric Education Center, 1990.

Other Hispanics, primarily in New Mexico and Southern Colorado (15%), Puerto Ricans (11%), and other Latin American immigrants and refugees (8%). The proportion of U.S. elders who are Hispanic is expected to grow from about 5 percent to more than 11 percent by 2050 (38).

According to the 1980 U.S. census, over 70 percent of Hispanics live in four states: California (25%), Texas (21%), Florida (13.5%), and New York (11%). Hispanic elders live predominantly in cities: 91 percent compared with 83 percent of older African Americans and 72 percent of older Anglo Americans. Over 57 percent of Hispanic elders were born in the United States (39).

Compared with other ethnic elders, Hispanics are more likely to live with other family members, particularly in multigenerational households headed by adult children. The tendency for elders to live with children during old age is reflected in the lower rate of admission for these persons to long-term care facilities. Only 3 percent of Hispanic elders at any given time live in nursing homes, including only 10 percent of those older than age 75 (40).

Spanish is the preferred language for the overwhelming majority of Hispanic elders. Limited English proficiency has been identified as a barrier to health services, benefits, and health promotion campaigns. More than 50 percent of older Hispanics are estimated to be functionally illiterate in both Spanish and English. Cubans tend to have the most formal education; Mexican-Americans, the least (39).

Hispanic elders do not belong to only one or even to several cohorts characterized by experiences shared by all. Table 20.7 suggests a few of the major events and conditions that directly or indirectly have affected the lives of older Mexican Americans, Puerto Ricans, and Cubans (41).

Health Status

Health studies featuring adequate samples of elderly Hispanics and protocols that identify Hispanics are too few to yield more than tentative conclusions about the mortality, health, and health-related beliefs and practices of older Hispanics. Many studies contain serious research limitations, including indiscriminate lumping of Hispanic and non-Hispanic subjects, inconsistency and incompleteness, and misleading generalizations.

Sorlie et al (42) recently published the most comprehensive analysis of mortality by Hispanic status in the United States. This study compared all-cause and cause-specific mortality rates between Hispanic and non-Hispanic groups and estimated the effect of family income, place of birth, and place of residence. The researchers analyzed data from 1979 to 1987 that involved 700,000 noninstitutionalized individuals aged 25 years or older, including 40,000 Hispanics. The findings confirmed several previous studies. When data were adjusted for age, Hispanics were shown to have lower mortality from all causes, compared with non-Hispanics, lower mortality from cancer, lower mortality from cardiovascular disease, higher mortality from diabetes, and higher mortality from homicide among men. After adjustment for differences in annual family income, the relative mortality ratios were lower for Hispanics than for non-Hispanics.

A study of mortality among first-generation Cubans, Puerto Ricans, and Mexican Americans (43) revealed that Puerto Ricans had the highest age-adjusted death rates and Cuban-born the lowest, which suggests an inverse relationship between socioeconomic status and mortality among the three main Hispanic divisions.

Morbidity patterns among Hispanics in general mirror those of the larger U.S. population. NIDDM is two to four times more prevalent among Mexican Americans and Puerto Ricans than it is among Anglo Americans. The rate among Cubans is slightly higher than it is among Anglo Americans. Among Hispanics older than age 50, at least 10 percent to 15 percent of cases of NIDDM will remain undiagnosed. The high incidence of type II diabetes among Mexican Americans has been associated with socioeconomic factors, obesity, diet, and Native American genetic admixture (44,45).

On the basis of a review of recent morbidity studies,

Table 20.8. Disease-Related Risks for Hispanics Compared with Risk for Total U.S. Geriatric Population.

Type of Risk	Relative Risk Among Hispanics
NIDDM	Increased
Obesity	Increased
Proteinuria	Increased
End-stage renal disease	Increased
Retinopathy	Increased
Gallstone disease	Increased
Neuropathy	No difference
Heart disease	No difference
Myocardial infarction	No difference
Hypertension	Increased
Stroke	No difference
Lipid disorders	Increased
Breast cancer	Decreased
Liver cancer	Increased
Lung cancer	No difference
Pancreatic cancer	Increased
Stomach cancer	Increased
Cervical cancer	Increased
Prostatic cancer	No difference

NIDDM = non-insulin-dependent diabetes mellitus.
Reprinted with permission from Villa ML, Cuellar J, Gamel N, Yeo G. Aging and health: Hispanic American elders. 2nd ed. SGEC Working Paper, Series 5. Stanford: Stanford Geriatric Education Center, 1993.

Villa et al (39) summarized the probable differences in relative disease-related risks for Hispanic elders compared with risks for the total older U.S. population (Table 20.8). Alcohol abuse, particularly among Mexican American males, has been linked to higher rates in that group for cirrhosis and motor vehicle accident-related trauma. In general, reported alcohol consumption among Hispanic men and, especially, women is lower than it is among Anglo Americans (46).

Acquired immunodeficiency syndrome (AIDS) has become a major health threat among Hispanics. In 1989, 15 percent of all reported AIDS cases were among Hispanics—almost twice the Hispanic representation in the U.S. population (47). Although less than 7 percent of cases among persons older than age 70 were Hispanic, clinicians should be alert to the possibility of AIDS in greater numbers of older people.

Higher rates of depression and depressive affect have been reported among Hispanic elders, but the data are only suggestive because of limitations imposed by language, culturally-biased mental status measures, and cultural differences in beliefs related to mental conditions. Much mental illness among the Hispanic elderly goes unrecognized and untreated because it often presents differently, and the services of mental health professionals are not sought. Older Hispanics are more likely than Anglo American individuals to regard the symptoms of mental illness as the result of moral failings or supernatural intervention.

Shrout et al (48) recently compared mental health characteristics of island Puerto Ricans to three groups from the Los Angeles Epidemiologic Catchment Area Study: Mexican American immigrants, U.S.-born Mexican Americans, and non-Hispanic whites. The Diagnostic Interview Schedule was used to gather both diagnostic and symptom scale information about affective disorders, alcohol abuse, somatization, and phobic and psychotic disorders. Mexican American immigrants showed the fewest mental health problems of all groups. Puerto Ricans expressed more somatization disorders, but showed fewer affective and alcohol disorders than U.S.-born Mexican Americans or non-Hispanic whites.

Health Beliefs

Within the large Hispanic category, two major cultural variants have evolved. Cubans and Puerto Ricans comprise one variant, sharing with other Caribbean groups affinities with the African Hispanic mulatto tradition. The second major variant is the Mexican and Central/South American Indo-Hispanic mestizo tradition characteristic of the Southwest and West Coast.

Despite great variation within and between these traditions, several unifying cultural themes are expressed that may affect health behavior and relations with health care providers. These themes are briefly summarized below.

Familismo

The family is of paramount importance in the lives of most Hispanics. The primacy of "la familia" encourages cooperation, mutual assistance, sharing within large kinship networks, and subordination of competition and individualism. Care of ill family members traditionally has been assumed by daughters, mothers, and other female relatives. Assumptions by health care providers that specific elderly Hispanic clients "will be cared for" by family members may be premature, however, because the positive ideal of "la familia" is not always realized, particularly in urban settings. Research on family supports for older Hispanics suggests that elders often receive less aid from family members than they expect.

Jerarquismo

Hispanic social relationships most often are conducted in terms of relative positions occupied in vertical social structures, in contrast to egalitarian and individualistic relational models. Matriarchal households are appearing more frequently in all groups. In families, older persons generally have more authority than younger members do; greater value is assigned to *machismo*, i.e., men generally garner more authority, respect, and control of resources than do women. The cultural response exhibited by many traditionally oriented Hispanic adult and elderly women is *marianismo*, the long-suffering mother.

Presentismo

More value may be given to a present-time orientation toward issues and concerns than it is to past or future perspectives. Manifestations of this attitude may include a focus on short-term planning, crisis management, and immediate gratification instead of long-term planning, problem prevention, and delayed gratification. Consequences of centering activities in the present may include delaying health care treatment until later stages of a disease manifest and indifference to health promotion and disease prevention strategies.

Personalismo

Hispanic individuals historically have managed their interpersonal relations primarily in terms of the whole person (one's personality, self-worth, and inner qualities) rather than on impersonal role expectations. "Rather than trusting or respecting a certain person . . . on the basis of past achievements or future possibilities, Hispanic *personalismo* emphasizes the building of *confianza* (trust), *respeto* (respect), *orgullo* (pride), and *dignidad* (dignity), which were very important in the delivery of health care . . . through formal but friendly interaction over a period of time (39).

Espiritismo

Hispanic cultures traditionally have regarded illness as the outcome of physical imbalances, powerful human emotions, social disharmony, or supernatural forces (including God's will, magical acts, and evil spirits). Exploration-era Spanish medicine (including Hippocratic humoral pathology—source of the hot-cold syndrome), Catholicism, and African and Latin American Indian religious beliefs and practices (including shamanism and herbalism) have all contributed to a perspective that incorporates scientific, folk, and popular components (49–51).

Folk illnesses that may afflict Hispanic elderly but that may not be revealed to allopathic health practitioners include

susto (spiritual fright): restlessness, anxiety, or generalized physical or behavioral disturbances triggered by unexpected events or shocks that separate body from soul.

empacho: digestive distress caused by eating hot foods and drinking cold liquids, and undigested foods adhering to or blocking the digestive tract.

mal de aire: generalized body pains from exposure to cold weather when the body is hot (and vice versa).

latido: stomach pains, loss of appetite, and constipation resulting from loneliness, depression, or malnourishment.

ataques de nervios: nervous breakdown characterized by *histeria* (great agitation, crying, fainting) sometimes resulting from *susto*.

Depending on their heritage and the nature of their illnesses, Hispanic elders may also seek relief from herbs or other *remedios*, church healing rites, or traditional healers. In the sphere of Mexican American culture, the dominant traditional healing system is *curanderismo*, a syncretic blend of Catholic and indigenous beliefs and practices carried out by the *curandera/o* in nonpublic healing sessions. Today curanderismo is more actively maintained in some areas (e.g., south Texas) than in others (e.g., southern California and Colorado). Puerto Rican *espiritismo* is a Euro-American healing cult focused on communicating with spirits and purifying the soul. Its healers are called *espiritistas*. In Cuba and among some Cuban Americans, a healing system known as *santeria* is practiced, which blends African and Catholic elements. Its practitioners are called *santeros*.

Geriatric Syndromes

Research on Hispanic populations is too meager to conclude whether any typical geriatric syndromes are more prevalent or problematic among this ethnic group. A constellation of disease conditions (including NIDDM, obesity, and hypertension) appears with markedly greater frequently among some Hispanic groups, especially Mexican Americans. Risk increases with age, and genetics and nutrition are associated factors (52,53).

"Most comparisons of [self-reported] functional status have shown Hispanic elders to be at a disadvantage compared to others in the United States" (39). However, cultural differences in perceptions and definitions of health may predispose fewer Hispanics to rate their health as excellent or good than do matched samples of non-Hispanics (53). Studies of one condition that affects functional status—hip fracture—indicate that Hispanic women (but not Hispanic men) are at lower risk for hip fracture than are Anglo American women (54).

Angel and Angel (55) analyzed data from the 1988 National Survey of Hispanic Elderly People to measure the impact of age at migration and of social contacts on the self-assessed health, functional disability, and life satisfaction of elderly Cuban Americans, Mexican Americans, and Puerto Ricans in the United States. They concluded that the difficulties associated with immigration late in life undermine an older person's morale and interfere with the ability to perform basic activities of daily living. Older Cuban Americans, in particular, appear to benefit from residence in ethnic enclaves in which they virtually duplicate their culture of origin.

Further research is also needed to clarify why symptoms, signs, and ill-defined conditions continue to be a leading reported cause of death among older Mexican Americans, especially for those older than 75 years. It has been postulated that the higher than normal use of this category for mortality "may be due to lack of access to health care among the economically disadvantaged and/or avoidance of conventional medical care" (39).

Russians and Other Eastern European Immigrants

Demography and History

Since 1975, emigration from the former Soviet Union has increased dramatically. Approximately 200,000 Russians now reside in the United States. About two-thirds are Jewish; the remaining one-third are often from other persecuted religious groups (e.g., fundamentalist Protestant, or Russian Orthodox) (56). The female-to-male ratio is 2:1. Unlike many other recent immigrants, about 20 percent of this population is already older than 65 years of age. Because the former Soviet Union considered the family, rather than the individual, to be the unit of emigration, older emigrants left home as much or more for the sake of the family as for their own personal desire for freedom or economic improvement. Recent immigrants are likely to have depleted their resources in the effort to relocate. Many emigrés were professionals in their homeland and are experiencing a profound change in status and independence, as well as in location, culture, and language. Most immigrants are from Russia or the Ukraine and have settled in major urban areas in the United States. As political and economic instability continues in those regions, there is little cause to anticipate a slowing of emigration, though its ethnic and religious makeup is likely to diversify.

Table 20.9 depicts the major historic events that shaped the lives of these people. They have intimate, first-hand experience with two world wars, political revolutions, religious persecution, and famine.

Health Status

The major health problems of older Russians are similar to those of their American-born counterparts: diabetes, atherosclerosis, and arthritis, although Russians typically report a higher level of dysfunction from these diseases. Arthritis and the disabilities accompanying it seem especially vexing to those who experienced persecution and hard labor in Siberia. They believe "the cold got in my bones and will never come out" (personal communication). In addition, Russians, like other recent immigrants, have a higher prevalence of tuberculosis than do U.S.-born Anglo American elders.

Health Beliefs

Health beliefs and behaviors for this group have been shaped by their having to learn to manipulate a large,

Table 20.9 Cohort Experiences for Russians and Other Eastern European Immigrants.

	Historic Experience			
	1900–1920	1920–1940	1940–1960	1960–Present
	World War I	Famine	World War II	1968 – Uprising in Czechoslovakia; increased dissidence in Soviet Union
	February and October Revolutions	Collectivization of agriculture	Death of Stalin	1980 – Gorbachev; rise of glasnost and perestroyka
			Consolidation of Soviet influence in Eastern Europe	1986 – Chernobyl nuclear meltdown
				1989 – Collapse of Soviet influence in Eastern Europe
Current Age of Cohort (yr)	Life Stage at Historic Experience			
	1900–1920	1920–1940	1940–1960	1960–Present
85+	Child–adolescent	Young adult	Middle-aged	Elder
75–85	Child	Adolescent–young adult	Young adult–middle-aged	Middle-aged–Elder
65–75		Child, adolescent	Adolescent–young adults	Adults–Young Elder
55–65		Child	Adolescent	Young adult–middle-aged

Adapted from Morioka-Douglas N, Yeo G. Aging and health: Asian and Pacific Island American elders. SGEC Working Paper, series 3. Stanford: Stanford Geriatric Education Center, 1990.

state-run bureaucracy to obtain benefits. Russians are "accustomed to literally having to make noise to receive care in Russia; they have been described as pushy, manipulative and abrasive" (56). Personal quality of care is important, and Russians often seek a personal recommendation for a specialist in the hope that this will guarantee being taken seriously.

Many medications are available over the counter in Russia, and immigrants have access to them through community networks in the United States. Some of these, particularly pills for "liver ailments," a common folk diagnosis for various symptoms, have no known American equivalent. Research into the content of these medications is needed to know whether they are safe or efficacious. Moreover, medications considered outmoded in the U.S. (e.g., reserpine) are still in common use in Russia. Russians may prefer to have their illnesses treated with these older, more familiar preparations.

Geriatric Syndromes

Little is known about the prevalence of the typical geriatric problem list (dementia, depression, falls, incontinence, and malnutrition) among this recently immigrated population. Many clinicians have noted that Russian patients tend to somaticize greatly (57), seek physical explanations for the distress they feel about relocating, and express physical pain out of proportion to specific disease activity or stimuli. This arises, in part, as an adaptive response designed to elicit attention from a large and indifferent state medical bureaucracy.

Russian immigrants are likely to be very resistant to hearing a psychosocial explanation of their ills. Again, this arises out of their experience with the Soviet state system, which used the diagnoses of mental illness and psychiatric hospitalization as tools of political repression. In addition, Soviet psychiatry tended to emphasize biologic rather than psychodynamic explanations of illness. Thus, the physician may need great patience to diagnose and appropriately treat major depression in these individuals.

Older Russian immigrants are faced with the daunting task of simultaneously acculturating and aging. Some survival skills that brought them through decades of extreme hardship in Europe serve well in the U.S.; others must be adapted to negotiate with a new and very different environment.

References

1. Bureau of the Census and National Institute on Aging. Profiles of America's elderly. No. 3. Washington DC: U.S. Government Printing Office, 1993.
2. Gelfand DE. Ethnicity and aging. Annu Rev Gerontol Geriatr 1981;2:91–117.
3. Barker JC. Cultural diversity—changing the context of medical practice. West J Med 1992;157:248–254.
4. Rosenthal CJ. Family supports in later life: does ethnicity make a difference? Gerontologist 1986;26:19–24.
5. Chester B, Holtan N. Working with refugee survivors of torture. West J Med 1992;157:301–304.
6. Putsch RW. Cross-cultural communication: the special case of interpreters in health care. JAMA 1985;254:3344–3348.
7. Miles TP, Bernard MA. Morbidity, Disability, and Health Status of Black American Elderly. J Am Geriatr Assoc 1992;40:1047–1054.
8. National Center for Health Statistics. Health, United States, 1992. U.S. Department of Health and Human Services. DHHS Pub. No. (PHS) 93-1232. Hyattsville, MD: Public Health Service, 1993.
9. Health Resources and Services Administration. Minority Aging. U.S. Department of Health and Human Services. DHHS Pub. No. HRS-P-DV 90-4. Hyattsville, MD: Public Health Service, 1990.
10. Minkler M, Roe KM, Price M. The physical and emotional health of grandmothers raising grandchildren in the crack cocaine epidemic. Gerontologist 1992;32:752–761.
11. Greenberg M, Schneider D. Regions of Birth and Mortality of Blacks in the United States. Int J Epidemiol 1992;21:324–328.
12. Markides KS, Machalek R. Selective Survival, Aging, and Society. Arch Gerontol Geriatr 1984;3:207–221.
13. Nickens HW. The Health Status of Minority Populations in the United States. West J Med 1991;155:27–32.
14. Joint National Committee on Detection, Evaluation, and Treatment of High Blood Pressure. The Fifth Report of the Joint National Committee on Detection, Evaluation, and Treatment of High Blood Pressure (JNCV). Arch Intern Med 1993;153:149–208.
15. Grim CE, Wilson TW. Salt, slavery and survival. In: Fray J, Douglas JG, eds. Pathophysiology of hypertension in blacks. New York: Oxford University, 1993:1–47.
16. O'Brien TR, et al. Are racial differences in the prevalence of diabetes in adults explained by differences in obesity? JAMA 1989;262:1485–1488.
17. Robinson R, et al. Pathways to freedom. Philadelphia: Fox Chase Cancer Center, 1992.
18. Sterling T, Weikam JJ. Comparison of smoking-related risk factors among black and white males. J Am Ind Med 1989;15:319–333.
19. Matthews HF. Rootwork: description of an ethnomedical system in the American South. South Med J 1987;80:885–891.

20. Wilson MR. Glaucoma in blacks: where do we go from here? JAMA 1989;261:281–282.

21. Jones-Webb RJ, Snowden LR. Symptoms of depression among blacks and whites. Am J Public Health 1993;83:240–244.

22. Brown D, et al. Symptoms of depression among older African Americans: an analysis of gender differences. Gerontologist 1992;32:789–795.

23. Bryde JF. Indian students and guidance. Boston: Houghton Mifflin, 1972.

24. Zintz MV. Education across cultures. Dubuque: WC Brown, 1963.

25. Manson SM, Callaway D. Health and aging among American Indians: issues and challenges for the biobehavioral sciences. In: Manson SM, Dinges N, eds. Behavioral health issues among American Indians and Alaska Natives. Denver: University of Colorado Health Sciences Center, 1988:160–210.

26. U.S. Department of Health and Human Services. Report of the Secretary's Task Force on Black and Minority Health. Vol II. Crosscutting Issues in Minority Health. Washington, DC: U.S. Government Printing Officer, 1985.

27. Baron AE, Manson SM, Ackerson LM. Depressive symptomatology in older American Indians with chronic disease. In: Attkisson C, Zitch J, eds. Screening for Depression in Primary Care. New York: Routledge, Kane, 1990:217–231.

28. Baker FM, Kamikawa LM, Espino DS, Manson SM. Rehabilitation in ethnic minority elderly. In: Brody SJ, Pawlson LG, eds. Aging and rehabilitation. New York: Springer, 1990:186–207.

29. Morioka-Douglas N, Yeo G. Aging and health: Asian Pacific Island American elders, SGEC Working Paper, Series 3. Stanford: Stanford Geriatric Education Center, 1990.

30. Choi ESK, McGandy RB, Sadowski JA, et al. The prevalence of cardiovascular risk factors among elderly Chinese Americans. Arch Intern Med 1990;150:413–418.

31. Serby M, Chou JCY, Franssen EH. Dementia in an American-Chinese nursing home population. Am J Psychiatry 1987;144:811–812.

32. Bates SR, Hill L, Barrett-Connor E. Cardiovascular disease risk factors in an Indochinese population. Am J Prev Med 1989;5:15–20.

33. Muecke MA. Caring for Southeast Asian refugee patients in the USA. Am J Public Health 1983;73:431–438.

34. Anderson JN. Health and illness in Filipino immigrants. West J Med 1983;139:811–819.

35. Palafox N, Warren A. Cross-Cultural Caring. Honolulu: Transcultural Health Care Forum, 1980.

36. Hopper SV. The influence of ethnicity on the health of older women. Clin in Geriatr Med 1993;9:231–259.

37. Fowles D. A profile of older Americans: 1991. Washington, DC: American Association of Retired Persons, 1991.

38. Lopez C, Aguilera E. On the sidelines: Hispanic elderly and the continuum of care. Washington, DC: National Council of La Raza, 1991.

39. Villa ML, Cuellar J, Gamel N, Yeo G. Aging and health: Hispanic American elders. 2nd ed. SCEG Working Paper, Series 5. Stanford: Stanford Geriatric Education Center, 1993.

40. Cubillos HL. The Hispanic elderly: a demographic profile. Washington, DC: National Council of La Raza, 1987.

41. Yeo G, Hikoyeda N. Cohort analysis as a clinical and educational tool in ethnogeriatrics: historical profiles of Chinese, Filipino, Mexican, and African American elders. SCEG Working Paper, Series 12. Stanford: Stanford Geriatric Education Center, 1992.

42. Sorlie PD, Backlund E, Johnson NJ, Rogot E. Mortality by Hispanic status in the United States. JAMA 1993;270:2464–2468.

43. Rosenwaike I. Mortality differentials among persons born in Cuba, Mexico, and Puerto Rico residing in the United States, 1979–1981. Am J Public Health 1987;77:603–606.

44. Marshall JA, Hamman RF, Baxter J, et al. Ethnic differences in risk factors associated with the prevalence of non-insulin-dependent diabetes mellitus. The San Luis Valley Diabetes Study. Am J Epidemiol 1993;137:706–718.

45. Hanis CL, Hewett-Emmett D, Bertin TK, Schull WJ. Origins of US Hispanics. Implications for diabetes. Diabetes Care 1991;14:618–627.

46. Molgaard CA, Nakamura CM, Stanford EP, et al. Prevalence of Alcohol Consumption Among Older Persons. J Community Health 1990;15:239–251.

47. Marin G. AIDS prevention among Hispanics: needs, risk behaviors, and cultural values. Public Health Rep 1989;104:411–415.

48. Shrout PE, Canino GJ, Bird HR, et al. Mental health status among Puerto Ricans, Mexican Americans, and non-Hispanic whites. Am J Community Psychol 1992;20:729–752.

49. Kay MA. Health and illness in a Mexican American barrio. In: Spicer EH, ed. Ethnic medicine in the Southwest. Tucson: University of Arizona, 1977:99–166.

50. Madsen W. The Mexican Americans of South Texas. New York: Holt, Rinehart and Winston, 1964.

51. Rubel AJ, O'Nell CW, Collado-Ardon, R. Susto, a Folk Illness. Berkeley: University of California, 1984.

52. Hanis CL, Ferrell RE, Schull WJ. Hypertension and sources of blood pressure variability among Mexican Americans in Starr County, Texas. Int J Epidemiol 1985;14:231–238.

53. Bastida E, Gonzales G. Ethnic variations in measurement of physical health status: implications for long-term care. In: Barresi CM, Stull DE, eds. Ethnic elderly and long-term care. New York: Springer, 1993:22–35.

54. Bauer RL. Ethnic differences in hip fracture: a reduced incidence in Mexican Americans. Am J Epidemiol 1988;127:145–149.

55. Angel JL, Angel RJ. Age at migration, social connections, and well-being among elderly Hispanics. J Aging Health 1992;4:480–499.

56. Brod M, Heurtin-Roberts J. Cross-cultural medicine a decade

later: older Russians emigrés and medical care. West J Med 1992;157:333–336.

57. Kohn R, Flaherty JA, Levav I. Somatic symptoms among older Soviet immigrants: an exploratory study. Int J Soc Psychiatry 1989;35:350–360.

58. Hingley R. Russia: a concise history. 2nd ed. New York: Thames and Hudson, 1991.

59. Dmytryshyn B. USSR: a concise history. 2nd ed. New York: Scribner, 1971.

Chapter 21
Legal Aspects of Care

Frank H. Marsh

No law is quite appropriate for all.

Livy

In the past several years, no other area has received more attention in medical ethics and medical law than that involving the rights of elderly patients. The main focus of this attention touches on issues surrounding the concept of autonomy in the elderly patient and what this requires of physicians and other health care professionals. Because the dictates of this important principle are often unclear and misunderstood by some physicians that attend to the elderly, potential ethical and legal conflicts may arise between a physician and the patient, the patient's family, or both. Unless resolved, these conflicts can ultimately undermine the relationship itself and work against the best interests of the patient and possibly, promote civil litigation.

In this chapter, the rights that are vested in the elderly patient as an autonomous agent and the appropriate response by the physician to these rights are examined. The first part of the discussion addresses the right to autonomy and informed consent, followed by a look at the question of "presumed competency" and the use of elderly patients as research subjects. These rights are then examined in the context of treating the incompetent patient, with specific emphasis on the difficult issue of futile care and do-not-resuscitate (DNR) orders. The chapter closes with a discussion of the legal implications of physician-assisted suicide.

Informed Consent and the Autonomous Elderly Patient

A general rule of our legal system is that people are allowed to exercise self-determination. The right of self-determination extends to all areas of health care; patients have both the right and responsibility to make their own

decisions about what will or will not be done to their body. Unfortunately, the rule is compromised or ignored by some physicians treating the geriatric patient because self-determination and advanced age are seen as being antithetical. As a result, one of the most pressing needs of geriatric patients is a clearer understanding by their physicians of the right to make personal decisions concerning their own well-being and how this right is manifested through the doctrine of informed consent.

Few legal issues surrounding the medical profession are as much discussed and as little understood as informed consent. The basic premise is that informed consent must be the willing and uncoerced acceptance of a medical procedure by a competent patient after adequate disclosure by the physician of the nature of the procedure, its risks and benefits, and the alternatives to the procedure with their risks and benefits (1). This premise is not compromised by the advanced age of a patient. Physicians who withhold information from any competent adult patient, regardless of the patient's age, may be exposed to liability.

There are, however, a few specific situations in which the law permits a physician to withhold certain details from a patient if disclosure would likely have an adverse affect on the patient's health or well-being. A physician opting to withhold information must carefully document in what way the information, if revealed, would have substantial adverse impact on the patient. It is important to note, however, that this therapeutic privilege cannot be relied on by physicians to wrongfully withhold important information from a patient, nor can a request and authorization of relatives or surrogates not to disclose be used as a reason for invoking the nondisclosure privilege (2).

Treating Patients with Diminished Competence
One of the most vexing issues confronting physicians who care for the elderly patient is the situation in which

the patient is no longer competent or has only, at best, borderline competence to make personal diagnostic and treatment decisions. These problems are not confined to the elderly, dying patient. In fact, excess attention to issues of death and dying has diverted attention from the majority of elderly patients of diminished competence whose condition is not life-threatening.

Even though a fairly large body of literature exists concerning patients who lack the capacity to participate in the decision-making process, there still is considerable difficulty in defining what is meant by the term incompetency or incapacity. In addition, there is considerable confusion as to the appropriate procedure for making such a determination. Although the question of competency can be determined by the courts, it is customary practice in the medical profession for a patient's attending physician to make this judgment (3).

When approaching the question of patient incompetency, physicians should keep in mind that the law presumes that every adult patient possesses the mental capacity to give an informed consent (4). Because this presumption also applies to elderly patients, physicians are not required to show that a patient has the capacity to participate in the decision-making process. The presumption holds even though the elderly patient evinces periods of confusion or disorientation. Many physicians, however, unwittingly ignore the presumption by starting from the premise that the patient's capacity to give an informed consent must be established. The law does not require a physician to follow this procedure. Instead, before a patient can be denied the right to participate in the decision-making process, the presumption of his competency must be clearly overcome. This means that a physician need not undertake the time-consuming task of demonstrating competency in the patient but can make a straightforward determination that the patient *does not* have the ability to understand the nature and consequences of authorizing or refusing treatment.

This presumption is not lost, nor is it overcome, in the case of elderly patients who drift in and out of periods of lucidity. A consent obtained while such individuals are lucid is valid, providing that the patient has the mental ability to understand the nature and consequences of consent (5). An important caveat here is that because consent obtained during a lucid phase is valid, the withdrawal of

consent during a lucid phase is also valid and should be respected. Sometimes, however, elderly patients who are confused may not realize they are incapable of giving consent. When this is the case, the physician must be prepared to prove at a later date that the patient lacked the mental capacity to understand the nature and consequences of his decision.

Using Elderly Persons as Research Subjects

The use of elderly patients in research has always been a delicate issue for clinician-investigators because of the stringent requirements of informed consent. Before an Institutional Review Board may approve human research, federal regulations require a finding that appropriate additional safeguards have been included in the study to protect the rights and welfare of subjects who are likely to be vulnerable to coercion or undue influence (6). Individuals specifically protected by these regulations include elderly patients who suffer from acute or severe physical or mental illness, or those who are economically or educationally disadvantaged.

The legal questions here are mainly concerned with disclosure of information and the actual consent given by the elderly patient-subject. Unfortunately, virtually no case law exists on the basis of which legal standards for consent to research and the disclosure of information, as distinguished from practice, can be defined (7). In other words, the requirements that apply to a patient who, for example, is about to undergo an operation or receive chemotherapy, are the same ones applied in all areas of research. However, in the case of enrolling elderly patients in a study, the informed consent process must be altered and amended to meet the particular situation. In this respect, the general disclosure statements required in consent forms by the Department of Health and Human Services and the Food and Drug Administration in all government-funded research are not always helpful or sufficient.

Many clinicians still believe that once an Institutional Review Board approves and signs off on the content of the consent form, an ethical and legal informed consent may be achieved when the form is signed by the patient or the patient's surrogate. This belief is a serious mistake. The written document is only part of the process of informing the subject and obtaining permission to participate. An informed consent form proves only that consent occurred; it does not prove that consent was informed. Instead, the process of communication and the explanation of the contents, regardless of how much time is consumed, is what legally satisfies the informed feature of consent (8).

Obtaining the consent itself from a prospective elderly subject also may present formidable legal problems for the clinician-investigator. The most prudent course for the clinician-investigator to follow is to avoid elderly persons of questionable competency as research subjects, regardless of the importance of the study. Although these individuals may initially give an effective consent when they are competent, the fact that they may slip in and out of states of lucidity may challenge the legal effectiveness of that consent, a prospect that may cause future problems for the investigator (9).

Federal regulations, however, do permit a legally authorized representative to consent on behalf of the elderly patient. According to the federal regulations, a legally authorized representative is "An individual or judicial or other body authorized under applicable law to consent on behalf of a prospective subject to the subject's participation in the procedure(s) involved in the research" (10).

Permission granted by a spouse or next of kin is not valid legally unless these individuals are legally authorized to act on behalf of the elderly patient. In addition, an elderly patient does not necessarily lose the right to consent to research because a guardian or conservator has been appointed to look after the person's affairs. To give a legally effective consent for research, the appointment of the guardian or conservator must include specific authority to do so.

Futile Care and Do-Not-Resuscitate Orders

During the past 3 years, debates over the meaning of futility and the issuance of DNR orders have surfaced both in frequency and in intensity. Even though many studies indicate that elderly patients with certain conditions rarely, if ever, survive cardiopulmonary resuscitation (CPR) (11), there is still a strong tendency by physicians and hospitals to regard the idea of futility as a concept with ambiguous overtones when it applies to medical treatment. The improbabilities associated with predicting outcomes in certain areas of medicine drastically affect the notion that there can be a clear understanding of what is futile care in other areas of medicine. In this context exists an important misunderstanding regarding CPR and the elderly patient. Specifically, physicians and hospitals are inclined to believe that CPR is futile only in situations in which it would be useless to employ other life-prolonging treatments (12). This perception is erroneous and is one of the central reasons for the difficulties in reaching a useful consensus for a definitive meaning of futile care.

Because futile care is viewed as a vague notion without empirical content, many physicians find themselves hopelessly trapped into administering CPR either because consent for a DNR order was sought and refused, or because the patient has previously specifically indicated through an advance directive that everything be done regardless of the medical condition. In both cases, administering futile care is a result of physicians no longer being willing to make certain decisions unilaterally, even though this authority has always been accorded to them by law. Physicians should not permit their exclusive authority to determine what beneficial treatment is available to meet the patient's needs to be compromised by the demands of the autonomous patient, the patient's family, or both. Both the fiduciary duties of the physician and the dictates of the doctrine of informed consent preclude any obligations on behalf of the physician to determine patient's preferences with respect to futile treatment (13).

Two rationales generally are offered by physicians in support of a decision that CPR would be futile: 1) the intervention is based on a value judgment, that is, the quality of the patient's life, either before or after CPR, is unacceptable, or the medical intervention cannot possibly achieve the patient's goals; or 2) the intervention will be unsuccessful and thus would be of no medical benefit (12). When the quality of a patient's life is the controlling factor in a decision to forego CPR, the physician is always obligated to seek the patient's input and consent before issuing the DNR order. This approach, however, is quite different from a judgment by the physician that CPR is futile because it offers no medical benefit to the patient. Although the latter judgment is also value laden, it is derived solely from the diagnostic and prognostic medical expertise of the treating physician, which is independent of the subjective interests, goals, and desires of the patient. Physicians serve no useful purpose by offering the choice of CPR when the procedure would be futile as defined by the second rationale (14). In these situations, it is legally proper for the treating physician to issue a DNR order.

Although a patient has every right to expect a physician to do everything possible for the patient's benefit, the physician is legally obligated only to preserve life by using the skills and means ordinarily employed by other physicians in similar cases (15). The physician is not legally obligated to exercise futile or extraordinary care, and failure to do so will not subject the physician to civil or criminal liability. It is the duty of the physician to treat patients only in conformity with professional medical standards that give rise to the patient's right to ordinary treatment, which right, in turn, includes informed consent (16). The duty of care does not extend to administering futile treatment because, in such situations, no ordinary treatment choice exists on behalf of the patient, nor does a right to extraordinary treatment exist.

In the development of the informed consent doctrine, the courts have focused on promoting the patient's well-being and protecting the patient's right of self-determination. This doctrine traditionally has required disclosure of enough information to allow the patient to make an informed decision. However, the doctrine has been limited to situations that call either for a decision to undergo treatment or to refuse treatment. In a case involving a DNR order, the patient's consent would be required only when CPR might be, or definitely would be, of some benefit to the patient. In this situation the patient's right to choose would exist. However, if all treatment alternatives, including CPR, are futile, the patient has no real choice, and there is no need for disclosure of information (17). It is ludicrous to suggest that futile administration of CPR provides a patient with a meaningful treatment choice under the informed consent doctrine.

Physician Liability for Rendering Futile Care

Most physicians point to the threat of civil liability as the justification for their unwillingness to enter a DNR order when they believe that CPR would be futile, but substantial case law supports the proposition that there is no liability for entering a DNR order in those circumstances. Actually liability for not offering or providing futile care is remote; a physician has greater liability exposure if futile care is provided (18).

The circumstances under which a physician could be liable in a malpractice action for entering a DNR order following a determination that CPR would be futile are no different from those in any other treatment context. Potential liability would not arise from the entry of the DNR order, but from the decision that CPR would be futile, if subsequently the decision about CPR was shown to be incorrect. The physician will not be found to be negligent so long as the decision that CPR would be futile is in accord with acceptable medical knowledge regarding the ineffectiveness of CPR as a life-saving or life-prolonging treatment for patients in similar conditions (19). For this reason, hospital medical staffs should adopt guidelines for issuing unilateral DNR orders that are based on profiles of patients for whom CPR is futile. So long as these guidelines are regularly updated in accord with new studies in this area, a physician who enters a DNR order pursuant to the guidelines should not be found liable in malpractice for such a decision.

Physician-Assisted Suicide

Suicide among the elderly is a problem of considerable magnitude in America. Of a total of 25,000 to 30,000 cases of suicide reported every year, 25 percent are committed by people older than 60 years of age (20). Unfortunately, the high rate of suicide among the elderly is used by advocates of rational suicide to promote physician-assisted suicide for elderly people who are terminally ill or who are suffering from an incurable affliction, even though the fraction of elderly suicide victims in this category is only 2 percent to 4 percent (21).

A person's desire to end a painful terminal illness is understandable, but physicians who assist in the process are treading dangerous waters. Approximately twenty-five states expressly prohibit assisted suicide by statute and another twelve states make some types of assisted suicide a form of murder or manslaughter (22). In addition, almost all of the living will statutes in the United States state that assisting patient suicide is not permitted under the statute (22). Complying with a legally effective living will is not, however, an act of physician-assisted suicide. There is a clear distinction between terminating the medical treatment of a terminally ill or catastrophically injured patient and helping someone to commit suicide. The two acts are causally different. In the first instance, an underlying fatal pathology must exist if allowing to die is even possible. In the second, killing provides its own fatal pathology, in that a lethal injection is necessary to precipitate death (23).

An important question often raised by physicians is whether sedating a patient from whom ventilation is withdrawn is legally permissible when it is known that the sedation will, in all probability, hasten and increase the patient's risk of death. Although there is a fine line between a dose that will sedate a very sick patient and a dose that will kill the patient, sedating the patient is not an act of physician-assisted suicide. Nor is termination of ventilatory support from a patient who might live for an indefinite duration if the support had not been withdrawn considered as assisted suicide (24). The idea that rejection of life-saving medical treatment by competent patients constitutes suicide has been uniformly rejected by legal authorities (24).

The main question that seems to produce ambiguous responses both in medicine and in the public sector is whether the right to die includes the right to assisted suicide. At first glance, the idea of a right to die seems difficult to overcome, let alone dismissed from consideration. If such a right exists, the next logical step would embrace a patient's right to demand help in committing suicide. There is, however, no constitutional "right to die." As set forth in the landmark case of *Cruzan* v. *Director, Missouri Department of Health*, what the competent adult patient does possess is "a constitutionally protected right to refuse life-saving hydration and nutrition" (25). This right of refusal, however, is not an absolute or fundamental right but must be weighed against the undeniable interest a state has in the protection and preservation of human life, an interest that includes among other things, the banning of assisted suicide. It is highly unlikely that the U.S. Supreme Court will pronounce any constitutional support for assisted suicide in the foreseeable future and will leave the matter to individual state legislatures. Physicians contemplating assisted suicide should become familiar with the state laws in which they practice with

regard to criminal penalties for one who assists another in suicide.

References

1. Appelbaum PS, Lidz CW, Meisel A. Informed consent: legal theory and clinical practice. Oxford: Oxford University, 1987:12–16.
2. Rozovsky FA. Consent to treatment: a practical guide. 2nd ed. Boston: Little, Brown, 1988:70–71.
3. Rosovsky FA. Consent to treatment: a practical guide. 2nd ed. Boston: Little, Brown, 1988:17–18.
4. Gottlieb RA. Preserving personal autonomy for the elderly. J Leg Med 1987;8:1.
5. Rozovsky FA. Consent to treatment: a practical guide. 2nd ed. Boston: Little, Brown, 1988:14–15.
6. 45 CFR § 46.111 (HHS) (1981); 21 CFR § 56.111 (FDA) (1981).
7. Levine R. Ethics and regulations of clinical research. 2nd ed. Baltimore: Urban & Schwarzenburg, 1986.
8. Maloney DM. Protection of human research subjects. New York: Plenum, 1984.
9. Rozovsky FA. Consent to treatment: a practical guide. 2nd ed. Boston: Little, Brown, 1988:566–567.
10. 45 CFR § 46.102 (HHS) (1981); 21 CFR § 50.31 (FDA) (1981).
11. Taffet W, Teasdale M, Luchi BA. In-hospital cardiopulmonary resuscitation. JAMA 1988;260:2069.
12. Tomlinson T, Brody HA. Ethics and communication in do-not-resuscitate orders. N Engl J Med 1988;318:43.
13. Stanley A. The Appleton consensus. J Med Ethics 1989;15:132.
14. Fadden R, Beauchamp T. A theory of informed consent. Oxford: Oxford University, 1986:38–39.
15. 61 AM Jur 2d. Physicians, surgeons and other healers. § 205:337–338 (1989).
16. King J. The law of medical malpractice. St. Paul: West, 1977:152–155.
17. Katz J, Capron A. Catastrophic diseases: who decides what? New York: Russell Sage, 1977:30–33.
18. Marsh FH, Staver A. Physician authority for unilateral DNR orders. J Leg Med 1991;12:144–149.
19. *William* v. *Lemon*, 194 Ga App 249; 390 SE2d 89, 90 (1990).
20. Society for The Right to Die. Refusal of treatment legislation, New York: Society for the Right to Die, 1991.
21. Hendin H, Klerman G. Physician-assisted suicide: the dangers of legalization. Am J Psychiatry 1993;150:143–145.
22. Kamisar Y. Are laws against suicide unconstitutional? Hastings Cent Rep 1993;23(3):32–41.
23. Callahan D. The troubled dream of life: living with mortality. New York: Simon & Schuster 1993:ch. 2.
24. March FH, Staver A. Physician authority for unilateral DNR orders. J Leg Med 1991;12:144–149.
25. *Cruzan* v. *Director, Missouri Department of Health*, 497 US § 261, 280 (1990).

Part III   Geriatric Syndromes

Chapter 22
Acute Confusional State

Lawrence A. Meredith and Christopher M. Filley

I'm not confused, I'm just well-mixed.

Robert Frost

Acute confusional state (ACS) may be defined most simply as a rapidly evolving disorder of neurobehavioral function characterized by altered attention. This common problem presents an important, sometimes difficult, diagnostic dilemma to physicians in all fields of medicine. In the geriatric population, ACS can present special challenges because of the prevalence and, often, multifactorial etiology of confusion in the elderly (1–5). The generally reversible nature of the ACS makes the prompt and accurate diagnosis of this syndrome far from a purely academic exercise.

Like many disorders in medicine, a variety of terms has been applied over time to the syndrome of ACS. The word "delirium" has been historically popular and still dominates much of the literature, especially within the psychiatric realm. Misunderstandings with this concept can arise because many physicians and lay persons associate delirium with an agitated or hyperaroused state (as is the case with the classic delirium tremens) and may fail to recognize the clinical significance of the more common lethargy or somnolence associated with acute confusion. "Toxic-metabolic encephalopathy," a descriptive term popular among practitioners of internal medicine, offers advantages because the most common etiologies of acute confusion are, in fact, toxic or metabolic; this term, however, is unnecessarily restrictive because there are many other causes of confusion. The description "acute organic brain syndrome" is nonspecific and should be avoided. ACS is preferred, therefore, and is used in this chapter.

Clinical Manifestations

ACS may be conceptualized as a disorder of attention (6). Most, if not all neuropsychological manifestations of ACS can be traced to this fundamental dysfunction. Other clinical manifestations that arise in association with the attentional impairment include increased distractibility, various perceptual abnormalities, disruption of the sleep-wake cycle, and variable disturbances of arousal (7–14).

Because the process of attention is so basic to other cognitive processes, specific assessment of higher cerebral function in ACS, including memory, language, visuospatial skills, abstract reasoning, writing (15), and calculations shows variable degrees of impairment (16). Confusion, the inability to maintain a coherent train of thought, dominates the examination and often precludes the adequate performance of any specific neurobehavioral task. In fact, once the presence of a confusional state has been established, detailed neuropsychological testing becomes very difficult and of limited value.

The perceptual distortions associated with confusional states usually take the form of illusions, which are misinterpretations of sensory information (8). Frank hallucinations occur rarely and usually involve the visual modality (8). Disturbances of arousal are most often manifested as hypoarousal; less common but more dramatic is the hyperaroused or agitated patient who presents additional management challenges. For example, although it is always best to avoid sedative medications and physical restraints (which may tend to further propagate confusion and agitation), safety consideration sometimes mandate this solution in the agitated patient. Many patients with ACS can experience striking fluctuations in level of consciousness (8).

Disruption of the sleep-wake cycle often goes with disturbances of arousal (9). A common scenario involves the elderly hospitalized patient who is somnolent or sleeping during the daytime, only to show increasing agitation and confusion during the night. The tendency toward "sundowning" can probably be explained as a result of decreased environmental stimulation and disruption of sleep-wake cycles, which play on already disordered systems of arousal and attention. Not only is the sleep-wake cycle vulnerable in ACS, but the disruption itself can represent a significant precipitating cause for confusion, and thus create a potentially vicious cycle of somnolence, agitation, and confusion.

Pathophysiology of Acute Confusion

The neuroanatomic substrates that underlie arousal and attention are complex and poorly understood. Likewise, the pathophysiologic changes involved in the disruption of this delicate balance are equally difficult to delineate. Patients who die in states of acute confusion may show little or no clear pathologic changes in the brain at autopsy (8), which reflects that in many cases the changes in brain function during acute confusion are reversible and functional, not structural. Cases in which there is clear structural pathology, as in right middle cerebral arterial infarctions (17), demonstrate that key areas of the brain subserve the mechanisms of attention and arousal.

The concept of "state" as compared with "channel" systems for information flow in the brain is useful for better understanding of how attention can be disrupted (18). State systems involve diffuse projection pathways from subcortical structures to wide areas of cerebral cortex that influence the background cortical tone of the individual. Each of these projection systems employs a particular neurotransmitter and thus is susceptible to pharmacologic manipulation. A good example is the cholinergic projection system from the basal forebrain, which provides the major source of cholinergic input to the cerebral cortex and hippocampus, and which is thought to play a role in facilitating memory. This system appears to be selectively damaged in some dementing illnesses such as Alzheimer's disease and may be temporarily disrupted by anticholinergic medications, which so commonly cause confusion and memory dysfunction. Other examples of diffuse systems involved in the maintenance of attention and arousal include adrenergic, serotonergic, and dopaminergic pathways from the brain stem, as well as projections from the reticular activating system and thalamus (19).

Channel systems involve the simultaneous processing of various components of information into parallel channels that involve different neuroanatomical substrates. For example, in the visual system, different neural networks are involved more or less independently in the parallel processing of form, color, and movement. The distributed neuronal networks occupy overlapping but distinct anatomical localizations. Discrete pathological events can disrupt one neuronal network while leaving neighboring networks relatively intact, and thereby interfere with the processing of a particular component of visual information. For instance, certain discrete lesions in the ventral visual association cortices can give rise to achromatopsia, the loss of color vision, while leaving intact mechanisms responsible for the detection of form and movement.

In a similar vein, several cortical regions appear critical to the distributed networks involved with different components of attention (20–22). These regions include the prefrontal (23,24), cingulate (25), and parietal (18) cortices, each of which appear to play distinct and complementary roles in maintaining and controlling attention. As a general rule, the right hemisphere appears dominant for many aspects of attention (18). Whereas lesions in the attentional network of the left hemisphere can be apparently compensated by the right hemisphere, the reverse is not true. This difference may explain the propensity for patients with lesions of the right hemisphere to develop neglect of the contralateral hemispace, whereas the association between lesions of the left hemisphere and contralateral hemispatial neglect is not nearly so robust.

Differential Diagnosis of Acute Confusion

Several diverse entities can be occasionally misinterpreted as ACS. The most important of these neurologic and psychiatric disorders include dementia, aphasia, schizophrenia, mania, depression, and hysteria. Because of the divergent treatments and prognoses involved with these disorders and the general reversible nature of ACS, early proper diagnosis may prove critical.

Dementia

Both the demented and the acutely confused patient may appear disoriented, irrational, and confused, but the distinction is usually not difficult if one remembers that dysfunction of attention is primary to acute confusion. Demented patients often demonstrate relatively intact attentional mechanisms while showing profound deficits in memory encoding and recall. Patients with dementia do not have fluctuations in level of consciousness, but do display prominent memory loss and other cognitive impairments. In addition, dementia is a chronic, not acute, syndrome. A potential difficulty can arise, however, when an otherwise minor medical problem, such as a urinary tract infection, unmasks a previously unrecognized dementia by superimposing ACS onto a less resilient nervous system. Careful and sympathetic history-taking from close family members can often reveal an otherwise subtle dementing process that was underway before ACS began.

Aphasia

A nonfluent or mute patient is not generally mislabeled as confused. However, patients with fluent or "receptive" aphasias may appear quite confused to the naive examiner, especially if the patient's comprehension is significantly impaired. Patients with Wernicke's aphasia, usually a result of infarction in the distribution of a posterior branch of the left middle cerebral artery, may produce fluent nonsense speech and comprehend nothing of what is said to them. Unlike patients with nonfluent aphasia, such as Broca's aphasia, who typically have contralateral hemiparesis, those with fluent aphasia have a posterior lesion that may result in no elemental neurologic deficits. In such cases, careful attention to mental status examination is especially crucial.

Occasionally, the frustration and anxiety associated with this communication deficit can cause considerable agitation, and thus further cloud the clinical picture. Another helpful clue in diagnosing aphasia is the presence of paraphasic errors. These involve the substitution of letters or whole words (e.g., "treen" for "train" or "table" for "chair") or sometimes the creation of new words (neologisms, e.g., "shipenfick"). Generally intact attentional mechanisms and the use of nonlinguistic communication (i.e., gestures) in these aphasic patients usually leave little doubt as to the diagnosis.

Schizophrenia and Other Psychiatric Disorders

In patients presenting with very limited historic information, acute psychosis, whether caused by schizophrenia or mania, may be difficult to distinguish from ACS. Irrational thought processes, hallucinations, and disturbances of attention can all be present to varying degrees in both acute psychosis and confusional states. However, observing the particular pattern of clinical features can usually clarify this distinction without great difficulty.

The presence of paranoid delusions, prominent auditory hallucinations, younger age, and any history of previous psychiatric illness tend to favor a psychiatric disorder. A good general rule is that auditory hallucinations suggest psychiatric disease, whereas visual hallucinations imply a neurologic disorder. As seen in mildly demented patients, those with borderline psychiatric functioning may decompensate with relatively minor insults to the brain, and thus produce a mixed picture of acute confusion and psychiatric symptoms.

Patients with severe depression may demonstrate somnolence, apathy, and poor cognitive processing reminiscent of demented patients. In depressed patients with pseudodementia, other symptoms of depression such as dysphoria, suicidal ideation, insomnia, anorexia, and weight loss can be useful. A normal electroencephalogram (EEG) in patients with depression, hysterical confusion, or other psychiatric disorders can be extremely useful to distinguish them from those with acute confusion, who demonstrate characteristic background slowing on the EEG (26).

Etiologies of Acute Confusion

As a general point, it should be remembered that the etiology of ACS is often multifactorial. This generalization is particularly true in the elderly population. In the young adult with acute confusion, a single etiologic entity can often be identified, but in the elderly, confused patient, this is frequently difficult or impossible. Thus, the geriatric patient, often with many medical problems requiring multiple medications, can provide a unique challenge to the judgment and insight of the investigating physician.

The list of specific etiologies that can contribute to ACS is varied, long, and constantly expanding. Some of the major categories include medications and drugs, toxic-metabolic disorders, systemic or central nervous system

Table 22.1. Common Etiologies of ACS in the Elderly.

Medication and drug toxicity
Metabolic disorders
  Azotemia
  Hyponatremia
  Volume depletion
  Hypoglycemia
  Hyperthyroidism
  Hypercalcemia
  Cushing's syndrome
Infection
  CNS
  Systemic
Cardiogenic disorders
  Acute myocardial infarction
  Arrhythmia
  Congestive heart failure
Neurologic disorders
  Stroke
  Trauma
  Tumors
Anesthesia or surgery
Pain
Change of environment

(CNS) infections, structural lesions of the brain, postsurgical and anesthesia-related events, and various other neurologic disorders such as seizures, head trauma, demyelination, ischemia, and hydrocephalus. The major categories will be disussed in greater detail below. Table 22.1 summarizes the common etiologies of ACS in the elderly.

Medications and Drugs

Medications and drugs are without doubt the most frequent cause of ACS (11). In teenagers and young adults, illicit recreational drug abuse is notorious for causing acute confusion, whereas in the elderly, prescription drugs are the more likely culprit. A complete list of every medication and drug that has been shown to cause or exacerbate acute confusion would be impractical and not particularly useful because of the enormous number of centrally active substances implicated in acute confusion, and because, in any individual patient, almost no medication can be considered absolutely free of potential adverse cognitive effects. Nevertheless, a necessarily incomplete list of medications and drugs that have been commonly

associated with acute confusion is provided in Table 22.2. Because idiosyncratic reactions to any medication can occur, it is paramount that any recent change in a confused patient's medical regimen be carefully scrutinized.

Disorders of Metabolism

Metabolic derangements represent another major category of etiologies commonly leading to an acute confusional state (11). Elderly patients are more vulnerable to the cognitive effects of toxic-metabolic disorders and are also more likely to harbor the medical disorders that lead to these derangements. Dysfunction in most of the major organ systems, including renal, hepatic, cardiac, pulmonary, and endocrine, can lead to acute encephalopathy and associated confusion. The fact that dysfunction of organ systems which have diverse functions can lead to a similar state of disordered arousal, attention, and complex cognitive processing demonstrates the exquisite sensitivity of the brain to perturbations in the body's internal milieu. Fortunately, routine laboratory tests such as chemistry panels, urinalysis, arterial blood gases, and liver function tests can conveniently rule out many of these common problems. Although nonspecific, the presence of asterixis on physical examination or triphasic waves on EEG can be helpful in suggesting a metabolic-toxic etiology for acute confusion.

Table 22.2. Common Medications and Drugs Associated with Acute Confusion.

Alcohol
Anticholinergics (trihexyphenidyl, benztropine)
Antihistamines (hydroxyzine, diphenhydramine, promethazine)
Barbiturates (pentobarbital, phenobarbital)
Benzodiazepines (diazepam, lorazepam)
Beta blockers (propranolol)
Digitalis preparations (digoxin)
Dopamine agonists (pergolide, bromocriptine)
Hallucinogens (LSD, PCP)
H_2 blockers (cimetidine, ranitidine)
Levodopa-carbidopa
Lidocaine (intravenous)
Narcotics (morphine, codeine, meperidine)
Neuroleptics (haloperidol, clozapine)
Stimulants (cocaine, amphetamine)
Theophylline

LSD = lysergic acid diethylamide; PCP = phencyclidine.

Infections

Both CNS and systemic infection remain important causes of acute confusion. Infections of the CNS, in particular, are often life-threatening emergencies that demand urgent attention. Full-blown bacterial meningitis with the characteristic symptoms of fever, headache, meningismus, and confusion is usually easy to recognize. A delay of only a few hours between the presentation of this illness and initiation of adequate antibiotic therapy can spell the difference between a good outcome and disaster.

However, the symptoms of meningeal irritation may be less reliable in elderly patients. Ironically, early diagnosis and treatment is even more critical for these patients because they have a potentially less vigorous immune defense. Most cases of aseptic (viral) meningitis and viral encephalitis are self-limited and the treatment is supportive. However, encephalitis caused by herpes simplex virus is an important exception. Treatment with intravenous acyclovir must begin early to be of significant benefit in this life-threatening illness. Herpes simplex encephalitis presents with a rapidly progressive ACS often accompanied by headache, fever, meningismus, and seizures of temporal lobe origin. The presence of erythrocytes as well as lymphocytes in the cerebrospinal fluid (CSF), enhanced medial temporal lobe lesions on magnetic resonance imaging (MRI) or computerized tomography (CT), frank seizures or focal spiking on EEG, and prominent focal findings are helpful in recognizing this disease. Identification of viral antigen using the polymerase chain reaction (PCR) techniques on CSF has recently been of increasing, although still limited, usefulness. Brain biopsy is recommended by some for definitive diagnosis, but recognition of clinical features is usually sufficiently accurate to avoid this invasive procedure.

Much more common in producing confusion in the elderly are primary infections outside the CNS. Infections of the urinary tract, lungs, decubitus ulcers, sinuses, and other sites that might have little or no effect on the cognitive processes of a young adult may produce significant confusion in geriatric patients, even without particularly high fevers or other metabolic derangement. A careful survey for any evidence of infection should be included in the evaluation of any confused patient, especially in the elderly.

Structural Lesions

Structural lesions of the brain, whether from invasive processes such as neoplasms or ischemic destruction from embolic infarction, are well known to cloud consciousness and impair attention. Many of these lesions disclose themselves by distinctive focal signs such as hemiplegia or hemianopsia and are beyond the scope of this discussion. There are, however, certain regions of the brain in which destructive lesions may present with acute confusion without other clear localizing signs. Right parietal vascular lesions, most often secondary to embolic infarction in the distribution of a posterior branch of the right middle cerebral artery, are well known to cause ACS (17). The dramatic syndrome of left hemispatial neglect so often associated with right parietal lesions may or may not be clinically evident in these cases. Other important regions of the brain in which lesions are known to impair attention without obvious focal signs include the medial frontal lobes (25) and the inferior temporo-occipital regions (27). These observations emphasize the variety of brain regions involved with maintenance of attention and the need for prompt brain imaging in cases of unexplained acute confusion.

Postsurgical Confusion

For decades, surgeons and anesthesiologists have witnessed the tendency of postsurgical patients to exhibit acute confusion, ranging in severity from mild to profound (28). Again, the elderly and those with multiple medical problems are most at risk. Potential factors contributing to the common occurrence of postsurgical confusion are many, and they are often difficult to identify with certainty. Included are direct effects of anesthesia (especially when sedatives, analgesics, or anticholinergic medications (29) are used), hypoxia or hypotensive ischemia (sometimes unrecognized or undocumented), poorly controlled pain, metabolic derangements, fever, disruption of sleep-wake cycles, and disorienting, unfamiliar environments. With the judicious use of medications (including adequate pain control), adequate preparation, when possible, before surgery, and supportive care, most cases of postsurgical confusion will spontaneously resolve (30). Failure of post surgical confusion to clear quickly should prompt a thorough search for an accurate diagnosis of the underlying factors responsible for the cognitive dysfunction.

Other Neurologic Disorders

Many common neurologic disorders can present with acute confusion. Postictal confusion is the rule after a generalized tonic-clonic seizure. Other types of epilepsy, particularly complex partial seizures, can cloud consciousness during the ictus itself and not show tonic-clonic movements, automatisms, urinary incontinence, or other obvious features usually associated with seizure activity. The elderly are particularly predisposed to "absence status," which presents as acute confusion and a fluctuating level of consciousness. The presence of continuous seizure activity, whether complex partial or absence status, can usually be easily verified by EEG (9). More difficult to diagnose are cases of postictal confusion in which the seizure goes unobserved or is subtle. A history of previous seizure activity, epileptogenic activity on the EEG, and observation of the patient for any evidence of recurrent seizure activity can be helpful in the evaluation of possible postictal confusion, which, if found, is self-limited and should clear within minutes or hours. However, repeated subtle or subclinical seizures missed on routine EEG and that produce prolonged states of ictal and postictal confusion can be a very difficult (and fortunately, rare) diagnosis. If seizure activity is suspected as a source of acute confusion, initiation of appropriate anticonvulsant therapy is usually prudent.

ACS associated with various degrees of head trauma is very common and probably underestimated in clinical significance (31). Any impairment in neurobehavioral function as a result of head trauma represents damage to the brain. In the elderly, ACS from traumatic brain injury can follow seemingly trivial blows to the head. Moreover, because even mild head injuries can occasionally lead to serious intracranial complications such as subdural or epidural hematoma, all patients with post-traumatic confusion should be examined for focal signs and closely observed for any evidence of deterioration. Patients who fail to return quickly to baseline or display other worrisome signs such as evidence of skull fractures or major trauma in other systems should receive emergent brain imaging. CT scanning is usually preferable to MRI in acute cases because it clearly delineates bony anatomy and can be obtained more quickly in most settings. The postconcussion syndrome, characterized by various combinations of headache, irritability, impaired attention, insomnia, and depression can persist for months or years after head trauma (31).

Several other neurologic entities can occasionally present with acute confusion, although additional associated symptoms are usually prominent. Acute obstructive hydrocephalus or increased intracranial pressure from any source can lead to somnolence and confusion. These syndromes usually produce other symptoms such as papilledema, ataxia, and gait disturbance. Wernicke's encephalopathy, characterized by the triad of acute confusion, various forms of ophthalmoplegia, and gait ataxia is a neurologic emergency that must be promptly treated with thiamine to prevent progression to often disabling Korsakoff's amnesia (32).

Workup of Acute Confusion

In considering the diagnostic workup for patients with acute confusion, one should remember that a combination of factors is often responsible, particularly in the elderly. Thus, the investigation of ACS may not uncover one specific cause, but may reveal a constellation of medication combinations, metabolic derangements, environmental changes, and underlying vulnerabilities that have conspired to produce a cumulative effect on the patient's attention and consciousness. Nevertheless, a careful systematic search for possible offending agents and underlying disorders should be undertaken with the same urgency as is warranted in other potentially life-threatening emergencies.

A complete history and physical examination should be performed, with particular scrutiny applied to any recent changes or additions in the patient's medications. Because the patient is often unable to provide a detailed and accurate history, careful physical examination is of even greater importance to look for any underlying medical disorder. Although some elements of the neurologic examination can be compromised by the patient's inattention (e.g., detailed sensory testing), the importance of a thorough neurological examination to discover any evidence of focal signs should not be underestimated.

Routine blood tests can be useful in ruling out many

underlying disorders, particularly those that involve metabolic disturbances. The tests should routinely include electrolytes (especially sodium), a complete blood count (CBC), liver function tests, blood urea nitrogen (BUN) and creatinine, calcium, magnesium, and glucose. Chest x-rays, electrocardiogram (ECG), urinalysis, toxicology screens, and serum concentrations of any known or suspected medications should always be obtained. Pulse oximetry is often useful for quickly determining an approximate level of serum oxygen saturation, but obtaining arterial blood gas values can provide additional valuable information on acid-base status. Arterial ammonia levels, carboxyhemoglobin levels, and thyroid function tests are also sometimes useful and should be obtained in appropriate cases.

Emergent brain imaging with CT or MRI is indicated to rule out acute infarction, intracranial hemorrhage, edema, herniation, and other potentially life-threatening neurologic emergencies. A delay in diagnosis of even a few hours can sometimes be fatal. Usually noncontrasted studies are sufficient to rule out serious pathology during the acute phase of illness.

Once mass effect or increased intracranial pressure has been excluded by brain imaging, lumbar puncture is usually indicated to look for CNS infection. The absence of high fever, meningismus, and headache should not dissuade the physician from obtaining CSF in the severely confused patient because these associated symptoms are variable and sometimes unreliable, especially in the elderly or immunocompromised patient. CSF should be routinely sent for cell counts, glucose, protein, and culture, and some fluid should be saved for additional special tests or cultures that may later be determined useful.

Although sometimes less available in the acute setting, EEG can be quite useful in the evaluation of confusion (9,26). Background slowing of the alpha rhythm on the EEG usually roughly correlates with the degree of the patient's cognitive impairment. Thus, patients who appear confused as a result of depression, mania, schizophrenia, hysteria, or malingering usually have essentially normal EEGs. The presence of triphasic waves in EEG is commonly associated with hepatic encephalopathy and other metabolic derangements. The presence of epileptogenic activity or frank electrographic seizures can be extremely helpful in directing diagnosis and treatment.

Detailed neuropsychologic assessment is typically very difficult in patients with acute confusion, particularly in moderate and severe cases. The data obtained from such attempts are of debatable value, given the pervasive effects of inattention and the patient's often rapidly fluctuating level of arousal. The time and expense necessary for detailed neuropsychologic testing is probably best reserved for subacute and chronic neurobehavioral disorders.

Management of Acute Confusion

The management goals for acutely confused patients are twofold. First, it is critical to provide symptomatic relief and guard the patient's safety. Second, the underlying precipitating factors should be corrected, if possible, before any neurologic damage becomes permanent. Both these efforts should proceed simultaneously. Table 22.3 summarizes the workup and management of ACS in the elderly.

In cases of mild acute confusion, simple environmental manipulations may succeed in significantly improving symptoms. Changes might include the continual presence of a close family member and the use of clocks, calendars, and other aids to the patient's orientation. A night light or other source of low-level illumination is useful at night to help prevent confusion and disorientation from unexpected awakenings. Daytime alertness and orientation

Table 22.3. Management of ACS in the Elderly.

Ensure patient safety
Sedation (see Table 22.4)
Physical restraints (when absolutely necessary)
Search for underlying cause
Complete history and physical examination
Routine laboratory tests
Brain imaging (CT, MRI)
Lumbar puncture
EEG
Special tests as indicated
Provide helpful environmental manipulations
Night light
Familiar family members
TV or radio during daytime
Clocks, calendars

CT = computed tomography; EEG = electroencephalogram; MRI = magnetic resonance imaging.

can be encouraged by the appropriate use of television or radio. Intensive-care psychosis is probably a variant of ACS precipitated in part by the bright lights and noisy activity that continually dominate the intensive care unit (33).

The use of sedating medication should be kept to a minimum and specific choices made with caution. For most cases of acute confusion that require sedation, haloperidol is usually the drug of choice. Intramuscular injections in incremental doses beginning with 0.5 to 1.0 mg provide prompt blood levels with minimal toxicity. Dystonia and other extrapyramidal side effects should be watched for and treated if necessary. Anticholinergic medications used to treat extrapyramidal side effects should be used with caution because they are well known to increase confusion. Benzodiazepines and barbiturates should generally be avoided because of possible increase in the patient's confusion and paradoxical agitation. An important exception is the use of benzodiazepines in cases of delirium tremens, alcohol withdrawal, and benzodiazepine withdrawal. The general axiom "start low and go slow" should be remembered in prescribing psychoactive medication to elderly patients. An initial dose of approximately one-half the usual adult dosage is often prudent. Table 22.4 summarizes the use of medications to help manage the symptoms of ACS.

Reversing the underlying source(s) of acute confusion should always remain a major goal of treatment. This may require thoughtful liaison between different medical disciplines. Often, the simple reduction or elimination of a medication (e.g., diazepam prescribed for anxiety) can result in a gratifying recovery. In other cases, more complex procedures are required.

Conclusion

This chapter describes ACS as a neurobehavioral disorder that results from a large number of insults disrupting the diffuse attentional system of the brain. Although many questions about the cerebral organization of attention remain, the most important practical point is that most cases of ACS can be partially or completely reversed if they are recognized early and treated appropriately. On the other hand, prolonged confusion in the elderly may be a marker for future cognitive decline and a less favorable functional outcome (34–36). The persistence of neurobehavioral deficits that linger long after the onset of acute confusion in the elderly often represents the unmasking of an underlying dementing process.

The outlook for most patients with ACS will likely improve with expanding knowledge of the attentional system of the brain in health and disease. ACS illustrates how insights into the structure and function of the brain can lead to improvements in diagnosis, treatment, and prognosis. In broader terms, ACS provides an instructive model for considering the special vulnerabilities of the elderly patient and emphasizes that the physician needs to remain aware of the myriad problems to which the elderly are prone.

Table 22.4. Medication for the Treatment of Acute Confusion.

1. Haloperidol—0.5–2.0 mg IM. Use the lowest effective dose and repeat every 1–4 hours as necessary; higher doses may be necessary for severely agitated patients; watch for "extrapyramidal" and anticholinergic side-effects; the elderly, especially women are at greater risk for tardive dyskinesia, usually with prolonged high dose treatment.
2. Lorazepam—0.5–2.0 mg IM or IV. (Repeat every 1–4 hours as necessary, not to exceed approximately 10 mg per day; watch for respiratory depression, ataxia and excessive somnolence; longer-acting benzodiazepines such as clorazepate or chlordiazepoxide are indicated for alcohol or benzodiazepine withdrawal).
3. Chloral hydrate—1000–2000 mg PO at bedtime, as necessary for insomnia. A safe medication useful for helping to restore disturbed sleep-wake cycles.

References

1. Francis J. Delirium in older patients. J Am Geriatr Soc 1992;40:829–838.
2. Francis J. Delusions, delirium and cognitive impairment: the challenge of clinical heterogeneity. J Am Geriatr Soc 1992;40:848–849.
3. Liston EH. Delirium in the aged. Psychiatr Clin North Am 1982;5:49–66.
4. Tueth MJ, Cheong JA. Delirium: diagnosis and treatment in the older patient. Geriatrics 1993;48:75–80.
5. Francis J, Martin D, Kapoor W. A prospective study of delirium in hospitalized elderly. JAMA 1990;263:1097–1101.
6. Geschwind N. Disorders of attention: a frontier in neuropsychology. Philos Trans R Soc Lond 1982;298:173–185.

7. Lipowski ZJ. Delirium: acute brain failure in man. Springfield, IL: Thomas, 1980.

8. Taylor D, Lewis S. Delirium. J Neurol Neurosurg Psychiatry 1993;56:742–751.

9. Strub RL. Acute confusional state. In: Benson DF, Blumer D, eds. Psychiatric aspects of neurologic disease. vol. 2. New York: Grune and Stratton, 1982:1–23.

10. Liptzin B, Levkoff SE, Gottlieb GL, Johnson JC. Delirium. J Neuropsychiatry Clin Neurosci 1993;5:154–160.

11. Lipowski ZJ. Delirium in the elderly patient. N Engl J Med 1989;320:578–582.

12. Cummings JL. Acute confusional states. In: Cummings JL. Clinical neuropsychiatry. Orlando: Grune and Stratton, 1985;68–74.

13. Levkoff SE, Besdine RW, Wetle T. Acute confusional states (delirium) in the hospitalized elderly. In: Eisdorfer C, ed. Annu Rev Gerontol Geriatr New York: Springer, 1986:1–25.

14. American Psychiatric Association. Diagnostic and statistical manual of mental disorders. 3rd ed. rev. Washington, D.C.: American Psychiatric Association, 1987:103.

15. Chedru F, Geschwind N. Writing disturbances in acute confusional states. Neuropsychologia 1972;10:343–353.

16. Chedru F, Geschwind N. Disorders of higher cortical function in acute confusional states. Cortex 1972;8:395–411.

17. Mesulam MM, Waxman SG, Geschwind N, Sabin TD. Acute confusional states with right middle cerebral artery infarctions. J Neurol Neurosurg Psychiatry 1976;39:84–89.

18. Mesulam M-M. Attention, confusional states, and neglect. In: Mesulam M-M, ed. Principles of behavioral neurology. Philadelphia: Davis, 1985:125–168.

19. Plum F, Posner JB. The diagnosis of stupor and coma. Philadelphia: Davis, 1982:1–30.

20. Cohen RM, Semple WE, Gross M, et al. Functional localization of sustained attention: comparison to sensory stimulation in the absence of instruction. Neuropsychiatr Neuropsychol Behav Neurol 1988;1:3–20.

21. Pardo JV, Fox PT, Raichle ME. Localization of a human system for sustained attention by positron emission tomography. Nature 1991;349:61–64.

22. Roland PE. Cortical regulation of selective attention in man: a regional cerebral blood flow study. J Neurophysiol 1982;48:1059–1078.

23. Stuss DT, Benson DF. Neuropsychological studies of the frontal lobes. Psychol Bull 1984;95:3–28.

24. Wilkins AJ, Shallice T, McCarthy R. Frontal lesions and sustained attention. Neuropsychologia 1987;25:359–365.

25. Amyes EW, Nielsen JM. Clinicopathologic study of vascular lesions of the anterior cingulate region. Bull Los Angeles Neurol Soc 1955;20:112–130.

26. Obrecht R, Okhomina FOA, Scott DF, Value of EEG in acute confusional states. J Neurol Neurosurg Psychiatry 1979;42:75–77.

27. Medina JL, Rubino FA, Ross E. Agitated delirium caused by infarctions of the hippocampal formation and fusiform and lingual gyri: a case report. Neurology 1974;24:1181–1183.

28. Seibert C. Recognition, management and prevention of neuropsychological dysfunction after operation. Int Anesthesiol Clin 1986;24:39–58.

29. Tune L, Carr S, Cooper T, Klug B, Golinger RC. Association of anticholinergic activity of prescribed medications with postoperative delirium. J Neuropsychiatry Clin Neurosci 1993;5:208–210.

30. Williams-Russo P, Urquhart BL, Sharrock NE, Charlson ME. Post-operative delirium: predictors and prognosis in elderly orthopedic patients. J Am Geriatr Soc 1992:40:759–767.

31. Alexander MP. Traumatic brain injury. In: Benson DF, Blumer D, eds. Psychiatric aspects of neurologic disease. vol 2. New York: Grune and Stratton, 1982:219–248.

32. Victor M, Adams RD, Collins GH. The Wernicke-Korsakoff syndrome and related neurologic disorders due to alcoholism and malnutrition. 2nd ed. Philadelphia: Davis, 1989.

33. Easton C, MacKenzie F. Sensory-perceptual alterations: delirium in the intensive care unit. Heart Lung 1988;17:229–237.

34. Francis J, Kapoor WN. Prognosis after hospital discharge of older medical patients with delirium. J Am Geriatr Soc 1992;40:601–606.

35. Levkoff SE, Evans DA, Liptzin B, et al. Delirium. The occurrence and persistence of symptoms among elderly hospitalized patients. Arch Intern Med 1992;152:334–340.

36. Rockwood K. The occurrence and duration of symptoms in elderly patients with delirium. J Gerontol 1992;48:M162–M166.

Chapter 23
Falls

Sylvia K. Oboler

Age has a good mind and sorry shanks.

Pietro Aretino
Letter to Bernardo Tasso

Falls constitute a serious threat to the health and independence of the elderly. This chapter reviews the epidemiology of falls, discusses both intrinsic and extrinsic causes of falls in the elderly, describes the approach to evaluating a patient who falls, suggests treatment options for many of the causes of falls, and reviews attempts to prevent falls by identifying at-risk patients and planning interventions for them.

The definition currently used by those involved in research is that falls are events that lead to the conscious subject "unintentionally coming to rest on the ground or at some lower level, not as a result of a major intrinsic event or overwhelming hazard" (1). This definition excludes major medical events such as stroke, syncope, seizure, or environmental hazards that would cause even young, healthy persons to fall, such as being pushed or being hit by a vehicle.

Even with a standard definition, evaluating falls in the elderly remains a complex issue for several reasons. First, falls are episodic. Both the conditions that cause or contribute to falls and the memory of a fall may be absent when a patient seeks medical care. In a prospective study of falls in ambulatory patients older than 59 years, as many as 32 percent of patients with a confirmed fall during the 12-month follow-up did not recall the fall (2). Second, the cause of falls is frequently multifactorial. An individual patient may have multiple co-existing diseases and multiple medications that contribute to a fall. In a prospective evaluation of long-term care patients who fell, patients had a mean of 2.1 active medical problems for which recommendations were given (3). The additive effects of apparently trivial abnormalities may result in a fall. Third, the interaction between physical activity, dis-

ability, and falling is complex, with the causes and site of falls changing as the frail elderly decrease physical activity and exposure to environmental hazards (4).

Epidemiology of Falls

Incidence of Falls

Community-living elderly

A number of recent studies found that about one-third of community-living elderly patients fell in a given year, with an annual incidence of 279 to 387 per 1000 (1,4–9). In all these studies, women were more likely than men to fall; the annual incidence of falls for men ranged 201 to 291 per 1000; the incidence for women was 335 to 402 per 1000. The association of age with falls has been confusing. In a prospective community study, the highest fall rate for women was in the age 65 to 69 group, but in men it was in the age 80 to 92 group; the fall rate for both women and men over age 80 was similar (4).

Up to one-half of those who fall have repeated episodes. In a prospective study of community-dwellers over age 75, 46 percent of those who fell had a single fall, 29 percent fell twice, and 25 percent fell at least three times during a year (1). Other prospective studies of community-living elders show that 39 percent to 57 percent of those who fall have repeated falls (4,10).

The majority of falls among independent elderly occur at home (4,8,11). In one prospective study evaluating patients who sought medical attention after a fall, 54 percent of patients were in or around their homes, of whom 42 percent were in the bedroom, 34 percent in the bathroom, 9 percent in the kitchen, 5 percent on stairs, 4 percent in the living room, and 6 percent in other areas (11). Most falls occur during activities that only mildly or moderately displace the person's center of gravity, such as getting up or sitting down, bending or reaching, or stepping up or down; only about 4 percent of falls are associated with clearly hazardous activities such as climbing on ladders or chairs or participating in sports (1).

Institutionalized elderly

The reported incidence of falls for institutionalized elderly is much higher than that for community-dwellers, probably because the individuals have poorer health and because institutions have better reporting mechanisms. In acute care hospitals, the annual incidence of falls ranges from 620 to 2900 per 1000 beds (5). Most falls in the hospital occur in the patient's room, with 41 percent near the bed, 14 percent near the bathroom, 29 percent in the bathroom, and 4 percent near the doorway (12). Over half of ambulatory nursing home residents fall each year. The incidence of falls in long-term care facilities ranges from 680 to 3770 per 1000 beds (3,5,13,14); a recent prospective study in a combined residential/skilled care facility found 1260 falls per 1000 beds (3). From 36 percent to 69 percent of nursing home residents who fall are likely to be repeat fallers (3,13,15).

Mortality of Falls

In adults older than age 75, injury is the sixth leading cause of death, with most deaths related to falls (16). About 9500 deaths per year among patients older than 65 years are attributed to falls. In the age group older than 85, one-fifth of fatal falls occur in nursing homes (16). In a community-based study of elderly patients with fall-related injuries, 2.2 percent of the patients died (17). Deaths were attributed to hip fracture in 45 percent of women and in 43 percent of men; men were more likely than women to have brain injury (14 percent versus 5 percent) and less likely to have fracture other than hip fracture (7 percent versus 13 percent).

In addition to direct fatal outcomes, falls are associated with excess mortality that cannot be attributed to the injuries sustained. Patients seen in an emergency department for falls at home had twice the expected death rate in 1 year (18). Another study in a British general practice compared patients who fell at home with age- and sex-matched controls (19). At 1 year, the death rate in the fallers was five times that of controls. An important predictor of outcome is the "long lie" (remaining on the ground more than 1 hour after a fall) (20). Complications of the long lie include hypothermia, bronchopneumonia, and dehydration; mortality as high as 50 percent in 6 months has been reported (19). Thus a fall for an elderly patient appears to be a marker for ill health.

Morbidity of Falls

Although the mortality of falls in the elderly is significant, the morbidity is even greater. The elderly are more susceptible to fall-related injuries than are the young because of increased frequency of falls, decreased soft tissue mass, and diminished bone strength (21). The severity of falls has been described in several community-based studies, with serious injury reported in 11 percent to 21 percent of patients and fractures in 4 percent to 5 percent of patients (1,2,8). Identifying patients with fall injuries from hospital and emergency room records shows that 31 percent to 42 percent of patients required hospitalization, and that 29 percent to 30 percent of fall injuries were fractures (17,22). Similar data are described for falls in long-term care settings. In 651 falls during a period of 5 years in one residential care facility, 54 percent of patients had no injury, 28 percent had trivial soft tissue injury, 11 percent had severe soft tissue injury, and 6 percent had fractures (13). Of fall-related fractures in these varied settings, hip fractures account for 20 percent to 30 percent of fractures, followed by upper extremity fractures for 14 percent to 45 percent of patients; rib or trunk fractures in 20 percent to 24 percent, lower extremity fractures in 10 percent to 25 percent, and skull fractures in 0 percent to 7 percent of patients.

In these studies, 5 percent to 6 percent of falls resulted in fractures, with approximately 20 percent of the fractures being hip fractures; thus, only 1 percent of falls resulted in hip fracture. However, the morbidity from hip fractures is substantial. The elderly account for about 85 percent of the 200,000 hip fractures per year in the U.S. (16). In-hospital mortality for hip fracture ranges from 0 percent to 16 percent depending on age, comorbid conditions, type of fracture, and type of treatment (23). One-year mortality has been reported as high as 45 percent (23). Ambulation outcomes after surgery for hip fracture in the elderly depend primarily on prefracture functional status. In one follow-up study, 60 percent to 70 percent of patients who were good ambulators before fracture recovered their function, but only 20 percent to 30 percent of patients who were poor ambulators before fracture were able to walk again (24).

In addition to physical injury, psychologic injury from falls can be substantial. Families identify falls as contributing to 40 percent of decisions to place relatives in a nursing home (20). Many patients who have fallen restrict their activities in what has been called "post-fall syndrome." At a retirement home, ambulatory residents who fell were twice as likely to restrict activities than were controls (25). In a community study, 48 percent of patients who fell reported fear of falling and 26 percent curtailed activities such as shopping or housecleaning because of fear of falling (1). When interviewed 2 months after an emergency room visit for a fall, 20 percent of patients reported restricting their usual activities, and 46 percent reported fear of falling (22); 5 months later, 12 percent reported continuing to restrict activity, and 22 percent described fear of falling.

Causes of Falls

Maintaining stability is a complex activity that requires intact neurologic, musculoskeletal, and cardiovascular systems to interact with the environment. Both age-related changes and acute and chronic disease states can contribute to dysfunction. Age-related changes include changes in balance with increased sway and slow response to postural perturbation, changes in gait with decreased step length and height, decreased velocity, and increased double stance time, changes in vision with decreased visual acuity, color and depth perception (especially in low light), changes in hearing, changes in proprioception, and changes in blood pressure regulation with decreased baroreceptor sensitivity and decreased heart rate response (26–28). Researchers have divided the causes of falls into intrinsic (patient-related) causes and extrinsic (environment-related) causes.

Intrinsic Causes of Falls

The list of diseases that can contribute to falls is long. Among studies that report a distribution of causes, there is little consistency, except a finding that environment is the leading cause. Table 23.1 shows some of the leading intrinsic causes divided into neurologic, musculoskeletal, cardiovascular, metabolic, and drug-related causes. Diz-

Table 23.1. Intrinsic Causes of Falls in the Elderly.

Neurologic
  Dizziness
  Vertigo
  Drop attacks
  TIAs/CVAs
  Dementia
  Seizures
  Parkinsonism
  Gait disorders
  Myelopathy
  Peripheral neuropathy
  Multiple sensory deficits
  Vision
  Hearing
Musculoskeletal
  Osteoarthritis
  Muscle weakness
  Myopathy
  Foot disorders
Cardiovascular
  Orthostatic hypotension
  Arrhythmias
  Aortic stenosis
  Carotid sinus hypersensitivity
  Vasodepressor syncope
Metabolic
  Hypoglcemia
  Anemia
  Hypoxemia
  Thyroid diseases
Drugs
  Sedatives/hypnotics
  Antidepressants
  Antipsychotics
  Vasodilators
  Diuretics

CVA = cerebrovascular accident; TIA = transient ischemic attack.

ziness and vertigo are common in the elderly and were identified in one study by 13 percent of the community-dwelling patients who fell (1). Drop attacks are poorly-understood episodes described as "a sudden, unexpected fall to the ground usually while standing or walking, and often following head or neck turning, in an otherwise well elder individual who vigorously denies loss of consciousness" (29). Earlier studies identified drop attacks in as much as 10 percent of falls, but recent studies have not found them so common. Dementia has been associated with both falls and fractures (1,14,30,31). During a 3-year prospective study of 157 ambulatory patients with Alzheimer's disease, 50 percent fell or became nonambulatory, and the annual fracture rate of 69 per 1000 was three times that of the general population (30). Seizures are usually excluded from fall studies, but history of a seizure disorder was the strongest predictor of more than two falls in a 1-year follow-up (10). Balance and gait disorders are important contributors to falls (1,7,10,31). In one study, parkinsonism was the most potent risk factor for multiple falls (10). Previous stroke, especially with hemiparesis, also contributes to falls (7). Falls are associated with both structural and functional changes in vision (1,10) and with proprioceptive changes associated with peripheral neuropathies (10). Musculoskeletal problems, particulary osteoarthritis, and foot disorders such as bunions and callouses have been associated with falls in several studies (1,7,10). In one recent study, generalized weakness was the most common identified intrinsic cause of falls (3).

Cardiovascular disease is a frequent cause of syncope in the elderly population (32,33), but less commonly causes falls. Orthostatic hypotension related to volume depletion, autonomic dysfunction, and drug effects accounts for 3 percent to 23 percent of falls (3,5). Twenty percent of patients 75 years of age and older who had orthostatic symptoms had fallen because of dizziness (34). A study looking at orthostatic symptoms and hypotension found that subjective postural dizziness was associated with recent falls, but objective postural hypotension was not (35). Postprandial hypotension is also a frequent finding in the elderly and may contribute to falls (36). Both ventricular and supraventricular arrhythmias are so common in the elderly that it is often difficult to attribute symptoms to an abnormal rhythm. Carotid sinus hypersensitivity is uncommon, but mainly found in elderly patients. Vasodepressor or vasovagal syncope in the elderly usually presents as situational syncope such as micturition, defecation, or cough syncope. In one study, vasodepressor syncope was more common in the elderly than arrhythmias or aortic stenosis (33). Metabolic causes for falls such as hypoglycemia, anemia, hypoxemia, and thyroid disease are not frequently implicated.

Any drug that affects alertness, decreases cerebral perfusion, or decreases blood pressure can contribute to falls. In practice, the drugs most frequently implicated in falls include centrally-acting drugs such as sedatives, antidepressants and antipsychotics, and blood pressure medications, including diuretics and vasodilators. In a case-control trial in a long-term care facility, fall risk was more often associated with drugs than with diagnoses (37). Significant association with falling was demonstrated for antidepressants, sedatives, nonsteroidal anti-inflammatory drugs (NSAIDs), vasodilators and tranquilizers, but *not* for hypotensives, cardiac drugs, and diuretics. Combinations were particularly risky, with the three-drug regimen of sedative + diuretic + NSAID having an odds ratio for falling of 17.8. For community-living elderly using benzodiazepines, continuous use doubled the risk of falling compared with that for nonusers, with intermittent use resulting in intermediate risk (38). Risk of hip fracture increases with use of long half-life (but not short half-life) benzodiazepines and with tricyclics and phenothiazines (39,40). The increased risk of falls with antidepressants does not appear to be a result of anticholinergic side effects; in a recent study, serotonin uptake blockers were as much associated with falls as were tricyclics (41). Unexpectedly, light to moderate alcohol use in the elderly does *not* appear to increase risk for falls or fall injuries (1,4,10,42,43), and "further efforts at reducing these injuries should concentrate on other modifiable risk factors" (42).

Extrinsic Causes of Falls

In most series, environmental causes of falls comprise the single largest etiologic group, accounting for as much as 30 percent to 50 percent of falls (1,3,5). In the home, hazards may relate to furniture, floors, lighting, stairways, walkways, and other obstructions (44,45). In addition to tripping on loose carpets, electric cords, or furniture, elderly patients may fall over unexpected obstructions such as pets or their own ill-fitting clothing or footwear. Improper use of assistive devices, such as not setting wheelchair locks, also contributes to falls. In the hospital and nursing home, some of the same problems with furniture, such as improper height of bed, chair or toilet, can occur. Highly waxed floors and poorly fitting pajamas or slippers may be more of a problem in institutions than they are in the home. Falls in the hospital are associated with patient disorientation and are most likely to occur shortly after the patient's admission or transfer (14). The practice of using mechanical restraints to protect patients from falls and fall-related injuries is not beneficial; evidence in nursing homes shows that restraint use has increased both falls and fall-related fractures (46).

Evaluation of the Elderly Patient Who Falls

A fall should be approached as a symptom of underlying disease. After assessing for injury, the physician must investigate the cause of the fall and understand that multiple etiologies are likely. Table 23.2 summarizes the important aspects of the workup of the elderly patient who has fallen.

Patient History

The patient's history should focus on an accurate description of the fall event, medical conditions that may have contributed to the etiology, and prescription and over-the-counter medications. If possible, a family member or witness should be interviewed. Of particular importance in describing the event is the patient's symptoms: dizziness or vertigo suggestive of a central or vestibular cause; dyspnea, chest pain or palpitations suggestive of a cardiovascular etiology; postural dizziness suggestive of orthostasis; or loss of consciousness suggestive of a neurologic or cardiac cause. The common "I tripped" or "my legs gave out" should not be considered adequate explanation of a fall. The patient's activity at the time should be determined: falls while climbing a ladder, reaching to an upper shelf, or running to catch a bus have very different prognoses from falls that occur while dressing or getting out of bed. The location of the fall (on the stairs or in the bathroom) may suggest the need for an environmental intervention.

Physical Examination

The physical examination of the patient who has fallen should focus on the organ systems likely to be involved. Orthostatic changes in blood pressure and pulse should be measured, and postural symptoms even without significant blood pressure drop should be noted. Vision and hearing should be assessed. Cardiac examination should focus on rhythm and murmurs. The musculoskeletal exam should address evidence of osteoarthritis and orthopedic deformities such as scoliosis and leg length discrepancies, as well as foot abnormalities and footwear. A complete neurologic examination is the most important part of the evaluation and should include a formal, objective assessment of cognition, such as a mini-mental status exam, as well as examination of motor and sensory reflexes, and cerebellar and posterior column function. There are instruments for formal assessment of gait and balance (47), but many prefer to use the simple "get up and go" test (48). In this test, the patient is seated in a straight-backed, high-seat chair with arm rests located 3 meters from a wall, and is asked to rise, stand still momentarily, walk toward the wall, turn around without touching the wall, walk back to the chair, turn around, and sit down. The test is scored on a 5-point scale, from 1 = normal to 5 = severely abnormal.

Laboratory Tests

No studies specifically address the most appropriate labo-

Table 23.2. Evaluation of the Elderly Patient Who Falls.

History
    Description of fall
        Symptoms
        Location
        Activity
    Medications
    Interview family/witness
Physical examination
    Postural blood pressure and symptoms
    Vision
    Hearing
    Cardiac rhythm, murmurs
    Musculoskeletal exam
        Strength
        Deformities
    Neurologic exam
        Mental status
        Balance, gait
        "Get up and go"
Laboratory tests
    Complete blood count
    Electrolytes
    Plasma glucose
    Renal function
    Urinalysis
    Stool for occult blood
    Chest x-ray
    Resting electrocardiogram

ratory evaluation for a patient who falls. However, laboratory tests frequently performed (more for their high yield in this age group than for their specific indication regarding falls) include complete blood count, serum electrolytes and renal function, plasma glucose, urinalysis, stool for occult blood, chest x-ray, and resting electrocardiogram. A recent prospective study of 79 residential care patients evaluated after a fall by a nurse practitioner also included hepatic enzymes, serologic test for syphilis, and free thyroxine index and detected new, significant problems in 82 percent of the patients but "relatively few findings that required treatment or monitoring were detected from laboratory tests alone." Almost all findings came from the patient's focused history and physical examination (3).

The usefulness of ambulatory cardiac (Holter) monitoring in evaluating the patient who falls has been studied (49). Residential care patients who fell were compared with controls on 24-hour Holter monitoring; all had supraventricular arrhythmias and 82 percent of both groups had ventricular arrhythmias with no significant difference in high-grade arrhythmias. Thus, routine Holter monitoring is not recommended unless the patient's history, cardiac examination, or resting ECG suggests cardiac arrhythmia as the likely etiology of the fall.

Indications for Admission

Most patients who fall, and even many patients with definite syncope, do not require hospital admission. Patients who should be admitted include those with a fracture (mainly hip) requiring surgery or stabilization, patients with multiple syncopal episodes, patients who live alone and for whom appropriate care can not be arranged, and patients whose initial evaluation suggests a serious cause for the fall, such as arrhythmia or myocardial ischemia, first seizure, hemodynamically significant bleeding, pulmonary embolus, or infection.

Treatment of Falls

Treatment of falls is directed toward preventing recurrence. An identified intrinsic cause can often be treated. When an extrinsic cause contributes, the environment may be modified.

Interventions for Intrinsic Falls

If drugs can be implicated in contributing to a patient's fall, the most obvious course is to adjust the patient's drug regimen. The person's entire medication list should be reviewed with the goal of eliminating all nonessential drugs and minimizing the doses of the rest. Particular attention should be paid to avoiding sedating the patient with long-acting benzodiazepines during the day.

Postural hypotension can be avoided by paying attention to the patient's hydration, especially during heat waves; using support stockings, elevating the head of the bed to avoid nocturnal diuresis, and considering caffeine for postprandial hypotension. Mineralocorticoids are occasionally recommended, but fluid retention and congestive heart failure are so common in the elderly that this is often not practical. If possible, autonomic dysfunction should be addressed by controlling a patient's diabetes and having the patient avoid alcohol. Micturition syncope can be helped by having patients sit while urinating or by providing bedside urinals. Carotid sinus syncope can be helped by having the patient not wear neckties or tight collars and by having the patient avoid extreme neck rotation.

Cardiac arrhythmias should be treated selectively. Symptomatic bradyarrhythmias may be treated with pacemakers. For other arrhythmias, the risks and benefits of antiarrhythmic therapy should be carefully weighed. Even in the very elderly, aortic stenosis may be treated with valvuloplasty or valve replacement. Vision can be improved with corrective lenses or cataract surgery, and hearing aids may improve function. Gait may be improved with physical therapy and walking aids. Since weakness is such a common component of falls, many patients should benefit from a physical therapy evaluation, both to improve strength and to ensure correct use of mobility aids.

Interventions for Extrinsic Falls

Making the home environment safe for the elderly involves cooperation of the patient, family, and health provider. Published checklists for home hazard assessment, which can be used by visiting nurses, family members or patients, are available (20,44,45,50). Table 23.3 summarizes some of the important areas for evaluation. The home environment must be assessed for safety with the

Table 23.3. Home Checklist for Fall Prevention.

Area	Problems
General household	
Lighting	Dim, glare, inaccessible switches
Carpets, rugs	Torn, slippery, deep pile
Furniture	Obstructing path, unstable, chairs with no arm rests or low backs
Appliances	Cords in path
Kitchen	
Cabinets, shelves	Too high, frequently used items inaccessible
Floor	Wet, waxed
Bathroom	
Bathtub, shower	Slippery, no grab bars
Toilet	Seat too low
Towel racks	Unstable
Stairways	
Height	Stair rise too high
Handrails	Missing, too short
Condition	Slippery, steps not clearly marked
Outdoors	
Walks, driveway	Holes, uneven surface, water/ice buildup
Lawns	Holes, uneven surface

realization that the elderly may use household items for purposes other than which they were designed. For example, towel racks may be used as grab bars and should be securely fastened, and chairs or tables may be leaned on and therefore must be stable. However, unless the patient perceives a situation as hazardous, he or she may be unwilling to correct it (51). In the hospital or nursing home, attention to patient orientation and flexible staffing patterns may help with fall prevention.

Prevention of Falls

Most prevention efforts have focused on secondary prevention—identifying and correcting the cause of a fall so that it does not recur. Primary prevention efforts currently center on identifying at-risk patients. Several studies have addressed risk factors for falls in community-living elderly. In community-dwellers 75 years of age or older, who were followed for 1 year, by far the strongest predictor of falls was use of sedatives, followed by cognitive impairment, lower extremity disability, palmomental reflex, abnormal balance and gait, and foot problems (1). In another study of patients 70 years of

age or older, risk factors were different for men and women: the strongest predictors for women were previous stroke and use of three or more drugs, and for men the inability to rise from a chair, knee arthritis, and increased body sway (7). Another study of patients 65 years of age or older found dizziness, frequent physical activity, days with activity limited because of ill health, trouble walking 400 meters, or bending down the most predictive of falls (4). A prospective study of patients who had fallen once showed that the strongest predictors of recurrent falls were Parkinson's disease, previous fall with injury, difficulty standing up from a chair, history of arthritis, poor tandem gait, and more than two falls in the previous year (10). One group was able to develop a predictive equation for falls on the basis of three factors: number of prescription medications, hip weakness, and low balance score (52).

Similar factors have been shown to predispose the institutionalized elderly to falls. A fall-risk score using nine factors (mobility score, distant vision, hearing, orthostatic blood pressure, back extension, morale score, mental status score, admission activities of daily living (ADL) score, and postadmission medications) at admission to an intermediate care facility predicted the risk of a patient falling during the first 3 months—patients with a low score had no falls and all patients with a high score had falls (53). Another study of falls during 1 year in a hostel for the aged determined that falls were related to impaired cognition, abnormal reaction to push or pressure, history of palpitation, and abnormal stepping (31).

Although the magnitude of risk conferred by these conditions varies among the studies, a consistent pattern allows identification of the patients at highest risk for falls: *those with multiple medications, especially sedatives, and those with dementia, weakness from arthritis or neurolgic disease, and those with gait or foot abnormalities.* Large-scale studies to determine whether targeting these high-risk patients for intervention actually prevents falls or improves outcome are ongoing.

Two recent, randomized studies provide insight into how difficult proving benefit in reducing falls may be when more fit and confident elders engage in risky activities. In the first study, residential care patients who fell were randomized to a postfall assessment or a control group (3). A nurse practitioner performed a detailed history and physical examination, standard laboratory tests, and an environmental assessment, and then provided the primary physician with diagnoses and recommendations. Ninety percent of the patients had at least one identified active problem, with a mean of 2.1 problems and 2.8 recommendations per patient. In a 2-year follow-up period, the intervention patients were no less likely to fall than were the control patients (81% versus 84%), but the intervention patients had significantly fewer hospitalizations (46% versus 62%), fewer admissions per patient (0.7 versus 1.25), and fewer hospital days per patient (5.9 versus 12.3). The study conclusion was that "although falls may not be easily prevented . . . falls indicate the presence of important treatable conditions and that some of the disability and costs associated with falls may be obviated by a thorough assessment" (3).

In another study involving 16 senior centers that enrolled adults older than age 60, subjects were randomized to four different groups: classes offering "stand-up/step-up" exercise three times per week; a weekly cognitive-behavioral class focusing on fall prevention, relaxation, and reaction time training; a class with both exercise and cognitive training; and a control class with weekly health discussions unrelated to fall prevention (9). During 1 year, neither the rate of falls nor the time to first fall was improved by any intervention compared with that of the control group; however, the exercise program was highly attractive to seniors, and led to the conclusion that "fall prevention is a difficult task and that interventions that elders enjoy may not produce the desired outcomes" (9).

An alternative approach focuses not on preventing falls, but on reducing the injury from a fall. Recently, a randomized trial of external hip protectors for patients in a nursing home showed a 53 percent reduction in hip fractures, and no hip fractures during a fall with direct trauma to the hip when the resident was wearing a hip protector (54).

Despite the absence of prospective data showing that intervention improves outcome, the U.S. Preventive Services Task Force decided to address falls in the elderly (55). On the basis of clinical judgment, the task force recommended that

> Elderly patients or those responsible for older persons should be advised to inspect the home for adequate lighting, to remove or repair floor struc-

tures that predispose to tripping, and to install handrails and traction strips in stairways and bathtubs. Clinicians caring for older persons should periodically test visual acuity, counsel patients with medical conditions affecting mobility, and monitor the use of drugs associated with falls. Older patients who lack medical contraindications should be counseled to engage in exercise programs to maintain and improve mobility and flexibility.

Summary

Falls affect about one-third of community-dwelling elderly and more than half the institutionalized elderly. Morbidity of falls is both physical, with about 5 percent of falls resulting in a fracture, and 1 percent of falls resulting in hip fracture, and psychologic, with decreased activity after a fall. Both intrinsic and environmental causes of falls can be identified, frequently in combination. Although the most appropriate prevention strategies have yet to be determined, patients who are at risk for falls because of medications, cognitive impairment, and neuromuscular abnormalities should be identified and targeted for intervention.

References

1. Tinetti ME, Speechley M, Ginter SF. Risk factors for falls among elderly persons living in the community. New Engl J Med 1988;319:1701–1707.
2. Cummings SR, Nevitt MC, Kidd S. Forgetting falls. The limited accuracy of recall of falls in the elderly. J Am Geriatr Soc 1988;36:613–616.
3. Rubenstein LZ, Robbins AS, Josephson KR, et al. The value of assessing falls in an elderly population. A randomized clinical trial. Ann Intern Med 1990;113:308–316.
4. O'Loughlin JL, Robitaille Y, Boivin J-F, Suissa S. Incidence of and risk factors for falls and injurious falls among the community-dwelling elderly. Am J Epidemiol 1993;137:342–354.
5. Rubenstein LZ, Robbins AS, Schulman BL, et al. Falls and instability in the elderly. J Am Geriatr Soc 1988;36:266–278.
6. Ebrahim S, Dallosso H, Morgan K, et al. Causes of ill health among a random sample of old and very old people: possibilities for prevention. J R Coll Physicians 1988;22:105–107.
7. Campbell AJ, Borrie MJ, Spears GF. Risk factors for falls in a community-based prospective study of people 70 years and older. J Gerontol 1989;44:M112–M117.

8. Hale WA, Delaney MJ, McGaghie WC. Characteristics and predictors of falls in elderly patients. J Fam Pract 1992;34:577–581.

9. Reinsch S, MacRae P, Lachenbruch PA, Tobis JS. Attempts to prevent falls and injury: a prospective community study. Gerontologist 1992;32:450–456.

10. Nevitt MC, Cummings SR, Kidd S, Black D. Risk factors for recurrent nonsyncopal falls. A prospective study. JAMA 1989;261:2663–2668.

11. DeVito CA, Lambert DA, Sattin RW, et al. Fall injuries among the elderly. Community-based surveillance. J Am Geriatr Soc 1988;36:1029–1035.

12. Morgan VR, Mathison JH, Rice JC, Clemmer DI. Hospital falls: a persistent problem. Am J Public Health 1985;75:775–777.

13. Gryfe CI, Amies A, Ashley MJ. A longitudinal study of falls in an elderly population: I. Incidence and morbidity. Age Ageing 1977;6:201–210.

14. vanDijk PTM, Meulenberg OGRM, vandeSande HJ, Habbema JDF. Falls in dementia patients. Gerontologist 1993;33:200–204.

15. Jantti PO, Pyykko VI, Hervonen ALJ. Falls among elderly nursing home residents. Public Health 1993;107:89–96.

16. Baker SP, Harvey AH. Fall injuries in the elderly. Clin Geriatr Med 1985;1:501–512.

17. Sattin RW, Huber DAL, DeVito CA, et al. The incidence of fall injury events among the elderly in a defined population. Am J Epidemiol 1990;131:1028–1037.

18. Morfitt JM. Falls in old people at home: intrinsic versus environmental factors in causation. Public Health (Lond) 1983;97:115–120.

19. Wild D, Nayak USL, Isaacs B. How dangerous are falls in old people at home? BMJ 1981;282:266–268.

20. Kellog International Work Group on the prevention of falls by the elderly: the prevention of falls in later life. Dan Med Bull 1987;34(suppl):1–24.

21. Melton LJ III, Riggs BL. Risk factors for injury after a fall. Clin Geriatr Med 1985;1:525–539.

22. Grisso JA, Schwarz DF, Wolfson V, et al. The impact of falls in an inner-city elderly African-American population. J Am Geriatr Soc 1992;40:673–678.

23. Kenzora JE, McCarthy RE, Lowell JD, Sledge CB. Hip fracture mortality. Relation to age, treatment, preoperative illness, time of surgery, and complications. Clin Orthop 1984;186:45–56.

24. McCown PL, Miller WA. Long-term follow-up of hip fractures. South Med J 1976;69:1540–1542.

25. Vellas B, Cayla F, Bocquet H, et al. Prospective study of restriction of activity in old people after falls. Age Ageing 1987;16:189–193.

26. Sudarsky L. Geriatrics: gait disorders in the elderly. New Engl J Med 1990;322:1441–1446.

27. Lipsitz LA. Orthostatic hypotension in the elderly. New Engl J Med 1989;321:952–957.

28. Wolfson LI, Whipple R, Amerman P, et al. Gait and balance in the elderly. Two functional capacities that link sensory and motor ability to falls. Clin Geriatr Med 1985;1:649–659.

29. Lipsitz LA. The drop attack: a common geriatric symptom. J Am Geriatr Soc 1983;31:617–620.

30. Buchner DM, Larson EB. Falls and fractures in patients with Alzheimer-type dementia. JAMA 1987;257:1492–1495.

31. Clark RD, Lord SR, Webster IW. Clinical parameters associated with falls in an elderly population. Gerontology 1993;39:117–123.

32. Kapoor W, Snustad D, Peterson J, et al. Syncope in the elderly. Am J Med 1986;80:419–428.

33. Lipsitz LA, Pluchino FC, Wei JY, Rowe JW. Syncope in institutionalized elderly: the impact of multiple pathological conditions and situational stress. J Chronic Dis 1986;39:619–630.

34. Sixt E, Landahl S. Postural disturbances in a 75-year-old population: I. Prevalence and functional consequences. Age Ageing 1987;16:393–398.

35. Ensrud KE, Nevitt MC, Yunis C, et al. Postural hypotension and postural dizziness in elderly women. The study of osteoporotic fractures. Arch Intern Med 1992;152:1058–1064.

36. Peitzman SJ, Berger SR. Postprandial blood pressure decrease in well elderly persons. Arch Intern Med 1989;149:286–288.

37. Granek E, Baker SP, Abbey H, et al. Medications and diagnoses in relation to falls in a long-term care facility. J Am Geriatr Soc 1987;35:503–511.

38. Sorock GS, Shimkin EE. Benzodiazepine sedatives and the risk of falling in a community-dwelling elderly cohort. Arch Intern Med 1988;148:2441–2444.

39. Ray WA, Griffin MR, Schaffner W, et al. Psychotropic drug use and the risk of hip fracture. New Engl J Med 1987;316:363–369.

40. Ray WA, Griffin MR, Malcolm E. Cyclic antidepressants and the risk of hip fracture. Arch Intern Med 1991;151:754–756.

41. Ruthazer R, Lipsitz LA. Antidepressants and falls among elderly people in long-term care. Am J Public Health 1993;83:746–749.

42. Nelson DE, Sattin RW, Langlois JA, et al. Alcohol as a risk factor for fall injury events among elderly persons living in the community. J Am Geriatr Soc 1992;40:658–661.

43. Felson DT, Kiel DP, Anderson JJ, Kannel WB. Alcohol consumption and hip fractures: the Framingham study. Am J Epidemiol 1988;128:1102–1110.

44. Tideiksaar R. Preventing falls: Home hazard checklists to help older patients protect themselves. Geriatrics 1986;41:26–28.

45. Hindmarsh JJ, Estes Jr EH. Falls in older persons. Causes and interventions. Arch Intern Med 1989;149:2217–2222.

46. Tinetti ME, Lui WL, Ginter SF. Mechanical restraint use and fall-related injuries among residents of skilled nursing facilities. Ann Intern Med 1992;116:369–374.

47. Tinetti ME. Performance-oriented assessment of mobility problems in elderly patients. J Am Geriatr Soc 1986;34:119–126.

48. Mathias S, Nayak USL, Isaacs B. Balance in elderly patients: The "get-up and go" test. Arch Phys Med Rehabil 1986;67:387–389.

49. Rosado JA, Rubenstein LZ, Robbins AS, et al. The value of

Holter monitoring in evaluating the elderly patient who falls. J Am Geriatr Soc 1989;37:430–434.

50. Beck JC. Geriatrics review syllabus. New York: American Geriatrics Society, 1991:491–493.

51. Isaacs B. Clinical and laboratory studies of falls in old people. Prospects for prevention. Clin Geriatr Med 1985;1:513–524.

52. Robbins AS, Rubenstein LZ, Josephson KR, et al. Predictors of falls among elderly people. Results of two population-based studies. Arch Intern Med 1989;149:1628–1633.

53. Tinetti ME, Williams TF, Mayewski R. Fall risk index for elderly patients based on number of chronic disabilities. Am J Med 1986;80:429–434.

54. Lauritzen JB, Petersen MM, Lund B. Effect of external hip protectors on hip fractures. Lancet 1993;341:11–13.

55. U.S. Preventive Services Task Force. Guide to clinical preventive services. Baltimore: Williams & Wilkins, 1989:321–329.

Chapter 24
Hypotension, Dizziness, and Syncope

Scott L. Mader

Once I looked into the mirror and saw my father's tired eyes look back at me; reaching to smooth a vagrant hair, Mother's wrinkled hand. Age came upon me unaware.

Helen Rul Lawler

Hypotension, particularly that which occurs after standing or eating, is an important and generally reversible condition in older persons. Hypotension can cause dizziness and syncope, which are common clinical problems in older patients. This chapter reviews the age- and disease-related changes in physiology that can predispose to hypotension and cerebral hypoperfusion. The clinical problems of orthostatic hypotension, postprandial hypotension, dizziness, and syncope are also reviewed.

Aging as a Risk Factor

Some known, age-associated changes in physiology would be expected to favor development of hypotension and cerebral symptoms after elderly persons experience cardiovascular stressors (1). Changes occur in arterial compliance and venous system tortuosity with age. Cardiac hypertrophy may impair diastolic filling. Renal sodium conservation is impaired and neurohypophyseal release of vasopressin is blunted after standing. Renin, angiotensin, and aldosterone levels are lower in elderly subjects. The change in heart rate after hypotensive maneuvers, and sensitivity or maximal heart rate during exercise or isoproterenol infusion is decreased. For any decrease in blood pressure (BP), elderly persons are also more likely to become symptomatic because of the high likelihood of cerebral vascular disease and the shift in cerebral autoregulation that occurs with hypertension, another common problem seen in the elderly (2).

Other age-related changes decrease the likelihood of hypotension. The vasoconstrictor response of blood vessels to alpha-adrenergic agonists probably does not change with normal aging. This is in contrast to beta-adrenergic mediated vasodilation, which is impaired despite an intact response to non-receptor-mediated vasodilators such as nitroglycerin. Plasma norepinephrine levels increase with age under both basal and stress conditions such as standing, isometric exercise, or cold stimulation. These changes suggest that vasoconstriction would be enhanced in elderly persons after standing. In addition, aging is associated with decreased heart rate variability, which may protect against vasovagal events (3).

Clinical data suggest that the balance of these age-related changes is toward increased risk of hypotension. Diuretic-induced volume depletion causes orthostatic hypotension in elderly subjects but not in younger controls (4). Postprandial BP declines occur in healthy elderly subjects, but not in younger controls (5). Older surgical patients are more susceptible to nitroprusside-induced hypotension (6). Therefore, hypotension and decreased cerebral perfusion leading to dizziness and syncope are likely to occur in elderly patients in the presence of a physiologic stressor.

Hypotension

Two common causes of episodic hypotension in older patients are orthostatic hypotension (OH) and postprandial hypotension (PPH). These episodes can be associated with dizziness, presyncope, syncope, falls, cerebral vascular symptoms, and myocardial infarction. Hypotension is often the result of interactions between acute and chronic disease, and between long-standing and new medications.

Epidemiology

The prevalence of OH depends on the patient group studied and the definition used. Most studies use the definition of an OH as a fall in systolic BP of at least 20 mm Hg after standing, with or without symptoms. Elderly subjects with no medical problems or medications have a very low prevalence of OH (6%) (7). In inpatient, outpatient, and nursing home surveys, from 11 percent to 33 percent of elderly subjects have significant falls in BP after standing. Therefore, OH can be anticipated in patient populations in which risk factors are present. Conversely, this finding should not be expected in otherwise healthy elderly persons.

The epidemiology of PPH has been less well studied. Some degree of postprandial BP decrease occurs in healthy elderly but not young subjects (5). In one nursing home study of 113 residents, 96 percent of residents had a reduction in systolic BP after eating. Thirty-six percent had a reduction in systolic BP of 20 mm Hg or more, 11 percent had a reduction in systolic BP of less than 100 mm Hg, and 2 subjects developed symptoms—angina, and transient ischemic attack (TIA) (8).

Differential Diagnosis

There are many causes of orthostatic hypotension. Table 24.1 shows some common and uncommon diagnostic categories found in older persons. Many medications associ-

Table 24.1. Differential Diagnosis of Orthostatic Hypotension.

Common
  Medications, dehydration, blood loss, anemia, hypokalemia,
    bed rest, deconditioning, malnutrition
Neurologic
  Central—cerebral vascular accidents, tumors, Parkinson's
    disease, depression, dementia
  Peripheral—peripheral neuropathy (diabetes, uremic, viral,
    amyloid), sympathectomy
Cardiovascular
  Cardiac—hypertrophic cardiomyopathy, aortic stenosis, mitral
    valve prolapse
  Vascular—large varicose veins
Endocrine/renal
  Adrenal insufficiency
  Pheochromocytoma
  Hypoaldosteronism, renal salt wasting
  Diabetes insipidus
Less common
  Idiopathic orthostatic hypotension
  Multiple system atrophy
  Tumor-associated (carcinoid, bradykinin)
  Baroreceptor destruction (neck radiation, surgery)

ated with hypotension are commonly used by elderly persons. These medications can cause OH or PPH by multiple mechanisms including a decrease in intravascular volume, vasodilation, impairment of autonomic reflexes, or central nervous system depression and include antihypertensives, antiadrenergics, antiparkinsonian agents, antianginals, antiarrhythmics, anticholinergics, antidepressants, diuretics, narcotics, neuroleptics, sedatives, and alcohol. Old age alone is not a sufficient explanation for OH, although some degree of PPH can be seen in otherwise healthy older subjects. Elderly patients who are found to have OH or significant PPH usually have multiple contributing factors.

Idiopathic orthostatic hypotension (IOH) and multiple system atrophy (MSA or Shy-Drager syndrome) are uncommon causes of OH in elderly persons. These disorders should be considered for patients who have supine hypertension and impressive OH in the absence of other conditions or medications known to be associated with OH.

The reason for the increased risk of PPH with aging is unknown. Carbohydrate ingestion and, especially, glucose appear to cause the greatest decrease in BP (9). Fructose ingestion, which does not stimulate insulin release, does not cause PPH. Fat, protein, or water ingestion cause little or no change in BP according to some studies. Possible mechanisms for BP changes include impairments in baroreflex function or sympathetic nervous system response, excessive vasodilation to adenosine, insulin, or gastrointestinal peptides, or excessive postprandial splanchnic blood pooling during digestion.

Evaluation

All elderly patients should have postural BP determinations as part of routine assessment and whenever potentially hypotensive medications are started (1). Patients who complain of dizziness, syncope, falls, TIA, or other cerebral symptoms should always be evaluated for OH, even in the absence of a clear-cut postural component. These recommendations are supported by a study that evaluated 80 patients with history of TIA who received a first or second opinion regarding diagnosis and management (10). The study found that 16 percent of patients had significant orthostatic hypotension, which reproduced their TIA symptoms. Of note, none of these patients recalled having had BP checked in the standing position, even though many of them had easily identifiable risk factors for orthostasis. Symptoms such as angina or TIA that occur after meals should prompt an evaluation of BP after the patient has eaten (8).

Patient history should focus on previous medical and surgical problems, medications, alcohol use, and dietary intake of salt, water, and calories. An autonomic, neurologic, cardiovascular, and endocrine review of systems should be performed. The autonomic review of systems is often confusing in older persons because of the large number of positive responses in this population (presence of constipation, urinary difficulties, sexual dysfunction, night blindness). However, a negative review of systems is helpful to rule out significant autonomic dysfunction.

The physical examination should begin with the BP determination. We use the mean of the second and third supine readings after 5 minutes of rest as our baseline. The subject stands, and time 0 is when the person is upright. Pulse is determined for 15 seconds and BP is subsequently measured 1 minute after the patient has been standing. For screening purposes, a 1-minute reading is sufficient. However, if the patient is being evaluated for symptoms, a reading at 3 minutes, 5 minutes, and after walking or climbing stairs may be useful. A greater difference in BP is seen when supine-to-standing, rather than sitting-to-standing readings are compared. OH is diagnosed if there is a 20 mm Hg or more decrease in systolic pressure or a 10 mm Hg or more decrease in diastolic pressure. A single OH determination can be misleading because serial determinations in patients can be variable (2). If symptoms compatible with cerebral hypoperfusion occur without a significant change in BP, these subjects may have orthostatic cerebral hypoperfusion (11), which occurs particularly in patients with carotid stenoses.

Measuring change in BP after a meal is more difficult. Studies on PPH have shown that maximal BP decline occurs approximately 1 hour after the subject begins the meal, although this can be variable. Whether an accurate BP reading can be ascertained by having a patient come to the office 1 hour after eating is unknown; studies measure BP continuously by having the patient in the sitting position throughout the meal period. Ambulatory BP monitoring or home measurement by family or visiting nurse may be needed.

An assessment of volume by examination of jugular venous pressure should be performed. The carotid arteries should be examined for the presence of bruits. Auscultation of the heart should be done while the patient is supine, as well as standing, because the murmurs of idiopathic hypertrophic cardiomyopathy or mitral valve prolapse may be more prominent when the subject is standing. A psychiatric and neurological examination should assess for depression, cognitive impairment, previous stroke, Parkinson's disease, and peripheral neuropathy.

Initial laboratory assessment need not be extensive. A complete blood count (CBC), electrolytes, blood urea nitrogen (BUN), creatinine, glucose, albumin, calcium, phosphorus, urinalysis with specific gravity, and electrocardiogram (ECG) should be performed. More extensive testing should be limited to patients who have suggestive abnormalities on history, physical, or laboratory screening. Additional tests that may be useful include echocardiogram, cosyntropin stimulation test, and urine electrolytes. Autonomic function testing, adrenergic drug infusions, or supine/standing plasma catecholamines are occasionally helpful (12).

Treatment

For PPH, medications should be reviewed as described below. It may be beneficial to not give potentially hypotensive medications near mealtimes. Smaller meals with less carbohydrate decrease the risk of hypotension. Eating with the legs in a nondependent position is associated with less PPH. Use of support stockings to help prevent PPH has not been studied. The addition of a caffeinated beverage at the end of the meal may also mitigate postprandial decline (13). For more difficult cases of PPH, octreotide, the synthetic analog of somatostatin, has proven to be useful (14).

Patients with OH may have a specific etiology, and this should be addressed. However, most older persons have multiple causative factors, some that are correctable and some that are fixed deficits (1,2,15). The initial steps are to 1) evaluate medications, 2) increase fluid, salt, and nutritional intake, 3) increase activity level, and 4) educate the patient about the condition. Medications can be reduced, changed, or stopped completely. Patients with hypertension and OH can be treated with beta-adrenergic antagonists or vasodilator agents (calcium channel blockers, angiotensin-converting enzyme (ACE) inhibitors). The following agents should be avoided in treating hypertensive patients with OH: diuretics, central sympatholytic agents (alpha methyldopa) or peripheral alpha-adrenergic blockers (prazosin). For patients with depression, nortriptyline or the serotonin reuptake inhibitors are less commonly associated with OH.

In some instances, it may be difficult to stop the offending medications. In these cases, treatment strategies including salt tablets, head of bed elevation, and fludrocortisone may be instituted before or while continuing the offending medication. Another useful measure is to increase salt intake. Many older persons follow a low-salt diet even in the absence of a history of hypertension. Salting food with one packet of salt (approximately 1 gm) at each meal can improve BP tolerance and food intake in these patients. Exercise and reconditioning are extremely important. Patients who spend most of the time in bed will continue to have OH despite other treatment measures. Prestanding and standing isometric exercise of the arms, legs, and abdominal muscles decrease blood pooling and can improve BP tolerance.

Education is important so that patients and families understand the cause and management of symptoms. Patients should be instructed to rise slowly from lying down to sitting, and to wait a few minutes before standing. Patients should stand only when there is support available to prevent falling. Isometric tensing of the legs, arms, and abdominal muscles decreases venous pooling and helps maintain BP when changing positions or during prolonged standing. A urinal or bedside commode should be provided so that patients do not have to walk to the bathroom. Patients should be instructed to take extra salt and fluid during times of volume stress, such as extreme heat, febrile illness, and gastroenteritis.

For patients who do not respond to these simple measures, additional treatments are available. Head-up tilt at night is effective and often easier with older patients who may sleep alone. This is best done with books or blocks under the legs at the head of the bed. The bed can be raised in small increments to tolerance.

Salt tablets (1 gm) can be prescribed for patients with poor oral salt intake. (1 gm NaCl is 17 mEq of Na; treatment can start at 2 gm bid and increase to 10 gm/day [170 mEq] if necessary and tolerated.) Fludrocortisone acetate, which acts by promoting salt retention and sensitizing blood vessels to catecholamines, is an effective treatment (0.1 mg qd and increased weekly to 0.5 mg bid). The most common side effect is hypokalemia (which can exacerbate OH), mild dependent edema, and supine hypertension. Adequate salt intake must be part of this regimen.

Support hose are a widely recommended therapy for OH but they are difficult for patients to pull up and are only really effective when waist-high fitted stockings are used. Other therapies are available, including a variety of medications and cardiac tachypacing. These therapies are best considered after consultation (15).

Dizziness

The complaint of dizziness is frequent among elderly persons. Dizziness is the third most common reason why patients aged 65 and older visit family physicians, the fifth most common reason why this age group visits general internists, and the most common presenting complaint of those aged 75 years and older (16). Dizziness is implicated in as much as 25 percent of falls and restricts activity in as many as one-third of subjects. An understanding of the differential diagnosis, workup, and management of this symptom is important to provide optimal care for elderly patients.

Epidemiology

The prevalence of the complaint of dizziness has been reported to be as high as 90 percent in the elderly. However, recent studies found prevalence rates that ranged from 5 percent for persons aged 65 to 69 years to 20 percent for those 85 years and older (17). Another group found the lifetime prevalence of dizziness that was severe enough to see a physician or take a medication was 30 percent (18). In this study, the 1-year incidence was 18 percent. The study found four clinical characteristics that were significantly related to dizziness: multiple neurosensory deficits, presence of cardiovascular risks, depressive symptoms, and the perception of being nervous. The general symptom of dizziness was not associated with increased risk of death or institutionalization after 1 year of follow-up.

When patients say they are dizzy, the symptom can generally be categorized as vertigo, presyncope, imbalance, or nonspecific lightheadedness (19). The study by Drachman and Hart (19) reported on 125 referred patients of unstated age. The top three diagnoses were peripheral vestibular disorders (38%), hyperventilation (23%), and multiple sensory deficits (13%). The patients with multisensory deficits tended to be older and generally had combinations of peripheral neuropathy, cervical spondylosis, and visual impairments. Only 9 percent had an undetermined cause.

Sloane and Baloh reported on 116 patients over age 70 who had been referred for dizziness to a neuro-otology clinic (20). This study found that 46 percent of the subjects had peripheral vestibular disorders, 19 percent had cerebrovascular disorders, 7 percent had other central disorders (cerebellar atrophy, previously diagnosed acoustic neuroma, drug toxicity), and 15 percent had other disorders (anxiety/depression, multiple sensory deficits, vasovagal attack, cardiac arrhythmia, post cataract surgery). No cause was determined for 14 percent of the subjects. Half the patients with peripheral vestibular disorders were believed to have benign positional vertigo.

These studies provide important information on patients referred to specialty clinics for evaluation of dizziness. However, in a nonreferral population, the distribution of diagnoses may be different.

Evaluation

Because dizziness is a symptom that cannot be measured objectively, the patient's history is essential (16). Sloane and Baloh claimed that the patient's clinical history provided the key diagnostic data in 70 percent of cases (20). After the patient's initial description, the physician should ask the following questions:

1. How many kinds of dizziness does the patient have? (It is not uncommon to find more than one type. Forty percent of patients have characteristics from more than one category.)

2. What does the patient mean by the term "dizzy" (vertigo—sense of rotation or being pushed, presyncope/impending faint, imbalance—sensation localized to the body, relieved by sitting or lying down, ill-defined lightheadedness—cerebral sensation of wooziness, floating, swimming, visual)?

3. What is the symptom pattern (acute, recurrent, positional, or continuous)? Are all episodes the same?

4. Are there any associated symptoms (hearing loss, tinnitus, nausea, sweating)?

5. What medications (including alcohol) does the patient take, or has taken recently (aspirinlike agents, anticonvulsants, antidepressants, aminoglycosides, vasodilators, antihypertensives, glaucoma medications)?

6. What diseases does the patient have, and has there been any recent acute illness, especially viral?

7. What is the patient's level of function and how has this been affected? Are there positions or movements the patient tries to avoid?

Table 24.2 lists the common differential diagnoses of vertigo (16,21). The physician needs to determine whether a patient's vertigo is related to peripheral neurologic dysfunction (e.g., labyrinth) or central neurologic dysfunction (e.g., brain stem, cerebellum). Vertigo of peripheral origin is generally worst at onset, aggravated by position, and often has associated tinnitus or hearing changes. The onset of vertigo in relationship to recent events helps suggest a diagnosis. Symptoms after a viral illness suggest vestibular neuronitis. Symptoms after other systemic

Table 24.2. Differential Diagnosis of Dizziness.

Vertigo
    Benign positional vertigo (idiopathic, post-traumatic, post-viral)
    Other peripheral vertigo (post-viral, post-traumatic, drug/toxin, Ménière's, hypothyroid, syphilitic, tumor)
    Central vertigo (vascular, drug/toxin, multiple sclerosis/demyelinating disorders, tumor, seizure)
Presyncope (see Tables 24.1 and 24.4)
    Hyperventilation
Imbalance
    Medication toxicity
    Multiple sensory impairments
    Cervical spine disease
    Muscle weakness, unstable joints
    Neurologic disease–previous CVA, cerebellar degeneration, peripheral neuropathy, myelopathy, parkinsonism
Ill-defined lightheadedness
    Medications, visual disorders, previous CVA, hyperventilation, psychiatric disorders, carbon monoxide intoxication

CVA = cardiovascular accident.

illnesses suggest acute toxic labyrinthitis. Symptoms after head trauma, whiplash, or loud noise suggest traumatic etiology. Symptoms without the above precipitants suggest a peripheral vascular event. Vertigo that is associated with Valsalva maneuver or sneeze suggests the infrequent possibility of a fistulous tract in the labyrinth. Vertigo that is episodic and associated with hearing loss suggests Ménière's disease.

A special category of peripheral vertigo is benign positional vertigo (BPV), which is almost always caused by a peripheral vestibular disturbance, although in rare cases can be associated with a central lesion (22). BPV is important to recognize because in most patients, the symptoms are self-limited and extensive workup is not necessary. About half the cases are idiopathic, but can be secondary to infectious or traumatic insults. The main historic features of BPV are that symptoms occur only with change in position, and after a change in position, the symptoms last less than 1 minute. This allows BPV to be distinguished from other conditions causing vertigo in which the sensation of rotation is generally continous but exacerbated by movement. BPV is an episodic condition, lasting weeks to months, and can recur. It is often precipitated by lying down, rolling over in bed, or during sudden head movements.

Vertigo of central origin often has other neurologic findings referable to the brain stem or cerebellum such as visual changes (diplopia or blindness) and cerebellar signs, and other indications of brain stem involvement. The vertigo is more likely continuous, only variably affected by position, and may not be maximal at onset. Primary brain tumors or metastatic brain tumors are uncommon causes of vertigo. Even acoustic neuroma does not typically present as vertigo. Hearing loss, tinnitus and, frequently, neurologic abnormalities occur first. Multiple sclerosis can occur in elderly persons but is unusual. Seizures rarely present with dizziness or vertigo as the sole manifestation.

If the problem is not vertigo, the next line of questioning is to determine whether the problem is one of an impending faint. This category includes patients with OH, hyperventilation, and cardiac disorders (see syncope). Hyperventilation is usually associated with lightheadedness and circumoral and digital paresthesias.

If the patient describes imbalance, questions should fo-

cus on vision (glaucoma or refractive error), hearing, arthritis of neck or extremities, alcohol use, and symptoms of peripheral neuropathy. The effect of support while walking (holding the elbow or carrying a cane) is important, as marked improvement in stability with only minimal support is characteristic of multiple sensory deficit. The possibility of Parkinson's disease should be considered. Dilated cerebral ventricles or a midline cerebellar tumor can also produce these symptoms without other specific neurologic findings.

The final category is ill-defined lightheadedness. Generally, this type of symptom usually does not suggest a serious underlying disorder. Lightheadedness may be secondary to medication, hyperventilation, or a previous stroke. In the winter months in conjunction with headache, carbon monoxide poisoning should be considered. Affective or anxiety disorders can also be associated with complaints of chronic lightheadedness.

The physical examination should be tailored to the patient's history. Time spent on a careful history can save time on the physical examination. Some of the following tests may be useful in evaluating the dizzy patient whose etiology is unclear from the history.

- Screening orthostatic BP supine and after the patient has been standing for 1 minute. Additional readings should be performed if the history is suggestive or unclear.
- Head turning (side to side and up/down)
- Hyperventilation
- Valsalva
- Carotid sinus stimulation (see syncope)
- Ear inspection and hearing testing
- Neurologic examination including:

  Evidence of previous stroke or parkinsonian features

  Sensory examination including joint position and vibration sense

  Cerebellar testing (past pointing suggests vestibular lesion; intention tremor and abnormal alternating movements suggest cerebellar dysfunction)

  Romberg

  Gait assessment

  Hallpike maneuver (see Table 24.3)

Laboratory testing depends on the working diagnosis and the site of presentation. In the emergency room, routine glucose determination (for hypoglycemia) and cardiac

Table 24.3. Hallpike Maneuver.

The Hallpike maneuver can be useful for assessment of some patients with vertigo. Rapid movements of the head and neck should be done with care, and are not always necessary.

Performance

1. The patient begins in a sitting position on the examination table.
2. The examiner quickly places the patient down with the patient's head hanging over the back of the table at approximately a 30 degree angle, with the patient's face turned 45 degrees to the right.
3. The patient is observed for nystagmus (eyes must be open and not fixed on a target), asked about vertigo, and asked about reproduction of symptoms. The patient's head is held in place for 1 minute. The patient is brought back to the sitting position and again observed for 1 minute.
4. The test is then repeated with the patient's head at 45 degrees to the other side. If vertigo is reproduced, the test should be repeated 2 or 3 times on the side that caused the greatest symptoms to see whether the nystagmus and symptoms fatigue.

Interpretation (if the patient has BPV)

1. After the patient is placed in the supine, head-turned position, there will be a short latency of 5–15 seconds, then the patient will complain of severe vertigo, and J-shaped, rotatory nystagmus will be observed. This will fade in less than 1 minute.
2. In the sitting position, the patient may again experience a transient vertigo and nystagmus.
3. When tested on the other side, only 20% of patients have recurrent symptoms and findings.
4. The vertigo will fatigue with repeated testing.

Additional Points

1. During remissions or mild episodes of BPV, the Hallpike maneuver may be negative, and the diagnosis will have to be made on patient history alone.
2. A central lesion should be suspected if:
   a. Vertigo is dissociated from the nystagmus
   b. The nystagmus begins immediately on positioning
   c. The nystagmus is primarily horizontal or vertical
   d. Nystagmus lasts longer than 1 minute
   e. Vertigo does not fatigue on repeated testing.

BPV = benign positional vertigo.
SOURCE: Leigh RJ, Zee DS. The neurology of eye movements. Philadelphia: Davis, 1983:207–213.

rhythm monitoring were useful in patients over age 45 who presented with dizziness (23). With acute vertigo, a computerized tomography (CT) scan to rule out a cerebrovascular event should be considered.

In less acute settings, testing of patients with vertigo should include glucose (to exclude hyperglycemia), thyroid function tests, and serological tests for syphilis as potentially reversible causes. In cases in which the diagnosis remains unclear, and symptoms are not resolving or causing functional impairment, consultation with an ear, nose, and throat subspecialist (ENT) or neurologist should be considered. If there is evidence for a central lesion, a CT scan thru the petrous pyramids or a magnetic resonance imaging (MRI) scan may be considered, although many asymptomatic elderly have abnormal findings on MRI (24). Imaging techniques are not usually necessary and are best ordered after consultation with a subspecialist.

Patients with presyncope should be evaluated in a similar fashion to patients with hypotension or syncope. Patients with a balance problem should have testing dictated by their history and physical findings. Those with lightheadedness should have drug levels performed, if appropriate.

Treatment

If an elderly patient without a previous history of vertigo develops an acute episode of moderate or severe vertigo, hospital admission for observation and symptom control should be considered. Because of the difficulty in separating peripheral from central neurologic findings, any new episode of acute vertigo in an elderly patient should be considered a cerebrovascular event until proven otherwise. Treatment of symptoms associated with acute vertigo are usually treated with medications possessing anticholinergic and antiemetic properties. A good initial choice is promethazine, which has both characteristics. Promethazine can be given orally, rectally, or intramuscularly in a dose of 12.5 to 50 mg. A benzodiazepine may also be useful adjunctive therapy. For patients with mild or moderate bouts of vertigo, promethazine can be used if nausea is present, and meclizine if nausea is not present. One should start with a low dose of either drug (12.5 mg) at bedtime and gradually titrate to tolerance. The scopalamine patch may cause severe anticholinergic toxicity in older patients and should not be used. In general, medication should be used for only short periods of time. Chronic therapy is rarely beneficial. Exercises have been developed to shorten the duration and impact of benign positional vertigo, and they may be useful for patients willing to perform them (25).

For those with presyncope, the specific etiology should be addressed (e.g., orthostatic hypotension, hyperventilation). For patients with balance problems or multisensory deficit, a referral to physical therapy for gait evaluation, strengthening, and gait assist device is important, as is formal assessment of vision and hearing. Appropriate treatment of patients with ill-defined lightheadedness begins with discontinuation of any offending medications and also includes ophthalmological assessment. Psychiatric evaluation is appropriate if other features suggest a psychiatric disorder. Physical therapy and exercise programs may be useful. Reassurance and regular follow-up are important.

Syncope

Syncope is a common and potentially dangerous problem for the elderly person. Syncope accounts for approximately 3 percent of emergency room visits and 1 percent of medical admissions to a general hospital (26). The causes of syncope differ in young, old, and old old patients. A syncopal episode can lead to acute injury, subsequent fear, and functional limitation. Therefore, its proper evaluation and management is essential to maintain maximum patient independence.

The term syncope is used to denote a transient loss of consciousness and postural tone that resolves spontaneously, without resuscitative intervention and without residual symptoms. This disorder needs to be differentiated from other states of altered consciousness such as cardiac arrest, coma, and seizure.

Epidemiology

Syncope is common in patients of all ages. In younger individuals, 37 percent have had a syncopal episode. A study of elderly nursing home residents showed a 23 percent incidence of syncope during a 10-year period, a 1-year incidence of 6 percent, and a recurrence rate of 30 percent (27).

Two studies provide data on the causes of syncope in young, old, and old old patients. Kapoor et al. evaluated 210 patients aged 60 years and older from emergency rooms, clinics, and inpatient services and compared them

with 190 younger patients with syncope (28). The mean ages of the two groups were 71 years and 39 years, respectively. Cardiac causes (especially ventricular tachycardia, sick sinus syndrome, carotid hypersensitivity, aortic stenosis, myocardial infarction) were twice as common in the old group as in the younger group (34% versus 17%). Noncardiac causes (especially vasovagal and psychiatric) were more common in the young group (38% versus 27%). Unknown causes were approximately equal. In the young group, the leading causes (in order) were vasovagal, orthostatic hypotension, situational, and ventricular tachycardia. Leading causes in the older group (in order) were ventricular tachycardia, orthostatic hypotension, situational stress, sick sinus syndrome, aortic stenosis, drug-induced syncope, and TIA. Approximately one-third of patients from both groups sustained trauma, but trauma was more likely to be serious in the elderly subjects.

Lipsitz et al reported on 97 institutionalized elderly with syncope, with data collected during a 3-year period (29). The mean age of this group, 87 years, was substantially older than Kapoor's group. This study divided the causes of syncope into three groups: specific diseases, situational stressors, and unknown. The most common specific diseases were myocardial infarction, aortic stenosis, and volume depletion. The most common situational stressors were hypotension induced by drugs, eating, defecation, and postural changes. Multivariate analysis identified five independent factors: coronary artery disease, functional impairment, postural BP reduction, aortic stenosis, and insulin therapy. Syncope patients were much more likely than controls to have multiple factors.

The prognosis for younger patients with syncope depends on etiology. The highest 2-year mortality occurs in patients with cardiac causes, with lower rates for noncardiac and unknown causes. In elderly nursing home residents, the presence or absence of syncope does not appear to alter mortality.

Evaluation

Initial evaluation for syncope begins with the patient's history. If an observer was present at the time of the episode, the person should be questioned because a patient's report of loss of consciousness is not always accurate. However, patients should be allowed to describe the event in their own words. Table 24.4 shows the differential diagnosis to keep in mind when beginning the evaluation. The following information should be obtained.

1. How many times has this occurred? (Recurrent episodes are common.) Has there been near syncope as well as syncope?

2. What has been the patient's general health in the past few days? Has the patient been eating, and taking fluids and medications in the usual manner? (These questions may uncover subtle illnesses, such as diarrhea, that in combination with a usual medical regimen may result in hypotension.)

3. How did the episode begin? Were there any associated symptoms? What activities was the patient engaged in

Table 24.4. Differential Diagnosis of Syncope.

Reflex
   Vasovagal
   Carotid sinus
   Cough
   Defecation
   Micturition
   Swallowing
Hypotensive
   Multiple diseases and impairments
   Medication
   Orthostatic
   Postprandial
   Volume depletion
Cardiac
   Arrhythmias
   Valvular disease
   Myocardial infarction
   Cardiomyopathy (dilated or hypertrophic)
   Pulmonary hypertension/embolism
   Aortic dissection
   Atrial myxoma
Central nervous system
   Seizure
   TIA
   Tumor
   Subclavian steal
   Psychiatric
Abnormal blood composition
   Anemia
   Hyperventilation
   Hypoglycemia
   Hypoxia

TIA = transient ischemic attack.

(shaving [carotid sinus], defecation, recent meal or medication [hypotension], climbing stairs [hypoxia, aortic stenosis], chest pain [angina or myocardial infarction], palpitations [arrhythmia])?

4. What occurred during the episode? Was there incontinence or tonic-clonic movements to suggest seizure? Was there any injury?

5. How did the episode end? (Slow onset and slow recovery suggests hyperventilation or hypoglycemia; sudden onset but slow recovery (>15 min) suggests a seizure disorder, TIA, or head trauma; sudden onset and offset suggests hypotension, outflow obstruction, or arrhythmia) (30).

The patient's history should include a careful review of medications, alcohol use, and use of eye drops (31). Past medical records may reveal cardiovascular and neurologic risk factors.

The physical examination should include BP measurement in both arms to rule out subclavian steal syndrome or aortic dissection as well as provide an orthostatic BP measurement. If the patient's history is suggestive, BP should also be measured after the patient has been walking, climbing stairs, or eating. A careful cardiopulmonary examination should be done to check for volume status, aortic stenosis, hypertropic cardiomyopathy, pulmonary embolism, or pulmonary hypertension. Stool guaiac and careful neurologic examination should be performed.

Laboratory testing should include CBC, blood chemistries, urinalysis for specific gravity, and an ECG. Frequent ectopic beats, bradycardia, abnormal PR interval, long QT interval, conduction delay, or bundle branch block may suggest a rhythm disturbance as an etiology. However, even in patients with bifascicular or trifascicular block, syncope is more commonly caused by another etiology than complete heart block (32).

With this data base, the diagnosis will be apparent in one-third of patients, and the workup or treatment can proceed accordingly. If the diagnosis is unclear, and there is no obvious cause for a hypotensive stressor, other testing should be considered. Carotid sinus massage can be performed to test for carotid sinus hypersensitivity (33). This maneuver is generally safe, but should not be performed in patients who have carotid bruits, cerebral vascular disease, or digitalis toxicity. There are rare reports of asystole, complete heart block, and stroke in elderly patients after carotid sinus massage and some authors recommend having intravenous access and atropine immediately available, and resuscitation equipment nearby. In patients with risk factors for complications from carotid sinus massage, Holter monitoring should be considered. Carotid sinus massage, when appropriate, can be performed as follows. With an ECG running, a baseline BP is taken. The carotid bifurcation is gently massaged for 5 seconds, the ECG observed and the BP checked. The test is then repeated on the opposite side. Criteria for abnormal response include symptoms, sinus pause of 3 seconds or longer, or systolic BP decline of more than 50 mm Hg or less than 90 mm Hg. Some investigators also perform this test while the patient is upright, but in this position a symptomatic response may not always represent the actual cause of the patient's syncope (34).

For patients with suspected defecation/micturition syncope or digitalis toxicity, the Valsalva maneuver can be performed. The patient forces air against a closed glottis for 15 seconds under ECG monitoring looking for excessive bradycardia. Holter monitoring and echocardiography are the most useful additional tests because of the high prevalence of rhythm disturbances, and valvular and myocardial disease in the elderly (28,29).

Prolonged ambulatory Holter monitoring, transtelephonic event monitoring, treadmill testing, cardiac catheterization, signal-averaged ECG, electrophysiology studies, and tilt-table testing may ultimately be useful but should be performed in conjunction with a cardiologist (35). A potential cause for syncope may be identified in some patients with electrophysiologic testing, particularly in the presence of coronary artery disease, abnormal ejection fraction, or bundle branch block (36).

Head CT scanning and EEG are very low-yield studies in patients who do not have clinical evidence of a cerebrovascular event or seizure (26).

Treatment

The goal of treatment is to prevent recurrence. If a specific etiology is defined, appropriate treatment options can be discussed. If no specific disorder is identified, careful consideration should be given to the possibility of multiple causes. Empiric therapy with pacemakers, digoxin,

antiarrhythmics, or antiseizure medications does not appear to reduce subsequent syncope rates (37,38). The following interventions may be useful:

- Medications should be reviewed, and those for which therapeutic benefit is unclear or that have a hypotensive effect should be tapered or discontinued.
- A regular exercise program should be initiated with supervision.
- Small, frequent meals should be given with liberal water and salt intake.
- Extreme neck rotation and tight collars should be avoided.
- Urination and showering should be performed while sitting.
- Prolonged, quiet standing should be avoided. If any symptoms develop, the patient should assume a supine or sitting position.
- Hypotensive stressors should be avoided (hot tubs, sauna).
- After prolonged supine or sitting position, the patient should perform isometric exercises of the upper and lower extremities, and patients should be cautioned to stand slowly with support assistance.

Patients should be monitored carefully and further episodes reported immediately. Caregivers or spouses should be trained to take a pulse so they can check rate and strength of pulse wave during subsequent episodes, if witnessed. Patients should be instructed not to drive until their evaluation is completed. It is important to remember that the cause of syncope remains unknown in approximately one-third of patients after evaluation.

References

1. Mader SL. Orthostatic hypotension. Med Clin North Am 1989;73:1337–1349.
2. Lipsitz LA. Orthostatic hypotension in the elderly. N Engl J Med 1989;321:952–957.
3. Lipsitz LA, Mietus J, Moody GB, Goldberger AL. Spectral characteristics of heart rate variability before and during postural tilt. Relations to aging and risk of syncope. Circulation 1990;81:1803–1810.
4. Shannon RP, Wei JY, Rosa RM, et al. The effect of age and sodium depletion on cardiovascular response to orthostasis. Hypertension 1986;8:438–443.
5. Mader SL. Effects of meals and time of day on postural blood pressure responses in healthy young and elderly subjects. Arch Intern Med 1989;149:2757–2760.

6. Wood M, Hyman S, Wood AJJ. A clinical study of sensitivity to sodium nitroprusside during controlled hypotensive anesthesia in young and elderly patients. Anesth Analg 1987;66:132–136.

7. Mader SL, Josephson KR, Rubenstein LZ. Low prevalence of postural hypotension among community-dwelling elderly. JAMA 1987;258:1511–1514.

8. Vaitkevicius PV, Esserwein DM, Maynard AK, et al. Frequency and importance of postprandial blood pressure reduction in elderly nursing-home patients. Ann Intern Med 1991;115:865–870.

9. Jansen RWMM, Lipsitz, LA. Postprandial hypotension: Epidemiology, pathophysiology, and clinical management. Ann Int Med 1995;122:286–295.

10. Dobkin BH. Orthostatic hypotension as a risk factor for symptomatic occlusive cerebrovascular disease. Neurology 1989;39:30–34.

11. Stark RJ, Wodak J. Primary orthostatic cerebral ischemia. J Neurol Neurosurg Psychiatry 1983;46:883–891.

12. Schatz IJ. Orthostatic hypotension I and II. Arch Intern Med 1984;144:773–777, 1037–1041.

13. Heseltine D, Dakkak M, Woodhouse K, et al. The effect of caffeine on postprandial hypotension in the elderly. J Am Geriatr Soc 1991;39:160–164.

14. Jansen RWMM, de Meijer PHEM, van Lier HJJ, Hoefnagels WHL. Influence of octreotide (SMS 201-995) and insulin administration on the course of blood pressure after an oral glucose load in hypertensive elderly subjects. J Am Geriatr Soc 1989;37:1135–1139.

15. Ahmad RAS, Watson RDS. Treatment of postural hypotension. A review. Drugs 1990;39:74–85.

16. Baloh RW. Dizziness in older people. J Am Geriatr Soc 1992;40:713–721.

17. Hale WE, Perkins LL, May FE, et al. Symptom prevalence in the elderly J Am Geriatr Soc 1986;34:333–340.

18. Sloane P, Blazer D, George LK. Dizziness in a community elderly population. J Am Geriatr Soc 1989;37:101–108.

19. Drachman DA, Hart CW. An approach to the dizzy patient. Neurology 1972;22:323–334.

20. Sloane PD, Baloh RW. Persistent dizziness in geriatric patients. J Am Geriatr Soc 1989;37:1031–1038.

21. Leigh RJ, Zee DS. *The neurology of eye movements.* Philadelphia: Davis, 1983:207–213.

22. Baloh RW, Honrubia V, Jacobson K. Benign positional vertigo: clinical and oculographic features in 240 cases. Neurology 1987;37:371–378.

23. Herr RD, Zun L, Mathews JJ. A directed approach to the dizzy patient. Ann Emerg Med 1989;18:664–672.

24. Day JJ, Freer CE, Dixon AK, et al. Magnetic resonance imaging of the brain and brain-stem in elderly patients with dizziness. Age Ageing 1990;19:144–150.

25. Brandt T, Daroff RB. Physical therapy for benign paroxysmal positional vertigo. Arch Otolaryngol 1980;106:484–485.

26. Kapoor WN. Evaluation and outcome of patients with syncope. Medicine 1990;69:160–175.

27. Lipsitz LA, Wei JY, Rowe JW. Syncope in an elderly, institutionalized population: prevalence, incidence, and associated risk. Q J Med 1985;55:45–54.

28. Kapoor W, Snustad D, Peterson J, et al. Syncope in the elderly. Am J Med 1986;80:419–428.

29. Lipsitz LA, Pluchino FC, Wey JY, Rowe JW. Syncope in institutionalized elderly: impact of multiple pathological conditions and situational stress. J Chronic Dis 1986;39:619–630.

30. Moss AJ. Evaluation of the syncopal patient. Hosp Med 1985;21:165–178.

31. Davidson E, Fuchs J, Rotenberg Z, et al. Drug-related syncope. Clin Cardiol 1989;12:577–580.

32. McAnulty JH, Rahimtoola SH, Murphy E, et al. Natural history of "high-risk" bundle branch block: final report of a prospective study. N Engl J Med 1982;307:137–143.

33. Schweitzer P, Teichholz LE. Carotid sinus massage. Its diagnostic and therapeutic value in arrhythmias. Am J Med 1985;78:645–654.

34. McIntosh S, Da Costa D, Kenny RA. Outcome of an integrated approach to the investigation of dizziness, falls and syncope in elderly patients referred to a "syncope" clinic. Age Ageing 1993;22:53–88.

35. Manolis AS. Syncope in the elderly. Compr Ther 1989;15:31–42.

36. Sugrue DD, Holmes DR, Gersh BJ, et al. Impact of intercardiac electrophysicologic testing on management of elderly patients with recurrent syncope or near syncope. J Am Geriatr Soc 1987;35:1079–1083.

37. Rattes MF, Klein GJ, Sharma AD, et al. Efficacy of empirical cardiac pacing in syncope of unknown cause. Can Med Assoc J 1989;140:381–385.

38. Aronow WS, Mercando AD, Epstein S. Prevalence of arrhythmias detected by 24-hour ambulatory electrocardiography and value of antiarrhythmic therapy in elderly patients with unexplained syncope. Am J Cardiol 1992;70:408–410.

Chapter 25
Fractures in the Elderly

Kenneth J. Koval and Joseph D. Zuckerman

Old age is no place for sissies.

Bette Davis

Fractures in the elderly remain a medical and surgical challenge. More than any other age group, this growing segment of the population requires fracture management tailored to the specific needs of the patient. Fracture management should be based on not only the fracture pattern and location, but also the preinjury status of the patient. One must avoid a "triumph of technology over reason," and at the same time try to achieve the goal of full restoration of preinjury function. This chapter reviews general concepts in fracture management and the more common fractures seen in the elderly: femoral neck, intertrochanteric, and subtrochanteric hip fractures; ankle fractures; proximal humerus fractures; distal radius fractures; vertebral compression fractures; and pathologic fractures.

Preinjury Status

The goal of fracture treatment for any patient is to return the patient to the prefracture level of function. It is particularly important in the elderly to obtain a detailed history of preinjury function to establish an appropriate treatment plan. The treatment goals of an independent, community walker with an intertrochanteric fracture differ from that of an institutionalized nonwalker. The former requires aggressive surgical treatment and rehabilitation; the latter patient should have a much less aggressive approach, probably consisting of early mobilization from bed to wheelchair. In each case, return to preinjury function is achieved but with significantly different approaches.

Systemic Disease

The elderly fracture patient often has pre-existing medical problems that affect fracture management. Cardiopulmonary disease affects the patient's ability to tolerate prolonged recumbency, undergo surgery, and participate in rehabilitation. Neurological disorders such as Alzheimer's disease, Parkinson's disease, and residual from a previous cerebrovascular accident must be considered when the physician plans the type of fracture management. For instance, a treatment plan that requires a high degree of patient cooperation is inappropriate for a patient with senile dementia.

Endocrine problems, particularly diabetes, are common in the elderly. Diabetic patients generally have vascular compromise caused by small vessel disease and are immunosuppressed. Vascular compromise increases the risk of wound complications such as skin slough, and immunosuppression increases the risk of infection. Fracture union has been shown to be significantly prolonged in diabetic patients, especially in fractures treated surgically (1). Therefore, nonoperative treatment of selected fractures may be preferred in these patients.

Vascular insufficiency, either arterial or venous, also presents management difficulties. Venous insufficiency is manifested by peripheral edema, skin discoloration, and ulcer formation, particularly around the malleoli. Arterial insufficiency is manifested by shiny, atrophic skin, absent hair, and diminished or absent pulses. Both vascular conditions affect fracture union and wound healing. In addition, these patients have fragile skin that is susceptible to breakdown even in a well-padded cast.

Osteopenia

Osteopenia is frequently present in the elderly. Osteopenia is a decreased bone mass, caused by either osteoporosis (decreased bone density with normal bone mineralization) or osteomalacia (decreased bone matrix mineralization with or without a change in bone density.) The presence of severe osteopenia necessitates a comprehensive medical evaluation to identify treatable causes such as hyperparathyroidism, nutritional deficiencies, Cushing's disease, renal disease, and tumors. Senile osteoporosis is the most common etiology of osteopenia in the elderly. Significant risk factors include female sex (especially postmenopausal), northern European ancestry, physical inactivity, multiparity, and excessive alcohol intake.

Osteomalacia in the elderly is often a result of nutritional deficiencies (low calcium and high phosphate intake) and may be more common than generally recognized. Malabsorption syndromes, aberrant states of defects in calcium, vitamin D and phosphorus metabolism, hypophosphatasia, and excessive use of medications such as phosphate-binding antacids and phenytoin (Dilantin) can result in osteomalacia.

Tumors can create significant local osteopenia secondary to replacement of bone mass by neoplasm. The most common tumors affecting bone in the elderly are multiple myeloma and metastases from prostate, breast, thyroid, lung, and renal carcinomas.

Osteopenia affects fracture treatment because it decreases the potential for the surgeon to achieve stable enough fixation to allow early range of motion and ambulation. Screws may provide suboptimal fixation in osteoporotic bone secondary to decreased pull-out strength. One can enhance implant fixation through the use of methylmethacrylate (bone cement).

Multiple Trauma Patients

Recent studies strongly support early surgical stabilization of long-bone fractures (particularly femoral shaft fractures) in polytrauma patients (2). Operative stabilization of long-bone fractures within 24 to 48 hours of injury has been shown to decrease the incidence of adult respiratory distress syndrome (ARDS), duration of ventilatory support, length of stay in the intensive care unit, and cost of hospitalization. The risk of pulmonary complications in the polytrauma patient can be significantly greater in the elderly, secondary to pre-existing pulmonary disease. Therefore, one should stabilize all long-bone fractures as soon as possible to allow early patient mobilization. The importance of age as a prognostic indicator in multiple trauma patients is reflected by the fact that the injury severity score (ISS) LD50 (the score associated with a 50% mortality rate) significantly decreases with increasing age (3).

Open Fractures

Open fractures (the bone is exposed to the outside environment) represent severe injuries associated with an increased risk of infection and nonunion. Open fractures in the elderly, particularly those of the lower extremities, should be treated as limb-threatening injuries. Pre-existing vascular insufficiency, immunocompromise, underlying diabetes mellitus, atherosclerosis, and osteopenia increase the risk of treatment complications. To optimize treatment results, one must adhere to the basic principles of open fracture management: meticulous debridement of soft tissue and bone, fracture stabilization, and soft-tissue coverage with early bone grafting, when appropriate.

Intra-Articular Fractures

Intra-articular fractures require an anatomic reduction to prevent post-traumatic arthritis, and fixation stable enough to allow early range of motion. Early joint motion has been demonstrated to promote articular cartilage healing (4). Intra-articular fractures involving an arthritic joint are generally unique to the elderly and may require primary prosthetic replacement. A displaced femoral neck fracture in a patient with an arthritic hip is an indication for a primary total hip arthroplasty. This procedure is also appropriate for comminuted proximal humerus fractures with associated glenohumeral arthritis.

Hip Fractures

Hip fractures are a common and often devastating injury in the elderly, with an impact that extends far beyond the fracture to the domains of medicine, rehabilitation, psychiatry, social work, and medical economics. Fractures of the proximal femur continue to consume a major portion of national health-care resources. Despite improvements in patient care, including advances in operative technique and implant technology, the number of hip fractures has increased each year, making it difficult to keep pace with this growing health-care problem. With the aging of the U.S. population, the annual number of hip fractures is projected to double by the year 2050 (5).

Management of the Patient with Hip Fracture

The treatment of choice for most hip fracture patients is operative stabilization, followed by early mobilization. Historically, nonoperative management has resulted in an unacceptable rate of mortality, medical morbidity, and fracture malunion and nonunion. Nonoperative management, however, may be appropriate in selected patients (demented nonambulators) who experience minimal discomfort from the injury. These patients should have early bed-to-chair mobilization to avoid the complications of prolonged bed rest, such as decubiti, urinary tract infections, deep venous thrombosis, and pulmonary insufficiency.

Preoperative Assessment Imaging Studies

The standard radiographic examination of the hip should include an anteroposterior (AP) view of the hip and pelvis and a cross-table lateral view. The AP view of the pelvis allows comparison with the nonfractured side, which

may be helpful in identifying minimally displaced or impacted fractures. A cross-table lateral is preferred over the frog lateral because the frog lateral requires abduction, flexion, and external rotation of the affected lower extremity. This position is poorly tolerated by hip fracture patients and may result in fracture displacement. In difficult-to-identify fractures, an internal rotation view of the hip may be helpful because it permits visualization of the entire femoral neck.

When a hip fracture is suspected but not apparent on standard radiographs, a technetium bone scan or magnetic resonance imaging (MRI) should be obtained. The bone scan is a sensitive indicator of unrecognized hip fractures, although in the elderly it may require 2 to 3 days to become positive. MRI has been shown to be as accurate as bone scanning in the assessment of occult fractures of the hip and can be reliably performed within 24 hours of injury (6) (Figure 25.1).

Timing of Surgery

In general, hip fracture surgery should be performed as soon as possible after injury. However, one must first stabilize all comorbid medical conditions, particularly cardiopulmonary conditions and fluid and electrolyte imbalances. Delays of 24 hours or more to achieve medical stabilization have not been shown to increase morbid-

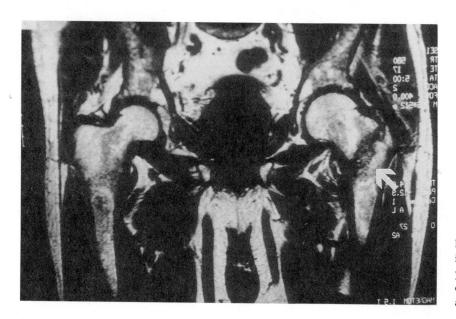

Fig. 25.1. MRI of a left intertrochanteric hip fracture in an 80-year-old woman, taken within 24 hours of injury. The fracture was not apparent on plain radiographs.

ity or mortality. Rather, surgical treatment of medically unstable patients significantly increases the mortality risk. Kenzora et al reported that a surgical delay of less than 1 week, which permitted medical stabilization, was not associated with increased mortality (7). Sexson and Lehner found that early surgery was detrimental to medically unstable elderly hip fracture patients (8).

Anesthetic Considerations

The choice of anesthesia (regional versus general) has not been shown to affect the incidence of postoperative morbidity or mortality in elderly hip fracture patients. In a prospective randomized, multicenter study of 538 geriatric hip fracture patients, Davis et al reported no difference in short- or long-term mortality for patients whose surgery was performed under general or spinal anesthesia (9). These findings were supported by Valentin and colleagues in a prospective series of 578 elderly hip fracture patients (10).

Postoperative Mobilization

Postoperative management remains controversial. Some authors recommend restricted weight-bearing until there is radiographic evidence of fracture healing; others advocate immediate, unrestricted weight-bearing. Biomechanical data has demonstrated that nonweight-bearing walking places significant stresses across the hip as a result of muscular contraction at the hip and knee. In addition, the simple act of moving onto a bedpan in bed places forces across the hip that are greater than body weight. Therefore, attempts at unloading the hip by nonweight-bearing ambulation are not realistic. Also, geriatric patients have great difficulty walking with restricted weight-bearing, and this results in significant limitations in their ability to become ambulatory. Therefore, our approach has been to allow weight-bearing, as much as it can be tolerated by the patient, for most geriatric hip fracture patients.

Functional Recovery

Successful treatment of geriatric hip fracture patients is frequently determined on the basis of the patients who are able to regain their prefracture level of function. This level of function, however, is often quite difficult to achieve. Among patients who were functionally independent and living at home before hip fracture, 15 percent to 40 percent require institutionalized care for more than 1 year after fracture. Only 50 percent to 60 percent of patients regain their prefracture ambulatory status within a year after fracture. Studies have tried to identify the factors that affect the patient's ability to regain prefracture ambulatory status after hip fracture. The important factors identified include sex, age, the presence of pre-existing dementia, and prefracture ambulatory status (11,12).

To achieve functional independence, a person must be able to perform certain activities of daily living (ADLs). The functions necessary for community dwelling have been identified and divided into two categories: basic activities of daily living (BADLs) and instrumental activities of daily living (IADLs). BADLs include bathing, feeding, toileting, and dressing; IADLs include food preparation, food shopping, laundry, banking, housework, and use of public transportation. Most patients with hip surgery require assistance in performing ADLs. Of patients who were independent in ADLs before fracture, only 20 percent to 35 percent regain their prefracture ADL independence. The factors reported to be predictive of recovery of function in ADLs are younger age, absence of dementia or delirium in nondemented patients, and a strong social network (13).

Femoral Neck Fractures

Femoral neck fractures are intracapsular fractures occurring in the proximal femur between the femoral head and intertrochanteric line. Most femoral neck fractures result from of a simple fall. The intracapsular location of femoral neck fractures has important implications for fracture healing and the development of femoral head osteonecrosis (bone death). The blood supply for the femoral head arises from the medial and lateral femoral circumflex arteries that form an extracapsular arterial ring at the base of the femoral neck. The ring gives rise to ascending branches that traverse the neck proximally and form an intracapsular ring at the junction of the femoral head and neck. Because the blood supply is distally based, displaced femoral neck fractures may result in its disruption.

Different classification systems the most popular of which was devised by Garden, have been used for femoral neck fractures (14). This classification divides femoral neck fractures into four types on the basis of the degree of displacement. Type I is an incomplete, impacted (stable) fracture; type II is a complete fracture without displacement; type III is a complete fracture with partial displacement; and type IV is a complete fracture with total displacement of the fragments. Radiographically differentiating the four different types is often difficult and, therefore, a simpler system has evolved in which types I and II are considered nondisplaced fractures and types III and IV are considered displaced fractures (Figure 25.2A and B).

The clinical presentation of patients with femoral neck fractures depends primarily on the type of fracture. Patients with nondisplaced or impacted fractures may be ambulatory with minimal hip/groin discomfort and complain of mild pain only at the extremes of hip motion. Patients with displaced fractures are usually much more symptomatic; they are unable to stand or ambulate, and the affected lower extremity is externally rotated and shortened. Any motion of the hip is painful.

Impacted and nondisplaced femoral neck fractures should be internally stabilized with multiple lag screws or pins placed in parallel (Figure 25.3). Some authors have recommended nonoperative management of impacted femoral neck fractures because there is some stability secondary to bone interdigitation at the fracture site. However, Bentley found a disimpaction rate of 8 percent to 15 percent in his series of patients (15).

Nonsurgical treatment of impacted fractures usually includes a prolonged period of toe-touch, weight-bearing ambulation, which is poorly tolerated by the elderly.

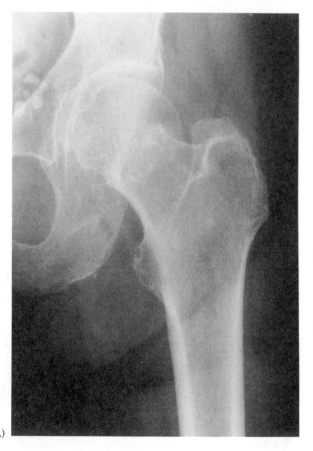

(A)

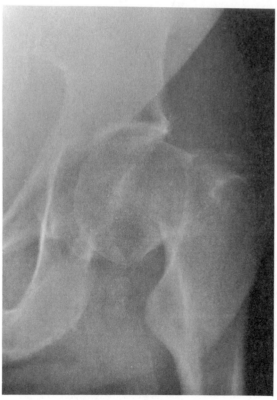

(B)

Fig. 25.2A,B. An impacted (stable) femoral neck fracture (A) and a displaced femoral neck fracture (B).

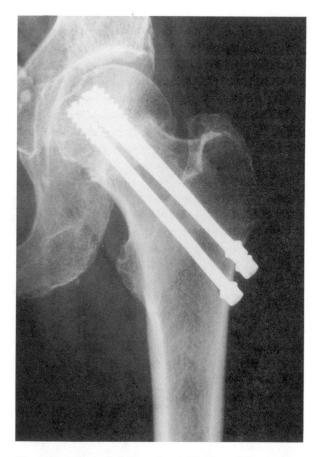

Fig. 25.3. An impacted femoral neck fracture stabilized with three parallel cancellous screws.

Nondisplaced fractures that are not impacted do not have the inherent stability of impacted fractures and have a high risk of displacement. Nonunion and osteonecrosis are uncommon complications after treatment of non-displaced fractures, with nonunion occurring in less than 5 percent of cases, and osteonecrosis in less than 8 percent (16).

Treatment of displaced femoral neck fractures remains controversial. Most authors advocate closed or open reduction and internal fixation in younger active patients and primary prosthetic replacement in older, less active patients (Figure 25.4). When fracture stabilization is used, achieving anatomic reduction is probably the most important factor to avoid healing complications. Prompt reduction of displaced fractures has been advocated, but

has not been consistently shown to decrease the incidence of osteonecrosis or nonunion. If a closed reduction is unacceptable, open reduction (with direct fracture manipulation) may be required. Internal fixation of displaced fractures most commonly uses multiple lag screws or pins.

Nonunion and osteonecrosis continue to be problems after displaced femoral neck fracture. The incidence of nonunion has ranged from 10 percent to 30 percent and, for osteonecrosis, 15 percent to 33 percent (16). The need for reoperation after internal fixation of displaced frac-

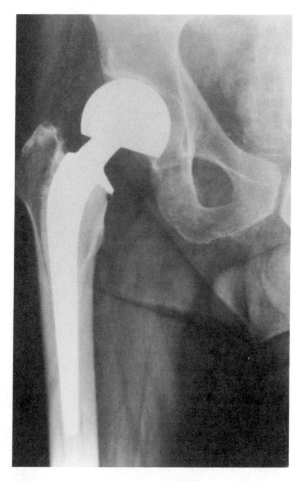

Fig. 25.4. A cemented hemiarthroplasty of the hip was the treatment of choice for a displaced femoral neck fracture in a 75-year-old man.

tures has been variable, with approximately one-third of patients with osteonecrosis and three-fourths of patients with nonunion or early fixation failure requiring additional surgery.

Hemiarthroplasty (femoral head and neck replacement) is a treatment alternative that has been advocated for older, less active patients with displaced femoral neck fractures. Historically, only a one-piece prosthesis was available for use in the treatment of these fractures. Although successful in select patient populations, use of these prostheses has been associated with increased rates of acetabular cartilage erosion and femoral stem loosening, which results in groin and thigh pain. The availability and use of methylmethacrylate has reduced the incidence of femoral stem loosening, but acetabular wear has remained a problem. Newer devices, such as the bipolar prosthesis (a two-piece prosthesis), have been introduced to lower the incidence of acetabular erosion. However, controversy remains over the efficacy of these expensive implants (17).

The results of primary, cemented, total hip replacement after femoral neck fracture have been disappointing (18). Nevertheless, primary total hip arthroplasty has a place in the treatment of acute femoral neck fractures for patients with pre-existing acetabular disease (rheumatoid arthritis, osteoarthritis, Paget's disease). In these situations, the results can be expected to be comparable with those reported for elective total hip arthroplasty. The results of secondary total hip replacement performed after failed internal fixation of a femoral neck fracture are reported to be similar to those obtained after primary arthroplasty for femoral neck fracture.

Intertrochanteric Hip Fractures

The intertrochanteric region is extracapsular, consisting of the transitional bone between the femoral neck and shaft, and includes the greater and lesser trochanters. The bone in this region is primarily cancellous bone and serves to transmit and distribute stresses. The trochanters provide insertion for some of the important muscles of the gluteal region. The abductors and short external rotators insert onto the greater trochanter. The iliopsoas inserts onto the lesser trochanter. The calcar femorale is a vertical wall of dense bone that extends from the posteromedial aspect of the femoral shaft to the posterior portion of the femoral neck. It forms an internal trabecular strut within the inferior portion of the neck and intertrochanteric region and acts as a strong conduit for stresses. The cancellous bone in this area is well vascularized. Consequently, the problems of nonunion and osteonecrosis encountered with intracapsular femoral neck fractures are rarely a problem after intertrochanteric fractures.

Intertrochanteric fractures occur with approximately the same frequency as femoral neck fractures in patients with similar demographic characteristics. Early reports indicated that patients who suffered intertrochanteric fractures were approximately 10 years older than patients with femoral neck fractures. However, recent reports have not supported these data. The female-to-male ratio for this injury ranges from 2:1 to 8:1. Mortality rates for patients with intertrochanteric fractures are comparable with those reported for femoral neck fractures.

Of the many classification systems devised for intertrochanteric hip fractures, the one most commonly used is that introduced by Evans and formulated on the basis of the stability of the fracture pattern and the possibility for converting an unstable fracture to a stable reduction (19). Evans recognized that the key to a stable reduction was to restore posteromedial cortical continuity (Figure 25.5A and B). In stable fracture patterns, the posteromedial cortex remains intact and a stable reduction can be obtained. Unstable fracture patterns are characterized by comminution (fragmentation) of the posteromedial cortex.

The treatment of choice for the vast majority of intertrochanteric hip fractures is surgery. Fracture reduction is performed by using manual traction and manipulation on a fracture table with fluoroscopy to assess fracture reduction. If an acceptable closed reduction cannot be obtained after a few attempts at gentle manipulation and traction, more forceful manipulation should not be used. Rather, an open reduction is preferable. With limited fracture exposure and release of traction, the fragments can usually be manipulated into an acceptable position.

The sliding hip screw is the implant most commonly used for fixation of intertrochanteric hip fractures (20,21) (Figure 25.6). This device consists of a large screw that provides fixation in the femoral head and neck and a

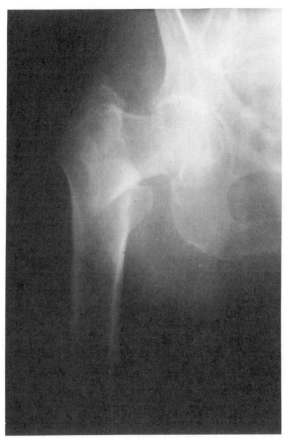

(A)

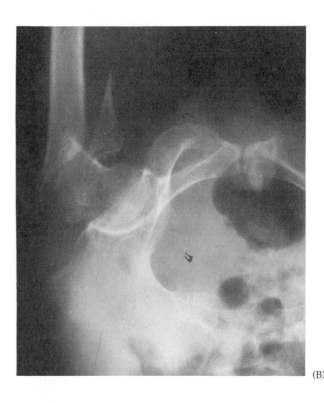

(B)

Fig. 25.5A,B. A stable intertrochanteric hip fracture (A) and an unstable intertrochanteric fracture (B). In stable fracture patterns, the posteromedial cortex remains intact and a stable reduction can be obtained. Unstable fracture patterns are characterized by comminution (fragmentation) of the posteromedial cortex.

sideplate and barrel attached to the femoral shaft that allows the screw to telescope within the barrel. The most important aspect of sliding hip screw insertion is secure placement of the screw within the femoral head and neck. The screw should be positioned within 1 cm of the subchondral bone. A central position within the femoral head and neck is usually recommended.

Prosthetic replacement for intertrochanteric fractures has been used successfully to treat postoperative loss of fixation when repeat open reduction and internal fixation is not possible or desirable. Primary prosthetic replacement for comminuted, unstable fractures has been used successfully in a limited number of patients. The disadvantages of this approach, however, include a larger,

more extensive surgical procedure and the potential for dislocation. Indications for its use in the treatment of acute intertrochanteric fractures remain undefined. Prosthetic replacement does not appear to offer any advantage over a properly inserted sliding hip screw.

Subtrochanteric Fractures

Subtrochanteric fractures comprise about 15 percent of all proximal femur fractures. Subtrochanteric fractures start at or below the lesser trochanter and involve the proximal femoral shaft. They are usually seen in three types of patients: young patients who suffer high energy trauma; older patients with weakened bone whose fractures result

tures, comminution results in loss of medial cortical continuity. These fractures are at highest risk for healing complications and implant failure.

The treatment of choice for most subtrochanteric fractures is surgery. The implant most commonly used for fracture fixation is the intramedullary nail (Figure 25.7). Most nonpathologic subtrochanteric fractures can be stabilized by intramedullary nails, regardless of the fracture pattern or amount of comminution (22). Favorable mechanical characteristics of intramedullary nails have eliminated the need for surgically reconstituting the medial femoral cortex. High rates of union have been reported in large series of subtrochanteric femur fractures treated with intramedullary nails.

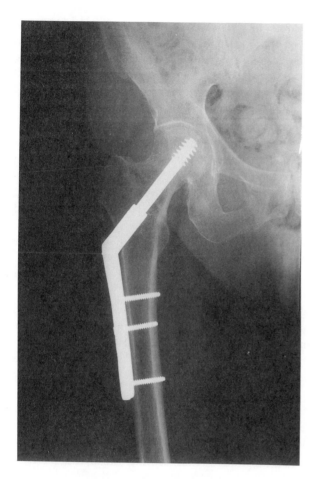

Fig. 25.6. A sliding hip screw used for stabilization of a stable intertrochanteric hip fracture.

from a minor fall; and older patients with pathologic or impending pathologic fractures from metastatic lesions. The subtrochanteric area is subjected to some of the highest biomechanical forces in the body. The medial and posteromedial cortex is a site of high compressive forces, and the lateral cortex experiences high tensile stresses. Stress distribution has important implications in fracture fixation and healing.

Various classification systems have been proposed, but none have been universally accepted. As noted in intertrochanteric fractures, fracture stability depends on the presence or absence of posteromedial continuity. In stable fractures, medial and posteromedial cortical support is intact or can be re-established. In unstable frac-

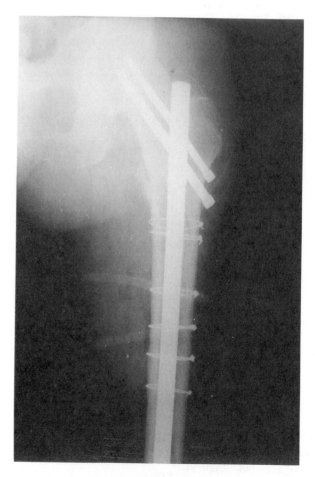

Fig. 25.7. A subtrochanteric hip fracture stabilized with an intramedullary nail and cerclage wires.

Sliding hip screws have been used with success, particularly in low-energy, subtrochanteric fractures in the elderly. One series reported a 95 percent union rate (23). For this device to function optimally, the sliding component of the device must cross the fracture site; therefore, subtrochanteric and intertrochanteric fractures are most suitable for this implant.

Postoperative management depends on the fracture pattern and the type of fixation. Subtrochanteric or intertrochanteric fractures treated with a sliding hip screw that allows impaction at the fracture site can allow weight-bearing. Stable fractures treated with intramedullary devices can also allow early weight-bearing. Fractures with medial comminution or segmental comminution must be protected, regardless of the internal fixation device, for at least 6 to 8 weeks until early healing is evident.

Ankle Fractures

The ankle joint is a modified hinge joint consisting of the talus, medial malleolus, and lateral malleolus. The lateral malleolus projects about 1 cm distal and posterior to the medial malleolus. Uniting these osseous structures are the medial and the lateral collateral ligaments and the ligaments of the tibiofibular syndesmosis. The deltoid ligament is a thick triangular band consisting of superficial and deep fibers. The superficial fibers attach to the navicular, the sustentaculum tali, and the talus. The stronger, deeper fibers attach to the medial surface of the talus. The lateral collateral ligament is comprised of three ligaments: (1) the anterior talofibular ligament that runs from the anterior margin of the lateral malleolus to the anterior talus, (2) the calcaneofibular ligament that extends from the tip of the fibula to the calcaneus and (3) the posterior talofibular ligament that originates on the medial surface of the lateral malleolus and inserts on the posterior lateral aspect of the talus. The most distal portions of the tibia and the fibula are joined together at the syndesmosis by four ligaments (the anterior inferior tibiofibular ligament, the posterior inferior tibiofibular ligament, the inferior transverse ligament, and the interosseous ligament).

The clinical examination of a patient with a suspected ankle fracture should include palpation of all structures surrounding the ankle. Swelling, tenderness, and ecchymosis can be present with injury to either ligament or bone, but their location may aid in differentiation. A neurovascular exam is mandatory. The patient may be able to bear weight on a stable fracture but rarely on an unstable fracture. If the injury is unstable, there is often clinical ankle deformity.

Radiographic evaluation should include an anteroposterior, lateral, and oblique view. The exact level of the fibula and medial malleolus fractures varies with the mechanism of injury. Rupture of the deltoid ligament must be suspected if there is a displaced fibula fracture, no medial malleolus fracture, but displacement of the talus from under the distal tibia (Figure 25.8).

The treatment goal for patients with an ankle fracture is to restore and maintain the tibiotalar relation with a congruous articular surface. If these goals are not achieved, post-traumatic arthritis may result. Stable injuries, such as nondisplaced isolated medial or lateral malleolar fractures requiring no reduction, should be immobilized in a bulky dressing, splinted to accommodate postinjury swelling, and the patient instructed to keep the leg elevated. Once swelling has subsided, a below-the-knee cast should be applied, with the foot and ankle in a neutral position and the patient allowed to bear weight. The cast should be removed after 6 weeks, and the patient started on physical therapy.

Unstable injuries or those associated with displacement of the talus require reduction. Talar shift from under the distal tibia, even slight, may cause joint incongruity and eventual degenerative changes (24). Unstable fractures treated nonoperatively require use of a long leg cast for 6 to 8 weeks and physical therapy thereafter. The primary indication for operative treatment is the inability to obtain or maintain an anatomic position of the talus, tibia, and fibula. Studies that compare closed versus open reduction are difficult to interpret because often the ankle treated surgically had a more severe injury.

Operative fixation of ankle fractures involves the use of plates and screws (Figure 25.9). The timing of surgery depends on soft-tissue swelling and the presence or absence of fracture blisters. At surgery, the skin should be handled atraumatically with little or no dissection of the subcutaneous tissues because the blood supply to the skin

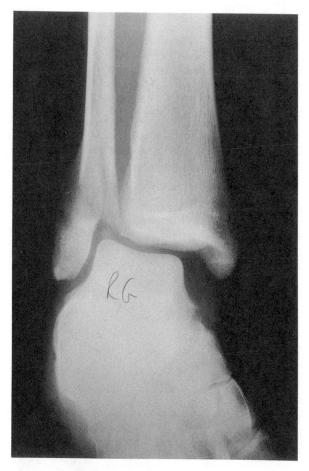

Fig. 25.8. An unstable ankle fracture with shift of the talus from under the distal tibia. There is a fibula fracture laterally and deltoid ligament rupture medially.

stable ankle fractures in patients older than age 60 (26). Only patients with a satisfactory fracture reduction were included. Patient satisfaction with regard to pain, deformity, and stability was significantly higher in the operative group. The study concluded that operative treatment was preferable to nonoperative treatment for displaced ankle fracture in the elderly.

Proximal Humerus Fractures

Proximal humerus fractures are common injuries in the elderly, reaching peaks of 112 and 439 fractures per 100,000 person-years in men and women, respectively, for

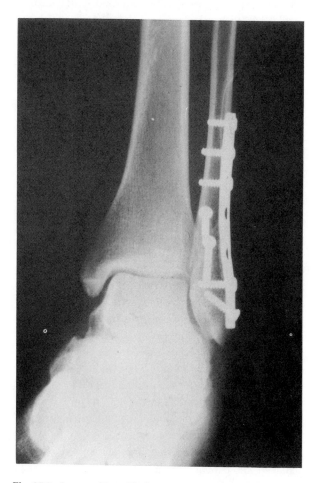

Fig. 25.9. An unstable ankle fracture stabilized laterally with plate and screws. With fibula stabilization, there is usually no need for deltoid ligament repair.

in this area is poor, and the possibility of skin slough and necrosis is high in the elderly patient.

Two recent studies reported the results of treatment of unstable ankle fractures in the elderly. Beauchamp et al compared operative and nonoperative treatment of displaced ankle fractures in patients older than age 50 (25). Operative management achieved better fracture position but was associated with a high complication rate in women, primarily because osteoporosis resulted in fixation failure. Two years or more after the injury, however, the study found no significant difference in function between the two groups. On the other hand, Ali et al compared nonoperative and operative treatment of un-the 80 years and older age groups. In people aged 75 and older, the proximal humerus is the third most common site of fracture and most often occurs after minimal trauma, such as a fall from a standing height.

The classification of proximal humerus fractures currently in use was described by Neer (27). Neer divided the proximal humerus into four anatomic segments: the humeral head (with the articular surface), the greater tuberosity, the lesser tuberosity, and the humeral shaft. He considered a segment significantly displaced (a separate part) if it were displaced at least 1 cm or angulated at least 45 degrees from its anatomic position. Thus, proximal humerus fractures can be described as minimally displaced (one-part), or as two-, three-, or four-part fractures. In addition, there are fracture-dislocations in which the humeral head is dislocated from the glenoid. Anterior fracture-dislocations are always associated with greater tuberosity displacement; posterior fracture-dislocations always have displacement of the lesser tuberosity. Articular surface fractures make up the final group in this classification.

The Neer classification is useful because it forms a basis for proximal humerus fracture treatment. Minimally displaced fractures account for 80 percent to 85 percent of all proximal humerus fractures and are usually stabilized by the intact surrounding soft tissue and periosteum. Early range of motion exercises can be instituted after a brief period of immobilization. There are four types of two-part fractures. Displaced anatomic neck fractures have a high risk of osteonecrosis; prosthetic replacement is usually indicated. Isolated lesser tuberosity displacements usually do not require operative treatment, unless the fragment contains a large portion of the articular surface or blocks internal rotation. Isolated greater tuberosity displaced fractures may be associated with longitudinal rotator cuff tears, and require open reduction, internal fixation, and rotator cuff repair (Figure 25.10).

Displaced surgical neck fractures can be impacted and angulated, separated, or comminuted. One can attempt a closed reduction, with the patient sedated or under anesthesia. If an acceptable and stable reduction is achieved, the patient's shoulder should be immobilized for about 3 weeks and followed by range-of-motion exercises. If the reduction is unacceptable or unstable, surgical intervention is necessary.

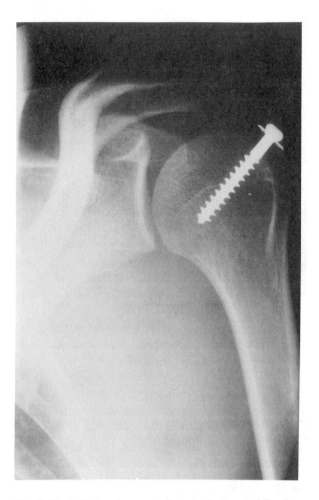

Fig. 25.10. A displaced greater tuberosity fracture stabilized with a screw and washer.

Reported results of closed treatment of three- and four-part fractures have generally been poor. Neer examined three- and four-part fractures and fracture-dislocations treated with closed reduction and reported satisfactory results in only 3 of 31 patients (28). These results were confirmed by others in both retrospective and prospective studies. The type of operative treatment in displaced three-part fractures depends on fracture comminution and bone quality: internal fixation for simpler fractures in patients with good bone quality, and prosthetic replacement for comminuted fractures in osteopenic bone.

Prosthetic replacement is recommended for four-part fractures and fracture-dislocations (Figure 25.11). The re-

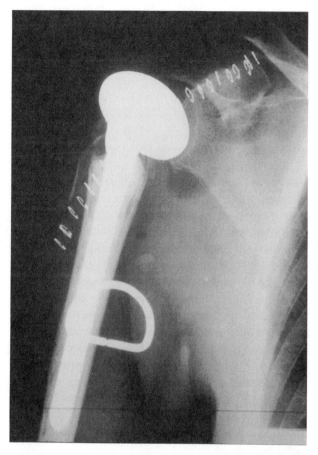

Fig. 25.11. A cemented hemiarthroplasty of the shoulder was used to treat a comminuted four-part proximal humerus fracture in a 75-year-old woman.

sults of open reduction and internal fixation in four-part fractures have been poor secondary to fixation failure or development of osteonecrosis. Other indications for hemiarthroplasty include chronic fracture problems such as painful malunion with articular incongruity, osteonecrosis with subchondral collapse and pain, and nonunion of surgical neck fractures with small, osteoporotic head fragments.

Regardless of the treatment method, elderly patients with displaced proximal humerus fractures require prolonged, supervised physical therapy to optimize functional result. Patients with minimally displaced fractures usually have a good result. Adequately reduced two-part fractures can also be expected to give good functional

results. Poor results may be related to inadequate rotator cuff repair or fracture nonunion or malunion. Results for prosthetic replacement are good in terms of pain relief, but functional results are variable. In general, younger male patients do better after prosthetic replacement. This may be related to better compliance with physical therapy.

Distal Radius Fractures

Distal radius fractures have long been recognized as common fractures in the elderly. Population-based studies of fracture frequency and distribution have shown that the rate of distal radius fracture increases dramatically with age, particularly for women (29). The age-related rate changes parallel similar increases seen with proximal femur and proximal humerus fractures and have been attributed to the effects of osteoporosis. Other factors, such as the increased tendency of the elderly to fall because of poor eyesight, impaired coordination, and decreased muscular strength, have been implicated.

Many classification systems have been described for distal radius fractures. Most are based on fracture geometry, degrees of displacement and comminution, and involvement of the radiocarpal or distal radioulnar joint (30). In general, stable fractures have minimal comminution and displacement. Unstable fractures have marked comminution, radial shortening (usually more than 10 mm), and angulation of the distal radial fragment. The more severe fractures are intra-articular, involving the radiocarpal and distal radioulnar joints. Comminuted, intra-articular fractures account for 15 percent to 25 percent of adult distal radius fractures and have a poorer prognosis.

Closed reduction and application of cast, splint, or both is the treatment of choice for most distal radius fractures. Most of these fractures can be successfully treated by closed means with manipulative fracture reduction performed under local or regional anesthesia. If closed reduction is successful, a short or long arm cast should be applied and maintained for 6 weeks, followed by physical therapy. Reduction of comminuted fractures can be difficult to maintain, and may require repeat manipulation at 1 to 2 weeks. If closed reduction is unsuccessful, operative intervention is necessary. Many operative methods have

325

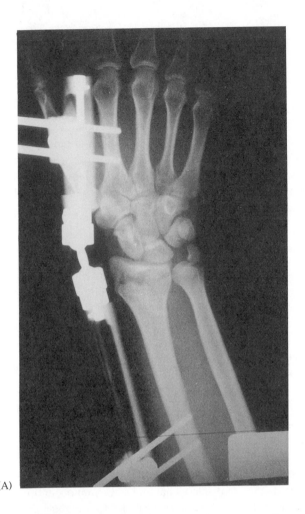

(A)

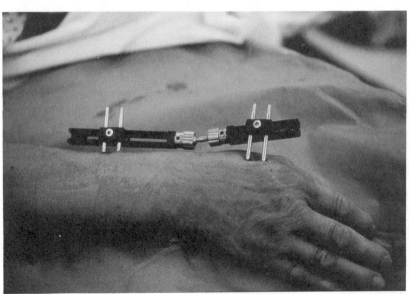

(B)

Fig. 25.12A,B. Radiograph (A) and clinical photograph (B) of a patient with a displaced distal radius fracture treated with an external fixator.

326

been advocated, including open reduction with internal fixation, external fixation, and percutaneous pins incorporated in a plaster cast (Figure 25.12A and B).

The results of distal radius fracture treatment vary and depend on the fracture type and the reduction achieved. Minimally displaced fractures do well with nonoperative treatment and one can expect a good functional result. The treatment results after displaced distal radius fracture are variable. Studying internal and external fixation techniques, authors have reported good to excellent results in 70 percent to 90 percent of patients with comminuted, unstable fractures (31). Surgeons who perform external skeletal fixation claim that this form of treatment achieves a more anatomic radial length than does conventional closed treatment, yet is less invasive than formal internal fixation.

Vertebral Compression Fractures

The vertebral compression fracture has become almost synonymous with osteoporosis (Figure 25.13). Jensen and co-workers estimated that 44 percent of women older than age 70 have vertebral compression fractures (32). Older patients with vertebral compression fractures have an increased risk for sustaining hip fractures and distal radius fractures.

Vertebral compression fractures often result from a relatively atraumatic event, such as rising up from a chair or lifting a light object. These fractures usually occur in the thoracolumbar spine, between T-8 and L-2. When vertebral collapse occurs over several segments, a thoracic kyphosis (hunchback deformity) results. Multiple compression fractures may also result in scoliosis; scoliosis in older women has been implicated as a marker for osteoporosis (33).

Vertebral compression fractures may present as incidental radiographic findings; however, most are associated with the acute onset of pain. The pain is usually located in the middle to lower thoracic spine or in the upper lumbar spine, but can be referred to the lumbosacral area. Neurological deficit is rare after these fractures. In fact, if a neurological deficit is present, one should consider metastatic disease, infection, or Paget's disease.

On physical examination, spinal range of motion is usu-

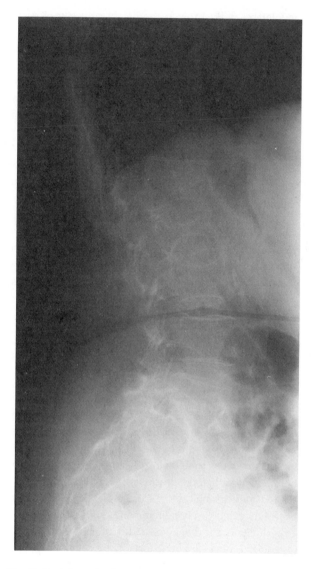

Fig. 25.13. A lateral radiograph of the lumbar spine in an 85-year-old woman with multiple vertebral compression fractures.

ally decreased; with multiple fractures, a kyphotic deformity may be present. Patient height may be affected by as much as 1 cm per vertebra if collapse is significant. Deep palpation and percussion usually elicits pain; however, there may not be significant tenderness over the spinous processes because the fracture is located anteriorly in the vertebral body.

Radiographic evaluation should include a standing AP

and lateral radiograph. If the height of a symptomatic vertebra is one-third less than the adjacent vertebrae, a fracture is present. The lateral radiograph may show an increased thoracic kyphosis. Fractures above T-6 are unusual, and other diagnoses should be considered. A bone scan can be helpful in differentiating old fractures from acute ones if uncertainty remains after clinical evaluation.

Nonoperative symptomatic management is the mainstay of treatment for vertebral compression fractures. A short length of bed rest may be necessary to alleviate acute symptoms, but prolonged bed rest should be avoided because it increases bone loss. Analgesics, muscle relaxants, and heat generally provide symptomatic relief. After the acute discomfort subsides, progressive ambulation should be instituted. A corset may prove helpful during the initial period of mobilization, but body casts and orthoses are not recommended because they are poorly tolerated. After a few weeks, a back exercise program should be started. Most fractures can be expected to heal uneventfully.

Pathologic Fractures

Pathologic fractures and impending pathologic fractures are common in the elderly. Primary tumor sites that commonly metastasize to bone include prostate, breast, lung, kidney, thyroid, and stomach. Common primary bone tumors not of bone cell origin are myeloma and lymphoma. Pathologic processes involving bone are described radiographically as osteolytic or osteoblastic. Osteolytic refers to a bone-removing process that appears as a hole in the bone on radiographic examination. Osteoblastic refers to a bone-forming process that appears as increased density on radiographic examination. Most metastases are either osteolytic or mixed osteolytic-osteoblastic. Pure osteoblastic lesions are seen in prostatic adenocarcinoma, Hodgkin's disease, and carcinoid tumor. Although these osteoblastic lesions are radiodense, they weaken the bone's structural integrity by disrupting the normal cortical anatomy and stress transmission. They predispose to pathologic fracture just slightly less often than osteolytic processes.

Bony metastases are most commonly found in the axial skeleton and proximal region of long bones. The proximal femur is by far the most commonly affected long bone.

Other frequent locations include the femoral shaft, acetabulum, and humerus.

Long-bone skeletal metastases usually present with pain, often before the lesion becomes radiographically detectable. Pain associated with a large lesion may represent microfracture and indicate an impending fracture. Hypercalcemia may be present as a result of rapid bone destruction by tumor. Hypercalcemia can be treated by calcium diuresis using saline, loop diuretics, or chemotherapeutic agents such as mithramycin, steroids, or neutral phosphates.

The treatment of pathologic fractures caused by bony metastases is palliative. Resection for cure is done for the rare, isolated metastasis of an occult primary thyroid or renal carcinoma. Primary treatment goals are pain relief and return to function of the involved extremity. Radiation therapy is often used to treat painful metastatic lesions. However, radiation produces a hyperemic response in the bone, maximal at 10 to 14 days, that actually weakens the bone and makes it more susceptible to pathologic fracture. Radiation also disrupts the normal fracture healing process by interrupting the radiosensitive chondrogenesis step required for callus formation (34).

Nonoperative management of pathologic fractures involves limb immobilization. In the upper extremity, this results in the loss of use of one arm; for the lower extremity, this often results in bed rest, traction, or both. Bed rest is poorly tolerated by elderly patients because they often suffer complications of recumbency such as pneumonia, thromboembolic problems, and decubitus ulcers. Two complications of prolonged bed rest specific to patients with metastatic disease are disseminated intravascular coagulopathy and malignant hypercalcemia. Fracture nonunion is common, particularly when radiotherapy is used to control pain and tumor progression. Therefore, operative stabilization of pathologic fractures of the lower extremities is recommended for any patient who is medically able to undergo surgery and whose life expectancy is greater than 1 month. Operative fixation is also recommended for upper extremity pathologic fractures to allow use of the extremity, which may be necessary for walking or ADLs.

Before the physician proceeds with operative intervention, a thorough medical and orthopedic evaluation of the patient is necessary to avoid iatrogenic fracture through an unrecognized pathologic lesion while positioning the anesthetized patient. A preoperative total body bone scan is needed with standard radiographs of any suspicious areas.

Prophylactic internal fixation of impending pathologic fractures remains controversial. Most orthopedists currently use the indications for prophylactic internal fixation outlined by Harrington: 1) a destructive lesion involving more than 50 percent of the cortical bone circumference, 2) a lytic lesion of the proximal femur larger than 2.5 cm, 3) a lesion of the proximal femur associated with avulsion of the lesser trochanter, and 4) a lesion of any size with persisting pain despite adequate radiotherapy (35). Prophylactic internal fixation of humeral metastases is generally not recommended because of the lower risk of fracture than with lower extremity metastases. However, in patients who bear weight through the humerus by using a walker, cane, or crutches, one should consider prophylactic internal fixation.

Results of operative fixation of pathologic fractures and impending pathologic fractures are good in terms of pain relief, patient mobilization, and return of function. Harrington, using internal fixation with adjunctive methylmethacrylate (bone cement) for pathologic fractures and impending fractures, reported that 85 percent of patients had satisfactory pain relief and 94 percent of patients who were ambulatory before fracture regained their ability to walk (36). These results have been supported by other authors studying function for both the upper and lower extremities.

References

1. Loder RT. The influence of diabetes mellitus on the healing of closed fractures. Clin Orthop 1988;232:210–216.
2. Johnson KD, Cadambi A, Seibert GB. Incidence of adult respiratory distress syndrome in patients with multiple skeletal injuries: effect of early operative stabilization of fractures. J Trauma 1985;25:375–377.
3. Bull JP. The injury severity score of road traffic casualties in relation to morbidity, time of death, hospital treatment time and disability. Accid Anal Prev 1975;7:249–255.
4. Salter RB, Dimonds DF, Malcolm BW, et al. The biological effect of continuous passive motion on the healing of full-thickness defects in articular cartilage. An experimental investigation in the rabbit. J Bone Joint Surg 1980;62A:1232–1251.
5. Brody JA. Commentary: prospects for an ageing population. Nature 1985;315:463–466.
6. Rizzo PF, Gould ES, Lyden JP, Asnis SE. Diagnosis of occult fractures about the hip. Magnetic resonance imaging compared with bone-scanning. J Bone Joint Surg 1993;75A:395–401.
7. Kenzora JE, McCarthy RE, Lowell JD, Sledge CB. Hip fracture mortality. Clin Orthop 1984;186:45–56.
8. Sexson SB, Lehner JT. Factors affecting hip fracture mortality. J Orthop Trauma 1988;1:298–305.
9. Davis FM, Woolner DF, Frampton C, et al. Prospective, multi-centre trial of mortality following general or spinal anaesthesia for hip fracture surgery in the elderly. Br J Anaesth 1987;59:1080–1088.
10. Valentin N, Lomholt B, Jensen JS, et al. Spinal or general anaesthesia for surgery of the fractured hip? Br J Anaesth 1986;58:284–291.
11. Magaziner J, Simonisick EM, Kashner TM, et al. Predictors of functional recovery one year following hospital discharge for hip fracture: a prospective study. J Gerontol 1990;45:101–107.
12. Miller CW. Survival and ambulation following hip fracture. J Bone Joint Surg 1978;60A:430–434.
13. Cummings SR, Phillips SL, Wheat ME, et al. Recovery of function after hip fracture. The role of social supports. J Am Geriatr Soc 1988;36:801–806.
14. Garden RS. Low-angle fixation in fractures of the femoral neck. J Bone Joint Surg 1961;43B:647–663.
15. Bentley G. Treatment of nondisplaced fractures of the femoral neck. Clin Orthop 1980;152:93–101.
16. Barnes R, Brown JT, Garden RS, Nicoll EA. Subcapital fractures of the femur. J Bone Joint Surg 1976;58B:2–24.
17. Drinker H, Murray WR. The universal proximal femoral endoprosthesis. A short-term comparison with conventional hemiarthroplasty. J Bone Joint Surg 1979;61A:1167–1174.
18. Greenough CG, Jones JR. Primary total hip replacements for displaced subcapital fracture of the femur. J Bone Joint Surg 1988;70B:639–643.
19. Evans EM. The treatment of trochanteric fractures of the femur. J Bone Joint Surg 1949;31B:190–203.
20. Mulholland RC, Gunn DR. Sliding screw plate fixation of intertrochanteric femoral fractures. J Trauma 1972;12:581–591.
21. Wolfgang GL, Bryant MH, O'Neill JP. Treatment of intertrochanteric fracture of the femur using sliding screw plate fixation. Clin Orthop 1982;163:148–158.
22. Wiss DA, Brien WW. Subtrochanteric fractures of the femur. Results of treatment by interlocking nailing. Clin Orthop 1992;283:231–236.
23. Mullaji AB, Thomas TL. Low-energy subtrochanteric fractures in elderly patients: results of fixation with the sliding hip screw plate. J Trauma 1993;34:56–61.
24. Ramsey PL, Hamilton W. Changes in tibiotalar area of contact caused by lateral talar shift. J Bone Joint Surg 1976;58A:356–357.
25. Beauchamp CG, Clay NR, Thexton PW. Displaced ankle frac-

tures in patients over 50 years of age. J Bone Joint Surg 1983;65B:329–332.

26. Ali MS, McLaren AN, Routholamin E, O'Connor BT. Ankle fractures in the elderly: nonoperative or operative treatment. J Orthop Trauma 1987;1:275–280.

27. Neer CS II. Displaced proximal humeral fractures: Part I. Classification and evaluation. J Bone Joint Surg 1970; 52A:1077–1089.

28. Neer CS II. Displaced proximal humeral fractures: Part II. Treatment of three-part and four-part displacement. J Bone Joint Surg 1970;52A:1090–1103.

29. Alffram P, Bauer G. Epidemiology of fractures of the forearm. J Bone Joint Surg 1962;44A:105–114.

30. Fryckman G. Fractures of the distal radius including sequelae. Acta Orthop Scand Suppl 1967;180:1–153.

31. Cooney WP, Linscheid RL, Dobyns JH. External pin fixation for unstable Colles' fractures. J Bone Joint Surg 1979; 61A:840–845.

32. Jensen GF, Christiansen C, Boesen J, et al. Epidemiology of post-menopausal spinal and long bone fractures. Clin Orthop 1982;166:75–81.

33. Healey JH, and Lane JM. Structural scoliosis in osteoporotic women. Clin Orthop 1985;95:216–223.

34. Bonarigo BC, Rubin P. Nonunion of pathologic fracture after radiation therapy. Radiology 1967;88:889–898.

35. Harrington KD. Impending pathologic fractures from metastatic malignancy: evaluation and management. American Association of Orthopedic Surgeons Instructional Course Lectures 1986;35:357–381.

36. Harrington KD, Sim FH, Enis JE, et al. Methylmethacrylate as an adjunct in internal fixation of pathologic fractures. J Bone Joint Surg 1976;58A:1047–1055.

Chapter 26

Urinary Incontinence and Catheters in the Elderly Male and Female

Richard R. Augspurger

As men draw near the common goal
Can anything be sadder
Than he who, master of his soul,
Is servant to his bladder?

Anonymous
The Speculum, Melbourne, 1938

As the proportion of Americans over the age of 65 increases, one of the greatest challenges for the U.S. health care system will be the management of urinary incontinence. Urinary incontinence can be defined as the involuntary loss of urine of sufficient amounts to cause psychologic, economic, or health problems. Urinary incontinence is a common major medical problem in the elderly.

It is estimated that 15 percent to 30 percent of community-dwelling elderly experience urinary incontinence. In 5 percent to 10 percent of these individuals, the incontinence is of sufficient quantity to soak their clothes and thus require pads (1,2). The institutionalized elderly have a much higher incidence (40% to 60%) of urinary incontinence (3).

The cost of management of the incontinent patient is significant. A highly conservative estimate of cost based on 1987 dollars is $10.3 billion (4). These costs include both the direct cost (diagnosis, treatment and rehabilitation) and indirect costs (lost productivity and time). The breakdown of cost is $3.3 billion in nursing homes and $7.0 billion in community care. The total figure exceeds the combined amount spent annually for coronary artery bypass surgery and renal dialysis (1).

The psychosocial impact of incontinence is great, not only for the patient, but also on the families and caregivers. Urinary incontinence can produce social isolation through the avoidance of contacts with family and friends. It contributes to depression, decreases self-esteem, and is yet another area in which the elderly expe-

rience loss of control over their lives. Significant stress is often placed on caregivers. Incontinence is a major factor contributing to the admission of the elderly to nursing homes.

The medical consequences of urinary incontinence are also important. Urinary incontinence can result in skin breakdown and decubitus ulcers, and the necessity of placing urethral catheters. Infection and stones associated with catheters and balanitis associated with external collecting devices all lead to increased morbidity and mortality in the elderly. The lowest estimates of cost for indwelling catheter management is $2.90 per day; however, there is a threefold increase in mortality and significant rise in morbidity with catheters, which increases the cost to $2,888 per year (3).

Urinary incontinence should not be accepted as a normal part of aging. Too often, this has been a neglected area of medical care in the United States. Until now, urologists have not shown much interest and have not participated in the evaluation and care of the elderly segment of the population (3). Elderly persons are likely to minimize or deny their urinary incontinence, and less than one-fifth of affected elderly individuals seek medical care. Those who seek help find that only one-third of physicians will institute even the most rudimentary evaluation (2).

Because urinary incontinence has a major impact on medical, psychologic, and economic well-being of the elderly, and on others, the First Clinical Practice Guidelines (developed by the U.S. Department of Health and Human Services) addressed the diagnosis and management of urinary incontinence. The guidelines were published in 1992 (6).

Two-thirds of the incontinent population can be significantly improved with appropriate treatment; the other one-third can benefit from palliative measures (1). It appears to be cost efficient to evaluate all incontinent elderly so that appropriate treatment can be instituted. Thus, better education of the elderly and the medical community that urinary incontinence is not a normal process of aging is needed. This chapter addresses the pathophysiology, diagnosis, and management of urinary incontinence in the elderly as one step in the educational process.

Anatomy and Neurourology

The bladder is a smooth muscle storage organ of the urinary tract. Urine produced in the kidneys passes down the ureters to enter the bladder. As urine enters the bladder, the bladder muscle relaxes to accommodate 450 to 500 ml of urine. The urine does not leak out of the urethra because of the sphincter mechanisms. There are two sphincters: the internal sphincter, which is smooth muscle, and the external sphincter, which is skeletal and smooth muscle (Figure 26.1). At capacity, voiding occurs voluntarily. The detrusor contracts, the proximal sphincter funnels open, and the distal sphincter relaxes, allowing urine to pass from the bladder.

The normal processes of urine storage and voiding are under the control of the central nervous system (CNS). Several theories of neurologic control have been proposed (7). The main reflex center for the bladder (Figure 26.2) appears to be located in the mesencephalic-reticular formation, the brain stem micturition center (BSMC). A less dominant center, the spinal cord micturition center (SCMC), also plays a role.

Sensory, proprioceptive fibers arising in the bladder pass by way of the pelvic nerves and the posterior columns to the BSMC. Motor fibers originating in the BSMC travel via the reticulospinal tracts to the detrusor motor nucleus in the intermediolateral grey cell column of the sacral spinal cord (S-2 to S-4). From the detrusor motor nucleus, parasympathetic fibers traverse the pelvic nerves, synapse in the pelvic ganglia, and innervate the detrusor muscle. The neurotransmitter is the cholinergic agent acetylcholine (Figure 26.3). Suprasacral interruption of the pathway releases the SCMC from inhibition. Thus, a low-capacity bladder with unsustained, uninhibited contractions of the detrusor muscle develops.

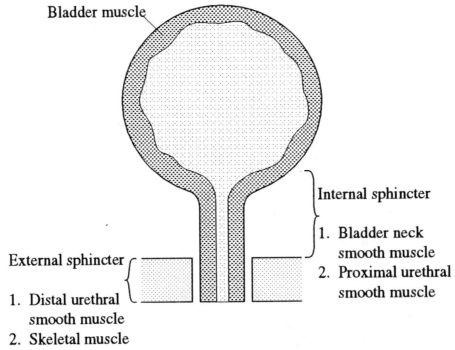

Fig. 26.1. Schematic diagram of the bladder and urinary sphincter. The internal sphincter consists of bladder neck smooth muscle and the proximal urethral smooth muscle. The external sphincter consists of the distal urethral smooth muscle and skeletal, striate, external sphincter.

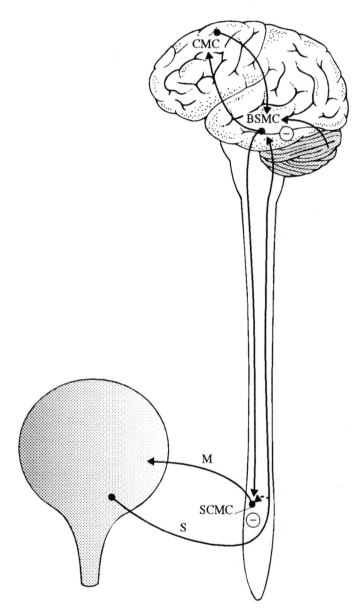

Fig. 26.2. The reflex arcs associated with micturition—motor neuron (M); sensory neuron (S); cortical micturition center (CMC); brain stem micturition center (BSMC); sacral cord micturition center (SCMC).

Supraspinal areas modulate the detrusor reflex through inputs on the BSMC (see Figure 26.2). The detrusor motor area is located in the prefrontal portion. Fibers pass via the internal capsule to synapse at BSMC. Other CNS areas, the thalmus, basal ganglia, and cerebellum, have input into the BSMC. The overall effect is one of inhibition

of the detrusor reflex; therefore, interruption of these pathways results in loss of voluntary control over the detrusor reflex. This is characterized by a sustained, uninhibited detrusor contraction.

Sympathetic innervation of the bladder (see Figure 26.3) originates in the thoracolumbar spinal cord (T-10 to

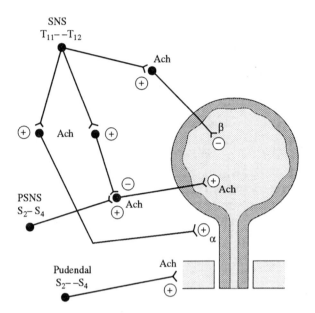

Fig. 26.3. Diagram of the dual innervation of the bladder by the sympathetic nervous system (SNS) and the parasympathetic nervous system (PSNS). The neurotransmitters, acetycholine (Ach), norephinephrine (α, β) are indicated; $-$ = inhibitory effect; $+$ = stimulating effect.

L-2). The efferent fibers pass via the hypogastric nerve and synapse in the inferior mesenteric, hypogastric, and pelvic ganglia. The dome of the bladder is innervated primarily by beta-adrenergic fibers, with the bladder neck innervated by alpha-adrenergic fibers. Stimulation of the beta-adrenergic fiber results in detrusor muscle relaxation; stimulation of alpha-adrenergic fibers causes contraction and tightening of the bladder neck.

Thus, storage of urine is a sympathetic response that occurs with tightening of the bladder neck and relaxation of the dome during alpha- and beta-adrenergic stimulation. Voiding is under parasympathetic control, with contraction of the detrusor and relaxation of the sphincters. An understanding of the neuropharmacologic principles aids in the understanding of the side effects of medicines and the selection of the appropriate medicines used for the treatment of urinary incontinence.

The striate (skeletal) external sphincter is under voluntary control. It is more highly developed in males than in females. Motor fibers arise in the pudendal motor area in the medial aspect of the central sulcus. Fibers pass through the internal capsule and corticospinal tract to synapse on the pudendal motor nucleus in the ventral grey of the sacral spinal cord (see Figure 26.3). Motor fibers pass by way of the pudendal nerve to the external striate sphincter. Suprasacral interruption of this pathway produces spasticity in the striate external sphincter.

There is a reciprocal innervation between the striate external sphincter and the detrusor muscle. Thus, a detrusor contraction produces reflex relaxation to the striate external sphincter and vice versa. To maintain a sustained, coordinated detrusor contraction and relaxation of the external sphincter, an intact spinal cord to the level of the BSMC is required. Any lesion below the BSMC can produce dyscoordination between the dome of the bladder and sphincter, and result in detrusor-sphincter dyssynergia.

Pathophysiology

With the normal aging process, changes occur in the lower urinary tract. Although there is a lack of definitive data, it appears that with aging, the ability to postpone voiding, compliance of the urethra and bladder, and the length and closing pressure of the urethra decrease. In contrast, uninhibited detrusor contractions and residual urine increase. The elderly, unlike younger individuals, excrete two-thirds of daily ingested fluid after 8 P.M. or 9 P.M. This, along with the higher incidence of sleep disorders in elderly persons, leads to nocturia, even in the normal elderly (1).

In themselves, these age-related changes do not cause urinary incontinence; they are also present in normal, continent elderly patients. They do, however, reduce the ability of the lower urinary tract to withstand further insults. The elderly have a constricted physiologic reserve. Thus, when disease is present, the weakest link in the system reflects the symptoms of presentation. Often this link is the urinary tract, and urinary incontinence or retention are the presenting symptoms (8).

From these changes, two important principles arise: 1) incontinence in the elderly is more likely to be caused by a precipitant outside the lower urinary tract, and 2) reversal of the precipitant frequently is sufficient to restore continence, even if any underlying urologic abnormality is not corrected (1).

Urinary incontinence occurs when the intravesical pressure exceeds the bladder outlet resistance. Any condition in which the bladder, bladder outlet, or both fail to function results in incontinence. Urinary incontinence in the elderly can be divided into two categories—transient and established.

The causes of transient incontinence can be recalled by the mnemonic DIAPPERS (Table 26.1). (1) Because transient incontinence occurs commonly, and correcting the underlying condition will, in most cases, restore continence, transient causes of incontinence need to be addressed in the evaluation of all incontinent elderly patients.

One major area of transient incontinence is the iatrogenic-induced incontinence secondary to pharmacotherapy. Many elderly patients are taking one or more medications, many of which have significant side effects on the bladder (Table 26.2) (9). A thorough drug history for the patient must be obtained. Many elderly also take over-the-counter cold preparations that contain alpha-adrenergic agents. The drugs may, therefore, cause bladder neck contraction and failure to empty the bladder. Often, the elderly do not volunteer a history of over-the-counter drug use because these medicines have not been prescribed by their physicians.

Table 26.1. Common Causes of Transient Incontinence.

Mnemonic Designation	Cause
D	Delirium or confusional state
I	Infection, urinary (symptomatic)
A	Atrophic urethritis or vaginitis
P	Pharmaceuticals
	Sedative hypnotics, especially long-acting agents
	Loop diuretics
	Anticholinergic agents
	Antipsychotics
	Antidepressants
	Antihistamines
	Antiparkinsonian medications
	Antiarrhythmics
	Opiates
	Alpha-adrenergic agonists and antagonists
	Calcium channel blockers
P	Psychologic disorders, especially depression
E	Endocrine disorders (e.g., hypercalcemia, hyperglycemia)
R	Restricted mobility
S	Stool impaction

SOURCE: Reproduced by permission from Resnick NM, Yalla SV. Aging and its effect on the bladder. Semin Urol 1987;5:82.

Table 26.2. Drugs and Their Effects on the Bladder.

Drug Class	Effect
Diuretics	Increased urinary output
Anticholinergics	Decreased bladder contractility; urinary retention
Sedatives/hypnotics	Some decreased attention to bladder cues
Antipsychotics	
Antidepressants	
Antiarrhythmics	
Alpha-adrenergic agents	
Agonists	
Antiallergy medications	Bladder neck closure; urinary retention
Cold medications	
Antagonists	Relaxation of bladder neck; incontinence
Antihypertensives	
Beta blockers	Bladder neck closure; urinary retention
Calcium channel blockers	Decreased bladder contractility; urinary retention
Narcotics	Decreased bladder contractility; urinary retention
Nonsteroidal anti-inflammatory agents	Decreased bladder contractility; urinary retention

Established incontinence, can also result from a failure to empty the bladder or a failure to store urine. Failure to empty the bladder can be a result of decreased bladder contractility, increased bladder outlet resistance (obstruction), or both. This combination results in urinary retention and overflow incontinence and accounts for 7 percent to 11 percent of total cause. In the male patient, this most commonly results from prostate hypertrophy (see Chapter 46) or urethral strictures. In the female, diabetes with resultant diabetic neuropathy and flaccid neurogenic bladder, is the more common cause. The diagnosis is made by the findings of an elevated residual urine, large bladder capacity (>900 ml), and decreased sensation of bladder filling.

Failure to store urine can have various etiologies. Functionally, it results from increased bladder pressure, decreased bladder outlet resistance, or a combination of both. The two main areas are stress incontinence and detrusor instability.

Stress urinary incontinence accounts for 3 percent to 10 percent of cause in females, but it is rare in males. Stress incontinence is characterized by leakage of urine associated with the sudden increase in intra-abdominal pressure, as happens with coughing, sneezing, or laughing. Diagnosis is made by objective demonstration of hypermobility of the bladder neck and urethra, associated leakage of urine, and stoppage of the incontinence with elevation of the bladder neck.

Detrusor instability is the most common cause of urinary incontinence and accounts for 40 percent to 60 percent of total cause. The etiology of abnormal bladder contractions is often unclear. They can occur with normal aging, in the presence of bladder outlet obstruction, or with loss of cortical inhibition of the voiding reflex commonly associated with parkinsonism, cerebrovascular accident, and dementia. Diagnosis is made by demonstrating an involuntary rise in bladder pressure greater than 15 cm of water on cystometry. This is often associated with a smaller than normal bladder capacity. A subset of this group is an uninhibited detrusor contraction but with impaired contractility (DHIC) (1). The condition is defined as uncontrolled detrusor contraction with impaired bladder emptying, leaving over one-third of bladder contents as residual urine. This diagnosis is likely, provided bladder outlet obstruction, spinal cord lesion,

detrusor-sphincter dyssynergia, fecal impaction, bladder suppressants, and volitional inhibition of the detrusor have been excluded. DHIC can be difficult to diagnose as it is the great mimic of other types of incontinence. In males, the symptoms of bladder incontinence secondary to prostate hypertrophy are similar to DHIC. In females, DHIC mimics stress incontinence. It is believed to be the most common cause of incontinence in the institutionalized elderly (1).

Evaluation

The elderly incontinent patient is not often provided the same thorough evaluation given younger individuals, not only because the elderly patient minimizes his or her symptoms but also because there appears to be a lack of awareness in the medical community of the significance of incontinence in the elderly. Because incontinence is not a consequence of aging and because many causes are readily treatable, a large number of the incontinent elderly would benefit from a basic urologic evaluation. An extensive, costly urodynamic assessment is not necessary in most cases, but the evaluation needs to be comprehensive enough to determine whether readily reversible causes of incontinence exist. Several authors have proposed screening protocols that allow identification of 70 percent to 90 percent of the treatable causes of incontinence (5,9,10). In general, this can be accomplished by using the approach outlined in Table 26.3. Another practical approach to the evaluation of urinary incontinence can be found in the U.S. Department of Health and Human Sciences Clinical Practice Guidelines (6).

In taking the patient's history, the physician must allow adequate time to gather information from the patient's family and caregivers. The key elements in the history are

Table 26.3. Screening Protocol for Evaluation of Urinary Incontinence.

Take thorough medical history
Perform physical examination
Evaluate urine analysis, including culture and
  sensitivity
Determine postvoid residual urine
Perform cystometric studies using water or CO_2
Observe for stress incontinence

related to potentially reversible conditions. Irritative symptoms of dysuria, frequency, and urgency suggest possible urinary tract infection or atrophic vaginitis or urethritis. Leakage with cough, sneezing, or activity has a high correlation with the findings of stress incontinence on physical examination. Urinary frequency must be evaluated with regard to both volume and time. A voiding diary in which time, fluid intake, urinary output, and episodes of incontinence are recorded for 24 to 48 hours is often helpful. High-volume frequency can be caused by diuretics or diabetic glucosuria; low-volume frequency, especially when associated with urgency, is often related to an unstable bladder. However, one-third of the elderly with detrusor instability give no history of urgency.

Nocturia without daytime frequency relates to the inability of elderly to excrete urine during the day. Bedwetting, voiding frequent small amounts, and incontinence may suggest overflow incontinence or urinary retention. Decreased flow rates, a complaint primarily of males, can be caused by bladder outlet obstruction or poor bladder contractility and must be differentiated.

Other important aspects of the patient's history include 1) identifying all prescription and over-the-counter medicines that the patient has at home; 2) assessing surgical history, including gynecologic, urologic, colorectal, and neurosurgical procedures; 3) determining whether neurologic disease exists, such as stroke, Parkinson's disease, or spinal stenosis; and 4) assessing changes in mobility and limitations in activities. In the cognitively impaired patient, much information will need to be provided by the caregiver.

During the history-taking and physical examination, attention should be directed to the patient's mental capacity, psychologic and behavioral disturbances, and mobility and manual dexterity. The lower abdomen should be palpated for bladder distention. Pelvic and rectal examinations are needed to evaluate for fecal impaction, pelvic masses, presence of pelvic prolapse, and size and consistency of the prostate. A limited urologic-neurologic examination should evaluate sensation in the perineal area (S-2 to S-4 distribution), anal sphincter tone, and presence of the bulbocavernosus and anal reflexes.

The minimal laboratory tests performed should be a urine analysis and urine culture and sensitivity. At times, plasma electrolytes, blood urea nitrogen (BUN), and serum creatinine, along with a fasting blood sugar evaluation, can be helpful. An intravenous pyelogram (IVP) and voiding cystogram should be done only when indicated by the initial evaluation.

The final steps in the evaluation are catheterization for measurement of postvoid residual urine, and a simple cystometrogram, using water or CO_2. Castleden and colleagues believe that the treatment of elderly incontinent patients without cystometry is analogous to treating a patient with cardiac arrhythmia without an electrocardiogram (ECG) (11). The cystometrogram gives the volume-pressure status of the bladder. This can be easily performed at the patient's bedside with a catheter tip syringe and sterile water for irrigation. The plunger is removed from the syringe, and the syringe is connected to the catheter. With the syringe held 15 cm above the pubis, water is instilled in 50-ml increments and the pressure is recorded. (The patient is instructed not to urinate.) The first sensations of bladder filling and fullness are noted. Any sudden rise in bladder pressure or leakage around the catheter that the patient cannot inhibit confirms the diagnosis of detrusor instability (Figure 26.4). The cystometrogram documents uninhibited detrusor contractions and gives information about bladder compliance, sensation, and, in some settings, capacity.

At the end of the test, the bladder is filled and the catheter is removed. Observation for leakage during coughing and sneezing when the patient is in the supine position and the upright positions tests for stress incontinence. The patient then is asked to urinate so that the force and caliber of the stream can be observed, flow rates can be determined, and voided volume can be recorded.

These tests can identify 70 percent to 90 percent of the causes of incontinence so that appropriate therapy can be instituted. Cystoscopy should be done when indicated for hematuria, suspected bladder tumor, interstitial cystitis, or persistent urinary tract infections. Sophisticated urodynamic evaluations (e.g., urethral pressure profiles, multichemical studies with fluoroscopy) should be reserved for patients who are at unacceptable risk for empiric therapy, fail to respond to therapy, have complicating comorbidity, or who require surgical intervention. Because of the high incidence of DHIC and because there is medical capability to safely perform complex urodynamic testing on frail elderly persons, male patients

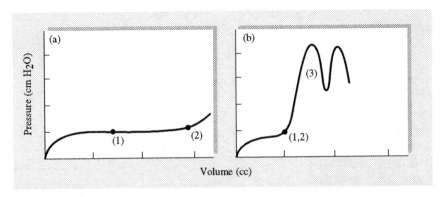

Fig. 26.4. A. A normal cystometrogram. First sensation to urinate (1); sensation of bladder fullness (2). B. Abnormal cystometrogram demonstrating detrusor instability with uninhibited detrusor contraction and a low-volume bladder (3) with leakage around the catheter.

with poor urine flow rate, women with stress incontinence only (those who would be treated surgically), or patients with equivocal diagnoses should have comprehensive evaluation (12).

Treatment

Therapy for urinary incontinence depends on the cause of the condition. Algorithms for the management of the various types of incontinence can be found in the Clinical Practice Guidelines (6). An example of the management algorithm for the nursing home frail, elderly patient who has incontinence is shown in Figure 26.5. First, the causes of transient incontinence should be identified because they are often easily reversed. Delirium and underlying medical causes, such as congestive heart failure or urinary tract infection, should be recognized and treated. Urinary tract infections should be treated with antibiotics, although the relationship between asymptomatic bacteriuria and incontinence has not been clearly established. Atrophic vaginitis and urethritis should be treated with topical or oral estrogens. Drug-induced incontinence is modified by stopping or changing drug therapy. Restricted mobility can be helped by changes in environment, such as the use of a bedpan or bedside commode and clothing that allows easier access with elastic bands in place of buttons. Treatment for fecal impaction should be instituted.

General methods such as behavior therapy, timed voiding, bladder retraining, prompted voiding, electrical stimulation, and biofeedback are available (see discussion of the treatment of detrusor instability). The use of an indwelling catheter should be avoided, if possible.

The elderly are particularly susceptible to the side effects of uropharmacologic therapy, thus limiting its usefulness. Therefore, initial doses should be about one-half the recommended dosage. In the elderly, the effectiveness of some treatment regimens has not been proved through controlled clinical trials.

As noted, failure to empty the bladder can result from poor bladder contractility or from the presence of bladder outlet obstruction. By far the most common cause of urinary retention in males is bladder outlet obstruction secondary to prostate hypertrophy see Chapter 46).

In patients who have a noncontractible bladder without outlet obstruction, pharmacotherapy can be directed at decreasing bladder outlet resistance. The lack of clinical efficacy of the oral cholinergic agonist bethanechol (Duvoid) has been demonstrated in several clinical studies that have measured changes in cystometrics and decrease in residual urines (13). An oral dose of 200 mg is required in a denervated bladder to produce the same effect as a subcutaneous dose of 5 mg (13).

Bladder outlet resistance can be decreased through alpha-adrenergic blockade. The most common alpha blocker used today is terazosin (Hytrin). The starting

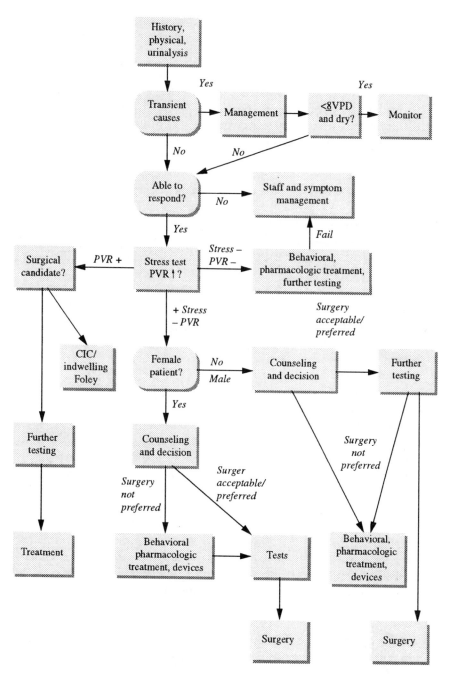

Fig. 26.5. Algorithm for the management of incontinence in nursing home patients or frail, elderly patients. (Reproduced from Urinary Incontinence Guideline Panel. Urinary incontinence in adults: quick reference guide for clinicians. AHCPR Pub. No. 92-0041. Rockville, MD: Agency for Health Care Policy and Research, Public Health Service, US Department of Health and Human Services, 1992.)

dose is 2 mg at bedtime slowly increased to 10 mg, if needed. Two other drugs used are phenoxybenzamine (Dibenzyline) 10 mg/day, which can be increased to a maximum dose of 60 mg/day, and prazosin (Minipress) 2 to 3 mg/day, which can be increased to a maximum dose of 20 mg/day in divided doses. Several side effects of these drugs may occur in the elderly, especially orthostatic hypotension, reflex tachycardia, nasal congestion, and sedation. Therefore, caution should be used with these drugs.

The mainstay of treatment of urinary retention is clean, intermittent self-catheterization. If patients have good use of their hands (this can be tested by the patient's ability to write his or her name), they can usually perform intermittent self-catheterization. The technique is well known (Table 26.4). A minimum schedule of three to four times a day must be maintained, and catheterized volume of 350 to 500 ml is the maximal acceptable amount. If larger volumes are obtained, the frequency of the catheterization should be increased. For cognitively impaired persons, the caregiver should be trained to assist, and a schedule that will provide continence, prevent infection, and avoid taxing the caregiver should be developed. Other forms of therapy for special situations are available (Table 26.5).

Stress urinary incontinence is the failure to store bladder urine and can be treated several ways. If atrophic vaginitis is present, oral or local estrogens can help restore the normal urethral mucosa and enhance the alpha-adrenergic effect. For mild stress incontinence, alpha-adrenergic stimulants, such as ephedrine 25 to 50 mg four times a day, phenylpropanolamine 50 mg three times a day, or imipramine (Tofranil) 10 to 25 mg three to four times a day, are effective in some cases. However, most patients with moderate or severe stress incontinence do not show a complete response, and incontinence persists.

Table 26.4. Technique of Clean, Intermittent Catheterization.

Wash catheter and hands with soap and water
Clean meatus with soap and water
Apply water-soluble lubricant to catheter tip
Insert catheter until urine returns
Empty bladder completely
Remove catheter and wash and rinse with water; dry
Store catheter until next use

Table 26.5. Treatment of Failure of Bladder to Empty.

Increase intravesical pressure/bladder contractility
　External compression with Credé or Valsalva maneuver
　Pharmacotherapy
　　Increase contractility with cholinergic medications (e.g., bethanechol); prostaglandins
　　Block inhibition with alpha-adrenergic antagonists
　Electrical stimulation
　　Direct-bladder pacemaker
　　Spinal cord-nerve roots
　Reduction cystoplasty
Decrease bladder outlet resistance
　Surgical treatment of anatomic obstruction (transurethral prostate resection; repair of urethral sphincter)
　Smooth muscle sphincter
　　Pharmacotherapy with alpha-adrenergic antagonists; beta-adrenergic agonists
　　Surgery (incision of bladder neck; Y-V plasty of bladder neck)
　Striate sphincter
　　Pharmacotherapy with skeletal muscle relaxants; alpha-adrenergic antagonists
　　Biofeedback
　　Surgery (urethral dilation; external sphincterotomy; pudendal nerve interruption)
Circumvention
　Intermittent self-catheterization
　Continuous catheterization
　Urinary diversion

Biofeedback training has been employed using vaginal cones to monitor the effectiveness of Kegel exercises and is a useful tool in teaching the exercises. Long-term results are variable. Electrical stimulation has not been sufficiently studied to determine its efficacy in the management of stress incontinence (6).

The mainstay of treatment is the bladder neck suspension procedure. This can be performed as an open abdominal surgical procedure (the Marshall-Marchetti-Krantz operation), vaginal endoscopy with minimal invasion (the Raz procedure), or laparoscopically. If the patient is not a candidate for surgery, pessaries (doughnut-shaped devices that are inserted into the vagina to elevate the bladder neck and compress the urethra against the pubis) can be employed with moderate success.

Detrusor instability, which accounts for 40 percent to 60 percent of cases of incontinence, can be approached multimodally. One of the cornerstones of treatment is behavioral therapy, which includes bladder retraining, biofeedback, habit training, timed voidings, electrical stimulation, and prompted voidings.

For the cognitively impaired patient, good success can be achieved with timed or prompted voiding. With timed voiding, the patient keeps a diary to document the time interval between voidings and incontinence episodes. Once the interval is established, a toileting schedule is developed. The patient is taken to the toilet on a fixed voiding schedule. With habit training, the time interval is initially fixed and then adjusted during treatment. With prompted voiding, the patient is asked about the need to urinate at fixed time intervals. When he or she gives a positive response, the patient is taken to the bathroom. Cognitively impaired patients will show a response to treatment, but once treatment is stopped, most of these patients revert to pretreatment levels of incontinence (14).

The ambulatory individual with higher cognitive levels can be treated through bladder retraining (bladder drill) and biofeedback, with or without the use of pharmacotherapy. Success rates approach 75 percent to 90 percent (15,16). In bladder retraining, the patient urinates on a mandatory, predetermined schedule at the risk of incontinence. The intervals between voiding are then gradually increased. In a second option, the patient can urinate on a self-determined schedule. Initially, the patient keeps a voiding diary for volume voided and for time interval. The patient then tries to extend the interval by 30 minutes or by a volume of 30 to 60 ml. At the end of 1 month, the voiding diary is rechecked to determine progress.

During biofeedback, certain parameters are monitored, such as changes in cystometry or sphincter electromyography (EMG) recordings. The patient then attempts to inhibit the abnormal detrusor contraction or relax the external sphincter with visual or auditory stimuli as a guide to success. Electrical stimulation of pelvic muscles, pelvic viscera, or the nerve supply is used to manage detrusor instability. Stimulation of pelvic floor muscles can produce reflex inhibition of the detrusor muscle. Stimulation of the afferent nerves facilitates storage by modifying bladder sensation. Adverse reactions are primarily pain and discomfort. The effectiveness of electrical stimulation is not known, however, and further research is needed (6).

Mainstay of treatment for bladder instability has been pharmacotherapy (17). Drugs that inhibit the detrusor contraction have been used most frequently. Anticholinergic medicines such as propantheline bromide (Probanthine) in doses of 15 to 30 mg four times a day; oxybutynin chloride (Ditropan), which also has a direct smooth muscle relaxant effect, in doses of 5 mg three to four times a day; and atropine in doses of 0.4 mg four times a day, exert their effect by blocking the acetylcholine-induced stimulation of the postganglionic, parasympathetic cholinergic receptor sites on the bladder smooth muscles. Other agents that act directly on bladder smooth muscle by producing relaxation are dicyclomine hydrochloride (Bentyl) 20 mg three to four times a day, and flavoxate hydrochloride (Urispas) 100 to 200 mg three to four times a day.

Tricyclic antidepressants such as imipramine (Tofranil) and nortriptyline (Pamelar) act through both a weak antimuscarinic effect and a strong, direct inhibiting effect on bladder smooth muscle. The initial dose is 25 mg at bedtime, which can be increased to a maximum of 150 mg. Tricyclic antidepressants may also be given in divided doses. (This author has found that antidepressants are the most useful drug category for treatment of detrusor instability in the elderly.)

Once incontinence is controlled, the use of behavioral modification and pharmacotherapy may allow slow tapering of medications. Most bladder regimens take 6 to 12 months to achieve long-lasting results. If detrusor contractions persist, other more invasive procedures can be used (Table 26.6).

When sphincter incompetence is present (e.g., postprostatectomy incontinence in men, neurologic lesions affecting the urethra and periurethral muscles, or nonfunctional fibrotic urethra in females), alpha-adrenergic medicines (see the treatment of stress incontinence) can be used. Limited success is usually achieved. Another option is implantation of an artificial urinary sphincter. This device is made up of three components: an occlusive cuff that can be placed around the urethra, a pressure balloon reservoir that controls the pressure in the cuff, and a pump that is placed in the labia or scrotum that controls the device (Figure 26.6). The artificial urinary sphincter has a success rate of 75 percent to 90 percent in selected elderly patients. The present reliability is much improved over that of earlier models.

341

Table 26.6. Treatment of Failure of Bladder to Store Urine.

Decrease bladder contractility
  Pharmacotherapy
    Anticholinergic medications
    Smooth muscle relaxants
  Surgery
    Hydrodilatation
    Nerve interruption (subarachnoid block; selective sacral
      rhizotomy; peripheral bladder denervation; cystolysis)
    Augmentation cystoplasty
Increase sphincter resistance
  Pharmacotherapy
    Alpha-adrenergic agonist
    Beta-adrenergic antagonists
    Antihistamines
  Surgery
  Urethral or urethrovesical suspension
  Reconstruction of proximal urethra
  Urethral plication
  Periurethral injection of bulking agents
  Urethral compression
  Artificial urinary sphincter
Circumvention
  Urinary diversion

Injection of periurethral bulking agents such as polyref, collagen or fat are being studied. Periurethral injection of collagen (Contigen) is currently approved by the Food and Drug Administration for sphincteric insufficiency, (type III stress incontinence in females), post-prostatectomy incontinence in males, and certain neurologic incontinence. The initial success at 1 year approaches 70 percent to 80 percent of patients improved or cured (18). The injection can be accomplished under local anesthesia as an outpatient procedure.

Despite the many modalities available, many elderly individuals remain incontinent. Palliative procedures can be very helpful to prevent scalding of the skin and skin breakdown, protect clothing and bedding, and prevent odor. Such procedures include the use of absorbent pads, pants, undergarments, and, for male patients, external collecting devices. As a last resort, an indwelling Foley catheter can be used. However, use of an indwelling Foley catheter should be discouraged, even though this is the "simple solution." Lower urinary tract infections are common in chronically ill elderly patients who are maintained on catheter drainage. The elderly also experience more

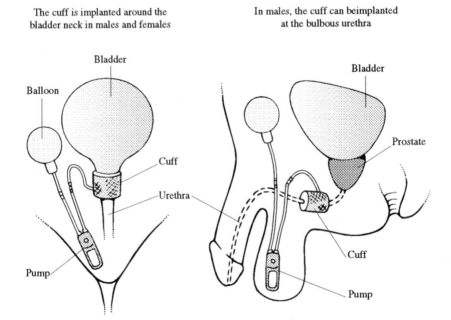

The cuff is implanted around the bladder neck in males and females

In males, the cuff can beimplanted at the bulbous urethra

Fig. 26.6. The American Medical Systems artificial urinary sphincter.

severe catheter-associated complications (19). Late complications include stones, sepsis, and in males, epididymitis, periurethral abscess and fistula formation, and stricture formation.

With catheterization, bacteriuria will develop in 50 percent of patients within 2 weeks and in 100 percent of patients within 6 weeks. Trauma to the bladder mucosa allows the bacteria access to the bladder wall, and infection begins. Any agent that increases trauma to the bladder mucosa, such as changes of the catheter, detrusor spasms, catheter blockage with overdistention of the bladder, irrigations, and stones, will promote infection (20).

Management of the indwelling catheter aims at minimizing infection. The use of prophylactic antibiotics, bladder irrigations, bladder instillations, and frequent catheter changes have all been unsuccessful in eliminating bacteriuria, encrustation, and obstruction. These measures are worth abandoning, because they lead to increased trauma to the mucosa and a potentially higher incidence of infection. More effective measures include making sure the patient takes in adequate fluid, avoiding catheter manipulation, and exchanging the catheter when urine flow is decreased or when infection is suspected (20).

The physician, caregiver, and patients are often in need of information and resource aids. Several organizations have been established to promote the treatment of urinary incontinence:

HIP (Help for Incontinent People), Inc.
P.O. Box 544
Union, SC 29379

The Simon Foundation
P.O. Box 815
Wilmette, IL 60091

Continence Restored, Inc.
785 Park Ave.
New York, NY 10021

Conclusions

Through better education, both the elderly population and the medical community should accept that inconti-

nence is not an inevitable consequence of aging. More incontinent elderly patients should be encouraged to seek evaluation so that appropriate treatment can be instituted. The physician must keep in mind that incontinence in the elderly is often caused by precipitants outside the urinary tract and that by correcting the precipitant, incontinence can be reduced (1). With appropriate treatment, urinary incontinence can be controlled, the quality of life of the elderly can be improved, and health care expenditures for the condition can be decreased.

References

1. Resnick NM, Yalla SV. Aging and its effect on the bladder. Semin Urol 1987;5:82.
2. Diokno AC, Brock BM, Herzogar AT, et al. Prevalence of urologic symptoms of the noninstitutionalized elderly. J Urol 1985;133:179A. Abstract.
3. Ouslander JG, Kane RL. The costs of urinary incontinence in nursing homes. Med Care 1984;22:69.
4. Hu TW. Impact of urinary incontinence on health care costs. J Am Geriatr Soc 1990;38:292–295.
5. Rohner TJ, Iquo JF. Urinary incontinence in the elderly. AUA Update Series 1986;2(26):1.
6. Urinary Incontinence Guidelines Panel. Urinary incontinence in adults: clinical practice guidelines. Washington, DC: US Department of Health and Human Services, 1992.
7. Wein AJ, Raezer DM. Physiology of micturition. In: Krane RJ, Siroky MB, eds. Clinical neuro-urology. Boston: Little, Brown, 1979:1.
8. DuBeau CE, Resnick NM. Evaluation of the causes and severity of geriatric incontinence: A critical appraisal. Urol Clin North Am 1991;18:243–256.
9. Badlani GH, Smith AD. Pharmacotherapy of voiding dysfunction in the elderly. Semin Urol 1987;5:120.
10. Ouslander JG, Staskin S, Orzeck S, et al. Diagnostic tests for geriatric incontinence. World J Urol 1986;4:16.
11. Castleden CM, Duffin HM, Aswen NH. Clinical and urodynamic studies in 100 elderly incontinent patients. BMJ 1981;282:1103.
12. Resnick NM. Geriatric urinary incontinence. AUA Update Series 1992;2(9):66–71.
13. Wein AJ. Drug treatment of voiding dysfunction. Part I. Evaluation of drugs: treatment of emptying failure. AUA Update Series 1988;7(14):106.
14. Schnelle JF. Management of geriatric incontinence in nursing homes. J Appl Behav Anal 1983;16:235.
15. Jarvis GJ. A controlled trial of bladder drill and drug therapy in the management of detrusor instability. Br J Urol 1981;53:565.
16. Cardozo L, Stanton SL, Hafner S, et al. Biofeedback in the treatment of detrusor instability. Br J Urol 1978;50:250.
17. Wein AJ. Drug treatment of voiding dysfunction. Part II.

Drug treatment of storage failure. AUA Update Series 1988;7(15):114.

18. Overview of treatment of urinary incontinence with contigen Bard collagen implant. CR Bard 1993.

19. Warren JW, Muncie HL Jr, Bergquist EJ, et al. Sequelae and management of urinary infections in the patient requiring chronic catheterization. J Urol 1981;125:1.

20. Seiler WO, Stahelin HB. Practical management of catheter associated UTIs. Geriatrics 1988;43:43.

Chapter 27
Pressure Ulcers

Matthew Rydberg and Dennis W. Jahnigen

Old age and sickness bring out the essential characteristics of a man.

Felix Frankfurter

Pressure ulcers are a significant problem among debilitated elderly persons. They are a source of extensive morbidity and contribute to health care costs. Although usually requiring hospitalization or nursing home care, pressure ulcers may develop among home-bound patients or require ongoing treatment after patients are discharged from the hospital. The chief factor for treatment and prevention is relief of pressure. Randomized controlled trials in the treatment of pressure ulcers are few, but new data indicating effective regimens for treatment of the pressure ulcer and associated complications are emerging. The terms "bedsore," "decubitus ulcer," "decubitus," "pressure sore" and "pressure ulcer" are used interchangeably, but the preferred terms are "pressure sore" or "pressure ulcer" because they emphasize the primary pathophysiologic mechanism of development.

Epidemiology

Prevalence and incidence of pressure ulcers vary according to the population studied (Table 27.1). Community studies of elderly patients indicate an incidence of pressure ulcers of approximately 2 percent during a 10-year span; most occur in bed-bound patients. The incidence of newly developing ulcers in acute care hospitals ranges from 1 percent to 3 percent for each hospital episode (1). Because nursing home patients have greater risk factors and comorbidity, rates of pressure ulcer development are 20 percent during a 2-year period. The rates are highest for bed- or chair-bound patients (1). Pressure sores are markers of underlying debility. They are associated with

an increased morbidity and mortality and are expensive and labor-intensive to treat.

Costs of Care

Added treatment costs per patient for pressure ulcers are estimated at $400 to $40,000, depending on the stage of the sores (2). A recent study revealed daily nursing home treatment using saline gauze clean technique costs $25.90/day for nursing time and supply costs. (3). Specialized beds also increase costs. More difficult to quantitate are costs of associated complications such as pain, infection, and psychological factors of depression and humiliation. Medicare hospital data from 1987 indicated that for 122,000 patients discharged with a primary or secondary diagnosis of pressure ulcer, the total hospital charges were $1.5 billion.

Morbidity and Mortality

Pressure ulcers are markers for serious underlying illnesses and have associated morbidity and mortality. In nursing home patients who develop new pressure sores, mortality increases by 60 percent to 80 percent. The 2-year mortality for those who develop ulcers exceeds 50 percent (4). It is estimated that 60,000 persons die annually from ulcer-related complications such as sepsis and osteomyelitis. Nearly all stage I and stage II ulcers heal, but only half of stage III or stage IV ulcers heal, even in the best therapeutic environments (5).

Pathophysiology

Four physical factors have been implicated in the development of pressure ulcers: pressure, friction, shearing forces, and moisture. Pressure is the single most important etiology for the development of pressure ulcers. Cap-

Table 27.1. Prevalence and Incidence of Pressure Ulcers.

Population	Prevalence (%)	Incidence (%)
Acute care hospitals		
All patients	3–11	1–3 during hospitalization
Bed- and chair-bound	28	8 during hospitalization
Nursing homes	3–11	12 during 6-month length of stay
Community	0.04–0.09 (all ages)	1.8 among 55- to 75-year-old patients during 10-year period

SOURCES: Allman RM. Epidemiology of pressure sores in different populations. Decubitus 1989;2:30–33. Goode P, Allman R. The prevention and management of pressure ulcers. Med Clin North Am 1989;73:1511–1522.

illary filling pressure is approximately 32 mm Hg. Subcutaneous tissues, including muscle, appear more susceptible to the effects of pressure than does surface tissue. Continuous pressure of 70 mm Hg for 2 hours can result in ischemia to subcutaneous tissues. With prolonged pressure, tissue ischemia progresses to vessel leak, hemorrhage, and interstitial edema caused by the release of lytic enzymes. Fibrin deposition and microvascular thrombosis follow. Eventually epidermal and dermal necrosis result. The point of maximum damage is often deep, directly over a bony prominence; therefore, pressure sores should be thought of as a pyramid with only the tip evident at the skin and a potentially large base of damage in the subcutaneous tissues. More than 90 percent of all pressure ulcers occur over the lower body, with the sacrum, the trochanters, the iliac crest, the ischial tuberosities, and the lateral malleoli representing the most common locations.

Shear forces are generated when skin is fixed to an exterior surface, but the subcutaneous tissues are subjected to lateral forces. The net result is a stretch of the subcutaneous tissues, which are less elastic than the epidermis and dermis. Penetrating capillaries appear to be more susceptible to shear forces. Patients in a semi-Fowler's position often exert high shear force on the capillaries overlying the sacrum because the skin adheres to the bed surface and gravity pulls the pelvis downward.

Abrading skin across a surface can result in heat and friction that can denude the stratum corneum. Transfers can involve inadvertently dragging a patient across the bed or bed sheet, a common cause of this type of injury.

Moisture causes tissue maceration and acts as a chemical irritant to open skin. Diarrhea with ileal contents can cause rapid irritation of skin. Fecal incontinence can also result in superinfection or bacterial contamination of an open ulcer. Fecal incontinence appears to be an independent risk factor delaying healing of pressure sores (6,7).

Normal aging is associated with decreased proliferation of epidermal tissue, degeneration of small dermal vessels, and decreased cutaneous pain and pressure sensation (8). Associated with the decreased sensation are fewer spontaneous movements while the patient sleeps. In one study, 90 percent of geriatric patients with fewer than 20 nocturnal spontaneous movements developed pressure ulcers (9).

Several nutritional risk factors for development of pressure ulcers have been identified, such as low levels of ascorbic acid and zinc and hypoalbuminemia. Among hospital patients whose serum albumin falls by 1 gm/dL, the odds ratio for developing a pressure ulcer is 5.1 (10).

Clinical Manifestations

Although the diagnosis of a pressure ulcer is often obvious, for atypical ulcers a differential diagnosis should be considered, such as stasis or ischemic ulcers, vasculitic processes, malignancies, fungal infections, and other dermatologic disorders.

Assessment

Unfortunately, several systems of pressure sore classification are used, which causes confusion in communicating with other health professionals and in evaluating clinical trials and interventions. The 1989 National Pressure Ulcer Advisory Panel Consensus Conference devised a classification system that is easy to use and has become the most accepted classification system (11) (Table 27.2).

Accurate stage assessment as well as indicating the number, size, and location of ulcers is crucial to the evaluation of subsequent treatments. While assessing the stage, the physician should keep in mind the potential for more

Table 27.2. Staging of Pressure Ulcers.

Stage	Involvement
I	Nonblanching erythema of intact skin
II	Partial-thickness skin loss involving epidermis or dermis
III	Full-thickness skin loss involving subcutaneous tissue that may extend to, but not through, the underlying fascia
IV	Full-thickness lesions extended through the fascia into underlying muscle or bone

Table 27.3. Risk Factors for Development of Pressure Ulcers.

Condition	Odds Ratio	Confidence Interval	Reference
Ambulation difficulty	3.3	2.0–5.3	22
Urinary incontinence	2.5	1.6–4.0	22
Diabetes mellitus	1.7	1.2–2.5	22
Feeding dependence	2.2	1.5–5.31	22
Male gender	1.9	1.2–3.6	22
Fecal incontinence	3.2	1.1–8.8	10
Fall in serum albumin of 1 gm/DL	3.0	1.3–7.1	10

SOURCE: Allman RM, Laprade CA, Noel LB. Pressure sores among hospitalized patients. Ann Intern Med 1986;105:337–342 and Brandeis G, Ooi W, Hossain M, et al. A longitudinal study of risk factors associated with the formation of pressure ulcers in nursing homes. J Am Geriatr Soc 1994;Apr;42(4):388–393.

extensive deep tissue involvement than is apparent on the skin surface. Even if treated promptly, an ulcer may rapidly worsen for a few days as a result of the initial injury.

Risk Factors

A number of risk factors for pressure sores have been identified (Table 27.3). Methods of risk assessment have been developed to identify patients who may benefit from special preventive measures. These scales are primarily useful in hospital or inpatient settings, but may also be useful for outpatients. The Norton scale (12) (Table 27.4) assesses the patient's general physical condition, level of consciousness, activity, mobility, and continence. However, this scale has been criticized for vague terminology and lack of assessment of nutritional status. The Braden scale (13), developed to overcome the drawbacks of the Norton scale, has six categories: sensory perception, activity, mobility, moisture, nutrition, and friction and shear. The first five categories contain ratings scales of 1 to 4, and the sixth category is rated from 1 to 3. At a rating of 16, the scale had 100 percent sensitivity and 90 percent specificity for predicting the presence of pressure sores (13). The Braden assessment tool may replace the Norton scale because it provides more accurate assessment of risks and thus enables the physician to take more concerted preventive measures.

Complications of Pressure Ulcers

Pressure ulcers are associated with many complications, including cellulitis, osteomyelitis, pyarthrosis, and sepsis. In one study, the mortality from sepsis associated with pressure sores approaches 100 percent. (14) Treatment

Table 27.4. Norton Scale for Risk Assessment of Developing Pressure Ulcers.

Category	Rating	
General physical condition	4	Good
	3	Fair
	2	Poor
	1	Very poor
Mental state	4	Alert
	3	Apathetic
	2	Confused
	1	Stuporous
Activity	4	Ambulant
	3	Ambulant with help
	2	Chair-bound
	1	Confined to bed
Mobility	4	Full
	3	Slightly limited
	2	Very limited
	1	Immobile
Incontinence	4	Not incontinent
	3	Occasionally incontinent
	2	Usually incontinent of urine
	1	Incontinent of urine and feces

SOURCE: Norton D. An investigation of geriatric nursing problems in hospital. 2nd ed. Edinburgh: Churchill Livingstone, 1975:193–238.

requires broad-spectrum, intravenous antibiotics. In addition to infectious complications, sinus tract formation, heterotopic calcification, and amyloid can occur from pressure ulcers.

Diagnostic Approach

Accurate diagnosis and assessment of the stage of the pressure sore are essential first steps. Comorbid and contributing factors should also be evaluated. If the patient's underlying condition is terminal, healing is not likely and attention should be turned to comfort, pain relief, and prevention of further ulcers. If the patient's underlying condition is reversible, complete resolution of the ulcer is a reasonable objective. Outpatients with ulcers require the physician to determine whether adequate resources exist for home treatment. Capable caregivers are essential because pressure ulcers require frequent repositioning of the patient and, often, several changes of dressings per day.

Prevention and Treatment

Pressure Relief

Without pressure relief, healing will not occur. The patient's mobility should be improved and sedation avoided if possible. An order should be written prohibiting the position that places the ulcer under pressure (e.g., a patient with a sacral ulcer should be prohibited from being in the supine position). Rotating patients in 30-degree oblique positions at intervals of 2 hours or less will keep all 5 common ulcer sites (sacrum, trochanters, ischial; tuberosities, heel and lateral malleoli) pressure-free. Heel and elbow protectors, sheepskins, chair cushions, foam mattress overlays, and air mattresses all reduce pressure and are economical. However, overlays do not reliably reduce pressure below capillary filling pressures of 32 mm Hg, and should not take the place of repositioning every 2 hours.

Doughnut cushions increase ischemia to the center of the cushion-free area and can worsen ulcers or delay healing and should be avoided. Massage of pressure ulcers should also be avoided because it adds mechanical trauma to an open wound.

Attention should be directed to avoiding friction and shear forces. The semi-Fowler position should not be used because it produces high shear over the sacrum. Repositioning should be done with draw sheets, and transfers should avoid dragging the patient across any surfaces. Counterpositioning of the patient's lower extremities can prevent shear forces. Sheepskins and other fabric overlays can also help prevent external tissue fixation to mattresses.

Low-air-loss and air-fluidized beds are becoming more widely used in hospital and nursing home settings. Air-fluidized beds contain ceramic beads covered by a polyester sheet. Warm air is forced through the beads, which gives them the characteristics of fluid. Pressures are below capillary filling pressures. Low-air-loss beds have multiple sections that are inflated with air. Because they are fitted to a regular hospital bed frame, they allow elevation of the head of the bed and adjustment to bed height. Air-fluidized beds do not provide these measures.

Both types of beds have been involved in a small number of controlled, randomized trials studying healing techniques. Air-fluidized therapy in an acute care hospital was found to be beneficial for ulcers of 7.8 cm^2 or larger but not for smaller ulcers (15). Follow-up, however, was only for a median of 13 days (range, 4 to 77 days) and only 13 percent of patients healed their largest ulcer during the study. In this study, the bed cost was $80/day. Low-air-loss beds were recently compared with conventional techniques and were found to produce a faster rate of healing: 9.5 mm^2/day versus 2.5 mm^2/day (7). The overall healing rate was not statistically significant between the two groups, although the trend favored the low-air-loss beds. Nine of the 41 conventionally treated patients progressed or worsened, but none of those treated with specialized beds progressed. The air-fluidized beds and low-air-loss beds have not been directly compared in a randomized trial. Given the significant cost of these beds, it seems reasonable to consider their use for patients with larger complicated ulcers or for patients who progress on adequate conventional treatment. It is unlikely that the beds will become routinely used in the outpatient or home setting.

Moisture Control

Perineal moisture can be an initiating factor in ulcer development. If skin is intact, absorbent adult diapers with frequent changes are adequate. For skin disruption, a temporary bladder catheter may be necessary while aggressive treatment takes place. Fecal incontinence appears to be worse than urinary incontinence (6,7), probably because of increased alkalinity of effluent and infection from coliform bacteria. Constipating medicines, rectal tubes, or rectal collecting pouches may be necessary. As always, reversible causes for incontinence should be looked for and treated.

Debridement of the Wound Surface

Adequate re-epithelialization requires a wound free of necrotic tissue and eschar. Several methods of debridement exist—enzymatic, wet-to-dry gauze dressings, and surgery.

Topical cleansing agents should be used as an adjunct to debridement to clean grossly decontaminated wounds. Topical cleansing agents must be used with care. Full-strength sodium hypochlorite solution, hydrogen peroxide, and povidone iodine, although antimicrobial, are toxic to fibroblasts and epithelial tissues. However, concentrations of 0.1% povidone iodine and 0.5% sodium hypochlorite that retain antimicrobial action but are not toxic to granulation tissue (16). Normal saline can be effective as a cleansing agent. Injection of saline under pressure can be done easily at the patient's bedside or in the office by syringe injection through a pliable 20-gauge IV catheter, or with use of a dental irrigator. Iodine and other red-colored antiseptics should be avoided because they hurt; stain surrounding tissues, which makes inflammation difficult to discern; and impair epithelialization. Antacids, cornstarch, molasses, and honey should not be used on open wounds.

Enzymatic debridement with collagenase, fibrinolysin, deoxyribonuclease or streptokinase generally requires two or three applications per day and is not effective with hard eschar. Results appear within 2 weeks. Saline wet-to-damp dressings are the most appropriate form of debridement. As the gauze dries it adheres to tissue; when removed, it pulls off surface necrotic tissue and bacteria. Unfortunately, new epithelial tissue is also removed. Wet-to-dry dressing changes can be quite painful to the patient and thus should be moistened before removal. Premedication of the patient with narcotics may be necessary.

Stage III and stage IV ulcers should be evaluated by a surgeon because they will likely require surgical debridement under general anesthesia. In some patients, a myocutaneous flap can be indicated, but poor overall prognosis often precludes this choice.

Heel ulcers are frequently far worse than they appear on the skin surface. A deep purple blister can be a sign of very severe subcutaneous tissue damage. Heel ulcers can be very difficult to heal because of associated vascular insufficiency; extremity amputation is often the unfortunate outcome. For patients with lower extremity ulcers, noninvasive assessment of the vascular supply can help determine likelihood of healing. Debridement should be stopped when granulation tissue is present.

Treatment of Infection

All pressure ulcers have bacteria on the wound surface, and routine cultures are unnecessary and can be misleading. Worsening ulcers may indicate infection because infected wounds do not re-epithelialize or granulate. The microorganisms involved are often polymicrobial with gram-negative rods, such as *Peudomonas aeruginosa*, *Proteus mirabilis*, *Escherichia coli*, or gram-positive cocci, such as *Staphylococcus aureus*, and anaerobes. The use of saline dressings in usually effective in eliminating surface infections. Topical antibiotics can be helpful in reducing cell counts but are associated with the development of resistant organisms. Topical metronidazole appears to be helpful when clinical suspicion of anaerobic infection (foul smelling and purulent ulcers) exists. When a clean base of granulation tissue is present, topical antimicrobials should be stopped.

Systemic antibiotics are necessary only for complications of pressure ulcers such as cellulitis, osteomyelitis, or sepsis. These organisms should be covered by an empiric antibiotic regimen until cultures confirm the etiologic bacteria and sensitivities, at which point the regimen can be adjusted appropriately. A tetanus booster is advisable if the patient's immunization status is not known or the patient has not had a booster for 10 years.

Physiologic Dressing

Once the wound is adequately debrided, a warm moist environment will stimulate wound healing (Table 27.5). Physiologic dressings help prevent wound recontamination but usually disrupt the fragile epithelial layer each time they are changed. Gauze dressings kept continuously moist with saline or various occlusive dressings should be used. Each dressing has advantages, disadvantages, and indications for use. Few direct com-

Table 27.5. Physiologic Dressings.

Modality	Indication	Considerations
Saline continuously moist gauze	Stage II ulcers* Stage III ulcers Stage IV ulcers	Can be done as clean technique; must keep continuously moist to prevent debriding healthy epithelial tissue; time consuming
Hydrocolloids	Low to moderate exudate wounds	Often leak and are messy; poor retention; possible maceration; may damage periwound tissue; higher materials cost than saline gauze
Polyurethane films	Superficial wounds with little or no exudate	Difficult to apply; poor exudate retention nonabsorbent; easily disrupted and removed from wound site
Biodressings and hydrogels		Nonadhesive; desiccate easily; generally not recommended for pressure ulcers

*Efficacy not confirmed by research (see text).

parison studies of these dressings exist. Saline-moist dressings require change every 8 hours, which allows frequent visualization of the wound. They are primarily indicated for stage III and stage IV ulcers and also for any ulcer in which there is a question of nonviable tissue.

Whether to use hydrocolloids or saline gauze dressings for stage II ulcers is not resolved by research literature. A recent study from Iowa revealed equal effectiveness for hydrocolloids and clean technique saline gauze dressings. Using the material cost and labor costs for the nursing home studied, the researchers calculated an overall daily cost of $15.90 for hydrocolloids and $25.31 for saline (3). The overall healing rates were comparable. Since costs vary from one region to another, and from one institution to another, cost analysis must be individualized.

Hydrocolloids are easy to apply, have good retention on low to moderate exudative wounds, are absorbent, and are water and gas impermeable. They require changing only every 3 days. However, once disrupted, they require replacement because the seal is lost. Hydrocolloids interact with the wound exudate to form a gel that promotes epithelialization and granulation. Hydrocolloids should not be used on stage III or IV ulcers or when nonviable tissue may exist in ulcers. Polyurethane films are occasionally useful for superficial wounds because they are transparent, thereby allowing visualization of the wound. However, they are nonabsorbent, which makes them useless on exudative wounds, and they adhere poorly.

Unfortunately, few randomized studies have compared different modalities. Gorse found hydrocolloid dressings more effective than wet-to-dry dressings (17). However, once the ulcer is adequately debrided, wet-to-dry dressings with any agent will retard re-epithelialization because removal of the dry gauze results in epithelial tissue damage. Xakellis (3) found that hydrocolloids and continually moist saline gauze dressings are equally effective, with healing rates of over 80 percent for each treatment group. Currently the size, stage and location, and cost differences dictate which modality is preferred.

Surgical treatments for larger ulcers include split thickness skin grafts, remodeling bony prominences, and myocutaneous flaps. The efficacy of surgery compared with nonsurgical modalities in the treatment of pressure ulcers is not concretely established. However, aging itself is not a contraindication to surgery.

Other Considerations and Newer Interventions

Careful attention should be paid to any comorbid medical conditions of the patient. Hypoxia, anemia, hyperglycemia, and peripheral edema should be corrected. Because patients with pressure ulcers are often malnourished, nutritional status should be assessed and optimized. The pressure ulcer itself can contribute to hypoproteinemia by leakage of huge amounts of protein-rich exudate. Protein and total calorie intake must be adequate for new tissue growth and may require supplementation either orally or parenterally. Supplemental water-soluble vitamins are advisable. Patients with femoral neck fractures who have low leucocyte vitamin C levels have nearly 50 percent risk of developing a pressure sore, according to one study (18). As a result, supplementation with 500mg vitamin C taken twice a day is recommended (19). Zinc is essential for normal healing but, in excessive amounts, impairs healing (20). Serum zinc levels should be assayed an supplements prescribed as necessary.

Several new modalities are expected to play larger roles in the future. Use of growth factors is entering human trials because animal studies have indicated promising results. The first randomized controlled trial was reported by Robson and colleagues (21). In this trial, basic fibroblast growth factor (bFGF) was compared with placebo. The number of patients evaluated was small, but the researchers found a trend in favor of bFGF for healing of pressure ulcers. However, the effect was not statistically different. There were no adverse effects from bFGF and no antibody formations against bFGF. Biopsies revealed increased numbers of fibroblasts, which indicated histologic confirmation of bFGF efficacy. As more experience is gained with the optimal use of growth factors, larger trials will be conducted to determine efficacy. Until efficacy is determined, growth factors will remain experimental and should not be routinely used.

The use of electricity to stimulate wound healing has been known, although poorly understood, since the mid-1900s. Wood and colleagues recently reported their data on pulsed, low-intensity, direct current for chronic (present for more than 5 weeks without improvement) stage II and stage III ulcers (22). This study demonstrated dramatic healing rates with treatments three times a week. The authors hypothesize that microamperage, direct current treatments increase the calcium influx into pressure sores. Calcium stimulates fibroblasts and keratinocytes and leads to improved revascularization and epithelialization. Growth factor receptors were also upgraded. Because this treatment is painless and simple to perform, it may find more widespread use.

Monitoring the Condition of the Ulcer

Skilled observation of the pressure ulcer in any setting is critical to successful healing. The person performing the daily dressing changes must be able to detect any worsening of the wound. Weekly evaluations by a skilled nursing home nurse or the physcian is essential. For stage III and stage IV ulcers, a surgeon with interest in pressure ulcers should be part of the team from the beginning because such wounds often require surgical debridement or may be amenable to surgical closure (23).

Ulcers that fail to heal should prompt re-evaluation of the treatment process. Unrelieved pressure, local infection, or worsening underlying condition are three major causes of nonhealing ulcers. Ulcers that are worsening with home care mandate hospitalization and inpatient care.

Summary

An awareness of risk factors, precipitating events, and treatment principles provides a rational approach to prevention and treatment of pressure ulcers. Vigilance is required, because even 1 day of inadequate treatment can greatly delay healing. Although pressure ulcers are a marker of poor medical condition, many ulcers can be healed. Their prevention and management is a team effort involving patient, nurse, primary care physician, and surgeon.

References

1. Allman RM. Epidemiology of pressure sores in different populations. Decubitus 1989;2:30–33.
2. Ebbs P. The economics of pressure ulcer prevention. Decubitus 1989;2:32–38.
3. Xakellis G, Chrischilles EA. Hydrocolloid versus saline gauze dressings in treating pressure ulcers: a cost effectiveness analysis. *Arch Phys Med Rehabil* 1992;73:463–469.
4. Brandeis G, Morris J, Nash D, Lipschitz L. The epidemiology and natural history of pressure ulcers in elderly nursing home residents. JAMA 1990;264:2905–2909.
5. Bennett RG, Ballawtoni MF, Ouslander JG. Air-fluidized bed treatment of nursing home patients with pressure sores. J Am Geriatr Soc 1989;37:235–242.
6. Goode P, Allman R. The prevention and management of pressure ulcers. Med Clin North Am 1989;73:1511–1524.
7. Ferrell BA, Osterweil D, Christenson P. A randomized trial of low-air-loss beds for treatment of pressure ulcers. JAMA 1993;269:494–497.
8. Levine J, Simpson M, McDonald RJ. Pressure sores: a plan for primary care prevention. Geriatrics 1989;44:75–90.
9. Exton-Smith AN, Sherwin RW. The prevention of pressure sores: Significance of spontaneous bodily movements. Lancet 1961;1:1124–1126.
10. Allman RM, Laprade CA, Noel LB. Pressure sores among hospitalized patients. *Ann Intern Med* 1986;105:337–342.
11. National Pressure Ulcer Advisory Panel: Pressure ulcer prevalence, cost and risk assessment: consensus development conference statement. Decubitus 1989;2:24–28.
12. Norton D. An investigation of geriatric nursing problems in hospital. 2nd ed. Edinburgh: Churchill Livingstone 1975: 193–238.
13. Bergstrom N, Braden B, Laguzza A, Holman V. The Braden scale for predicting pressure sore risk. Nurs Res 1987;36:205–210.
14. Galpin JE, Chao AW, Boyer AS, et al. Sepsis associated with decubitus ulcers. Am J Med 1976;61:346–350.
15. Allman RM, Walker J, Hart M, Laprade C, Noel L, Smith C. Air fluidized beds or conventional therapy for pressure sores. Ann Intern Med 1987;107:641–648.

16. Lineaweaver W, Howard R, Sovey D, et al. Topical antimicrobial toxicity. Arch Surg 1985;120:267.

17. Gorse G, Messner R. Improved pressure sore healing with hydrocolloid dressings. *Arch Dermatol* 1987;123:766–771.

18. Goode HF, Burns E, Walker B. Vitamin C depletion and pressure sores in elderly persons with femoral neck fracture. *BMJ J* 1992;305:925–927.

19. Taylor TV, Rimmer S, Day B, Butcher J, Dymock I. Ascorbic Acid Supplementation in the Treatment of Pressure Sores. *Lancet* 1974;2:544–546.

20. Norris JR, Reynolds RE. The effect of oral zinc sulfate therapy on Decubitus Ulcers. *J Am Geriatr Soc* 1971;19:793–797.

21. Robson MC, Phillips CG, Lawrence WT, et al. The safety and effect of topically applied recombinant basic fibroblast

22. Wood JM, Evans PEZD, Schallreuter KU, et al. A multicenter study on the use of pulsed low intensity direct current for healing chronic stage II and stage III decubitus ulcers. Arch Dermatol 1993;Aug;129(8):999–1009.

23. Brandeis G, Ooi W, Hossain M, et al. A longitudinal study of risk factors associated with the formation of pressure ulcers in nursing homes. J Am Geriatr Soc 1994;Apr;42(4):388–393.

Suggested Readings

Agency for Health Care Policy and Research. Preventing pressure ulcers: Clinical practice guideline. AHCPR No. 92-0047.

Agency for Health Care Policy and Research. Treatment of pressure ulcers: Clinical practice guideline. AHCPR No. 95-00652.

Allmon RM. Pressure ulcers among the elderly. N Engl J Med 1989;320:850–853.

Hagisawa S, Ferguson-Pell MW, Palmieri VR, Cochran GV. Pressure sores: a biomechanical test for early detection of tissue damage. Arch Phys med Rehab 1988;69:668–671.

Moody B, Fanale J, Thompson M, et al. Impact of staff education of pressure sore development in elderly hospitalized patients. Arch Intern Med 1988;148:2241–2243.

Mulder GD, LaPan M. Decubitus ulcers: update on new approaches to treatment. Geriatrics 1988;43:37–50.

Perez, ED. Pressure ulcers updated guidelines for treatment and prevention. Geriatrics 1993;48:39–44.

Reuler JB, Cooney TG. The pressure sore: pathophysiology and principles of management. Ann Int Med 1981;94:661–666.

Seiler W, Stahelin H. Decubitus ulcers: preventive techniques for the elderly patient. Geriatrics 1985;40:53–60.

Seiler W, Stahelin H. Decubitus ulcers: treatment through five therapeutic principles. Geriatrics 1985;40:32–40.

Shea JO. Pressure sores classification and management. Clin Orthop 1975;112:89–100.

Yarkony GM, Kirk PM, Roth EJ, et al. Classification of pressure ulcers. Arch Dermatol 1990;126:1218–1219.

Yoshikawa TT. Pneumonia, UTI, and decubiti in the nursing home: optimal management. Geriatrics 1989;44:32–34, 37–40.

Chapter 28
Hearing Loss and Tinnitus

Jerome G. Alpiner and Vivyenne Roche

There is no medicine against old age.

Nigerian Proverb

The ability to communicate is essential for participation in everyday living activities. When a person cannot hear adequately, communication breakdowns occur: for example, in participating in a religious service, in understanding a physician's comments and recommendations, in misunderstanding family members and friends (which precipitates friction), and in "bluffing" through the day's activities. If one considers all the hearing one does from arising in the morning until retiring at night, it becomes apparent that quality of life heavily depends on hearing. Millions of persons have a reduced quality of life because of hearing loss (Table 28.1).

Age-Related Hearing Loss

It is important to consider the changes that occur with aging which affect hearing loss. These changes can be considered anatomically in terms of the outer, middle, and inner ear (Figure 28.1).

Outer Ear
Loss of skin elasticity and muscle tone contribute to the physical enlargement of the outer ear. Loss of elasticity can lead to difficulties with audiological testing and placement of hearing aids. External earphone placement may also lead to collapse of the external auditory canal and some conductive hearing loss.

Middle Ear
Despite loss of elasticity, muscle atrophy (1), and age-related structural changes in the auditory membrane (2),

no associated, significant, conductive hearing impairment occurs. Arthritic changes occur in the joints of the middle ear but no significant transmission deficits.

Inner Ear
Histological changes cause significant age-related hearing defects. Atrophic changes involve the membranous labyrinth including afferent and efferent nerve fibers. There is a decrease in the number of auditory neurons in the eighth cranial nerve and the central auditory pathways. This slow progression results, in part, in the bilateral, high-frequency, sensorineural hearing loss known as presbycusis.

Although data suggest that hearing loss progresses with age, there is great individual variability; thus, age alone is not the only predictor of hearing thresholds. Hearing loss is more common in men than in women. Rosenhall (3) suggests that elderly patients develop hearing loss irrespective of noise exposure. Elderly patients achieve poorer word recognition scores when compared with younger persons with similar hearing losses of 60 decibels (dB) or more (4).

Types of Hearing Loss

There are three major types of hearing loss: conductive sensorineural, and mixed.

Conductive Hearing Loss
The anatomic site of conductive hearing loss extends from the external ear to the tympanic membrane that divides the outer from the middle ear. This type of loss is usually amenable to medical or surgical treatment. Causes of conductive hearing loss include excessive cerumen, cholesteatoma, trauma, otosclerosis, rheumatoid arthritis, and Paget's disease.

Sensorineural Hearing Loss

The pathological sites of sensorineural hearing loss occur in the cochlea and in the auditory branch of the eighth cranial nerve. This type of loss is usually permanent.

Table 28.1. Hearing Loss Highlights.

1. The 2 most common causes of hearing loss for adults are presbycusis and noise exposure.
2. An estimated 9.4 million persons (nearly 1/3 of the approximately 30 million persons in the U.S. age 65 and older) have significant hearing problems.
3. Presbycusis is generally defined as hearing loss caused by the aging process.
4. Presbycusis trends are demonstrated by data from the National Center for Health Statistics (1987)
   Age 45–64, 14% have hearing loss
   Age 65+, 30% have hearing loss
   Age 75+, 35% have hearing loss
5. Persons in frequent contact with senior citizens are likely to encounter these individuals' frustrations because of their hearing impairment.
6. "Testing patients for hearing loss is a crucial diagnostic area that many physicians overlook." This quote comes from a recent issue of the Medical Tribune (cited in the Hearing Journal [March 1994]). According to the article, by the year 2000, an estimated 40 million Americans will be hearing-impaired.

Common causes of sensorineural hearing loss are presbycusis, noise exposure, ototoxic drugs, and Ménière's disease.

Mixed Hearing Loss

A mixed hearing loss pattern can be caused by both conductive and sensorineural factors. An additional factor, central auditory problems, should also be considered. These are problems of language processing in which the patient is able to hear, with or without amplification, but is unable to fully comprehend what is said and has difficulty responding normally.

Etiology of Presbycusis

Schuknecht and Gasek (5) reported in 1993 that the previous concept of four pathologic types of presbycusis was still confirmed. The four types are sensory, neural, strial, and cochlear conductive presbycusis. These types and their clinical manifestations are presented in Table 28.2. Sensory presbycusis results in an abrupt, high-tone hearing loss, strial presbycusis in a flat threshold audiogram, and neural presbycusis in a reduction in word recognition or understanding. A gradually decreasing, linear audiometric pattern in which there is no major pathologic

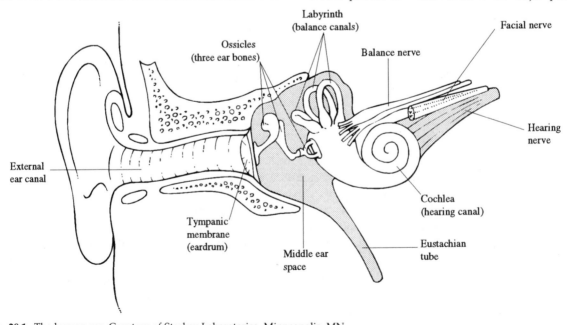

Fig. 28.1. The human ear. Courtesy of Starkey Laboratories, Minneapolis, MN.

Table 28.2. Types of Presbycusis.

Type	Pathologic Findings	Audiogram
1. Sensory	Loss of hair cells	Abrupt high-tone loss
2. Strial	Decrease in nutritive supply	Flat threshold
3. Neural	Nerve degeneration and atrophy	Reduction in word recognition
4. Cochlear conductive	Alterations in cochlear duct	Gradual linear decreasing audiogram

finding is identified as cochlear conductive presbycusis, which is caused by alterations in the cochlear duct. These four types frequently present as a mixed picture, not as a single entity (6). Reversible causes of hearing loss should be excluded before the diagnosis of presbycusis is made.

Examination to Screen for Hearing Loss

Screening for hearing loss should be done in the physician's office as part of the patient's routine annual examination (Table 28.3). Important aspects of the medical history should include noise exposure, use of ototoxic medications, family history, rapidity of onset, and asymmetrical hearing loss. Information regarding tinnitus, vertigo, and previous surgery should also be obtained. Hearing handicap assessment scales such as the Alpiner-Meline Aural Rehabilitation Screening Scale (7) and the Denver Scale of Communication Function—Modified (8) (Figures 28.2 and 28.3) can be used to identify the impact of hearing loss on the patient. A neurological evaluation should also be part of the process.

Useful Screening Procedures

Assessment should be preceded by an otoscopic examination with removal of cerumen as necessary. Cerumen can account for deficits as great as 40 dB. Cerumen should be removed by gentle curettage rather than irrigation because irrigation may damage the middle ear if perforations are present.

Weber & Rinne tuning fork tests should be performed using 256 and 512 hertz (Hz). These two tests may help to differentiate sensorineural from conductive hearing loss if gross abnormalities are present. Normal air conduction and sound is louder than bone conduction but the opposite occurs in the presence of conductive impairment.

Rinne Test

Hold the tuning fork over the patient's external ear canal and ask the patient to listen to the tone; then place the base of the fork on the mastoid bone and ask which tone is louder.

Weber Test

Place the vibrating tuning fork on the center of the patient's forehead, and ask where the tone originates. Normally the tone is heard midline, but in the presence of unilateral sensorineural hearing loss, the tone is heard louder in the better ear.

The handheld audioscope is a reliable, sensitive, and easily used tool for measuring hearing acuity. Testing may be done at 40 and 60 dB levels at 500, 1000, and 4000 Hz. The patient should be referred to an audiologist if there is failure to hear these tones in either or both ears. Formal audiological evaluation may then be conducted, with appropriate rehabilitative recommendations and hearing aid recommendations initiated, depending on the severity and type of hearing loss.

Table 28.3. Physician's Annual Clinic Screening for Patient Hearing Status*.

Evaluation
  Patient history and physical examination
  Otoscopic examination
  Alpiner-Meline and Denver assessment scales
  Weber and Rinne tests
  Handheld audioscope
Referral to audiologist
  Hearing loss detected
Referral to otolaryngologist
  Sudden-onset hearing loss
  Unilateral or asymmetrical deafness
  Abnormal neurological findings relative to auditory
    mechanism

*Physician's screening time, 15 minutes; patient's form completion time, 15 minutes.

**Alpiner-Meline Aural Rehabilitation (AMAR0
Screening Scale**

Name: _____

Birthday: _____ Age: _____ SSN: _____

Hearing Aid Status:
(Circle one)   NONE ITE BODY NONE EYEGLASS MONAURAL NINAURAL

Number of Years of hearing aid use: _____
Occupation: _____
Audiologist: _____ Date of Screening: _____

PART I: SELF ASSESSMENT OF HEARING HANDICAP

(Choose One)   A = Always U = Usually S = Sometimes R = Rarely N = Never

1. I feel like I am isolated from things because of my hearing loss.	A U S R N	+ −
2. I feel very frustrated when I can not understand a conversation.	A U S R N	+ −
3. My hearing loss has affected my life.	A U S R N	+ −
4. I tend to avoid people because of my hearing loss.	A U S R N	+ −
5. People in general are tolerant of my hearing loss.	A U S R N	+ −
6. My hearing loss has affected my relationship with my spouse.	A U S R N	+ −
7. I try to hide my hearing loss from my co-workers.	A U S R N	+ −
8. My hearing loss has interfered with job performance.	A U S R N	+ −
9. I feel more pressure at work because of my hearing loss.	A U S R N	+ −

PART I PROBLEMS _____

Fig. 28.2. Alpiner-Meline Aural Rehabilitation (AMAR) screening scale. (Reproduced by permission from Alpiner JG, Meline NC, Cotton AD. An aural rehabilitation screening scale: self assessment, auditory aptitude, and visual aptitude. J Acad Rehabil Audiol 1991;24:75–83.)

Audiology Evaluation

An audiology evaluation determines the degree of the patient's hearing loss, the severity of the loss, and whether the loss is conductive, sensorineural, or mixed. An audiogram can specify the impact of the hearing loss on the person's ability to hear. An audiology case history should be taken to evaluate the client more completely in terms of hearing loss and to make recommendations that will help minimize communication problems. Several ba-

sic procedures are performed in the audiologist's routine evaluation. These tests include immittance testing, pure-tone air and bone conduction assessment, and speech audiometry—speech reception thresholds (SRTs), and word recognition.

Figure 28.4 shows an audiogram. The audiogram depicts hearing within normal limits in the lower frequencies, sloping to a severe high-frequency hearing loss, caused by presbycusis, for the right ear. The patient's audiogram indicates there will be some difficulty hearing

The Denver Scale of Communication Function – Modified

Specific Difficulty Listening Situations

1. I have trouble hearing the radio or television unless I turn the volume on very loud. Comments:
   - _____ 1. Definitely agree
   - _____ 2. Slightly agree
   - _____ 3. Irrelevant
   - _____ 4. Slightly disagree
   - _____ 5. definitly disagree

2. If someone calls me when my back is turned. I do not always hear him. Comments:
   - _____ 1. Definitely agree
   - _____ 2. Slightly agree
   - _____ 3. Irrelevant
   - _____ 4. Slightly disagree
   - _____ 5. definitly disagree

3. If someone calls me from another room. I have much trouble hearing. Comments:
   - _____ 1. Definitely agree
   - _____ 2. Slightly agree
   - _____ 3. Irrelevant
   - _____ 4. Slightly disagree
   - _____ 5. definitly disagree

4. When I sit talking with my friends in a quite room. I have a great deal of difficulty hearing. Comments:
   - _____ 1. Definitely agree
   - _____ 2. Slightly agree
   - _____ 3. Irrelevant
   - _____ 4. Slightly disagree
   - _____ 5. definitly disagree

5. When I use the phone. I have much difficulty hearing. Comments:
   - _____ 1. Definitely agree
   - _____ 2. Slightly agree
   - _____ 3. Irrelevant
   - _____ 4. Slightly disagree
   - _____ 5. definitly disagree

6. When I play cards, understanding my partner gives me much difficulty. Comments:
   - _____ 1. Definitely agree
   - _____ 2. Slightly agree
   - _____ 3. Irrelevant
   - _____ 4. Slightly disagree
   - _____ 5. definitly disagree

7. At lectures or discussions I have much difficulty hearing the speaker. Comments:
   - _____ 1. Definitely agree
   - _____ 2. Slightly agree
   - _____ 3. Irrelevant
   - _____ 4. Slightly disagree
   - _____ 5. definitly disagree

8. In church when the minister gives the sermon, I have much difficulty. Comments:
   - _____ 1. Definitely agree
   - _____ 2. Slightly agree
   - _____ 3. Irrelevant
   - _____ 4. Slightly disagree
   - _____ 5. definitly disagree

9. When a movie is shown, I have much difficulty hearing what is said. Comments:
   - _____ 1. Definitely agree
   - _____ 2. Slightly agree
   - _____ 3. Irrelevant
   - _____ 4. Slightly disagree
   - _____ 5. definitly disagree

10. I have difficulty understanding announcements sent through the loudspeaker even when the speaker is in the same room. Comments:
    - _____ 1. Definitely agree
    - _____ 2. Slightly agree
    - _____ 3. Irrelevant
    - _____ 4. Slightly disagree
    - _____ 5. definitly disagree

11. I have trouble understanding messages sent over the intercom. Comments:
    - _____ 1. Definitely agree
    - _____ 2. Slightly agree
    - _____ 3. Irrelevant
    - _____ 4. Slightly disagree
    - _____ 5. definitly disagree

Fig. 28.3. The Denver scale of communication Function–Modified. (Reproduced by permission from Kaplan H, Feely J, Brown J. A modified Denver scale: test-retest reliability. J Acad Rehabil Audiol 1978;11:15–32.)

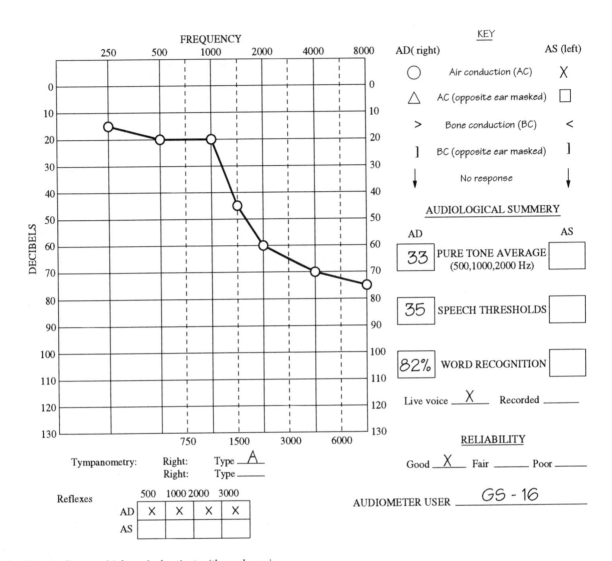

Fig. 28.4. Audiogram (right ear) of patient with presbycusis.

/s/, /f/, and voiceless /th/ sounds, resulting in word recognition difficulties. The pure-tone average indicates a mild hearing loss in speech frequencies, which is verified by the similar speech reception threshold. The patient's word recognition score is reduced. Normal ear pressure is represented by a type A tympanogram. Normal reflexes are reported for the frequencies 500 through 4000 Hz. There appear to be no problems that require medical/surgical treatment, but the patient is a candidate for hearing aids to help improve communication function.

The first step in the audiology evaluation process is an otoscopic examination of the patient's external auditory canal to rule out excessive cerumen or other problems. Second, acoustic immittance tests determine the resting pressure in the middle ear. Normal pressure exists when the air pressure in the middle ear is essentially similar to air pressure outside the head. Acoustic reflex testing of the middle ear may be of diagnostic significance relative to disorders of the auditory system.

Specific frequencies are tested on the audiogram because speech in our language is basically a conglomeration of frequencies or pitches. The numerical level

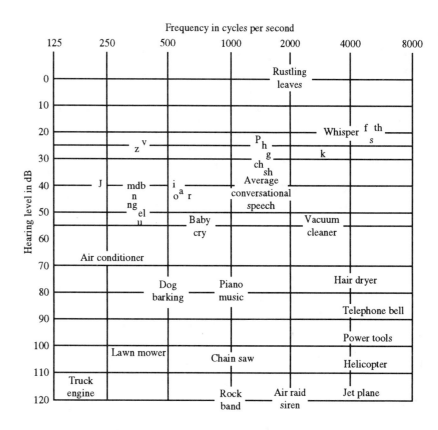

Fig. 28.5. Frequency spectrum of familiar sounds. (Reproduced by permission from Northern JL, Downs MP. What is hearing loss? Hearing in children. Baltimore: Williams & Wilkins, 1984;7. Copyright © 1984, Williams & Wilkins Co.)

indicated for each frequency represents the threshold (the lowest level), stated in dB, at which an individual is able to hear by the normal route of hearing: external (outer) ear to middle ear to inner ear to auditory (eight cranial) nerve to auditory temporal lobe.

Figure 28.5 demonstrates the importance of frequency in understanding speech. A classic statement made by many seniors is "I can hear you but I don't understand all of the words." Note that lower frequencies are responsible for certain sounds, such as the vowel sounds and consonants /v/, /z/, /m/, and /ng/. High frequencies are responsible for other sounds such as /f/, voiceless /th/ (as in *th*umb), /s/, and /k/. The general pattern of hearing loss in presbycusis is one in which the higher frequencies deteriorate first. Presbycusis usually occurs gradually and individuals may not realize that a hearing loss exists because low frequency sounds can still be heard normally. Consider, for example, the sentence "I am going fishing next Thursday if the sun shines." With a

high frequency hearing loss, the sentence may be heard as: I am going . . . ing nex . . . ursday i . . . the . . . un . . . ines. Thus, the person "hears but doesn't understand."

If one shouts to this person, speech is louder but not necessarily clearer. This process of evaluaton is termed word recognition ability. On the audiogram the score is given in terms of a percentage. Word recognition scores are classified as indicated in Table 28.4.

The matter of loudness is considered independently of clarity. Regardless of the percentage of clarity, if speech is

Table 28.4. Classification of Word Recognition Scores.

Percentage	Classification
90–100	Normal or good
75–89	Slight difficulty
60–74	Moderate difficulty
50–59	Poor ability
Below 50	Very poor ability

Table 28.5. Categories of Hearing Loss, by Numerical Threshold Score.

Hearing Threshold Level (dB)	Hearing Difficulty	Clinical Picture of Hearing
−10–26	Within normal limits	No difficulty
27–40	Mild loss	Faint speech
41–55	Moderate loss	Loud speech
56–70	Moderately severe loss	Very loud speech
71–90	Severe loss	Very little
90+	Profound loss	Hear nothing

not sufficiently loud, it will not be heard. On the left side of the audiogram (see Figure 28.4), hearing level (loudness) is presented in dB. Hearing loss is generally classified by averaging the pure-tone thresholds at 500, 1000, and 2000 Hz (primary speech frequencies). The scale in Table 28.5 categorizes the amount of hearing loss on the basis of numerical threshold scores.

Concomitant Clinical Problems

Tinnitus

Tinnitus may be defined as "head noise, conscious sound that originates in one's head" (9) or the "perception of

---

TINNITUS QUESTIONNAIRE

Date of Onset _____   Related to Specific Incident: _____

IS TINNITUS: _____   CONSTANT_____   INTERMITTENT

IS TINNITUS: _____ UNILATERAL _____ BILATERAL

DESCRIPTION OF TINNITUS: _____ RINGING _____ BUZZING _____ HISSING
_____ PULSING _____ POPPING _____ WIND_____ ROARING _____ INSECTS
_____ CLICKING _____OTHER: _____

IS THE TINNITUS;

1.   MASKED BY ENVIRONMENTAL SOUNDS?   ____ YES ____ NO
2.   INTERFERING WITH SLEEP?   ____ YES ____ NO
3.   AGGRAVATED BY ANY STIMULI?   ____ YES ____ NO
     __ NOISE __ CAFFEINE __ ALCOHOL __ OTHER: _____
4.   INTERFERING WITH DAILY ACTIVITIES?   ____ YES ____ NO
5.   HANDICAPPING YOU IN ANY WAY?   ____ YES ____ NO

6.   INTERFERING WITH FAMILY RELATIONSHIPS?   ____ YES ____ NO

COMMENTS: _____

	SUBJECTIVE DEGREE OF PROBLEM			
	MILD		MODERATE	SEVERE
PATIENT'S IMPRESSION	1	2	3	4	5
EXAMINER'S IMPRESSION	1	2	3	4	5

DATE _____ EXAMINER _____

PATIENT'S NAME _____ AGE: _____

Fig. 28.6. Tinnitus questionnaire.

sound in the absence of environmental input" (10). Tinnitus appears in a variety of forms: tonal or noise, steady or pulsating, intermittent or continuous. It can localize to one ear or be heard in both ears. Tinnitus may be subjective (heard by the patient) or objective (heard by the examiner). Objective tinnitus is rare and is thought to be caused by vascular or muscular problems. Individuals with subjective tinnitus report a variety of different noises: high-pitched ringing, cricketlike sound, rushing water, hissing, clicking, wind, and buzzing. Figure 28.6 is an example of a tinnitus questionnaire used to determine the nature and extent of the problem. The two most common causes of subjective tinnitus are noise-induced damage to the fine hair receptors of the cochlear nerve and age-related alterations in the hearing apparatus (11). Goodhill (12) points out that tinnitus is a symptom, not a disease; it may be associated with numerous diseases and conditions.

Rosenhall and Karlsson (13) reported on a study of 674 persons in an investigation of tinnitus in old age. From 8 percent to 15 percent of the subjects had continuous tinnitus, and 20 percent to 42 percent had occasional tinnitus. The prevalence of tinnitus was about equal for men and women. There were significant correlations between tinnitus and occupational noise exposure. In a U.S. National Health Examination Survey, approximately 30 percent of respondents age 55 years or older had mild tinnitus, and another 10 percent suffered from severe tinnitus (14).

It is important to assess the impact of tinnitus on an individual's well-being. Medically treatable tinnitus must first be ruled out during the evaluation process. In most situations in which tinnitus is not medically reversible, effort should be directed to determine the subjective impact of the problem. Table 28.6 outlines the causes and factors associated with tinnitus; Table 28.7 lists suggestions for interventions in chronic tinnitus.

Ototoxic Medications
Drug-induced ototoxicity has been well documented in the literature with permanent and transient deficits described. The cochlea, the vestibular apparatus, or both may be affected. Cochlear toxicity results in tinnitus, hearing loss, or both. Drugs selectively damage different parts of the cochlea. Damage to the basal section results in

high-frequency hearing loss, and apical cochlear involvement results in low-frequency hearing loss. Vestibular toxicity is manifested by vertigo, nausea, vomiting, and ataxia, which occurs at a later stage. Certain risk factors make patients more susceptible to damage: renal impairment, dehydration, hepatic disease, cumulative doses of drugs, previous exposure to ototoxic drugs, and use of more than one ototoxic agent.

A simple pneumonic may help as a quick checklist for a physician seeing a patient with new-onset hearing loss or tinnitus: **T** = Tricyclics, **A** = Antibiotics or aspirin, **L** = Loop diuretics, **C** = Cisplatin or carboplatin.

Table 28.6. Causes and Associated Factors of Tinnitus.

Conditions that cause tinnitus
  Aging
  Noise-induced damage
  Ototoxicity
  Stress
  Hypertension
  Hyperthyroidism
  Vascular abnormalities
  Familial hyperlipidemia
  Hypercholesterolemia
  Hypertriglyceridemia
  Ménière's disease
  Acoustic neuroma
  Temporomandibular joint dysfunction
Drugs and other substances that aggravate or cause tinnitus
  Caffeine
  Aspirin and combined drugs
  Antimicrobials
  Atropine sulfate
  Chloroquine
  Quinidine sulfate
  Quinine sulfate
  Antidepressants (Nortriptyline)
  Nicotine
  Antihistamines and combinations
  Nonsteroidal anti-inflammatory drugs
  Antihypertensives
  Cyclobenzaprine
  Ergot and ergotamine derivatives
  Mechlorethamine
Recreational and job activities that cause noise-induced tinnitus
  Power tool use (boat motors, lawnmowers, saws)
  Motorcycle and racetrack riding
  Firearm use (hunting, target practice)
  Headphone abuse

SOURCE: Reproduced by permission from Ross V, Echevarria KH, Robinson B. Geriatric tinnitus. J Gerontol Nurs 1991;17:6–11

Table 28.7. Chronic Tinnitus Interventions.

Correct physical problems
  Remove ear wax or foreign bodies, itching, or inflammation
  Evaluate hypertension
  Improve acoustics to promote healthy hearing
  Wear noise-protective ear plugs
  Check dental and temporomandibular joint problems
Avoid ototoxic substances in foods, drinks, and drugs
  Delete quinine, aspirin, and anti-inflammatory drug compounds
  Delete caffeine, chocolate, tea, and alcohol
  Reassure elderly that tinnitus is not life-threatening
Teach simple home masking measures to relieve tinnitus
  Radio tuned between stations
  Clocks that tick
  Soft, pleasant, distracting music
  Semi-elevated head position to sleep
Recommend evaluation for properly fitted hearing aid; may relieve tinnitus even if hearing loss is mild
Sophisticated, commercial tinnitus maskers and instruments are matched to individualized pitch of tinnitus
Teach relaxation training to cope with stress and promote sleep; combined with biofeedback, this has been proved to be beneficial for long-term tinnitus sufferers
Contact local self-help tinnitus support groups (for information, contact the American Tinnitus Association, PO Box 5, Portland, OR 97207)

SOURCE: Reproduced by permission from Ross V, Echevarria KH, Robinson, B. Geriatric tinnitus. J Gerontol Nurs 1991;17:6–11

Tricyclics

A prevalence of 1 percent of tinnitus is described for patients taking tricyclics. Tinnitus may subside despite continued therapy.

Antibiotics

Aminoglycosides, erythromycin, and vancomycin can all cause hearing loss.

Aminoglycosides can cause cochlear and vestibular damage to varying degrees depending on which drug is prescribed. Most ototoxicity is associated with parenteral administration, but ototoxicity has also followed topical, oral, and irrigation use, especially neomycin. Streptomycin and gentamicin predominantly damage the vestibular system, neomycin is more toxic to the cochlear system, and tobramycin affects both systems equally. Serial audiometry helps detect early ototoxicity because high-

frequency hearing is affected first and may go unnoticed by the patient.

Erythromycin typically causes sudden-onset hearing loss that affects all frequencies. Symptoms diminish with discontinuation of the drug.

Vancomycin has been reported to cause permanent damage, but in these reports concurrent aminoglycoside therapy was administered; thus permanent damage may be a cumulative effect.

Aspirin

Tinnitus, high-frequency hearing loss, and occasionally vertigo are common features of toxicity. Marked patient variability occurs. Salicylate ototoxicity is almost always reversible in 48 to 72 hours, but permanent loss has been reported.

Loop Diuretics

Furosemide, ethacrynic acid, and bumetanide can cause bilateral, high-tone hearing loss, which is normally transient but may be permanent. Although furosemide is widely prescribed, the incidence of ototoxicity is less than 0.2 percent in patients who receive less than 80 mg intravenously. The likelihood of toxicity is increased when large parenteral doses are rapidly administered. The effects occur in less than 30 minutes after intravenous administration.

Cisplatin

Tinnitus and hearing loss occur frequently in patients taking cisplatin. Patients with previous hearing loss are at increased risk. Because the effects can be permanent, the drug should be discontinued.

In addition to the well-known or frequently encountered ototoxic drugs discussed here, many other drugs can cause hearing loss. When a patient presents with new-onset hearing loss, sufficient evaluation should take place to exlude medication as a cause.

Hearing Aids

The major contribution to improved communication is amplification (hearing aids). For several years, new technologies have produced hearing aids that deliver speech

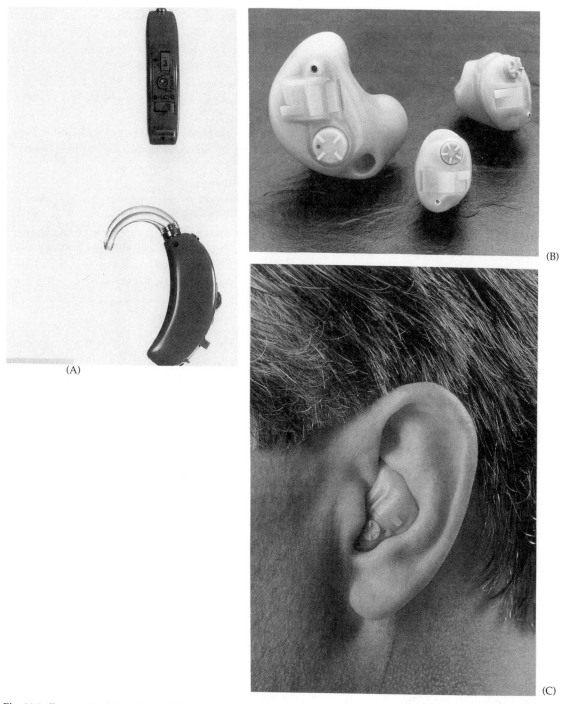

(A)

(B)

(C)

Fig. 28.7. Types of hearing aids. A. Behind-the-ear hearing aid, front and side views. B. In-the-ear hearing aids (various sizes). C. Full in-the-ear hearing aid.

and other auditory stimuli to individuals in a clearer and more pleasing manner. Although hearing aids are not the same as "new ears," hearing is improved in a significant manner. For some persons, a period of adjustment may be necessary to become accustomed to amplified sounds (15) (Alpiner & Vaughn, 1990). Two hearing aids (binaural amplification) are recommended. Binaural hearing aids tend to make speech clearer and to allow for better localization of speech and environmental sounds.

Fortunately, the belief of years ago that hearing aids will not help those with nerve-type hearing loss has largely diminished. In 1993, 1,677,196 hearing aids were dispensed in the United States (16). Sadly, only about 20 percent of individuals who need hearing aids wear them. Some reasons for this situation are 1) lack of awareness that hearing loss exists, 2) belief that hearing aids cost too much money, 3) belief that hearing aids are a sign of old age, 4) belief that hearing aids will not help, and 5) a feeling of being unprepared emotionally (17). The need for professional consultation to deal with these feelings is essential if physicians are to fulfill their responsibilities to hearing-impaired persons by improving their quality of life.

There are two major types of hearing aids: those worn behind the ear (over the ear), and those worn in the ear (Figure 28.7). There are several variations of in-the-ear hearing aids, generally categorized by size from in-the-canal to full in-the-ear. In 1993, about 79 percent of hearing aid sales were in-the-ear type, and about 20 percent were behind-the-ear style. (Less than 1 percent of hearing aid sales were a third type, the eyeglass or body type.)

The process of evaluation for a hearing aid is comprehensive, referral to certified audiologists (certification in audiology by the American Speech-Language-Hearing Association) is of utmost importance. At present there is no national standard for credentials for those who may dispense hearing aids. In some states, there are no credentialling requirements.

Hearing aid costs vary considerably, another reason to recommend that patients seek professional consultation. For example, one may purchase a very basic in-the-ear hearing aid for $500; an elaborate, programmable hearing aid costs $2000. The price is double for binaural amplification. We need to realize that improving the quality of life is worth the price for properly fitted hearing aids pro-

vided by qualified professionals who service their patients. For persons who have severe financial limitations, organizations can help. One major national organization to whom patients may be referred is:

> Hear Now
> 9745 E. Hampden Avenue, Suite 300
> Denver, CO 80231-4923

In 1993, this organization provided almost 1000 hearing aids nationally at no cost to financially eligible persons.

Aural Rehabilitation

Aural rehabilitation is one aspect of the total process of audiology. Aural rehabilitation is also called rehabilitative audiology and audiologic rehabilitation. Major components of aural rehabilitation (18) (Alpiner, 1982) are:

1. Selecting hearing aids, assistive devices, or both to make available to the patient as much undistorted sensory information as possible.

Table 28.8. Hearing Aid Care.

Taking care of your hearing aids everyday will help to keep them from breaking down. Here is a list of *Do's* and *Dont's* that you should follow:

Do's
1. Clean your hearing aids with a dry cloth every night before retiring.
2. Remove the battery or open the battery drawer every night.
3. Remove the hearing aids before bathing, showering, shaving, or swimming. Keep the hearing aids dry.
4. Remove the batteries if the hearing aids are to be stored for any length of time. Batteries could cause corrosion.
5. Turn the hearing aids off when inserting or removing from your ears to avoid feedback.

Dont's
1. Expose your hearing aids to intense heat or cold.
2. Subject your hearing aids to excessive humidity or perspiration.
3. Leave your hearing aids where they may be picked up by animals or small children.
4. Stick pins, paper clips, or anything in the hearing aid openings.
5. Attempt to repair your hearing aids yourself.
6. Take your hearing aids apart to examine them. Curiosity killed the cat, and it also voids the warranty.

SOURCE: Reprinted with permission from Alpiner JG, Hansen EM. Your new hearing aids: care and use. Denver: Department of Veterans Affairs Medical Center, 1993 (unpublished pamphlet)

Table 28.9. Conversational Tips.

Conversational tips (for speaking with individuals with a hearing impairment)
1. Speak naturally and pronounce words clearly.
2. Orient the listener to the topic. (Especially important if they enter in the middle of a conversation, or if there is a change of topic)
3. Speak one person at a time.
4. Do not overexaggerate lip movements.
5. Do not use distracting gestures.
6. Do not cover your mouth or turn away when speaking.
Communication repair strategies (when the hearing-impaired person does not understand)
1. Repeat the message clearly and slowly.
2. Shorten the message—use main or primary subject words.
3. Rephrase the message
    If the person exhibits decreased word recognition ability, this may be more effective than repeating.
    If words or sounds are missed the first time they are said, they may also be missed the second time. Certain sounds may fall below the person's level of hearing, thus they may be unable to "pick out" those sounds.
4. Utilize written material—spell out words that are not understood, give demonstrations when providing instructions.
Other tips
    Do not assume that if a person is wearing a hearing aid, that you should talk louder.
    Do not assume that a hearing aid has restored the individual's hearing to "normal."
    The more you talk with a hearing-impaired individual, the easier it will become for the listener to understand you.

SOURCE: Reproduced by permission from Alpiner JG, Hansen EM. Your new hearing aids: care and use. Denver: Department of Veterans Affairs Medical Center, 1993 (unpublished pamphlet)

2. Counseling patients, family members, and significant others about hearing loss.

3. Providing patients with assertiveness communication training regarding coping with the environment.

4. Pre- and postassessment procedures to determine feelings, attitudes, and specific situational difficulties.

Judgments should be made on the basis of responses of patients to the items in the Alpiner-Meline and Denver assessment scales (see Figures 28.2 and 28.3).

Aural rehabilitation can be seen as a broad-based process in which all these aspects need to be considered. Alpiner and Meline (19) present additional aspects which should be considered:

1. Review basic anatomy and physiology of the hearing mechanism as it pertains to patients.

2. Discuss the importance of interpersonal relationships in terms of everyday communication.

3. Provide listening training, emphasizing the effects of distance, noise, and visibility.

4. Reinforce individual patient's progress and the importance of establishing a stress-free communication environment complemented by personal confidence in effective communication skills.

Physicians should provide patients with information on how to care for their hearing aids and with specific strategies to use in coping with everyday life. Tables 28.8 (20) and 28.9 (20) are examples that may be helpful in dealing with hearing-impaired patients.

Summary and Conclusion

In this chapter a general understanding of hearing loss and tinnitus has been presented with an overview of the major aspects of hearing and how physicians may identify patients who have hearing loss. Follow-up procedures for referral to audiology after the physician has completed any necessary medical or surgical treatment, and diagnostic and rehabilitative procedures of audiology have been described. The importance of adequate communication has also been discussed. The role and responsibility of the physician in recognizing a patient's hearing loss and facilitating the process to minimize the effects of a patient's hearing loss have been emphasized. The outome should bring an improved quality of life to the hearing-impaired patient.

References

1. Schuknecht H, Presbycusis. Laryngoscope 1995;65:419–420.
2. Jerger J, Jerger S, Mauldin L. Studies in impedance audiometry: normal and sensorineural ears. Arch Otolaryngol 1972;96:513–523.
3. Rosenhall U, Pederson J, Svanborg A. Presbycusis and noise induced hearing loss. Ear Hear 1990;11:257–263.
4. Bess F, Townsend T. Word discrimination for listeners with flat sensorineural hearing losses. J Speech Hear Disord 1977;42:232–237.
5. Schuknecht HF, Gacek MR. Cochlear pathology in presbycusis. Ann Otol Rhinol Laryngol 1993;102:1–16.
6. Corso JF. Support for Corso's hearing loss model relating aging and noise exposure. Audiology 1992;31:162–167.
7. Alpiner JG, Meline NC, Cotton AD. An aural rehabilitation screening scale: self-assessment, auditory apitude, and visual

aptitude. J Acad Rehab Audiol 1991;24:75–83.

8. Kaplan H, Feeley J, Brown J. A modified Denver scale: test retest reliability. J Acad Rehab Audiol 1978;11:15–32.

9. Sullivan M, Katon M, Dobie W, et al. Disabling tinnitus-association with affective disorders. Gen Hosp Psychiatry 1988;10:258–291.

10. Forte V, Turner A, Liu P. Objective timmitus associated with abnormal mastoid emissary vein. J Otolaryngol. 1989; 18(5):232–235.

11. Ross V, Echevarria KH, Robinson B. Geriatric tinnitus. J. Gerontol Nurs 1991;17:6–11.

12. Goodhill V. Deafness, tinnitus and dizziness in the aged. In Rossman I, Clinical geriatrics. Philadelphia: Lippincott, 1986.

13. Rosenhall U, Karlsson AK. Tinnitus in old age. Scandinavian Audiology 1991;20(3):165–171.

14. Leske MC. Prevalence estimates of communication disorders in the U.S.; language, hearing and vestibular disorders. ASHA 1981;23:229–237.

15. Alpiner JG, Vaugn GR. Hearing, Aging, Technology. International journal of aging and technology 1988;2(1):15–20.

16. Kirkwood DH. The economy + FDA = the media add up to an off year for hearing aid sales. Hear J 1993;46:7–14.

17. Alpiner JG, Kaufman KJ, Hanavan PC. Overview of rehabilitative audiology. In Alpiner JG, McCarthy PA. Rehabilitative audiology: children and adults. Baltimore: Williams & Wilkins, 1993.

18. Alpiner JG. Rehabilitation of the geriatric client. In: Alpiner JG. Handbook of adult rehabilitative audiology. Baltimore: Williams and Wilkins, 1982.

19. Alpiner JG, Meline NC. A self-assessment scale of hearing handicap. Paper presented to annual convention of Alabama Speech and Hearing Association: Birmingham, 1989.

20. Alpiner JG, Hansen EM. Your new hearing aids: care and use. Denver: Department of Veterans Affairs Medical Center, 1993 (unpublished pamphlet).

Suggested Readings

Brummet RE, Fox KE. Aminoglycoside-induced hearing loss in humans. Antimicrob Agents Chemother 1989;33:797–800.

Corso JF. Support for Corso's hearing loss model relating aging and noise exposure. Audiology 1992;31:162–167.

Gates GA, Cooper JG, Kannel WB, Miller NJ. Hearing in the elderly: the Framingham Report, 1983–1985. Ear Hear 1990;11:247–256.

Lesar TS. Disorders of the eyes, nose and throat. In JT Dipiro, RL Talbert, PE Hayes, et al. *Pharmacology: A Pathophysiologic Approach.* New York: Elsevier, 1989.

Lichtenstein MJ. Hearing and visual impairments. Clin Geriatr Med 1992;8:173–182.

Mader S. Hearing impairment in elderly persons. J Am Geriatr Soc 1984;32:548–553.

Moore RD, Smith CR, Lietman PS. Risk factors for the development of auditory toxicity in patients receiving aminoglycosides. J Infect Dis 1984;149:23–30.

Northern JL, Downs MP. *Hearing in Children.* Baltimore: Williams & Wilkins, 1984.

Prescod SV. *A Standard Dictionary of Audiology.* Santa Monica, CA: Vanguard, 1986.

Schacht J. Molecular mechanism of drug-induced hearing loss. Hear Res 1986;22:297–304.

Schweitzer VG, Olsen NR. Ototoxic effect of erythromycin therapy. Arch Otolaryngol 1984;110:258–260.

Voek S, Gallager C, Langer E, Drinka P. Hearing loss in the nursing home. J Am Gerontol Soc 1990;38:141–145.

Chapter 29
The Aging Eye

Roger H.S. Langston

Old men's eyes are like old men's memories; they are strongest for things a long way off.

George Eliot

Aging brings a number of changes to the eye and to the life of the elderly patient. Some changes are natural annoyances that must be tolerated, and some represent significant diseases. A large portion of the geriatrician's work is to interpret and explain these changes to patients. Blindness is a problem clearly associated with increasing age, and many elderly patients naturally fear this outcome when any new ocular symptoms develop. This chapter outlines some of the more common, normal, aging changes and some common diseases of the aging eye.

Common Ophthalmic Symptoms

Diminished vision is by its nature a potentially serious symptom usually caused by changes that occur in the eye, although it can be caused by problems in the visual pathways or occipital cortex. In decreased vision, sudden change is always an indication of significant disease. Slowly progressive loss may result from a fairly benign problem, such as the need for a change in prescription lenses, the development of cataract, or from more serious conditions. If the patient maintains good vision under some circumstances (for example, maintaining good near vision but losing distance vision) the problem is much less likely to be serious than if vision is decreased under all circumstances (Figure 29.1).

Fluctuations in vision associated with lighting are fairly common with aging and are generally caused by a cataract or other opacity in the ocular media. With age, the pupil tends to become smaller and the iris less reactive to changes in lighting. In addition, the lens of the eye darkens and may develop some opacities. The retina also becomes less sensitive. All these changes cause the elderly patient to have problems in adapting to very bright illumination or to dim illumination. Fluctuations in vision, especially darkening of vision, which occur independent of lighting conditions, are more sinister and often are due to carotid or vertebral transient ischemic attacks (TIA) or, occasionally, to elevated intraocular or intracranial pressure.

When a patient complains of poor vision, it is important to ascertain whether this is present in one or both eyes, at near or far distance, and with or without glasses. A description of how the patient noticed the visual change can be helpful. For example, a patient may think he or she has sustained a sudden loss of vision when, covering one eye, the person discovers that the vision is poor in the other eye; the vision loss, in fact, may have been slowly progressive but suddenly noticed. Similarly, most patients are not ordinarily conscious of their visual fields, and if they have a transient loss of the left visual field resulting from a TIA, for example, they may interpret this as a loss of vision in the left eye, unless they checked the vision in each eye separately. In this example, the distinction is significant in differentiating between ocular or carotid artery disease and cerebrocortical or vertebral artery disease. Patients who notice difficulty with reading may have poor near vision, but the complaint also can be caused by a scotoma from ocular or cerebral disease, by dyslexia from a stroke, or by diminished mental faculties from Alzheimer's disease or other dementia states.

A scotoma, or loss of part of the visual field, always represents serious disease and warrants prompt evaluation. Uniocular scotomas are commonly caused by glaucoma or retinal disease. Binocular scotomas are commonly a result of stroke or cerebral tumors.

Photopsia (flashing lights in the visual field) can be caused by migraine, but in the elderly, this symptom is commonly caused by vitreous traction, which may be

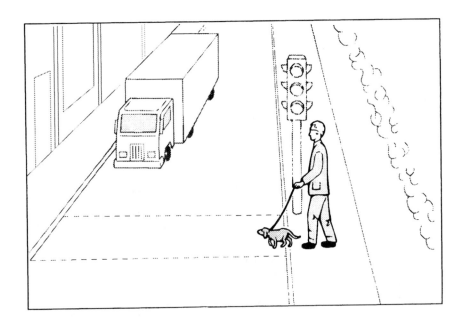

Fig. 29.1. In normal vision, the central area shows the truck and the traffic light. The dog and person are in sharp focus. Peripheral objects are seen in less detail.

associated with developing retinal detachment. Photopsia requires ophthalmic evaluation.

Metamorphopsia, or distorted vision, is usually related to retinal disease, especially macular disease, although it can be caused by a cataract or by corneal disease. In the elderly patient, metamorphopsia should be reason for a prompt ophthalmologic examination because it may indicate retinal pathology that is treatable only if detected early.

Diplopia (double vision) is pathologic. Binocular diplopia implies a misalignment of the eyes. Its onset in the elderly most frequently results from an extraocular muscle palsy caused by diabetes or vascular occlusion, although it has a wide variety of causes ranging from tumor to myasthenia gravis. Monocular diplopia is almost always caused by cataract or other opacity in the eye.

Burning, stinging, itching, and dryness are common ocular symptoms associated with irritation of the conjunctiva and cornea. In the absence of any visual symptoms, ocular inflammation, or discharge, tear substitutes may be used for temporary relief. Itching, which is worsened by rubbing the eyes, is suggestive of an allergy.

Foreign-body sensation in the eye may be associated with corneal disease and warrants an evaluation with a slit lamp because corneal tissue is delicate and damage can easily lead to loss of vision.

Deep pain in the eye itself is a serious symptom. It usually represents significant intraocular inflammation, which is potentially vision-threatening. Ocular inflammation usually also causes photophobia, that is, pain when the eye is exposed to light. Nonophthalmic problems in the distribution of the trigeminal nerve, caused by dental or sinus disease, for example, occasionally lead to referred pain in the eye.

Headache, even headache behind the eyes, is rarely related to ocular disease, unless it is associated with a concurrent decrease in vision. A brow ache or headache can develop from fatigue caused by prolonged use of the eyes when driving, reading, and so forth, but there will be a clear relationship between the headache and these activities. Often, headache is easily relieved by a change in lens prescription or even by reassurance that the headache does not represent ocular disease.

In any elderly patient with headache, especially if there are associated symptoms of scalp tenderness, painful chewing, proximal myalgias, or weight loss, the diagnosis of temporal arteritis should be considered. This condition can lead to sudden, permanent visual loss if it is not treated with systemic corticosteroids.

Presbyopia

The shape of the lens of the eye can be altered by the action of the ciliary muscles, which allows a change in focus from distance to close. This is called accommodation. In a young child, the near point of accommodation is almost at the nose. With age, however, the lens becomes progressively harder and denser, and its shape is less able to change, which leads to a progressive inability to focus on near objects and, for the average person, leads to a need for reading glasses at about age 45. The process is progressive, and stronger reading glasses become necessary over time; reading material must be held closer to the eyes. Stronger reading glasses also have a narrower working range. For this reason, most persons are happiest when they do not change eyeglass prescriptions until they clearly need to because of fatigue with near work.

In addition to bifocals and trifocals, "progressive" or "graduated" multifocal lenses are made. These lenses have the advantage that, if the appropriate portion of the lens is used, any object at any distance can be brought into a clear focus. This is particularly of value when the wearer cannot adjust distance from the object viewed. The disadvantage of these lenses is that the area of the spectacle lens that focuses a given distance is quite small and requires that the patient adjust head position to use the lenses comfortably.

Ultraviolet Radiation Exposure

Currently, considerable commercial attention is focused on the advisability of ultraviolet (UV) protection for the eyes. The scientific basis for this is limited. Animal experiments show UV radiation can cause cataracts (1). Several studies have shown an indirect relationship between UV exposure and incidence of cataract in certain populations (2). A dose-response relationship between (UV-B) exposure and cortical cataract has been demonstrated in an epidemiologic study of 838 Chesapeake Bay watermen (3). The same study did not show a relationship between UV exposure and macular degeneration of the retina although other studies have suggested a relationship (4).

Most persons are exposed to a relatively small percent of ambient UV radiation that is scattered, as in blue light. A sky with a clear horizon for 360 degrees gives maxi-

Table 29.1. Percentage of Surface Reflectivity of UV-B Light.

Grass and soil	1–5
Water	3–13
Sand and concrete	7–18
Snow	80–88

mum exposure, but this exposure is diminished by buildings, trees, and the like and is also reduced about 15 percent by one's eyebrows, eyelashes, and nose. Exposure to UV-B radiation can be reduced 50 percent more if a person wears a hat outdoors, and can be reduced by approximately 95 percent if a person has close-fitting plastic spectacles without a special UV filter (5).

Ultraviolet radiation exposure is not a practical problem indoors because there is a substantial difference in reflectivity of various surfaces to UV light (Table 29.1) (6). The difference in reflectivity is a strong argument for a person to wear protective lenses when in the snow or at the beach.

Cataract

In addition to becoming harder and denser with age, the lens of the eye also tends to become somewhat opaque. This is called cataract. Although some cataracts are associated with diseases, such as diabetes, or with drug toxicity (e.g., oral corticosteroids), most cataracts are age-related ("senile") cataracts. Cataracts are very common with aging; the incidence of vision decrease caused by cataracts in the United States has been found to be 18 percent from ages 65 to 74 and 46 percent from ages 75 to 85 (7).

Cigarette smoking appears to increase the risk of cataract (8) as does extended exposure to UV light (3). Aspirin usage does not appear to protect against cataract (9).

Generally, the only symptom caused by cataracts is blurred vision (Figure 29.2); however, depending on the type of cataract, the blurring may be worse at distance or at close range. In all cases, cataract leads to increasing problems with glare; vision is ordinarily best in a moderately lit room and is worse in bright sunlight, when the person looks at someone in a doorway or against a window with light behind the person, or when the person tries to see a traffic light against a bright sky. These exam-

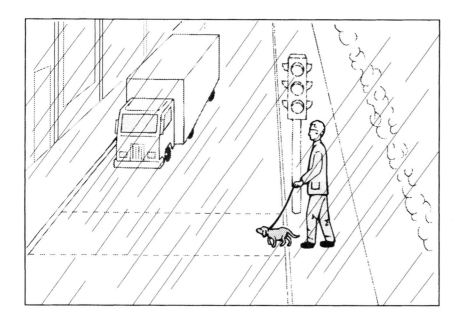

Fig. 29.2. Cataract leads to a diffuse blurring or fogging of vision, particularly when light shines towards the eye.

ples suggest why patients with developing cataracts may function perfectly well in their own homes but find their lifestyles substantially compromised. A cataract is best seen with a slit lamp microscope through the patient's dilated pupil, but it can also be visualized with an ophthalmoscope as a dark opacity in the red reflex from the retina.

Patients are often concerned about when the cataract should be removed. In rare cases, a cataract may need to be removed for medical reasons, but in more than 99 percent of cases, the only reason to remove a cataract is to permit the patient to see better. Because the results of cataract surgery are the same regardless of when it is performed, the patient can decide when to have surgery on the basis of how he or she is functioning. Surgery is appropriate when the patient's lifestyle is affected. Clearly, this will be different for the active, driving, working patient than for the bedridden, nursing home resident.

Modern cataract surgery with intraocular lens implantation is ordinarily successful. Over 95 percent of patients with otherwise normal eyes achieve reading- and driving-quality vision. The surgery is usually performed in an outpatient setting and requires minimal postoperative restrictions. (A description of the current procedure is

sometimes useful for an apprehensive patient who remembers a grandparent in bed for a week with sandbags around the head after cataract surgery.)

Since the 1970s, the routine of cataract surgery has been to replace the cataractous lens with one made of polymethyl methacrylate plastic. These lens implants are available in various focusing powers. Hence, at the time of surgery, the patient and surgeon have the opportunity to select a new lens that will make the patient nearsighted or farsighted. Ordinarily, the choice is for a lens that balances with the unoperated eye and that minimizes refractive error (need for glasses) of the patient. The calculations for replacement lens power are based on empirically derived formulae using past experience with several thousand patients. Since any given individual patient may deviate slightly from the norm of the equation, it is not possible to promise a patient perfect vision without glasses. Most patients do have good vision without glasses but need some spectacle correction to get maximum vision.

Since 1987, a limited number of multifocal lenses, based on diffraction optics, have been implemented. These lenses possess two focusing powers simultaneously and can focus both distant and near objects (10). If the lens power is correct for the patient, the distance image will be sufficiently out of focus for the patient to ignore it when he is looking at a near object, and vice versa. However, the difficulty in selecting exactly the correct lens power for a patient and problems with diminished contrast sensitivity with these lenses have limited their general acceptance.

Patients often wonder whether their cataract can be removed by a laser. In fact, cataract surgery is performed with a knife and other surgical instruments, not with a laser. However, after cataract surgery, a portion of patients will develop a clouding of a membrane in the eye, the posterior capsule, and some blurring of vision. If this happens, a hole can be cut in the membrane with a laser in the office. The clouding of the posterior capsule could be called an "after cataract" or "secondary cataract"; these are not very useful terms, but they explain the advertisements one sees for laser cataract surgery centers.

Cataract surgery is the single most frequently performed operation in the age group using Medicare, with more than 1 million operations per year being performed in the United States. The large number has led to concern about unnecessary surgery being performed. Part of the concern relates to the fact that the patient's visual acuity, as tested in the office with a Snellen chart, often does not reflect the patient's visual function in the real world. As a result, a number of tests of contrast sensitivity and glare sensitivity have been devised. By and large, the value of these tests is in justifying a clinical decision made on the basis of the patient's history and examination of the eye.

Because the temporary strategy of requiring precertification for cataract surgery for Medicare patients did not demonstrate a significant amount of unnecessary surgery, this approach was abandoned. Recently, the Federal Agency for Health Care Policy and Research has produced several versions of *Clinical Practice Guidelines, Cataract in Adults: Management of Functional Impairment* intended for use by ophthalmologists, other health care workers, and patients. These are available from

AHCPR Publications Clearinghouse, P.O. Box 8547, Silver Spring, MD, 20907

Other strategies to deal with the huge financial burden of cataract surgery (approximately 12 percent of the Medicare budget) include the progressive ratcheting down of reimbursement schedules to hospitals and surgeons and the bundling of more pre- and postoperative services. As yet, no attempts have been made in the U.S. to limit patient access.

Tear Deficiency

The cornea is not a naturally wettable surface. Although the tear film contains wetting agents and stabilizers (chiefly mucin and lipids), there is a definite tendency for the tear film to break up and for the cornea to dry. Continuous production of tears by the ocular adnexa and spreading of the tears over the cornea by blinking of the eyelids is necessary to keep the cornea comfortable and healthy.

Aging generally causes diminished tear secretion, that is, a decrease in the quality and quantity of the tears produced in a resting, nonirritated state. Although this is rarely severe enough to cause vision loss from corneal scarring, it commonly leads to a chronic feeling of dryness and burning in the eyes. The symptoms tend to be worse in artificial heat and when the humidity is low and are often exacerbated by reading, watching television, or driving, because of a person's decreased blinking rate during these activities. Dust, smoke, and fumes also increase irritation caused by tear deficiency.

Most patients with a tear deficiency find treatment less than satisfactory. Controlling the environment is difficult, and tear substitutes have a transient effect. Although ointments give more relief, they blur vision. Often, the most a physician can do is to reassure the patient that the problem is not vision-threatening, although this advice may not be possible for patients with a severe tear deficiency associated with ocular pemphigoid and certain other pathologic states. A decrease in vision in a patient with tear deficiency is cause for prompt referral to an ophthalmologist because the tear deficient eye is particularly susceptible to infection.

Eyelid Ptosis

With age, the skin of the lids becomes thinner and wrinkled, and the subcutaneous tissues and ligaments become more lax. This leads to drooping lids. In the upper lid, the ptosis is usually a cosmetic concern, but occasionally, the lid will droop enough to cover part of the pupil and interfere with the upper visual field. (In such cases, third-party medical insurance payers may cover the cost of correction.) In the lower lid, the laxity may lead to senile ectropion, in which the lid tends to fall away from the eye, which causes chronic tearing. This often causes the patient to wipe constantly at the eyes, exacerbating the problem. The patient with lid laxity should blot tears gently, pushing the lid up and in rather than wiping laterally, which tends to increase the problem. Although senile ectropion is unlikely to be vision-threatening, the chronic tearing and irritation of the exposed conjunctiva can be very annoying to the patient. The definitive treatment is lid surgery. Both ptosis of the upper lid and ectropion of the lower lid can result from pathologic processes such as third- or fifth-nerve palsies or tumors of the skin or meibomian glands.

Vitreous Floaters and Retinal Detachment

The major cavity of the eye, behind the lens and in front of the retina, contains a gel formed largely of collagen fibrils and hyaluronic acid. This is the vitreous humor (the modern term is vitreous body). With advancing years, the gel normally separates into a watery component and clumps and strands of collagen. These are seen by patients as black specks and strands, often initially interpreted as being a fly or something else in the external environment. These "floaters" tend to come and go, but eventually move forward in the eye and settle out of the axis of vision and thus become less noticeable to the patient. They are innocuous, but annoying. As part of the same aging process, the collagen fibrils shrink and pull away from the retina. As they do so, they stimulate the retina and produce photopsia, usually in the periphery of the vision. Rarely, the retina will tear when the vitreous pulls on it, and a retinal detachment can occur as fluid leaks through the tear. In this case, the patient will have the sensation of a dark curtain or shade coming in from the periphery and obscuring vision.

A retinal detachment is unlikely to be seen with the ordinary handheld ophthalmoscope because detachments usually start in the peripheral retina beyond the area that can be visualized with this instrument.

Any patient with a dramatic increase in floaters or photopsia should be warned about retinal detachment.

An ophthalmologic examination should be performed promptly, since retinal detachment surgery is more successful when treated in its early stages.

A retinal tear without detachment can often be sealed off to prevent further damage with the use of a laser in the office. Small detachments may be managed with a combination of laser treatment and injections of intraocular air or other gases. More extensive or longer standing detachments will require a trip to the operating room. Retinal detachment surgery is usually successful. One series shows a reattachment rate of 94 percent, with 56 percent of patients regaining 20/50 (daytime driving) vision or better (11).

Macular Degeneration

Only one portion of the retina is capable of high-grade, fine, discriminatory vision such as that needed for reading and driving. This is the macula. It subserves the central few degrees of the visual field. The remaining retina is capable only of perceiving relatively large objects. Unfortunately, the macula is prone to degenerative changes with aging. In the United States, macular degeneration is the leading cause of permanent blindness (i.e., vision of 20/200 or less) in patients over age 65. Its prevalence in the Framingham study was 9 percent (12).

The visual result of macular degeneration is a central scotoma, a small spot in the center of the vision in which objects are not seen well (Figure 29.3). Ordinarily, this is slowly progressive. At first, patients may have trouble only when reading; they may miss or confuse some letters in the words. Progressively, the scotoma enlarges, so that all central vision is gone, and activities such as reading and driving become impossible. Patients are not able to see the face of the person talking to them and have to recognize people by their voices. This is devastating to the elderly patient, especially because the condition is almost never treatable and is never reversible. Although the rate of change in macular degeneration is usually slow, it is always progressive. It may be asymmetric, but is generally bilateral.

The only positive factor in this condition is that it is never completely blinding. The process is largely confined to the macular region, and the rest of the retina remains normal. Experience shows that most patients

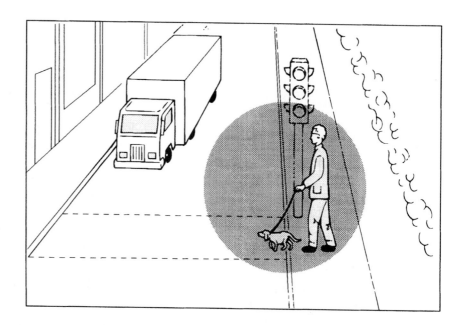

Fig. 29.3. In macular degeneration, approximately 10 degrees of the central visual field is lost. Only peripheral vision remains, and that region is not seen in detail.

with macular degeneration maintain the ability to dress and groom themselves and generally function fairly well in a controlled, familiar environment such as their own homes. They usually do need assistance when away from familiar areas.

The diagnosis of macular degeneration is made with the ophthalmoscope. The earliest changes are drusen, yellowish spots in the macula, and clumping and dispersion of the retinal pigment epithelium. Later, the entire macula may be atrophic and scarred.

The vast majority of patients with age-related macular degeneration have a so-called dry form of the condition, which is untreatable. A few patients will develop vascular nets underneath the neurosensory retina, which can be treated with laser therapy to retard the progress of the disease. Because this possibility exists, all patients with macular degeneration should be examined by an ophthalmologist at least once.

Although magnifying lenses have limited value in macular degeneration, a low-vision clinic or sight center is often useful to the patient by offering various low-vision aids as well as counseling and support.

There is growing evidence that visible and UV radiation can damage the retina over time. It may be particularly sensible for patients with macular degeneration to avoid direct exposure to bright sunlight and to wear tinted sunglasses to exclude blue and ultraviolet light when they are outdoors (13).

Diabetic Retinopathy

Diabetics are much more likely to develop cataracts or glaucoma than are nondiabetics. However, the major threat to vision in diabetics is diabetic retinopathy. It is a serious problem, secondary only to macular degeneration, as a cause of permanent blindness in the United States.

The duration of the diabetes is the most important determinant of retinopathy. Retinopathy is rare in insulin-dependent diabetics who have had diabetes for 5 years or less; it occurs in 27 percent of patients who have had the disease for 5 to 10 years, and in 71 percent of patients with diabetes for more than 10 years. Patients who have had diabetes for 30 years have an incidence of 95 percent. The figures are about half these percentages for non-insulin-dependent diabetics (14).

The presence of diabetic retinopathy is strongly correlated with diabetic renal disease (proteinuria and elevated blood urea nitrogen). There is good evidence that hyperglycemia causes diabetic retinopathy; the recent Diabetes Complication Control Trial (DCCT) demonstrated that tight control of blood sugar delays the onset and progression of retinopathy.

Table 29.2. Diabetic Retinopathy Study*.

Risk	With Photocoagulation (%)	Without Photocoagulation (%)
NVD less than 1/2 DD with hemorrhage	4	26
NVD more than 1/2 DD without hemorrhage	8	26
NVD more than 1/2 DD with hemorrhage	20	37
NVE more than 1/2 DD with hemorrhage	7	30

*Eyes with less than 5/200 vision after 2-year follow-up.
DD = disk diameter; hemorrhage = preretinal or vitreous hemorrhage; NVD = neovascularization arising on or within 1 disk diameter of optic disk; NVE = neovascularization arising elsewhere.
SOURCE: Diabetic Retinopathy Study Group. Four risk factors for severe visual loss in diabetic retinopathy. The third report from the Diabetic Retinopathy Study. Arch Ophthalmol 1979;96:158.

The earliest visible changes of diabetic retinopathy are capillary microaneurysms, first on the venous side then on the arterial side. As the condition progresses, hemorrhages and exudates occur. The hemorrhages may be round or splinter shaped. (If predominantly the latter, systemic hypertensive disease should be considered.) These changes are often called background diabetic retinopathy (BDR). There may be associated macular edema that decreases vision in severe cases. As the disease progresses, the normal retinal circulation is altered, which leads to areas of retinal hypoxia that are believed to stimulate a vasoproliferative response and cause the neovascularization of proliferative diabetic retinopathy (PDR) (15). The new vessels may be associated with fibrous proliferation, as well as extensive hemorrhaging into the retina and vitreous humor, with both tractional and rhegmatogenous retinal detachments.

One of the great triumphs of ophthalmology in the past several decades has been the recognition, through national collaborative studies sponsored by the National Institutes of Health, of the appropriate treatment for diabetic retinopathy to interrupt this sequence of events and thus preserve vision for most diabetics. The treatment is retinal photocoagulation, in which areas of neovascularization and areas of hypoxia or the peripheral retina are diffusely ablated with a laser. The panretinal photocoagulation (PR) probably improves the oxygen flow through the remaining retinal circulation and decreases the production of vasoproliferative factors. For high-risk patients, this treatment dramatically reduces the risk of blindness (Table 29.2) (16). Other treatments include grid photocoagulation for diabetic macular edema and vitrectomy for diabetic vitreous hemorrhages.

Fairly well-defined protocols have been established for deciding who is an appropriate candidate for treatment. Hence, diabetic screening should be done on an annual basis by an ophthalmologist who is familiar with these protocols.

Carotid Artery Insufficiency

Because early diagnosis of carotid artery insufficiency and institution of anticoagulant therapy or endarterectomy can substantially improve the morbidity and mortality of this condition (17), it is important to maintain a high index of suspicion.

Two-thirds of patients with carotid occlusive disease present with ocular symptoms. About half these patients will have clearly associated neurologic symptoms on the contralateral side, but half will have ocular symptoms only. Amaurosis fugax is the hallmark symptom—the patient experiences a sudden, painless, transient loss of vision (usually less than 15 minutes), which clears gradually. Ordinarily, the loss is unilateral and caused by diminished flow in the ophthalmic artery. Very rarely, the patient with carotid artery disease experiences a contralateral homonymous field defect as a result of involvement of the middle cerebral artery. More usually, bilateral symptoms relate to the vertebral-basilar system.

Unilateral carotid occlusive disease can have a protective effect on the diabetic with hypertensive retinopathy. Hence, this condition should be considered in any patient with obviously asymmetric retinopathy.

Patients with significant carotid occlusive disease may demonstrate a carotid bruit, but Doppler ultrasonography is usually needed as a first step in evaluating the patient for carotid endarterectomy. Approximately one-third of patients who have TIAs will have a completed stroke within 5 years.

Glaucoma

Glaucoma is a disease primarily associated with aging; it is unusual in persons under the age of 40 but occurs with increasing frequency as persons grow older. Approximately 11.5 million people in the U.S. have glaucoma (18).

By definition, glaucoma is a disease manifest by increased pressure in the eye, which leads to damage to the optic nerve and to loss of vision. If untreated, glaucoma leads to progressive and irreversible loss, first of peripheral vision and, finally, of central vision (Figure 29.4). With treatment, the damage and visual loss can ordinarily be arrested; however, an optic nerve that has been damaged by glaucoma is more susceptible to further damage. Therefore, it is important to detect glaucoma in its early stages.

Because patients are not aware of intraocular pressure, and self-monitoring devices do not exist, it is advisable that all adults have an annual intraocular pressure check as part of their complete eye examination. This is especially indicated for blacks, diabetic patients, and persons with a family history of glaucoma, all of whom are more likely to develop glaucoma as they become older.

The diagnosis of glaucoma is made on the basis of increased cupping of the optic nerve head associated with characteristic visual-field defects. If the disease is detected early, the only manifestation may be an elevated intraocular pressure, although elevated pressure alone usually is not diagnostic, as the general population shows a wide variation in intraocular pressure. If the patient falls into a high-risk group (for example, a patient with diabetes), the ophthalmologist may elect to treat solely on the basis of a suspiciously high pressure.

Advanced glaucoma leads to a loss of the peripheral visual field. Some patients may maintain a small central field that allows them to read or watch television quite well. However, they remain disabled by the peripheral field loss because it limits their ability to walk or, for example, to notice someone entering a room, unless they happen to be looking directly at the doorway. (An impression of the effect of this deficit can be achieved by looking through a tube of cardboard or rolled paper and attempting to walk about, even in a familiar room.)

Glaucoma is ordinarily treated with topical medications. Beta-blockers such as timolol are the first line of treatment, and miotics such as pilocarpine are used if further treatment is needed. The latter is less satisfactory because its use leads to problems with pupil adaptation to changing lighting conditions, especially in patients with some cataract. Epinephrine compounds have been found

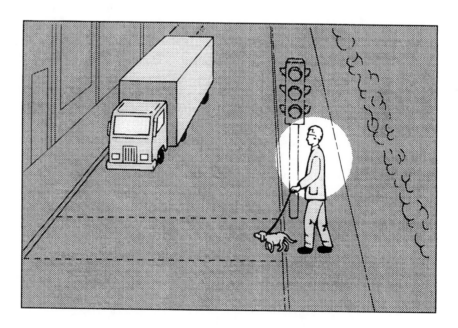

Fig. 29.4. In advanced glaucoma, only the object of immediate regard is in view. The rest is restricted.

useful. Oral carbonic anhydrase inhibitors, laser treatment, or surgery may be necessary if topical medications do not control the pressure.

Regular use of medication is critical to prevent further eye damage in patients with glaucoma. Elderly, forgetful, and confused patients often require some help and support to remember to take medications. This is especially true because the medication is prophylactic, and there is no obvious visual benefit noticed by the patient.

The medications used for glaucoma have considerable systemic side effects. For example, beta-blockers can exacerbate asthma, bradycardia, cardiac arrhythmias, hypotension, and impotence. Pilocarpine stimulates a cholinergic response in the gastrointestinal system with salivation, vomiting, cramps, and diarrhea, though this is relatively unusual. Carbonic anhydrase inhibitors not infrequently lead to anorexia, paresthesias, weight loss, impotence, renal stones, and depression.

Presently, a collaborative multicenter trial is under way in the U.S. to compare early surgery with medical treatment of chronic open-angle glaucoma. The rationale for this study is the common observation that some patients continue to have progressive damage from glaucoma in spite of an apparently adequate medical regimen, probably a result of problems with compliance with their glaucoma medication regimen.

Low Vision Service

Many sight-impaired patients are only partially blind and can benefit from a variety of low vision aids. These devices, such as convex lenses, telescopes, or closed-circuit television, improve visual performance by magnification, other nonoptical devices, such as large print books, reading stands, and electronic reading scanners with voice output, simplify visual tasks. The evaluation of the patient and an introduction to appropriate aids is often not available in the ophthalmologist's office. However, a local ophthalmological society can usually identify appropriate resources. It is important for the patient to have this experience in a supportive environment as the circumstances are by nature trying, expectations may be unrealistic, and the first step to rehabilitation should be a positive one.

To improve reading, magnification is usually necessary for the sight-impaired. The value of increasing the pa-

tient's lens strength is limited because only a certain amount of magnification can be achieved and most people find it uncomfortable to read at the necessary close range and to hold the material as steadily as needed. Consequently, hand magnifiers or stand magnifiers are often preferable, although this makes reading a two-handed task. The stooped posture required by these devices can be relieved somewhat by the use of a reading stand. The maximum useful magnification of hand magnifiers is limited by the fact that the visual field decreases as the magnification increases—thus, a person could read a sentence one letter at a time, but the task is difficult and unpleasant. To a certain extent, the problem of size of field can be solved by using closed-circuit television. These devices also have the advantage of being able to vary contrast and black-white polarity as each patient needs. However, these devices are not yet readily portable.

Another value of low vision services is in counseling the patient about ways that have proved effective in dealing with the disability. This can speed rehabilitation and also let the patient know that he or she is not alone in this plight.

Social Aspects of Vision Loss

The major effect of diminishing vision in elderly patients is loss of independence. Sight-impaired patients need help with many activities, such as driving, reading, hobbies, and work—activities that had given them pleasure and reinforced feelings of competence and personal value. Some patients may have to give up some of these activities entirely and learn to rely on others more than they have in the past. Consequently, these patients need to maintain, and even improve, their social skills. For some patients, this comes easily; for others, it is difficult, either because of ingrained personality traits or because of concomitant disabilities, especially deafness. In all cases, however, patients need a network of support to keep from withdrawing and becoming despondent.

Many sight-impaired patients are reluctant to ask for help for fear of being a burden or being taken advantage of. It is important, therefore, that they be in an environment that is automatically supportive. This may be a nursing home or retirement facility, but support can often be effectively arranged at home if services are scheduled and reliable, and if communication is regular. The arrangement of supports is generally beyond the responsibility of the physician, but he or she should be aware of the facilities available in the community so that referral can be made for patients and their families to the local sight center and social service agencies. In addition to the practical benefits (free phone directory assistance, Meals-on-Wheels, and so on), these efforts help patients to understand that they are not alone and that the community cares about them.

References

1. Pigman S, Yulo T, Schulz J. Possible roles of near UV light in the cataractous process. Exp Eye Res 1974;13:462.
2. Hollows F, Moran D. Cataract—the ultraviolet risk factor. Lancet 1981;2:1249.
3. Taylor HR, West SK, Rosenthal FS, et al. Effect of ultraviolet radiation on cataract formation. N Engl J Med 1988;319:1429.
4. Munoz B, West S, Bressler N, et al. Blue light and risk of age-related macular degeneration. Invest Ophthalmol 1990;32(suppl):49.
5. Rosenthal FS, Bakalian AE, Taylor HR. The effect of prescription eye wear on ocular exposure to ultraviolet radiation. Am J Pub Health 1986;76:1216.
6. Sliney DH. Physical factors in cataractogenesis: ambient ultraviolet radiation and temperature. Invest Ophthalmol Vis Sci 1986;27:781.
7. Kahn HA. The Framingham eye study: Outline and major prevalence findings. Am J Epidemiol 1977;106:17.
8. West S, Munoz B, Emmett EA, et al. Cigarette smoking and risk of nuclear cataracts. Arch Ophthalmol 1989;107:1166.
9. West SK, Munoz BE, Newland HS, et al. Lack of evidence for aspiring use and prevention of cataract. Arch Ophthalmol 1987;105:1229.
10. Ellingson FT. Explanation of 3M diffractive intraocular lenses. J Cataract Refract Surg 1990;16:997.
11. Hilton GF, Norton EWD, Curtin TV, et al. Retinal detachment surgery: a comparison of diathermy and cryosurgery. Bibl Ophthalmol 1969;79:440.
12. Framingham Monography. Surv Ophthalmol 1980;24(suppl):355.
13. Marshall J. Radiation and the aging eye. Ophthalmic Physiol Opt 1985;51:241.
14. Yanko L, Goldbourt U, Michaelson IC, et al. Prevalence and 15-year incidence of retinopathy and associated characteristics in middle-aged and elderly diabetic men. Br J Ophthalmol 1983;67:759.
15. Michaelson IC. Retinal circulation in man and animals. In: Retinal circulation in man and animals. Springfield, IL: Thomas, 1954:117–131.
16. Diabetic Retinopathy Study Group. Four risk factors for severe visual loss in diabetic retinopathy: The third report from the Diabetic Retinopathy Study. Arch Ophthalmol 1979;96:1518.
17. Frank G. Comparison of anticoagulation and surgical treatments of TIA and consolidation of recent national history and treatment studies. Stroke 1971;2:369.
18. National Advisory Eye Council. Vision research: a national plan, 1983–1987. vol 1. Bethesda, MD: National Institutes of Health, 1983.

Chapter 30
Oral and Dental Problems in the Elderly

Douglas B. Berkey and Jeffrey Astroth

Old fellows like ye'ersilf an' me make a bluff about th' advantages iv age. But we know there's nawthin' in it. We have wisdom, but we wud rather have hair. We have expeeryence, but we wud thrade all iv its lessons f'r hope an' teeth.

Finley Peter Dunne
"Books," Mr. Dooley Says

Men and women, by genetic design, are not intended to exit this world in a toothless (edentulous) state. Older adults should be able to enjoy a functioning, esthetic, and pain-free mouth. To provide the best medical care of patients, the physician must be aware of problems related to the oral cavity and work in collaboration with dental colleagues to maximize dental function and minimize tooth loss. The physician should more fully understand 1) how oral conditions may significantly influence general health and well-being, 2) the prevalence of oral problems and what can be done about them, 3) dental utilization patterns for older adults and how the medical team can help with this issue, 4) how to perform oral screening examination, and 5) how to interact with dental professionals in a referral and consultative fashion regarding medical-dental geriatric problems.

Systemic disease, the complications of therapeutic interventions, physical deficits, and cognitive impairments may act individually or in concert to undermine oral health. Because each problem has the potential for a significant deleterious impact on the mouth and ultimately to the patient's general well-being, the health care provider should view these health compromises as red flags requiring attention. If the practitioner properly identifies a dental problem, the dental team can be involved to provide an acceptable intermediate or long-term intervention. Knowledge-based interaction and coordinated referral between the medical and dental members of the health care team are essential in achieving and preserving oral health in the elderly population.

Quality of Life

Studies have reported that the elderly place significant importance on the role of oral health as a necessary condition for good quality of life (1). The importance of oral health includes the issues of chewing ability and food selection, esthetic appearance, and distinct speech. The loss of posterior teeth results in the reduction of occlusal tooth contacts and is negatively correlated with chewing efficiency (2). Further, Veterans Administration research indicates that individuals select food on the basis of the perceived ease of mastication (3,4). Therefore, a shift in dietary intake and, by implication, nutrition can be associated with a poorly perceived chewing ability.

The loss of posterior teeth or anterior teeth may also obviously influence an individual's appearance. If posterior teeth are lost and not replaced, the necessary support of the facial musculature may be compromised; this condition is known as a loss in the vertical dimension of occlusion. Typically, the individual elder will appear to have a vertically collapsed facial profile with poor lip support and associated angular cheilitis. Fixed dental bridgework, removable partial dentures, and complete dentures are therapeutic modalities designed to reestablish fully functional dentition at proper jaw relationships.

When anterior teeth are missing without suitable replacement, not only esthetics but also phonetics can be compromised. Distinct speech patterns are formed through the coordinated efforts of the lips, tongue, palate, and anterior teeth. Prosthodontic therapy to replace missing anterior teeth or to replace dysfunctional existing prostheses may enhance the desired incisive capacity of the anterior teeth during mastication. In addition, dental restoration of the anterior teeth can facilitate acceptable facial appearance and proper speaking ability.

Problems with chewing ability, esthetics, and speech are often well tolerated in the elderly population. However, it has been suggested that these problems may negatively alter the image and dignity of the affected individuals (5). In the eyes of family, friends, and health care workers, these elders may be perceived as lacking self-esteem and adequate quality of life. Proper oral evaluation, timely referral, and subsequent dental care have the potential to greatly improve the individual elder's quality of life and to reverse the misconceptions and presumptions of caretakers and health care workers.

Sequelae of Dental Problems and Treatment Solutions

Dental Caries

Problems

Bacterial plaque constitutes the etiologic agent in the formation of dental caries. These microorganisms thrive in an environment of readily metabolized carbohydrates, such as sucrose and other refined sugars. When these organisms are allowed to remain in contact with tooth structure because of poor oral hygiene, they are capable of significant acid production that demineralizes enamel, dentin, and cementum. This demineralization can occur within minutes of eating a sucrose-rich food. Coronal caries is defined as the destruction of the enamel-covered crown portion of the tooth; root caries is initiated in cementum or dentin, the structural components of the tooth root (Figure 30.1).

Historically, dental caries have not been a significant problem for the elderly population. However, national dental survey findings indicate a trend of increasing prevalence of decayed teeth in the 65 years or older age group (6–8). Caries prevalence is expected to increase over the next 3 decades for three reasons. First, there is greater retention in the number of teeth in the elderly population. Root canal therapy, long-term filling materials, sophisticated crown and bridge techniques, and periodontal therapy are responsible for saving teeth that in

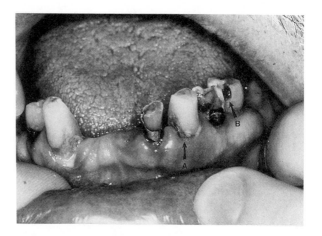

Fig. 30.1. Extensive root and coronal caries. A. root caries; B. coronal caries.

the past were routinely extracted. However, retained teeth are susceptible to dental caries. Second, the elderly are living longer. As the life span of our aged population continues to expand, the potential for tooth decay increases if teeth are subjected to poor dietary and oral hygiene habits for longer periods of time. Third, prevention strategies, such as drinking fluoridated water, using toothpaste with fluoride, and seeking preventive dental care have led to a dramatic decline in decay rates in younger populations. These individuals will enter old age with many more teeth than their predecessors.

Root caries are especially prevalent in the elderly. Research indicates that the frequency rate is 3.75 times greater in the elderly compared with that for younger age groups (8). In addition, the rate per tooth has been determined to be five times greater in those older than 65 years of age (8). Though much of root caries in the elderly can be attributed to poor oral hygiene and diets rich in readily metabolized sugars, there are several other notable predisposing factors. First, many elders demonstrate recession of the gingival (gum) tissues. Exposure of the root surfaces of the teeth allows microorganisms the opportunity to attack protective cementum and the underlying dentin. These structures are more vulnerable to dental decay because they are less mineralized than enamel. Banting et al reported that among a group of institutionalized older adults, 90 percent showed gingival recession and 83 percent had some root caries (9). Second, any condition or therapy that reduces salivary flow will significantly increase the likelihood of root caries and possibly periodontal disease. A dry mouth caused entirely by normal physiologic aging is not supported in the research literature (10,11). Rather, the side effects of various classes of medications, as previously mentioned, may be important causes of dry mouth. Polypharmacy and resulting interactions may increasingly suppress salivary flow rates. Radiation therapy to the head and neck areas may also permanently damage salivary glands and prevent the normal production and discharge of protective saliva.

Solutions

The key to controlling dental caries in the elderly rests firmly in the area of prevention. Adequate oral hygiene is fundamental. The teeth require brushing with a fluoride-containing toothpaste twice each day. Some technique for cleaning between the teeth is likewise essential, for example, the use of floss, toothpicks, or rubber tips. For those individuals with functional deficits (e.g., stroke, arthritis, or Parkinson's disease) simply grasping a thin toothbrush handle may be a major challenge. Handles are easily modified using aluminum foil or small rubber balls (Figure 30.2). For the cognitively impaired individual, often oral hygiene must be provided by a health care worker, family member, or friend. Access to the teeth for brushing may require the use of tongue depressors wrapped with gauze to literally separate the posterior teeth. Whatever the situation, effective and daily oral hygiene is essential.

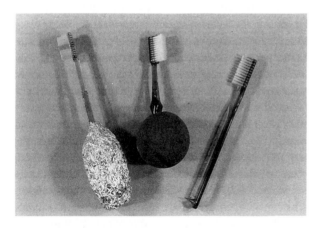

Fig. 30.2. Example of modified handles to aid effective toothbrushing.

Educating elders about the consequences of eating foods rich in highly refined carbohydrates may go a long way in preventing coronal and root decay. Dried fruits, soft drinks, mints, and other hard candies are often consumed without thought of the sugar content.

For elderly patients with significant caries, or those at risk of developing caries (e.g., after radiation therapy), additional fluoride therapy is suggested. Formulations include topical rinses and gels that can greatly fortify tooth structures. The use of fluoride solutions at bedtime have been shown to be very effective in preventing new dental caries and in initiating remineralization of existing carious lesions, thus causing a halt to the decay process (12). After 2 weeks of daily use, the concentration of intraoral fluoride reaches an equilibrium point and remains relatively constant between daily applications (13). Wescott et al reported a complete reduction of teeth lost to caries and a near total reduction of new caries in postradiation and institutionalized patients taking daily fluoride applications (14).

For elders with xerostomia, three therapeutic strategies should be considered. First, sucking on sugar-free mints or hard candies may help to stimulate salivary flow. Second, artificial saliva substitutes are commercially available in over-the-counter preparations. Although these seem efficacious, many patients object to the transitory nature of these preparations and the sensation they produce in the oral cavity. Water is the saliva-substitute of choice in many cases. Third, Fox et al suggest the use of the sialogogue pilocarpine hydrochloride (5mg three times a day) for xerostomia associated with Sjögren's syndrome, head and neck radiation therapy, or of unknown etiology (15). Pilocarpine was recently approved by the Food and Drug Administration for this use. It is important to note that its drug interactions are generally unknown at this time.

In terms of new innovations in restorative dentistry, materials that contain fluoride are now available to fill cavities. These materials combine plastics and a fluoride-containing glass isonomer compound. Used to restore root carious lesions, these fillings are tooth-colored, easily placed, and reportedly resistant to recurrent decay (Figure 30.3). The caries resistance may be a direct function of the slow release of fluoride ions from the filling material.

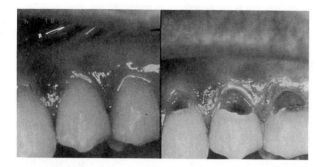

Fig. 30.3. Before and after restoration of root caries with fluoride-containing tooth-colored material. (Courtesy of Fuji Corporation)

Periodontal Disease

Problems

Although much of dental therapy in the past has been directed toward the treatment of dental caries, periodontal disease, which affects the bone and soft tissues supporting the teeth, remains a major etiologic component for the loss of adult teeth. A variety of microorganisms work in concert to create the inflammation of gingival tissue and the destruction of alveolar bone, the hallmarks of periodontal disease. The bacteria propagating the disease are abundant in the dental plaque typically found along the junction of tooth and gingival tissue. Calculus deposits (tartar) along the inside of the lower anterior teeth and the outside of the upper posterior teeth are common contributors to the gingival inflammation. Often characterized as asymptomatic and progressive, periodontal disease may show periods of rapid bone destruction, followed by periods of quiescence.

The clinician can identify periodontal disease by recognizing halitosis, tooth mobility, gingival recession, and edematous, reddish to blue gingival tissue that bleeds with little provocation (Figure 30.4). The elderly population appears to be at significant risk. Data collected in a 1985 to 1986 national survey suggest that 88 percent of the dentate elderly clearly show signs of gingival recession, and approximately one-half of the population demonstrate gingival bleeding (8).

Solutions

A primary strategy for addressing periodontal disease is meticulous oral hygiene. Brushing, interproximal clean-

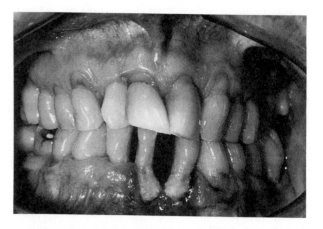

Fig. 30.4. Gingivitis and attachment loss associated with advanced periodontitis on lower incisors.

ing, and rinsing with chemotherapeutic agents can effectively control the progression of moderate disease. Surgical and nonsurgical (scaling, root planing) therapies have been developed and successfully implemented as treatment approaches for many patients. However, for the physically or cognitively compromised older patient, daily oral hygiene and chemotherapeutic regimens may be the treatment of choice. A recent advance in chemotherapeutic agents has been the use of 12% chlorhexidine oral rinses. Chlorhexidine is an efficacious, bacteriocidal agent, available by prescription, that has been shown to significantly reduce the occurrence and severity of gingivitis, which is usually a precursor to irreversible periodontal bone loss. Older adults at risk should be encouraged to use an appropriate chemotherapeutic agent on a daily basis to facilitate prevention or to control periodontal disease.

Tooth Loss

Problems

In the past, edentulism was considered a natural and unpreventable consequence of aging. However, there has been a dramatic alteration of this perception. Public awareness, education, increased access to dental care, emphasis on prevention, and community fluoridation of drinking water supplies have contributed to a significant decline in edentulism. Before 1957, the prevalence of edentulism in the United States for individuals 65 years of age and older was 60 percent (16,17). By 1986, national studies reported a reduction to 41 percent in total tooth loss (8,17). When the results are stratified by age, the 65- to 69-year-olds showed 32 percent edentulism, and those older than 80 years had a 49 percent prevalence rate (8).

Many adverse outcomes are associated with total tooth loss. From a functional standpoint, the occlusion of dentures must be precise and accurately refined to provide even the 20 percent efficiency dentures can furnish compared with natural dentition. For persons without dentures or teeth, foods that are difficult to chew may be routinely avoided, such as vegetables and meat. From an external viewpoint, an individual without teeth appears to have a collapsed facial musculature, a protruded lower jaw, loss of lip support, and a general hollow, sunken facial appearance. Elders without teeth may feel old and useless and lack a sense of wholeness and self-esteem. Often these individuals complain of their appearance, but remain resistant to dental therapy without the encouragement of family, friends, or the medical team. A referral to the dentist can be the beginning of a renewed interest in socialization and vigor for life for an isolated elder.

Solutions

Modern dentistry has refined many useful techniques for replacing missing teeth. When some of the natural teeth remain, fixed bridgework or removable partial dentures may be fabricated to restore the oral cavity to normal form and function. For individuals without natural teeth, complete dentures or modifications of dentures continue to represent the treatment option of choice.

Complete Dentures

Problems

Complete dentures without semi-rigid fixation to the underlying tissues will always be a poor substitute for natural dentition. The potential for tissue trauma, poor masticatory ability, unacceptable esthetics, and candidal infestation of the acrylic denture bases are among the many and varied problems that accompany denture wearing (Figure 30.5).

A fundamental problem, well documented by Tallgren, is the phenomenon of residual ridge resorption of the bone supporting the denture bases (Figure 30.6) (18). This

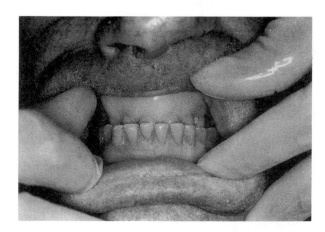

Fig. 30.5. Extremely worn dentures with associated poor fit and impaired masticatory function.

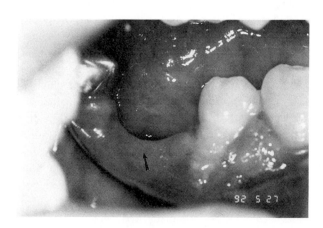

Fig. 30.6. Example of mandibular ridge bone resorption as a result of tooth extractions.

continual process is responsible for the poor fit of most dentures after a few years of use. Lack of stability and retention of denture bases typically compromise masticatory function, speech ability, and general appearance. The continual bony ridge changes coupled with the normal wearing down of prosthetic teeth can also head to obvious loss of the vertical dimension of occlusion (i.e., apparent loss of facial height) (5).

Solutions

Dentures should be maintained very much like natural

dentition. Because denture sores often go unnoticed, a dental examination of the denture patient should be completed at least once a year. Often a simple denture adjustment can greatly improve the individual's ability to use the dentures effectively. For ill-fitting, nonfunctional dentures, the option to remake or reline the dentures should be explored. The denture wearer can also be educated at the annual examination. Specifically, proper care and cleansing of the dentures should be stressed. Brushing the dentures twice daily with a commercial denture toothpaste or simple soap and water removes food debris and dental plaque. In addition, the dentures should be soaked in a commercially available denture cleanser for at least 12 minutes each day to destroy the microorganisms, including candida yeast cells, that typically inhabit the denture acrylic (plastic). Denture hygiene is especially important because candidiasis beneath the denture bases is the most common cause of a denture sore mouth. The reddish, edematous nature of the oral mucosa under a denture base is the most common manifestation of this condition. No adverse outcomes have been measured from a patient's failure to remove dentures at night before sleeping, although most practitioners suggest allowing the oral tissues adequate rest at some point during each 24-hour period. Infrequent removal of dentures may produce such problems as papillary hyperplasia, epulis fissuratum, and other inflammatory responses.

Not all complete dentures must be supported totally by the underlying mucosa. Overdentures are a special type of complete denture fabricated to fit over retained teeth that have undergone root canal therapy. The benefits are improved stability and retention of the denture, preservation of the supporting alveolar bone, and proprioception provided by the periodontal ligament lining the bony socket of the retained tooth root.

This same principle applies to the newest of prosthetic innovations: dental implants. These titanium root-form, intrabony implants provide all the benefits of overdentures. Research conducted worldwide now confirms the fact that dental implants have more than a 90 percent success rate (19). Complete dentures can be fastened to dental implants with greatly improved masticatory efficiency (Figure 30.7). Comparison of maximum biting force between standard complete dentures and implant-retained dentures showed a mean increase of

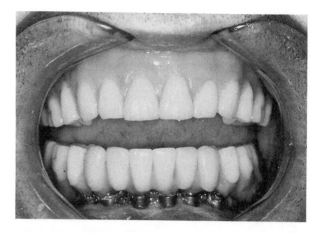

Fig. 30.7. Typical mandibular denture stabilized and retained by intraosseous dental implants.

12.0 lbs, a 47 percent increase, of biting force after implant therapy (20).

Other new developments in denture therapies include reline materials used in the dental office, adult day care, or long-term care facility. Semi-permanent (2 years' duration) reline preparations allow the dentist to perform a valuable service in less than 1 hour. The required equipment can easily be transported to the desired site. Additional adjuncts to improving the function of complete dentures are denture adhesives. Commercially available creams, pastes, and powders are effective agents to help retain and stabilize dentures. No adverse consequences have been substantiated with their usage, although most individuals complain of the messy nature of the materials. Caution should be exercised if an elder is using a home reline or home repair kit or adhesive gauze pads. The repair and reline kits available over-the-counter are typically misused and may result in poorer fitting, more traumatic prostheses. Adhesive gauze pads, designed to retain and stabilize dentures, may or may not be changed daily as recommended. If left inside the denture base, these pads become a nidus for candidal infections and reinfection and set up a cycle of inflammation in the oral tissues that continues unresolved.

Use of Dental Services

If no pain or deformity exists, pathologic oral conditions

may persist for years in the elderly without being evaluated by a dentist. The 1985 to 1986 national dental survey reported that only 37.5 percent of those older than 65 years of age had seen the dentist within the previous year (8). If these findings are stratified by dentition status, 54.5 percent of individuals with teeth had a dental visit, but only 13.0 percent of denture wearers sought annual dental care. Perhaps the most disturbing revelation from these data is the fact that almost half the denture wearers had not seen a dentist for more than 5 years. The potential for oral pathology, dysfunctional prostheses, facial collapse, and compromised mastication in this group of elders should be a major concern to the geriatric care team. Many dental services are not covered under any Medicare, Medicaid, or private insurance plans (only 17 percent are covered for persons age 65 and older) (21). Although for some elderly lack of insurance coverage presents no substantial financial hardship, the situation represents a major barrier to care for 28 percent of older Americans who are poor or near poor (e.g., below 150% percent of poverty threshhold) (22).

The need for dental care seems to be only a fair predictor of the demand for dental care in view of the fact that oral problems are usually distributed throughout the socioeconomic strata of the elderly. As Bailit and Wilson suggest, most public health specialists consider the lack of perceived need for dental care to be a more substantive reason for the low use of dental care services by the elderly (23). Another plausible explanation is the substitution of medical visits for dental visits because of more critical medical concerns and conditions. Poor access to dental services may also hinder use. Access may be influenced by any or all the following factors: lack of accessible, affordable transportation; general financial barriers; and lack of committed providers in long-term care facilities, adult day care centers, and home-bound settings. Whatever the reasons for poor rates of use of dental care, early diagnosis and treatment of oral pathology, dental caries, and periodontal disease remain essential to the maintenance of adequate general health and decent quality of life.

Physician's Role in Oral Assessment

Many elderly patients are unaware or apathetic about pathologic conditions that present in the oral cavity. Broken or chipped teeth may not cause notable irritation or pain; teeth with periapical or periodontal lesions may be asymptomatic; draining fistulas and soft tissue lesions may be tolerated without complaint or simply exist unnoticed for months or longer. The physician can play an invaluable role in uncovering oral problems and encouraging patients to seek appropriate dental care. Analysis of a recent survey of more than 12,000 noninstitutionalized U.S. citizens showed that only 13.3 percent of the group older than 65 years of age reported ever having had an oral examination for cancer (24). Respondents stated that 23 percent to 35 percent of such examinations were performed by physicians or as part of a routine physical examination (24).

Because more elderly persons seek regular medical care than dental care (75 percent versus 60 percent), the physician may have the initial or only opportunity to evaluate conditions in the patient's oral cavity (25). In fact, a panel of health care experts recently endorsed routine oral cavity examination by physicians for all individuals older than age 65 (26). Two expert panels also advocate physician-initiated oral hygiene instruction as an essential element of periodic health counseling of adults (26). Assessment provided by direct questioning and oral examinations should be used to identify oral problems that need resolution.

Assessment

The dental interview should include questions regarding past dental experience and the date of last dental evaluation. The elderly often ignore symptoms that they view as inconsequential or mildly disruptive. Through the use of specific questioning strategies, however, the practitioner can gather pertinent information about the patient's oral cavity. The physician's decision to refer a patient to the dentist may often be made simply on the basis of the patient's history. As a rule of thumb, any geriatric patient who has not visited the dentist within 1 year should be referred for dental evaluation.

Suggested questioning (closed-ended format) should be directed toward general mouth discomfort, pain or irritation in any soft tissue area of the mouth, mouth dryness, bad breath, altered taste sensation, pain/clicking or popping in the temporomandibular joints, difficulty in chewing or biting, and bleeding gums (27). For patients with some or all of their remaining dentition, the physician should ask questions regarding toothaches, loose teeth, missing fillings or crowns (caps), broken teeth with or without irritation, and food entrapment between teeth. The interviewer should question geriatric individuals wearing partial or full removable dentures about the comfort, efficiency, stability, and retention of the prosthesis. A word of caution: many elders report that their dentures function adequately even though oral tissues may be traumatized and the stability and retention of the dentures are severely compromised.

Examination

Although discomfort may motivate most elders to seek dental care, pain may or may not be present during routine office evaluation. Therefore, the physician or medical staff member should be proficient in providing a thorough extraoral/intraoral examination. The extraoral examination should begin with the skin of the head and neck. Even a cursory inspection may uncover epidermal lesions suggestive of basal cell carcinoma, the prevalence of which significantly increases with age. Further examination should evaluate skeletal form (facial profile, symmetry, and jaw position); the neck by digital palpation to assess lymphadenopathy associated with preauricular, parotid, submandibular, posterior cervical, and supraclavicular nodes; ears for referred mandibular pain, or myofascial pain dysfunction syndrome; paranasal sinuses for referred pain to the maxillary molars and bicuspids; breath to check poor oral hygiene resulting in halitosis, chronic periodontal disease, or abscessed tooth; parotid gland for enlargement or tenderness; and the temporomandibular joints and associated musculature for tenderness, crepitus, clicking, deviation of the mandible upon opening and closing, or trismus.

To assess pain or dysfunction in these joints, a simple two-part examination should be performed. The physician can evaluate externally the temporomandibular joints by digitally compressing the skin of the patient's face approximately 1 inch anterior to the external auditory meatus. With the fingers in position, ask the patient to open widely and evaluate the presence of pain, clicking, or grating in the joint apparatus. The second part of this examination is performed by placing the tips of the

little fingers into the external auditory meatus so that the fleshy side of the digit is against the posterior element of the joint capsule (i.e., finger-tips positioned anteriorly in the ear canal). Pain, clicking, or grating on full opening of the mandible may indicate temporomandibular pathology. Referral to a dentist is suggested when findings are clinically notable.

The intraoral examination should begin with a careful inspection of the patient's lips for any ulcerated or discolored lesions suggestive of malignant change. The lips should be evaluated using bidigital palpation to determine the presence or absence of lumps or bumps beneath the epithelium. The examiner should also assess the angles of the mouth for compromised epithelial integrity, salivary drooling, and evidence of inflammation caused primarily by *Candida albicans*. These features, typically termed angular cheilosis, may indicate a collapsed facial profile and unsupported facial musculature that result from worn-down natural dentition or worn-out dentures. Proper vertical support for the facial musculature can be achieved only by restoring the occlusion of the posterior teeth, natural or artificial. If the vermilion borders of the lips disappear when the patient closes teeth together, the probability is extremely high that the patient has lost vertical facial support. Again, in general, the bite needs to be assessed by the dentist.

A thorough intraoral examination requires excellent visualization of oral structures. Any removable prosthesis (e.g., complete or partial dentures) should be removed. This may be accomplished by the use of tongue depressors, 2 × 2 gauze squares, and a good light source. The following sequence is suggested for the intraoral examination: 1) turn the buccal mucosa of the cheeks toward the light source for good inspection; 2) examine all surfaces (dorsal, ventral, lateral sides) of the tongue by wrapping a 2 × 2 gauze around the end of the tongue and asking the patient to stick the tongue out of the mouth (Figure 30.8); 3) while the gauze is around the patient's tongue, check the floor of the patient's mouth because the tongue and floor of the mouth are the most common sites for intraoral squamous cell carcinoma; 4) after removing the gauze, palpate the floor of the patient's mouth by placing a finger in the mouth and one hand under the chin and lower jaw—any lump or bump of unknown origin should be evaluated by a dentist; and 5) carefully illuminate and inspect

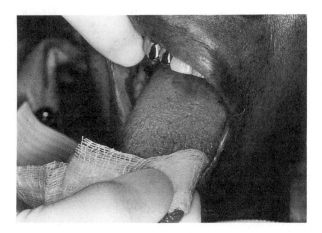

Fig. 30.8. Manipulation of the tongue with gauze to facilitate a thorough oral examination.

the patient's palate and oropharynx. Any red, white, or red-white mucosal lesion (sore, ulcer, or growth), painful or not, of unknown duration should be considered cancerous until proved otherwise. An assessment of the relative dryness of the patient's mouth should also be made. If a pool of saliva does not form in the floor of the mouth during examination, the patient is likely to have salivary dysfunction. Visual assessment also includes inspection of the alveolar mucosa apical to the tooth roots for swelling, fistulous tracts or both; the periodontium for gingival inflammation, bleeding, or purulent exudate; the teeth for lost fillings and crowns, gross caries (especially on exposed root surfaces), and mobility, tenderness, or pain; and removable prostheses for faulty speech patterns, poor fit, discomfort, and general defects (e.g., missing teeth, broken prostheses, or sharp, rough edges).

Geriatric Problems: Medical-Dental Considerations

The dentist may contact the physician to better understand the implications of systemic diseases on oral health and how to more safely manage the frail or functionally dependent geriatric patient.

Oral Cancer
Oral cancer continues to be a significant threat to the elderly. Within the United States, 5 percent of male malig-

nancies and 2 percent of female malignancies have been attributable to oral carcinomas (28,29). Survival is greatly reduced in patients with advanced disease at diagnosis. As Figure 30.9 graphically depicts, oral cancer increases with age (28). When lesions are small and localized, about 75 percent of oral cancer patients survive for 5 years, but prognosis drops to 40 percent with regional stage and to 17 percent with distant stage involvement (29). Early detection and referral are extremely important.

Clinical presentations of oral cancer might include tissue enlargement or thickening; red or white plaques that cannot be rubbed off the tissue; other discolorations, such as dark brown or black patches suggesting melanoma; ulceration that persists beyond 2 weeks after alleviating possible irritants; chronic numbness, pain, or sore throat; repeated bleeding; tongue or jaw movement restriction; dry mouth; or loose teeth or notable change in the fit of removable prostheses. Persistent changes in color, texture, or surface elevation should be considered malignant unless proven otherwise. Cofactors associated with the incidence of oral cancer include age, tobacco use, and alcohol consumption (30,31). Therefore, the alert physician or other nondental health care provider plays a crucial role in recognizing these typically asymptomatic lesions and making referrals when appropriate.

Cardiac Disease
Medications associated with controlling hypertension and heart disease may negatively impact oral health. Antihypertensive medications such as diuretic and alpha$_2$ agonists classically produce reduced salivary flow. Because saliva reduces the numbers of microorganisms in the oral cavity, both dental caries and periodontal diseases may be accelerated in patients receiving these medications. Reduced salivary flow also tends to compromise the proper fit and comfort of both complete and partial dentures.

Older patients who are taking medications to control heart rate, rhythm, and contractility may be at risk for adverse effects caused by local anesthetics containing epinephrine used in dentistry. A commonly asked question is which anesthetic is appropriate for the elderly patient with heart or circulatory conditions. The American Heart Association guideline states that no more than 0.04 mg of epinephrine should be administered at a single

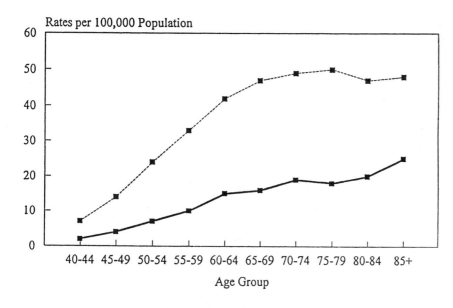

Fig. 30.9. Incidence and mortality rates per 100,000 population for cancer of the buccal cavity and pharynx.

dental appointment for patients with a history of myocardial disease (32). The most commonly used epinephrine-containing local anesthetics are 2% lidocaine with 1:100,000 epinephrine (2 capsules maximum) and 0.5% bupivacaine with 1:20,000 epinephrine (4 capsules maximum). An additional local anesthetic, 2% mepivacaine with 1:20,000 levonordefrin, is commonly used because the vasoconstrictor (levenordefrin) exhibits less potential for raising blood pressure than does epinephrine. All vasoconstrictors are used to prolong the effect of local anesthesia by limiting the entry of the anesthetic into the circulation. However, extreme caution must be exercised in administering the vasoconstrictor-containing local anesthetics to patients with a history of hypertension, atherosclerotic heart disease (ASHD), cerebral vascular insufficiency, and heart block. Also at risk of significant blood pressure fluctuations are patients taking monoamine oxidase (MAO) inhibitors, tricyclic antidepressants, and phenothiazines. Perhaps the best approach to addressing this issue is simply to use a local anesthetic such as 3% mepivacaine without a vasoconstrictor, especially if prolonged anesthesia is not necessary.

Many elderly patients tolerate a variety of dental interventions without local anesthesia; therefore, prolonged use of local anesthetics is seldom required. Geriatric dosage reductions are recommended on the basis of the 70 percent or greater decrease in lidocaine metabolism that occurs from the third to seventh decade of life (33). In general, because of diverse individual variation in drug metabolism, specific dosage reductions should be individualized for the geriatric population (Table 30.1).

Elderly patients actively taking anticoagulants are clearly at risk for excessive bleeding if dental surgical interventions are required. Medications that place the geriatric patient at greatest risk are aspirin and other nonsteroidal anti-inflammatory drugs (NSAIDS) (prolonged bleeding time for 1 week after last dose), warfarin (4 to 5 days of prolonged anticoagulation after last dose), and heparin (active for 5 hours after intravenous dose or 1 day after subcutaneous dose). Consultations between physician and dentist is paramount to the proper management of these patients.

Diabetes Mellitus

The geriatric diabetic patient does not effectively resist infection in the oral cavity. Recent research suggests that poorly controlled insulin-dependent diabetes mellitus patients are susceptible to significantly more loss of gingival attachment, loss of supporting bone around

Table 30.1. Local Anesthetics Used for Dental Procedures.

Agent	Amount of Injection (mg)[a]	Vasoconstrictor	Amount of Injection (mg)	Maximum Number[b]
Lidocaine 2%	36	1 : 100,000 epinephrine	0.018	8 (4.4 mg/kg)
Mepivacaine 2%	36	1 : 20,000 levonordefrin	0.09	8 (4.4 mg/kg)
Mepivacaine 3%	36	none	none	5.5 (4.4 mg/kg)
Bupivacaine 0.5%	9	1 : 200,000 epinephrine	0.009	10 (1.3 mg/kg)

[a] 1.8-ml cartridge.
[b] For 70-kg healthy adult.
SOURCE: Reproduced by permission from Berkey DB, Shay K. General dental care for the elderly. In: Baum BJ, ed. Clinics in geriatric medicine. Philadelphia: Saunders, 1992:591.

the teeth, generalized gingivitis, and gingival pocket bleeding than are controlled insulin-dependent patients (34,35). In addition, postsurgical healing for simple dental extractions may be compromised. A coordinated decision between physician and dentist is essential to determine whether antibiotic therapy may be required to enhance healing. For more complex procedures, such as multiple tooth extractions, periodontal surgery, or both, the ability of the patient to maintain a proper diet during healing may be compromised. Consequently, management of the patient's nutritional requirements, healing potential, and control of postoperative infection must involve a coordinated effort of both medical and dental care providers.

Head and Neck Cancer with Radiation Therapy

The patient who has head or neck cancer treated with radiation may experience severely reduced salivary flow. Typically, the effects of the radiation are permanent and the likelihood that these patients will develop rampant root caries or other complications is extremely high. Consultation with the dental team before the patient undergoes radiation therapy is mandatory for pretherapy and posttherapy management of this potential problem. Dental surgical consultations and preventive dental strategies (i.e., topical fluoride therapy and saliva substitutes) are essential considerations.

Long-Term Corticosteroid Therapy

An elderly patient may be taking a long-term course of corticosteroids for chronic obstructive lung disease, severe arthritis, or myeloproliferative disorders. Corticosteroid therapy may result in two dental problems. First, patients demonstrate considerable susceptibility to

oral infection from *candida albicans* and the oral mucosa may be especially prone to trauma from ill-fitting dentures. Second, because dental interventions may be particularly stressful for an elderly patient, he or she can be at risk of acute adrenal insufficiency. Management should be individualized for each patient according to the specific corticosteroid regimen. Routine dental procedures such as examinations, cleanings, fillings, and removable prosthodontic procedures may require only modest or no change in drug therapy. Conversely, complex procedures such as prolonged crown or bridgework, extractions, periodontal surgery, or root canal therapy mandate the adjustment of steroid dosages on the basis of recommendations of the physician.

Prevention of Infective Bacterial Endocarditis

The high prevalence of cardiac conditions in this age group should highlight the need for better understanding of dental issues. The prevention of infective endocarditis is the major concern associated with rheumatic heart disease and cardiac murmurs. Dentists should routinely consult with physicians regarding the need for antibiotic prophylaxis in patients with murmurs and conditions such as mitral valve prolapse (MVP). Transient bacteremias occur after procedures as commonplace as brushing and flossing. For surgical dental interventions, the incidence of procedurally induced bacteremia is considerable (Table 30.2). Patients with valvular or other structural heart disease are at risk of developing subacute bacterial endocarditis. The *Journal of the American Medical Association* has published guidelines for the administration of prophylactic antibiotic coverage for patients at risk. Any dental procedure that may induce gingival or

Table 30.2. Incidence of Procedurally Induced Bacteremia in Oral and Dental Procedures.

Procedure	Positive Blood Cultures (%)
Chewing	12–51
Brushing	24–26
Flossing	20
Oral irrigation device	7–50
Oral prophylaxis	28–40
Subgingival scaling	8–84
Gingivectomy	32–83
Periodontal flap surgery	50–88
Extraction	12–86

SOURCE: Reproduced by permission from Berkey DB, Shay K. General dental care for the elderly. In: Baum BJ, ed. Clinics in geriatric medicine. Philadelphia: Saunders, 1992:594.

Table 30.3. Antibiotic Prophylaxis for Prevention of Infective Bacterial Endocarditis after Dental Procedures.

Antibiotic	Dose and Regimen
Amoxicillin	3 gm 1 h before procedure, 1.5 gm 6 h after initial dose
For patients allergic to penicillin antibiotics:	
Oral erythromycin ethylsuccinate	800 mg 2 h before procedure, 400 mg 6 h after initial dose
or	
Oral erythromycin stearate	1 gm 2 h before procedure, 500 mg 6 h after initial dose
or	
Oral clindamycin	300 mg 1 h before procedure, 150 mg 6 h after initial dose

SOURCE: Reproduced by permission from Dajani AS, Bisno AL, Chung KJ, et al. Prevention of bacterial endocarditis. Recommendations by the American Heart Association. JAMA 1990;264:2919.

mucosal bleeding (e.g., professional cleanings, surgical interventions, incision and drainage of infected tissues, and intraligamentary injections) should be preceded by antibiotic therapy in patients having previous history of bacterial endocarditis; most congenital malformations of the heart; rheumatic and other acquired valvular dysfunction; hypertrophic cardiomyopathy; and mitral valve prolapse with regurgitation (36).

A dentist should always contact the patient's physician when uncertainty exists regarding the appropriateness, duration, or choice of antibiotic. Table 30.3 presents the recommendations of the American Heart Association for prophylactic antibiotic coverage for patients at risk of infective bacterial endocarditis.

Patients with Prosthetic Joint Replacements

Although most septic prosthetic joints are the result of staphylococci organisms that rarely inhabit the oral cavity, oral pathogens possess the capability to infect prosthetic joint replacements. Because of this inherent microbial capability, invasive dental procedures could result in a potentially infective bacteremia. The American Dental Association and the American Academy of Oral Medicine suggest that the decision to provide prophylactic antibiotic therapy for this class of dental patients be made on the basis of dentist-physician consultation (37). Each patient must be assessed individually. The consultation between orthopedic surgeon and dentist should be completed before any invasive dental treatment for the

patient (38). In addition, patients with prosthetic joints who acquire dental infections should be aggressively treated with antibiotics (37). Commonly, diabetic patients and patients with a history of rheumatoid joint disease receive insurance coverage for extractions and periodontal surgery. Although orthopedic surgeons vary in their antibiotic of choice, Jaspers and Little report oral cephalosporins to be the preferred drugs (39).

Polypharmacy

Many geriatric patients typically consume 10 to 12 prescription medications every day. Though the medical indications for therapy may be appropriate, the interaction between medications and salivary production and flow can be considerable. Classes of chemotherapeutic agents that may induce reduced salivary flow include analgesics, anticonvulsants, antiemetics, antihistamines, antihypertensives, antinauseants, antiparkinsonian agents, antipruritics, antispasmodics, and appetite suppressants. The xerostomic effects of these medications compromise the saliva's natural ability to dilute and cleanse the oral cavity of opportunistic microorganisms. Elderly patients taking one or more xerostomic-inducing medications are at risk for developing significant root caries and possibly peri-odontal disease in the same manner as happens with irra-diated patients. The geriatric individual wearing an oral prosthesis (e.g., full or partial denture), may also experi-ence trauma to the oral mucosa and difficulty in maintain-ing proper denture retention. Saliva is essential in providing a layer of lubrication between the prosthesis and oral mucosa and thereby minimize tissue trauma. Saliva is also essential in providing a liquid medium that ensures the seal of the prostheses against the mucosal tissues, which enhances stability and retention of the dentures.

In the course of dental care, most dental practitioners will have occasion to prescribe additional medications for their elderly patients. For example, the anxious patient may require a sedative/hypnotic preparation, infections may require antibiotic therapy, and pain medication may be indicated after oral or periodontal surgery. Therefore, if the treating dentist has need to prescribe medication beyond what the older adult is currently taking, a consul-tation with the patient's physician remains the best course of action.

Functional Deficits

Poststroke paralysis, Parkinson's disease, and joint de-formities of arthritis represent a class of physical impair-ments that greatly affect a patient's ability to care for the oral cavity. All such patients should be thoroughly evalu-ated to assess their ability to perform adequate oral hygiene. Typically, these patients have considerable difficulty holding a toothbrush, effectively positioning the toothbrush, and performing any adjunctive hygiene procedures such as flossing.

Cognitive Impairments

Clearly, the cognitively impaired patient represents a con-siderable challenge to both physician and dentist. The practitioner's inability to communicate with the patient may compromise the simplest of dental interventions. The patient with Alzheimer's disease or the severely de-pressed patient may be incapable of providing an accu-rate medical history, discussing a chief complaint, understanding oral hygiene instructions, or the rationale for care. Typically, care of the oral cavity is neglected. Without the dedicated help of a friend, family member, or caretaker, these patients may receive no oral health care. The patient's ability to understand dental interventions may also be totally compromised, and informed consent must be obtained from individuals empowered to make decisions for the patient. Management of the patient with Alzheimer's disease often requires a team approach to perform even the most rudimentary oral examination. Dental care treatment plans and management techniques must be coordinated between the medical and dental teams. Proactive dental interventions and coordinated management regimens have the potential to provide ad-equate oral health as one aspect of quality of life for the cognitively impaired elder.

Summary

Oral health is an important criterion for successful aging. The physician can play an important role in helping to maintain or improve the oral health status of older adults by understanding dental problem etiologies and treat-ment interventions, encouraging better use of dental serv-ices, performing routine dental screening exams and oral health education during physician visits, and seeking ac-tive involvement with dental colleagues to better manage geriatric medical-dental patient concerns.

References

1. Berkey DB, Call RL, Loupe, MJ. Oral health perceptions and self-esteem in non-institutionalized older adults. Gerodontics 1985;1:213–216.
2. Manly RS, Shiere FR. The effect of dental deficiency on mas-tication and food preference. Oral Surg Oral Med Oral Pathol 1950;3:674–685.
3. Wayler AH, Muench ME, Kapur KK, Chauncey HH. Masti-catory performance and food acceptability in persons with removable partial dentures, full dentures and intact natural dentition. J Gerontol 1984;39:284–289.
4. Chauncey HH, Muench ME, Kapur KK, Wayler AH. The effect of the loss of teeth on diet and nutrition. Int Dent J 1984;34:98–104.
5. Gordon SR. Oral and dental problems. In: Schrier RW, ed. Geriatric medicine. Philadelphia: Saunders, 1990:129–137.
6. National Center for Health Statistics. Decayed, missing, and filled teeth in adults, United States, 1960–1962. Series 11, No. 23. DHEW Publ. No. 1000. Washington, DC: Public Health Service, 1967.
7. National Center for Health Statistics. Decayed, missing, and

filled teeth among persons 1–74 years, United States. Series 11, No. 223, DHHS Publ. No. 81-1673. Hyattsville, MD: Public Health Service, 1981.

8. National Institute for Dental Research. Oral health of United States adults. The national survey of oral health in US-employed adults and seniors: 1985–1986. DHHS Publ. No. 87–2868. Washington, DC: National Institutes of Health, 1987.

9. Banting DW, Ellen RP, Fillery ED. Prevalence of root surface caries among institutionalized older persons. Community Dent Oral Epidemiol 1980;8:84–88.

10. Baum BJ. Evaluation of stimulated parotid saliva flow rate in different age groups. J Dent Res 1981;60:1292–1296.

11. Atkinson JC, Fox PC. Salivary gland dysfunction. In: Baum BJ, ed. Clinics in geriatric medicine. Philadelphia: Saunders, 1992:499–511.

12. Billings RJ, Brown LR, Kaster AG. Contemporary treatment strategies for root surface dental caries. Gerodontics 1985; 1:20–27.

13. Duckworth RM, Morgan SN, Murray AM. Fluoride in saliva and plaque following use of fluoride-containing mouthwashes. J Dent Res 1987;66:1730–1734.

14. Wescott WB, Starcke EN, Shannon, IL. Chemical protection against post-irradiation dental caries. Oral Surg Oral Med Oral Pathol 1975;40:709–719.

15. Fox PC, Atkinson JC, Macynski A, et al. Pilocarpine for treatment of salivary hypofunction: a six-month trial. J Dent Res 1989;68:315.

16. Bureau of Economic Research and Statistics. Utilization of dental services by the elderly population. Chicago: American Dental Association, 1979.

17. National Center for Health Statistics. Edentulous Persons, United States, 1971. Vital and Health Statistics, Series 10, No. 89. DHEW Publ. No. (HRA)74–1516. Washington, DC: Public Health Service, 1974.

18. Tallgren A. The continuing reduction of the residual alveolar ridges in complete denture wearers: a mixed-longitudinal study covering 25 years. J Prosthet Dent 1972;27:120–132.

19. Adell R, Lekholm U, Rockler B, Branemark, PI. A 15-year study of osseointegrated implants in the treatment of the edentulous jaw. Int J Oral Surg 1981;10:387–416.

20. Carr AB, Laney WR. Maximum occlusal force levels in patients with osseointegrated oral implant prostheses and patient with complete dentures. Int J Oral Maxillofacs Implants 1987;2:101–108.

21. Olsen, ED. Dental insurance and senior Americans. J Am Coll Dent 1991;58:22–25.

22. Moon M. The economic situation of older Americans: Emerging wealth and continuing hardship. In: Maddox G, Lawton P (eds). Varieties in Aging: Annual Review of Gerontology

and Geriatrics. New York: Springer, 1988.

23. Bailit HL, Wilson AA. Dental services in the elderly population. In: Holm-Pedersen P, Loe H, eds. Geriatric dentistry. Copenhagen: Munksgaard, 1986:386–392.

24. Centers for Disease Control and Prevention. Examinations for oral cancer–United States, 1992. MMWR 1994;43(11):198–200.

25. Burt BA, Ekland SA. The public served by dentistry. In: Dentistry, dental practice, and the community. 4th ed. Philadelphia: Saunders, 1992:11–22.

26. Sox, HC. Preventive health services in adults. N Engl J Med 1994;330:1589–1595.

27. Berkey DB, Shay K. General dental care for the elderly. In: Baum BJ, ed. Clinics in geriatric medicine. Philadelphia: Saunders, 1992:579–597.

28. Bhasker SN. Synopsis of oral pathology. 5th ed. St. Louis: Mosby, 1977.

29. Shklar G. Oral pathology in the aging individual. In: Toga CJ, Nandy K, Chauncey HH, eds. Geriatric dentistry. Lexington, MA: Lexington Books, 1979:127–145.

30. Katz RV, Meskin LH: The epidemiology of oral diseases in older adults. In: Holm-Pedersen P, Loe H, eds. Geriatric dentistry. Copenhagen: Munksgaard, 1986;221–237.

31. Graham S, Dayal H, Rohrer T, et al. Dentition, diet, tobacco, and alcohol in the epidemiology of oral cancer. J Natl Cancer Inst 1977;59:1611–1618.

32. American Heart Association Council on Dental Therapeutics. ADA and American Heart Association joint report: management of dental problems in patients with cardiovascular disease. J Am Dent Assoc 1964;68:533–535.

33. Malamed SF. Handbook of Local Anesthesia, 2nd ed. St. Louis: Mosby, 1986.

34. Safkan-Seppala B, Ainamo J. Periodontal conditions in insulin-dependent diabetes mellitus. J Clin Periodontol 1992; 19:24–29.

35. Seppala B, Ainamo J. A site-by-site follow-up study on the effect of controlled versus poorly controlled insulin-dependent diabetes mellitus. J Clin Periodontol 1994;21:161–165.

36. Dajani As, Bisno AL, Chung KJ, et al. Prevention of bacterial endocarditis. Recommendations by the American Heart Association. JAMA 1990;264:2919–2922.

37. American Dental Association Council on Dental Therapeutics. Management of dental patients with prosthetic joints. J Am Dent Assoc 1990;121:537–538.

38. Shrout MK, Scarbrough F, Powell BJ. Dental care and the prosthetic joint patient: a survey of orthopedic surgeons and general dentists. J Am Dent Assoc 1994;125:429–434.

39. Jaspers MT, Little JW. Prophylactic antibiotic coverage in patients with total arthroplasty: current practice. J Am Dent Assoc 1985;111:943–948.

Chapter 31
Lower Extremity Problems in the Elderly

Jeffrey M. Robbins

Forty years on, growing older and older,
Shorter in wind, as in memory long,
Feeble of foot, and rheumatic of shoulder
What will it help you that once you were strong?

E. E. Bowen, 1836–1901
English Schoolmaster

Barring any congenital defects, the human foot is essentially normal at birth. Modern society mandates that the foot be shod and placed on hard, flat, unyielding surfaces for growth, development, work, and recreation. The result is progressive pedal deformity in many cases. It has been estimated that 85 percent to 95 percent of all people over the age of 65 suffer from some type of painful foot condition severe enough to limit ambulation. The rate of physical decline increases once an individual loses the ability to walk (1).

The human foot is subjected to considerable trauma. Macrotrauma in the form of severe trauma (sprains, strains, contusions, lacerations) and microtrauma (walking, running, inappropriate shoe gear) play a role in the development of foot deformity. The key to successful aging is the prevention of pathology and the preservation of function. The clinician must recognize that pedal pathology is most often slowly progressive in nature. The identification of the early signs and symptoms of foot deformity is essential for the prevention of painful deformity and the preservation of optimal function through timely podiatric intervention.

Scope of Podiatric Medical Practice

Podiatric medical practice involves the management, both medically and surgically, of foot and ankle conditions. This includes the pedal manifestations of systemic diseases but not the systemic disease itself. The components of podiatric practice include podiatric primary medicine, podiatric orthopedics and biomechanics, and podiatric surgery. Specialty residency training and recognized board certification exist for primary podiatric medicine, podiatric orthopedics and biomechanics, and podiatric surgery. In addition, board certification is available in podiatric public health.

Podiatric Primary Medicine
Podiatric primary medicine was defined in 1991 by the American Board of Primary Orthopedics and Primary Podiatric Medicine as the podiatric medical specialty concerned with the comprehensive and continuous foot care of individuals and families. It integrates the biological, clinical, and behavioral sciences and is not limited by age, sex, or disease entity. Primary podiatric medicine encompasses first contact, continuous care, long-term care, comprehensive care, and competence in scientific podiatric and general medicine.

Podiatric Orthopedics and Biomechanics
Podiatric orthopedics and biomechanics is defined as the podiatric medical specialty concerned with the mechanic function of the foot and lower extremity. It attempts to control foot and lower extremity function to optimize ambulation and limit deformity. The podiatric physician uses biomechanic foot orthoses, accommodative foot orthoses, appropriate shoe gear and shoe modifications, exercise, and other nonsurgical methods to control foot function and prevent deformity.

Podiatric Surgery
Podiatric surgery is defined as the specialty of podiatric medicine concerned with the operative management of pedal pathology.

Pedal Manifestations of Systemic Disease
Most elderly patients present with one or more chronic

degenerative conditions. The most common of the disease states that result in pedal complications are diabetes, cardiovascular diseases, peripheral vascular diseases, and the arthritides. Each of these common conditions can result in pedal pathology, which places the patient at great potential risk if the conditions are not managed properly (2).

Diabetes

The biostatistics of diabetic foot disease speaks for the absolute necessity of early podiatric preventive interventions. Of approximately 35,000 nontraumatic amputations, 17,000 to 26,000 (50% to 75%) have been a result of diabetes. In diabetic patients who have undergone an amputation, an additional 67 percent will have another limb amputation within 5 years. The overall survival rate for diabetics with gangrene is 45 percent (3–5).

The four pedal manifestations of diabetes are, ischemia, neuropathy, immunopathy, and infection. These four complications are interrelated and negatively synergistic.

Ischemia

The ischemia associated with diabetes is atherosclerotic in nature. It is generally present in diabetics at an earlier age than it is in the nondiabetic population, but the pathologic process is essentially identical (4,20). The major pedal complication of greatest concern is gangrene, which is intimately associated with neuropathy, immunopathy, and infection.

Whether the ischemia associated with diabetes is macrovascular or microvascular is controversial. Evidence exists to support both viewpoints, and both entities must be considered when examining the diabetic patient (3–5,20). This is especially true for the patient with microvascular disease, which is readily apparent in a patient with nonpalpable pulses because the circulation to the digits is diminished. However, in the patient with palpable pedal pulses the possibility of small vessel disease should not be dismissed without an assessment of the digital circulation. This can be accomplished by performing toe pressures with use of the photoplethysmograph probe and a digital cuff. Toe pressures are generally 5 to 10 mm Hg less than brachial pressures. Pressures less than 30 mm Hg indicate a serious decrease in blood flow (6,7).

Diabetic Neuropathy

The second pedal complication of diabetes is neuropathy. Diabetic neuropathy can be further divided into sensory, motor, autonomic, and neuroarthropathy.

Sensory Neuropathy Sensory neuropathy can result in a number of symptom complexes. The gradual loss of sensation in the foot is the most limb-threatening. The insensitive foot has lost its protective sense and is vulnerable to foot trauma that often goes unnoticed until signs of infection are present. Distal symmetrical polyneuropathy presents in the lower extremity with symptoms such as pain, burning, pruritis, numbness, and tingling. The distribution of these symptoms is generally stocking and glove. Symptoms are more profound in the evening (8).

Motor neuropathy Acute diabetic motor neuropathy in the form of mononeuropathy multiplex (proximal amyotrophic neuropathy) is rare and involves asymmetrical proximal muscle weakness that leads to gait disturbances. More commonly, chronic distal symmetrical polyneuropathy exhibits motor manifestations that result in small muscle wasting and absent reflexes in the lower extremity (8).

Diabetic autonomic neuropathy The manifestations of autonomic neuropathy in the diabetic patient affect the gastrointestinal, cardiovascular, thermoregulatory, and genitourinary systems. The major lower extremity manifestation is anhydrosis, which leads to chronic xerosis (dry skin) that has a propensity to crack and fissure. This condition sets up an ideal breeding ground for both bacterial and fungal infection.

Neuroarthropathy The diabetic patient with severe sensory neuropathy is susceptible to neuroarthropathy (Charcot's foot). This is a progressive, destructive arthritis mainly of joints of the midfoot, although metatarsal, phalangeal, and ankle joints can also be invovled (9). One or more joints may be involved. In the poorly controlled diabetic, the disease state is a continuous cycle of trauma–sensory neuropathy, followed by joint degeneration, subluxation, joint fractures, and osteochondral fragmentation. Later, joint debris is absorbed and subchondral osteoporosis with adjacent sclerosis occurs. Autonomic neuropathy may play a role in neuroarthritis by causing an increase in blood flow to the area, which leads to active bone resorption. Early in this process the midfoot may look slightly swollen, erythematous, and be warm to the touch. As this process develops, the midfoot collapses and forms a "rocker bottom" appearance (Figure 31.1).

Immunopathy

The chronic hyperglycemic state is also said to impair the immunologic response. It is theorized that the chronic hyperglycemic state interferes with the macrophages and other phagocytizing leukocytes. The result is decreased ability to fight infection (10,11).

Infection

The diabetic patient is especially susceptible to foot infections caused by combinations of concomitant ischemia, neuropathy, and immunopathy. Whether hyperglycemia causes the infection or the infection causes the blood sugar to rise has not been definitively determined. Strict glycemic control has been suggested as the best defense against all manifestations and is an essential factor in resolving foot infections (10,11).

Diabetic Ulceration

Probably the most common pedal infection associated with diabetes is the diabetic ulcer that has become secondarily infected (Figure 31.2). Initially presenting under or over a prominent bony structure such as metatarsal heads, hammer digit, or the heel, the ulceration, once infected, can involve soft tissue and bone and result in gangrene and amputation.

Peripheral Vascular Disease

Generally, the first symptom of peripheral vascular disease is intermittent claudication. Pain that is reproducible walking the same distance and that is relieved with standing rest, is the criterion used to differentiate this symptom from other causes of leg pain. The most common site is the calf, followed by the arch, thigh, and buttocks. Intermittent claudication is a symptom, not a diagnosis. The underlying diagnosis is occlusive vascular disease, most commonly atherosclerosis. In severe arterial disease, pain in the foot at rest, especially at night, is a common finding. Placing the foot in a dependent position may provide temporary relief. If pain is severe enough to limit ambulation, referral to a vascular surgeon is warranted. See also chapter 37.

Arterial Disease

Lower extremity arterial disease is usually a chronic insidious, progressive, degenerative problem caused by genetic factors as well as preventable factors. Genetic factors may predispose a patient to arterial disease; however, diet, exercise, and smoking are controllable preventable risk factors for arterial disease. The patient with arterial occlusive disease presents with clinical signs (Table 31.1).

As the most distal appendage from the heart, the foot is vulnerable to the effects of reduced circulation (Figure 31.3). Simple lacerations and injuries to the foot can become limb-threatening infections because of the lack of blood flow that not only reduces nutrition to distal tissues and the immune response system, but also decreases

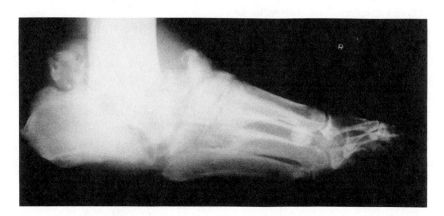

Fig. 31.1. X-ray of a Charcot's foot with complete destruction and collapse of the midfoot.

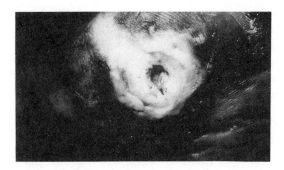

Fig. 31.2. Diabetic neurotrophic ulceration. Notice the characteristic hyperkeratotic tissue surrounding the ulcer.

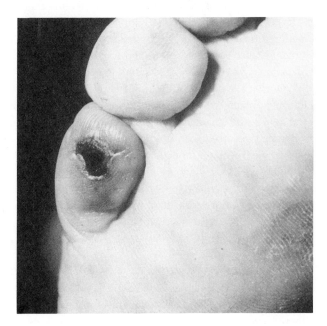

Fig. 31.3. Blue toe syndrome, micro emboli to the fifth digit from a proximal occlusion.

Table 31.1. Pedal Signs of Arterial Disease.

Absent or barely palpable pulses (dorsalis pedis and posterior tibial)
Pallor on elevation
Rubor on dependency
Capillary filling time >5 seconds in the elevated position
Thin, shiny, dry skin
Ankle–arm index less than 1.0

the amount of antibiotic treatment that can be delivered to the site.

Effects of Smoking

The general public is well aware that cigarette smoking, both active and passive, causes heart disease and lung cancer. However, according to the 1990 Surgeon General's Report on cigarette smoking (12), only 15.6 percent of patients are aware of the relationship of cigarette smoking and peripheral vascular disease. Cigarette smoking has such a profound effect on the peripheral vasculature that it is considered the single most important risk factor (and preventable cause) of occlusive vascular disease. It is theorized that cigarette smoke damages arterial intima and causes relative hypoxia. Once damaged, the tunica intima is more susceptible to the formation of atheroma (12).

Patients with arterial disease should be seen on a regular schedule for both primary care and secondary prevention. Regular care for nails and hyperkeratotic lesions is mandatory for this risk group. The prescription and fabrication of accommodative orthotic devices can help to maintain safe ambulation and protect sites of irritation. The use of pentoxifylline and walking programs has been used to encourage the development of collateral circulation. In some cases, surgical intervention may be necessary for pedal pathology if conservative methods fail and if the patient has acceptable circulation for healing (13).

Venous Diseases

The venous diseases most often affecting the lower extremity include varicose veins, superficial thrombophlebitis, deep thrombophlebitis, and chronic venous insufficiency. The venous system is divided into three components: the superficial venous system, the communicating venous system, and the deep venous system. Each system has bicuspid valves that allow blood to flow back in a cephalic direction only. When valves are damaged, they lose their ability to stop retrograde flow, and distal edema results. Valvular incompetence can result from varicose veins, superficial thrombophlebitis, deep vein thrombosis, pregnancy, and certain abdominal masses (14,15).

Varicose veins Varicose veins of the lower extremity are

dilated, tortuous, superficial veins that protrude. Symptoms include aching, swelling, a feeling of heaviness, and pruritis. The exact etiology is unclear, but inherent weakness of the superficial veins, a genetic predisposition, and pregnancy seem to play important roles in development. Complications of varicose veins include stasis dermatitis, cellulitis, venous ulceration, brawny edema, and induration (14–16).

Management of varicosities includes light to medium support hose and elevation for mild cases, pneumatic compression pumps and moderate to heavy support hose for moderate cases, and referral for vein stripping in severe cases that do not respond to other conservative therapies (14–16).

Superficial thrombophlebitis Trauma and prolonged inactivity can cause a tender red cord along the course of a varicose or other superficial vein. The area, directly over the vein, is slightly warm, red, and edematous. Treatment includes warm moist packs, nonsteroidal anti-inflammatory drugs (NSAIDs), and elevation and support hose for mild cases, and bed rest in addition to intermittent warm packs and elevation if the thrombosis is more extensive (14–16).

Deep vein thrombosis Deep vein thrombosis is a medical emergency that requires immediate hospitalization. Patients generally present with severe leg pain, generalized lower extremity edema distal to the occlusion, elevated systemic temperature, and constitutional symptoms. The most life-threatening complication is pulmonary embolism (14–16).

Chronic venous insufficiency A complication of deep venous thrombosis is the destruction of the venous valves that prevent blood from retrograde flow distally. Once this occurs, a symptom complex develops, progressively known as chronic venous insufficiency, postphlebitic syndrome, or chronic venous stasis. Because of stasis of blood in the distal tissues, several complications can occur. Soft, puffy, transient edema generally occurs at the end of the day. The edema will respond if treated early, but allowed to progress unchecked, it will ultimately become indurated and resistant to compression therapy. Stasis dermatitis results from chronic stasis of venous blood and results in the deposition of hemosiderin in the lower leg and a characteristic eczema. This creates a brown skin discoloration and scaling type dermatitis. Induration is

the hard type of edema that is a result of subcutaneous fibrosis secondary to chronic edema. Ulceration of the lower leg is also common in venous stasis. It is most commonly found just above the medial malleolus. Pain is an inconsistent finding in chronic venous insufficiency. It is most commonly associated with a feeling of heaviness secondary to the physical congestion in the lower extremity.

Management of chronic venous insufficiency is directed at reducing edema and induration with moist compresses and compression therapies, topical medications for any dermatitis, and wound care for ulceration (15,16).

Lymphedema

Lymphedema is a form of lower-extremity edema that results from obstruction of the lymph system. The obstruction can be inflammatory, noninflammatory, or congenital. Because both the venous and lymphatic systems work against gravity, prolonged standing taxes these systems. During the course of the day even properly functioning lymphatic systems will leak some fluid into the distal tissues and cause a very mild edema. This edema is very quickly reversed with simple elevation. In the early stages of obstructive lymphedema, the edema is reversible with elevation, but as the obstructive process progresses, the edema requires more aggressive treatment such as compression therapy in the form of over-the-counter support hose, custom support hose, and compression pumping (15,16).

Vasospastic Disorders

The arterioles and capillaries of the digits have their own means of regulating flow, independent of arterial flow. Although capillaries have no real capacity to constrict, the arterioles act as valves to control blood flow to the capillaries. Vasospasticity is the result of sympathetic neuromuscular stimulation from several different causes, such as mental stimulation, endocrine stimulation, external cold stimulation, previous cold injury, and repetitive microtrauma (17).

The most commonly diagnosed vasospastic disease is Raynaud's syndrome, characterized by color changes to fingers, toes, or both on exposure to cold. The initial color change is white and occurs while the part is exposed to cold. This stage is generally pain free. Color then changes to red, representing rebound arteriolar vasodilatation, and blue, representing venous dilatation. Pain, burning and, pruritis symptoms are noticed during these two color changes.

Raynaud's syndrome is divided into two entities: 1) Raynaud's disease, which is characterized by Raynaud's symptoms in the absence of a secondary causal condition; and 2) Raynaud's phenomena, which is characterized by Raynaud's symptoms associated with a secondary disorder such as rheumatoid arthritis, systemic lupus erythematosus, scleroderma, or arteriosclerosis obliterans (15,17).

Treatment for Raynaud's syndrome is focused on prevention and, for Raynaud's phenomena, in the control of the secondary disorders. Patients are instructed to keep their feet warm and protected from the cold. Prolonged exposure to cold, especially damp, cold environments, should be avoided. Shoes, boots, and socks should be loose fitting. Calcium channel blockers such as nefedipine and diltiazem have been found to be effective in preventing and treating vasospastic episodes. Biofeedback has been used to treat Raynaud's disease and allows the patients to regulate their own digital blood flow through muscular relaxation. For intractable cases that fail to respond to conservative therapies, sympathectomy may be considered (15–17).

Acrocyanosis Acrocyanosis is a vasospastic disorder characterized by a bluish discoloration seen year round, although it is generally worse in colder weather. This condition can be primary and idiopathic or secondary to a connective tissue disease. Patients present with blue discoloration to hands and feet that are cold. The condition has usually been present for years.

Management includes the use of appropriate warm clothing for protection, avoidance of cold, control of psychogenic factors (if present), and control of underlying connective tissue disease (15–17).

Livedo reticularis Patients with livedo reticularis present with a reddish-blue discoloration in a mottled or reticular pattern on the extremities and, sometimes, the trunk. This condition can present in a primary or idiopathic type or secondary to a connective tissue disorder. Although this condition is generally benign, a severe form called livedo vasculitis can present with cutaneous ulcers (15–17).

Pedal Manifestations of the Arthritides

The foot is especially susceptible to the effects of the various arthritides. Regardless of the basic etiology, the trauma the foot is subjected to–from flat, hard, unyeilding surfaces, ill fitting shoes, abnormal foot biomechanics, progressive foot deformities, and obesity–potentiates the degenerative effects of the arthritides.

Rheumatoid Arthritis

Rheumatoid arthritis (RA) is a chronic, systemic, inflammatory disorder affecting joints and other organ systems. The disorder may be mild or severe and typically presents with exacerbations and remissions that ultimately result in progressive joint destruction. This disorder is highly variable in presentation and severity and generally manifests itself in the fourth decade of life (1,18,19,21). Although inconsistent, symptoms include morning stiffness, joint pain, limitation of motion, and signs of inflammation (heat, warmth). The joint symptoms may be preceded by generalized systemic symptoms such as fatigue, anorexia, weight loss, weakness, and generalized aching and stiffness. Lower extremity involvement can be seen in the metatarsal, phalangeal, ankle, and knee joints. Common foot deformities of RA include hallux valgus, subluxation of the metatarsal heads, lateral deviation of the toes, and hammering of the toes, clawing of the toes, or both.

X-ray changes of RA can involve the entire foot but usually not the distal interphalangeal joints. Fusiform, soft-tissue swelling may be present. Juxta-articular osteopenia, uniform narrowing of the joint spaces, and bone erosions occur near the attachments of the joint capsule. The erosions are usually found on the medial margins of the metatarsal heads, although erosions of the lateral aspect of the fifth metatarsal head is often an early sign. Calcaneal spur formation at both the retrocalcaneal bursa and at the attachment of the plantar aponeurosis is common (18,19,21).

Treatment for the pedal complications of RA include accommodative palliation for the foot, surgical correction of existing deformities if they are severe enough to limit ambulation, and the traditional progressive treatment protocols for the systemic condition (1,18,19,21). Shoe modifications and foot orthosis to limit or retard progression of deformities, accommodate existing lesions, and generally maintain optimum ambulation are discussed later.

Osteoarthritis

Osteoarthritis, osteoarthrosis, or degenerative joint disease is the most common of the arthritides affecting the foot. Symptoms include pain and stiffness that develop slowly and progress to joint enlargement and loss of joint motion. Pain occurs after use of the joint and is relieved with rest. Pain on passive range of motion with joint crepitus is common as the disease progresses. Heberden's nodes at the distal interphalangeal joint and Bouchard's nodes at the proximal interphalangeal joints may be seen and represent dorsolateral and medial osteophytes. The disease can be seen in most people 65 years of age and older.

Characteristic changes of osteoarthritis include osteophyte spur formation at joint margins, cyst formation in juxtaarticular bone, and secondary synovitis that can become chronic and result in gross deformity and subluxation of joints. X-ray changes include joint space narrowing of distal interphalangeal joints, subchondral sclerosis, and osteophyte formation at the margins of joints. Common deformities of the foot are hallux valgus, saddle bone deformity, hammer toe syndrome, digital spur formations at various sites, and calcaneal spur formation.

Treatment includes periodic debridement of painful lesions, reduction of trauma to the foot by use of appropriate foot gear, accommodative orthotics to control progression of deformities, and surgical correction of existing deformities if conservative therapy fails and the deformities are severe enough to limit ambulation (1,18,19,21).

Diffuse Idiopathic Skeletal Hyperostosis

Diffuse idiopathic skeletal hyperostosis (DISH) is a common skeletal disorder of the elderly and produces both spinal and extraspinal changes. It is seen in 5 percent to 10 percent of the population older than 65 years. This disorder may confuse the diagnosis of RA or osteoarthritis because of the tendency to develop bony proliferation enthesopathies at the attachments of ligaments and tendons. Common sites in the foot include the tarsal and metatarsal areas and calcaneal spurs (18).

Gout

Gout is a uric acid crystal deposition disorder that affects joints, periarticular tissues, and the kidneys. The most commonly affected joint is the first metatarsal phalangeal joint (MPJ) (75% of initial cases). Manifestations of the gout syndrome include acute, recurrent, severe articular and periarticular inflammation of the first MPJ, tophaceous deposits or accumulations of uric acid crystal in various tissues, and renal complications.

An acute gouty attack is characterized by a sudden severe swelling with erythema and pain of the first MPJ or, on occasions, of other joints such as the heel, ankle, and knee. The pain is so severe that the patient may say that even the bed sheet causes severe pain. The condition is self-limiting and usually subsides with a few days to 2 weeks.

Definitive diagnosis can only be made from examination of the joint aspirate, which will demonstrate negatively birefringent crystals (18). Serum uric acid levels have not been found to be a good predictor of gout. X-ray findings early in the disease may show only soft-tissue swelling, but chronic gout will display round bony erosions with a sclerotic margin. Erosions may be intraarticular or periarticular with a thin overhanging edge of bone. Joint spaces are usually maintained until late in the disease.

Treatment of gout includes addressing the immediate acute episode and then the systemic condition. Acute gouty attacks can be treated with 0.5 to 0.6 mg of colchicine per hour until symptoms resolve or gastric upset occurs. The total dose should not exceed 6 to 8 mg/day. Colchicine can also be given intravenously, which usually negates gastrointestinal complications. Other NSAIDs can also be used to treat acute gouty arthritis. The most popular today is 50 mg of indomethacin given 3 to 4 times daily.

In some cases of chronic gout, the first MPJ becomes chronically enlarged and shoe modifications and foot orthosis may be necessary to improve function. Surgical intervention may be considered if severe deformity limits the patient's ability to ambulate (18–21).

Structural and Biomechanic Deformities

Structural deformities are common in the elderly. A lifetime of weight bearing on hard surfaces, degenerative joint disease, and possible genetic predisposition results in progressive deformation of the foot. In addition, improperly fitted shoe gear adds another etiologic factor.

Hallux Valgus

Deformity of the first ray (hallux and first MPJ) can occur in three planes. In the transverse plane, the hallux can deviate laterally and the first MPJ migrates medially. In the frontal plane, the hallux rotates in a valgus position. In the sagittal plane, the first ray may be dorsiflexed or plantarflexed.

Abnormal foot function causes compensatory muscular stabilization that results in this progressive deformity. When the first MPJ becomes prominent, a bursal sac may develop medially and become inflamed and painful (Figure 31.4). Arthritis in the first MPJ can result in painful range of motion, restricted range of motion, or joint fusion that makes ambulating difficult.

Tailor's Bunion

The fifth ray can also undergo deformation and result in a medial migration of the fifth toe and a lateral migration of the fifth metatarsal. The fifth MPJ is then subjected to the development of painful bursitis, joint arthritis, and loss of normal range of motion and function.

Treatments include conservative accommodation that attempts to arrest and retard the progression of deformity and relieve pain. Surgical intervention may be appropriate when conservative methods fail to provide pain relief and acceptable functional ambulation. Although the elderly have an increased incidence of structural deformities of the foot, primary and secondary preventive interventions should be directed toward young and middle-aged groups to prevent this progressive deformity. Controlling the function of the foot on unyielding surfaces helps to slow the progression of structural deformities (18,19).

Hyperkeratosis

One of the great ironies of the aging foot is that although aging muscle tissue is replaced with fat in most parts of the body, the plantar fat pad that protects the foot from pressure and friction associated with ambulation, atrophies or migrates distally and effectively reduces the protection under the metatarsal heads. This leads to increased pressure and friction to the osseous structures and overlying skin and produces hyperkeratotic tissue. Later, the subcutaneous tissues develop adventitious bursa that act as an additional buffer to protect the underlying bone. As this condition progresses, local nerves can hypertrophy within the soft tissues and capsular structures and cause entrapments and painful ambulation.

The presenting symptom of most hyperkeratotic lesions is pain and discomfort. Hyperkeratotic tissue, by itself, is not painful. The underlying bursitis or neuroma

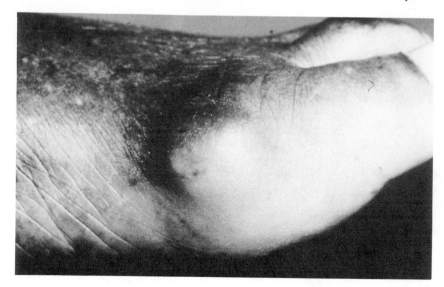

Fig. 31.4. Inflamed bursal sac overlying the medial aspect of the first metatarsal phalangeal joint.

or neuritis is responsible for the pain associated with hyperkeratotic lesions (19,20).

Hammer Digit Syndromes

Years of improper foot biomechanics commonly cause progressive deformities to the digits in the elderly. Three distinct types of deformity have been identified–hammer toe, claw toe, and mallet toe. The hammer toe exhibits dorsiflexion of the proximal phalanx on the metatarsal head, plantarflexion of the middle phalanx on the proximal phalanx, and the distal phalanx neither dorsiflexed nor plantarflexed (Figure 31.5). The claw toe differs from the hammer toe in that the distal phalanx is also plantarflexed (Figure 31.6). The mallet toe appears straight except for the distal phalanx, which is plantarflexed (Figure 31.7).

Helomas

Deformities of the toes, coupled with shoe pressure and osteophyte formation, can result in painful lesions of the digits and are referred to as helomas (corns). Helomas are areas of hyperkerotic tissue that occur over these bony

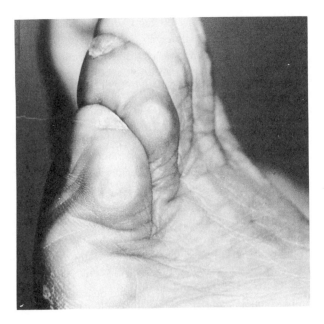

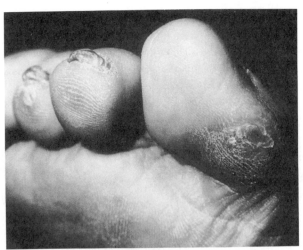

Fig. 31.6. Claw toe 4 and 5 with overlying heloma durum.

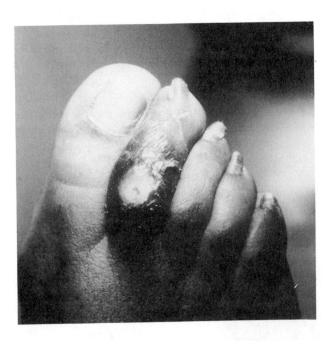

Fig. 31.5. Hammer toe second digit with joint inflammation and small ulceration dorsally.

Fig. 31.7. Mallet toe with overlying hyperkeratotic tissue of the distal aspect. A hyperkeratotic lesion is seen over the medial plantar aspect of the interphalangeal joint of the hallux.

projections and prominences. Histologically, the stratum corneum is hypertrophic in a conic shape, with the apex toward the basement membrane (19). As a result of constant trauma, sublesional bursa and nerve impingement are common (Figure 31.8).

Table 31.2. Heloma Descriptions, Locations, and Treatments.

Name	Location	Description	Treatment
Heloma durum	Dorsal aspect of the (DIPJ) and (PIPJ), and over other bony prominences	Hard, circumscribed area of hyperkeratosis	1. Conservative: regular palliation and paddings, latex shields 2. Surgical correction of underlying pathology
Heloma molle	Medial or lateral aspect of the digits	Macerated hyperkeratosis	1. Conservative: regular palliation and paddings, latex shields 2. Surgical correction of underlying pathology
Heloma vasculare	Dorsal aspect of the DIPJ and PIPJ and over other bony prominences	Blood vessles found within the heloma itself	1. Conservative: gentle debridement 2. Surgical removal
Heloma miliare	Dorsal or plantar foot	Small plug not related to bone; may be related to shoes and or xerosis	1. Conservative: debridement followed by use of emollients 2. Change of shoe gear or spot stretching of shoe
Heloma neuro vasculare	Dorsal aspect of the DIPJ and PIPJ and over other bony prominences	Both nerves and blood vessles found within the heloma itself	1. Conservative: gentle debridement 2. Surgical removal

DIPJ = distal interphalangeal joint; PIPJ = proximal interphalangeal joint.

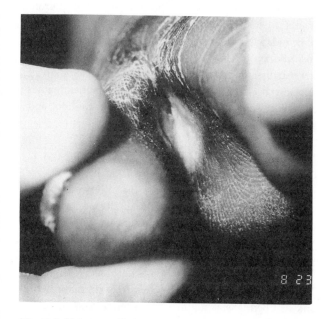

Fig. 31.8. Heloma molle between digits 4 and 5 with hyperkeratotic tissue formation on adjacent sides.

Tylomata

Tyloma (calluses) are accumulations of hyperkeratotic tissue found under or over areas of intermittent pressure and friction. They are commonly found over bony prominence, the plantar areas under the metatarsal heads, base of the fifth metatarsal, and the heel. These lesions can range from very mild to severe, and they may significantly limit the patient's ambulation. In the compromised patient, these lesions can lead to ulceration.

Intractable Plantar Keratoma

Often a conic-shaped keratotic plug may be found within a tyloma. This especially hard, painful lesion forms in response to excessive pressure from hypertrophied or prominent bony structures. Called an intractable plantar keratosis because of its resistance to conservative treatment, these lesions can be very painful (Figure 31.9).

Treatment for plantar hyperkeratotic conditions includes periodic debridement, accommodative or biomechanic orthoses, and surgery if conservative therapy fails to control pain and limits ambulation (20).

401

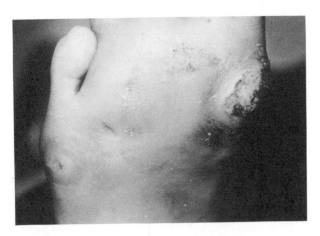

Fig. 31.9. Intractable plantar keratosis sub 5 metatarsal head. Notice the nucleated core in the center of the lesion. Preulcerative keratosis sub 1 metatarsal head.

Heel Spur Syndrome and Plantar Fasciitis

Heel pain is a common presenting complaint of the elderly. The usual causes are lack of shock absorption, atrophy of the plantar fat pad, and plantar fascial strain (19,20). Heel spur syndrome is a symptom complex characterized by morning pain and stiffness of the heel and posterior plantar fascia, which improves with weight-bearing after the patient arises in the morning, but becomes progressively more painful by the end of the day. Returning to weight-bearing after short periods of rest during the day can cause the pain and stiffness to return.

Presumably, the etiology of this symptom complex involves a chronic inflammatory process of the insertion of the plantar fascia at the inferior anterior calcaneous (Figure 31.10). Chronic inflammation develops because of abnormal foot mechanics and lack of shock absorption. It has been suggested that an adventitious bursa develops under the plantar fascia, or that small fibers tear off the insertion of the plantar fascia at its insertion and result in inflammatory changes (19,20). Left untreated, symptoms can continue to progress from minor discomfort to profound pain that can limit the patient's ability to ambulate.

Treatment for heel spur syndrome and plantar fasciitis is directed toward pain relief and control of the mechanical causes. Physical modalities such as ultrasound and electrical stimulation, padding and tapping, NSAIDs, steroid injections, and orthotics are conservative thera-

pies. Surgical intervention is considered after all conservative therapy has failed to relieve symptoms.

Neuroma

Shoes and abnormal biomechanics of the foot can result in excessive irritation to the nerves of the foot. This results in a benign hypertrophy of the nerve and can cause distal pain and burning, tingling, or both in the areas served by the involved nerve. The most commonly affected nerve is the intermetatarsal nerve in the third inner space, but any nerve subjected to chronic irritation can be affected (19,20).

Treatment for neuroma is directed toward pain relief and reducing the size of the neuroma by decreasing the trauma to the nerve. Physical modalities such as ultrasound and electrical stimulation, padding and tapping, NSAIDs, steroid injections, and orthotics are conservative therapies. Surgical intervention is considered after all conservative therapy has failed to relieve symptoms.

Onychology and Dermatology

The foot is subjected to significant microtrauma from shoes and supporting surfaces. Even well-fitting shoes contact nail and skin structures of the foot and contribute to nail and skin changes. The shoe is an excellent environment for both fungal and bacterial growth. It is warm and dark and, with the perspiration of the foot, it is also moist. In addition, the shoe is the only article of clothing that is not usually laundered. Even if the foot is cleaned daily, it is placed back into a "dirty" shoe. We recommend either a daily antifungal foot powder applied to the foot and shoe or a weekly disinfectant spray to the shoes.

Nail Conditions

Onychomycosis is a common condition in the elderly population and results from the invasion by a dermatophyte to the nail and nail bed. The most common organisms causing onychomycosis are *Trichophyton rubrum, T. mentagrophytes,* and *Candida albicans* (19–21) (Figure 31.11).

Several types of onychomycosis have been identified. Total dystrophic onychomycosis affects the entire nail and nail bed. Distal subungual onychomycosis involves first the distal and sometimes lateral aspects of the nail and nail bed. Left untreated, this condition can progress

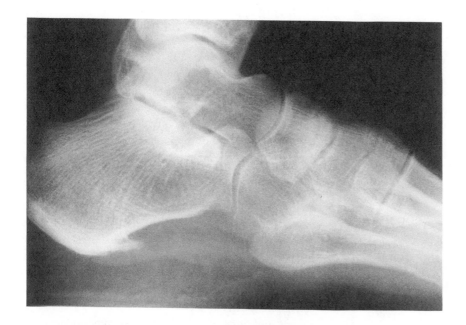

Fig. 31.10. Inferior calcaneal spur formation.

to total dystrophic onychomycosis. Proximal subungual onychomycosis begins at the proximal nail fold and nail bed and progresses distally if left untreated. This type is seen commonly in human immunodeficiency virus (HIV)-positive patients. Superficial white onychomycosis affects the superior aspect of the nail and may not affect the nail bed in any way.

Conservative treatment for mycotic nail conditions are directed toward controlling the infection, reducing painful nail thickness, and preventing secondary skin infections. This can be accomplished with periodic debridement and the use of topical antifungal creams and powders. Definitive treatment of mycotic nail disorders requires the use of either oral antifungal agents, permanent surgical removal, or both of these measures. More aggressive therapies should be considered only when conservative measures fail to control the infection (20,21).

Onychocryptosis and Paronychia

Ingrown toe nails are a common presenting podiatric complaint in all patient populations. Any nail margin may become ingrown; however, the most frequently involved are the hallux nails. The condition can be caused by ill-fitting shoes, onychomycosis, familial incurvated nails (Figure 31.12), improper self-trimming (Figure 31.13), and other trauma. The nail of the involved margin

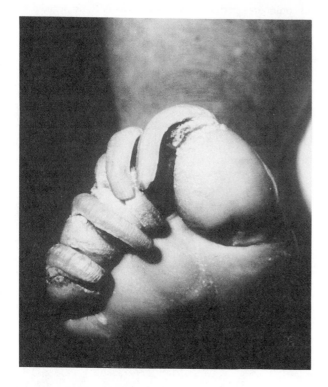

Fig. 31.11. Onychomycosis: hypertrophic, dystrophic, discolored, elongated nails. Notice the subungual debris representing infection of the nail bed.

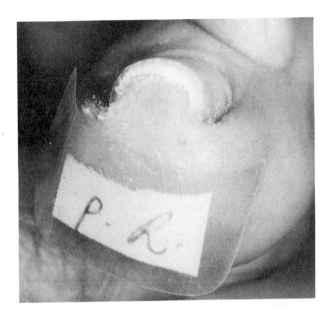

Fig. 31.12. Familial onychocryptosis.

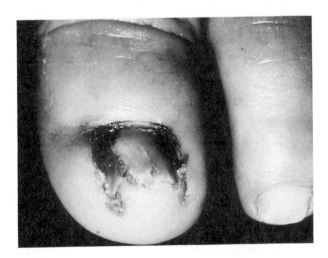

Fig. 31.13. Onychocryptosis and paronychia due to improper trimming of nail margins.

lacerates the tissues in the nail groove and results in a paronychia. The nail causes severe pain and discomfort and acts as a foreign body, which requires removal. Treatment involves incision, draining the paronychia, and removing the nail spicule. Antibiotics are usually not needed once the nail spicule is removed. Permanent sur-

gical correction is indicated if the condition recurs or becomes chronic.

This condition is generally benign and is easily treated unless complicated by a systemic condition that places the patient at risk, such as diabetes, peripheral vascular disease, immunocompromising conditions, neuropathies, or other conditions that interfere with the healing process. In these cases or if there is cellulitus, an antibiotic can be used in addition to removing the nail spicule. In the nondiabetic population, the most common causes are *Staphylococcus* and *Streptococcus*. In the diabetic population, the infection is more likely to be polymicrobial. In these patients, the use of broad-spectrum antibiotics such as amoxicillin-clavulanate potassium combinations or clindamycin can be used empirically until culture results are completed (10,11,13).

Foot Infections (Tinea Pedis)

Fungal infections of the foot are classified as acute or chronic tinea pedis. Acute tinea pedis is characterized by macerated web spaces (Figure 31.14), vesicles, pruritis (which can be severe at times), fissures, and erythema. The causative organism is usually *T. mentagrophytes*. Severe pruritis can cause excoriation and can lead to secondary bacterial infections. Chronic tinea pedis is characterized by a moccasin-type distribution of scaling and dry skin (Figure 31.15). The web spaces may also be involved. The causative organism is usually *T. rubrum*. Although the diagnosis is most often made clinically, cultures and a

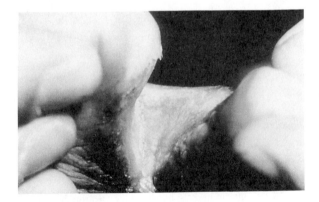

Fig. 31.14. Acute tinea pedis: macerated web space with erosion.

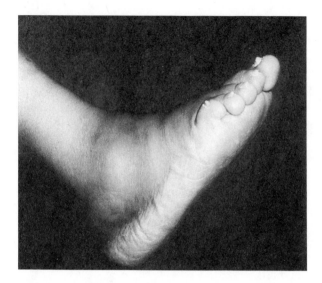

Fig. 31.15. Chronic tinea pedis: dry, scaly skin in moccasin distribution.

potassium hydroxide preparation may be used for definitive diagnosis.

Treatment for acute tinea pedis involves the use of commonly available topical antifungal agents and local skin care consisting of warm saline soaks (except for diabetic and other compromised patients), proper foot hygiene, and avoidance of trauma, which could result in secondary bacterial infection. With acute vesicular or pustular tinea, a short course of an oral agent, such as griseofulvin, may be used. If a secondary bacterial infection is suspected, an oral antibiotic for directed toward *Staphylococcus* and *Streptococcus* may be considered. Chronic tinea is treated much like acute tinea but generally for longer periods of time. After resolution, preventive measures should be given to the patient to prevent recurrence. These include instruction in proper foot hygiene, antifungal foot powder to use on a daily basis, and disinfective spray to use in shoes at least once weekly (19–21).

Xerosis

Excessively dry skin can lead to complications in the elderly. The decrease in skin turgor seen commonly in the elderly can lead to fissuring if skin becomes excessively dry. Left untreated, fissures can become infected. Prevention of excessive dryness is easily accomplished with the use of emollients. Over-the-counter preparations are readily available and should be recommended to all patients with xerosis (20,21).

Pedal Ulceration

One of the most frustrating conditions of the foot and lower extremity is ulceration. As a breakdown of the dermis and subcutaneous tissues, the foot ulcer can extend to deeper structures such as muscle and bone if not addressed immediately (Figure 31.16). Ulcers are caused by excessive pressure over bony prominences. Pressure causes a relative local ischemia to the skin and subcutaneous tissues (Figure 31.17). Once the skin is broken down, the opportunity for pathogenic bacteria to cause infection is high. Commonly, lower extremity ulcers are caused or complicated by conditions such as diabetes, neuropathy, and arterial and venous peripheral vascular diseases which necessitates primary and secondary preventive intervention whenever possible. Medicare has recently established a shoe program for diabetics that provides either molded or extra-depth shoes and multidensity inserts for the shoes to prevent ulceration and the all-too-common subsequent complications, such as amputations, that follow.

Management of lower extremity ulceration is a team effort. The underlying systemic condition must be carefully controlled. Failure to maintain blood sugar control

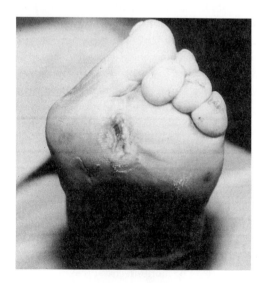

Fig. 31.16. Deep plantar ulceration sub 2 metatarsal head.

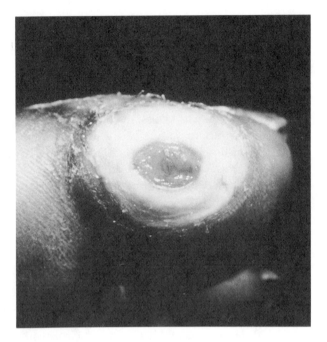

Fig. 31.17. Ulceration from chronic irritation of the medial aspect of the first interphalangeal joint.

in a diabetic or to re-establish blood flow in arteriosclerosis obliterans will result in uniformly poor results.

Infection must be definitively established with appropriate aerobic and anaerobic cultures for deep ulcers. Clean wounds with no clinical signs of infection need not be cultured. Any open wound will have bacteria, but if the bacteria are not causing infection, the wound need not be treated (11). For diabetic patients, immunocompromised patients, or other patients unable to muster an immune response, the normal signs of infection may be absent. In those patients, because of the propensity to polymicrobial infection the use of broad-spectrum antibiotics such as amoxicillin-clavulanate potassium combinations or clindamycin can be used empirically until culture results are completed. Local wound care involves appropriate debridement of necrotic tissue, keeping the wound clean and moist, and protecting it from further trauma. The use of occlusive and nonocclusive membranes has been suggested to aid in debridement and wound management. Newer, nonocclusive dressings may be more effective for skin ulceration (22).

Once the ulceration has healed, it should be considered chronic and a potential problem. Tertiary preventive interventions to prevent reulceration should be instituted. Appropriate shoes and multidensity inserts (Figure 31.18) that redistribute weight away from the ulcer site will help to maintain the patient's ambulation and prevent further breakdown of tissues.

Bone and Joint Infections

Both acute and chronic ulceration can result in osteomyelitis or bone infection. This type of infection can very quickly spread to other parts of the foot and leg. It is generally managed with intravenous antibiotics and surgical debridement of all infected tissues, although in some cases antibiotic therapy alone can be used if the condition is mild (21).

Shoe Gear and Foot Orthoses

With the exception of congenital and inherited foot deformities, we were all born with normal feet. Society has progressively changed natural surfaces and forced man to protect his feet from both environmental elements and flat, hard surfaces. The original purpose of the shoe was to

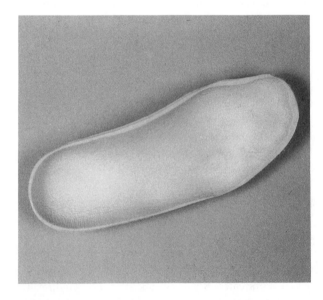

Fig. 31.18. Molded multidensity inserts for protection from excessive plantar pressure.

protect the foot and allow it to function within the environment. Today, however, style and fashion overshadow the original purpose. Functional shoes are available, but they are not considered fashionable and are not promoted by shoe manufacturers and retail shoe stores. One rarely finds an advertisement for an orthopedic oxford.

The shoe is not a primary etiologic agent in the development of structural foot deformities, but improperly fitted and inappropriate foot gear do contribute to the progression of foot deformities such as bunions, hammer toes, ingrown toenails, and neuromas. Once these deformities have developed, they must be accommodated, and this limits shoe style choices. Ideally, the clinician should be able to recommend appropriate shoes to patients at the first sign of a progressive foot deformity as a form of secondary prevention (23,24).

Components of the Shoe

A basic understanding of the components of the shoe is necessary before the clinician can recommend a shoe that suits the patient's needs.

The Last

The last is the model over which the shoe is constructed. Lasts are available in several different shapes to accommodate different foot structures. Most shoes today are made over an adducted last that adducts the forefoot on the rearfoot. When viewed from the sole of the shoe, a definitive right and left shoe shape is seen. These are also known as inflare lasts. Abducted lasts have the forefoot abducted on the rearfoot and are known as outflare lasts. These also have a definitive right and left shoe. Straight lasts have no abductory or adductory deviation; thus, the right and left shoe look the same. Children's prescription shoes are often straight last orthopedic oxfords. Bunion last shoes are designed to accommodate prominent first metatarsal heads in hallux valgus deformity. Combination last shoes (also known as slender heel last shoes) are designed to have different heel and forefoot widths. Having a foot that has a narrow heel and wider forefoot is one of the most common shoe-fit problems for women. Because most shoe stores do not carry combination last shoes, or if they do, they have few size variations, these patients are forced to buy shoes that fit the heel but are too tight in the forefoot. The heel must be snug in the shoe to keep the shoe on when the patient walks (23–26).

The Vamp

The vamp is the upper forepart of the shoe. This area is also known as the toe box. The toe box must be high enough to accommodate any forefoot deformities in the elderly.

The Outsole

The sole of the shoe plays an essential role in protecting the elderly foot from the supporting surface. Many materials are used to sole shoes, such as leather, rubber, crepe, and composite materials. The sole needs to be flexible enough to bend with the foot when the patient walks but sturdy enough to protect the plantar surface of the foot.

The Counter

One of the most important components of the shoe, which serves to control foot motion, is the counter. The counter is the back portion of the shoe that hugs the heel medially, laterally, and posteriorly. It should be rigid enough to stabilize the heel and maintain the shape of the shoe.

The Heel

Heel strike is the most significant shock that the shoe must absorb. As such, the heel serves to absorb heel strike and protect the foot. It also serves a fashion function, especially in women's shoes. Materials used in heels include leather, wood, plastic, or composite materials (25,26).

Types of Shoes

There are seven basic shoe designs. They include the moccasin, sandal, oxford, pump, monk, mule, and boot. The moccasin is the oldest form of foot gear and is essentially one piece of material wrapped around the foot. The sandal is a sole that is secured to the foot with straps or thongs. The oxford is a low-cut shoe that laces. The pump is a laceless shoe that must fit snugly to the foot to remain on the foot while the person walks. The monk is also a laceless shoe. It has a strap across the instep to secure it to the foot. The mule is a backless, slip-on type of shoe. The clog is an example of a mule-type shoe. The boot is a style of high foot gear that can vary in height from above the ankle to over the knee. The boot was originally used for military protection from the elements and for battle (23,25,26).

Advice to the Patient About Shoes

Shoes should be purchased late in the day or early evening after a full day of weight-bearing. This allows for proper fit over normal orthostatic edema or edema from other causes. Shoes should feel snug, but not tight, and should not be expected to stretch significantly with wear. The counter of the shoe should be firm, and the toe box should be high enough to accommodate any digital lesions. The sole should be flexible enough to allow for propulsive walking and strong enough to protect the foot from the shock of hard surfaces. Take time and walk in the shoes for 10 to 15 minutes, and notice any areas of irritation. This is especially important for the patient with neuropathy who may not have enough feeling to protect from traumatic friction injury.

Patients should be discouraged from using bedroom slippers for all-day ambulation, even at home. Slippers are designed for a short walk, from bedroom to bathroom, for example, not for general ambulation or prolonged standing.

Foot Orthoses

Foot orthoses are used to accommodate and control foot function within the shoe. Plantar deformities such as heel spur syndrome, medial longitudinal arch pain, and sublesional bursitis under bony prominence usually respond well to foot orthoses. Both soft and rigid materials are used, and the choice depends on the conditions being treated. Often combination devices of semi-rigid materials to control function and softer materials to accommodate lesions are used for the elderly (Figure 31.19).

Molded Shoes and Extra-Depth Shoes

If commercially available shoes do not adequately accommodate foot deformities, a molded shoe should be considered. Molded shoes are fabricated from a last made from a plaster cast of the patient's foot. This allows for custom accommodation of specific deformities; however, because ambulation is a dynamic activity and the casting proce-

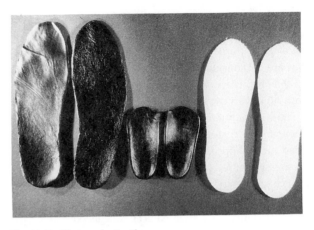

Fig. 31.19. Various foot orthoses.

dures are static, it is not uncommon for the patient to need several adjustment visits before proper fit is achieved. Extra-depth shoes are also available. They should be tried before molded shoes are prescribed.

Prevention of Podiatric Problems

Preventing pedal pathology is significantly easier than treating it. Patient education is directed toward enabling the patient to make voluntary changes in behavior to prevent disease and to allow for self-diagnosis and treatment of minor problems.

Routine Hygiene

The foot should be washed daily. It should be dried by patting, not rubbing, and dried carefully between the toes. For elderly patients who have trouble bending, the use of a back brush may allow the patient to wash the feet. If feet are excessively dry, an emollient or hand lotion should be used to moisturize the skin; if feet are excessively moist, foot powders should be used on the feet and in the shoe. (If these measures fail to control excessive dryness or moisture, the patient should contact the podiatrist or physician.) Feet should be inspected daily for irritations or injuries to skin, including spreading the toes to look for signs of problems. A mirror can be used to see the bottom of the foot, if needed. Corns and calluses in the elderly should be trimmed only by a podiatrist or physician.

Nail Care

Nails should be cut straight across when they are soft after bathing, and the edges should be filed to follow the normal contour of the toe. Thick brittle nails or nails that are difficult to trim should be cared for by a podiatrist or physician. The patient should not cut down into nail grooves. Ingrown nails should be treated by a podiatrist or physician.

First Aid For Minor Injuries

Prompt attention should be given to any cut, scrape, abrasion, or burn to the lower extremity. Any minor wound should be washed with a mild soap-and-water solution or Epsom-salt solution (1 quart warm water plus 2 tablespoons Epsom salts). An antiseptic cream or ointment should be applied and the wound should be covered with an adhesive strip bandage. If the wound does not improve within 24 to 48 hours, the patient should see the podiatrist or health care specialist.

Counseling for the Compromised Patient

It is essential that patients suffering from chronic degenerative diseases such as diabetes, peripheral vascular disease, and other disorders that decrease the patient's ability to heal, be directed to inspect their feet each day.

References

1. Helfand AE. Public health and podiatric medicine. Baltimore: Williams & Wilkins, 1987.
2. Levy LA. Clarifying the role of podiatrists as primary care providers. J Am Podiatry Assoc 1979;69:466–468.
3. Gibbons G, Freeman D. Vascular evaluation and treatment of the diabetic. In: Harkless LB, Dennis KJ, eds. Clinics in podiatric medicine and surgery. The diabetic foot. Philadelphia: Saunders, 1987.
4. Ritz G, Friedman S, Osbourne A. Diabetes and peripheral vascular disease. In: Robbins JM, ed. Clinics in podiatric medicine and surgery. Peripheral vascular disease in the lower extremity. Philadelphia: Saunders, 1992.
5. Kilo C. Vascular complications of diabetes. Cardiovasc Rev Rep 1987;8.
6. Hoffman A. Evaluation of arterial blood flow in the lower extremity. In: Robbins JM, ed. Clinics in podiatric medicine and surgery. Peripheral vascular disease in the lower extremity. Philadelphia: Saunders, 1992:19–56.
7. Hodgson KJ, Sumner DS. Noninvasive assessment of lower extremity arterial disease. Ann Vasc Surg 1988;2.
8. Weber G, Cardile MA. Diabetic neuropathies. In: Weber G, ed. Clinics in podiatric medicine and surgery. Neurologic disorders affecting the lower extremity. II. Philadelphia: Saunders, 1990.
9. Frykberg R. Osteoarthropathy. In: Harkless LB, Dennis KJ, eds. Clinics in podiatric medicine and surgery. The diabetic foot. Philadelphia: Saunders, 1987.
10. Joseph WS. Treatment of lower exteremity infections in diabetics. J Am Podiatr Med Assoc 1992;82.
11. Joseph WS. Handbook of lower extremity infections. New York: Churchill-Livingstone, 1990.
12. Department of Health and Human Services. Reducing the health consequences of smoking: 25 years of progress. A report of the surgeon General. DHHS Publication No. (CDC) 89-8411. Washington, DC: Department of Health and Human Services, 1989.
13. Kushner D. Primary podiatric care of the vascularly compromised foot. In: Robbins JM, ed. Clinics in podiatric medicine and surgery. Peripheral vascular disease in the lower extremity. Philadelphia: Saunders, 1992.
14. Baele HR. Venous disease. In: Robbins JM, ed. Clinics in podiatric medicine and surgery. Peripheral vascular disease in the lower extremity. Philadelphia: Saunders, 1992.
15. Fairbairn JF, Juergens JL, Spittell JA. Peripheral vascular disease. 5th ed. Philadelphia: Saunders, 1980.
16. Spittell J. Clinical vascular disease. Philadelphia: Davis, 1983.
17. Kidawa A. Vasospastic disorders. In: Robbins JM, ed. Clinics in podiatric medicine and surgery. Peripheral vascular disease in the lower extremity. Philadelphia: Saunders, 1992:139–150.
18. Rodnan GP, Schumacher HR, eds. Primer on the rheumatic diseases. 8th ed. Atlanta: Arthritis Foundation, 1983.
19. Yale J. Podiatric medicine. 3rd ed. Baltimore: Williams & Wilkins, 1987.
20. Levy L, Hetherington V, ed. Principles and practice of podiatric medicine. New York: Churchill-Livingstone, 1990.
21. Robbins JM. Primary care podiatric medicine. Philadelphia: Saunders, 1994.
22. Carr RD, Lalagos DE, Upman PJ. Comparative study of occlusive wound dressings on full thickness wounds in domestic pigs. Wounds 1989;1.
23. Schuster RO. The effects of modern footgear. J Am Podiatr Med Assoc 1978;68.
24. Rossi WA. Shoes and the shoe industry–Reality Versus Illusion. J Am Podiatr Med Assoc 1978;68.
25. The art and science of footwear manufacturing. Arlington, VA: American Footwear Industries Association, 1974.
26. Miller RG, ed. Manual of shoemaking. Bristol, UK: Clarks, 1989.

Chapter 32
Sexual Function in Older Persons

Margaret-Mary G. Wilson, Fran E. Kaiser, and John E. Morley

So, lively brisk old fellow, don't let age get you down. White hairs or not, you can still be a lover.

Goethe

The persistence of ageism and negative stereotyping of older persons serves to reinforce the myth that sexual decline is an integral component of the aging process. Sociocultural attitudes within most societies have led to expectation of this sexual decline as a norm. Thus, until very recently, sexual activity in older persons had traditionally been considered inappropriate, even immoral or representing deviant behavior (1–3). These factors hindered objective appraisal of issues surrounding sexuality in the older person, and undoubtedly affected the physician's approach to effective evaluation of sexual function in their patients.

Kinsey et al (4), in 1948, reported in his subjects a reduction in coital frequency to once every 10 weeks by the age of 80 years. The Starr-Weiner report found that 55 percent of men over 60 years of age had sexual intercourse only once a week, and that 7 percent of the total population studied was sexually inactive. Females aged 60 to 91 years had a coital frequency of 1.4 times a week (5). Pfeiffer et al (6) found that 95 percent of men aged 46 to 50 years of age had sexual intercourse at least once a week. In men older than the age of 66 years, this frequency was maintained by only 28 percent and total sexual inactivity was recorded for 24 percent. Four decades after initial reports by Kinsey et al, Bretschneider (7) reported a coital frequency of at least once weekly for 29 percent of men older than 80 years, which demonstrates a significant increase in sexual activity within this age group. Thus, although these studies are often cited to support a reduction in sexual activity with increasing age, they also show that reduction is not a universal, inevitable accompaniment of aging.

Further negating the ageist theory of sexual decline was the demonstration of an increase in sexual activity with age in 13 percent of the subjects studied by Pfeiffer et al (6). Their findings highlight that age is no longer an adequate explanation for sexual dysfunction in the older person. Confounding the purity of most of these studies, however, is the fact that coital frequency or ability were usually the primary indexes used to assess sexual function. This introduced a significant bias, because normal sexual function, unlike coitus, which is strictly a physiologic process, depends on several factors. The interplay within the individual among social, cultural, psychological, physiological, biological, and hormonal factors determines sexuality, and ultimately, sexual function.

The current geriatric population has its origins in the pre–World War II era, and is thus permeated with sexual attitudes, concepts, and sociocultural expectations in keeping with that period. Sexuality in the elderly thus remains shrouded in negative myths, and is not an issue often raised for open discussion. Consequently, sexual dysfunction is frequently unrecognized as a substantive, pathologic process (8,9). Several studies have clearly dissociated a decline in sexual ability from aging by demonstrating that the etiology of sexual dysfunction is very often linked to disease, therapeutic intervention, or clearly identifiable psychological and sociocultural factors (6–13).

An accurate appraisal of sexual function in the older person must take into consideration the separate influences of health problems, disease, quality of life of the individual, and the availability of a social network that provides a platform for sexual expression. Normal expression of sexuality often depends on the existence of a functioning social relationship between partners. This may be compromised for various reasons within the geriatric population and some older patients may engage in masturbation as their sole sexual outlet. The physician should not perceive this as abnormal, unless the patient expresses concern. The influence of ageist or sexist misconceptions and prevailing sociocultural norms and attitudes cannot be overemphasized. Of paramount importance is realization that sexuality is an integral part of self, and caters to the individual's lifelong need for emotional and physical intimacy. Expression of sexuality should not be compromised by age.

Changes in Sexual Function with Aging

Physiological Factors

The study by Masters and Johnson of the human sexual response clearly defined four separate phases (Table 32.1). Although they studied only small numbers of young older people, their data suggested that each of these phases is vulnerable to alteration by the aging process. During the excitement phase, there is a reduction in scrotal vasocongestion and testicular elevation. Women experience decreased breast and genital vasocongestion, reduced vaginal secretions, and a lesser degree of uterine elevation. Older men tend to experience a longer plateau phase with diminished pre-ejaculatory secretions. Orgasms in both sexes are of shorter duration. Men have fewer prostatic and urethral contractions, and women experience fewer and weaker uterine and vaginal contractions. In some women, spastic and painful uterine contractions may occur. These changes may diminish the pleasure derived from orgasms. After orgasm, women return more rapidly to the prearousal stage, and men experience more rapid detumescence and testicular descent than they did during their younger years. In older men, the refractory period, during which men are incapable of physical sexual arousal, is significantly prolonged. In spite of these changes, a significant proportion of elderly patients report continued sexual satisfaction and pleasure (14).

Libido, the necessary initiating stimulus of sexual intercourse, is variably affected by age. Various studies have shown decreased, increased, or unchanged libido with advancing age (4–7). The precise mechanism by which libido is maintained remains ill-defined, though testosterone is thought to play an important role in both men and women (15–17). Testosterone withdrawal has been shown to reduce both libido and erectile capacity; high-dose testosterone replacement in hypogonadal males increases libido and the frequency of erections (18,19). With advancing age, there is a decrease in testicular size and a reduction in the number of Leydig cells. This is, in part, presumed to be the cause of reduced serum testosterone and bioavailable testosterone (BT) levels detected in older men.

Testosterone response to human chorionic gonadotropin (HCG) is also attenuated with age (20,21). Several studies have highlighted the presence of secondary hypogonadism in a notable proportion of older men, which occurs independently of sexual function. Such men exhibit a reduced luteinizing hormone (LH) response to gonadotropin-releasing hormone (GnRH) and altered LH pulsatility, which suggests defects at both the pituitary and hypothalamic levels. The reduction in serum testosterone and BT that occurs in men with advancing age is now believed to be predominantly caused by hypothalamic-pituitary failure (22). These changes may adversely affect sexual potency.

Table 32.1. Changes in the Human Sexual Response with Aging.

Phase	Male	Female
Excitement	Reduced scrotal vasocongestion Decreased testicular elevation Delayed penile erection	Reduced breast and genital vasocongestion Diminished vaginal secretions Delayed arousal
Plateau	Prolonged Diminished pre-ejaculatory secretions	Reduced elevation of the uterus and labia majora
Orgasm	Short duration Reduction in prostatic and urethral contractions	Short duration Fewer and weaker uterine and vaginal contractions
Resolution	Rapid detumescence and testicular descent Prolonged refractory period	Rapid reversion to prearousal stage

A decrease in the compliance of type 3 collagen fibers in the corpora, secondary to increased collagen crosslinking, has also been implicated in the onset of erectile failure with aging. The decrease contributes to a diminution in both the frequency and tumescence of penile erections (23).

Studies exploring parallel changes in older women tend not to dissociate peri- and postmenopausal reproductive changes from changes in sexuality and sexual function, probably because symptoms of sexual dysfunction may be triggered by the onset of menopause. The climacteric comprises multiple symptoms of diverse etiologies, including loss of libido for some women. Ovarian failure is the underlying event (24). In the perimenopausal period, plasma production and clearance rates of estrogens are reduced, and estrone replaces estradiol as the dominant circulating estrogen (25). In postmenopausal women, these are derived predominantly from peripheral conversion of adrenal precursors, with the ovary serving only as a minor source (25,26). Degenerative changes in the granulosa and theca cells result in reduced inhibin secretion, and cause an increase in follicle-stimulating hormone (FSH) levels. As estradiol levels fall, there is also an increase in LH levels, although this occurs later and is of lesser magnitude (27). Pulsed secretion of these hormones is maintained and clearance rates are unchanged. The gonadotropin response to GnRH is exaggerated, unless illness intervenes (28).

Estrogen deficiency is linked to a significant proportion of menopausal symptoms that reflect on sexual function and include symptoms arising from urogenital and breast atrophy (29,30). The etiology of psychosomatic symptoms and changes in mood and libido is less clear. Reasons for a decrease in libido in females have not been clearly elucidated. Current studies have failed to show a significant correlation between estrogen levels and libido. Progestogens may decrease libido, but available data are not convincing (31,32).

A positive correlation has been identified between coital frequency in females and serum testosterone levels (33). Cyproterone acetate, an antiandrogenic compound, has been shown to reduce libido in a significant proportion of women; consequently, libidinal problems have been treated with a combination of testosterone and estrogen implants with variable success (34–37).

Testosterone replacement therapy in women after total abdominal hysterectomy and bilateral salpingooophorectomy has also resulted in increased libido (38). Estrogen supplementation in isolation, however, has not been shown to have much effect in restoring libido (39).

Psychosocial Factors

The psychological changes that occur with aging also influence sexual function. Psychosocial stressors are often the factors that complete the transition from altered physiology to pathology (40). Aging may result in the development of a negative body image and altered perception of self. This is more common in personality types with elevated neuroticism, and has been correlated with a reduction in libido and decreased sexual satisfaction (41). Marital and relationship problems constitute the bulk of social stressors that compromise sexual function. Chronic illness, death of a spouse, intramarital discord, or the deterioration of a supportive social network may all result in a negative impact on sexual function (42).

Variations in sexual function have also been described between socioeconomic groups in elderly men. Educated middle-class, and upper-class men tend to continue sexual activity, in spite of erectile dysfunction. They usually employ alternative sexual techniques, such as mutual masturbation and oral sex. Men in lower socioeconomic groups use these techniques less frequently, with most discontinuing sexual intercourse once vaginal intromission becomes impossible (43).

Subtle psychological processes compromised by age may also exert an influence on sexual function. The older person has relatively impaired image rotation and activation, the process by which visual memories are accessed and activated. Sexual imagery, be it real or fantasized, is a significant component of sexual activity and may be compromised by this defect (44). Distractor suppression has also been assessed in the older individual. Older people process distracting stimuli normally, but have a reduced ability to engage inhibitory mechanisms in rejection of such stimuli (45). It is reasonable to postulate that this may influence their capacity for focused sexual concentration during coitus.

The appraisal of sexual function in older persons from the psychosocial standpoint must allow for the cultural ideology within the geriatric population. Male dominance, female submissiveness, and the rejection of alternative sexual lifestyles, such as homosexuality, are attitudes that remain deeply entrenched within some older cohorts. Recognition of a deviation from such norms within the individual's experience may present as an intrapsychic conflict and, in itself, may adversely affect sexual function (46). However, a proportion of older persons have coped with alternative lifestyles since early adulthood without experiencing any form of psychosocial distress.

Sexual Dysfunction in the Older Man

The Circuitry of Penile Erection

A penile erection may result from either cortical or local stimuli, and both factors often operate synergistically. Cortical stimuli comprised visual imagery that may be enhanced by erotic thought. Efferent impulses are conveyed via the thoracolumbar outflow to the hypogastric plexus. Local stimulation of the penis sends impulses through the pudendal nerve to the erectile center, which is located in the second to fourth sacral segments of the spinal cord. The efferent limb of this reflex is the nervi erigentes (47) (Figure 32.1). Excitation of either polysynaptic pathway should result in arterial dilatation

and sinusoidal filling, with a reduction in venous outflow (48). Nitric oxide, vasoactive intestinal peptide, and various prostaglandins facilitate the relaxation of vascular smooth muscle to accommodate the increase in blood volume. Release of these neurotransmitters depends on cholinergic mediated stimulation of muscarinic receptors (13,47).

Impotence

Impotence is defined as the inability to achieve or maintain an erection in at least 75 percent of attempts at coitus. The incidence increases with age, exceeding 50 percent in men over the age of 75 years (4). The etiology is often multifactorial, with vascular causes predominating. Neurologic disease and medication are also often implicated (Table 32.2). The high frequency of impotence in older men is related to these factors. The incidence of atherosclerosis of the penile arteries increases with age (47). This usually coexists with atherosclerosis elsewhere in the vascular tree, and often serves as an index of increased risk of ischemic heart disease and cerebrovascular disease (49). Venous leakage from the corpora cavernosa in older men may also contribute to erectile failure (50). This may be induced by local ischemia secondary to atheromatous changes; however, defects in type 3 colla-

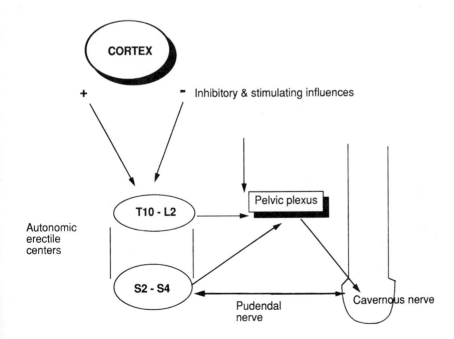

Fig. 32.1. Penile erection: A schematic of neurologic pathways.

Table 32.2. Causes of Impotence.

Vascular
    Penile atherosclerosis
    Venous leaks
    Arteriovenous malformations
Drugs*
Neurologic
    Autonomic neuropathy
    Cerebrovascular disease
    Dementia
    Myelopathy
    Demyelinating disease
    Complex partial seizures
Endocrine
    Diabetes mellitus
    Hypogonadism
    Hyperprolactinemia
    Thyrotoxicosis
    Hypothyroidism
    Cushing's disease
Psychogenic
    Endogenous depression
    Primary performance anxiety
    Situational depression/anxiety
Chronic Illness

*See Table 32.3.

gen of the tunica albuginea have also been implicated (23,51).

Impotence occurs frequently as an adverse effect of drugs (4,11) (Table 32.3). All antihypertensives, including the newer calcium channel blockers and angiotensin-converting enzyme inhibitors, are associated with impotence through various mechanisms (52). Thiazide diuretics, often used in the elderly, may produce impotence by critically lowering penile blood flow and are also known to reduce serum testosterone via a reduction in zinc levels (10–12,53). Digoxin, a commonly used antiarrhythmic agent, is known to alter the metabolism of sex hormones and may result in impotence (52). Prostaglandin inhibition induced by nonsteroidal anti-inflammatory drugs may also impair erectile function (54). A wide range of antipsychotic and antiparkinsonian agents have also been implicated, usually resulting in impotence as a result of their anticholinergic and antidopaminergic properties. Other frequently used drugs, including type 2 histamine receptor blockers, antihistamines, tranquilizers, and cytotoxic agents have also

been implicated (52,55). Several recreational drugs may affect erectile function.

The effect of alcohol on sexual ability is well recognized. Although alcohol increases libido, it has a direct inhibitory effect on erectile ability (12). This usually returns to normal after the alcohol load has been excreted. Chronic alcohol abuse, however, may lead to permanent impotence through its attendant complications of autonomic and sensory neuropathies or hypogonadism (55).

Nicotine, a well-established risk factor for atherosclerosis, may critically reduce penile blood flow. This may result from atherogenic changes within the penile vasculature (56). Alternative mechanisms through which nicotine induces impotence may also exist. Erections resulting from cavernosal nerve stimulation in animals can be inhibited by nicotine, and cigarette smoking has been

Table 32.3. Drugs Implicated in Impotence.

Antihypertensives
    Diuretics
    Beta blockers
    Methyldopa
    Prazosin
    Clonidine
    Reserpine
    Calcium channel blockers
    Angiotensin-converting enzyme inhibitors
Centrally Active Agents
    Phenothiazines
    Butyrophenones
    Tricyclic antidepressants
    Monoamine oxidase inhibitors
    Lithium
    Barbiturates
    Benzodiazepines
Antiandrogens
    Digoxin
    GnRH agonists
    H_2-receptor blockers
    Spironolactone
    Ketoconazole
    Cancer chemotherapeutic agents
Analgesics
    Nonsteroidal anti-inflammatory drugs
    Opiates
Recreational Drugs
    Alcohol
    Nicotine
    Morphine and derivatives

noted to counteract the effect of papaverine on penile tumescence (57,58).

The use of opiates may produce hyperprolactinemia and direct inhibition of the hypothalamic-pituitary-gonadal axis and result in impotence (55). The multifactorial basis of impotence is an important consideration in presumed drug-related erectile failure. Quite often, in diseases such as hypertension, atherosclerosis, and psychoses, both the disease and the medication may be implicated. In such cases, if these factors are considered in isolation, removal or control of the presumed etiologic factor may not result in restoration of potency.

Secondary hypogonadism may be found in as many as 60 percent of normal older men (22). This compromises libido to a greater extent than it compromises erectile capacity. Secondary hypogonadism is rarely the primary cause of impotence; it often acts in concert with other factors (47). Hyperprolactinemia, though known to cause impotence, does so rarely (59).

The diagnosis of thyroid disease in the elderly is often fraught with difficulty. Hyperthyroidism may result in elevated sex hormone-binding globulin (SHBG) levels and, consequently, reduced bioavailable testosterone (BT). This may result in impotence as a presenting symptom in thyroid disease (10). Hypothyroidism and Cushing's disease are associated with hypogonadism and may also predispose to accelerated atherosclerosis, which may involve the penile vasculature (10,60).

Erectile function may be compromised in over 90 percent of diabetic men (13). This is usually a result of interplay among vascular, neurogenic, and psychogenic factors. The penile brachial index has been found to be markedly reduced in some diabetic patients (13,62). Changes in nerve latency, penile dorsal nerve conduction, autonomic function, and nitric oxide have also been identified (62–64). Hyperprolactinemia, which may occur in diabetics also plays a role (65).

Neurologic disease of varying etiology, including vascular, neurogenic, traumatic, and degenerative, may also predispose to impotence (66,67). Autonomic neuropathy, which occurs with increasing frequency in older persons, is an important contributor to impotence (68).

Psychological disorders, coexisting with chronic disease, may facilitate the development of impotence (69). This may explain the development of erectile failure in chronic disease without demonstrable genital pathology. Depression has been shown to reduce testosterone and LH levels and may alter autonomic function (55,70). Anxiety is well known to reduce sexual arousal (71,72). This is often primary performance anxiety that arises from concerns over sexual ability; however, anxiety linked to nonsexual events, such as may occur after a myocardial infarction, can also lead to impotence (47,52). The fear of experiencing a repeat infarct may deter resumption of sexual intercourse. This situation usually stems from inadequate health education and counseling.

Psychosocial concerns, such as bereavement, intramarital discord, increasing isolation with advancing age, or the stress of coping with chronic illness in one or both partners, may also serve to inhibit sexual arousal. Psychological problems resulting in impotence were previously thought to have deep-seated origins, and were thought to be linked to childhood events or conflicts. This may still hold true, but for the larger proportion of elderly patients, psychological issues can often be related to recent events or stressors and may be addressed quite easily, once understood. Well-defined psychological syndromes are recognized. The widower's syndrome refers to the conflict that arises when a recently bereaved older man enters into a new relationship. The sexual component of this relationship may evoke feelings of guilt and disloyalty toward his deceased partner. A subconscious desire to repress his sexuality presents as impotence (47).

Disorders of Ejaculation

Ejaculatory disorders are another form of sexual dysfunction in men (73). Anejaculation and retrograde ejaculation can frequently be attributed to underlying organic disease such as transverse myelitis, multiple sclerosis, and diabetic neuropathy. Any form of injury to the spinal cord, ranging from trauma to complicated retroperitoneal lymph node dissection, can affect ejaculation (74). In the older man, retrograde ejaculation frequently complicates transurethral retrograde prostatectomy (75).

The prevalence of premature ejaculation far exceeds that of the other ejaculatory disorders in younger men, although its prevalence in the older man remains unknown. Anxiety may play a major etiologic role, but this has been found to vary significantly with the individual.

As yet unidentified organic or cognitive factors may also be important (76,77). A distinction has been drawn between primary (PPE) and secondary premature ejaculators (SPE). The former group consists of patients who have a lifelong history of this disorder. The latter group, in which premature ejaculation presents as a complication of previously normal sexual function, is more likely to include the older man. This cohort of patients often have coexisting erectile disorders and reduced libido (78).

Sexual Dysfunction in the Older Woman

In women, anatomic indexes reflecting the ability to achieve satisfactory sexual intercourse are more covert than they are in men. Dyspareunia, defined as difficult or painful sexual intercourse, is often the presenting symptom of sexual dysfunction. This is commonly caused by urogenital disease, but quite often may be an indirect consequence of systemic disease or psychopathology (Table 32.4). Available data suggest that a significant proportion of older women may be affected, but precise figures are difficult to obtain because most women consider this a very sensitive issue and tend not to discuss it with professional care providers (79).

Postmenopausal vaginal atrophy, a common cause of dyspareunia in older women, results in a relatively dry and poorly lubricated mucosa and makes the mucosa

Table 32.4. Causes of Dyspareunia in the Older Woman.

Vaginal atrophy
Inflammation
  Vulvovaginitis
  Cervicitis
  Urethritis
  Cystitis
  Pelvic inflammatory disease
Pelvic and gynecologic neoplasms
Athritides
Connective tissue diseases
  Sjögren's syndrome
  Progressive systemic sclerosis
Miscellaneous
  Postoperative vaginal adhesions and scarring
  Radiation injury
  Chronic inflammatory bowel disease
  Anorectal diseases
  Psychogenic

more susceptible to friction injuries during coitus and reduces natural immunity to local disease (7,80). Dyspareunia can also result from local disease of the vulva and vagina, interstitial cystitis, chronic pelvic inflammation, or gynecological neoplasms. Surgical procedures or radiation therapy, complicated by pelvic adhesions or vaginal vault fibrosis, can predispose to dyspareunia (81). Endometriosis, the presence of functioning extrauterine endometrial tissue, is a frequent cause of dyspareunia in younger women. The onset of natural or artificial menopause is often thought to constitute an effective treatment modality. However, symptomatic endometriosis has been described in postmenopausal women (82,83). This can occur even in the absence of hormone replacement therapy, which is known to reactivate dormant endometriosis.

Psychiatric illness, psychological problems, stressful social circumstances, and relationship problems can also precipitate dyspareunia (81). Women with Crohn's disease may experience this symptom, especially if they have complicating perianal disease or fistula formation. The frequent occurrence of candidiasis in these patients may also cause considerable discomfort during sexual intercourse (84). Skeletal disorders have also been implicated with dyspareunia resulting from sacral nerve root compression secondary to lumbosacral osteoarthroses and exostosis formation after pelvic fractures (85,86). Iatrogenic dyspareunia may complicate the initiation of Kegel's pelvic floor exercises, often carried out to prevent or control stress incontinence. This is attributed to muscular overexertion of the levator ani muscles and consequent localized myalgia (87).

Urinary incontinence is common in older women and 25 percent experience intracoital incontinence, which may inhibit sexual desire and response (88,89). The older woman may also experience postcoital dysuria resulting from repeated penile stimulation of the posterior bladder wall and subsequent irritation of the atrophic urovesical mucosa (90). These symptoms often serve as a deterrent to sexual intercourse, provoking reactive depression, extreme anxiety, or loss of libido.

In the United States, more than 33 percent of women older than age 60 have had a hysterectomy. Theoretic complications following removal of the uterus include increased vaginal ballooning and reduced vasocongestion (91). Few studies, however, have demonstrated this consequence of a hysterectomy. Organic dyspareunia is more likely to result from surgical complications of this procedure and may result in vaginal scarring or fibrosis and significant shortening of the vault (92). In practice, sexual dysfunction after hysterectomy is usually psychological, arising from issues that revolve around concepts of altered body image and diminished femininity (80). These mythical beliefs may be dispelled by appropriate education and counseling. Breast surgery may give rise to similar concerns. Postmastectomy patients have been shown to experience a decrease in the frequency of sexual intercourse and orgasms. Reduced nipple sensitivity in some women may contribute to this consequence of mastectomy (93).

Diabetes mellitus, a common cause of impotence in men, has also been linked to organic sexual dysfunction in women. Loss of libido and anorgasmia occur with increased frequency in older women with type II diabetes. This correlates positively with duration of the disease. Reduced vaginal secretions secondary to abnormal vasocongestion occur in some diabetics and interfer-with effective intromission during coitus (94). Postmortem histologic studies have identified neurovascular degenerative changes in the clitoris, which may inhibit sexual arousal (95). The precise mechanism for these changes remains unknown. The mental and physical stress of coping with diabetes, as with any other chronic illness, may further compromise sexual function by reducing libido.

A significant number of women admit to the inability to reach orgasm. The perception of anorgasmia as a manifestation of sexual dysfunction varies with the individual. In some women, failure to attain orgasm does not detract from the sexual satisfaction obtained from shared physical intimacy. Others find anorgasmia frustrating and consider it a marker of sexual inadequacy. In a significant proportion of cases, anorgasmia may be attributed to a paucity of sexual knowledge, poor communication between partners, or performance anxiety. This is often easily rectified by appropriate sex education and counseling (96).

Women may experience psychological syndromes similar to those found in men. Widows who remarry have an increased incidence of dyspareunia, in the absence of identifiable organic risk factors other than vaginal atrophy (80).

Psychiatric disorders, particularly when associated with depression, severe behavioral changes, or reduced cognitive function, may result in sexual dysfunction in one or both partners. This spectrum of problems is well represented in dementia. The partner subject to intense caregiver stress may experience a decline in sexual dysfunction. Signficant role changes occur as dementia progresses. As the affected partner becomes increasingly dependent, a once equal social partnership is transformed into a facsimile of a parent-child relationship, and assumption of these new roles may notably distort the sexual content and dimensions of the relationship. Persisting in sexual intercourse with a confused and disorientated partner may convert the sexual act from a function dependent on mutual consent to an act of near-coercion (97). Furthermore, a pathologic increase in libido and sexually inappropriate behavior can occur in some patients with dementia and introduce added problems (98).

Evaluation of Sexual Dysfunction

Skillful history-taking is crucial in the detection of symptoms of sexual dysfunction. Symptoms are rarely volunteered by the patient and often lurk beneath seemingly trivial complaints. Consequently, they may remain completely unaddressed by the unsuspecting physician. A sexual history should form part of the routine clinical evaluation of the older patient. The current approach by most physicians reflects the lack of awareness and formal training in dealing with these issues. Personal beliefs, unwarranted embarrassment, and undue reticence on the part of either the patient or physician often prevent effective communication. Specific details of the sexual problem should be obtained, with particular emphasis on the duration, severity, and rate of progression of each symptom. Inquiry should be made into the patient's libido, erectile function, and ability to attain orgasm. To a large extent, sexual function is individualized; thus, obtaining a sexual history enables meaningful comparison and assists in effective evaluation. The presence of associated medical illnesses may provide important etiologic clues. Cardiovascular, neurologic, and endocrine diseases would be of particular interest. A detailed drug history, which should include nonprescription medication, recreational drugs such as nicotine or alcohol, and drugs of abuse, is essential. The patient's social or marital relationships should be discussed, if deemed relevant.

Physical examination may offer helpful diagnostic clues. Signs of peripheral neuropathy, hypogonadism, atherosclerotic vascular disease or thyroid dysfunction may suggest an underlying cause. Simple bedside tests, such as the demonstration of orthostatic hypotension, an impaired response to the Valsalva maneuver or an absent bulbocavernosus reflex indicate underlying autonomic neuropathy.

A genital examination must be carried out. The penis should be assessed for structural abnormalities. Peyronie's disease, in which spontaneous fibrosis of the penile shaft occurs, leads to abnormal curvature of the penis, which interferes with efficient vaginal intromission. The meatal orifice should also be inspected. Hypospadias, in which the urethra opens on the underside of the penis or perineum, is a developmental anomaly that presents in childhood. The older patient, however, may present with erectile failure as a complication of attempted surgical repair (99). In a proportion of patients, hypospadias serves as a phenotypic marker of underlying abnormal androgen metabolism or receptor defects, and further investigations may be indicated (100). The scrotum should be examined for evidence of testicular atrophy or softening, as may occur in chronic liver disease or alcoholism. Firm, atrophic testes suggest Klinefelter's syndrome. Examination of the prostate for enlargement, nodularity, or tenderness assists in the exclusion of prostatitis, prostatic hypertrophy, and neoplastic changes.

In women, a pelvic examination, which should include digital and speculum studies, is mandatory. Introital erythema suggestive of vulvovaginitis, vaginal atrophy, vault scarring, and pelvic inflammatory disease or neoplasms are readily detectable.

A Folstein's mini-mental status examination and a Yesavage geriatric depression score may be obtained to assist in psychiatric evaluation, should this eventually prove necessary (101,102).

Routine laboratory investigations should include thyroid function tests, blood glucose, and fructosamine levels. Serum gonadotropin and prolactin levels should also be measured. Testosterone and bioavailable testosterone assays are helpful in both sexes, often assisting in the differentiation of androgen deficiency syndrome from psychogenic sexual desire disorders in females (103). Hyperprolactinemia or a biochemical profile suggestive of secondary hypogonadism necessitates exclusion of a pituitary neoplasm. Visual field perimetry and magnetic resonance imaging or a computerized tomographic scan may be employed for this purpose.

Formal autonomic function tests are useful in the assessment of diabetics. The Valsalva index and the sympathetic skin response have been shown to be sensitive indexes in the identification of diabetic patients with autonomic dysfunction (104).

Nocturnal penile tumescence (NPT) rigidity monitoring has fallen out of favor in the assessment of older men with erectile failure. Accurate interpretation is precluded by variable results of questionable significance. Furthermore, reduced NPT is not uncommon in older men with normal sexual function. This investigation is probably best reserved for investigation of the younger man with suspected psychogenic impotence, in whom the monitoring is of proven value (47).

Penile duplex ultrasonography and pulsed Doppler waveform analysis are useful in the assessment of penile arterial perfusion if arteriogenic impotence is suspected (105). These investigations have proved superior to estimation of the penile brachial index (PBI), which involves comparison of the penile and brachial blood pressures. This was thought to reflect the integrity of the penile vasculature, but has been found to be inaccurate and poorly reproducible. Significant inter- and intraobserver variation has also been demonstrated (106). These measures may be useful in the diagnosis of the pelvic steal syndrome, which occurs in the presence of a partially occluded penile artery and which refers to erectile failure as a result of exercise-induced vasodilatation and subsequent redistribution and diversion of blood from the penile circulation (47,107). It is yet to be determined how closely these findings, demonstrated under experimental conditions, mirror the precise events that occur during sexual intercourse.

Failure to maintain an erection after intracorporeal injection of prostaglandin E1 (PGE-1) or papaverine suggests venous leaks. Specialized studies such as pharmacocavernosometry and cavernosography may be used to confirm this abnormality (108,109). Color-coded duplex ultrasonography is also useful in this regard (110). Invasive angiographic studies are rarely indicated in the investigation of vascular impotence.

Neurologic studies that are occasionally employed include dorsal penile nerve conduction studies, assessment of pudendal somatosensory evoked potentials, and biothesiometric studies (13,111,112). Failure to identify an organic cause of sexual dysfunction may be considered an indication for formal neuropsychiatric evaluation.

Management of Sexual Dysfunction

The management of sexual dysfunction is usually initiated by the primary care physician. Properly focused evaluation attempts to identify patients that require referral for specialized management, and facilitates selection of appropriate therapeutic options (Table 32.5). Initial therapy should address readily reversible factors. Drugs known to cause impotence should be withdrawn. Patients with hyperprolactinemia may benefit from bromocriptine, and optimizing therapy of associated illnesses such as thyroid disease and diabetes mellitus may be helpful.

Creating a nonjudgmental ambience devoid of moralizing permits free expression of anxieties and concerns that may surround sexual issues. Patients should not be dis-

Table 32.5. Therapeutic Modalities in Impotence.

Sex therapy and counseling
Pharmacologic
  Testosterone replacement
  Intracavernosal injections
    Prostaglandin E-1
    Papaverine
    Phentolamine
Mechanical vacuum tumescent devices
Penile prostheses implantation
  Malleable rods
  Hinged prostheses
  Inflatable hydraulic prostheses
Surgery
  Penile venoablation
  Penile arterial revascularization
  Deep dorsal vein arterialization
  Percutaneous transluminal angioplasty

couraged from broadening their sexual horizons, if this may improve their sexual function. Alternative sexual positions and practices, which may increase sexual satisfaction in the individual patient, should be explored. Sexual dysfunction should be addressed as a couple-oriented problem only if relevant to the individual's particular social circumstances.

The appreciation of sexuality as it pertains to the older person has resulted in renewed interest in the treatment of impotence. An abundance of therapeutic options now exist. As the treatment of impotence varies with the individual, the onus rests with the physician to decide on the most appropriate therapeutic modality.

Older men with hypogonadism have been shown to benefit from testosterone replacement therapy. Although this has a greater effect on increasing libido, a significant qualitative improvement in erectile function has been reported (113). Intramuscular and dermal preparations are usually preferred because these significantly reduce the incidence of hepatotoxicity. Regardless of the route of administration, testosterone therapy mandates serial monitoring of hemoglobin and liver function tests because secondary polycythemia and hepatic dysfunction are acknowledged adverse effects. Rectal digital examinations should be done every 3 to 6 months to assess prostate size because testosterone therapy may predispose to worsening benign prostatic hypertrophy. A prostate-specific antigen (PSA) profile performed periodically while the patient is undergoing testosterone therapy may be advisable because some evidence suggests that pharmacologic testosterone therapy may increase the risk of prostatic cancer (53,107). Added advantages of testosterone repletion in the older man include an increase in muscle strength, which may further enhance sexual ability. Testosterone replacement has also been shown to result in an improved lipid profile, as evidenced by a reduction in serum cholesterol levels. High-density lipoproteins are unaffected (114,115).

Other modes of therapy that are not specifically directed at a particular etiology are also available. Intracavernosal injection of vasoactive drugs for the treatment of erectile failure is accepted as a standard therapeutic procedure and may improve erectile function, regardless of the underlying cause. A high rate of patient and partner satisfaction have been reported. The fact that self-injection can be carried out positively influences patient acceptability and compliance (116), although in some patients this procedure may have the paradoxical effect of reducing sexual desire by detracting from the spontaneity of sexual intercourse. Penile pain may occur immediately after injection and is thought to be related to the acidity of the drug medium. This side effect may be prevented by increasing the pH of the drug-carriage solutions. The addition of sodium bicarbonate has been found useful for this purpose (117). Other short-term side effects are bruising, hematoma formation, urethral bleeding, and priapism. Fibrosis of the corpora and penile fibrosis may complicate repeated injections (118).

Pharmacologic agents used most commonly for intracavernosal injections are papaverine, PGE-1, and phentolamine. PGE-1 may be the agent of choice because it has been shown to have fewer side effects and produces erections of longer duration, although slower onset of action may be a drawback (119). Combined therapy with all three agents has been tried and is purported to have an additive effect on improving erectile quality without an attendant increase in side effects (120). Vasoactive intestinal peptide has been used, but the degree of penile rigidity produced is usually inadequate for vaginal intromission (121). The identification of calcitonin-gene-related-peptide (CGRP) as a putative neurotransmitter involved in penile erection led to exploration of its therapeutic potential in impotence. Properly controlled trials are yet to be carried out, but initial reports suggest that the combination of CGRP and PGE-1 may be more effective and less painful than any of the other agents used in isolation (122). On the basis of research to establish the role of nitric oxide in achieving penile erections, intracavernosal sodium nitroprusside was studied with unimpressive results. Only mild increases in penile tumescence were achieved, and severe hypotension occurred frequently (123).

Pharmacologic alternatives to intracavernosal injections have been studied. Yohimbine, an alpha$_2$-adrenergic antagonist derived from the bark of the yohimbine tree, was widely publicized as an aphrodisiac. These claims remain largely unsubstantiated as its efficacy has not been proven and clinical use is precluded by prohibitive side effects, which include hepatotoxicity and systemic hypertension (47,124). Pentoxyfilline, which reduces erythro-

cyte membrane rigidity, is of proven benefit in some patients with vasculogenic impotence (125). Other drugs include fluoxetine, a serotonin reuptake inhibitor, minoxidil, and topical nitrates, all of which have been tried with variable success (126–128).

For patients who fail to respond to pharmacotherapy or for those who do not wish to inject themselves, the use of vacuum tumescent devices is a justifiable option. These devices generate negative pressure through a plastic cylinder placed over the penis and encourage increased perfusion which results in a functional erection. Penile rigidity may be maintained for as long as 30 minutes with the aid of a constricting band placed over the base of the penis, before the device is removed. Side effects of repeated use include penile pain, bruising, and diminished ejaculation. Nonetheless, studies have confirmed the relative efficacy and safety of these devices (129,130). The noninvasive nature of this technique constitutes an added advantage.

Of the available surgical options, penile prosthesis insertion is most favored. Semirigid and inflatable varieties are available and have been found to be of comparable efficacy, although the semirigid varieties are less expensive and easier to use (131). A major disadvantage of inflatable devices is the low, 5-year durability rate of approximately 50 percent, which exposes the patient to the possibility of repeat surgery and its attendant risks and complications (132).

Arterial or venous surgery is rarely indicated in the management of vasculogenic impotence. Penile venoablation or venous surgery is used in the management of impotence associated with venous leaks for selected patients who fail to respond to intracavernosal vasoactive therapy and retain unimpaired arterial perfusion (133,134). Other surgical techniques include arterial revascularization and deep dorsal vein arterialization; however, the results are relatively poor (135,136). Percutaneous transluminal angioplasty has been used in younger men with moderate atherogenic stenosis of the penile vasculature (137). Data pertaining to the older man are currently unavailable.

Despite the uncertain etiology, several relatively successful treatment modalities are available for the treatment of premature ejaculation. Sex therapy and sensuality training are important in the management of this condition. The patient should be instructed in the pause-squeeze sexual technique, which is designed to prolong the period between intromission and ejaculation. This method is of proven efficacy and has become established as the initial treatment of choice, before drug therapy (73). Pharmacologic agents used with varying results include low-dose clomipramine and fluoxetine, both of which selectively inhibit 5-hydroxytryptamine uptake (129,138). For patients with coexisting erectile failure, combined therapy with intracavernosal papaverine and phentolamine may correct both premature ejaculation and impotence (139).

Management of sexual dysfunction in the older woman follows essentially the same principles as those applied to men. Thus, identification and treatment of etiological factors, sex education and counseling, where appropriate, and optimization of the medical management of associated illnesses are usually the initial steps. Identification of a specific organic urogenital disease necessitates definitive management.

Vaginal atrophy, a relatively common cause of dyspareunia, responds to the application of topical estrogens. Women prescribed hormone-replacement therapy for coexistent perimenopausal symptoms also experience regression of dyspareunia related to urogenital atrophy. Estrogens increase vaginal secretions and improve the integrity of vaginal tissue, which facilitates intromission during sexual intercourse and reduces the chances of friction injury. The physician should be aware that systemic side effects of estrogen therapy can occur with topical application because of transmucosal absorption (140,141). The effect of estrogens on other climacteric symptoms, such as sleep disturbances and mood lability, reinforces the patient's perception of improved health. This may positively influence libido and sexual activity. Hormone-replacement therapy in the older woman has been shown to be cardioprotective. It also retards the onset and progression of osteoporosis. The resultant reduction in frailty and morbidity constitutes important permissive factors in the retention of normal sexual function (140,141).

The treatment of women who experience intracoital incontinence varies with the mechanism of urinary loss identified. Detrusor muscle instability is usually managed with anticholinergic drugs such as oxybutinin; stress in-

continence responds to bladder and pelvic floor muscle exercises. Ideally, in multiparous women and after childbirth or pelvic surgery, these exercises should be instituted as preventive measures (142,143).

Vulvar vestibulitis syndrome (VVS) describes the combination of dyspareunia, introital erythema, and tenderness. Acute cases usually have a readily identifiable cause, inflammatory or otherwise, which is readily amenable to appropriate treatment. Chronic VVS has been described. The etiology remains unknown, but is presumed to be multifactorial. Treatment is symptomatic and directed mainly at pain relief. Topical xylocaine, acupuncture, and hypnotherapy have been tried. Some patients fail to respond and, in such cases, oral antiviral therapy or interferon has proved beneficial (144). The relevance of this condition to the older woman is not known.

In a proportion of women with sexual dysfunction, surgical intervention is occasionally indicated. Severe urinary incontinence and dyspareunia resulting from conditions such as uterovaginal prolapse may require pelvic floor repair. A variety of uterine suspension surgical procedures have been designed to correct fixed uterine retroversion in symptomatic patients. Laparoscopic methods are currently favored and are relatively free of significant operative morbidity (145).

It is imperative to recognize and address psychological and relationship issues that may contribute to sexual dysfunction. Appropriate sex education and counseling are pivotal aspects of effective management. Ideal treatment of the patient with sexual dysfunction should involve a multidisciplinary team with readily accessible avenues for psychological counseling and neuropsychiatric evaluation. Behavioral and sex therapy should complement formal medical management. Instruction in specific techniques to improve sexual arousal and performance may be appropriate. Marriage or relationship counseling may improve communication between partners and assist in the resolution of interpersonal conflict.

Before surgery such as hysterectomy, mastectomy, or other operations that may impair the individual's perception of self, psychological counseling should be carried out and the issue of sexuality specifically addressed. Similarly, difficulty with sexual arousal and response should be anticipated after surgery and managed accordingly.

Patient support groups and self-help groups often assist the individual in the development of a positive body image, which serves to improve self-esteem and enhance sexuality.

The attitude of the physician is of utmost importance in the appraisal of sexual function in the older patient. Current management of sexual disorders hinges substantially on the extrapolation of research findings from the younger population. In constructing management and therapeutic strategies, the physician must not fall prey to the vagaries of ageism, because there is a significant possibility that the clinical presentation of sexual dysfunction in the older patient may be at variance with universally accepted sexual syndromes. Detection of such areas of controversy should serve as the initiating stimulus for further research in an attempt to improve understanding and refine current management techniques of sexual dysfunction within the context of geriatric medicine.

References

1. Bishop JM, Krause DR. Depictions of aging and old age on Saturday morning television. Gerontologist 1984;24:91–94.
2. Arluke EA, Levin J, Suchwalko J. Sexuality and romance in advice books for the elderly. Gerontologist 1984;24:415–419.
3. Gupta K. Sexual dysfunction in elderly women. Clin Geriatr Med 1990;6(1):197–203.
4. Kinsey AC, Pomeroy WB, Martin CE. Sexual behavior in the human male. Philadelphia: Saunders, 1948.
5. Starr BD, Weiner MB. The Starr-Weiner report on sex and sexuality in the mature years. New York: Stein and Day, 1981.
6. Pfeiffer E, Verwoerdt A, Wang HS. Sexual behavior in aged men and women. Arch Gen Psychiatry 1968;19:735–758.
7. Bretschneider JG, McCoy L. Sexual interest and behavior in healthy 80–120-year-olds. Arch Sex Behav 1988;17:109–129.
8. Persson G. Sexuality in a 70-year-old urban population. J Psychosomatic Res 1980;24:335–342.
9. The portrayal of elders in magazine cartoons. Gerontologist 1979;19:408–412.
10. Morley JE. Impotence. Am J Med 1986;80:897–906.
11. Slag MF, Morley JE, Elson MK, et al. Impotence in medical clinic outpatients. JAMA 1983;249:1736.
12. Kaiser FE, Viosca SP, Morley JE, et al. Impotence and aging: clinical and hormonal factors. J Am Geriatric Soc 1988;36:511–519.
13. Kaiser FE, Korenman SG. Impotence in diabetic men. Am J Med 1988;85(suppl 5A):147–152.
14. Masters WH, Johnson VE. Human sexual response. Boston: Little Brown, 1966.
15. Salmon JJ, Geist SH. Effects of androgens on libido in women. J Clin Endocrinol Metab 1943;3:235–238.
16. Schiavi RC, Schreiner-Engel P, Mandeli J, et al. Healthy aging and male sexual function. Am J Psychiatry 1990;147:766–771.
17. Sherwin BB, Gelfand MM, Brender W. Androgen enhances sexual motivation in females: a prospective crossover study of sex steroid administration in surgical menopause. Psychosom Med 1984;47:339.
18. Skakkeback N, Bancroft J, Davidson DW, et al. Androgen replacement with oral testosterone undecanoate in hypogonadal men: a double-blind controlled study. Clin Endocrinol 1981;14:49–55.
19. Davidson JM, Chen JJ, Crapo L, et al. Hormonal changes and sexual function in aging men. J Clin Endocrinol Metab 1983;57:71–77.
20. Morley JE, Kaiser FE. Testicular function in the aging male. In: Armbrecht HJ, ed. Endocrine function and aging. New York: Springer-Verlag, 1990:99–174.
21. Neaves WB, Johnson L, Parker CR, et al. Leydig cell numbers, sperm production and serum gonadotropin levels in aging men. J Clin Endocrinol Metab 1984;59:756–763.
22. Korenman SG, Morley JE, Mooradian AD, et al. Secondary hypogonadism in older men: its relation to impotence. J Clin Endocrinol Metab 1990;71:963–969.
23. Pradma-Nathan H, Boyd SD, Cheung D. The biochemical effects of aging, diabetes and ischemia on corporal and tunica collagen. J Urol 1991;145:342.
24. Rakoff AE, Nowroozi K. The female climacteric. In: Greenblatt RB, ed. Geriatric endocrinology. vol 5. New York: Raven, 1978:165–90.
25. Judd HL. Hormonal dynamics associated with the menopause. Clin Obstet Gynecol 1976;19:775–788.
26. Siiteri PK, Macdonald PC. Role of extraglandular estrogen in human endocrinology. In: Gareep RO, Astwood E, eds. Endocrinology handbook of physiology 2. Washington, DC: American Physiology Society, 1973:615–629.
27. Sherman BM, West JH, Korenman SG. The menopausal transition: analysis of LH, FSH, estradiol and progesterone concentrations during menstrual cycles of older women. J Clin Endocrinol Metab 1982;42:629–636.
28. Scaglia H, Medina M, Pinto-Ferreira AI, et al. Pituitary LH and FSH secretion and responsiveness in women of old age. Acta Endocrinol 1976;81:673–679.
29. Strathy JM, Coulam CB, Spelsburg TC. Comparison of estrogen receptors in human premenopausal and postmenopausal uteri. Am J Obstet Gynecol 1982;142:372–376.
30. Hasselquist MB, Goldberg N, Schroeter A, Spelsberg TC. Isolation and characteristics of the estrogen receptor in human skin. J Clin Endocrinol Metab 1980;50:76–82.
31. Koster A. Change of life anticipations and emotional experiences among middle aged Danish women. Health Care Women Int 1991;12:1–13.
32. Morrell MJ, Dixon JM, Carter SM. The influence of age and ovulatory status on sexual arousability in women. Am J Obstet Gynecol 1984;148:66–71.

33. Mead M. Cultural determination of sexual behavior. In: Young WC, Corner GW, eds. Sex and internal secretions. Baltimore: Williams & Wilkins, 1969:1433–1476.

34. Appelt H. The effects of antiandrogen treatment on the sexuality of hirsute women. Presented at the Seventh World Congress of psychosomatic medicine. Hamburg, Germany, 1983.

35. Studd JWW, Collins WP, Charkravati S. Estradiol and testosterone implants in the treatment of psychosexual problems in the postmenopausal woman. Br J Obstet Gynaecol 177;84:314–316.

36. Dow MGT, Hart DM, Forrest CA. Hormonal treatments of sexual unresponsiveness in postmenopausal women. Br J Obstet Gynaecol 1983;90:361–366.

37. Burger H, Hailes J, Nelson J, Menelaus M. Effect of combined implants of estradiol and testosterone on libido in postmenopausal women. BMJ 1987;294:936–937.

38. Sherwin BB, Gelfand MM, Brender W. Androgen enhances sexual motivation in females: a prospective crossover study of sex steroid administration in surgical menopause. Psychosom Med 1984;47:339.

39. Campbell S. Double-blind psychometric studies on the effect of natural estrogens on postmenopausal women. In: Campbell S, ed. Management of menopause and postmenopause years. Lancaster, England: MTP press, 1976:149.

40. Kaplan HS. Sex, intimacy and the aging process. J Am Acad Psychoanalysis 1990;18:185–205.

41. Costa PT, Fagan PJ, Piedmont RL, et al. The five-factor model of personality and sexual functioning in outpatient men and women. Psychiatr Med 1992;10:199–215.

42. Catalan J, Hawton K, Day A. Couples referred to a sexual dysfunction clinic. Psychological and physical morbidity. Br J Psychiatry. 1990;156:61–67.

43. Cogen R, Steiman W. Sexual function and practice in elderly men of lower socioeconomic status. J Fam Pract 1990;31:162–166.

44. Dror IE, Kosslyn SM. Mental imagery and aging. Psychol Aging 1994;9:90–102.

45. Kane MJ, Hasher L, Stoltzfus ER, et al. Inhibitory attentional mechanisms and aging. Psychol Aging 1994;103–112.

46. Leavitt SC. Sexual idealogy in a Papua, New Guinea Society. Soc Sci Med 1994;33:897–907.

47. Morley JE, Kaiser FE. Impotence: the internist's approach to diagnosis and treatment. Adv Intern Med 1993;38:151–168.

48. Krane RJ, Goldstein I, deTejada IS. Impotence. N Engl J Med 1989;321:1648–1659.

49. Morley JE, Korenman SG, Kaiser FE, et al. Relationship of penile brachial pressure index to myocardial infarction and cerebrovascular accidents in older males. Am J Med 1988;84:445–448.

50. Raifer J, Rosciszewski A, Mehringer M. Prevalence of corporeal venous leakage in impotent men. J Urol 1988;140:69–73.

51. Tudonu T. My views about the applied anatomy of the penis and the physiopathology of erection. Arch Ital Urol 1989;61:249–273.

52. Kaiser FE. Sexuality and impotence in the aging man. Clin Geriatr Med 1991;7:63–73.

53. Billington CJ, Shafer RB, Krezouski PA, et al. Zinc status and impotence. In: Morley JE, Glick Z, Rubenstein LZ, eds. Geriatric nutrition. New York: Raven, 1990:441–448.

54. Milier L, Rogers JC, Sire DE. Indomethacin associated sexual dysfunction. J Fam Pract 1989;29:210–211.

55. Morley JE, Kaiser FE. Impotence in elderly men. Drugs Aging 1992;2:330–334.

56. Padma-Norton H, Goldstein I, Krane RJ. Vascular effects of chronic cigarette smoking. Presented at the Second World Meeting on impotence. Prague, Czechoslovakia, June 16–20, 1986.

57. Jeureman KP, Lue TF, Fournier GR Jr, et al. Haemodynamics of papaverine and phentolamine induced penile erections. J Urol 1986;136:158–163.

58. Giena S, Reichert AL, Leao PP, et al. Impact of cigarette smoking on papaverine-induced erections. J Urol 1987;138:438–439.

59. Leonard MP, Nickel CJ, Morales A. Hyperprolactinaemia and impotence: why, when and how to investigate. J Urol 1989;142:992–994.

60. Luton JP, Thiebot P, Valcke JC, et al. Reversible gonadotropin deficiency in males with Cushing's disease. J Clin Endocrinol Metab 1977;45:488–495.

61. Gaskell P. The importance of penile blood pressure in cases of impotence. Can Med Assoc J 1971;105:1047–1051.

62. Lin JT, Bradley WE. Penile neuropathy in insulin-dependent diabetes mellitus. J Urol 1985;133:213–215.

63. Metha AJ, Viosca SP, Korenman SG, et al. Peripheral nerve conduction studies and bulbocavernosus reflex in the investigation of impotence. Arch Phys Med Rehabil 1986;67:332–335.

64. Saenz de Tejada I, Goldstein I, Azadozoi K, et al. Impaired neurogenic and endothelium mediated relaxation of penile smooth muscle from diabetic men with impotence. N Engl J Med 1989;320:1025–1030.

65. Mooradian AD, Morley JE, Billington CJ, et al. Hyperprolactinaemia in male diabetics. Postgrad Med J 1985;61:11–15.

66. Lundberg PO. Sexual dysfunction in multiple sclerosis. Sexuality Disability 1978;1:218–222.

67. Blumer D, Walker AE. Sexual behavior in temporal lobe epilepsy. Arch Neurol 1967;16:37–43.

68. Bemermans BLH, Meuleman EJH, Anten BWM, et al. Penile sensory disorders in erectile dysfunction. J Urol 1991;146:777–782.

69. Zeiss RA, Delmonico RL, Zeiss AM, et al. Psychological disorders and sexual dysfunction in elders. Clin Geriatr Med 1991;17:133–151.

70. Yesavage JA, Davidson J, Widrow L, et al. Plasma testosterone levels, depression, sexuality and age. Biol Psychiatr 1988;20:199–228.

71. Hale VE, Strassberg DS. The role of anxiety on sexual arousal. Arch Sex Behav 1990;19:569–581.

72. Beck JG, Barlow DH. The effects of anxiety and attentional

focus on sexual responding. 1. Physiological patterns in erectile dysfunction. Behav Res Ther 1986;24:9–18.

73. St. Lawrence JS, Madakasira S. Evaluation and treatment of premature ejaculation: a critical review. Int J Psychiatr Med 1992;22:77–97.

74. Witt MA, Grantmyre JE. Ejaculatory failure. World J Urol 1993;11:89–95.

75. Hershlag A, Schiff SF, Decherney AH. Retrograde ejaculation. Human reproduction. 1991;6:255–258.

76. Strassberg DS, Mahoney JM, Schaugaard M, Hale VE. The role of anxiety in premature ejaculation: a psychophysiological model. Arch Sex Behav. 1990;19:251–257.

77. Rowland DL, Haensel SM, Blom JH, Slob AK. Penile sensitivity in men with premature ejaculation and erectile dysfunction. J Sex Marital Ther 1993;19:189–197.

78. Cooper AJ, Cernovsky ZZ, Colussi K. Some clinical and psychometric characteristics of primary and secondary premature ejaculators. J Sex Marital Ther 1993;19:276–288.

79. Sarazin SK, Seymour SF. Causes and treatment options for women with dyspareunia. Nurs Pract 1991;16:30, 35–38, 41.

80. Roughan PA, Kaiser FE, Morley JE. Sexuality and the older woman. Clin Geriatr Med 1993;9:87–106.

81. Dewitt DE. Dyspareunia: tracing the cause. Postgrad Med 1991;89:67–68, 70, 73.

82. Petros JG, Spirito N, Gosshein R. Endometriosis causing colon obstruction in two postmenopausal women. Mount Sinai J Med 1992;59:362–365.

83. DePriest PD, Banks ER, Powell DE, et al. Endometrioid carcinoma of the ovary and endometriosis: the association in postmenopausal women. Gynecol Oncol 1992;47:71–75.

84. Moody G, Probert CS, Srivastava EM, et al. Sexual dysfunction among women with Crohn's disease: a hidden problem. Digestion 1992;52:179–183.

85. Wilkes RA, Seymour N. Dyspareunia due to exostoses formation after pelvic fracture. Br J Obstet Gynaecol 1993;100:1050–1051.

86. Browning JE. Mechanically induced pelvic pain and organic dysfunction in a patient without low back pain. J Manip Physiol Ther 1990;13:406–411.

87. Delancey JO, Sampselle CM, Punch MR. Kegel dyspareunia: levator ani myalgia caused by overexertion. Obstet Gynecol 1993;82(suppl):658–658.

88. Sutherst JR. Sexual dysfunction and urinary incontinence. Br J Obstet Gynaecol 1979;86:338–398.

89. Hilton P. Urinary incontinence during sexual intercourse: a common but rarely volunteered symptom. Br J Obstet Gynaecol 1988;95:377–381.

90. Cardozo LD. Sex and the bladder. BMJ 1988;296:587–588.

91. Morgan S. Sexuality after hysterectomy and castration. Women Health 1978;3:5–10.

92. Morley JE. Sexual function and the aging woman. In: Morley JE, Korenman SG, eds. Endocrinology and metabolism in the elderly. Boston: Blackwell Science, 1992:307–321.

93. Frank D, Dornbush RL, Webster SL, Kolodny RC. Mastec-

94. Jensen SB. Sexual relationships in couples with a diabetic partner. J Sex Marital Ther 1985;11:259–270.

95. Rostlapil J, Zrustova M. Etiology of female sexual disorders. Diabetes Outlook 1978;13:6–10.

96. McCabe MP, Delaney SM. An elevation of therapeutic programs for the treatment of secondary inorgasmia in females. Arch Sex Behav 1992;21:69–89.

97. Kaiser FE, Morley JE. Sexuality and dementia. In: Morris J, ed. Handbook of dementing illnesses. New York: Marcel Dekker, 1994:539–548.

98. Rabins PV, Mac NL, Lucas MJ. The impact of dementia on the family. JAMA 1982;248:333–335.

99. Secrest CL, Jordan GH, Winslow BH, et al. Repair of the complications of hypospadias surgery. J Urol 1993;150:1415–1418.

100. Eberle J, Uberreiter S, Radmayr C, et al. Posterior hypospadias: long-term follow-up after reconstructive surgery in the male direction. J Urol 1993;150:1474–1477.

101. Folstein M, Anthony JC, Parbad I, et al. The meaning of cognitive impairment in the elderly. J Am Geriatr Soc 1985;33:228–235.

102. Yesavage JA, Brink TL. Development and validation of a geriatric depression screening scale: a preliminary report. J Psychiatr Res 1983;17:37–49.

103. Kaplan HS, Owett T. The female androgen deficiency syndrome. J Sex Marital Ther 1993;19:13–24.

104. Zgur T, Vodusek DB, Kizan M, et al. Autonomic system dysfunction in moderate diabetic polyneuropathy assessed by sympathetic skin response and the Valsalva index. Electromyog Clin Neurophysiol 1993;33:433–439.

105. Robinson LQ, Woodcock JP, Stephenson TP. Duplex scanning in suspected vasculogenic impotence: a worthwhile exercise. Br J Urol 1989;63:432–436.

106. Aitchison M, Aitchison J, Carter R. Is the penile brachial index a reproducible and useful measurement? Br J Urol 1990;66:202–204.

107. Morley JE, Kaiser FE. Sexual function with advancing age. Med Clin North Am 1989;73:1483–1495.

108. Williams G, Mulcahy J, Hartnell G, et al. Diagnosis and treatment of venous leakage: a curable cause of impotence. Br J Urol 1989;64:93–97.

109. Rudnick J, Bodecker R, Weidner W. Significance of the intracavernosal pharmacological injection test, pharmacocavernosography, artificial erection and cavernosometry in the diagnosis of venous leakage. Urol Int 1991;46:338–343.

110. Schwartz ZAN, Lowe M, Berger RE, et al. Assessment of normal and abnormal erectile function: color, Doppler flow sonography versus conventional techniques. Radiology 1991;180:105–109.

111. Lehman TP, Jacobs JA. Etiology of diabetic impotence. J Urol 1983;129:291–294.

112. Lin JT, Bradley WE. Penile neuropathy in insulin dependent diabetes mellitus. J Urol 1985;133:213–215.

113. Korenman SG, Viosca S, Garza D, et al. Androgen therapy of hypogonadal men with transdermal testosterone systems. Am J Med 1987;83:471–478.

114. Morley JE, Perry III HM, Kaiser FE. Effect of testosterone replacement therapy in old hypogonadal males. J Am Geriatric Soc 1993;41:149–152.

115. Tenover JS. The effects of testosterone supplementation in the aging male. J Clin Endocrinol Metab 1992;75:1092.

116. Chiang HS, Wen TC, Wu CC, Chiang WH. Intracavernous self-injection therapy for the treatment of erectile dysfunction. J Formosa Med Assoc 1992;91:898–901.

117. Moriel EZ, Raifer J. Sodium bicarbonate alleviates penile pain induced by intracavernous injections for erectile dysfunction. J Urol 1993;149:1299–1300.

118. Mooradian AD, Morley JE, Kaiser FE, et al. The role of biweekly intracavernous injection of papaverine in the treatment of erectile dysfunction. West J Med 1989;151:515–517.

119. Chen JK, Hwang TI, Yang CR. Comparison of effects following the intracorporeal injection of papaverine and prostaglandin E1. Br J Urol 1992;69:404–407.

120. Gorieir FE, McClure RD, Weissman RM, et al. Experience with triple drug therapy in a pharmacological erection program. J Urol 1993;150:1833.

121. Roy JB, Petrone RL, Said SI. A clinical trial of intracavernous vasoactive intestinal peptide to induce penile erection. J Urol 1990;143:302–304.

122. Stief CG, Wetterauer U, Schaebsdau FH, Jonas U. Calcitonin-gene-related-peptide: a possible role in human penile erection and its therapeutic application in impotent patients. J Urol 1991;146:1010–1014.

123. Brock G, Breza J, Lue TF. Intracavernous sodium nitroprusside: inappropriate impotence treatment. J Urol 1993;150:864–867.

124. Morales A, Condra MS, Owen JE, et al. Oral and transcutaneous pharmacological agents in the treatment of impotence. Urol Clin North Am 1988;15:87–93.

125. Korenman SG, Mooradian Ad, Kaiser FE, et al. Treatment of vasculogenic sexual dysfunction with pentoxyfilline. Clin Res 1988;36:123A.

126. Radomski SB, Herschorn S, Rangaswamy S. Topical minoxidil in the treatment of male erectile dysfunction. J Urol 1994;151:1238.

127. Meyttoff HH, Rosenkilde P, Bodker A. Noninvasive management of impotence with transcutaneous nitroglycerin. Br J Urol 1992;69:88–90.

128. Power-Smith P. Beneficial sexual side effects from fluoxetine. Br J Psychiatr 1994;164:249–250.

129. Van Thillo EL, Delaere KP. The vacuum erection device. A noninvasive treatment for impotence. Acta Urol Belgica 1992;60:9–13.

130. Cookson MS, Nadig PW. Long-term results with vacuum constriction devices. J Urol 1993;149:290–294.

131. Lange PH, Duffy M, Braatz GA, et al. A comparison of functional and cosmetic results among different penile prostheses. J Urol 1984;131:301A.

132. Kabahn JN, Kessler R. Five-year follow-up of the Scott inflatable penile prosthesis. J Urol 1988;140:1428–1430.

133. Knispel HH. Penile venous surgery in impotence: results in highly selected cases. Urol Int 1991;47:144–148.

134. Muller SC, Schild H, Fritz T, Witzsch U. Percutaneous transpenile and retrograde venous occlusion for the treatment of venous leak impotence. Eur Urol 1991;19:101–103.

135. Michal V, Kramer R, Pospical J. Direct arterial anastomoses on corpora cavernosa of the penis in the therapy of erectile impotence. Rozhi Chir 1973;52:587–590.

136. Sarramon JP, Janssen T, Rischmann P, et al. Deep dorsal vein arterialization in vascular impotence. Eur Urol 1994;25:29–33.

137. Mielecki T, Marchinak R, Drelichowski S. Results of the treatment of vascular induced impotence using PTA. Rontgenblatter 1990;43:435–438.

138. Segraves RT, Saran A, Segraves K, Naguire E. Clomipramine versus placebo in the management of premature ejaculation: a pilot study. J Sex Marital Ther 1993;19:198–200.

139. Fein RL. Intracavernous medication for treatment of premature ejaculation. Urology 1990;35:301–303.

140. Morley JE, Korenman SG, Kaiser FE. The menopause. In: Morley JE, Korenman SG, eds. Endocrinology and metabolism in the elderly. Boston: Blackwell Science, 1992:322–335.

141. Kaiser FE, Morley JE. The menopause and beyond. In: Cassel KC, Riesenberg DE, Sorenson LB, Walsh JR, eds. Geriatric medicine. New York: Springer-Verlag, 1990:279–290.

142. Segraves RT. Psychiatric drugs and inhibited female orgasm. J Sex Marital Ther 1988;14:202–207.

143. Cardozo LD. Sexually induced urinary incontinence. BMJ 1988;296:587–588.

144. Secor RM, Fertitta L. Vulvar vestibulitis syndrome. Nurs Pract 1992;3:161–168.

145. Perry CP, Sarria C. Minimal-incision Pereyra needle uterine suspension. J Laparoendosc Surg 1991;1:151–155.

Part IV Common Diseases and Disorders

Chapter 33
Coronary Artery Disease in the Elderly

Eugene E. Wolfel

You're not as young as you used to be. But you're not as old as you're going to be. So watch it!

Irish Toast

The elderly population in the United States is becoming an increasing larger percentage of the total number of patients with coronary artery disease. This is a reflection of growing numbers of elderly in the United States as well as the increasing prevalence of heart disease in older people. Seventy-two percent of all cardiovascular deaths in the United States occur in patients over age 65, with 69 percent related to complications from coronary heart disease (1). Despite decreases in overall cardiovascular mortality in the United States, the morbidity and mortality of coronary artery disease remains high in the elderly population (2). In addition, the influence of underlying cardiac disease in the elderly on quality of life issues such as exercise capacity, independent living, and economic factors, both individual and societal, is tremendous. Because of several unique physiologic and psychosocial issues in the elderly population, the diagnosis and management of coronary artery disease has become a major focus in the general health care of elderly patients. Unfortunately, little information has come from large clinical trials on coronary artery disease to determine the efficacy and safety of different management strategies for elderly patients (3). Most care for older patients with coronary artery disease is based on information from small clinical studies of elderly patients, extrapolations of studies performed with younger patients, or on intuitive deductions from knowledge of the interactions between the normal aging process and the pathophysiology of coronary artery disease (4–6).

In this chapter, elderly is defined as persons age 65 years or older, although some discussion of the advanced elderly (≥75 years) is also provided. A comprehensive discussion of epidemiology, risk factors, and the diagnosis and management of chronic coronary artery disease including medical therapy, percutaneous transluminal coronary angioplasty (PTCA), and coronary bypass surgery (CABG) is presented. In addition, the management of elderly patients with acute myocardial infarction is reviewed with special reference to the role of thrombolytic therapy and acute interventional procedures for these patients.

Epidemiology

Coronary atherosclerosis is an extremely common finding at autopsy in elderly patients, with an incidence of 46 percent in the sixth decade and 84 percent in the ninth decade of life (7). Autopsy material from routine cases in Olmstead, Minnesota has shown that 60 percent of all patients older than age 60 had at least one coronary artery with a 75 percent to 100 percent occlusion (8). Pomerance showed that 48.5 percent of patients with congestive heart failure older than age 75 had autopsy evidence of significant coronary artery disease (9). In a series of routine autopsies of patients older than 90 years of age, Waller and Roberts reported significant coronary artery disease in 39 of 40 patients (10). The severity of coronary atherosclerosis varied and was related to serum cholesterol in these patients. These data suggest that coronary atherosclerosis may not be a necessary consequence of aging but may be related to coronary risk.

The high incidence of coronary disease in elderly persons at autopsy contrasts sharply with the clinical incidence of disease. At age 70, 15 percent of men and 9 percent of women have clinical evidence of coronary artery disease, but at age 80, the incidence reaches 20 percent in both genders (1). Results from the Framingham Study in patients age 65 to 74 reported an incidence of 20 percent in men and 15 percent in women (11). However, the prevalence of coronary artery disease in the elderly is quite high, with a 50 percent prevalence for ages 65 to 74 years and a 60 percent prevalence for those older than 75 years of age (12). Compared with a younger population, the prevalence of coronary artery disease in the elderly is similar for men and women. The discrepancy between autopsy evidence and clinical evidence of coronary artery disease is partially related to the underdetection of the disease in this population. The subtle presentation of coronary disease in the elderly, along with episodes of silent ischemia and infarction, contribute to the lower rate of detection for this population.

Coronary Risk Factors

The decline in cardiovascular mortality in the last decade has been less noted in the elderly population. Although the mortality rate from acute myocardial infarction decreased by 23 percent in patients aged 55 to 64 years, the mortality decreased only 12 percent in patients aged 65 to 74 years (2). In addition, the mortality rates in women were higher and decreased less than those for men. In younger patients, the decline in cardiovascular mortality has been attributed not only to better medical care of known cardiac disease, but also to reductions in coronary risk factors. Although coronary risk factors in the elderly have been recognized, the importance of risk factor modification to change the morbidity and mortality of coronary artery disease has not been determined. The Framingham Study clearly showed that several risk factors retain their predictive values for an increased cardiac event rate in the elderly population (Table 33.1). In addition, high and low levels of risk have been determined. Two percent of subsequent coronary artery disease cases were found in the lowest decile of risk factors; 25 percent of cases in men and 37 percent of cases in women were found in the highest risk decile (13).

The relative importance of several known coronary risk factors changes with age (14). Although cigarette smoking has been shown to carry significant coronary risk for younger persons, it is less predictive than other risk factors in the elderly (15). However, elderly women who continue to smoke have an increased risk of cardiac events (14). Quitting smoking returned the rate of clinical coronary disease to the rate of nonsmokers within 1 year.

Table 33.1. Framingham Study Risk Factors for Coronary Artery Disease in the Elderly.

Major Risk Factors	Optimal Risk[a]	Poor Risk[b]
Elevated SBP	SBP = 105	SBP = 195
Decreased HDL	Chol = 185	Chol = 385
Elevated LDL	Normal glucose	Elevated glucose
High chol/HDL	Nonsmoker	Smoker
LVH on ECG	Negative LVH on ECG	Positive LVH on ECG
Diabetes (women)		

[a] At age 70, only 10% men and 9% women developed clinical coronary disease.
[b] At age 70, 82% men and 68% women developed coronary disease.
Chol = total cholesterol; ECG = electrocardiogram; HDL = high-density lipoprotein; LDL = low-density lipoprotein; LVH = left ventricular hypertrophy; SBP = systolic blood pressure.
SOURCE: Gordon T, Castelli WP, Hjortland MC, et al. Predicting coronary heart disease in middle-aged and older persons: the Framingham Study. JAMA 1977;238:497 and Castelli WP. Risk factors in the elderly: a view from Framingham. Am J Geriatr Cardiol 1993;3:8.

Systolic blood pressure elevation is a significant risk for cardiovascular disease, specifically for coronary artery disease in the elderly. Levels greater than 180 mm Hg are associated with a striking increase in coronary risk. Left ventricular hypertrophy (LVH) on electrocardiogram (ECG) is an independent risk factor and probably reflects elevation in both systolic and diastolic blood pressure with evidence of end-organ damage. Diabetes mellitus nearly doubles the coronary risk in men and is an even stronger risk factor for coronary disease in women (14).

Serum lipid abnormalities also appear to influence cardiovascular risk in elderly patients. The importance of total serum cholesterol in predicting overall mortality as well as cardiovascular mortality for elderly patients remains controversial. In a recent analysis of the Framingham Study, an elevated total serum cholesterol predicted an increase in overall mortality only for patients in the 40- and 50-year age groups (Figure 33.1). This applied to both men and women. Total mortality rose with age whether the patient's serum cholesterol level was less than 200 mg/dL or 280 mg/dL or higher (16). Total serum cholesterol had similar predictive value related to cardiovascular mortality. Other studies report some continued role for an elevated serum cholesterol in

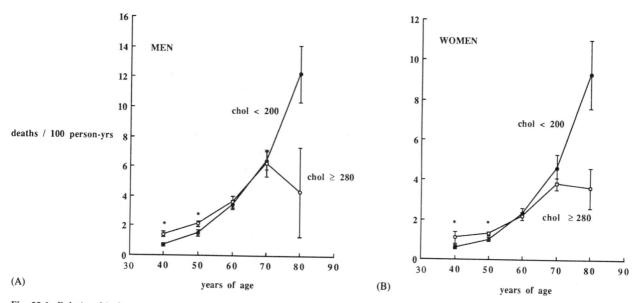

Fig. 33.1. Relationship between overall mortality and serum cholesterol in men (A) and women (B) aged 40–80 years in the Framingham Study. $p < 0.05$ between highest and lowest total serum cholesterol quartiles. (Figures derived from data in Kronmal RA, Cain KC, Ye Z, Omenn GS. Total serum cholesterol levels and mortality risks as a function of age: a report based on the Framingham data. Arch Intern Med 1993;153:1065.)

predicting cardiovascular risk in the elderly with a retained risk from 60 to 80 years of age (17). However, most studies suggest that the lipoprotein subfractions have greater predictive value in elderly patients.

High levels of low-density lipoprotein (LDL) and low levels of high-density lipoprotein (HDL) and an elevated LDL/HDL ratio or total cholesterol to HDL ratio have the major impact on cardiovascular risk. The effects of aging on serum lipids may explain the change in hierarchy of cardiac risk in the various lipid measurements (18). Serum cholesterol does not rise after age 60 in men, although it continues to rise until age 70 in women. At advanced age (≥90 years), women have higher cholesterol values than men. LDL rises until age 60 and begins to decline by age 70, with women having higher LDL levels than men at advanced age. The protective effects of HDL do not appear to decline with age in men; however, HDL does decrease in elderly women, although their levels remain higher than those in men. Triglycerides also decline after age 50 in men but continue to increase in women, so that at age 70, women have higher levels than men. These lipid changes with aging in women may explain why the incidence and prevalence of coronary ar-

tery disease in elderly women is similar to men, unlike the situation for younger age groups in which there is a striking preponderance for coronary artery disease in men.

Although several coronary risk factors have been well delineated in the elderly, the role and safety of risk factor modification is not well defined. Despite evidence that systolic hypertension is strongly associated with both stroke and myocardial infarction (MI) in the elderly, there is minimal direct evidence that aggressive treatment decreases the risk of MI and sudden death. The type of drug therapy used may influence the impact of blood pressure on these outcomes. At the present time, it seems reasonable to lower systolic blood pressure below 160 mm Hg and diastolic blood pressure below 95 mm Hg with antihypertensive agents because the risks of therapy are relatively low. Control of diabetes, especially in elderly women, may also modify coronary risk. Smoking cessation clearly reduces the cardiac risk although the risk of lung cancer and lung disease may not be affected in elderly patients. Weight reduction and an increase in physical activity has an effect on several risk factors and is recommended.

The relative importance of aggressive lipid-lowering

431

therapy in the elderly remains uncertain. In younger patients, primary preventive therapy with both cholestyramine and gemfibrozil in patients with elevated serum cholesterol have demonstrated a reduction in cardiovascular mortality and nonfatal MI (19,20). These improvements resulted from both reductions in LDL and increases in HDL. Neither study demonstrated a decrease in total mortality, and neither study included patients older than 60 years of age. It is unclear whether these results can be extrapolated to the elderly because the predictive value of lipid abnormalities changes with age and elderly patients have a potentially greater risk of drug toxicity. In a recent study of 431 elderly patients (mean age, 71 yrs) with elevated serum cholesterol, lovastatin resulted in a 17 percent to 20 percent fall in total cholesterol, a 24 percent to 28 percent fall in LDL, a 4 percent to 10 percent fall in triglycerides, and a 7 percent to 9 percent increase in HDL (21). These changes occurred with a low incidence of side effects. The impact on cardiac morbidity and mortality was not reported. Because of the uncertainty of the risk-benefit ratio of aggressive lipid lowering therapy in the elderly, current recommendations suggest a less aggressive approach, especially for patients older than age 70 (22,23). Secondary causes of elevated serum cholesterol should be excluded before any lipid modifying therapy is considered. These disorders include hypothyroidism, uncontrolled diabetes, obstructive liver disease, and nephrotic syndrome.

The first line of therapy should be diet modification. The Step I diet recommended by the National Cholesterol Education Program should be the initial step in lowering LDL. This diet consists of 8 percent to 10 percent of total calories from saturated fat, 30 percent or less of calories from total fat, and less than 300 mg/day of cholesterol. Lack of response after 12 weeks requires advancing to a Step II diet in which less than 7 percent of total calories are obtained from saturated fat with less than 200 mg/day of cholesterol. The diet must maintain adequate nutritional balance in elderly persons for general overall health. Dietary intervention needs to be supplemented with patient information and procedures to monitor adherence.

For patients with the highest degree of risk (LDL ≥ 160 mg/dL and total cholesterol ≥240 mg/dL with an associated low HDL) and no comorbid illnesses that would increase the risk of drug toxicity, pharmacological therapy can be attempted. Because there is no current data to support a benefit in cardiovascular mortality and morbidity with lipid-lowering therapy in the elderly, caution is required to avoid serious adverse effects from this therapy. More aggressive therapy should probably be reserved for patients with significant lipid abnormalities and known coronary artery disease. The potential physiologic, psychological, and social impact of aggressive coronary risk factor modification needs to be balanced with the potential improvement in longevity and the prevention of debilitating cardiovascular disorders in the elderly patient.

Diagnosis

Angina is the most common presenting symptom of coronary artery disease in the elderly patient. Angina occurs in 80 percent of this population, yet the history of classic exertional angina may be difficult to obtain. Many elderly patients have limited physical activity and do not develop symptoms until late in the course of their disease, when angina at rest or nocturnal angina becomes the first severe symptom. The description of chest pain may also be misleading because of the patient's inability to remember details of a recent painful episode or because of confusion with other noncardiac medical disorders. Often, ischemic pain is thought to be the result of an arthritic problem in the shoulder or a gastrointestinal disorder such as peptic ulcer disease or esophagitis (24). The pattern of the chest pain syndrome and the factors precipitating its occurrence become the most important historic factors in determining whether ischemic pain is present. Dyspnea on exertion is a very common manifestation of coronary disease in the elderly. Aging causes an increase in stiffness of the left ventricle as well as an increase in end-diastolic volume with exercise (25). These factors make the aged heart more susceptible to developing significant intraventricular pressure elevation produced by myocardial ischemia, which causes dyspnea with activity. Congestive heart failure can often be the presenting complaint in elderly patients with underlying coronary disease. Other symptoms of myocardial ischemia in the elderly include weakness, unexplained diaphoresis, indigestion, and neck and shoulder pain.

Unstable angina, defined as angina at rest, new onset angina, or rapidly progressive angina, occurs more frequently in the elderly. In the Coronary Artery Surgery Study (CASS) 50 percent of all patients age 65 and older who had coronary artery disease had unstable angina compared with only 33 percent of patients younger than age 65. Coronary artery spasm may also contribute to anginal symptoms in the elderly. Vasomotor abnormalities in the coronary vascular bed may contribute to symptoms in elderly patients with known or suspected obstructive coronary disease who experience cold-induced angina, angina at rest, and angina occurring at a variable, unpredictable level of physical exertion. Silent ischemia occurs in elderly patients (26), but its incidence compared with that for younger patients is unknown. Patients with angina have been shown to have more frequent episodes of silent myocardial ischemia with activities of daily living (27). Although elderly patients have been shown to have a higher incidence of silent MI (28), it remains unproven whether they also have a higher incidence of silent ischemia.

Because the history of angina often can be confusing in the elderly patient, other evidence is frequently necessary to confirm the diagnosis of coronary artery disease. Physical examination is usually not helpful because most elderly patients have a fourth heart sound resulting from decreased ventricular compliance related to aging and a high prevalence of mitral valve murmurs caused by other cardiac disorders. The presence of carotid or peripheral arterial disease increases the likelihood of coronary disease, but does not confirm the diagnosis. The resting ECG is usually abnormal in 50 percent of elderly patients, and by itself, is not a specific indicator of coronary disease unless previous transmural MI is clearly demonstrated by the presence of Q waves. Echocardiography with Doppler recordings can be useful to exclude noncoronary causes of cardiac chest pain, including valvular aortic stenosis, hypertrophic cardiomyopathy, pericardial disease, pulmonary hypertension, and mitral valve prolapse. Resting regional LV wall motion abnormalities are a good predictor of coronary artery disease, but they do not provide evidence for the presence of active myocardial ischemia. Some provocative method to stress the myocardium is required to diagnose ischemia. A variety of diagnostic tests are available to determine whether an elderly patient

has coronary artery disease (Table 33.2). Each method has several advantages and disadvantages and the choice of test depends on the special needs of each individual patient.

Exercise testing has been the standard method employed in the initial diagnosis of stable coronary artery disease. Usually, a treadmill is used, with standard protocols modified for the decreased exercise capacity of elderly patients. The Modified Bruce protocol with three-minute stages (1.7 mph/0% grade; 1.7 mph/5% grade; 1.7 mph/10% grade; 2.5 mph/12% grade to the remainder of the standard Bruce protocol) or the modified Naughton protocol with two-minute stages (1.0 mph/0% grade; 1.5 mph/0% grade; 2.0 mph/3.5% grade; 2.0 mph/7.0% grade; 2.0 mph/10.5% grade; 3.0 mph/7.5% grade; 3.0 mph/10% grade; 3.0 mph/12.5% grade) are most often used because of the low energy requirement and the gradual increase in workload. The ECG response to graded exercise has remained the most common variable analyzed to detect myocardial ischemia.

The diagnostic accuracy of ST-segment depression during exercise as an indicator of ischemia depends on the adequacy of the exercise response, the sensitivity and specificity of the test, and the prevalence of coronary artery disease in the population being studied. According to Bayes' theorem, the pretest likelihood of disease is a strong determinant of whether an abnormal exercise ECG truly represents coronary artery disease. The high prevalence of coronary disease in the elderly has a direct influence on the posttest likelihood of disease. Elderly men 60 to 69 years of age with noncardiac pain have a 28 percent pretest likelihood of disease compared with 14 percent for men age 40 to 49 years (28). The data are even more impressive in elderly women in whom a four- to sixfold greater likelihood of disease occurs with atypical symptoms, compared with that for younger women. The posttest likelihood of coronary disease in both elderly men and women with 1.0 to 1.5 mm of ST-segment depression is clearly greater than it is in younger patients (29). For men 60 to 69 years of age the posttest likelihood of disease with this degree of ST-segment depression is 23 percent for asymptomatic patients, 45 percent for patients with nonanginal chest pain, 81 percent for patients with atypical chest pain, and 97 percent for patients with typical angina. For women in this age group, the posttest

Table 33.2. Diagnostic Methods for Coronary Artery Disease in the Elderly[a].

Method	Advantages	Disadvantages
Exercise test	Comparable sensitivity to nonelderly patients; high posttest likelihood of disease with positive test defines high-risk subset of CAD	Requires good exercise effort; poor specificity, from abnormal resting ECG
Thallium		
Exercise	Increased predictive accuracy of exercise test; better risk stratification than exercise ECG	Requires good exercise effort; expensive; requires quantitative analysis; sensitivity and specificity undetermined
Dipyridamole[b]	Sensitivity and specificity greater than exercise test (sensitivity = 86%; specificity = 75%); low adverse effect rate; no increase with age; ability to rapidly reverse effect with aminophylline; results independent of exercise ability and medication	Trend toward increased side effects; worsening bronchospasm with asthma; expensive; requires quantitative analysis
Holter monitor	Detection of asymptomatic, silent ischemia; no exercise effort required; detection of arrhythmias and ST-segment changes; silent ischemia correlates with increased cardiac events	Requires normal resting ECG; sensitivity and specificity not defined; additional value over ETT not defined; requires patient compliance
Angiography	Definitive test for degree of coronary disease; allows ability for intervention	Increased incidence of adverse effects; expensive, invasive

[a] Diagnostic efficacy of exercise radionuclide angiography and stress echocardiography with either exercise or dobutamine has not been determined in the elderly.
[b] Sensitivity and specificity data from Lam JYT, Chaitman BR, Glaenzer M, et al. Safety and diagnostic accuracy of dipyridamole-thallium imaging in the elderly. J Am Coll Cardiol 1988;11:584.
CAD = coronary artery disease; ECG = electrocardiogram; ETT = exercise treadmill test.

likelihood of disease with 1.0 to 1.5 mm ST-segment depression is 15 percent for asymptomatic patients, 33 percent for patients with nonanginal chest pain, 72 percent for patients with atypical chest pain, and 95 percent for those with typical angina. Thus, for elderly patients, ST-segment analysis has the potential to be a more effective diagnostic tool than for younger patients, regardless of symptoms. Unfortunately, the sensitivity of the exercise test is often decreased because of the elderly patient's inability to attain an adequate heart rate response during exercise, because of limited ability to perform near-maximal exertion, as well as underlying cardiac conduction disease or autonomic disorders that result in chronotropic incompetence during exercise.

Difficulties also arise with the specificity of an abnormal ST-segment response during exercise testing in the elderly. Often, the patient's baseline ECG is abnormal, which greatly reduces the diagnostic accuracy of the test. The specificity of the test can be improved when other parameters such as angina, R-wave amplitude, and Q-wave depth are evaluated along with ST-segment depres-

sion. Other standard exercise variables, including exercise duration, time of onset of signs and symptoms suggestive of ischemia, blood pressure responses, and heart rate responses, also provides diagnostic and prognostic information. Variables that indicate a poorer prognosis and a high likelihood of either significant left main or severe, three-vessel coronary disease include early onset of ST-segment depression, persistence of these changes beyond 7 minutes in the recovery period, a drop in systolic blood pressure of more than 20 mm Hg during exercise, and widespread significant (≥ 2 mm) ST-segment depression. The presence of 1.0 mm or more of ST-segment depression in elderly patients, by itself, is a predictor of subsequent cardiac mortality in this age group (30).

Because of the problems with sensitivity and specificity of routine exercise testing in the diagnosis of coronary artery disease in elderly patients, radionuclide imaging has been used to improve diagnostic accuracy. Thallium scintigraphy, a method to determine myocardial perfusion, has increased the sensitivity of exercise testing from 58 percent with ST-segment analysis to 92 percent with combined imaging; specificity also improved from 82 percent to 92 percent (31).

Most of these studies have been performed in younger patients, and the sensitivity and specificity of thallium exercise tests in a large population of elderly patients is unknown. Abnormal thallium exercise tests in elderly men have been shown to influence the decision to proceed with coronary angiography (32), but little additional diagnostic value was obtained if the patient's routine exercise test was normal. Abnormal thallium images have been shown to predict a higher cardiac event rate in elderly patients. In a study of 449 patients with a mean age of 65 years, the risk for a future cardiac event within 2 years was less than 1 percent with normal images, 5 percent with a single perfusion abnormality, and 13 percent if multiple abnormalities were seen (33). Similarly, in a group of 120 patients, age of more than 70 years, the presence or absence of a thallium defect, and the treadmill exercise stage achieved with the Bruce protocol best predicted the low- and high-risk groups for a future cardiac event in a 3-year follow-up period (34). The annual cardiac event rate was less than 1 percent in the low-risk group and more than 15 percent in the high-risk group. Thus, thallium scintigraphy can be a useful additional test in the diagnosis and prognosis of coronary artery disease in the elderly and is most useful when the patient's resting ECG is abnormal, if the patient has equivocal ST-segment changes and chest pain during a standard exercise test, and if the patient cannot complete the exercise protocol.

The other radionuclide approach to improve the sensitivity and specificity of exercise testing for the diagnosis of coronary artery disease in elderly patients is exercise radionuclide ventriculography. A decrease or failure to increase global left ventricular ejection fraction (LVEF) during exercise by 5 percent or more compared with the resting level and the development of regional wall motion abnormalities have been used as diagnostic criteria for the presence of myocardial ischemia during exercise. Using these criteria, the sensitivity and specificity of the exercise test in predicting coronary artery disease has been substantially improved (31). Interpreting LV events during exercise is more complex in the elderly patient because of the effects of aging itself on ventricular function. The expected increase in overall LVEF to graded exercise is

clearly reduced in older persons without cardiac disease (35,36). Because the global LV systolic responses to exercise can be influenced by a variety of factors in the elderly, the specificity of an abnormal response appears to be diminished, which limits the usefulness of this test in the diagnosis of coronary artery disease. Postexercise echocardiography, with the major emphasis on regional wall motion analysis, may be a more useful imaging modality to evaluate elderly patients for myocardial ischemia. However, there is little information currently available to determine the diagnostic value of this technique in elderly patients.

The main limitation to exercise testing in the elderly is the inability of a large number of these patients to perform adequate exercise. Often, these patients have significant musculoskeletal, respiratory, or neurologic symptoms that limit exercise performance. Many of these patients cannot attain 85 percent of their age-predicted maximal heart rate, which decreases the sensitivity of the test. Thallium scintigraphy with intravenous dipyridamole has become a useful diagnostic test for these patients, and avoids the risks of coronary arteriography for all patients who cannot perform an exercise test. Dipyridamole is a coronary vasodilator that promotes vascular steal and produces a hypoperfused area of myocardium detectable by thallium scanning. Dipyridamole-thallium studies have a reported sensitivity of 90 percent and a specificity of 95 percent for younger patients with coronary artery disease (37). With abnormal scans that suggest ischemia, ischemic ST-segment depression occurred in only 10 percent to 15 percent of patients and angina has been reported to occur in about 20 percent of these patients (38). Despite maximal coronary vasodilation and the potential for major areas of relative hypoperfusion of myocardium supplied by diseased vessels, the technique is relatively safe (38,39). There is a less than 1 percent risk of major adverse events, including fatal and nonfatal MI. A 46.5 percent rate of minor side effects has been reported (38). These include acute bronchospasm, headache, chest pain, dizziness, nausea, and hypotension. Most adverse effects can be reversed with intravenous aminophylline.

The frequency of major and minor adverse effects is not influenced by advanced age (40), and elderly patients have been shown to have less hypotension and heart rate elevation compared with these factors for younger subjects (41). The diagnostic accuracy of dipyridamole-thallium imaging is not affected by beta-blocker therapy; only oral theophylline and recent caffeine ingestion reduce the pharmacologic action of dipyridamole and thus limit the sensitivity of the test for detecting myocardial ischemia. The sensitivity and specificity of dipyridamole-thallium testing in elderly patients are similar to the results for younger patients. In comparing 101 patients 70 years of age or older with 236 patients younger than age 70, the sensitivity for coronary disease was 86 percent and 83 percent in older and younger patients, respectively, and the specificity was 75 percent and 70 percent, respectively (40). An abnormal thallium scan after dipyridamole also predicts an increased cardiac event rate in elderly patients. In 149 elderly patients with a normal scan, there was a 5 percent rate for a cardiac event within 2 years; an abnormal scan was associated with a 35 percent rate for a cardiac event (42). Thus, this technique appears to be a relatively safe, effective means to diagnose and stratify for risk elderly patients with suspected coronary artery disease.

Twenty-four-hour ambulatory monitoring has been used to diagnose silent ischemia in patients with coronary artery disease. Horizontal or downsloping ST-segment depression of 1.0 mm or more sustained for more than 60 seconds has been found to have a sensitivity of 55 percent and a specificity of 100 percent for myocardial ischemia and coronary artery disease (27). The sensitivity of this test increases with longer periods of monitoring. In elderly patients with known coronary artery disease, evidence for silent ischemia on ambulatory ECG monitoring was associated with a doubling in the rate of new cardiac events (26). Because of the high prevalence of silent ischemia in patients with known coronary disease, this technique may be used to detect myocardial ischemia in elderly patients who are unable to perform an exercise test. However, the high prevalence of an abnormal resting ECG in the elderly may limit the usefulness of asymptomatic ST-segment depression as an indicator of myocardial ischemia.

Coronary arteriography remains the definitive test for the diagnosis of coronary artery disease. Data from CASS demonstrated that elderly patients had higher mortality and morbidity from this procedure compared with the results for younger patients (43). The death rate was 1.9 per 1000 patients, with the incidence of nonfatal MI at 7.9 per 1000, vascular complications at 8.4 per 1000, embolic complications at 1.9 per 1000, neurologic complications (including stroke) at 3.7 per 1000, ventricular fibrillation at 4.2 per 1000, and an incidence of 23.8 per 1000 patients for one or more complications. Except for vascular complications, all other adverse effects of coronary arteriography were more frequent in elderly patients. For these reasons, coronary arteriography should be reserved for elderly patients with more severe coronary artery disease, such as medically refractory angina, severe unstable angina, myocardial ischemia presenting as pulmonary edema, significant angina in the presence of LV dysfunction, and an abnormal noninvasive test for ischemia that suggests a high-risk status for future cardiac events. Because of the higher risks of coronary arteriography in the elderly patient, this test should not be routinely performed to exclude coronary artery disease in a stable patient with an atypical chest pain syndrome and a nondiagnostic noninvasive evaluation. In these patients, a therapeutic trial with sublingual nitroglycerin or empiric antianginal therapy may be warranted before exposing the patient to the increased risks of arteriography.

Medical Therapy

All elderly patients with presumed or diagnosed coronary artery disease and chronic stable angina should be initially treated with medical therapy. Because of the increased morbidity and mortality of mechanical procedures in this age group, both PTCA and CABG should be reserved for patients with refractory symptoms or more severe coronary disease. Anemia, hyperthyroidism, congestive heart failure, supraventricular and ventricular arrhythmias, and hypertension should be sought and treated because they contribute to an increase in myocardial oxygen demand and may precipitate angina in an otherwise asymptomatic patient. In the patient with chronic stable angina, sublingual nitroglycerin remains the initial treatment. Elderly patients are particularly susceptible to the vasodilating effects of this drug, and they need to be carefully instructed in its proper use. For many patients with arthritis or poor vision, the sublingual spray is easier to use than the standard, small, sublingual tablets. If symptoms occur frequently, maintenance antianginal drug therapy is required. The currently available antianginal drugs, their mechanisms of action, and their side effects are outlined in Tables 33.3 and 33.4. In general, elderly patients should be treated with lower doses of all antianginal medications because of the higher incidence of side effects (44).

Nitrates remain the initial therapy for most patients with chronic stable angina, as well as for patients with a component of vasospasm. The plasma half-life of nitrates is longer and the volume of distribution is larger in elderly patients which leads to increased venous smooth muscle responsiveness and is probably responsible for the increased frequency of side effects in these patients (45). Elderly patients are more sensitive to the vasodilating action of these drugs because of a decrease in plasma volume, a higher incidence of venous disease, a decreased sensitivity and responsiveness of the baroreceptor reflex, and a diminished cardiac response to catecholamine stimulation. Because of the development of nitrate tolerance, particularly with the longer-acting preparations, a nitrate-free interval during the day is required to ensure maximal effectiveness. Headache remains the most common side effect and usually improves

after several days of low-dose therapy. Elderly patients may also have more skin irritation from the topical preparations because of their transparent, fragile skin. Recently, isosorbide mononitrate has become available in single or twice-a-day formulations. This drug allows better patient compliance and has higher bioavailability than isosorbide dinitrate.

Beta blockers continue to be the most effective therapy for exertional angina because of their effects on reducing exercise heart rate, which lowers myocardial oxygen consumption. The response to beta blockade in the elderly patient is somewhat unpredictable. Achieving effective beta-blocking effects can be more difficult, despite the higher blood levels of these drugs in elderly patients, because of decreased metabolism. Elderly patients have a diminished chronotropic response to beta-adrenergic agonists, but the mechanism of attenuation of beta-blocking effects in some patients is unknown (46). Hydrophilic beta blockers (e.g., atenolol and nadolol) generally have fewer side effects than the lipophilic drugs (e.g., propranolol and metoprolol), but their doses must be decreased in patients with reduced creatinine clearance because these drugs are excreted primarily by the kidneys. Cardioselectivity is important in patients with diabetes, peripheral arterial disease, and LV dysfunction. Interac-

Table 33.3. Mechanism of Action for Medical Management of Angina in the Elderly.

Drug	Arterial Vasodilation	Venous Vasodilation	Coronary Vasodilation	Negative Inotropic	Negative Chronotropic	Negative Dromotropic[a]
Nitrates, NTG	+	+++	++	0	−[b]	0
Beta blockers	0	0	−[c]	++	+++	++
Calcium channel blockers						
Nifedipine	+++	0	+++	+	−[b]	+/−[d]
Amlodipine	+++	0	+++	+/−[e]	−[b]	+/−[d]
Felodipine	+++	0	+++	+/−[e]	−[b]	+/−[d]
Isradapine	+++	0	+++	+/−[e]	−[b]	+/−[d]
Nicardipine	+++	0	+++	+/−[e]	−[b]	+/−[d]
Verapamil	+	0	+++	++	++	++
Diltiazem	++	0	++	+	+	+

[a] Dromotropic properties refer to effects on left ventricular relaxation and filling.
[b] Both nitrates and dihydropyridine calcium channel blockers can increase heart rate by reflex sympathetic action.
[c] Beta blockade causes a reduction in coronary blood flow from lower myocardial oxygen consumption and has been reported to cause coronary vasoconstriction in some patients.
[d] Drug has been shown to have variable effects on left ventricular diastolic function.
[e] Drug is vasoselective, with more effects on vascular smooth muscle than on cardiac myocytes.
NTG = nitroglycerin; + = positive response (level of positive response); − = negative response; 0 = no response.

Table 33.4. Adverse Drug Effects of Medical Management of Angina in the Elderly.

Drug	Adverse Effects
Nitrates, nitroglycerin	Orthostatic hypotension, headache, syncope, skin rash, gastrointestinal distress
Beta blockers	Fatigue, depression, heart block, heart failure, symptomatic bradycardia, bronchospasm
Calcium channel blockers	
Dihydropyridine drugs*	Orthostatic hypotension, flushing, edema, syncope, reflex tachycardia, gastrointestinal distress
Verapamil	Constipation, heart block, symptomatic bradycardia, heart failure, hypotension
Diltiazem	heart block, edema, hypotension, constipation

*These drugs include nifedipine, amlodipine, felodipine, isradapine, and nicardipine.

tions of beta blockers with cimetidine and lidocaine necessitate a reduction in the dose or increase in the dosing interval of these drugs. In general, the dose of beta blocker should be titrated to produce a resting heart rate between 50 and 60 beats per minute (bpm) and a peak exercise heart rate of less than 100 bpm.

Calcium channel blockers are important agents in the therapy of both vasospastic and exertional angina. Most of these drugs are potent vasodilators, which explains both the therapeutic action and the common side effects of these medications. Elderly patients have decreased rates of hepatic metabolism and lower hepatic blood flow, which leads to decreased clearance and prolonged half-lives for these drugs (47). Thus, lower doses and longer dosing intervals are recommended with calcium channel blockers in elderly patients. The dihydropyridine drugs (nifedipine, amlodipine, felodipine, isradapine, and nicardipine) are more potent vasodilators and increase sympathetic stimulations by the baroreceptor reflex. This may not be desirable for patients with acute ischemic syndromes. Diltiazem and verapamil, drugs that tend to lower heart rate and do not enhance sympathetic stimulation, may be more appropriate. Although all calcium

channel blockers have intrinsic negative inotropic properties, the vasoselective agents (amlodipine, felodipine, isradapine, and nicardipine) may produce the same degree of vasodilation with less negative effects on cardiac contractility. Because both diltiazem and verapamil decrease cardiac electrical conduction, they should not be used in patients with underlying conduction abnormalities. In general, patients with decreased LV systolic function should not receive these drugs because of the possibility of precipitating congestive heart failure. Use of diltiazem after MI in patients with depressed cardiac function has also been shown to increase both mortality and the rate for a cardiac event (48). Because of the higher prevalence of conduction defects and LV dysfunction in the elderly, these patients are also more susceptible to the side effects of calcium blockers. Initial doses of these drugs should be lower for elderly patients, with more gradual titration to relief of symptoms or occurrence of side effects.

Combinations of antianginal drugs are reserved for patients with more severe symptoms. The risk of complications increases significantly in elderly patients on combination therapy; therefore, the initial dose of each drug should be low. The combination of beta blocker and verapamil should be avoided because of a high incidence of heart block or congestive heart failure. Diltiazem and beta blockers need to be administered cautiously and at low doses because combined use increases the frequency of atrioventricular block. The combination of dihydropyridine calcium channel blockers and nitrates should also be used cautiously because the combined vasodilatory effects of these drugs may result in orthostatic hypotension or syncope.

The treatment of unstable angina in the elderly probably does not differ from that for younger patients. Unfortunately, no clinical studies exist to determine the optimal therapy for unstable coronary syndromes in the elderly. This reflects the general paucity of data on therapy of coronary artery disease in large numbers of elderly patients (49). Initially, stabilization should be accomplished with intravenous nitroglycerin, beta blockers, and in some cases, calcium channel blockers. Aspirin has been shown to decrease the rate of infarction in patients with unstable angina and should be used early in the treatment course (50,51). Intravenous heparin has been shown to be more effective than aspirin alone in preventing refractory angina and MI in patients with unstable angina (52). In patients with significant ongoing symptoms and persistent ST-segment depression, heparin should be used instead of aspirin. The use of both agents increases the rate of serious bleeding and should probably be avoided for elderly patients.

Thrombolytic therapy has not been shown to be effective in patients with unstable angina and should be reserved only for patients with ST-segment elevation and probable transmural MI. Although intra-aortic balloon counterpulsation has been shown to be an effective means to increase coronary artery perfusion and prevent refractory angina in younger patients, this form of therapy should be used cautiously in elderly patients because of the higher morbidity from local vascular complications. Patients who have refractory symptoms require coronary arteriography to assess their candidacy for PTCA or CABG. Patients with persistent ST-segment depression, evidence for anterior circulation (left anterior descending artery) ischemia or ischemia associated with congestive heart failure probably should receive early arteriography. For patients with single-vessel disease, PTCA may be superior to medical therapy in preventing recurrent unstable angina and MI because patients with stable angina and single-vessel disease do better with PTCA (53). Many patients stabilize on medications and do not require intervention unless they have recurrent symptoms. In patients with three-vessel coronary disease and normal LV function, initial therapy with medications is appropriate. Results from two large randomized trials indicate that early CABG is not necessary for this group of patients with unstable angina because mortality and nonfatal MI rates were similar for both medical and surgical therapy (54,55). Patients with three-vessel disease and decreased LV function or those with refractory symptoms benefit from early surgical intervention. Patients with one- or two-vessel disease and selected patients with three-vessel disease may benefit from PTCA. However, the role of PTCA in elderly patients with unstable angina is unclear, but it may represent an alternative form of therapy at a lower risk than CABG. The restenosis rate of PTCA is generally greater for patients with unstable angina than it is for those with stable angina, which reduces the therapeutic advantage of this therapy.

Percutaneous Transluminal Coronary Angioplasty

Elderly patients who present with severe unstable coronary artery disease, who have evidence for extensive myocardium at risk on noninvasive testing, or who develop angina refractory to medical therapy become candidates for mechanical revascularization therapy. The risks of CABG are clearly higher in this patient population; the CASS registry data revealed a 4.6 percent mortality for patients from 65 to 69 years of age and a 9.5 percent mortality for patients 75 years or older (43). PTCA has been shown to be a very effective form of revascularization therapy for younger patients with coronary artery disease (56), and this therapy has been suggested as the preferred treatment for elderly patients with simple coronary disease (single- or two-vessel) and preserved ventricular function (57). Treatment of single-vessel coronary artery disease in younger patients with PTCA resulted in more effective angina relief and better performance on an exercise test (53). The possibility of more effective palliation of symptoms as well as a reduced need for antianginal medical therapy, which reduces the chance of side effects, makes PTCA a viable option for therapy of coronary disease in the elderly. Initial concern about inability to dilate calcified, hardened atherosclerotic plaques in elderly patients has not been realized. Early studies of PTCA reported a lower success rate than that for younger patients, but improved catheter technology, better patient selection, and greater operator experience resulted in comparable successful dilatation rates.

Although studies of PTCA in small numbers of elderly patients have reported excellent results (58,59), a review of the larger studies involving PTCA in the elderly will provide a better understanding of the role of this therapy in the management of coronary artery disease in this population. Pertinent data from six studies involving 2353 elderly patients are presented in Table 33.5. These patients were treated either at one institution (60–64) or as part of a multicenter registry (65). Most patients had single- or two-vessel coronary disease except for the study involving multivessel PTCA (60). The majority of patients had normal LV function although the percentage of patients with depressed LV dysfunction was higher than that in most series of PTCA in younger patients. The

Table 33.5. Summary of Large Trials Using PTCA in the Elderly.

	Bedotto (60)	Dorros (61)	NHLBI (65)	Mick (62)	Raizner (63)	Simpfendorfer (64)
No. patients	1373	109	486	142	119	124
Average age (yr)	69	76	71	82	70	74
Success rate (%)	96	89	80	94	81	90
Complications (%)[a]	3.2	15.0	7.0	16.0	7.4	12.0
Deaths (%)	1.6	1.8	3.2	2.0	0.8	0.0
MI (%)	1.4	4.6	4.6 (8.7)*	6.0	2.5	0.8
Emergency CABG (%)	0.8	0.9	5.3	0.0	4.1	4.0
LVEF < 0.40 (%)	13.6	2.7	22.0	11.0	NR	9.0
Extent of CAD (%)						
One-vessel	0.0	45.0	40.0	21.0	79.0	77.0
Two-vessel	42.5	55.0	35.0	43.0	18.0	11.0
Three-vessel	57.5	(multivessel)	25.0	34.0	3.0	9.0
Hospital stay (days)	NA	3.4	NA	9.0	NA	NA
Long-term follow-up						
Length of follow-up (mo)	32.5	23.0	24.0	40.0	18.0	28.6
Improvement (%)	92	92	77	72	91	NA
Restenosis rate (%)	36.3	17.0	20.0	12.0	39.0	21.0
Late deaths (%)	15.2	1.8	14.0	15.0	3.4	7.0
MI (%)	7.9	NA	NA	4.0	0.0	2.4
Late CABG (%)	15.8	NA	NA	8.0	2.5	13.0
Survival (%)	92.0 (1 yr)	96.0 (2 yr)	87.0 (1 yr)	92.0 (2 yr)	85.0 (2 yr)	93.0 (2 yr)

[a] Complications include arrhythmias, myocardial infarction, death, and emergency CABG.

[b] Data from patients ≥75 yr.

CABG = coronary artery bypass surgery; CAD = coronary artery disease; LVEF = left ventricular ejection fraction; MI = myocardial infarction; NA = not available; NHLBI = National Heart, Lung, and Blood Institute; PTCA = percutaneous transluminal coronary angioplasty.

initial success rate of dilatation of the coronary lesion varied from 80 percent to 96 percent, with a low rate of significant complications. Deaths and nonfatal MI occurred infrequently although at a higher rate than they occurred in younger patients. The need for emergency CABG varied from 0 percent to 5.3 percent. Long-term follow-up revealed a similar restenosis rate as that reported for younger patients (56). Overall survival was excellent although the need for CABG varied from 2.5 percent to 15.8 percent. Clinical improvement occurred in most elderly patients who underwent PTCA. The rate of

late MI and deaths occurred more frequently in the patient cohorts with a greater percentage of multivessel disease and LV dysfunction.

To better appreciate how the age of the patient influenced the results of PTCA, an analysis of the patient characteristics and outcomes in the National Heart, Lung, and Blood Institute (NHLBI) PTCA registry from 1985 to 1986 was performed (Figure 33.2). This represents a multicenter experience that would tend to minimize bias in patient selection. Patient characteristics and early and late outcomes of PTCA were compared for 1315 patients

Fig. 33.2. (A) Characteristics of elderly patients in the National Heart, Lung, and Blood Institute registry of percutaneous transluminal coronary angioplasty (PTCA), 1985–1986. $p < 0.05$ between elderly and nonelderly groups. N = 1315 (<65 yr); N = 394 (65–74 yr); and N = 92 (≥75 yr). (B) In-hospital complications after PTCA in elderly patients in the NHLBI registry, 1985–1986. CP = chest pain. $p < 0.05$ between elderly and nonelderly groups. (C) Long-term (2 yr) outcomes of PTCA in elderly compared with those of nonelderly patients in the NHLBI PTCA registry, 1985–1986. No Rx indicates no antianginal therapy. (Figures derived from data in Kelsey SF, Miller DP, Holubkov R, et al. Results of percutaneous transluminal coronary angioplasty in patients ≥65 years of age. Am J Cardiol 1990;66:1033.)

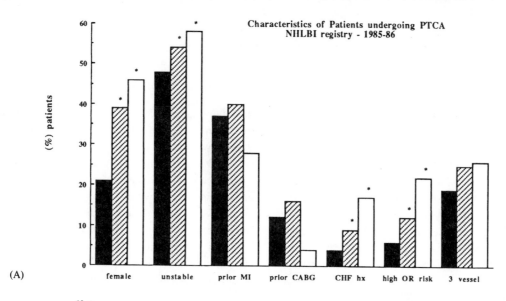

(A)

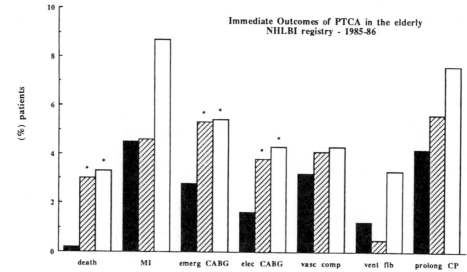

(B)

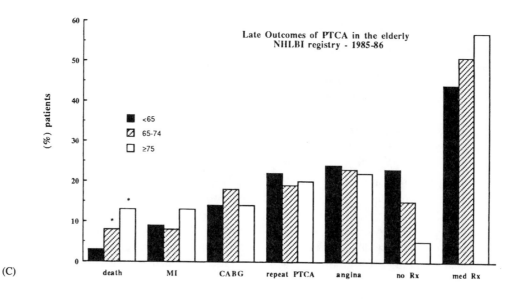

(C)

less than 65 years of age, 394 patients age 65 to 74, and 92 patients 75 years of age or older. There were greater numbers of women patients, more unstable angina, a greater history of congestive heart failure, and a greater risk for cardiac surgery with advancing age (Figure 33.2A). There was no difference between the groups in the percentage of all patients with three-vessel disease and a history of MI. Patients age 75 years or older were less likely to have had previous CABG. The early in-hospital complication rate was higher for elderly patients, with a greater number of deaths, MI, and emergency and elective CABG (see Figure 33.2B middle). The risk of MI was even greater for patients 75 years of age or older. There was no difference among the various age groups in vascular complications and the incidence of ventricular fibrillation. Prolonged chest pain after PTCA tended to be more frequent in the elderly patients.

Follow-up at 24 months revealed a higher mortality in both elderly age groups, but all other outcomes were similar, irrespective of age (Figure 33.2C). There was no difference in the need for CABG or repeat PTCA between younger and older patients. Fewer patients age 75 years or older were able to be maintained without antianginal therapy and older patients tended to need more medical therapy for their coronary artery disease. These results were similar to another large, single-center study that compared outcome after PTCA for patients across a comparable age range (66).

Although the mortality and complication rates of PTCA in the elderly are somewhat greater than those for younger patients, a comparison with outcomes after CABG is required to determine the optimal revascularization strategy for elderly patients. No large randomized studies that directly compare PTCA with CABG in elderly patients are available. A recent retrospective review of 195 octogenarian patients, 142 with CABG and 53 with PTCA, at the Cleveland Clinic demonstrated relatively low morbidity and mortality with either procedure (62). Patients undergoing PTCA had a tendency for a slightly lower mortality, and CABG patients had a 4 percent incidence of stroke and a 3 percent incidence of sepsis (Figure 33.3A). In fact, there were no neurologic complications in the PTCA group.

The long-term follow-up period was 40 months for the CABG group and 26 months for the PTCA group. During the follow-up period, there was no difference between the treatment groups in late deaths and MI (Figure 33.3B). Patients who had PTCA had a tendency for higher rates of late CABG and repeat PTCA, and patients who received CABG were more likely to be free of angina. Unfortunately, the patients were not comparable in each group – the PTCA patients had a higher likelihood of having single-vessel disease and normal LV systolic function, but a higher frequency of more severe angina. Data on outcomes after PTCA or CABG in a comparable group of elderly patients across a wider age range are not available.

The Bypass Angioplasty Revascularizaton Study (BARI) will address which therapy is optimal for patients to 80 years of age with multivessel disease approachable by either procedure. Currently, PTCA seems preferable to CABG for elderly patients with single- and, perhaps, two-vessel disease and stable ischemic symptoms. The hospital stay is shorter for PTCA and the cost about 50 percent less than that for CABG. The absence of significant neurologic complications with PTCA compared with those for CABG and the somewhat lower early mortality are also important factors in deciding on a therapy. PTCA as a primary treatment strategy for unstable angina in elderly patients has not been adequately evaluated. In a study of multivessel PTCA, patients with unstable angina had a tendency for a higher mortality than did patients with stable angina (60), but no comparison with mortality rates for CABG or medical therapy in a similar group of patients is available. (The use of PTCA as primary reperfusion therapy for acute transmural MI is discussed in the section on MI in the elderly.) Overall, PTCA has become an important form of therapy for elderly patients who have more advanced coronary artery disease and may be preferable to either medical therapy or CABG for carefully selected patients.

Coronary Artery Bypass Surgery

Early experience in the 1970s with CABG in the elderly indicated an increased surgical mortality of 3.7 percent to 19 percent. Because of the high number of surgical mortalities, CABG was performed mainly for elderly patients with symptoms refractory to medical therapy. With improvements in myocardial preservation techniques, the

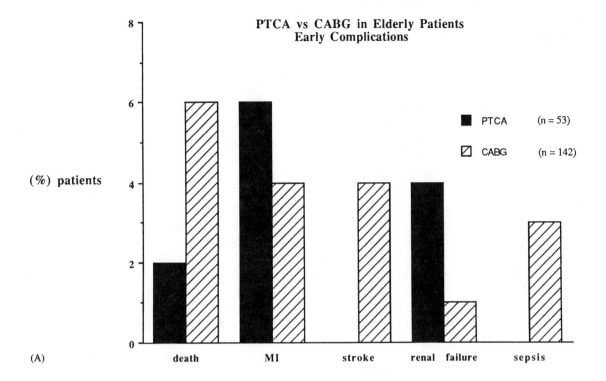

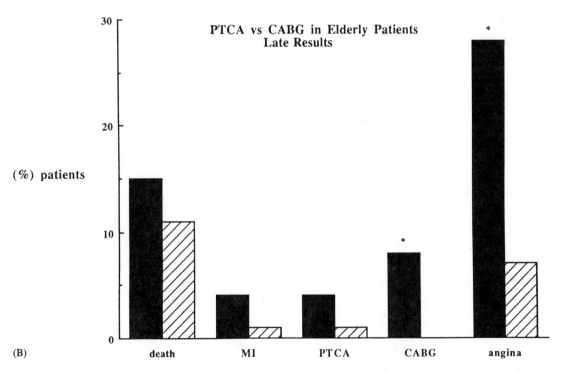

Fig. 33.3. (*A*) Comparison of in-hospital complications between coronary bypass surgery (CABG) and PTCA in nonrandomized octogenarians with coronary artery disease treated at the Cleveland Clinic. No significant differences between the two treatment groups. (*B*) Late results (CABG = 40 months; PTCA = 26 months) after either CABG or PTCA in patients ≥80 yr. $p < 0.05$ between CABG and PTCA. (Figures derived from data in Mick MJ, Simpfendorfer C, Arnold AZ, et al. Early and late results of coronary angioplasty and bypass in octogenarians. Am J Cardiol 1991;68:1316.)

surgical mortality for CABG in the elderly has dropped considerably. In carefully selected groups of low-risk patients, mortalities of 1.6 percent to 3 percent have been reported (67,68). Even after recent MI, elderly patients have undergone CABG with a mortality rate of only 6 percent. Thus, the indications for CABG for elderly patients have expanded to include not only medically refractory patients but also patients with multivessel disease who have indicators of a poorer outcome from either invasive or noninvasive studies. In these patients, the risks of CABG need to be balanced with the potential benefits in improved quality of life and enhanced longevity.

An evaluation of the risks from CABG in the elderly can be determined from the CASS registry (43). At various institutions, 1086 patients 65 years of age or older underwent CABG. The overall operative mortality in the elderly was 5.2 percent compared with 1.9 percent in patients younger than age 65. The mortality rate increased with age–4.6 percent for ages 65 to 69 years, 6.6 percent for ages 70 to 74 years, and 9.5 percent for patients older than age 75. Cardiogenic shock and refractory heart failure were the most frequent causes of death, and there were 9 cerebrovascular accidents in the 1086 patients (0.8%). Elderly patients also had longer hospital stays than did younger patients. The predictors of perioperative mortality in this elderly group were 70 percent or more stenosis of the left main coronary artery, LV end-diastolic pressure greater than 20 mm Hg, a history of current cigarette use, presence of rales on lung examination, and one or more associated medical problems. There was a tendency for a slightly higher mortality in women (6.9%) compared with that for men (4.7%). When all 7658 patients in the CASS registry were analyzed, age older than 65 years became an independent predictor of increased mortality, surpassed in importance only by the severity of congestive heart failure and left main coronary artery stenosis in a left dominant coronary circulation. One additional factor associated with a poor outcome of CABG in elderly patients was severe calcification of the ascending aorta, which was associated with a higher likelihood of neurologic complications and a higher mortality (67).

In addition to the CASS registry data, there has been a growing experience with CABG in patients older than 65 years of age. A summary of five major studies (68–72) reviewing the early complications of CABG in 8702 elderly patients is presented in Table 33.6. The early in-hospital death rate varied from 2.3 percent to 7.4 percent. The rate of MI ranged from 1.2 percent in the Cleveland Clinic series to 11.8 percent in the multicenter CASS registry. Of importance is the overall incidence of stroke which varied from 2.0 percent to 4.2 percent. The 5- to 6-year survival rate was 79 percent to 87 percent in this selected elderly group of patients.

A more detailed look at the Cleveland Clinic study (72) allows a comparison of patient demographics and postoperative complication rates among patients younger than age 65, age 65 to 74, and those 75 years of age or older (Figure 33.4). For elderly patients a greater percentage of women, more severe angina, more left main coronary artery stenoses, and a higher prevalence of diabetes, peripheral arterial disease, and previous cerebrovascular accidents were found than for patients younger than age 65 (Figure 33.4A). The percentage of patients with LV dysfunction and mutivessel coronary disease was similar for younger and elderly patients. Death (2.0% to 4.8%),

Table 33.6. Summary of Large Trials Using CABG in the Elderly.

	Bhattacharya (69)	CASS (71)	Elayda (70)	Loop (72)	Rahimtoola (68)
No. patients	597	1086	674	1275	5070
Age (yr)	≥70	≥65	≥70	≥70	≥65
Deaths (%)	2.7	5.0	7.4	5.8	2.3
MI (%)	1.5	11.8	7.1	1.2	1.0
Stroke (%)	2.0	2.4	4.2	2.5	2.3
Survival (%) (yr)	NA	79 (6)	NA	87 (5)	81 (5)

CABG = coronary artery bypass surgery; CASS = Coronary Artery Surgery Study; MI = myocardial infarction; NA = not available.

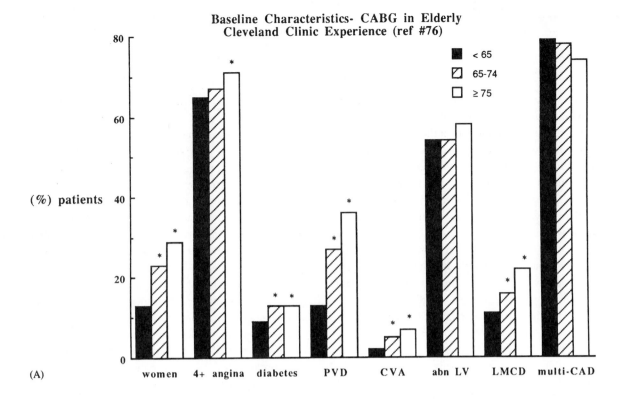

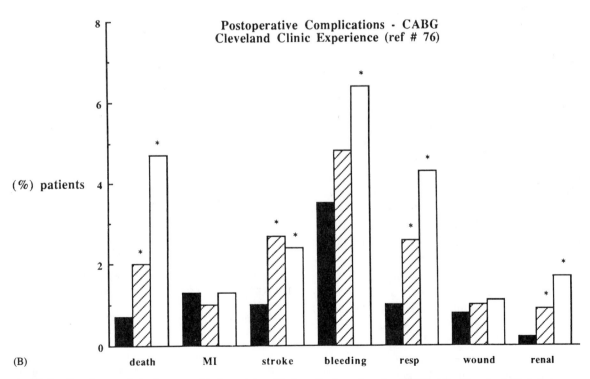

Fig. 33.4. (*A*) Baseline characteristics between elderly and nonelderly patients undergoing CABG at the Cleveland Clinic between 1976–1986. N = 17,996 (<65 yr); N = 4603 (65–74 yr); N = 467 (≥75 yr). PVD = peripheral arterial disease; CVA = previous cerebrovascular accident; LMCD = left main coronary artery disease. $p < 0.05$ between elderly and nonelderly groups. (*B*) Postoperative (in-hospital) complications in the same cohorts of patients undergoing CABG at the Cleveland Clinic. $p < 0.05$ between elderly and nonelderly groups. (Figures derived from data in Loop FD, Lytle BW, Cosgrove DM, et al. Coronary artery bypass graft surgery in the elderly. Indications and outcome. Cleve Clin J Med 1988;55:23.)

stroke (2.4%), bleeding, respiratory complications with prolonged intubation, and renal failure were more common in elderly patients, although all the event rates were relatively low (Figure 33.4B). In all cases, elderly patients 75 years of age or older had a higher complication rate than did patients 65 to 74 years of age. Interestingly, the incidence of perioperative MI and wound complications were similar between elderly and younger patients. Elderly patients had a higher postoperative incidence of atrial fibrillation in this study, and these patients had a lower long-term survival compared with that for patients 65 years of age or older without this rhythm. These data indicate that elderly patients have a higher complication rate after CABG than do younger patients, but in carefully selected patients with minimal comorbid medical conditions, as in this series, complication and mortality rates are not prohibitive. Long-term survival was returned to values expected for the given age group in the general population, which suggests a favorable outcome for survival in all age groups.

With the higher risk of perioperative mortality in elderly patients, CABG is probably indicated less often for prolongation of survival alone than it is for younger patients. Clearly, patients who are refractory to medical therapy should be considered for surgery, especially if their coronary anatomy is not ideal for PTCA. Patients who present with pulmonary edema secondary to severe global ischemia and who have normal LV systolic function at rest appear to benefit from CABG because they represent a high-risk group (73). For patients with other evidence of severe myocardial ischemia, either by clinical presentation or by noninvasive testing, CABG should be considered if multivessel coronary disease is discovered.

Does CABG prolong life for elderly patients? The results of three randomized trials of CABG showed that patients with three-vessel coronary disease and severe symptoms, LV dysfunction, or abnormal exercise performance have a lower mortality with surgical therapy (74–75). None of these randomized trials included elderly patients; therefore, the data from these studies cannot be extrapolated to this patient population. An analysis of medical versus surgical therapy was performed in 1491 patients older than age 65 in the CASS registry (71). The overall 6-year survival rate was 79 percent for the surgically treated group compared with 64 percent for the medically treated group. An analysis of survival in this study is shown in Table 33.7. Patients from age 65 to 75 who had two- or three-vessel disease, LV dysfunction, and more severe symptoms had a lower mortality with surgical therapy. Surgery alone was found to be an independent predictor of improved survival. Patients with left main coronary artery disease and a left dominant coronary circulation were excluded from this analysis.

The results of this study must be interpreted with caution because the baseline characteristics of the two groups differed. The medically treated group included more women, more patients with other significant medical problems, and more LV dysfunction, whereas the surgically treated group had more severe angina and more three-vessel disease. Despite these differences, the data does suggest that for high-risk elderly patients, CABG may prolong life. Low-risk patients with stable angina and normal LV function did not benefit from CABG, and these patients should be treated medically, unless they

Table 33.7. CASS Registry of CABG in the Elderly.

	Medical Therapy	Surgical Therapy
Survival (%, 6 yr)		
Overall	64	79[a]
65–69 yr	67	81[a]
70–74 yr	51	77[a]
≥75 yr	56	75
One-vessel CAD	81	82
Two-vessel CAD	70	89[a]
Three-vessel CAD	47	75[a]
Normal LV function	83	87
Low-risk group[b]	80	88
High-risk group[c]	33	62[a]

[a] $p < 0.05$ for between-group comparisons.
[b] Low-risk is defined as mild angina, good LV function, and no left main coronary disease.
[c] High-risk is defined as severe symptoms–usually unstable angina, LV dysfunction, and severe three-vessel and left main coronary disease.
CABG = coronary artery bypass surgery; CAD = coronary artery disease; CASS = Coronary Artery Surgery Study; LV = left ventricular.
SOURCE: Adapted from Gersch BJ, Kronmal RA, Schaff HV, et al. Comparison of coronary artery bypass surgery and medical therapy in patients 65 years of age and older: a nonrandomized study from the Coronary Artery Surgery Study (CASS) registry. N Engl J Med 1985;313:217.

develop refractory angina. No comparison of PTCA, CABG, and medical therapy for elderly patients is available to indicate whether alternative forms of revascularization therapy also favorably increase survival in high-risk patients.

Besides the favorable effects on angina relief and longevity, CABG has been shown to improve functional capacity in elderly patients. Twelve months after CABG, 74 percent of elderly patients showed marked improvement in functional status (77). Factors associated with a lower functional capacity after CABG in these elderly patients included postoperative complications, female gender, previous cardiac operation, advanced age, continued cigarette smoking, syncope, and greater number of comorbid conditions. Thus, CABG represents a viable treatment option for elderly patients with extensive coronary disease and indicators of either high clinical risk status, poor response to medical therapy, or unfavorable anatomy for PTCA. Although the mortality and complication rates are higher than those for younger patients, the risk-benefit ratio favors CABG in carefully selected elderly patients, with the expectation of relief of angina, improved functional status, and possibly improved survival.

Acute Myocardial Infarction

The incidence of acute MI remains high in the elderly population despite an overall decline in cardiovascular mortality in the United States (2). The mortality rate of acute MI in the elderly is also substantially higher than it is for younger patients. The in-hospital mortality of elderly patients with acute MI before thrombolytic therapy was begun was reported to vary from 20 percent to 43 percent with a 1-year mortality rate of 20 percent to 53 percent (78,79). With use of thrombolysis, the mortality of elderly patients with acute MI remains high, with a mortality rate of 12.3 percent for patients aged 65 to 74 and 17.8 percent for patients age 75 and older, compared with a mortality rate of less than 5 percent for patients younger than age 65 (79). The high mortality of elderly patients is caused by the subtle, early presentation of infarction, which causes a delay in diagnosis and therapy, a high incidence of LV dysfunction, and withholding of effective therapy to reperfuse jeopardized myocardium early in the

clinical course of an acute MI. In one series, only 12 percent of elderly patients received thrombolytic therapy compared with 39 percent of younger patients (80). Even in large clinical trials involving the use of thrombolytic therapy for acute MI, the mortality rate is consistently higher for elderly patients in the setting of effective and successful thrombolysis (81). Silent MI occurs in a significant number of elderly patients. Twenty-one percent of patients from a chronic care facility presented with a silent MI (82). The Framingham Study showed that 36 percent of men and 46 percent of women with a new MI on ECG had no symptoms, and a substantial number of these patients were older than 65 years of age (28). The history of a previous silent MI on ECG confers a three-fold risk of a future MI (83).

Diagnostic Aspects

The presenting symptoms of MI in the elderly can be quite atypical, especially in patients older than age 80 (84). Although several studies have shown that chest pain is still a common presenting symptom, the incidence of this symptom is lower than it is in younger patients (84,85). Dyspnea is a very common early manifestation of MI in the elderly (86). Other common presentations include mental confusion, syncope, neurologic disturbances, and gastrointestinal complaints. In contrast, diaphoresis is an uncommon manifestation of acute MI in the elderly. In addition to an inexact history, other factors can make the diagnosis of acute MI difficult in certain elderly patients. On ECG many patients have conduction defects that may mask the changes of acute transmural MI. The incidence of non-Q-wave MI appears to be higher in elderly patients, and the ECG changes may be subtle (79). Twenty percent of elderly patients with non-Q-wave MI have "microinfarctions" (87,88). These patients have normal total creatine phosphokinase (CPK) levels, but elevated CPK-MB fractions, and 20 percent of patients also developed a flip in the LDH_1/LDH_2 ratio, confirming that MI had occurred. These patients usually have a clinical course consistent with an MI and increased in-hospital morbidity and mortality.

Elderly patients with MI have an increased incidence of pericarditis, supraventricular and ventricular arrhythmias, myocardial rupture, conduction disturbances, congestive heart failure, cardiogenic shock, cerebrovascular accidents, pneumonia, phlebitis, and drug toxicity (78). The most common causes of death are severe congestive heart failure and shock, ventricular arrhythmias, sudden death, and myocardial rupture. The incidence of myocardial rupture in the elderly is much greater than that in younger patients, with a 28.6 percent incidence reported in one study (78). Elderly women with hypertension who have a first MI appear to be at a particularly high risk for this complication. Even with thrombolytic therapy, the incidence of myocardial rupture in elderly patients is quite high. In the Gruppo Italiano per lo Studio della Sopravvivenza Nell'Infarto Miocardico-2 (GISSI-2) study, in which streptokinase was compared with tissue plasminogen activator (tPA), the frequency of cardiac rupture in the patients who had in-hospital death was 19 percent for patients age 60 years or older, but rose to 86 percent for patients older than age 70 (81). Univariate predictors of survival in acute MI include age, previous infarction, diastolic hypertension, history of diabetes, history of congestive heart failure, presence of rales and a ventricular gallop, cardiomegaly on chest x-ray, Killip class (the presence or absence of rales and/or hypotension), and the use of diuretics or digoxin (79). The only multivariate predictor of survival after acute MI was Killip class, which indicates that LV function is the most important predictor of survival after acute MI in the elderly.

Therapy

Reperfusion therapy with either thrombolytic agents or PTCA has become the major focus to reduce morbidity and mortality in acute Q-wave MI. Most of the benefits from early reperfusion have been shown with large clinical trials using various thrombolytic agents. The three major thrombolytic agents are streptokinase, antistreplase (APSAC), and tissue plasminogen activator (tPA). All three agents have been proven to have favorable benefits on vessel patency after acute Q-wave MI (89). Streptokinase works by indirectly binding to plasminogen and has minimal fibrin-specific properties. APSAC has properties similar to those of streptokinase but can be given in a shorter time period. tPA directly binds to plasminogen and is fibrin specific. The plasma clearance rate of tPA is extremely short (4–8 min) compared with the rates for streptokinase and APSAC, which

increases the risk of reocclusion. Aspirin is usually given at the beginning of thrombolytic therapy, and intravenous heparin is usually started before the completion of administration of the lytic agent to prevent reocclusion of the coronary artery. This is particularly important with a short-acting drug such as tPA.

Several large clinical trials have evaluated the efficacy of various thrombolytic agents in reducing cardiac mortality in the setting of acute MI (90–95). Most of these trials included a sufficient number of elderly patients so that the effectiveness and safety of thrombolytic therapy in elderly patients with acute MI can be evaluated. Early experience with intravenous streptokinase in a small series of elderly patients was associated with a substantial risk of hemorrhagic complications, including cerebral hemorrhage (96). In larger series, however, the risks were much lower.

In the Second International Study of Infarct Survival (ISIS-2), in which streptokinase, with or without aspirin, was compared with placebo, there was a substantial reduction in cardiac mortality. In patients younger than 70 years, the mortality rate was 10.6 percent for the placebo group and 6.1 percent for the group receiving streptokinase and aspirin (Figure 33.5A). Patients age 70 or older had higher mortalities regardless of therapy; however, streptokinase and aspirin did reduce mortality in this age group – to 23.8 percent for placebo and to 15.8 percent for streptokinase and aspirin (94). Therapy was most effective if given within a few hours of the onset of chest pain, although some benefit was shown for therapy given as late as 24 hours after onset of symptoms.

GISSI-1 was a large, placebo-controlled, Italian study designed to test the benefits of intravenous streptokinase in acute MI (90,91). Streptokinase resulted in a reduction in mortality for patients younger than age 70 but not for patients age 70 or older (Figure 33.5B). Therapy was most effective if given within the first 3 hours after presentation.

GISSI-2 and the Global Utilization of Streptokinase and tPA for Occluded Coronary Arteries trial (GUSTO) were two large clinical trials that compared the efficacy of streptokinase with tPA as well as with adjunctive heparin therapy (92,93). In the GISSI-2 trial, streptokinase and tPA were equally effective for both younger and older patients (Figure 33.5C). The GUSTO trial compared the rapid ad-

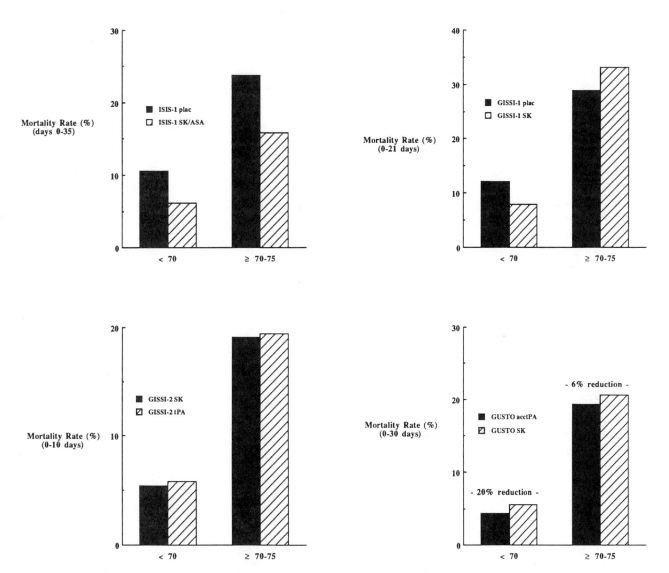

Fig. 33.5. Early mortality between elderly and nonelderly patients receiving thrombolytic therapy for acute myocardial infarction in several large clinical trials. Mortality in elderly patients was higher than that for nonelderly patients in all studies regardless of treatment. ISIS-1 (*A*) and GISSI-1 (*B*) were placebo-controlled trials; GISSI-2 (*C*) and GUSTO (*D*) were nonplacebo-controlled trials comparing various thrombolytic agents and regimens. (Figures derived from data in References 90–94.)

ministration of tPA (accelerated tPA) with different protocols of streptokinase (93). tPA by this method was somewhat more effective than was streptokinase at lowering mortality for younger patients, however, there were minimal differences seen in patients age 70 years or older (Figure 33.5D).

All studies demonstrated that thrombolytic therapy was effective for elderly patients and produced a definite decrease in mortality. Therapy was most effective if given within the first 4 hours and if patients had larger MIs. In elderly patients, the major concern is the risk of thrombolytic therapy compared with the benefits of early reperfusion of the involved coronary artery. Elderly patients were shown to have an increased risk of hemorrhage in all studies; however, the major concern was the risk of cerebral hemorrhage. The risk of

449

cerebrovascular accidents (CVAs) in all the major thrombolytic clinical trials is listed in Table 33.8. There appeared to be no significant risk of CVA in the ISIS-2 trial. In the Thrombolysis in Myocardial Infarction (TIMI) trials with tPA, cerebrovascular accidents and hemorrhage was increased with use of thrombolytic therapy (97). The risk increased with age and was much greater with 150 mg of the drug. Subsequently, the total dose was reduced to 100 mg, which resulted in some reduction in the rate of CVA. Both the GISSI-2 and GUSTO trials reported a higher risk of CVA with tPA, especially with older patients. Other analyses of the risk of CVA with thrombolytic therapy confirm a slightly increased risk with tPA (98,99). Heparin administration did not appear to influence the incidence of CVA in any of the studies. Despite the increased neurologic risk, thrombolytic therapy has been advocated for elderly patients because of the higher mortality compared with that for younger patients (100–102). Thrombolytic therapy has also been shown to be cost effective in the elderly (103).

It is important to follow the guidelines strictly and assess elderly patients for absolute and relative contraindications (Table 33.9). In general, streptokinase should be used instead of tPA because of the less proven benefit of tPA in older patients and the increased risk of cerebral hemorrhage. In elderly patients with large anterior infarctions, accelerated administration of tPA may be required to assure rapid vessel patency. When available, urgent PTCA may be the preferred therapy.

There is limited information on the role of primary PTCA in the management of acute MI in the elderly. Patients with contraindications to thrombolytic therapy, large anterior infarctions, cardiogenic shock, and the presence of previous CABG may benefit more from early PTCA than from lytic therapy. In the Primary Angioplasty Myocardial Infarction trial (PAMI), patients older than age 70 had fewer recurrent ischemic episodes, lower reinfarction rates, and decreased hemorrhagic strokes with PTCA compared with use of tPA (104). In this trial, 5 percent of patients had anatomy unsuitable for PTCA and were excluded from the trial. Other studies have shown comparable outcomes with primary PTCA versus lytic therapy in elderly patients with acute MI

Table 33.8. Risk of Cerebrovascular Accident with Thrombolytic Therapy in the Elderly Patient with Acute Myocardial Infarction, by Large Trials[a].

ISIS-2
0.7% incidence with SK/aspirin
0.8% incidence with placebo
no age-risk stratification

TIMI-2 (tPA) Age (yr)	total stroke (%)	Incidence (%)[b]	
		cerebral hemorrhage	cerebral infarction
>50	0.5	0.1	0.4
50–59	0.8	0.3	0.5
60–69	2.1[c]	1.1[c]	1.0[c]
≥70	2.6[c]	1.1[c]	1.5[c]

GISSI-2 Age (yr)	Total Stroke (%)	
	SK	tPA
≤70	0.8	0.9
>70	1.6	2.7[cd]

GUSTO Age (yr)	Total Stroke (%)	
	SK	Acc tPA
≤75	1.08	1.20
>75	3.05	3.93[cd]

[a] No data available from GISSI-1, ISIS-3, and GISSI-3 trials.
[b] Higher risk with 150 mg tPA.
[c] $p < 0.05$ vs younger age group.
[d] $p < 0.05$ vs other treatment group.
Acc tPA = accelerated tissue plasminogen activator; ISIS-2 = Second International Study of Infarct Survival; GISSI-2 = Gruppo Italiano per lo Studio della Sopravvivenza Nell'Infarto Miocardico-2; GUSTO = Global Utilization of Streptokinase and tPA for Occluded Coronary Arteries; SK = streptokinase; TIMI-2 = Thrombolysis in Myocardial Infarction-2; tPA = tissue plasminogen activator.

(105,106). Salvage PTCA after unsuccessful thrombolytic therapy was associated with high in-hospital mortality (34%) but patients with a patent infarct artery had a substantially improved outcome compared with that for patients with an occluded artery (105). In many hospitals, emergency PTCA as primary therapy for acute MI in the elderly is not available because of lack of facilities or delay in therapy.

Table 33.9. Thrombolytic Therapy for Acute Myocardial Infarction.

Eligibility–Chest pain or equivalent syndrome consistent with acute MI ≤ 12 hr onset with

    ≥1 mm ST elevation in ≥2 contiguous limb leads
    ≥2 mm ST elevation in ≥2 contiguous precordial leads
    New bundle branch block
    Cardiogenic shock (urgent cardiac catheterization and
       revascularization preferred unless not immediately available)
Contraindications*

Absolute	Relative
Altered consciousness	Active peptic ulcer disease
	History of CVA (ischemic or embolic)
Active internal bleeding	
Known spinal cord or cerebral	Current use of anticoagulants
AV malformation or tumor	
Recent head trauma	Major trauma or surgery
Known previous hemorrhagic CVA	(≥2 weeks, <2 months)
Intracranial or intraspinal surgery	History of uncontrolled
within 2 months	HTN (DBP > 100, +/– treated)
Trauma or surgery within 2 weeks	Subclavian or internal
(risk for bleeding in closed	jugular venous
space)	cannulation
Persistent BP > 200/120 mm Hg	
Known bleeding disorder	
Pregnancy	Patient (age ≥75 yr
Suspected aortic dissection	(less proven benefit;
Previous allergy to streptokinase	risk for CVA
(can use other thrombolytics)	hemorrhage– female, HTN, diabetes)

* CPR not a contraindication.
AV = atrioventricular; BP = blood pressure; CVA = cerebrovascular accident; CPR = cardiopulmonary resuscitation; DBP = diastolic blood pressure; HTN = hypertension; MI = myocardial infarction.
SOURCE: Modified from the National Heart Attack Alert Program, National Heart, Lung, and Blood Institute, 1993.

Thus, thrombolytic therapy, administered promptly to elderly patients felt to be at high risk for significant myocardial necrosis without major contraindications, remains the major approach to acute reperfusion therapy in acute MI. Aspirin should be used in combination with lytic therapy. Intravenous heparin should not be started immediately if streptokinase is used because of the long half-life of the lytic state and potential for an increased risk of bleeding. Heparin needs to be administered if tPA

is used because of its brief half-life and the potential for vessel reocclusion.

Elderly patients have a lower incidence of ventricular fibrillation at the onset of infarction, and because lidocaine toxicity is more common in the elderly, lidocaine prophylaxis is not indicated for this group of patients. If lidocaine is required for ventricular arrhythmias, the loading dose should be 50 to 75 mg followed by an infusion at 25 µg/kg/min. Plasma levels should be used to monitor therapy. Because many elderly patients have abnormal gas exchange, oxygen therapy is extremely important to increase oxygen delivery. All elderly patients should receive low-dose subcutaneous heparin because of the high risk for venous thromboembolic disease in all patients at bed rest during MI. Full-dose anticoagulation therapy is often given to patients with anterior MI because of the high risk of mural thrombus and possible embolization. Because anticoagulation carries a substantial risk for this age group, all elderly patients should receive an echocardiogram within the first 48 hours of admission. If a mural thrombus or large apical wall motion abnormality is visualized, full-dose anticoagulationt therapy is indicated, if no contraindications are present. In patients of advanced age (>80 years), the risks of this therapy may outweigh the benefits.

Acute beta-blocker therapy has been shown to improve mortality, prevent postinfarction angina, and prevent reinfarction, even with thrombolytic therapy. Therapy should be instituted with intravenous metoprolol at 5 mg every 5 minutes for three doses followed by oral drug. Hypotension, bradycardia, and severe acute heart failure are the major contraindications to using this therapy.

Management After Myocardial Infarction

The 1-year mortality after MI in the elderly is quite high (81,107); therefore, risk stratification is extremely important. Post-MI exercise testing should be performed because it is a safe and useful test to determine the risk for future cardiac events (108,109). The presence of significant ST-segment depression, an abnormal blood pressure response, or the development of angina is a strong predictor of mortality, even in the elderly population. Beta-blocker therapy has been shown in several large multicenter studies to decrease cardiac mortality after MI (110,111). In elderly patients, timolol has been shown to decrease mortality by 35.5 percent and reinfarction by 39.2 percent (112). Several studies suggest that beta blockade may be especially protective in the elderly population. Patients with non-Q-wave MI have been shown to have a higher early reinfarction rate, and diltiazem has been shown to reduce the risk of reinfarction by 51 percent and post-MI angina by 49 percent at 2 weeks after infarction (113). Since non-Q-wave MI seems to be more common in elderly patients, cautious use of diltiazem may play a role in reducing future cardiac events. Diltiazem and other calcium channel blockers have no role as secondary prevention drugs after Q-wave MI. In fact, patients with LV dysfunction have a worse outcome with diltiazem (48). Antiplatelet therapy with aspirin is recommended for both Q-wave and non-Q-wave MI. Risk stratification and secondary prevention strategies with these medications has become an important part of the management of MI in the elderly (114).

The indications for PTCA and CABG after MI in elderly patients depend on severity of symptoms, the degree of LV dysfunction, and the severity of underlying coronary disease. Surgery for acute complications of MI in the elderly has also been performed in selected patients with good results (115).

Cardiac rehabilitation is an important aspect of post-MI therapy in elderly patients. The elderly are especially sensitive to the deconditioning effects of bed rest and require early mobilization to prevent profound deterioration in functional capacity. The complications of orthostatic hypotension caused by relative hypovolemia and thrombophlebitis as a result of circulatory status can thus be prevented. Elderly patients are able to increase their functional capacity with regular exercise by increments similar to those for younger patients, although the elderly start at a lower functional capacity (116,117). There is no increased risk of appropriately prescribed exercise for the elderly cardiac patient, and the attainment of a lower heart rate and blood pressure during submaximal exercise results in less myocardial oxygen demand during activities of daily living, and thereby decreases the likelihood of cardiac symptoms.

References

1. Agner E. Epidemiology of coronary heart disease in the elderly patient. In Coodley EL, ed. Geriatric heart disease. Littleton, MA: PSG, 1985:114.
2. Gillum RF. Trends in acute myocardial infarction and coronary heart disease death in the United States. J Am Coll Cardiol 1994;23:1273.
3. Satler LF, Green CE, Wallace RB, Rackley CE. Coronary artery disease in the elderly. Am J Cardiol 1989;63:245.
4. Rogers WB, von Dohlen TW, Frank MJ. Management of coronary disease in the elderly. Clin Cardiol 1991;14:635.
5. Wenger NK, O'Rourke RA, Marcus FI. The care of elderly patients with cardiovascular disease. Ann Intern Med 1988;109:425.
6. Wenger NK. Cardiovascular disease in the elderly. Curr Probl Cardiol 1992;17:609.
7. Medalia LS, White PD. Disease of the aged: analysis of pathological observations in 1,251 autopsy protocols in old persons. JAMA 1952;149:1433.
8. Elreback L, Lie JT. Combined high incidence of coronary artery disease at autopsy in Olmstead County, Minnesota, 1950–1979. 1984; Circulation 70:345.
9. Pomerance A. Pathology of the heart with and without cardiac failure in the aged. Br Heart J 1965;27:697.
10. Waller BF, Roberts WC. Cardiovascular disease in the very elderly: analysis of 40 necropsy patients aged 90 years or over. Am J Cardiol 1983;51:403.
11. Kannel WB, Gordon T. Evaluation of cardiovascular risk in the elderly: the Framingham Study. Bull NY Acad Med 1978;45:573.
12. Kennedy RD. Epidemiology of heart disease in old age. Israel J Med Sci 1985;21:928.
13. Gordon T, Castelli WP, Hjortland MC, et al. Predicting coronary heart disease in middle-aged and older persons: the Framingham Study. JAMA 1977;238:497.
14. Castelli WP. Risk factors in the elderly: a view from Framingham. Am J Geriatr Cardiol 1993;3:8.
15. Kennedy RD, Andrews GR, Caird FI. Ischemic heart disease in the elderly. Br Heart J 1977;39:1121.
16. Kronmal RA, Cain KC, Ye Z, Omenn GS. Total serum cholesterol levels and mortality risk as a function of age: a report based on the Framingham data. Arch Intern Med 1993;153:1065.
17. Rubin SM, Sidney S, Black DM, et al. High blood cholesterol in elderly men and the excess risk for coronary heart disease. Ann Intern Med 1990;113:916.
18. Kreisberg RA, Kasim S. Cholesterol metabolism and aging. Am J Med 1987;82(suppl 1B):54.
19. Frick MH, Elo O, Haapa K, et al. Helsinki Heart Study: primary-prevention trial with gemfibrozil in middle-aged men with dyslipidemia. N Engl J Med 1987;317:1237.
20. Lipid Research Clinics Program. The Lipid Research Clinics Coronary Primary Prevention Trial results. JAMA 1984;241:351.

21. LaRosa JC, Applegate W, Crouse JR III, et al. Cholesterol lowering in the elderly. Results of the Cholesterol Reduction in the Seniors Program (CRISP) pilot study. Arch Intern Med 1994;154:529.

22. Denke MA, Grundy SM. Hypercholesterolemia in elderly persons: resolving the treatment dilemma. Ann Intern Med 1990;112:780.

23. Kafonek SD, Kwiterovich PO. Treatment of hypercholesterolemia in the elderly. Ann Intern Med 1990; 112:723.

24. Limacher MC. Clinical features of coronary heart disease in the elderly. Cardiovasc Clin 1992;22:63.

25. Wei JY. Age and the cardiovascular system. N Engl J Med 1992;327:1735.

26. Aronow WS, Epstein S. Usefulness of silent myocardial ischemia detected by ambulatory electrocardiographic monitoring in predicting new coronary events in elderly patients. Am J Cardiol 1988;62:1295.

27. Coy KM, Imperi GA, Lambert CR, et al. Silent myocardial ischemia during daily activities in asymptomatic men with positive exercise test response. Am J Cardiol 1987; 59:45.

28. Kannel WB, Abbott RD. Incidence and prognosis of unrecognized myocardial infarction: an update on the Framingham Study. N Engl J Med 1984;311:1144.

29. Diamond GA, Forrester JS. Analysis of probability as an aid in the clinical diagnosis of coronary disease. N Engl J Med 1979;300:1350.

30. Glover DR, Robinson CS, Murray RG. Diagnostic exercise testing in 104 patients over 65 years of age. Eur Heart J 1984;5(suppl E):59.

31. Beller G. Nuclear cardiology: current indications and clinical usefulness. Curr Probl Cardiol 1985;10:1.

32. Detry JMR, Melin JA, Derwael-Barchy C, et al. Role of exercise testing and stress thallium scintigraphy in the management of old men with suspected or documented coronary artery disease. Eur Heart J 1984;5(suppl E):75.

33. Iskandrian AS, Heo J, Decoskey D, et al. Use of exericse thallium-201 imaging for risk stratification of elderly patients with coronary artery disease. Am J Cardiol 1988; 61:269.

34. Hilton TC, Shaw LJ, Chaitman BR, et al. Prognostic significance of exercise thallium-201 testing in patients aged ≥70 years with known or suspected coronary artery disease. Am J Cardiol 1992;69:45.

35. Port S, Cobb FR, Coleman RE, et al. Effect of age on the response of the left ventricular ejection fraction to exercise. N Engl J Med 1980;303:1133.

36. Rodeheffer RJ, Gerstenblith G, Becker LG, et al. Exercise cardiac output is maintained with advancing age in healthy human subjects: cardiac dilatation and increased stroke volume compensate for a diminished heart rate. Circulation 1984;69:203.

37. Francisco DA, Collins SM, Go RT, et al. Tomographic thallium-201 myocardial perfusion scintigrams after maximal coronary artery vasodilation with intravenous dipyridamole: comparison of qualitative and quantitative approaches. Circulation 1982;66:370.

38. Ranhosky A, Kempthorne-Rawson J, et al. The safety of intravenous dipyridamole thallium myocardial perfusion imaging. Circulation 1990;81:1205.

39. Beller GA. Dipyridamole thallium 201 imaging. How safe is it? Circulation 1990;81:1425.

40. Lam JYT, Chaitman BR, Glaenzer M, et al. Safety and diagnostic accuracy of dipyridamole-thallium imaging in the elderly. J Am Coll Cardiol 1988;11:585.

41. Gerson MC, Moore EN, Ellis K. Systemic effects and safety of intravenous dipyridamole in elderly patients with suspected coronary artery disease. Am J Cardiol 1987;60:1399.

42. Shaw L, Chaitman BR, Hilton TC, et al. Prognostic value of dipyridamole thallium-201 imaging in elderly patients. J Am Coll Cardiol 1992;19:1390.

43. Gersh BJ, Kronmal RA, Frye RL, et al. Coronary arteriography and coronary artery bypass surgery: morbidity and mortality in patients age 65 years or older: a report from the Coronary Artery Surgery Study. Circulation 1983; 67:483.

44. Covinsky JD. New therapeutic modalities for the treatment of elderly patients with ischemic heart disease. Am J Med 1987;82(suppl 1B):41.

45. Alpert JS. Nitrate therapy in the elderly. Am J Cardiol 1990;65:23J.

46. Lakatta EG. Deficient neuroendocrine regulation of the cardiovascular system with advancing age in healthy humans. Circulation 1993;87:631.

47. Wei JY. Use of calcium entry blockers in elderly patients: Special considerations. Circulation 1989;80(suppl IV):IV-171.

48. Multicenter Diltiazem Postinfarction Trial Research Group. The effect of diltiazem on mortality and reinfarction after myocardial infarction. N Engl J Med 1988;319:385.

49. Yusuf S, Furberg CD. Are we biased in our approach to treating elderly patients with heart disease? Am J Cardiol 1991;68:954.

50. Cairns JA, Gent M, Singer J, et al. Aspirin, sulfinpyrazone, or both in unstable angina: results of a Canadian multicenter trial. N Engl J Med 1985;313:1369.

51. Lewis HD, Davis JW, Archibald DG, et al. Protective effects of aspirin against acute myocardial infarction and death in men with unstable angina: results of a Veterans Administration Cooperative Study. N Engl J Med 1983;309:396.

52. Theroux P, Ouimet H, McCans J, et al. Aspirin, heparin, or both to treat acute unstable angina. N Engl J Med 1988; 319:1105.

53. Parisi AF, Folland ED, Hartigan P. A comparison of angioplasty with medical therapy in the treatment of single-vessel coronary artery disease. N Engl J Med 1992; 326:10.

54. Luchi RJ, Scott SM, Deupree RH, et al. Comparison of medical and surgical treatment for unstable angina: results of a Veterans Administration Cooperative Study. N Engl J Med 1987;316:977.

55. National Cooperative Study Group. Unstable angina pectoris: National Cooperative Study Group to compare surgical and medical therapy. II. Am J Cardiol 1978;42:839.

56. Landau C, Lange RA, Hillis LD. Percutaneous transluminal coronary angioplasty. N Engl J Med 1994;330:981.

57. Gold S, Wong WF, Schatz IJ, Lanoie Blanchette P. Invasive treatment for coronary artery disease in the elderly. Arch Intern Med 1991;151:1085.

58. Jeroudi MO, Kleiman NS, Minor ST, et al. Percutaneous transluminal coronary angioplasty in octogenarians. Ann Intern Med 1990;113:423.

59. Taylor GJ, Rabinovich E, Mikell FL, et al. Percutaneous transluminal coronary angioplasty as palliation for patients considered poor surgical candidates. Am Heart J 1986; 111:840.

60. Bedotto JB, Rutherford BD, McConahay DR, et al. Results of multivessel percutaneous transluminal coronary angioplasty in persons aged 65 years and older. Am J Cardiol 1991;67:1051.

61. Dorros G, Janke L. Percutaneous transluminal coronary angioplasty in patients over the age of 70 years. Cathet Cardiovasc Diagn 1986;12:223.

62. Mick MJ, Simpfendorfer C, Arnold AZ, et al. Early and late results of coronary angioplasty and bypass in octogenarians. Am J Cardiol 1991;68:1316.

63. Raizner AE, Hust RG, Lewis JM, et al. Transluminal coronary angioplasty in the elderly. Am J Cardiol 1986; 57:29.

64. Simpfendorfer C, Raymond R, Schraider J, et al. Early and long-term results of percutaneous transluminal coronary angioplasty in patients 70 years of age and older with angina pectoris. Am J Cardiol 1988;62:959.

65. Kelsey SF, Miller DP, Holubkov R, et al. Results of percutaneous transluminal coronary angioplasty in patients ≥65 years of age (from the 1985 to 1986 National Heart, Lung, and Blood Institute's coronary angioplasty registry). Am J Cardiol 1990;66:1033.

66. Thompson RC, Holmes DR, Gersh BJ, et al. Percutaneous transluminal coronary angioplasty in the elderly: early and long-term results. J Am Coll Cardiol 1991;17:1245.

67. Knapp WS, Douglas JS Jr, Craver JM, et al. Efficacy of coronary artery bypass grafting in elderly patients with coronary artery disease. Am J Cardiol 1981;47:923.

68. Rahimtoola SH, Grunkemeier GL, Starr A. Ten-year survival after coronary artery bypass surgery for angina in patients aged 65 years and older. Circulation 1986;74:509.

69. Bhattacharya SK, Teskey JM Cohen M, et al. Risks and benefits of open-heart surgery in patients 70 years of age and older. Can J Surg 1984;27:150.

70. Elayda MA, Hall RJ, Gray AG, et al. Coronary revascularization in the elderly patient. J Am Coll Cardiol 1984;3:1398.

71. Gersh BJ, Kronmal RA, Schaff HV, et al. Comparison of coronary artery bypass surgery and medical therapy in patients 65 years of age and older: a nonrandomized study from the Coronary Artery Surgery Study (CASS) registry. N Engl J Med 1985;313:217.

72. Loop FD, Lytle BW, Cosgrove DM, et al. Coronary artery bypass graft surgery in the elderly. Indications and outcome. Cleve Clin J Med 1988;55:23.

73. Kunis R, Greenberg H, Yeoh CB, et al. Coronary revascularization for recurrent pulmonary edema in elderly patients with ischemic heart disease and preserved ventricular function. N Engl J Med 1985;313:1207.

74. CASS Principal Investigators. Coronary Artery Surgery Study (CASS): a randomized trial of coronary artery bypass surgery: survival data. Circulation 1983;68:939.

75. European Coronary Surgery Study Group. Long-term results of prospective randomized study of coronary artery bypass surgery in stable angina pectoris. Lancet 1982; 2:1173.

76. Murphy ML, Hultgren HN, Detre K, et al. Treatment of chronic stable angina: a preliminary report of survival data of the randomized Veterans' Administration Cooperative Study. N Engl J Med 1977;297:621.

77. Jaeger AA, Hlatky MA, Paul SM, Gortner SR. Functional capacity after cardiac surgery in elderly patients. J Am Coll Cardiol 1994;24:104.

78. Latting CA, Silverman ME. Acute myocardial infarction in hospitalized patients over 70. Am Heart J 1980;100:311.

79. Olmsted WL, Groden DL, Silverman ME. Prognosis in survivors of acute myocardial infarction occurring at age 70 years or older. Am J Cardiol 1987;60:971.

80. Weaver WD, Litwin PE, Martin JS, et al. Effect of age on use of thrombolytic therapy and mortality in acute myocardial infarction. J Am Coll Cardiol 1991;18:657.

81. Maggioni AP, Maseri A, Fresco C, et al. Age-related increase in mortality among patients with first myocardial infarctions treated with thrombolysis. N Engl J Med 1993; 329:1442.

82. Aronow WS. Prevalence of presenting symptoms of recognized acute myocardial infarction and of unrecognized healed myocardial infarction in elderly patients. Am J Cardiol 1987;60:1182.

83. Nadelmann J, Frishman WH, Ooi WL, et al. Prevalence, incidence and prognosis of recognized and unrecognized myocardial infarction in persons aged 75 years or older: the Bronx Aging Study. Am J Cardiol 1990;66:533.

84. Bayer AJ, Chadha JS, Farag RR, et al. Changing presentation of myocardial infarction with increasing age. J Am Geriatr Soc 1986;34:263.

85. Solomon CG, Lee TH, Cook EF, et al. Comparison of clinical presentation of acute myocardial infarction in patients older than 65 years of age to younger patients: the Multicenter Chest Pain Study experience. Am J Cardiol 1989;63:772.

86. Pathy MS. Clinical presentation of myocardial infarction in the elderly. Br Heart J 1967;29:190.

87. Heller GV, Blaustein AS, Wei JY. Implications of increased myocardial isoenzyme level in the presence of normal serum creatine kinase activity. Am J Cardiol 1983;51:24.

88. Hong RD, Licht JD, Wei JY. Elevated CK-MB with normal total creatine kinase in suspected myocardial infarction: associated clinical findings and early prognosis. Am Heart J 1986;111:1041.

89. Anderson HV, Willerson JT. Thrombolysis in acute myocardial infarction. N Engl J Med 1993;329:703.

90. GISSI Study Group. Effectiveness of intravenous thrombolytic treatment in acute myocardial infarction. Lancet 1986;1:297.

91. GISSI Study Group. Long-term effects of intravenous thrombolysis in acute myocardial infarction: final report of the GISSI Study. Lancet 1987;1:871.

92. GISSI-2 International Study Group. In-hospital mortality and clinical course of 20,891 patients with suspected acute myocardial infarction randomized between alteplase and streptokinase with or without heparin. Lancet 1990;336:71.

93. GUSTO Investigators. An international randomized trial comparing four thrombolytic strategies for acute myocardial infarction. N Engl J Med 1993;329:673.

94. ISIS-2 Collaborative Group. Randomized trial of intravenous streptokinase, oral aspirin, both, or neither among 17,187 cases of suspected acute myocardial infarction: ISIS-2. Lancet 1988;2:349.

95. ISIS-3 Collaborative Group. ISIS-3: a randomized comparison of streptokinase vs tissueplasminogen activator vs anistreplase and of aspirin plus heparin vs aspirin alone among 41,299 cases of suspected acute myocardial infarction. Lancet 1992;339:753.

96. Lew AS, Hod H, Cerek B, et al. Mortality and morbidity rates of patients older and younger than 75 years with acute myocardial infarction treated with intravenous streptokinase. Am J Cardiol 1987;59:1.

97. Gore JM, Sloan M, Price TR, et al. Intracerebral hemorrhage, cerebral infarction, and subdural hematoma after acute myocardial infarction and thrombolytic therapy in the Thrombolysis in Myocardial Infarction Study (TIMI). Circulation 1991;83:448.

98. DeJaegere PP, Arnold AA, Balk AH, Simoons ML. Intracranial hemorrhage in association with thrombolytic therapy: incidence and clinical predictive factors. J Am Coll Cardiol 1992;19:289.

99. Maggioni AP, Franzosi MG, Santoro E, et al. The risk of stroke in patients with acute myocardial infarction after thrombolytic and antithrombotic treatment. N Engl J Med 1992;327:1.

100. Muller DW, Topol EJ. Selection of patients with acute myocardial infarction for thrombolytic therapy. Ann Intern Med 1990;113:949.

101. Sleight P. Is there an age limit for thrombolytic therapy? Am J Cardiol 1993;72:30G.

102. Topol EJ, Califf RM. Thrombolytic therapy for elderly patients. N Engl J Med 1992;327:45.

103. Krumholz HM, Pasternak RC, Weinstein MC, et al. Cost effectiveness of thrombolytic therapy with streptokinase in elderly patients with suspected acute myocardial infarction. N Engl J Med 1992;327:7.

104. Grines CL. PAMI Investigators. A comparison of immediate angioplasty with thrombolytic therapy for acute myocardial infarction. N Engl J Med 1993;328:673.

105. Holland KJ, O'Neill WW, Bates ER, et al. Emergency percutaneous transluminal coronary angioplasty during acute myocardial infarction for patients more than 70 years of age. Am J Cardiol 1989;63:399.

106. Ribeiro EE, Lelio AS, Ellis SG, et al. Randomized trial of direct coronary angioplasty versus intravenous streptokinase in acute myocardial infarction. J Am Coll Cardiol 1993;22:376.

107. Smith SC, Gilpin E, Ahnve S, et al. Outlook after acute myocardial infarction in the very elderly compared with that in patients aged 65 to 75 years. J Am Coll Cardiol 1990;16:784.

108. Ciaroni S, Delonca J, Righetti A. Early exercise testing after acute myocardial infarction in the elderly: clinical evaluation and prognostic significance. Am Heart J 1993;126:304.

109. Froelicher VF, Perdue ST, Atwood JE, et al. Exercise testing of patients recovering from myocardial infarction. Curr Probl Cardiol 1986;11:370.

110. Beta-Blocker Heart Attack Trial Research Group: a randomized trial of propranolol in patients with acute myocardial infarction. JAMA 1982;247:1707.

111. Norwegian Multicenter Study Group. Timolol-induced reduction in mortality and reinfarction in patients surviving acute myocardial infarction. N Engl J Med 1981;304:801.

112. Gunderson T, Abrahamsen AM, Kjekshus J, et al. Timolol-related reduction in mortality and reinfarction in patients ages 65–75 years surviving acute myocardial infarction. Circulation 1982;66:1179.

113. Gibson RS, Boden WE, Theroux P, et al. Diltiazem and reinfarction in patients with non-Q-wave myocardial infarction: results of a double-blind, randomized, multicenter trial. N Engl J Med 1986;315:423.

114. Forman DE, Gutierrez Bernal JL, Wei JY. Management of acute myocardial infarction in the very elderly. Am J Med 1992;93:315.

115. Weintraub RM, Wei JY, Thurer RL. Surgical repair of remediable post infarction cardiogenic shock in the elderly: early and long-term results. J Am Geriatr Soc 1986;34:389.

116. Ades PA, Hanson JS, Gunther PG, et al. Exercise conditioning in the elderly coronary patient. J Am Geriatr Soc 1987;35:121.

117. Williams MA, Maresh CM, Esterbrooks DJ. Early exercise training in patients older than age 65 years compared with that in younger patients after acute myocardial infarction or coronary bypass grafting. Am J Cardiol 1985;55:263.

Chapter 34
Congestive Heart Failure in the Elderly

JoAnn Lindenfeld

I thought no more was needed
Youth to prolong
Than dumbbell and foil
To keep the body young.
Oh, who could have foretold
That the heart grows old?

W. B. Yeats
A Song

Congestive heart failure is an increasingly common cause of morbidity and mortality in the United States. It is a particular problem for the elderly because 75 percent of all patients with congestive heart failure are older than age 60 (1). The incidence of heart failure rises exponentially with age. New cases appear annually at the rate of 1.8 and 0.8 per 1000 in men and women aged 45 to 54 years, and the rate doubles with each succeeding decade (2). Although the incidence of heart failure in the elderly primarily reflects the increasing incidence of underlying diseases such as coronary artery disease and hypertensive heart disease, the occurrence of heart failure signals a particularly bad prognosis whatever the underlying disease. The annual mortality for all patients with heart failure is 10 percent to 20 percent; for those patients with symptoms of heart failure at rest (patients classified as New York Heart Association Class IV), the annual mortality is 50 percent (3). The economic impact of heart failure is enormous. The treatment of heart failure consumes approximately 6.5 percent of the total health care budget, and hospitalization costs for heart failure are greater than those for cancer or myocardial infarction (4).

Cardiovascular Changes with Aging

Because a number of cardiovascular diseases increase in frequency as a person ages, separating changes in the cardiovascular system that occur because of aging alone from those that result from underlying diseases is very difficult. Disease processes may affect cardiovascular function by involving the heart directly or by affecting other organ systems, which results in physical inactivity and cardiovascular deconditioning. Thus, although older studies reported a significant decline in cardiovascular function with age, recent studies done carefully to exclude underlying disease have reported less change solely on the basis of aging. Therefore, symptoms of congestive heart failure should not be attributed to age alone.

Age-related morphological changes in the myocardium are few (5,6). In general, experienced pathologists cannot discern age from microscopic examination of the myocardium. However, there is some progressive myocyte loss with age. Adaptation to this loss and to increased vascular stiffness by compensatory hypertrophy of myocytes may be impaired in the elderly (6). Macroscopic changes in the healthy elderly are nearly as subtle. Heart size is not changed by age alone. A gradual, mild increase in left ventricular wall thickness has been reported with aging but this finding is controversial (7,8). Systolic or contractile function does not appear to be significantly affected by aging (9). However, changes in diastolic function do occur and consist of a prolonged relaxation time and a decrease in early diastolic filling compensated for by an increase in late diastolic filling (the atrial portion of filling) (9,10).

Age-related changes in the vascular bed lead to a generalized increase in vascular stiffness (11). These changes appear first in the proximal aorta. Endothelial cells develop a progressive heterogeneity in size, shape, and axial orientation (9). Subendothelial calcium, lipids, and connective tissue also increase. There is gradual medial thickening with fragmentation of elastic tissue and calcification of the media. The thickening of the media in the proximal aorta is primarily caused by increased elastic lamina; the media of the distal aorta enlarges because of smooth muscle proliferation. The changes in the wall of the aorta lead to progressive dilation and elongation. Elasticity is lost and there is less contraction of the aorta during diastole. Thus, pulse pressure is increased and the left ventricle faces an increased load with the larger volume of blood in the aorta in systole. Changes in autonomic tone may exaggerate the increase in vascular stiffness. β-adrenergic (vasodilator) responsiveness of vessels tends to decrease with aging, but α-adrenergic (vasoconstrictor) responses are preserved (12).

Changes in β-adrenergic function also affect the heart. Resting heart rate does not change with age, but maximum heart rate declines by about one beat per year, primarily from a decrease in sinus node responsiveness to β-adrenergic stimulation (13). Maximum heart rate can be estimated by subtracting the patient's age from 220.

In addition to the effects of β-adrenergic subsensitivity on heart rate, aging is also associated with β-adrenergic subsensitivity for inotropic responses (14,15). The causes of decreased β-adrenergic responsiveness in the elderly are not completely understood. Plasma norepinephrine increases with age in humans as does sympathetic nerve activity (12,16,17). This may be the cause of the down-regulation of $β_1$-adrenergic receptors seen in the aging human heart and which is most prominent in women (18,19). Despite diminished maximum chronotropic and inotropic responses to circulating catecholamines, in one study resting and exercise cardiac output did not decrease in healthy elderly subjects who had been carefully screened to exclude heart disease (20). Cardiac output was maintained by the Frank-Starling mechanism with a larger rise in end-diastolic volume, a smaller decrease in end-systolic volume and, therefore, a smaller increase in ejection fraction and in heart rate than occurs in younger subjects (20). However, other studies have suggested that cardiac output does decline somewhat with age even in very healthy elderly subjects (21). The fall in cardiac output is caused by a decrease in stroke volume and in heart rate (a result at least in part from decreased β-adrenergic responsiveness) and by an increase in blood pressure and peripheral vascular resistance (21,22). The fall in cardiac output and a decrease in skeletal muscle oxygen uptake result in a marked fall in maximum oxygen consumption ($\dot{V}O_2$ max) with exercise. The decline in $\dot{V}O_2$ max and the abnormal diastolic function seen in the elderly can be significantly improved by regular exercise (21–23).

Decreased baroreceptor responsiveness accompanies aging (9). There is an attenuation of the baroreceptor reflex response with both hypo- and hypertension. In the normal individual, a fall in blood pressure is registered as a decrease in stretch of the baroreceptors in the carotid arteries and aorta. The response is a withdrawal of parasympathetic tone with an increase in heart rate and an increase in sympathetic activity which causes an additional increase in heart rate, an increase in inotropic effect, and vasoconstriction–all designed to maintain blood pressure and, thus, cerebral perfusion (24). This system allows the normal person to stand up with only modest increases in heart rate and little change in blood pressure. In the elderly, the baroreceptor reflex is attenuated. When the elderly person stands, heart rate does not increase as much as expected and the fall in stroke volume is greater than expected (25). However, most older people can maintain a normal blood pressure when standing because of a larger increase in peripheral vascular resistance (25,26). Baroreceptor attenuation is only manifest when there is an additional stress in the system such as volume depletion. The addition of even mild diuresis may result in significant orthostatic hypertension (26) (Figure 34.1). However, the sensitivity to orthostatic stress is also caused by a less vigorous stroke volume response to standing in the elderly (25). This may be due to β-adrenergic subsensitivity and the increased peripheral vascular resistance of the elderly (25).

The defect in baroreceptor function seems to be most closely related to the supine blood pressure–the higher the supine blood pressure, the more significant the baroreceptor defect. In some elderly subjects, eating may result in orthostatic hypotension, which can lead to syncope or angina. This is most severe in elderly patients with higher supine blood pressures (26,27). The exact cause of baroreceptor dysfunction in the elderly is not entirely clear and may be multifactorial, involving decreased vascular elasticity with decreased stretch of the baroreceptors, altered parasympathetic activity, and decreased cardiovascular responsiveness to β-adrenergic agonists (12). The age-related morphologic and physiologic alterations in the cardiovascular system are summarized in Table 34.1.

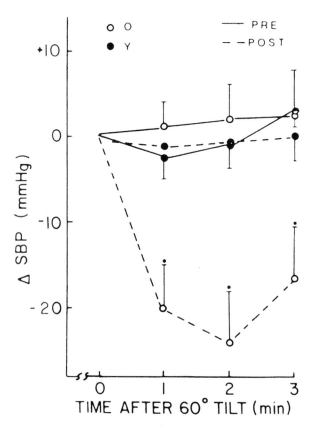

Fig. 34.1. Change in systolic blood pressure (SBP) during upright tilt (60°) in six young (Y) and six older (O) healthy adults before (PRE) and after (POST) modest diuresis. Asterisk indicates significant change from prediuresis values (p < 0.02). (Reproduced by permission from Shannon RP, Wei JU, Rosa RM, et al. The effect of age and sodium depletion on cardiovascular response to orthostasis. Hypertension 1986;8:438).

Definition and Etiology

Heart failure is not a disease itself but a syndrome—a complex of signs and symptoms. It is most often defined as the inability (caused by a cardiac abnormality) to meet the oxygen demands of the body. However, some patients are primarily limited by symptoms resulting from pulmonary venous or systemic venous congestion. Thus, it is reasonable to expand the definition of heart failure to include patients who have symptoms of inadequate oxygen delivery, symptoms of pulmonary or systemic venous congestion, or both. It is particularly important to realize that the complex of signs and symptoms recog-

Table 34.1. Morphologic and Physiologic Changes in the Cardiovascular System of the Elderly.

Morphologic
  Myocardial
    Loss of myocytes
    Decreased β-adrenergic receptors
  Vascular
    Increased heterogeneity of endothelial cells
    Increased subendothelial layer
    Increased smooth muscle cell layer with
      fragmentation of elastin
  Conduction System
    Loss of sinus node cells
Physiologic
  Decreased inotropic and chronotropic responses to
    β-adrenergic stimulation
  Decreased arterial and venodilation with β-adrenergic
    stimulation
  Increased blood pressure and vascular resistance
  Decreased early diastolic filling
  Abnormal baroreceptor function
  Decreased skeletal muscle oxygen uptake with exercise

nized as heart failure may result from a number of diseases that affect the heart in different ways. Pressure or volume overload of the myocardium, loss of myocardium, diminished contractility of myocardium, or restricted filling of the myocardium may result in heart failure individually or in combination. Table 34.2 lists the most common causes of heart failure in the elderly by disease process. Hypertension and ischemic heart disease, alone or in combination, are found in about 90 percent of the elderly with heart failure (1,2,28).

The prevalence of hypertension increases with age. The higher the systolic and diastolic pressures, the greater the cardiovascular morbidity and mortality, but in the elderly, elevated systolic pressure alone increases the risk of a major cardiovascular event (29). Hypertension is a risk factor for coronary artery disease, cerebral vascular event, renal failure, and peripheral vascular disease as well as for heart failure. The development of left ventricular hypertrophy may lead to diastolic dysfunction and restricted filling of the ventricle (30). Eventually, the pressure overload on the myocardium may result in decreased contractility and systolic dysfunction. It is now clear that the treatment of hypertension decreases the incidence of heart failure (31).

Atherosclerotic coronary artery disease also increases

Table 34.2. Common Causes of Heart Failure in the Elderly.

Ischemic heart disease
Hypertensive heart disease
Valvular heart disease
  Rheumatic
  Ischemic mitral regurgitation
  Calcific degenerative aortic stenosis
  Calcification of the mitral annulus
Cardiomyopathy
  Idiopathic
  Hypertrophic
  Restrictive (amyloid)
Cor pulmonale

---

in frequency with age and is the most important cause of heart failure in the elderly. Coronary artery disease may lead to systolic dysfunction and heart failure as a result of loss of myocardium after a myocardial infarction. In addition, ischemia may result in diastolic dysfunction. Dyspnea on exertion without angina is a much more common symptom of ischemia in the elderly than it is in younger patients (32). In fact, it has been suggested that aging is associated with a defect in the perception of angina (32). The presence of exercise-induced silent myocardial ischemia increases with age and is associated with an increased incidence of coronary events within 5 years (33).

Rheumatic heart disease is seen in elderly patients, but two other causes of valvular disease are more specific to the elderly. Calcific degenerative aortic stenosis is seen with increased frequency. Echocardiography is especially helpful in separating aortic stenosis from aortic sclerosis. Much less commonly, calcification of the mitral annulus may lead to significant mitral regurgitation. Because of the high frequency of coronary disease in the elderly, ischemic mitral regurgitation is a common problem.

Cardiomyopathies are generally divided into three types: congestive, hypertrophic, and restrictive (34). Idiopathic cardiomyopathy seems to be less common in older patients, but does occur (34). Hypertrophic cardiomyopathy is not common in the elderly, but as seen with idiopathic cardiomyopathy, it cannot be arbitrarily excluded. Although infrequent, restrictive cardiomyopathy may be seen more often in the elderly because of their increased incidence of amyloid heart disease. In pathologic studies, amyloid is seen frequently in

the cardiovascular system of the elderly. However, it only very rarely appears to be a cause of restrictive disease and heart failure. Senile amyloidosis with cardiovascular involvement occurs in three forms (35). *Senile atrial amyloidosis* consists of atrial amyloid deposits only. *Senile aortic amyloidosis* affects the medial layer of the aorta in the elderly. Clinical manifestations of these two forms of senile amyloidosis are few, although atrial amyloidosis may be associated with a slightly increased incidence of atrial fibrillation. The third form, *senile systemic amyloidosis* may involve the lungs, liver, and kidneys as well as the heart, including the ventricles. This form of amyloid results in clinical heart disease and is indistinguishable clinically from amyloid associated with multiple myeloma or primary systemic amyloidosis. In these patients who have immunoglobulin-derived amyloidosis, monoclonal immunoglobulin light chains are found in the serum or urine in 85 percent of patients. However, in 15 percent the light chains are not detected; only cardiac biopsy with immunohistochemistry can differentiate the types of amyloid protein (36). This differentiation is important because prognosis and treatment differ for senile systemic amyloidosis and immunoglobulin-derived amyloidosis (36).

Cor pulmonale is seen as frequently in the elderly as it is in younger patients. Abnormalities in diastolic function, baroreceptor function, β-adrenergic responsiveness, and blood pressure in the elderly make this age group much more likely to develop symptoms of heart failure when even mild heart disease or any other medical problem such as anemia, thyroid disease, or dysrhythmias is superimposed. Thus, it is not surprising that more than 50 percent of the elderly with symptoms of heart failure have normal systolic function (9).

Pathophysiology

An understanding of the patient with heart failure requires an understanding of the factors that determine cardiac performance, the compensatory mechanisms that occur when cardiac performance is inadequate, and the necessary balance between myocardial oxygen supply and demand.

Cardiac performance is determined by four major factors—preload, afterload, contractility, and heart rate (37).

As the resting length of myocardial fibers is increased, the force of contraction of these fibers increases. This is called the Frank-Starling effect. The length or stretch of the myocardial fibers is called the *preload*—the load on the heart before contraction. Because it is not possible to measure the length of myocardial fibers in a living patient, the intraventricular pressure at end-diastole (the end-diastolic pressure) is used as an estimate of the stretch or preload of the fibers. In a patient this relationship is often graphically shown by use of a left ventricular function curve in which a measure of the output of the heart is plotted against the end-diastolic pressure (Figure 34.2). As end-diastolic pressure increases, the cardiac output increases, but there is a point at which an increase in preload or end-diastolic pressure no longer results in an increase in cardiac output.

Afterload refers to the total load against which the heart must eject blood. The afterload is determined by a complex combination of factors but is best estimated by the myocardial wall stress, which is a function of the intraventricular pressure and the ventricular radius divided by the ventricular wall thickness during contraction.

wall stress = $P \times R / 2h$

where P = intraventricular pressure

R = the radius of the ventricle and

h = the thickness of the ventricular wall.

Thus, wall stress or afterload increases as the intraventricular pressure increases or as the ventricular radius increases; afterload decreases as the ventricular wall thickness increases. In actual practice, wall stress is difficult to measure and systemic vascular resistance is used as an estimate of afterload. As afterload or systemic resistance increases, cardiac output decreases; as systemic vascular resistance is decreased, cardiac output increases. The effect of a change in afterload or systemic vascular resistance is shown in the ventricular function curve (see Figure 34.2B). Systemic vascular resistance increases with age as a result of increased vascular stiffness.

Contractility is the intrinsic force of contraction of the myocardial fibers. Myocardial contractility can be changed by many factors. For example, it can be increased by β-adrenergic agonists such as isoproterenol or can it be decreased by disease that affect the myocardial fibers or

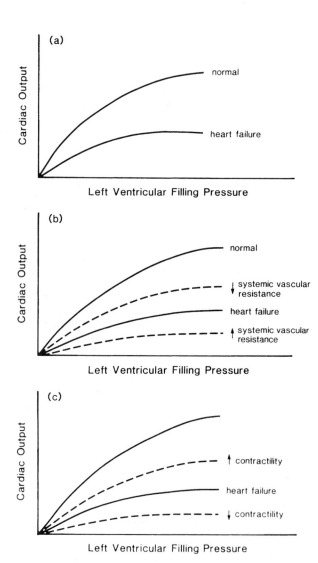

Fig. 34.2. Ventricular function curves. (*a*) normal ventricular function curve and the curve in a patient with heart failure. (*b*) the effects of increased and decreased systemic vascular resistance on the ventricular function curve in a patient with heart failure. (*c*) the effects of changes in contractility.

by drugs with negative inotropic effects such as verapamil. The effect of changes in contractility is shown in Figure 34.2C. If all other factors are held constant, cardiac output will increase as heart rate increases. Intrinsic contractility of myocytes appears to be normal in the elderly but the contractile response to β-adrenergic agents

460

is decreased and myocyte loss may occur. Typical ventricular function curves describing cardiac performance in a normal person and in patients with moderate and severe heart failure are shown in Figure 34.3. At any given level of ventricular filling, cardiac output is below normal. However, the determinants of cardiac performance operate in the same general direction.

A fall in cardiac output initiates a number of compensatory mechanisms, both acute and chronic (38,39). There is increased activity of the sympathetic nervous system. This results in an increased *heart rate*, increased contractility of the myocardium, and increased vascular tone. Increases in heart rate and contractility improve cardiac output, and increased vascular tone ensures that blood flow is maintained to vital organs such as the brain. In general, this response is a beneficial, but increased heart rate and contractility can increase myocardial oxygen demand and increased vascular resistance can increase afterload. At the same time, patients with heart failure caused by systolic dysfunction demonstrate a

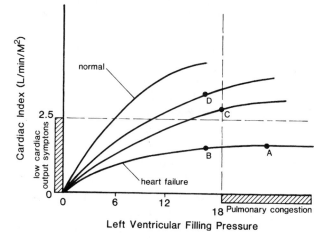

Fig. 34.3. Correlation of symptoms with hemodynamics and the effects of various therapeutic interventions in patients with heart failure as demonstrated by use of ventricular function curves. As cardiac index falls below 2.5 L/min/M² at rest, patients begin to note low output symptoms. Left ventricular filling pressures above 18 mm Hg are correlated with symptoms of pulmonary congestion. (Reproduced by permission from Miller RR. Ventricular afterload-reducing agents in congestive heart failure. In: Mason DT, ed. Congestive heart failure. New York: Yorke Medical Books, 1976:358).

down-regulation in myocardial β_1 receptors as well as other changes in the myocardial β-adrenergic system—perhaps a result of the chronically increased cardiac sympathetic activation of heart failure (40).

Activity of the renin-angiotensin-aldosterone axis also increases in patients with heart failure, especially after diuresis, and results in salt and water retention and vasoconstriction. With salt and water retention, preload is increased and, in turn, increases the contractility of the heart, but if preload increases too much, pulmonary venous congestion that results in dyspnea may occur. The angiotensin-converting enzyme (ACE) inhibitors decrease the formation of angiotensin II and aldosterone and thus reduce vasoconstriction and sodium retention. Since angiotensin II directly stimulates thirst and activation of the sympathetic nervous system, the ACE inhibitors decrease thirst and sympathetic activation in patients with heart failure (38). It is now known that the basic elements of the renin-angiotension system are synthesized in many tissues including vascular smooth muscle and the heart, and these local systems may be important in a number of processes such as vascular and myocardial hypertrophy (41).

However, specific alterations in local tissue renin-angiotension systems and their consequences in patients with heart failure are not completely understood. Arginine vasopressin is often elevated in the late stages of heart failure and results in vasoconstriction and water retention (38,39). Atrial natriuretic peptide (ANP), which is released by atrial stretch, is increased in patients with heart failure and promotes salt and water excretion and vasodilation. ANP also inhibits the release of renin and norepinephrine (39). Vasodilator prostaglandins, especially in the kidneys, are important in maintaining renal function. The use of nonsteroidal anti-inflammatory drugs (NSAIDs) blocks formation of the vasodilator prostaglandins and causes salt and water retention in patients with heart failure. Endothelin, a potent vasoconstrictor released by endothelial cells, is increased in heart failure, and the release of endothelium-derived relaxing factor is decreased in these patients (38). A number of other neurohormones are increased in heart failure, although their relative importance is not yet clear (39). Recently, it has been suggested that neurohormonal activation, although providing short-term benefit, contributes to the progressive decline in myocardial function seen in patients with systolic dysfunction. Treatment with ACE inhibitors and possibly with β-adrenergic blocking drugs slows this progression (38,40,42).

When cardiac dysfunction and salt and water retention continue, ventricular dilatation and hypertrophy may serve as an additional compensatory mechanisms. As the ventricle dilates, the end-diastolic volume increases. This serves to maintain resting cardiac output despite a decrease in ejection fraction. For example, if the normal ventricle has an end-diastolic volume of 100 mL and an ejection fraction of 60 percent, the stroke volume is 60 mL. If the ventricle dilates to an end-diastolic volume of 200 mL and the ejection fraction is 30 percent, the stroke volume is still 60 mL (43). However, as seen with other compensatory mechanisms, ventricular dilatation may be detrimental. As the ventricular radius increases, so does ventricular wall stress. If the ventricle becomes hypertrophic, wall stress may return to normal, but some disease processes limit myocardial hypertrophy.

There is a necessary balance between myocardial oxygen supply and demand. If demand increases without a concomitant increase in supply, myocardial function may worsen. Tachycardia, increased sympathetic activity, and ventricular dilatation may increase myocardial oxygen demands. Hypotension may limit myocardial oxygen supply. These factors assume particular importance for the patients with coronary artery disease because myocardial oxygen supply is already limited by obstruction of the coronary arteries.

Compensatory mechanisms in heart failure may not always be beneficial. With a sudden fall in cardiac output, compensatory mechanisms may serve to maintain perfusion of vital organs such as the heart and the brain and limiting flow to less vital organs. However, in the chronic situation, salt and water retention may lead to pulmonary congestion and edema, vasoconstriction, and tachycardia, all of which may impose an increased burden on the heart. In addition, chronic neurohormonal activation may cause some of the progressive myocardial dysfunction seen in these patients.

Signs and Symptoms

The symptoms of heart failure fall into two general cat-

egories—those of low output and those of pulmonary or systemic venous congestion or both. Signs of low output occur when blood flow and oxygen delivery to various organs is limited. If blood flow to skeletal muscle is not increased with exercise, muscle fatigue results; when blood flow to the brain is compromised, confusion and somnolence are seen. When ventricular end-diastolic pressure increases markedly, there is an increase in pulmonary venous pressure that causes pulmonary interstitial edema and dyspnea. Salt and water retention combined with failure of the right ventricle and elevated systemic venous pressure leads to peripheral edema and, if severe enough, to hepatic and splanchnic congestion. These symptoms can be better understood when superimposed on the ventricular function curve (see Figure 34.3). Most patients with heart failure have symptoms of low output and of pulmonary congestion. However, patients often are bothered more by one set of symptoms than another, depending on the underlying disease, the duration of the disease, the compensatory mechanisms, the level of activity, and the treatment. Symptoms of shortness of breath with exertion occur earlier in the elderly because of their underlying abnormalities in diastolic function, vascular stiffness, and the β-adrenergic hyporesponsiveness.

Early in heart failure symptoms may occur only with significant exercise; as heart failure progresses, symptoms may appear with mild exercise, and then when the person is at rest. This has led to a clinical classification of heart failure called the New York Heart Association Classification (Table 34.3). Dyspnea, the sensation of shortness of breath, is initially noted with exertion. Paroxysmal nocturnal dyspnea is the sudden onset of shortness of breath, which usually occurs 1 to 2 hours after the person is asleep. The patient is awakened suddenly and must sit or stand to relieve pulmonary congestion. This is often caused by the gradual reabsorption of fluid from the extremities during recumbency but may also be initiated by episodes of ischemia. Orthopnea is dyspnea provoked by lying down and which is relieved by sitting or standing. Nocturia is determined by several factors: an increase in cardiac output in the supine position, mobilization of fluid from the lower extremities, and a decrease in renal vasoconstriction with lying down.

A number of factors may obscure the symptoms of

Table 34.3. New York Heart Association Functional
Classification.

CLASS I	Patients with cardiac disease but without resulting limitations of physical activity. Ordinary physical activity does not cause undue fatigue, palpitation, dyspnea, or anginal pain.
CLASS II	Patients with cardiac disease resulting in slight limitation of physical activity. They are comfortable at rest. Ordinary physical activity results in fatigue, palpitation, dyspnea, or anginal pain.
CLASS III	Patients with cardiac disease resulting in marked limitation of physical activity. They are comfortable at rest. Less than ordinary physical activity causes fatigue, palpitation, dyspnea, or anginal pain.
CLASS IV	Patients with cardiac disease resulting in inability to carry on any physical activity without discomfort. Symptoms of cardiac insufficiency or of the anginal syndrome may be present even at rest. If any physical activity is undertaken, discomfort is increased.

heart failure in the elderly. Older patients often have several diseases—thus, dyspnea may be caused by lung disease and nocturia by benign prostatic hypertrophy. Limitations in physical activity may prevent recognition of exertional symptoms of heart failure. Elderly patients may have an altered respiratory drive and thus not report dyspnea, but rather a chronic, nonproductive cough or other complaint. Mental confusion is a common presenting sign of many serious illnesses in the aged and may make it difficult to obtain an adequate history (44).

The physical examination in heart failure is determined by the underlying disease and its severity as well as by compensatory mechanisms. The signs of heart failure are not substantially different for the older patient compared with those of the younger patient. There may be signs specific to the underlying disease, such as a murmur of mitral or aortic stenosis or the peripheral signs of endocarditis. However, the signs of critical aortic stenosis may be obscured in the elderly (45). A fourth heart sound is frequently heard in the elderly, which reflects the increased importance of the atrial kick in diastolic function, but does not necessarily indicate heart failure. However, a third heart sound is definitely abnormal in this age group and usually indicates heart failure. Rales and pleural effu-

sion may be found. If there is right ventricular failure, gallop sounds may be heard over the right ventricle—usually along the left sternal border or in the subxiphoid area. These are usually accompanied by jugular venous distension. As heart failure progresses, various degrees of edema, ascites, and hepatomegaly may occur. With severe heart failure, pulsus alternans or Cheyne-Stokes respiration may be observed.

Diagnosis

The diagnosis of heart failure is usually made by the appropriate signs and symptoms. The ECG is nonspecific but may give clues to the underlying diagnosis with Q waves suggestive of old myocardial infarction or findings suggesting left ventricular hypertrophy. The chest x-ray is often quite helpful to document pulmonary venous congestion and heart size. A number of other diagnostic tests can document underlying left ventricular dysfunction as well as provide clues to the specific disease process. Many patients who present with signs and symptoms of congestive heart failure have normal or near-normal systolic function (46). It is helpful to recognize the patients with diastolic dysfunction because their therapy is often different than that for patients with systolic dysfunction (47). Radionuclide and echocardiographic-Doppler studies can differentiate systolic from diastolic dysfunction. These studies may also show specific localized ventricular wall motion abnormalities and ventricular aneurysms that suggest coronary artery disease. The echocardiographic-Doppler studies provide evidence for valve pathology, myocardial hypertrophy, hypertrophic cardiomyopathy, and occasionally may suggest amyloid infiltration. Exercise testing, with or without the radionuclide thallium-201 or with sestaMIBI or echocardiography, can document underlying coronary artery disease. In elderly patients who cannot exercise, echocardiography or radionuclide scans can be performed with dobutamine, dipyridamole, or adenosine to detect coronary disease. In some patients, ambulatory ECG monitoring may suggest silent ischemia with ST-depression (32,33). Cardiac catheterization will define coronary artery disease and hemodynamics. Occasionally, myocardial biopsy is necessary to document infiltrative diseases of the myocardium.

Management

The approach to management of the patient with heart failure is outlined in Table 34.4. The first order of business is to diagnose underlying disease. In some cases, surgical therapy can correct underlying disease. Cardiac surgery, coronary angioplasty, and occasionally valvuloplasty are all feasible for many older patients. If surgical therapy is not appropriate, the next step is to correct any factors that may have precipitated heart failure (48). These are listed in Table 34.5. Hypertension should be treated (see Chapter 36) because the treatment of hypertension prevents the onset of heart failure in many patients (29,31). Thyrotoxicosis may exacerbate heart failure and ischemia in the elderly, but the diagnosis may not be obvious because the usual associated noncardiovascular findings of

Table 34.4. Management of the Patient with Heart Failure.

Diagnose underlying disease
Correct precipitating factors
Reduce workload of the heart
Restrict salt and water intake
Administer diuretics, vasodilators, digoxin
Administer intravenous therapy with dobutamine,
    nitroprusside, milrinone
Perform cardiac transplantation

Table 34.5. Precipitating Factors for Heart Failure.

Increased sodium intake
Medication noncompliance
Medication interactions
Concurrent infections
Anemia
Thyroid disease
Increased cardiac workload
    Hypertension
    Increased physical activity
    Emotional stress
Hypoxia
Pulmonary embolism
Arrhythmias
Drug effects
    Negative inotropic–β adrenergic blockers, calcium channel
      blockers, disopyramide, flecainide, amiodarone, alcohol
    Sodium retention–steroids, nonsteroidal anti-inflammatory
      drugs, cyclosporine
    Myocardial damage–anthracyclines

thyrotoxicosis may not be evident in the elderly patient. Anemia may impose a volume burden on the heart and decrease myocardial oxygen delivery. Endocarditis may be more subtle in the elderly than it is in the younger patient, and indeed, infections such as pneumonia or urinary tract infections may unmask moderate myocardial dysfunction by increasing myocardial oxygen demands. Arrhythmias such as atrial fibrillation should be controlled or converted to sinus rhythm as indicated. Loss of the atrial kick is a particular problem in the elderly because a greater proportion of ventricular filling occurs in this phase. As heart failure progresses, infections, arrhythmias, and pulmonary emboli occur with increasing frequency.

A number of physiologic changes associated with aging can alter the pharmacology of medications. These include decreased cardiac output, which decreases hepatic and renal blood flow; decreased albumin; decreased lean body mass; decreased hepatic metabolism; decreased autonomic and baroreceptor function; and decreased renal function. In addition, multiple diseases are often found in the elderly. This results in multiple medications and abnormal function for several organs, which confounds medical therapy. Thus, it is crucial to ask patients to bring all their medication bottles for inspection because prescriptions may be confused or duplicated. A number of medications may depress myocardial function or promote salt and water retention (Table 34.5). Although it is well known that alcohol may cause cardiomyopathy, it is less often appreciated that alcohol is a myocardial depressant and that moderate amounts may unmask latent myocardial dysfunction. Chapter 7 discusses the effects of aging on drug metabolism in more detail.

Once precipitating factors have been corrected, therapy is aimed at decreasing the workload of the heart. If the patient is obese, weight loss will be very helpful. Patients can be instructed to limit activity, but this can promote depression or feelings of isolation. Instead, one or two rest periods each day may be helpful. If possible, emotional causes of stress should also be eliminated. Controlling blood pressure may be particularly important for this age group (29).

Therapy is next directed to correct salt and water retention. A careful dietary history may reveal excess sodium intake. Canned and packaged foods that are high in sodium are often a major part of the diet of elderly people. If the sodium content of the diet is high, sodium should be restricted to 4 grams per day (equivalent to no added salt); however, especially in the elderly, one must be careful that the diet does not become so unpalatable that nutrition is compromised. If sodium restriction is not adequate to relieve symptoms of heart failure, diuretics are extremely valuable.

Four groups of diuretic drugs are used in the treatment of heart failure (Table 34.6). A mild diuretic, such as a thiazide, is often used first. Thiazides cause less natriuresis, and thus less volume depletion, than loop diuretics, but cause as much or more hypokalemia than loop diuretics (49). This may be a result of the longer duration of action of the thiazides. The natriuretic effect of thiazides decreases as the glomerular filtration rate (GFR) falls below 50mL/min and they are ineffective below a GFR of 35mL/min. GFR often is decreased in the elderly without an increase in serum creatinine because of loss of muscle mass.

If a thiazide is not potent enough, several loop diuretics are available. In general, the side effects of loop diuretics are similar to those of thiazides. Several factors make the elderly patient susceptible to diuretic-associated hypokalemia. Dietary sodium may be increased and dietary potassium decreased, and diuretic action may be prolonged by either diminished renal function or hepatic metabolism. ACE inhibitors decrease the incidence of hypokalemia in patients with heart failure. Changes in serum magnesium caused by diuretics follow changes in potassium. Diuretic-induced hyponatremia is also more common in the elderly population. Carbohydrate intolerance and hyperlipidemia are more problematic with thiazides than they are with loop diuretics. Hyperuricemia is common with both groups of diuretics, but is rarely symptomatic. The elderly patient is less able to maintain a normal standing blood pressure when there is volume depletion (see Figure 34.1).

Part of the diuretic effect of loop agents is an increase in medullary blood flow, which is mediated by prostaglandins. NSAIDs block prostaglandin synthesis and may significantly diminish the natriuretic effects of loop diuretics. In patients with very severe heart failure, NSAIDs may cause salt and water retention and azotemia.

Potassium-sparing diuretics are not generally used

Table 34.6. Diuretics.

Type	Max. Filtered Na Excreted (%)	Duration of Action of Oral Drug (hr)	Hypokalemia (%)	Usual Oral Dose (mg/day)
Thiazide				
Hydrochlorothiazide	5–8	6–12	5–30	25–100
Chlorothiazide	5–8	6–12	5–30	500–1000
Chlorthalidone	5–8	48–72	5–30	25–100
Metolazone	5–8	12–24	20–30+	5–10
Loop				
Furosemide	20–25	4–6	5–15	20–1000
Bumetanide	20–25	4–6	5–15	6–20
Ethacrynic acid	20–25	6–8	5–15	50–150
Potassium-sparing				
Spironolactone	2–3	72–96	K-sparing	25–100
Triamterene	2–3	7–9	K-sparing	100–300
Amiloride	2–3	24	K-sparing	5–10
Carbonic anhydrase inhibitors				
Acetazolamide	3–5	8–12	Unknown, but does occur	250–500

K = potassium; Na = sodium.

SOURCE: Modified from Puschett JB. Clinical pharmacologic implications in diuretic selection. Am J Cardiol 1986;57:6A.

alone in patients with heart failure because they are not potent natriuretic agents. They most often are combined with thiazides or loop diuretics to preserve potassium. They should be used carefully because the elderly are more susceptible to hyperkalemia and hypokalemia. If potassium-sparing diuretics are necessary, patients should be educated to avoid potassium supplements and potassium-containing salt substitutes (which may have 50 to 60 mEq of potassium per teaspoon). The combination of potassium-sparing diuretics and ACE inhibitors or NSAIDs should be avoided because life-threatening hyperkalemia can result.

Acetazolamide is used primarily for patients with heart failure when a metabolic alkalosis complicates diuretic therapy but significant salt and water retention persist. Often only a few doses are necessary to restore acid-base balance.

The therapeutic benefit of diuretics in heart failure is a decrease in salt and water retention and a decrease in preload, which results in fewer symptoms of pulmonary and systemic venous congestion. This is often demonstrated on a ventricular function curve as shown in Figure 34.3. However, some data suggest that diuretics may lead to an improvement in left ventricular function by one of several mechanisms—direct vasodilator action, improved oxygenation, a decrease in vascular rigidity, and a decrease in myocardial wall stress (50).

If moderate diuresis is not adequate, the next step is either administration of digitalis glycosides or use of vasodilators. The right choice depends on the underlying disease, the presence of atrial fibrillation, the patient's ability to take drugs frequently, the cost of the drugs, and the presence of associated diseases.

Digoxin has been used for years for the treatment of congestive heart failure. Its basic effect is to increase myocardial contractility, presumably through its effect on membrane Na+K+ATPase, but digoxin also improves baroreceptor function in patients with heart failure (51,52). Digoxin slows conduction through the atrioventricular node and is particularly useful for patients with atrial fibrillation and a rapid ventricular response. There has been considerable controversy about the value of digoxin in patients with heart failure and normal sinus rhythm. If patients have significant systolic dysfunction, there is a beneficial response to digoxin. A re-

cent study demonstrated that for stable patients with systolic dysfunction and heart failure who took ACE inhibitors, digoxin withdrawal caused an increased frequency of worsening heart failure and lower functional capacity and quality of life (53). Thus, digoxin appears to be indicated for patients with heart failure caused by systolic dysfunction.

Patients with diastolic dysfunction or restricted filling are not likely to have a beneficial response unless they have atrial fibrillation. Digoxin can be given once a day—a particular convenience for older patients—but a number of factors make digoxin more difficult to use in this age group. Lean body mass decreases with age, which lowers the volume of distribution for digoxin. Renal function gradually declines with age, which decreases elimination of digoxin. Thus, both the loading dose and maintenance dose of digoxin need to be decreased for the elderly. An average maintenance dose is 0.125 to 0.25 mg per day. Although data from animals suggest that the inotropic effects of digoxin may be less in the aged, it is not clear that this is true for humans. However, it does appear that older patients are more susceptible to the toxic effects of digoxin. This is probably primarily a result of their decreased dosage requirements, but may also be caused by the increased frequency of other factors that predispose to digoxin toxicity; for example, the larger number of drugs taken by older patients increases the possibility of drug interactions.

Factors that predispose a patient to digoxin toxicity are listed in Table 34.7. Hypokalemia is a particular problem, and potassium replacement is mandatory for patients on digoxin. Diuretic-induced hypomagnesemia may also predispose to digoxin toxicity. Patients with chronic lung disease seem to have an increased incidence of digoxin toxicity, perhaps because of hypoxia or because of other drugs that sensitize the myocardium to the effects of digoxin. Patients with hypothyroidism are resistant to the effects of digoxin. Patients with amyloid heart disease may be at particular risk for digoxin toxicity, perhaps because digoxin binds to the amyloid fibrils.

Toxicity is most often manifest as an increase in arrhythmias—these may be of any variety, but are often premature ventricular beats. Central nervous system symptoms such as confusion or hallucinations or gastrointestinal symptoms such as nausea or anorexia

Table 34.7. Predisposing Factors for Digoxin Toxicity.

Electrolyte abnormalities
  Hypokalemia
  Hypomagnesemia
  Hyponatremia
  Hyperkalemia
Renal failure
Pulmonary disease
Thyroid disease
Increasing age
Multiple drug therapy

may suggest digoxin toxicity. If manifestations of digoxin toxicity are life-threatening, digoxin antibodies are a rapid, safe therapy (51).

A number of drugs interact with digoxin to alter the pharmacokinetics or pharmacodynamics. Table 34.8 lists most drug interactions that affect the pharmacokinetics of digoxin. All drugs that affect sinus node or atrioventricular nodal function, alone or in combination with digoxin, may have greater than expected effects in the elderly.

In the past several years, significant developments have occurred in the use of vasodilators for heart failure. These drugs have been shown to improve symptoms, improve exercise capacity, and to prolong survival in elderly patients. Vasodilators can cause venous vasodilation, which increases venous capacitance or arteriolar vasodilation (which causes a decrease in systemic vascular resistance) or both. Vasodilators that affect both the veins and arterioles are called mixed vasodilators. The effects of a vasodilator affecting primarily the venous system are shown in Figure 34.3; the effects are similar to those of a diuretic. The effect of a mixed vasodilator is represented in Figure 34.3.

The most beneficial vasodilators for patients with heart failure are ACE inhibitors. These drugs result in consistent improvement in symptoms, exercise capacity, and mortality for patients with systolic dysfunction and heart failure (54–56). A recent study with enalapril for patients with class IV heart failure and an average age of 70 years demonstrated a substantial benefit in mortality (56). In another trial comparing captopril and lisinopril, the drugs were equally beneficial for older patients and younger patients (57). The most experience in treating heart failure

has been gained with use of captopril and enalapril, although a third ACE inhibitor, lisinopril, is approved by the Food and Drug Administration (FDA) for the treatment of heart failure. There does not appear to be a significant benefit of one ACE inhibitor over another, although only these three have FDA approval for heart failure. Captopril is not metabolized but is excreted by the kidneys. Its peak effect is in 1 to 2 hours and its duration of action is 4 to 6 hours. The average dose for patients with heart failure is 25 to 50 mg three times a day. Enalapril requires conversion to enalaprilat in the liver and enalaprilat is excreted by the kidneys. This prolongs its onset and duration of action. The average dose is 5 to 20 mg twice a day.

All ACE inhibitors may require less frequent dosing and lower doses for elderly patients with abnormalities in hepatic function, renal function, or both ACE inhibitors block the conversion of angiotensin I to angiotensin II and thus relieve vasoconstriction caused by angiotensin II. The decrease in angiotensin II decreases release of aldosterone, and thus decreases salt and water retention. ACE inhibitors also block the breakdown of bradykinin, which may have an additional beneficial effect. As seen with most drugs used for the treatment of heart failure, the benefits of ACE inhibitors gradually increase over a period of several weeks (58).

The major side effect of ACE inhibitors is hypotension. The hypotension is often asymptomatic but can be a serious problem. Patients most likely to develop serious hypotension are those with the most severe heart failure–particularly patients who have hyponatremia. Hypotension can be minimized by avoiding volume depletion. Patients with severe heart failure, systolic blood pressure less than 100 mm Hg, or hyponatremia should be started on a low dose of drug, 6.25 mg of captopril, 2.5 mg of enalapril, or 2.5 mg of lisinopril. Blood pressure should be monitored for 1 to 2 hours after the first dose of captopril and for 4 to 6 hours after the first dose of enalapril or lisinopril. Azotemia may develop in 5 percent to 15 percent of patients, and renal function should be evaluated after therapy is instituted. Neutropenia and proteinuria are rarely problems in patients who do not have collagen vascular disease. Dysgeusia, cough, and skin rash are more common when captopril is used. Cough is a difficult problem with all the ACE inhibitors

Table 34.8 Drug Interactions with Digoxin.

Drug	Effect on Digoxin Pharmacokinetics	Change in Digoxin (%)	Suggested Remedy
Cholestyramine	Absorption	25	Give digoxin 8 hr before cholestyramine or use digoxin capsules
Kaolin pectate; bran	Absorption	20	Separate by 2 hr
Antacids	Unknown	25	Separate by 2 hr
Neomycin; sulfasalazine; PAS	Unknown	18–22	Measure serum digoxin; increased digoxin dose if necessary
Erythromycin; tetracycline (10%)	Decreases intestinal metabolism	43–116	Measure serum digoxin; decrease dose; use digoxin capsules
Quinidine	Renal and nonrenal clearance; volume of distribution and bioavailability	100	Decrease digoxin by 50%; measure serum digoxin at 1 week
Verapamil	Renal and nonrenal clearance	70–100	Same as for quinidine
Amiodarone	Renal and nonrenal clearance	70–100	Same as for quinidine
Diltiazem	Unknown renal clearance	0–22	None
Spironolactone	Renal and nonrenal clearance	30	Measure serum digoxin
Triamterene	Nonrenal clearance	20	Measure serum digoxin

PAS = para-aminosalicylate.
SOURCE: Adapted from Marcus FI. Pharmacokinetic interactions between digoxin and other drugs. J Am Coll Cardiol 1985;5:82A.

and there is no effective treatment except discontinuation of the drug. Tolerance is not a significant problem with ACE inhibitors.

ACE inhibitors improve hypokalemia for many patients with heart failure. Thus, when an ACE inhibitor is instituted, potassium-sparing diuretics may need to be discontinued and potassium supplements may need to be modified. NSAIDs may worsen hyperkalemia and azotemia.

If patients cannot tolerate ACE inhibitors or if significant symptoms of heart failure remain after use of diuretics, digoxin, and ACE inhibitors, the combination of hydralazine and nitrates may offer additional improvement in exercise capacity (54). Nitrates in combination with hydralazine have been shown to improve mortality in patients with heart failure in the absence of ACE inhibitors (59).

Hydralazine is a direct-acting vasodilator that affects arterioles and thus decreases vascular resistance. Hydralazine, when used alone, has not proven to be efficacious in the long-term management of patients with heart failure. However, when combined with nitrates, hydralazine improves exercise capacity and survival. The appropriate dose of hydralazine varies widely among patients with heart failure, but effective doses seem to be 25 to 300 mg four times a day. Side effects of hydralazine at higher doses include hypotension, possible precipitation of ischemic events, and a lupus-like syndrome.

Nitrates have effects on both venous and arteriolar systems but are predominately venous vasodilators. Various forms of nitrates have been shown to be effective in reducing symptoms and prolonging exercise in patients with heart failure. Because oral nitrates undergo a significant first pass effect, large doses may be required. Tolerance develops quickly to the hemodynamic effects of nitrates. Transdermal patches should be used no longer than 12 hours a day and oral nitrates should be given no more frequently than every 8 hours; even this frequency may result in tolerance in some patients (60). Side effects of nitrates are few, primarily hypotension and headache, and these usually improve with subsequent doses.

Prazosin, a peripheral α_1-antagonist, has been widely used in the treatment of heart failure. However, tolerance appears to develop so commonly that long-term benefits in exercise capacity or mortality have not been demonstrated and this class of drug is rarely used for the treatment of heart failure.

Calcium channel blockers have vasodilator properties

and have thus been tried in patients with heart failure. Verapamil has significant negative inotropic potential and should not be used in patients with significant systolic dysfunction. Nifedipine and diltiazem have also not been shown to be beneficial for these patients and may actually worsen symptoms. Newer calcium channel blockers with fewer negative inotropic effects are currently being studied. The dihydropyridine, amlodipine, is apparently safe in patients with heart failure.

A number of drugs with inotropic or vasodilator effects, or both, are being evaluated in patients with heart failure. Amrinone and milrinone are phosphodiesterase inhibitors that have been approved for intravenous use in patients with heart failure. Their hemodynamic effects seem to be similar to dobutamine, but the onset and duration of action are significantly longer. Amrinone and milrinone did not prove to be effective with long-term oral use. Oral sympathomimetic drugs have not proven to be of benefit in chronic long-term use, at least in part because of the tolerance that develops. Bashinergic blocking agents, especially the third generation agents, bucindolol and carveditol, have been quite promising in the treatment of heart failure. Although still experimental, these drugs may soon be available for the treatment of heart failure.

Levodopa is converted to dopamine in the circulation. One study has demonstrated both a short- and long-term benefit. However, the drug is difficult to use, has a high incidence of side effects, and may result in vasoconstriction in some patients. It should probably be used only for patients with heart failure in extreme circumstances. Other dopamine analogues are in various stages of testing.

When heart failure is refractory, several steps should be taken. There should be a reconsideration of precipitating factors such as exacerbation of the underlying disease or drug interactions. Short-term dobutamine infusions may produce symptomatic improvement for several weeks. Heart transplantation may be of benefit in selected patients older than age 60.

References

1. Smith WM. Epidemiology of congestive heart failure. Am J Cardiol 1985;55:3A–8A.

2. McKee PA, Castelli WP, McNamara PM, Kannel WB. The natural history of congestive heart failure. N Engl J Med 1971;285:1441–1446.

3. Massie BM, Conway M. Survival of patients with congestive heart failure: past, present, and future prospects. Circulation 1987;75:11–19.

4. O'Connell JB, Bristow MR. Economic impact of congestive heart failure in the U.S. J Heart Lung Transplant 1994;13:S107–12.

5. Pomerance A. Pathology of the myocardium and valves. In: Caird FL, Dalle JLC, Kennedy RD, eds. Cardiology in old age. New York: Plenum, 1976: 11–53.

6. Olivetti G, Melissari M, Capasso JM, et al. Cardiomyopathy of the aging human heart. Myocyte loss and reactive cellular hypertrophy. Circ Res 1991;68:1560–1568.

7. Gerstenblith G, Frederiksen J, Yin FCP, et al. Echocardiographic assessment of a normal adult aging population. Circulation 1977;56:273–278.

8. Dannenberg AL, Levy D, Garrison RJ. Impact of age on echocardiographic left ventricular mass in a healthy population (The Framingham Study). Am J Cardiol 1989;64:1066–1068.

9. Wei JY. Age and the cardiovascular system. New Engl J Med 1992;327:1735–1739.

10. Kitzman DW, Sheikh KH, Beere PA, et al. Age-related alterations of Doppler left ventricular filling indexes in normal subjects are independent of left ventricular mass, heart rate, contractility, and loading conditions. J Am Coll Cardiol 1991;18:1243–1250.

11. Yin FCP. The aging vasculature and its effects on the heart. In: Weisfeldt ML, ed. The aging heart. New York: Raven, 1980:137–214.

12. Lakatta EG. Catecholamines and cardiovascular function in aging. Endocrinol Metab Clin North Am 1987;16:877–891.

13. Hossack K, Bruce RA. Maximal cardiac function in sedentary normal men and women: comparison of age-related changes. J Appl Physiol 1982;53:799–804.

14. White M, Leenen FH. Aging and cardiovascular responsiveness to beta-agonist in humans: Role of changes in beta-receptor responses versus baroreflex activity. Clin Pharm & Ther 1994;56:543–53.

15. Stratton JR, Cerqueria MD, Schwartz RS, et al. Differences in cardiovascular responses to isoproterenol in relation to age and exercise training in healthy men. Circulation 1992;86:504–512.

16. Poehlman ET, McAuliffe T, Danforth E Jr. Effects of age and level of physical activity on plasma norepinephrine kinetics. Am J Physiol 1990;258:E256–E262.

17. Ng AV, Callister R, Johnson DG, Seals DR. Age and gender influence muscle sympathetic nerve activity at rest in healthy humans. Hypertension 1993;21:498–503.

18. White M, Roden RL, Minski, W, et al. Age-related changes in β-adrenergic neuroeffector systems in the human heart. Circulation 1994;90:1225–38.

19. Lindenfeld J, White M, Roden RA, et al. Gender-related differences in age-associated down regulation of human ven-

tricular myocardial β-adrenergic receptors. Clin Res 1994;42:333A.

20. Rodeheffer RJ, Gerstenblith G, Becker LC, et al. Exercise cardiac output is maintained with advancing age in healthy human subjects: cardiac dilation and increased stroke volume compensate for a diminshed heart rate. Circulation 1984;69:203–213.

21. Ogawa T, Spina RJ, Wade HM, et al. Effects of aging, sex, and physical training on cardiovascular response to exercise. Circulation 1992;86:494–503.

22. Hagberg JM, Allen WK, Seals DR, et al. A hemodynamic comparison of young and older endurance athletes during exercise. J Appl Physiol 1985;58:2041–2046.

23. Levy WC, Cerquerira MD, Abrass IB, et al. Endurance exercise training augments diastolic filling at rest and during exercise in healthy young and older men. Circulation 1993;88:116–126.

24. Lindenfeld J. Syncope. In: Horwitz LD, Groves BM. Signs and symptoms in cardiology. New York: Lippincott 1985:51–96.

25. Shannon RP, Maher KA, Santinga JT, et al. Comparison of differences in the hemodynamic response to passive postural stress in healthy subjects >70 years and <30 years of age. Am J Cardiol 1991;67:1110–1116.

26. Shannon RP, Wei JY, Rosa RM, et al. The effect of age and sodium depletion on cardiovascular response to orthostasis. Hypertension. 1986;8:438–443.

27. Lipsitz LA, Nyquist RP, Wei JY, Rowe JW. Postprandial reduction in blood pressure in the elderly. N Engl J Med 1983;309:81–83.

28. Pomerance A. Pathology of the heart with and without cardiac failure in the aged. Br Heart J 1965;27:697–710.

29. SHEP Cooperative Research Group. Prevention of stroke by antiphypertensive drug treatment in older persons with isolated systolic hypertension. JAMA 1991;265:3255–3264.

30. Topol EJ, Traill TA, Fortuin NJ. Hypertensive hypertrophic cardiomyopathy of the elderly. N Engl J Med 1985;312:277–283.

31. The fifth report of the Joint National Committee on Detection, Evaluation and Treatment of High Blood Pressure (JNCV). Arch Intern Med 1993;153:154–183.

32. Umachandran V, Ranjadayalan K, Ambepityia G, et al. Aging, autonomic function and the perception of angina. Br Heart J 1991;66:15–18.

33. Fleg JL, Gerstenblith G, Zonderman AB, et al. Prevalence and prognostic significance of exercise-induced silent myocardial ischemia detected by thallium scintigraphy and electrocardiography in asymptomatic volunteers. Circulation 1990;81:428–436.

34. Shah PM, Abelmann WH, Gersh BJ. Cardiomyopathies in the elderly. J Am Coll Cardiol 1987;10:77A–79A.

35. Cornwell GG III, Kyoe RA, Westermark P, Pitkanen P. Frequency and distribution of senile cardiovascular amyloid: A clinicopathologic correlation. Am J Med 1983;75:618–623.

36. Olson LJ, Gertz MA, Edwards WD, et al. Senile cardiac amyloidosis with myocardial dysfunction: diagnosis by endomyocardial biopsy and immunohistochemistry. N Engl J Med 1987;317:738–742.

37. Braunwald E, Sonnenblick EH, Ross J Jr. Mechanisms of cardiac contraction and relaxation. In: Braunwald E, ed. Heart disease: a textbook of cardiovascular medicine. Philadelphia: Saunders, 1992:370–381.

38. Packer M. Pathophysiology of chronic heart failure. Lancet 1992;340:88–92.

39. Francis G. Neurohormones in congestive heart failure. Cardiol Rev 1993;1:278–289.

40. Bristow MR. Changes in myocardial and vascular receptors in heart failure. J Am Coll Cardiol 1993;22(suppl A):61–71.

41. Dzau VJ, Re RN. Evidence for the existence of renin in the heart. Circulation 1987;75(suppl):134–136.

42. The SOLVD Investigators. Effect of enalapril on the development of heart failure in asymptomatic patients with reduced left ventricular ejection fraction. N Engl J Med 1992;327:685–691.

43. Lindenfeld J, Hammermeister K. Cardiovascular disease. In: Schrier R, ed., Medicine: diagnosis and treatment. Boston: Little, Brown, 1988:55–56.

44. Howell TH. Causation of diagnostic errors in octogenarians: a clinico-pathological study. J Am Geriatr Soc 1966;14:41–47.

45. Wenger NK. Cardiovascular disease in the elderly. Curr Probl Cardiol 1992;17:611–690.

46. Soufer R, Wohlegelernter D, Vita Na, et al. Intact systolic left ventricular function in clinical congestive heart failure. Am J Cardiol 1985;55:1032–1036.

47. Bonow RO, Udelson JE. Left ventricular diastolic dysfunction as a cause of congestive heart failure. Mechanisms and management. Ann Intern Med 1992;117:502–510.

48. Sodeman WA, Burch GE. The precipitating causes of congestive heart failure. Am Heart J 1938;15:22–27.

49. Flamenbaum W. Diuretic use in the elderly: potential for diuretic-induced hypokalemia. Am J Cardiol 1986;57:38A–43A.

50. Wilson JR, Reichek N, Dunkman WB, Goldberg S. Effect of diuresis on the performance of the failing left ventricular in man. Am J Med 1981;80:234–239.

51. Smith TW. Digitalis glycosides. Orlando: Grune and Stratton, 1986:5–27.

52. Ferguson DW, Berg WJ, Sanders JS, et al. Sympathoinhibitory responses to digitalis glycosides in heart failure patients. Circulation 1989;80:65–77.

53. Packer M, Gheorghiade M, Young JB, et al. Withdrawal of digoxin from patients with chronic heart failure treated with angiotensin-converting enzyme inhibitors. N Engl J Med 1993;329:1–7.

54. Cohn JN, Johnson G, Ziesche S, et al. A comparison of enalapril with hydralazine-isosorbide dinitrate in the treatment of chronic congestive heart failure. N Engl J Med 1991;325:303–310.

55. The SOLVD Investigators. Effect of enalapril on survival in patients with reduced left ventricular ejection fraction and congestive heart failure. N Engl J Med 1991;325:292–302.

56. Consensus Trial Study Group. Effects of enalapril on mortality in severe congestive heart failure. Results of the Cooperative North Scandinavian Enalapril Survival Study (CONSENSUS). N Engl J Med 1987;316:1429–1435.

57. Giles TD, Fisher B, Rush JE. Lismopril and captopril in the treatment of heart failure in older patients. Comparison of a long and short acting angiotensin converting enzyme inhibitor. Am J Med 1988;85(suppl 3B):44–47.

58. Captopril Multicentre Research Group. A placebo controlled trial of captopril in refractory heart failure. J Am Coll Cardiol 1983;2:755–763.

59. Cohn JN, Archibald DG, Ziesche S, et al. Effect of vasodilator therapy on mortality in chronic congestive heart failure: results of a Veterans Administration Cooperative Study. N Engl J Med 1986;314:1547–1552.

60. Elkayam U. Tolerance to organic nitrates: evidence, mechanisms, clinical relevance, and strategies for prevention. Ann Intern Med 1991;114:667–677.

Chapter 35
Arrhythmias

David E. Mann

To keep the heart unwrinkled, to be hopeful, kindly, cheerful, reverent—that is to triumph over old age.

Thomas Bailey Aldrich

Aging affects the prevalence, severity, diagnosis, and treatment of cardiac arrhythmias. The prevalence of arrhythmias is increased in the elderly, not only because the incidence of heart disease increases with age (1), but also because aging has direct effects on the conduction system (2–4). Arrhythmias in the elderly often result in more severe symptoms than are present in the young. Older people tend to tolerate extremes of heart rate poorly, thus they are likely to experience myocardial ischemia, congestive heart failure, syncope, or death as the result of arrhythmias that might be better tolerated in the young. Diagnosis of suspected arrhythmias may be more difficult in the elderly because they have more trouble filling out Holter monitor diaries or operating transtelephonic event recorders than their younger counterparts (5). Treatment of arrhythmias in the aged can also be complicated because there is an increased incidence of antiarrhythmic drug side effects and drug interactions in these patients since they are often taking multiple medications (6).

Despite the challenges involved, caring for the elderly patient with arrhythmias can be a gratifying experience, thanks to recent, remarkable advances in the management of arrhythmias. Nearly all forms of supraventricular tachycardia can now be cured by catheter ablation. Permanent pacemakers have become much smaller and more "physiologic." Implantable cardioverter defibrillators are evolving to an eventual ease of implantation similar to that for pacemakers and hold promise to reduce sudden arrhythmic death—a common cause of death in adults (1,7,8). The geriatrician needs to keep abreast of this rapidly developing field so that he or she can choose the best therapy for each patient.

Certain principles should be followed in treating all arrhythmia patients—principles that ultimately derive from the maxim "primum non nocere." These principles are outlined in Table 35.1. Electrocardiographic documentation of an abnormal rhythm is important for diagnosis of arrhythmia, but correlation of the abnormal rhythm with the patient's symptoms is also usually necessary to determine whether treatment is justified. As an example, in a patient with syncope, a Holter monitor recording that shows asymptomatic episodes of sinus bradycardia does not establish that a similar episode of bradycardia resulted in syncope, and such a finding does not justify implantation of a permanent pacemaker. Even when symptoms do correlate with an arrhythmia, it does not always follow that treatment is mandatory. The need for treatment must be based on the severity of the patient's symptoms, the risk of the patient's arrhythmia, and the risk of treatment.

The goals of treatment should be defined. These may include prevention of symptoms directly related to the arrhythmia (such as palpitations or syncope), prevention of the sequelae of certain arrhythmias (in particular, treatment of atrial fibrillation to reduce the risk of systemic embolism), improvement in hemodynamic status (such as cardioversion of atrial fibrillation to restore the atrial kick in a patient with hypertrophic cardiomyopathy), or prevention of sudden death. In the case of acute or emergency management of arrhythmias, reasonably safe, effective, and well-established measures, such as electrical cardioversion, are available. Unfortunately the risk-benefit ratio of therapy for chronic or recurrent arrhythmias is mostly unknown, and is probably widely underestimated.

It is well known that the presence of premature ventricular contractions (PVCs) after myocardial infarction is associated with an increased risk of sudden cardiac death (9). It was commonly assumed 10 years ago that suppres-

Table 35.1. Principles of Arrhythmia Management.

1. Document arrhythmia electrocardiographically.
2. Correlate arrhythmia with symptoms, if any.
3. Determine goals of therapy.
4. Determine risk of arrhythmia.
5. Determine risk of therapy.
6. Decide if therapy is warranted on the basis of principles 3, 4, 5.

sion of PVCs was likely to result in a reduction in this risk. There was frequent use of antiarrhythmic drugs for this indication at the time, despite any scientific data supporting this use (10). The "PVC-suppression" hypothesis was soundly disproved by the Cardiac Arrhythmic Suppression Trials (CAST-I and CAST-II) (11,12) that showed increased mortality for patients in whom PVCs were suppressed by Class I antiarrhythmic drugs after myocardial infarction. As important as the CAST studies were in defining the risks of antiarrhythmic drug therapy, perhaps an even more important result was realization of the need for well-designed clinical trials to validate the use of antiarrhythmic drugs or nonpharmacologic therapy such as implantable cardioverter defibrillators in the treatment of arrhythmias. Fortunately, many such clinical trials are in progress.

Diagnostic Techniques

For patients with suspected symptomatic arrhythmias it is important to correlate symptoms with arrhythmias. Because the prevalence of arrhythmias is high in the elderly, one cannot assume that a documented asymptomatic arrhythmia is the true cause of a patient's symptoms. On the other hand, correlation of symptoms with arrhythmias can be frustrating and difficult in the elderly, and there may be some risk involved waiting for recurrence of symptoms while the patient carries an event recorder, especially when the symptom is recurrent syncope. In some cases, electrophysiologic testing, which can more directly document arrhythmias and conduction system disease, may be a quicker means to an answer; however, the physician must realize that nonspecific arrhythmias can be induced in the electrophysiology laboratory, possibly steering therapy in the wrong direction. Because electrophysiologic testing is an invasive

technique and thus carries some risk, some have used signal-averaged electrocardiography (SAECG) to select patients who are candidates for this test. SAECG can detect the substrate for re-entrant ventricular arrhythmias with high sensitivity and moderate specificity, and thus can predict which patients are likely to have inducible ventricular arrhythmias by electrophysiologic testing (13,14). As with any screening test, it is important to understand the strengths and limitations of SAECG before applying it in this fashion.

Electrocardiographic correlation of symptoms with arrhythmias still represents the gold standard in diagnosis of symptomatic arrhythmias. A variety of transtelephonic event recorders are available for long-term electrocardiographic monitoring. These can be used for months at a time, if needed, to document infrequent symptoms. Event recorders should be considered instead of Holter monitoring unless events occur daily or absolute quantification of arrhythmia frequency is required. In addition, event recorders require patient cooperation to activate; they may not be practical in patients unable or unwilling to use them. Besides documentation and diagnosis of specific arrhythmias, other testing to evaluate left ventricular function, to determine the presence of ischemia, and to detect the presence or absence of underlying structural heart disease is often needed for patients with arrhythmias, particularly those who present with ventricular arrhythmias or cardiac arrest.

Changes in the Conduction System with Aging

Although the prevalence of heart disease increases with age, the aging process itself affects the conduction system. Thus the "normal" heart rhythm of an octogenarian is not the same as that for a teenager.

With aging, there is loss of pacemaker cells in the sinus node, and loss of conduction fibers in the bundle branches, with replacement by fat and fibrous tissue (2–4). Sinus node dysfunction and atrioventricular block may merely represent extremes of this natural degenerative process. The conduction system may also be affected by amyloid deposition, which becomes increasingly common with age ("senile amyloidosis"), appearing in 10 percent of autopsies of patients over age 80 and in 50 percent of patients over age 90 (15). Studies have shown that with age there are also changes in the autonomic nervous system that may indirectly affect the heart rhythm. Although circulating catecholamines increase with age, there is decreased heart rate responsiveness to sympathetic stimulation, possibly because of decreased or altered beta receptors (16). Baroreceptor responsiveness and parasympathetic regulation also appear to be altered and result in a predictable decrease in respiratory sinus arrhythmia with age (17).

These natural processes cause several effects. Resting sinus rate slows with age, and there is a blunting of the heart rate increase that occurs with exercise (18). The incidence of first degree atrioventricular block, bundle branch block, and fascicular block increases with age (19–22). Other electrocardiographic abnormalities are more common with aging. ST-segment and T-wave abnormalities are common, although whether these represent primary changes in cellular repolarization with aging or the concomitant effect of frequently used drugs, such as digoxin and diuretics in older patients is not clear (23).

Ambulatory monitoring in the elderly reveals that premature atrial and ventricular complexes and short runs of atrial and ventricular tachycardia are very common, but sinus pauses exceeding 2 to 3 seconds are unusual (24–28). In Holter monitor recordings performed on 26 asymptomatic men older than age 70 without known heart disease, 77 percent had premature atrial and ventricular complexes, 12 percent had nonsustained ventricular tachycardia, and the longest sinus pause was 2.5 seconds during sleep (28). In contrast, in a similar study of young medical students, rare premature ventricular complexes were present in 50 percent (29).

To what degree the increased incidence of premature beats represents an increased prevalence of occult organic heart disease is unknown, but during follow-up in one study, there were no adverse effects in elderly patients with asymptomatic premature ventricular complexes (28). This suggests that in elderly subjects, just as in younger ones, the mere presence of premature ventricular complexes has no adverse effect on prognosis if normal left ventricular function exists (30). Incidental findings of premature ventricular complexes on Holter monitor recordings or electrocardiograms are likely to be frequent in the elderly and do not warrant treatment.

The incidence of atrial fibrillation increases with age,

probably because of an increased frequency of associated diseases such as hypertension and coronary artery disease (31,32). A few arrhythmias appear to decrease in incidence with age. The incidence of Wolff-Parkinson-White syndrome and supraventricular tachycardias caused by accessory atrioventricular pathways decreases with age, most likely because of degeneration of accessory pathways over time (33,34).

Bradyarrhythmias

Sinus Node Dysfunction

Sinus node dysfunction ("sick sinus syndrome") can occur in all age groups, but is most closely associated with old age. The causes of sinus node dysfunction are listed in Table 35.2. Most cases are associated with degenerative disease of the sinus node, and may arise from atherosclerosis involving the sinus node artery (35–37). Some commonly prescribed drugs may cause or worsen sinus node dysfunction. Avoidance of these drugs or correction of metabolic abnormalities may obviate the need for permanent pacing in some patients.

Changes in sinus node function occur with aging for

Table 35.2. Causes of Sinus Node Dysfunction.

Idiopathic/degenerative
Coronary artery disease
Cardiomyopathy (primary and secondary)
Inflammatory (pericarditis/myocarditis)
Surgical trauma
Metabolic
   Hypothyroidism
   Hypothermia
   Hyperkalemia
Autonomic Nervous System
   Neurocardiogenic syncope
   Hypersensitive carotid and related reflexes
   Dysautonomia
   Hypervagatonia
Drugs
   Beta-adrenergic blockers
   Calcium channel blockers
   Digitalis
   Other antiarrhythmic drugs
   Lithium
   Cimetidine
   Tricyclic antidepressants
   Phenothiazines

various reasons. Asymptomatic sinus bradycardia is thus a common finding in the elderly and is usually of little hemodynamic consequence (38). Sinus pauses in the *asymptomatic* patient are not an indication for pacing regardless of the length of the pauses (39). Sinus pauses during sleep are often physiologic and caused by enhanced vagal tone, but may also be a manifestation of a sleep disorder such as sleep apnea (40,41).

Abnormal sinus node function may result from loss of automaticity, when the sinus node fails to depolarize at an adequate rate (sinus bradycardia or sinus arrest), or sinoatrial exit block, when impulses from the sinus node fail to conduct out of the node into the atrium. Clinically, the distinction is often impossible to make; the end result of both problems is sinus pauses. Pauses longer than 3 seconds in duration may cause dizziness or syncope. These pauses may occur spontaneously or may follow the abrupt termination of tachycardia, usually atrial fibrillation or flutter. During tachycardia, the sinus node is suppressed. When tachycardia terminates, the sinus node must recover and begin depolarizing again. When the recovery time is prolonged, symptomatic pauses may result. This clinical picture has been termed the *brady-tachy syndrome* (35,42).

In the electrophysiology laboratory, mimicking this syndrome to test sinus node function is possible by rapidly pacing the right atrium with a catheter. At cessation of pacing, the recovery time of the sinus node can be measured. An abnormal sinus node recovery time is fairly specific for sinus node dysfunction, but a normal recovery time does not exclude sinus node problems (43,44). Thus, this test and other tests of sinus node function in the electrophysiology laboratory are rarely useful in evaluating patients with suspected sinus node dysfunction. Holter monitoring for 24 to 48 hours may detect abnormalities of sinus node function in patients with frequently occurring symptoms and can help correlate symptoms with the arrhythmia. Patient-activated transtelephonic event recorders with memory can be useful to document the cause of infrequently recurring symptoms.

Sinus node dysfunction is frequently associated with other abnormalities of cardiac conduction (45). Subsidiary cardiac pacemakers in the atrioventricular (AV) junction or ventricle may also be abnormal so that sinus pauses result in asystole. Atrial tachyarrhythmias, such as atrial fibrillation or flutter, may be present, sometimes with an abnormally slow ventricular response, which suggests associated abnormal AV node function. Such disease of the AV junction may not be manifested during electrocardiographic monitoring. Fear of this type of "occult" atrioventricular block has resulted in the rare use of atrial pacing alone to treat patients with sinus node dysfunction; instead, less physiologic ventricular pacing or more expensive dual chamber pacing is used. Nevertheless, in selected patients, single-chamber atrial pacing can be used successfully (46). Of relevance to patients with brady-tachy syndrome, it appears that the incidence of atrial fibrillation is reduced in patients who receive pacemakers that maintain A-V synchrony as opposed to single-chamber ventricular pacemakers (47).

Intrinsic sinus node dysfunction may be difficult to distinguish from abnormalities of the autonomic nervous system. In particular, it has recently been recognized that a large proportion of patients with syncope have the syndrome of neurocardiogenic syncope (48). This syndrome involves an abnormal response to upright posture, during which stretch receptors in the ventricle are inappropriately stimulated, possibly because of an increased inotropic state associated with increased circulating catecholamines. Normally, the stretch receptors are inhibited during upright posture, when the ventricle is relatively underfilled as a result of redistribution of blood volume to the lower extremities from the effects of gravity. The paradoxical stimulation of these receptors while the person is upright results in increased vagal tone and decreased sympathetic stimulation and causes bradycardia, vasodilatation, hypotension, and syncope or presyncope. Testing using a tilt table may elicit this response in susceptible patients (49). Of importance, despite marked sinus bradycardia or sinus arrest, permanent pacing is usually *not* helpful for this condition, probably because pacing does not affect the vasodilation that is a prominent feature of this syndrome (50).

Neurocardiogenic syncope is probably related to other forms of vasovagal syncope, such as the common faint, hypersensitive carotid sinus, micturition syncope, cough syncope, and deglutition syncope. Although more common in young persons, such forms of syncope can occur in the elderly and can be difficult to distinguish from intrinsic sinus node dysfunction. A history of symptoms that are posturally or situationally related and lack of evidence of sinus node dysfunction while the person is supine may be helpful in diagnosing neurocardiogenic syncope. Tilt testing may be necessary in some cases to make the diagnosis. It is probable that in the past, some permanent pacemakers were inserted inappropriately in patients with syncope and sinus pauses who were actually suffering from neurocardiogenic syncope. (For a more complete discussion of this syndrome and its treatment, see Chapter 24.)

Sinus node dysfunction, although a cause of morbidity, infrequently causes mortality. Deaths are caused by underlying heart disease, not bradyarrhythmias; in addition, the incidence of stroke is also quite high (51). Intervention with permanent pacing does not appear to lower mortality; it does, however, ameliorate symptoms (39,51–56). For this reason, permanent pacemakers are not recommended for asymptomatic patients with sinus node dysfunction. Their use should be reserved for patients in whom a definite connection between symptoms and sinus pauses can be established (57,58). In patients with the brady-tachy syndrome, drug therapy to suppress atrial fibrillation or flutter may prolong sinus pauses and make symptoms worse (42). In such a situation, permanent pacing may be necessary to give these drugs safely. Indications for permanent pacing are summarized in Table 35.3. In patients who have sustained tachyarrhythmias that require elective cardioversion and who have present or suspected sinus node dysfunction, temporary pacing (either transvenous or transcutaneous) should be used prophylactically to prevent postcardioversion asystole (59).

Atrioventricular Block

AV block is another common cause of symptomatic bradycardia in the elderly. AV block is frequently the result of degenerative fibrosis of the conduction system (4). Whether this is diffuse throughout the bundle branches (Lenegre's disease) or involves only the proximal bundle branches (Lev's disease) is a pathologic distinction of little clinical importance (60,61). Other causes of AV block include coronary artery disease, cardiomyopathy, valvular disease, bacterial endocarditis, and calcification of the AV groove (mitral annular calcification). Most drugs listed in Table 35.2 as causes of sinus node dysfunction can also cause or worsen AV block.

Indications for permanent pacing in patients with AV block are summarized in Table 35.3. Reversible causes of AV block (e.g., drugs, acute myocardial infarction) must first be excluded or corrected before permanent pacing is considered. First-degree AV block (PR interval > 0.2 sec) is a benign electrocardiographic finding and needs no intervention (21). Bundle branch block, including bifascicular block (right bundle branch block with either left anterior or left posterior fascicular block), has a low risk (1% to 2% per year) of progressing to complete heart block, even in an elderly subset of patients (19–22). Thus, permanent pacemakers are not indicated for asymptomatic patients with bifascicular block. For symptomatic patients with bundle branch block, further studies to establish a link between symptoms and intermittent heart block should be performed before permanent pacemaker implantation is considered.

Patients with second-degree AV block associated with symptoms should receive pacemakers. Pacing in asymptomatic patients with second-degree AV block is controversial. An attempt to localize the level of block in the conduction system should be made. Progressive prolongation of the PR interval before a blocked beat and shortening of the PR interval in the next conducted beat after the blocked beat is termed Mobitz I second-degree AV block (Wenckebach block) and is usually associated with block in the AV node.

Table 35.3. Indications for Permanent Pacing.

I. Sinus node dysfunction
  1. Documented symptomatic sinus bradycardia or pauses without reversible cause (e.g., drugs, metabolic abnormalities)
  2. Symptomatic sinus pauses in patients who require antiarrhythmic drug therapy (e.g., brady-tachy syndrome)
II. Atrioventricular block
  1. Complete AV block with one or more factors
      Heart rate <40 or pauses >3 sec
      Symptoms
      Congestive heart failure
      Requirement for antiarrhythmic drug therapy
  2. Symptomatic 2nd-degree AV block
  3. Asymptomatic infranodal 2nd-degree AV block (pacing probably indicated)

A pattern of isolated nonconducted beats without changes in the PR interval before or after each blocked beat is termed Mobitz II second-degree AV block, and is usually due to block distal to the AV node–that is, in the bundle of His or the bundle branches. Ratios of 2:1 or higher second-degree AV block may result from block in the AV node or distal to the AV node.

Another clue to the anatomic site of block is the QRS pattern of the conducted beats; a narrow QRS implies that block is probably in the AV node; a wide QRS (bundle branch block) implies that block is distal to the AV node. The distinction between AV nodal and infranodal second-degree AV block may be important clinically because the latter site of block is associated with a high rate of progression to complete heart block and a poor prognosis (62). Thus, pacing is usually not indicated for asymptomatic patients with second-degree AV block localized to the AV node, but pacing may be indicated for asymptomatic patients with infranodal second-degree AV block (57,58). Occasionally, electrophysiologic testing may be useful to establish unequivocally the site of block.

Complete (third-degree) AV block may be caused by disease in the AV node, the bundle of His, or both bundle branches. Atrioventricular nodal block is usually associated with a narrow QRS complex escape rhythm, which arises in the AV junction and is often well tolerated. Infranodal complete AV block is associated with a slower and less reliable ventricular escape rhythm (with a wide QRS complex) and is frequently poorly tolerated. The survival rate for patients with complete heart block before the use of pacemakers was poor (63,64). Implantation of permanent pacemakers allows a survival rate comparable with that of the population with normal heart beat, prevents recurrent syncope (Stokes-Adams attacks), and, in some cases, can improve congestive heart failure caused by or exacerbated by bradycardia or loss of AV synchrony (65).

In the elderly, permanent pacemakers are indicated in nearly all patients who present with complete AV block, with or without symptoms (57). Patients with the acute onset of third-degree AV block who are hemodynamically compromised need emergency temporary pacing. Atropine or isoproterenol can be administered until pacing can be instituted. In addition to the standard transvenous route for temporary pacing, transcutaneous pacing holds particular promise for the elderly because it can be instituted more quickly and is safer than transvenous pacing (66).

Tachyarrhythmias

Atrial Tachyarrhythmias

Premature atrial complexes are found in most elderly subjects undergoing Holter monitoring and are usually of no significance (24–28). Atrial fibrillation, atrial flutter, and atrial tachycardia are related arrhythmias, occurring most commonly in patients with atrial disease of any sort. Atrial fibrillation is the most common sustained tachyarrhythmia in older people, with a prevalence of 4 percent in patients over 55 years old (31,32). The most frequent underlying cardiovascular causes of atrial fibrillation are hypertension, valvular heart disease, and coronary artery disease (31). Atrial fibrillation may also be a presentation of acute pulmonary embolus, myocardial infarction, pericarditis, and occult hyperthyroidism (67). Atrial fibrillation is associated with twice the mortality of age-matched controls, and six times the risk of stroke (31,68,69). Although atrial fibrillation itself is not a lethal arrhythmia, the thromboembolic and hemodynamic sequelae of this arrhythmia can be quite devastating.

If atrial fibrillation cannot be prevented by pharmacologic means, then the question of chronic anticoagulation must be addressed. Although the risk of thromboembolism is greatest for patients with atrial fibrillation and rheumatic valvular disease, nearly all patients with atrial fibrillation are at increased risk for thromboembolic events (69). One exception may be patients younger than 60 years of age who have "lone" (i.e., without associated heart disease or hypertension) atrial fibrillation–a group not included in the scope of this book (70). Several studies support the routine use anticoagulation with warfarin (Coumadin) for all patients with atrial fibrillation (71–74). In patients with contraindications to warfarin, the use of low-dose aspirin is justified (73).

The goal of treatment of atrial fibrillation should be resumption and maintenance of sinus rhythm; or, if this is not feasible, control of the ventricular rate. Conversion to sinus rhythm may be accomplished with antiarrhythmic drugs or with electrical cardioversion–the latter with a higher success rate. There is a 1 percent to 2 percent risk of embolization associated with cardioversion, whether accomplished with drugs or electricity (75–77). Patients taking anticoagulants at the time of cardioversion have a lower risk of embolization (76,77). For atrial fibrillation of unknown duration or duration longer than 2 days, full anticoagulation with warfarin for at least 3 weeks should be instituted before cardioversion. Anticoagulation should then be continued for at least another 4 weeks because there may be a delay before mechanical atrial systole returns (78), which accounts for a small but definite occurrence of late embolization after cardioversion (77).

The decision to attempt cardioversion should be made on the basis of the duration of fibrillation, left atrial size, presence of mitral valve disease, patient age, results of previous attempts at cardioversion, and importance of restoring sinus rhythm in each patient (75). Generally, fibrillation lasting longer than 1 year, left atrial size larger than 4.5 cm (measured by echocardiogram), and mitral stenosis make maintenance of sinus rhythm for longer than 6 months unlikely (79). Older patients generally have more atrial disease, and thus the chance of successfully maintaining sinus rhythm decreases with age. Cardioversion generally should not be repeated for an elderly patient in whom previous cardioversion did not result in sinus rhythm lasting longer than 6 months. Clearly, more aggressive and repeated attempts may be made, despite these factors, when the ventricular response is difficult to control with drugs or when atrial fibrillation is associated with congestive heart failure or recurrent emboli.

Elective cardioversion of atrial fibrillation should be performed in the sedated or anesthetized patient, with initial energy levels of at least 100 J. Higher energies should be used if lower ones fail. Generally, if atrial fibrillation is caused by an acute process, such as pulmonary embolus, decompensated heart failure, or hyperthyroidism, treatment of the underlying disease should be performed first. The patient may be maintained in the hospital on heparin during this time, and spontaneous conversion to sinus rhythm may occur with improvement in the underlying cause of the arrhythmia.

Pharmacologic cardioversion can be achieved with various antiarrhythmic drugs, including class Ia (qui-

nidine, procainamide, disopyramide), class Ic (flecainide, propafenone), and class III (amiodarone, sotalol) agents. In general, rate control should be achieved first with digoxin or other AV nodal blocking drugs to avoid acceleration of the ventricular response caused by the anticholinergic effects of some of these drugs, particularly quinidine. Initiation of any of these drugs should occur in the hospital, with telemetry monitoring, because of the potential for proarrhythmia inherent in most, if not all, antiarrhythmic drugs. The same drugs can be used to maintain sinus rhythm following cardioversion.

Digoxin alone is not effective in conversion or maintenance of sinus rhythm (80). Quinidine has been considered standard therapy for conversion of atrial fibrillation and maintenance of sinus rhythm; however, a meta-analysis of studies of quinidine in atrial fibrillation revealed an excess mortality for patients on this drug compared with that for patients who had no therapy (81). We have found sotalol (80 to 160 mg every 12 hr) to be a well-tolerated drug for this purpose, with efficacy comparable with that of quinidine but with fewer side effects (82). Low-dose amiodarone (100 to 200 mg/day) is also useful for maintenance of sinus rhythm for patients who do not respond to other antiarrhythmic therapy (83).

To achieve rate control, AV nodal blocking drugs are used. These drugs include digoxin, verapamil, diltiazem, propranolol, and other beta blockers. The goal of treatment should be to achieve a heart rate less than 100 beats per minute (bpm) at rest and a rate with exercise that is commensurate with an expected exercise rate if the patient were in sinus rhythm. Rarely, catheter ablation of the AV node with permanent pacemaker implantation is required to achieve rate control in problematic cases (84).

Atrial flutter is usually associated with structural heart disease. Generally, rate control is more difficult to achieve with atrial flutter than it is with fibrillation. Patients usually present with 2:1 AV conduction and a resultant ventricular rate of 150 bpm. In most cases, a form of cardioversion should be attempted. Drugs used for conversion of atrial fibrillation can also be used for atrial flutter. Electrical cardioversion, with lower energy shocks than those used for atrial fibrillation, may be successful, with energy delivery starting at 25 J. Atrial flutter can also be converted in most cases with a pacing catheter in the right atrium, with pacing faster than the flutter rate (usually >300), which interrupts the re-entry circuit (85).

Recently, cure of atrial flutter using radiofrequency catheter ablation has been described (86). The technique involves destruction of a critical part of the flutter reentry circuit in the right atrium. Although preliminary data indicate a relatively high recurrence rate, it is likely this technique will be very useful for patients who have recurrent atrial flutter and who do not tolerate or fail antiarrhythmic drug therapy.

Atrial tachycardias may be caused by multiple mechanisms, including reentry, abnormal automaticity, and triggered activity (87,88). On electrocardiogram, there is usually a narrow QRS complex, regular rhythm, with evident P waves and PR interval shorter than the RP interval. The P wave morphology is not similar to sinus. These rhythms may be paroxysmal or incessant, the latter probably caused by abnormal automaticity. Incessant tachycardia may lead to cardiomyopathy and, thus, should be treated (89).

Use of intravenous adenosine usually results in transient AV block without termination of tachycardia. Rate control with AV nodal blocking drugs is difficult, as with atrial flutter. Antiarrhythmic drugs used to prevent atrial fibrillation can also be used in atrial tachycardia, but success may be poor. Radiofrequency catheter ablation has been used successfully to cure atrial tachycardia (90), and should be considered in drug refractory cases, particularly if tachycardia is incessant and tachycardia-induced cardiomyopathy is suspected because the latter may reverse with treatment of the tachycardia (89).

Multifocal atrial tachycardia (MAT) is an irregular atrial tachycardia characterized by multiple (≥3) P wave morphologies. MAT usually occurs in the setting of chronic lung disease and is related to right atrial distension and fibrosis. MAT must be distinguished from atrial fibrillation, which it resembles electrocardiographically. Treatment includes management of the underlying lung disease and calcium channel blockers such as verapamil (91,92). Digoxin is not useful for this arrhythmia (92).

Paroxysmal Supraventricular Tachycardia

Although the arrhythmias discussed in the preceding section are all supraventricular in origin, the designation *paroxysmal supraventricular tachycardia* (PSVT) is usually reserved for a distinct set of arrhythmias. PSVT is a regular, usually narrow, QRS complex (unless there is incidental bundle branch block) tachycardia during which there is a 1:1 atrial to ventricular relationship. The older term *paroxysmal atrial tachycardia* should be used only for arrhythmias arising in the atrium, i.e., true atrial tachycardia, if it is used at all. In most cases of PSVT, the mechanism is reentry involving the AV node as part of the circuit. Thus adenosine, which causes transient AV nodal block, is highly successful in interrupting reentry and terminating PSVT episodes acutely.

Most cases of PSVT are caused by abnormalities in the heart's conduction system and are probably congenital in origin. Elderly patients with PSVT commonly admit to a lifelong history of episodic palpitations. Occasionally, and somewhat inexplicably, PSVT presents late in life. Symptoms range from infrequent, brief episodes of palpitations to frequent, severely symptomatic, prolonged tachycardias that require emergency room treatment.

About 60 percent of PSVT is caused by AV nodal reentry (93). Current data suggest that the reentrant circuit involves the AV node itself (fast pathway) and another slowly conducting pathway that lies posterior to the AV node (slow pathway). During tachycardia, P waves are usually simultaneous with each QRS complex on electrocardiogram. For acute episodes, intravenous adenosine is very effective in terminating tachycardia, but other AV nodal blocking drugs can also be used. For chronic therapy nearly all antiarrhythmic drugs (except lidocainelike drugs) have been used to prevent AV nodal reentry tachycardia, although AV nodal blocking drugs such as digoxin, verapamil, and beta blockers are probably best tolerated long-term. It is now possible with radiofrequency catheter ablation to ablate the slow pathway with a success rate of more than 95 percent, and a low risk of complications. Catheter ablation is becoming the procedure of choice for this condition (94).

Overall, about 30 percent of cases of PSVT are caused by an accessory AV pathway (usually concealed, i.e., only able to conduct retrogradely from the ventricle to the atrium and thus not manifesting ECG signs of Wolff-Parkinson-White syndrome), but the incidence of this mechanism in the elderly is probably lower (33,93). The reentry circuit involves the atrium, AV node, ventricle, and accessory pathway retrogradely. During tachycardia, retrograde P waves are usually seen superimposed on the ST segment or T wave, with an RP interval shorter than the PR interval. Acute therapy is the same as for patients with AV nodal reentry–thus, there is no pressing need to identify the exact electrophysiologic mechanism of a narrow-complex tachycardia before treating it acutely. These patients and those with overt Wolff-Parkinson-White syndrome are all highly amenable to cure with catheter ablation (95). Atrial tachycardia makes up about 10 percent of cases of PSVT (93).

Ventricular Arrhythmias

The incidence of premature ventricular complexes (PVCs) increases with age (25,26). When they occur in patients with otherwise normal hearts, there is no prognostic significance (30). Although PVCs are associated with an increased risk of sudden death if underlying heart disease (particularly left ventricular dysfunction and congestive heart failure) is present (9), there is no evidence that suppression of PVCs improves survival–in fact, studies suggest the opposite (11,12). For patients after myocardial infarction, beta blockers have been shown to improve survival; however, it is not clear whether the survival rate relates to suppression of PVCs or to other actions of beta blockers (96,97). Preliminary data from trials of amiodarone (which has beta-blocking and numerous other effects) indicate a possible beneficial effect on survival after myocardial infarction, but more studies need to be done before routine recommendation of this potentially toxic drug can be made (98).

It is difficult to make recommendations on the treatment of nonsustained ventricular tachycardia. About 40 percent of patients with nonsustained ventricular tachycardia have inducible, sustained ventricular arrhythmias during electrophysiologic testing, and these patients have a poor prognosis (99). Nevertheless, because nonsustained ventricular tachycardia is prevalent, particularly in the elderly, it is difficult to recommend a very aggressive and expensive approach that uses electrophysiologic testing, especially because suppression of inducible arrhythmias in this patient group has not been shown to improve survival. Clinical studies examining this group are currently in progress. Our policy is not to treat these patients if they are asymptomatic. If symptoms are present, particularly syncope, we perform electrophysiologic testing. Patients with inducible, sustained arrhythmias are treated with drug therapy guided by electrophysiologic testing or an intracardiac defibrillator (ICD). Patients without inducible arrhythmias are treated with Holter monitor-guided, antiarrhythmic drug therapy, or are treated empirically with amiodarone.

Sustained ventricular tachycardia and ventricular fibrillation are both emergency situations and causes of sudden cardiac death. For acute episodes, such arrhythmias require immediate treatment. If a patient presents in sustained ventricular tachycardia that is well-tolerated hemodynamically, frequently such a rhythm is misdiagnosed as supraventricular tachycardia with aberrant conduction, and is inappropriately treated (100). Intravenous verapamil given in this situation is dangerous, often leading to hemodynamic collapse, ventricular fibrillation, or both (101,102). Adenosine may be safer, though rarely effective for ventricular tachycardia (103).

Electrocardiographic means to diagnosis a wide QRS complex tachycardia have been reviewed (100,104). In the elderly, *all* wide complex rhythms should be assumed to be ventricular tachycardia unless proven otherwise, and treated accordingly. Well-tolerated ventricular tachycardia can be treated with intravenous lidocaine or procainamide, followed by electrical cardioversion starting at 100 J if the rhythm persists. Hypotensive ventricular tachycardia or ventricular fibrillation require immediate electrical cardioversion or defibrillation with at least 200 J. Hemodynamic and ventilatory support using basic and advanced cardiac life support protocols are frequently necessary, but should not take the place of rapid electrical defibrillation. Unfortunately, overall survival of cardiac arrest in the elderly is poor (22 percent acute survival, 3.8 percent survive to hospital discharge); survivors are those whose initial arrhythmia is ventricular tachycardia or fibrillation as opposed to those who present with asystole or electrical-mechanical dissociation (105).

For those who survive, chronic treatment of these arrhythmias is generally recommended because of a high recurrence rate, estimated at about 30 percent per year (106,107). Antiarrhythmic drug therapy guided by the results of electrophysiologic testing has been widely used in this setting, although in only a small percentage of patients can a drug be found to render the arrhythmia noninducible (108). For patients who have both frequent PVCs (>10 per hour) on Holter monitoring and who show inducible ventricular tachycardia in the electrophysiology laboratory, either Holter monitor-guided or electrophysiologically guided drug testing appears to be equally effective, albeit with a high arrhythmia recurrence rate (109). The Class III drug sotalol seems to be associated with a lower rate of recurrence of arrhythmia than the Class I drugs (110). Empiric use of amiodarone in these patients has also been advocated (111,112).

The ICD has become the most frequently recommended therapy for patients who do not respond to drug therapy, and some consider it first-line therapy (113–115). This device automatically senses ventricular tachycardia or fibrillation and then delivers an internal shock via electrodes attached to the heart. Recent developments with this device include the ability to implant it without a thoracotomy, the incorporation of backup pacing and antitachycardia pacing in the generator, and sophisticated diagnostic features such as stored electrograms (116,117). Although the sudden-death mortality with this device is reduced to only 1 percent to 2 percent per year (114), the total mortality in some studies is about 10 percent per year, not dissimilar to some studies of antiarrhythmic drug therapy (109). It has been pointed out that patients with ICDs still die from progression of their underlying heart disease or develop incessant ventricular tachycardia and die in the hospital of "not-so-sudden" arrhythmic death (118,119). In addition, there are significant morbidity and lifestyle adjustments from ICDs. The sensing abilities of these devices are imperfect and lead to the not uncommon occurrence of inappropriate shocks. Shocks are painful and psychological trauma can occur. Trials comparing ICD and antiarrhythmic drug therapy for ventricular tachyarrhythmias are in progress.

Pacemaker Therapy

Over the years, pacemakers have become much more reliable and sophisticated. Routine features include the ability to program multiple function, telemetry of pacer functions, small size, and long battery life. The transvenous route is preferred to the epicardial route because of its ease of insertion and low complication rate.

One decision the physician must make is whether to use a single- or dual-chamber device. Dual-chamber pacing provides AV synchrony and preserves the atrial kick that may account for as much as 25 percent of the cardiac output at rest (120,121). AV synchrony is less important in increasing cardiac output with exercise; increased cardiac output with exercise is achieved primarily by increased heart rate (122,123). Many patients requiring a pacemaker have sinus node dysfunction and, thus, cannot increase their atrial rate normally with exercise. In this situation, a simple dual-chamber pacemaker will not provide the rate responsiveness necessary to increase cardiac output with exercise. Recently, single-chamber and dual-chamber rate-responsive pacemakers that use an independent sensor to detect exercise and increase the heart rate appropriately have been developed. The sensor may detect vibrations from exercise or other more physiologic parameters (124).

Because dual-chamber pacemakers and activity-sensing pacemakers have additional cost and complexity, candidates for these pacing modes should be selected carefully. Medicare guidelines discourage dual-chamber pacing use; nevertheless, in active patients, despite advanced age, studies suggest that dual-chamber pacing improves exercise tolerance and well-being both acutely and chronically (125–128). Thus, candidates for physiologic pacemakers should include active, ambulatory patients and patients who might benefit from maintenance of AV synchrony—those with congestive heart failure, hypertrophic cardiomyopathy, or aortic stenosis. Single-chamber, fixed rate ventricular pacing is appropriate in patients who are inactive or who have only intermittent bradycardia.

Antiarrhythmic Drugs

Specific guidelines for antiarrhythmic drug use in the elderly have not been well documented. There is an increased incidence of adverse drug reactions, which has resulted from altered pharmacokinetics with age and from increased use of polypharmacy (which may lead to

Table 35.4. Applications of Catheter Ablation.

Curative
  Success rates > 90%
    Supraventricular tachycardia caused by AV nodal reentry or
      accessory pathway
    WPW syndrome
    Idiopathic ventricular tachycardia
  Success rates < 90%
    Atrial flutter
    Atrial tachycardia
    Ventricular tachycardia caused by structural heart disease
Palliative
  Atrial fibrillation
    AV node ablation with pacer implant for rate control

WPW = Wolff-Parkinson-White syndrome.

drug interactions). Absorption, protein binding, volume of distribution, hepatic and renal blood flow, and glomerular filtration all change with age (129). Receptor changes may also alter the patients's sensitivity to drugs (6). Some of the specific changes in individual drugs have been reviewed (130).

Because of the sometimes unpredictable metabolism of drugs in the elderly, it is best to follow serum drug levels to avoid both toxic and subtherapeutic responses. The risk of toxicity is real with any of the antiarrhythmic drugs, especially in the elderly. Therefore, the prudent physician must expect a reasonable chance of benefit before prescribing any of these drugs.

Catheter Ablation

In the past few years, catheter ablation, using radio-frequency current, has become a widespread method for treatment of cardiac arrhythmias. With catheter ablation, the electrophysiologist can perform precise surgery—cutting accessory pathways and destroying arrhythmogenic foci that in the past were approachable only by major open heart surgery. Using radiofrequency energy, small (<5 mm) discrete lesions can be made in the endocardium (131). Although there is a risk of catheter-related complications, the cure rate for many types of arrhythmias is high (84,86,90,94,95,132,133). Arrhythmias amenable to catheter ablation are listed in Table 35.4, grouped by current success rates. In the near future, as catheter ablation is developed further, more arrhythmias

are expected to be amenable to cure, with success rates over 90 percent.

References

1. Shurtleff D. Some characteristics related to the incidence of cardiovascular disease and death: Framingham Study, 18-year follow up. In: Kannel WB, Gordon T, eds. The Framingham Study. An epidemiologic investigation of cardiovascular disease. Section 30. Washington, D.C.: U.S. Government Printing Office, 1974:1–40.
2. Erickson EE, Lev M. Aging changes in the human atrioventricular node, bundle and bundle branches. J Gerontol 1952;7:1–12.
3. Lev M. Aging changes in the human sinoatrial node. J Gerontol 1954;9:1–9.
4. Davies MJ. Pathology of the conduction system. In: Caird FI, Dall JLC, Kennedy RD. Cardiology in old age. New York: Plenum, 1976:57–80.
5. Dreifus LS. Clinical arrhythmias in the elderly: clinical aspects. Cardiol Clin 1986;4:273–283.
6. Goldberg PB, Roberts J. Pharmacologic basis for developing rational drug regimens for elderly patients. Med Clin North Am 1983;67:315–331.
7. Gordon T, Kannel WB. Premature mortality from coronary heart disease–the Framingham Study. JAMA 1971; 215:1617–1625.
8. Lown B. Sudden cardiac death: the major challenge confronting contemporary cardiology. Am J Cardiol 1979; 43:313–328.
9. Bigger JT, Fleiss JL, Kleiger R, et al. The relationships among ventricular arrhythmias, left ventricular dysfunction and mortality in the 2 years after myocardial infarction. Circulation 1984;69:250–258.
10. Morganroth J, Bigger JT, Anderson JL. Treatment of ventricular arrhythmias by United States cardiologists: a survey before the Cardiac Arrhythmia Suppression Trial (CAST) results were available. Am J Cardiol 1990;65:40–48.
11. Echt DS, Liebson PR, Mitchell B, et al. Mortality and morbidity in patients receiving encainide, flecainide or placebo. The Cardiac Arrhythmia Suppression Trial. New Engl J Med 1991;324:781–788.
12. CAST-II Investigators. Effect of the antiarrhythmic agent moricizine on survival after myocardial infarction. New Engl J Med 1992;327:227–233.
13. Kuchar DL, Thornburn CW, Sammel NL. Signal-averaged electrocardiograms for evaluation of recurrent syncope. Am J Cardiol 1986;58:949–953.
14. Turitto G, Fontaine JM, Ursell SN, et al. Value of the signal-averaged electrocardiogram as a predictor of the results of programmed ventricular stimulation in nonsustained ventricular tachycardia. Am J Cardiol 1988;61:1272–1278.
15. Pomerance A. Senile cardiac amyloidosis. Br Heart J 1965;27:711–718.

16. Rowe JW, Troen BR. Sympathetic nervous system and aging in man. Endocr Rev 1980;1:167–179.

17. Hrushesky WJM, Fader D, Schmitt O, et al. The respiratory sinus arrhythmia: a measure of cardiac age. Science 1984;224:1001–1004.

18. Kostis JB, Moreyra AE, Amendo MT, et al. The effect of age on heart rate in subjects free of heart disease. Circulation 1982;65:141–145.

19. Dhingra RC, Wyndham C, Amat-Y-Leon F, et al. Incidence and site of A-V block in patients with chronic bifascicular block. Circulation 1979;59:238–246.

20. Dhingra RC, Wyndham C, Deedwania PC, et al. Effect of age on atrioventricular conduction in patients with chronic bifascicular block. Am J Cardiol 1980;45:749–756.

21. Mymin D, Mathewson FAL, Tate RB, Manfreda J. The natural history of primary first-degree atrioventricular block. N Engl J Med 1986;315:1183–1187.

22. McAnulty JH, Rahimtoola SH, Murphy E, et al. Natural history of "high-risk" bundle-branch block: Final report of a prospective study. N Engl J Med 1982;307:137–143.

23. Mihalic MJ, Fisch C. Electrocardiographic findings in the aged. Am Heart J 1974;87:117–128.

24. Glasser SP, Clark PI, Applebaum HJ. Occurrence of frequent complex arrhythmias detected by ambulatory monitoring. Findings in an apparently healthy asymptomatic elderly population. Chest 1979;75:565–568.

25. Camm AJ, Evans KE, Ward DE, Martin A. The rhythm of the heart in active elderly subjects. Am Heart J 1980;99:598–603.

26. Fleg JL, Kennedy HL. Cardiac arrhythmias in a healthy elderly population: detection by 24-hour ambulatory electrocardiography. Chest 1982;81:302–307.

27. Kantelip J-P, Sage E, Duchene-Marullaz P. Findings on ambulatory electrocardiographic monitoring in subjects older than 80 years. Am J Cardiol 1986;57:398–401.

28. Wajngarten M, Grupi C, Bellotti GM, et al. Frequency and significance of cardiac rhythm disturbances in healthy elderly individuals. J Electrocardiol 1990;23:171–176.

29. Brodsky M, Wu D, Denes P, et al. Arrhythmias documented by 24-hour continuous electrocardiographic monitoring in 50 male medical students without apparent heart disease. Am J Cardiol 1977;39:390–395.

30. Kennedy HL, Whitlock JA, Sprague MK, et al. Long-term follow-up of asymptomatic healthy subjects with frequent and complex ventricular ectopy. N Engl J Med 1985; 312:193–197.

31. Kannel WB, Abbott RD, Savage DD, McNamara PM. Epidemiologic features of chronic atrial fibrillation. N Engl J Med 1982;306:1018–1022.

32. Kannel WB, Abbott RD, Savage DD, McNamara PM. Coronary heart disease and atrial fibrillation: the Framingham Study. Am Heart J 1983;106:389–396.

33. Klein GJ, Yee R, Sharma AD. Longitudinal electrophysiologic assessment of asymptomatic patients with the Wolff-Parkinson-White electrocardiographic pattern. N Engl J Med 1989;320:1229–1233.

34. Munger TM, Packer DL, Hammill SC, et al. A population study of the natural history of Wolff-Parkinson-White syndrome in Olmsted County, Minnesota, 1953–1989. Circulation 1993;87:866–873.

35. Kaplan BM, Langendorf R, Lev M, et al. Tachycardia-bradycardia syndrome ("sick sinus syndrome"). Am J Cardiol 1973;26:497–508.

36. Rasmussen K. Chronic sinus node disease: Natural course and indications for pacing. Eur Heart J 1981;2:455–459.

37. Shaw DB, Linker NJ, Heaver PA, et al. Chronic sinoatrial disorder (sick sinus syndrome): A possible result of cardiac ischemia. Br Heart J 1987;58:598–607.

38. Agruss NS, Rosin EY, Adolph RJ, Fowler NO. Significance of chronic sinus bradycardia in elderly people. Circulation 1972;46:924–930.

39. Mazuz M, Friedman HS. Significance of prolonged electrocardiographic pauses in sinoatrial disease: sick sinus syndrome. Am J Cardiol 1983;52:485–489.

40. Shepard JW Jr. Cardiopulmonary disorders during sleep: Diagnosis and management. Geriatrics 1987;42:51–60.

41. Otsuka K, Sadakane N, Ozawa T. Arrhythmogenic properties of disordered breathing during sleep in patients with cardiovascular disorders. Clin Cardiol 1987;10:771–782.

42. Moss AJ, Davis RJ. Brady-tachy syndrome. Prog Cardiovasc Dis 1974;16:439–454.

43. Mandel W, Hayakawa H, Danzig R, Marcus HS. Evaluation of sino-atrial node function in man by overdrive suppression. Circulation 1971;44:59–66.

44. Gann D, Tolentino A, Samet P. Electrophysiologic evaluation of elderly patients with sinus bradycardia. Ann Intern Med 1979;90:24–29.

45. Rosen KM, Loeb HS, Sinno MZ, et al. Cardiac conduction in patients with symptomatic sinus node disease. Circulation 1971;43:836–844.

46. Kallryd A, Kruse I, Ryden L. Atrial inhibited pacing in the sick sinus node syndrome: clinical value and the demand for rate responsiveness. PACE 1989;12:954–961.

47. Rosenqvist M, Brandt J, Schuller H. Long-term pacing in sinus node disease: effect of stimulation mode on cardiovascular morbidity and mortality. Am Heart J 1988;116:16–22.

48. Sra JS, Jazayeri MR, Dhala A, et al. Neurocardiogenic syncope. Diagnosis, mechanisms, and treatment. Cardiol Clin 1993;11:183–191.

49. Almquist A, Goldenberg IF, Milstein S, et al. Provocation of bradycardia and hypotension by isoproterenol and upright posture in patients with unexplained syncope. N Engl J Med 1989;320:346–351.

50. Sra JS, Jazayeri MR, Avitall B, et al. Comparison of cardiac pacing with drug therapy in the treatment of neurocardiogenic (vasovagal) syncope with bradycardia or asystole. N Engl J Med 1993;328:1085–1090.

51. Fairfax AJ, Lambert CD, Leatham A. Systemic embolism in chronic sinoatrial disorder. N Engl J Med 1976;295:190–192.

52. Rubenstein JJ, Schulman CL, Yurchak PM, DeSanctis R. Clinical spectrum of sick sinus syndrome. Circulation 1972;46:5–13.

53. Chokshi DS, Mascarenhas E, Samet P, Center S. Treatment of sinoatrial rhythm disturbances with permanent cardiac pacing. Am J Cardiol 1973;32:215–220.

54. Krishnaswami V, Geraci AR. Permanent pacing in disorders of sinus node function. Am Heart J 1975;89:579–585.

55. Wohl AJ, Blomqvist CG. Prognosis of patients permanently paced for sick sinus syndrome. Arch Intern Med 1976;136:406–408.

56. Gould L, Reddy CVR, Becker WH. The sick sinus syndrome. A study of 50 cases. J Electrocardiol 1978;11:11–14.

57. Frye RL, Collins JJ, DeSanctis R, et al. Guidelines for permanent pacemaker implantation, May 1984. Circulation 1984;70:331A–339A.

58. Phibbs B, Friedman HS, Graboys TB, et al. Indications for pacing in the treatment of bradyarrhythmias: report of an independent study group. JAMA 1984;252:1307–1311.

59. Ferrer MI. The sick sinus syndrome. Circulation 1973;47:635–641.

60. Lenegre J. Etiology and pathology of bilateral bundle branch block in relation to complete heart block. Prog Cardiovasc Dis 1964;6:409–444.

61. Lev M. The pathology of complete atrioventricular block. Prog Cardiovasc Dis 1964;6:317–326.

62. Dreifus LS, Watanabe Y, Haiat R, Kimbiris D. Atrioventricular block. Am J Cardiol 1971;28:371–380.

63. Rowe JC, White PD. Complete heart block: a follow-up study. Ann Intern Med 1958;49:260–270.

64. Edhag O, Swahn A. Prognosis of patients with complete heart block or arrhythmic syncope who were not treated with artificial pacemakers. Acta Med Scand 1976;200:457–463.

65. Simon AB, Zloto AE. Atrioventricular block: natural history after permanent ventricular pacing. Am J Cardiol 1978;41:500–507.

66. Zoll PM, Zoll RH, Falk RH, et al. External noninvasive temporary cardiac pacing: clinical trials. Circulation 1985;71:937–944.

67. Forfar JC, Miller HC, Toft AD. Occult thyrotoxicosis: a correctable cause of "idiopathic" atrial fibrillation. Am J Cardiol 1979;44:9–12.

68. Wolf PA, Dawber TR, Thomas HE Jr, Kannel WB. Epidemiologic assessment of chronic atrial fibrillation and risk of stroke: the Framingham Study. Neurology 1978;28:973–977.

69. Hinton RC, Kistler JP, Fallon JT, et al. Influence of etiology of atrial fibrillation on incidence of systemic embolism. Am J Cardiol 1977;40:509–513.

70. Kopecky SL, Gersh BJ, McGoon MD, et al. The natural history of lone atrial fibrillation: a population-based study over three decades. N Engl J Med 1987;317:669–674.

71. Petersen P, Boysen G, Godtfredsen J, et al. Placebo-controlled, randomised trial of warfarin and aspirin for prevention of thromboembolic complications in chronic trial fibrillation: the Copenhagen AFASAK study. Lancet 1989;1:175–179.

72. Boston Area Anticoagulation Trial for Atrial Fibrillation Investigators. The effect of low-dose warfarin on the risk of stroke in non-rheumatic atrial fibrillation. N Engl J Med 1990;323:1505–1511.

73. Stroke Prevention in Atrial Fibrillation Investigators. Stroke Prevention in Atrial Fibrillation Study. Final Results. Circulation 1991;84:527–539.

74. Connolly SJ, Laupacis A, Gent M, et al. Canadian Atrial Fibrillation Anticoagulation (CAFA) study. J Am Coll Cardiol 1991;18:349–355.

75. Goldman MJ. The management of chronic atrial fibrillation: indications for and method of conversion to sinus rhythm. Prog Cardiovasc Dis 1960;2:465–479.

76. Bjerkelund CJ, Orning OM. The efficacy of anticoagulant therapy in preventing embolism related to D.C. electrical cardioversion of atrial fibrillation. Am J Cardiol 1969;23:208–216.

77. Arnold AZ, Mick MJ, Mazurek RP, et al. Role of prophylactic anticoagulation for direct current cardioversion in patients with atrial fibrillation or atrial flutter. J Am Coll Cardiol 1992;19:851–855.

78. O'Neill PG, Puleo PR, Bolli R, Rokey R. Return of atrial mechanical function following electrical conversion of atrial dysrhythmias. Am Heart J 1990;120:353–359.

79. Henry WL, Morganroth J, Pearlman AS, et al. Relation between echocardiographically determined left atrial size and atrial fibrillation. Circulation 1976;53:273–279.

80. Falk RH, Knowlton AA, Bernard SA, et al. Digoxin for converting recent-onset atrial fibrillation to sinus rhythm. Ann Intern Med 1987;106:503–506.

81. Coplen SE, Antmann EM, Berlin JA, et al. Efficacy and safety of quinidine therapy for maintenance of sinus rhythm after cardioversion: A meta-analysis of randomized control trials. Circulation 1990;82:1106–1116.

82. Juul-Moller S, Edvardsson N, Rehnqvist-Ahlberg N. Sotalol versus quinidine for the maintenance of sinus rhythm after direct current conversion of atrial fibrillation. Circulation 1990;82:1932–1939.

83. Gold RL, Haffajee CI, Charos K, et al. Amiodarone for refractory atrial fibrillation. Am J Cardiol 1986;57:124–127.

84. Scheinman MM, Laks MM, DiMarco J, Plumb V. Current role of catheter ablative procedures in patients with cardiac arrhythmias. A report for health professionals from the Subcommittee on Electrocardiography and Electrophysiology, American Heart Association. Circulation 1991;83:2146–2153.

85. Waldo AL, MacLean WAH, Karp RB, et al. Entrainment and interruption of atrial flutter with atrial pacing: studies in man following open heart surgery. Circulation 1977;56:737–745.

86. Feld GK, Fleck P, Chen P-S, et al. Radiofrequency catheter ablation for the treatment of human type 1 atrial flutter. Identification of a critical zone in the reentrant circuit by

endocardial mapping techniques. Circulation 1992;86:1233–1240.

87. Scheinman MM, Basu D, Hollenberg M. Electrophysiologic studies in patients with persistent atrial tachycardia. Circulation 1976;50:266–269.

88. Wyndham CRC, Arnsdorf MF, Levitsky S, et al. Successful surgical excision of focal paroxysmal atrial tachycardia: observations in vivo and in vitro. Circulation 1980;62:1365–1372.

89. Gillette PC, Smith RT, Garson A, et al. Chronic supraventricular tachycardia: a curable cause of congestive cardiomyopathy. JAMA 1985;253:391–392.

90. Kay GN, Chong F, Epstein AE, et al. Radiofrequency ablation for treatment of primary atrial tachycardias. J Am Coll Cardiol 1993;21:901–909.

91. Shine KI, Kastor JA, Yurchak PM. Multifocal atrial tachycardia: Clinical and electrocardiographic features in 32 patients. N Engl J Med 1968;27:344–349.

92. Levine JH, Michael JR, Guarnieri T. Treatment of multifocal atrial tachycardia with verapamil. N Engl J Med 1985;312:21–25.

93. Josephson ME, Seides SF. Clinical cardiac electrophysiology: techniques and interpretations. Philadelphia: Lea & Febiger, 1979:147–190.

94. Jackman WM, Beckman KJ, McClelland JH, et al. Treatment of supraventricaular tachycardia due to atrioventricular nodal reentry by radiofrequency catheter ablation of slow-pathway conduction. N Engl J Med 1992;327:313–318.

95. Jackman WM, Wang X, Friday KJ, et al. Catheter ablation of accessory atrioventricular pathways (Wolff-Parkinson-White syndrome) by radiofrequency current. N Engl J Med 1991;324:1605–1611.

96. Beta-blocker Heart Attack Study Group. A randomized trial of propranolol in patients with acute myocardial infarction. I. Mortality results. JAMA 1982;247:1707–1714.

97. Danforth J, Ports TA. Using beta blockers after MI in the elderly. Geriatrics 1985;40:75–85.

98. Burkart F, Pfisterer M, Kiowski W, et al. Effect of antiarrhythmic therapy on mortality in survivors of myocardial infarction with asymptomatic complex ventricular arrhythmias: Basel Antiarrhythmic Study of Infarct Survival (BASIS). J Am Coll Cardiol 1990;16:1711–1718.

99. Wilber DJ, Olshansky B, Moran JF, Scanlon PJ. Electrophysiological testing and nonsustained ventricular tachycardia. Use and limitations in patients with coronary artery disease and impaired ventricular function. Circulation 1990;82:350–358.

100. Akhtar M, Shenasa M, Jazayeri M, et al. Wide QRS complex tachycardia. Reappraisal of a common clinical problem. Ann Intern Med 1988;109:905–912.

101. Stewart RB, Brady GH, Greene HL. Wide complex tachycardia: misdiagnosis and outcome after emergent therapy. Ann Intern Med 1986;104:766–771.

102. Buxton AE, Marchlinski FE, Doherty JU, et al. Hazards of intravenous verapamil for sustained ventricular tachycardia. Am J Cardiol 1987;59:1107–1110.

103. Rankin AC, Oldroyd KG, Chong E, et al. Value and limitations of adenosine in the diagnosis and treatment of narrow and broad complex tachycardias. Br Heart J 1989;62:195–203.

104. Wellens HJJ, Bar FWHM, Lie KI. The value of the electrocardiogram in the differential diagnosis of a tachycardia with a widened QRS complex. Am J Med 1976;64:27–33.

105. Murphy DJ, Murray AM, Robinson BE, Campion EW. Outcomes of cardiopulmonary resuscitation in the elderly. Ann Intern Med 1989;111:199–205.

106. Liberthson RR, Nagel EL, Hirschman JC, Nussenfeld SR. Pre-hospital ventricular defibrillation: prognosis and follow-up course. N Engl J Med 1974;291:317–321.

107. Schaffer WA, Cobb LA. Recurrent ventricular fibrillation and modes of death in survivors of out-of-hospital ventricular fibrillation. N Engl J Med 1975;293:259–262.

108. Wilber DF, Garan H, Finklestein D, et al. Out-of-hospital cardiac arrest. Use of electrophysiologic testing in the prediction of long-term outcome. N Engl J Med 1988;318:19–24.

109. Mason JW, for the Electrophysiologyic Study versus Electrocardiographic Monitoring investigators. A comparison of electrophysiologic testing with holter monitoring to predict antiarrhythmic-drug efficacy for ventricular tachyarrhythmias. N Engl J Med 1993;329:445–451.

110. Mason JW, for the Electrophysiologyic Study versus Electrocardiographic Monitoring investigators. A comparison of seven antiarrhythmic drugs in patients with ventricular tachyarrhythmias. N Engl J Med 1993;329:452–458.

111. Kay GN, Pryor DB, Lee KL, et al. Comparison of survival of amiodarone-treated patients with coronary artery disease and malignant ventricular arrhythmias with that of a control group with coronary artery disease. J Am Coll Cardiol 1987;9:877–881.

112. Herre JM, Sauve MJ, Malone P, et al. Long-term results of amiodarone therapy in patients with recurrent sustained ventricular tachycardia or ventricular fibrillation. J Am Coll Cardiol 1989;13:442–449.

113. Tchou PJ, Kadri N, Anderson J, et al. Automatic implantable cardioverter defibrillators and survival of patients with left ventricular dysfunction and malignant ventricular arrhythmias. Ann Intern Med 1988;109:529–534.

114. Winkle RA, Mead RH, Ruder MA, et al. Long-term outcome with the automatic implantable cardioverter-defibrillator. J Am Coll Cardiol 1989;13:1353–1361.

115. Fogoros R, Elson JJ, Bonnet CA, et al. Efficacy of the automatic implantable cardioverter-defibrillator in prolonging survival in patients with severe underlying cardiac disease. J Am Coll Cardiol 1990;16:381–386.

116. Hook BG, Marchlinski FE. Value of ventricular electrogram recordings in the diagnosis of arrhythmias precipitating electrical device shock therapy. J Am Coll Cardiol 1991;17:985–990.

117. Bardy GH, Hofer B, Johnson G, et al. Implantable transvenous cardioverter-defibrillators. Circulation 1993;87:1152–1168.

118. Guarnieri T, Levine JH, Griffith LSC, et al. When "sudden

death" is not so sudden: lessons learned from the automatic implantable defibrillator. Am Heart J 1988;115:205–207.

119. Kim SG, Fisher JD, Furman S, et al. Benefits of implantable defibrillators are overestimated by sudden death rates and better represented by the total arrhythmic death rate. J Am Coll Cardiol 1991;17:1587–1592.

120. Samet P, Bernstein WH, Nathan DA, Lopez A. Atrial contribution to cardiac output in complete heart block. Am J Cardiol 1965;16:1–10.

121. Benchimol A. Significance of the contribution of atrial systole to cardiac function in man. Am J Cardiol 1969;23:568–571.

122. Pehrsson SK. Influence of heart rate and AV synchronization on maximal work tolerance in patients treated with artificial pacemakers. Acta Med Scand 1983;214:311–315.

123. Fananapazir L, Bennett DH, Monks P. Atrial synchronized ventricular pacing: contribution of the chronotropic response to improved exercise performance. PACE 1983;6:601–608.

124. Benditt DG, Milstein S, Buetikofer J, et al. Sensor-triggered, rate-variable cardiac pacing. Ann Intern Med 1987;107:714–724.

125. Kappenberger L, Gloor HO, Babotai I, et al. Hemodynamic effects of atrial synchronization in acute and long-term ventricular pacing. PACE 1982;5:639–645.

126. Kruse I, Arnman K, Conradson T-B, Ryden L. A comparison of the acute and long-term hemodynamic effects of ventricular inhibited pacing. Circulation 1982;65:846–855.

127. Perrins EJ, Morley CA, Chan SL, Sutton R. Randomised controlled trial of physiological and ventricular pacing. Br Heart J 1983;50:112–117.

128. Kristensson B, Arnman K, Smedgard P, Ryden L. Physiological versus single-rate ventricular pacing: a double-blind cross-over study. PACE 1985;8:73–84.

129. Crooks J, O'Malley K, Stevenson IH. Pharmacokinetics in the elderly. Clin Pharmacokinet 1976;1:280–283.

130. Marcus FI, Ruskin JN, Surawicz B. Arrhythmias. J Am Coll Cardiol 1987;10:66A–72A.

131. Franklin JO, Langberg JJ, Oeff M, et al. Catheter ablation of canine myocardium with radiofrequency energy. PACE 1989;12:170–176.

132. Klein LS, Shin H-T, Hackett K, et al. Radiofrequency catheter ablation of ventricular tachycardia in patients without structural heart disease. Circulation 1992;85:1666–1674.

133. Morady F, Harvey M, Kalbfleisch SJ, et al. Radiofrequency catheter ablation of ventricular tachycardia in patients with coronary artery disease. Circulation 1993;87:363–372.

Chapter 36
Hypertension

Ray W. Gifford, Jr., Michael D. Cressman, and Raymond A. Borazanian

Within the past twenty years measurements of the blood pressure have come to constitute a part of the routine physical examination, and the frequency with which arterial hypertension has been found in persons of middle age or beyond has become commonly known not only to physicians but also to the laity.

John Phillips, MD
(a founder of the Cleveland Clinic Foundation)
The Ohio State Medical Journal, 1925

Hypertension and *elderly* are generally defined numerically. Although numerical definitions are not perfect and, indeed, are somewhat arbitrary, a discussion of hypertension in the elderly is difficult to present without definitions. In this chapter, *elderly* refers to an individual who is at least 65 years of age. Numerical classification of blood pressure levels defines differences with respect to cardiovascular risk between normal blood pressure and abnormal (hypertension) levels. Optimal blood pressure is categorized as systolic blood pressure (SBP) less than 120 mm Hg with a diastolic blood pressure (DBP) less than 80 mm Hg (120/80); normal pressures are defined as SBP less than 130 with DBP less than 85 mm Hg (1). Blood pressure levels higher than these measurements are categorized by types and stages of hypertension. For example, *isolated systolic hypertension* (ISH) is defined as SBP of 140 mm Hg or more with DBP less than 90 mm Hg; a measurement of 170/85 mm Hg would be defined as stage 2 ISH (1,2). A DBP average (of two or more readings taken on each of two or more occasions) of 90 mm Hg is defined as *diastolic hypertension* (1,2). When systolic and diastolic pressures fall into separate categories, the higher category is used to classify an individual's blood pressure status; thus, 160/92 mm Hg would be classified as stage 2 and 180/120 mm Hg as stage 4. The presence or absence of target-organ disease and other risk factors also affects classification. For example, a patient with blood pressure

of 142/94 mm Hg, left ventricular hypertrophy (LVH), and diabetes would be classified as having stage 1 hypertension with target-organ disease (LVH) and another major risk factor (diabetes). Specificity is important for risk classification and management. Categorization of blood pressure, including stages of hypertension, adopted by the 1993 report of the Joint National Committee on Detection, Evaluation, and Treatment of High Blood Pressure (JNCV) are shown in Table 36.1 (1).

Prevalence

The prevalence of hypertension in the U.S. population was estimated from data from the second and third National Health and Nutrition Examination Surveys (NHANES II and III) and other sources (3,4). In NHANES II and III, three blood pressure measurements were obtained in a civilian, noninstitutionalized population on a single occasion, and the average of these three measurements was used for analysis. Although the use of single-occasion measurements probably overestimates the true prevalence of hypertension, these data demonstrate that the prevalence of hypertension in individuals aged 65 to 74 years is high, but has fallen over the past 10 years (Table 36.2) (2,3). If a SBP 140 mm Hg or more and/or a DBP 90 mm Hg or more or reported use of antihypertensive medications is used to define hypertension, 71.8 percent of blacks and 52.9 percent of whites between the ages of 65 and 74 are hypertensive (2,3). The distribution of measured blood pressures in people age 60 years and older with hypertension is given in Table 36.3. Approximately half of elderly patients with hypertension have stage 1 (mild) hypertension (2,3). The prevalence of isolated systolic hypertension increases with age; thus, nearly 75 percent of hypertensive people 75 years of age and older have SBP 140 mm Hg or more and DBP less than 90 mm Hg (Table 36.3) (2,3).

Table 36.1. Classification of Blood Pressure for Adults Age 18 Years and Older[a].

Category	Systolic (mm Hg)	Diastolic (mm Hg)
Normal	<130	<85
High normal	130–139	85–89
Hypertension[b]		
Stage 1	140–159	90–99
Stage 2	160–179	100–109
Stage 3	180–209	110–119
Stage 4	≥210	≥120

[a] Subjects were not taking antihypertensive drugs and were not acutely ill.

[b] Based on the average of two or more readings taken at each of two or more visits after an initial screening.

SOURCE: Fifth report of the Joint National Committee on Detection, Evaluation, and Treatment of High Blood Pressure. Arch Intern Med 1993;153:154–183.

Risks of Hypertension in the Elderly

Cardiovascular risk increases as SBP or DBP rises (5). The graded risk associated with hypertension is present in both young and elderly individuals. In fact, the relationship of SBP and DBP to cardiovascular events is more pronounced for persons age 65 and older than it is for those aged 35 to 65 (6). Data from the Framingham Study indicate that SBP is a better predictor of coronary heart disease (CHD) risk than DBP is for individuals over 45 years of age (7). In addition, SBP was a better predictor of the risk of atherothrombotic brain infarction (ABI) than DBP in 65- to 74-year-old men in the Framingham cohort (8). Systolic and diastolic hypertension also increase the risk of congestive heart failure, aortic aneurysm, renal failure, and intermittent claudication (5). Cardiovascular mortality was increased fourfold in 65- to 74-year-old women and twofold in 65- to 74-year-old men with mild hypertension (140/90 to 160/95 mm Hg) when compared with age-matched normotensive women and men in the Framingham Study (9).

Cardiovascular risk is also increased in individuals with ISH. This has been demonstrated in the 1979 Blood Pressure Study of the Society of Actuaries, the Framingham Study, and the Chicago Stroke Study. In the Blood Pressure Study, individuals with ISH had a 51 percent excess mortality, in contrast to those with normal SBP and DBP (10). The risk of cardiovascular death dur-

Table 36.2. Trends in Hypertension Prevalence[a] by Gender and Ethnicity in the Civilian, Noninstitutionalized Population, Ages 65 to 74 years in 1976–1980 and 1988–1991.

Gender/Ethnic Group	1976–1980(%)	1988–1991(%)
Women	67.5	52.5
African Americans[b]	82.9	71.9
Whites[b]	66.2	51.2
Mexican Americans	–	53.1
Men	60.2	56.4
African Americans[b]	67.1	71.6
Whites[b]	59.2	54.9
Mexican Americans	–	56.9
Totals[c]	64.3	54.3
African Americans[b]	76.1	71.8
Whites[b]	63.1	52.9
Mexican Americans	–	54.9

[a] Defined as the average of three blood pressure measurements ≥140 mm Hg (systolic) and/or ≥90 mm Hg (diastolic) on a single occasion or on reported taking of antihypertensive medication. Estimates based on all sitting blood pressure measurements taken by physicians in the HANES mobile examination center.

[b] Non-Hispanics.

[c] Totals include racial and/or ethnic groups not shown separately.

SOURCE: Centers for Disease Control and Prevention. Second National Health and Nutrition Examination Survey (NHANES II) 1976–1980, Hispanic HANES 1982–1984, NHANES III 1988–1991. Hyattsville, MD: National Center for Health Statistics, 1992 and Report of the National High Blood Pressure Education Program Working Group on Hypertension in the Elderly. Hypertension 1994;23:275–285.

ing a 2-year follow-up of Framingham participants with ISH was increased from twofold to fivefold (11). Shekelle reported that the 3-year incidence of stroke in the Chicago Stroke Study was 2.5 times greater for individuals with ISH in contrast to those with normal SBP (12). Colandrea and colleagues noted that residents of a retirement community with ISH had twice the incidence of myocardial infarction (MI), three times the frequency of angina pectoris, three times the frequency of stroke, and a sevenfold increase in cardiovascular death rate than did age-matched normotensive residents (13).

Treatment Trials for Elderly Hypertensive Patients

Isolated Systolic Hypertension

The Systolic Hypertension in the Elderly Program (SHEP) was a multicenter, randomized, placebo-controlled, dou-

Table 36.3. Percentage Distribution of Blood Pressure Levels by JNCV Categories in the U.S. Population with Hypertension, Ages 60 and Older, by Sex.

			Hypertensive Stage		
Category	ISH	Controlled[a]	Stage 1	Stage 2	Stages 3, 4[b]
SBP (mm Hg)	≥140	<140	140–159	160–179	≥180
	and	and	or	or	or
DBP (mm Hg)	<90	<90	90–99	100–109	≥110
Total (All)[c]	64.8	25.6	49.6	18.2	6.5
Men					
Total[c]	63.3	21.8	54.9	18.1	5.1
60–74 yr	58.9	23.7	54.9	17.3	4.1
≥75 yr	74.6	16.9	55.1	20.2	7.8
Women					
Total[c]	65.9	28.2	46.0	18.3	7.5
60–74 yr	61.0	32.7	47.9	14.7	4.7
≥75 yr	73.7	21.1	43.0	24.0	11.9

[a] Controlled with medication.
[b] Stages 3 and 4 are collapsed because of insufficient sample size.
[c] Totals may not equal 100 percent because of rounding.
DBP = diastolic blood pressure; ISH = isolated systolic hypertension; SBP = systolic blood pressure.
SOURCE: Centers for Disease Control and Prevention. Third National Health and Nutrition Examination Survey (NHANES III) 1988–1991. Hyattsville, MD: National Center for Health Statistics, 1992. And the Report of the National High Blood Pressure Education Program Working Group Report on Hypertension in the Elderly. Hypertension 1994;23:275–285.

ble-blind trial conducted to determine whether antihypertensive drug treatment reduces the risk of nonfatal and fatal stroke in patients with isolated systolic hypertension (14). Participants were 60 years of age and older, with a mean age of 72 years. A total of 4736 patients with SBP from 160 to 219 mm Hg and DBP less than 90 mm Hg entered the study; the average SBP was 170 mm Hg and the average DBP was 77 mm Hg. The participants were randomly assigned to receive either placebo or active treatment consisting of 12.5 mg/day of chlorthalidone. This dose could be doubled, and 25 mg/day of atenolol or 0.05 mg/day of reserpine could be added as necessary to reach a goal SBP of less than 160 mm Hg and a reduction in SBP of at least 20 mm Hg.

The average follow-up was 4.5 years, during which the average SBP was 155 mm Hg for the placebo group and 143 mm Hg for the treated group; the average DBP was 72 and 68 mm Hg, respectively. The 5-year incidence of total stroke was 5.2 per 100 participants for active treatment and 8.2 per 100 for placebo, a reduction of 36 percent. The relative risk by proportional hazards regression analysis

was 0.64 ($p = 0.0003$). For the secondary end point of clinical nonfatal myocardial infarction plus coronary death, the relative risk was 0.73. Major cardiovascular events were reduced (relative risk 0.68). For deaths from all causes, the relative risk was 0.87. These results were observed even though approximately 35 percent of those assigned to placebo took antihypertensive medications before the end of the trial.

During the trial, 3.9 percent of the active treatment group had at least one serum potassium value less than 3.2 mEq/L, compared with 0.8 percent in the placebo group. Similarly, 5.3 percent of the active treatment group had at least one serum uric acid value greater than 10 mg/dL compared with 1.3 percent of the placebo group. Serum glucose values greater than 200 mg/dL were found in 9.3 percent of the active treatment group and in 7.6 percent of the placebo group, serum cholesterol values greater than 300 mg/dL were found in 13.2 percent of the active treatment group and in 11.0 percent of the placebo group, and serum sodium values less than 130 mEq/L were found in 4.1 percent of the active treatment group

Table 36.4. Entry Criteria, Blood Pressure at Entry, Goal Pressure, and Achieved Pressure in Seven Trials.

Category	Trials of Diastolic Hypertension Only					Trials Including ISH	
	HDFP	Australian	EWPHE	Coope and Warrender	STOP-Hypertension	MRC	SHEP
No. of patients	2376	582	840	884	1627	4396	4736
Age range (yr)	60–69	60–69	60–97	60–79	70–84	65–74	≥60
Blood pressure entry criteria							
Systolic	–	<200	160–239	170–280	180–230 or <180	160–209	160–219
Diastolic	≥90	95–109	90–119	105–120	90–120 or 105–120	<115	<90
Mean blood pressure at entry	170/101	165/101	182/101	197/99	195/102	185/91	170/77
Blood pressure goal							
Systolic	–	–	–	<170	<160	≤160 or ≤150[a]	<160 and >20 decrease
Diastolic	≤90 and >10 decrease	<90 then <80	<90	<105	<95	–	–
Treatment							
Initial	Chlorthalidone	Chlorothiazide	HCTZ + triamtrene	Atenolol	HCTZ + amiloride, atenolol, metoprolol, or pindolol	HCTZ + amiloride or atenolol	Chlorthalidone
Added	Reserpine or methyldopa; hydralazine; guanethidine	Various	Methyldopa	Bendrofluazide; methyldopa	Atenolol, metoprolol, or pindolol; HCTZ + amiloride	Atenolol; HCTZ	Atenolol; reserpine
Blood pressure obtained							
Treatment group	/81	143/87	149/85	162/77	167/87	152/79	143/68
Placebo group	/86[b]	155/94	172/94	180/88[c]	186/96	167/85	155/72

[a] If SBP was <180 mm Hg, goal was ≤150 mm Hg; if SBP was ≥180 mm Hg; goal was ≤160 mm Hg.
[b] Trial compared a stepped care regimen to referred care at usual sources in the community.
[c] Open-label trial that compared a treated group to an untreated group of controls.
DBP = diastolic blood pressure; EWPHE = European Working Party on Hypertension in the Elderly; HCTZ = hydrochlorothiazide; HDFP = Hypertension Detection and Follow-up Program; ISH = isolated systolic hypertension; MRC = Medical Research Council; SBP = systolic blood pressure; SHEP = Systolic Hypertension in the Elderly Program; STOP-Hypertension = Swedish Trial in Old Patients with Hypertension.
SOURCE: Gifford RW Jr, Borazanian RA. Treatment of hypertension in the elderly. In: Oreopoulos DG, Michelis MF, Herschorn S, eds. Nephrology and urology in the aged patient. The Netherlands: Kluwer, 1993:153–164. Reprinted by permission of Kluwer Academic Publishers.

and in 1.3 percent of the placebo group. These differences were all statistically significant. Compared with placebo, active treatment was associated with a slight increase in some adverse effects, but there was no evidence of increase in dementia or depression (14).

Diastolic Hypertension

Several studies have demonstrated the benefit of treating diastolic hypertension in the elderly (15,16). These are summarized in Tables 36.4 and 36.5. The design of the Hypertension Detection and Follow-up Program (HDFP) (17–19) was atypical because there was no true placebo-control group. It is possible that the apparent benefit of aggressive antihypertensive treatment delivered in stepped care (SC) centers was not a result of changes in blood pressure but a manifestation of the extra care that the SC patients received. However, data from other trials, some of which did include placebo groups, also demon-

strated benefits from aggressive antihypertensive treatment in elderly patients with diastolic hypertension (20–25).

Etiology and Pathophysiology

Isolated Systolic Hypertension

Isolated systolic hypertension is believed to be caused by loss of elasticity of the aorta and its major branches. This results from destruction of elastic fibers and deposition of collagen and calcium in the aortic media. Hallock and Benson (26) showed that closed aortic segments obtained at autopsy from individuals aged 71 to 78 generated higher pressures when filled with a given volume of saline solution than did aortic segments obtained from 20- to 24-year-old individuals. The implication of these studies is that a rigid aorta generates a higher SBP for a given stroke volume than does a more elastic aorta.

Table 36.5. Percentage of Change in Event Rates in Seven Trials.

	Trials of Diastolic Hypertension Only					Trials Including ISH	
Event	HDFP	Australian	EWPHE	Coope and Warrender	STOP-Hypertension	MRC	SHEP
Nonfatal							
Stroke	−41	−36	−35	−27	−38[a]	−30	−37[a]
MI	−37	+20	NA	+10	−16	NA	−33[a]
All cardiac	NA	−8	−9	−26	NA	−13	−40[a]
All cardiovascular	NA	−17	−36[a]	−26	NA	−25[a]	−36[a]
Fatal							
Stroke	−48	NA	−32	−70[a]	−73[a]	−12	−29[a]
Cardiac	−22	−75[b]	−38[a]	0	−25[b]	−22[b]	−20[b]
All cardiovascular	−22	−62	−27	−22	NA	−9	−20
All noncardiovascular	NA	+19	+21	NA	NA	+5	+5
Total deaths	−16	−26	−9	−3	−43[a]	−3	−13
All events							
Stroke	−45[a]	−33	−36[a]	−42[a]	−47[a]	−25[a]	−36[a]
Cardiac	−14[a]	−18	−20	−15	−13[c]	−19[b]	−27[a]
All cardiovascular	NA	−26	−34[a]	−23[a]	−40[a]	−17[a]	−32[a]

[a] $p < 0.05$.
[b] Ischemic heart disease.
[c] Myocardial infarction.

EWPHE = European Working Party on Hypertension in the Elderly; HDFP = Hypertension Detection and Follow-up Program; ISH = isolated systolic hypertension; MI = myocardial infarction; MRC = Medical Research Council; NA = not available; SHEP = Systolic Hypertension in the Elderly Program.

SOURCE: Gifford RW Jr, Borazanian RA. Treatment of hypertension in the elderly. In: Oreopoulous DG, Michelis MF, Herschorn S, eds. Nephrology and urology in the aged patient. The Netherlands: Kluwer, 1993:153–164. Reprinted by permission of Kluwer Academic Publishers.

Although the average SBP increases with age in most Western industrialized nations, the development of ISH is not a normal consequence of aging. Epidemiologic observations conducted in several nonindustrialized societies do not show an age-related rise in SBP (27). Individuals in these societies tend to consume low-sodium, high-potassium, low-fat diets and remain lean and physically active throughout life.

Systolic hypertension resulting from rigidity of large arteries should be accompanied by a reduction in DBP (if total peripheral resistance remains normal). Even if compensatory reduction in DBP occurs, cardiac work (CW) is increased because CW is the product of stroke volume (SV), heart rate (HR), and mean blood pressure during systole ($\overline{SBP}$), according to the simplified formula (28)

$$CW = SV \times HR \times \overline{SBP}.$$

For this reason, it is not surprising that certain complications of hypertension, such as congestive heart failure, are closely associated with elevation of SBP.

Elderly individuals with diastolic hypertension often have a disproportionate elevation in SBP. Participants 60 to 69 years of age in the HDFP had an average SBP that was 20 mm Hg higher than that in 30- to 49-year-old participants, even though the DBP was virtually identical (101 mm Hg) in both groups (29). Koch-Weser (30) defined disproportionate systolic hypertension as

$$SBP > (DBP - 15) \times 2.$$

Diastolic Hypertension

Diastolic hypertension may be defined as primary (idiopathic, essential) or secondary to diseases such as renal artery disease, renal parenchymal disease, primary aldosteronism, Cushing's syndrome, and pheochromocytoma. Although detailed studies defining the prevalence of the secondary forms of hypertension in the elderly have not been performed, most elderly patients with hypertension have primary hypertension. For this reason, detailed laboratory investigation to identify secondary causes of hypertension in an older individual is usually not required. However, it should be recognized that the sudden onset of hypertension after age 55 or the loss of control of previously controlled hypertension is an important clue to the presence of secondary hypertension.

In this situation, atherosclerotic renal artery disease should be strongly considered. This is particularly true if the hypertension is severe or resistant to standard triple-drug therapy and on physical examination the patient has evidence of generalized atherosclerosis. Severe bilateral renal artery stenosis or severe stenosis in the artery to a solitary kidney should be considered if a patient who develops acute renal failure during treatment with an angiotensin-converting enzyme (ACE) inhibitor (31).

The neurohumoral and hemodynamic characteristics of diastolic hypertension are somewhat different for young and elderly patients. Elderly patients with primary hypertension, as a group, have lower cardiac output, higher peripheral vascular resistance, lower blood volume, lower plasma renin activity (PRA), and higher plasma catecholamine levels. Messerli and coworkers (32) reported that 60 percent of 30 elderly patients with diastolic hypertension had echocardiographic evidence of LVH; however, LVH was present in only 10 percent of the younger patients. The reduced cardiac output in elderly patients was caused by a reduction in both stroke volume and heart rate. Total peripheral vascular resistance was 40 percent higher in the older group, and total and central blood volume were lower in these patients.

Baroreflex sensitivity is also decreased in the elderly (33). Baroreceptor reflexes are primarily responsible for buffering excessive changes in blood pressure and are important in modulating the hemodynamic adjustments required to maintain blood pressure with changes in body position. When a person rises from the supine position, blood pressure in the upper thorax and head tends to fall. This results in reduced stimulation of high pressure carotid sinus and aortic baroreceptors. Reduced neural activity is sensed by the nucleus tractus solatarius and leads to stimulation of the vasoconstrictor center in the medulla and an inhibitory vagal response. Total peripheral resistance rises, and heart rate increases. Dysfunction in any portion of this reflex arc or an abnormality in the peripheral arterioles can lead to an excessive fall in SBP and DBP when the patient is upright. Rutan et al (34) reported that 16.2 percent of 5201 men and women aged 65 years and older had asymptomatic decreases in SBP of 20 mm Hg or greater, decreases of DBP of 10 mm Hg or greater, or both within 3 minutes of assuming the upright posture. An additional 2 percent had symptoms associated with decreases in blood pressure when they stood up, notably dizziness. Orthostatic hypotension was associated significantly with difficulty walking, frequent falls, and histories of myocardial infarction and transient ischemic attacks. For this reason, blood pressures should always be measured in both the sitting (or supine) and standing positions in elderly patients before and during antihypertensive therapy. Peripherally acting sympatholytic agents such as guanethidine and guanadrel and alpha$_1$ blockers such as prazosin, terazosin, and doxazosin should be used with great caution in the elderly because they can aggravate orthostatic hypotension. Overzealous diuretic treatment with its risk of volume depletion can also lead to orthostatic hypotension in these individuals. It is also important to recognize that elderly patients are susceptible to postprandial reductions in supine blood pressure, which may be asymptomatic (35).

In summary, elderly hypertensive patients have, on average, lower cardiac output and higher total peripheral vascular resistance than do younger hypertensive patients. Blood volume and PRA levels also tend to be reduced for elderly persons compared with those factors for young hypertensive patients. Elderly hypertensive patients with reduced baroreflex sensitivity are predisposed to orthostatic hypotension, which can be exacerbated when certain antihypertensive drugs are administered.

Management Considerations

Evaluation

The goals of the initial evaluation of any patient with hypertension are to confirm the presence of high blood pressure, assess the patient's overall health, evaluate the status of target organs, determine whether other cardiovascular risk factors are present, and exclude secondary causes of high blood pressure (1,36). Repeated blood pressure measurements are required to document the presence of sustained hypertension because blood pressure, particularly SBP, is often quite labile in elderly patients. In addition, concern has been raised about the accuracy of indirect blood pressure measurements in elderly patients with significant sclerosis of the brachial artery. Messerli and coworkers noted that elderly patients with hypertension who were "Osler-positive" had indirect cuff blood

pressure measurements that were 10 to 54 mm Hg higher than direct intra-arterial pressure measurements (37).

A patient was classified as being Osler-positive if either the brachial artery or radial artery could definitely be palpated after the artery was occluded by increasing cuff pressure above SBP. Messerli found that 13 of 24 elderly hypertensive patients were Osler-positive. This spurious elevation in blood pressure, because of sclerosis of the large arteries, has been referred to as pseudohypertension. Other investigators have compared indirect measurements of blood pressure with direct arterial pressure measurements and found close correlations for SBP in patients as old as 81 years of age (38,39).

Irrespective of age, indirect blood pressure measurements overestimate DBP. Nevertheless, one should consider pseudohypertension when 1) blood pressure is elevated out of proportion to the degree of clinical evidence of target organ involvement, 2) blood pressure fails to respond to an appropriate antihypertensive regimen, or 3) symptoms suggestive of hypotension develop during drug treatment, despite persistence of measured blood pressure elevation.

Blood pressure should be measured at each visit while the patient is in the supine or sitting position and again 2 to 3 minutes after the patient assumes the standing position because elderly individuals are more likely than young patients to have significant orthostatic decreases in blood pressure and to develop symptoms of cerebral hypoperfusion that may include dizziness, unsteadiness, falls, and syncope (34). This tendency is particularly important when pharmacologic therapy is administered.

The patient's medical history and physical examination are used to detect associated conditions that frequently coexist with high blood pressure in the elderly. These conditions and the medications used to treat them may influence the choice of antihypertensive drugs. For example, agents with significant central nervous system (CNS) side effects (such as beta blockers or centrally acting sympatholytic agents) are best avoided for individuals with a history of depression or varying degrees of organic dementia. In addition, drugs such as the alpha$_1$ receptor-blockers (prazosin, terazosin, doxazosin) and the peripherally acting sympatholytic agents (guanethidine, guanadrel) should be avoided for individuals who have a history of stroke or evidence of significant extracranial or intracranial cerebrovascular disease and significant orthostatic hypotension before initiation of drug therapy.

The status of the patient's coronary circulation must be considered. Calcium antagonists and beta blockers are particularly useful in the treatment of hypertensive patients with angina pectoris. However, beta blockers, diltiazem, and verapamil may further impair myocardial contractility in individuals with ischemic, idiopathic, or hypertensive cardiomyopathy. Beta-adrenergic receptor-blockers should also be used with caution in patients with chronic obstructive pulmonary disease (COPD), particularly if a bronchospastic component is present. Renal blood flow and glomerular filtration rate (GFR) are often reduced in the elderly; for this reason, drugs with renal excretion should be used at a reduced dose. A large number of elderly hypertensive patients regularly use nonsteroidal anti-inflammatory drugs (NSAIDs) to treat various chronic arthropathies. These agents blunt the efficacy of most antihypertensive agents and may cause deterioration of renal function.

Treatment

Lifestyle Modifications

Lifestyle modifications should be tried first as an alternative to drug therapy for most elderly patients with hypertension (2). Although there is a general impression that elderly individuals will not exercise, alter their diets, or attempt to reduce body weight, data from the Minnesota Heart Health Program suggest that a significant number of older individuals will make recommended lifestyle changes (40). Applegate and colleagues (41) found that elderly patients randomly assigned to a 6-month program of weight reduction, sodium restriction, and increased activity lost an average of 2.1 kg, and experienced a reduction in SBP and DBP that was 4.2 to 4.9 mm Hg greater than that found in the control group.

Sodium intake can be very high in elderly patients, particularly in individuals who ingest large quantities of canned foods, processed meats, and snacks. Attempts to reduce sodium intake in these individuals are obviously desirable. Calcium intake is often inadequate in the elderly, and there has been increased enthusiasm for use of calcium supplements for the prevention of osteoporosis in postmenopausal women. Some reports suggest that oral calcium supplementation has a beneficial blood pressure-lowering effect (42). Some investigators advocate dietary supplementation of magnesium or potassium for the treatment of hypertension, as magnesium and potassium intake may be reduced in the elderly. However, one should recognize that the renal excretion of magnesium and potassium may be reduced in elderly patients with renal disease. Thus, this form of treatment is theoretically not without hazard. The JNCV report advocates insuring an adequate intake of calcium, potassium, and magnesium to meet minimum daily requirements, but found no convincing evidence that supplements of these minerals were beneficial in reducing blood pressure (1). With these limitations and precautions in mind, a 3- to 6-month trial of nonpharmacologic therapy is reasonable for elderly hypertensive patients, except when stage 2 to stage 4 (moderate to severe) diastolic hypertension or complications are present.

Daily alcohol intake should be limited to no more than two glasses of wine (8 ounces), two bottles of beer (24 ounces), or two shots of whiskey (2 ounces). Even though cigarette smoking and dietary saturated fat and cholesterol are not directly implicated in raising blood pressure, elderly patients with hypertension should also be advised to avoid cigarette smoking and to reduce dietary intake of saturated fat and cholesterol, especially if they have dyslipidemia (2).

Pharmacologic Therapy

If a trial of nonpharmacologic therapy proves unsuccessful, the clinician should proceed cautiously with pharmacologic therapy, keeping in mind that older patients are particularly susceptible to orthostatic hypotension. Therefore, blood pressure readings should be taken in the standing and seated positions at every visit. If there is a large orthostatic drop, the standing blood pressure should be used to guide dosing. As already discussed, older patients often are sensitive to antihypertensive drugs because they tend to have impaired baroreflexes, low plasma volume, and low cardiac output. Consequently, treatment should be started with one-half the usual adult dose, and increases in dosage should be made at intervals of no less than 3 weeks.

Older patients frequently take a variety of medications for conditions other than hypertension and thereby increase their risk for drug interactions. However, older participants in the HDFP had a lower incidence of side effects than did younger patients (43). At the end of 5 years, the cohort that was 60 to 69 years of age at baseline had an average diastolic pressure of 81 mm Hg, 80 percent of them were still receiving treatment, and 75 percent had achieved the goal DBP. This result was equal to or better than the record achieved by younger patients (18).

Diuretics The JNCV (1) notes that all classes of antihypertensive drugs have been shown to be effective in lowering blood pressure in older patients. It further notes, however, that only diuretics and beta blockers have been found to reduce morbidity and mortality in controlled trials and recommends that these drugs be given preference for this reason. Diuretics were used for elderly patients in the Australian trial (20), the HDFP (17–19), the European Working Party on High Blood Pressure in the Elderly study (21,22), the SHEP (14), the Medical Research Council (MRC) trial (25), and the Swedish Trial in Old Patients with Hypertension (STOP-Hypertension) trial (24).

Hydrochlorothiazide was given in combination with triamterene in the European Working Party on High Blood Pressure in the Elderly study (21,22). This combination was quite effective in preventing diuretic-induced hypokalemia, but a slight increase in serum uric acid and creatinine and a reduction in glucose tolerance were observed in the diuretic-treated patients. Martin and Milligan (44) reported that elderly patients receiving diuretics at the time of hospital admission had lower serum magnesium concentrations that did elderly hospitalized patients who were not receiving diuretics. Renal magnesium wasting was noted in hypomagnesemic subjects receiving either loop or thiazide-type diuretics. Whang and associates (45) noted that hypomagnesemia was relatively common in hospitalized patients receiving diuretics and digitalis. Because diuretics also cause hypokalemia, there is concern that the combination of hypokalemia and hypomagnesemia may increase the risk of digitalis-associated cardiac arrhythmias.

Despite these potential problems, diuretics are very useful agents because of their low cost, convenience, and proven efficacy. Patients with significant azotemia (serum creatinine above 2 to 3 mg/dL) may benefit from use of one of the newer thiazide-type diuretics such as indapamide or metolazone. Loop diuretics may be re-

quired in more severely azotemic individuals. These agents (furosemide, bumetanide, ethacrynic acid) generally require administration twice daily. The adverse metabolic effects of diuretics are dose-related (46) and should be less pronounced if the low doses currently recommended are used (1).

Some physicians routinely use a thiazide-potassium-sparing agent because of concern about the hypokalemic effect of the thiazides. There is, however, a risk of hyperkalemia, especially in elderly people receiving potassium-sparing diuretics such as amiloride, spironolactone, or triamterene and who also have renal insufficiency, diabetes mellitus, hyporeninemic hypoaldosteronism, or are receiving an NSAID, ACE inhibitor, or potassium supplement. Because the risk of hyperkalemia is real and the thiazide-potassium-sparing agents do not always prevent hypokalemia, the patient's serum potassium level must be monitored even if these agents are used. Our own preference is to reserve the use of thiazide-potassium-sparing drugs for those patients who develop diuretic-induced hypokalemia.

Beta Blockers Buhler and colleagues noted an inverse relationship between age and the blood pressure-lowering response to beta-blocker monotherapy; an adequate response occurred in only 20 percent of patients aged 60 and older compared with a 75 percent response rate for individuals younger than 40 years of age (47). The reduced antihypertensive response in the elderly may relate to low renin status, reduced beta-adrenergic receptor responsiveness, or the low cardiac output that has been described in these patients. However, many elderly individuals do respond to beta-blocker monotherapy, and these drugs are especially indicated in certain situations. In the Veterans Administration (VA) Trial of Single-Drug Therapy in Men (48), the beta blocker atenolol was among the most effective agents for elderly white men but was among the least effective for elderly black men. In a controlled clinical trial comparing atenolol, enalapril, and isradipine in elderly white hypertensive women, the efficacy of monotherapy in lowering the DBP to 90 mm Hg or less and greater than 10 mm Hg below baseline was 84 percent for atenolol, 71 percent for enalapril, and 80 percent for isradipine (49). Furthermore, the frequency of reported adverse symptoms differed little for these agents and was not excessive with the beta blocker.

Beta blockers are effective antianginal agents, and beta blockers without intrinsic sympathomimetric activity have been shown to reduce the incidence of reinfarction and sudden death after an MI (50–52). Anderson and coworkers (53) originally suggested that elderly patients did not benefit from postinfarction beta-blocker prophylaxis, on the basis of the results of their relatively small study with use of alprenolol. Both the larger Norwegian trial (using timolol) and the Beta Blocker Heart Attack Trial (using propranolol) have shown a favorable response in older individuals (50–52). For this reason, it is appropriate to treat a hypertensive patient who has had an MI with a beta blocker because the protective effect of beta blockade seems to persist for several years after initiation of treatment.

Absolute or relative contraindications to beta-blocker treatment, such as heart block greater than first degree, COPD, peripheral occlusive arterial disease, and diabetes mellitus, are more common in older persons than they are in younger individuals. Elderly individuals tend to have higher steady-state blood levels of beta blockers than do younger patients treated with equivalent doses of these drugs because both hepatic and renal clearance of drugs are reduced in the elderly. In general, it is reasonable to initiate therapy in the elderly with approximately one-half the usual recommended dose of beta blocker if one of these agents is used to treat hypertension.

Alpha₁ Receptor-Blockers Prazosin, terazosin, and doxazosin are postsynaptic alpha₁-receptor-blocking drugs that reduce blood pressure primarily by reducing peripheral vascular resistance. These agents also reduce preload as a result of their vasodilatory effects on the venous system. Although simultaneous reduction in preload and afterload is desirable for hypertensive patients with impaired myocardial pump function, there is a risk of orthostatic hypotension when these drugs are used to treat elderly patients with high blood pressure. For these reasons, alpha₁-receptor-blockers must be used with caution as first-line or as adjunctive agents.

Alpha-Beta Blocker Labetalol is a noncardioselective, beta-adrenergic receptor-blocker that also possesses postsynaptic alpha₁-receptor-blocking properties. The hemodynamic properties of labetalol for hypertensive patients differ somewhat from the profile of beta blockers that lack alpha₁-receptor-blocking activity. Beta blockers reduce blood pressure primarily by decreasing cardiac output. In contrast, the blood pressure-lowering effect of labetalol is mainly caused by a reduction in peripheral vascular resistance. Cardiac output generally does not change. Because elderly hypertensive patients tend to have low cardiac output and high peripheral vascular resistance (32), the hemodynamic profile of labetalol is theoretically desirable for the hypertensive elderly patient. There is a limited body of information detailing the safety and efficacy of labetalol treatment in elderly, hypertensive patients, but the drug appears to be effective and well tolerated (54). It is prudent to initiate labetalol administration in low doses (100 mg once to twice daily) because of the risk of orthostatic hypotension, which is a theoretical problem with any drug that blocks alpha₁ receptors.

Angiotensin-Converting Enzyme Inhibitors ACE inhibitors (captopril, enalapril, lisinopril, benazepril, cilazepril, fosinopril, perindopril, quinapril, ramipril, spirapril) have become popular antihypertensive agents in recent years. They reduce blood pressure by vasodilatation. Cardiac output may improve in patients with impaired myocardial pump function but does not change in individuals with normal cardiac output. The ACE inhibitors prevent the generation of the potent vasoconstrictor angiotensin II and also reduce angiotensin II-stimulated aldosterone secretion. The latter effect is responsible for the blunting of diuretic-induced hypokalemia, which has been observed when these agents are administered (55). Diuretics also increase the antihypertensive efficacy of these drugs. Tuck and associates found that low-dose captopril (25 mg twice daily) was effective as monotherapy in a group of elderly hypertensive patients (56). Forette and colleagues (57) were able to reduce blood pressure using enalapril to less than 160/90 mm Hg in 67 percent of elderly patients 75 to 97 years of age after a period of 8 weeks. Blood pressure fell below 160/90 mm Hg in 35 percent of patients receiving a placebo in this study. The VA trial found that captopril was only slightly more effective than placebo for elderly black men, but it reduced DBP to below 95 mm Hg in 62 percent of the elderly white men who took it (48).

There is evidence that the efficacy of the ACE inhibitors may be less for elderly persons than they are for young patients, although in the VA trial, race was a more impor-

496

tant factor than age (48). Lijnen and colleagues (58) found an inverse correlation between age and the reduction in SBP and DBP in hypertensive patients receiving captopril. Similarly, Vidt (59) noted that enalapril was more effective as monotherapy in patients younger than 55 years of age compared with older individuals. Corea and coworkers (60) compared the blood pressure-lowering effects of captopril (50 mg twice daily) to chlorthalidone (25 mg once daily) in 20 elderly patients. The two regimens were equally effective in reducing blood pressure and were well tolerated. However, chlorthalidone caused a 0.5 mEq/L decrease in serum potassium and a 5.5 mg/dL increase in fasting blood glucose. Captopril did not induce these biochemical changes.

The ACE inhibitors can cause acute renal failure in patients who have severe bilateral renal artery stenosis or severe stenosis in an artery to a solitary kidney (31). This is of concern in elderly patients, who have an increased prevalence of bilateral atherosclerotic renal artery disease. The ACE inhibitors can also cause hypotension in individuals who are volume depleted, are receiving diuretics, or who have high plasma renin levels because of renovascular hypertension. Rash and nonproductive cough are probably the most frequent symptomatic side effects of ACE inhibitor therapy. These agents are particularly useful in the treatment of hypertensive patients with low ejection fractions with or without chronic congestive heart failure (61,62). The cost of the ACE inhibitors may be prohibitive for many elderly patients who have limited incomes.

Calcium Antagonists The calcium antagonists include diltiazem, verapamil, and the dihydropyridines (nifedipine, nicardipine, isradipine, amlodipine, and felodipine). The dihydropyridines are the most potent vasodilating agents and may produce reflex tachycardia and profound blood pressure reduction after acute administration. The dihydropyridines do not produce any significant electrophysiologic effects on the heart and do not reduce cardiac output in vivo. In contrast, verapamil and, to a lesser extent, diltiazem have negative inotropic effects and suppress the cardiac conduction system. They are useful in the management of supraventricular tachyarrhythmias.

In the VA trial, diltiazem successfully lowered DBP to less than 95 mm Hg in more than 70 percent of the black patients, irrespective of age. In the white men, diltiazem was more effective for the elderly (72%) than it was for younger patients (58%) (48). Buhler and coworkers (47) noted that verapamil was more effective for elderly patients than it was for younger hypertensive individuals. Pool and associates (63) reported the results of a multicenter trial using diltiazem. Patients over age 60 had greater antihypertensive responses than did younger patients during the first 6 weeks of the trial, but by the end of 12 weeks, the age-related difference in efficacy was less apparent. It is of note, however, that enhanced efficacy of calcium antagonists in older individuals has not been confirmed in a number of other studies (64,65).

Verapamil and diltiazem should be used with caution in patients receiving beta blockers. Both classes of drugs reduce conduction through the atrioventricular node and reduce myocardial contractility. However, nifedipine has few electrophysiologic effects on the heart and does not usually produce a reduction in cardiac output. For these reasons, combination treatment with nifedipine and a beta blocker seems reasonable.

Side effects of the various calcium antagonists differ. The dihydropyridines and diltiazem can produce headache, palpitations, flushing, edema, and dizziness. Constipation is the most prominent side effect of verapamil. Verapamil and diltiazem are contraindicated for patients who have heart block greater than first degree. Calcium channel blockers have been used in combination with a variety of other antihypertensive agents including diuretics, centrally acting sympatholytic agents, and ACE inhibitors (66–68).

Alpha$_2$ Agonists Some centrally acting sympatholytic agents (clonidine, guanabenz, guanfacine, methyldopa) have been used to treat hypertension in elderly individuals for many years. These agents reduce blood pressure by stimulating alpha$_2$ receptors in the CNS. This results in a reduction of sympathetic outflow and a simultaneous reduction in plasma norepinephrine, blood pressure, and heart rate.

Fatigue, sedation, and dry mouth are the most frequent side effects associated with the centrally acting agents. These effects are particularly troublesome early in treatment but tend to diminish with time. The CNS side effects can be partially avoided by prescribing that most of the total daily dose of these drugs be taken 1 or 2 hours before bedtime. It is reasonable to initiate treatment with a single bedtime dose; if larger doses are required, we usually give approximately one-third of the dose in the morning and two-thirds before bedtime. It is prudent to avoid large doses of the centrally acting agents in the elderly. The reason for this is related to the possibility of a withdrawal rebound hypertension, which is characterized by a pheochromocytoma-like syndrome if the centrally acting agent (especially clonidine) is abruptly discontinued. This may occur in patients who forget to take their drugs or in those who cannot take medications because of an intercurrent illness. Concomitant administration of a diuretic has a dose-sparing effect with all of these agents, which minimizes side effects.

Clonidine is available in a transdermal formulation that provides constant drug delivery over a period of approximately 7 days. This method of administration seems to reduce the incidence of side effects generally seen in patients receiving oral clonidine. However, skin rash localized to the site of the patch can be a problem. The use of transdermal clonidine is theoretically attractive for individuals who have difficulty remembering to take medications daily.

Conclusions

The incidence of ISH or diastolic hypertension is very high for elderly individuals and is associated with an increased risk of cardiovascular disease. Treatment trials have demonstrated a reduction in strokes, myocardial infarctions, and cardiovascular deaths by treating ISH and diastolic hypertension. A number of trials have also demonstrated that elderly patients tolerate antihypertensive agents well.

The hemodynamic characteristics of essential hypertension differ between young and old hypertensive patients, which may influence the response to drug treatment. The clinician must also consider the influence of medication on conditions that coexist with hypertension in elderly patients and the large number of unrelated medications that elderly individuals often ingest.

Lifestyle modifications, particularly weight reduction for obese patients, moderate sodium restriction, and alcohol reduction are useful starting points for treatment of elderly patients with stage 1 ISH and diastolic hypertension. However, the patient must be followed closely to document the efficacy of nonpharmacologic maneuvers. Low doses of thiazide-type diuretics (e.g., 12.5 to 25 mg hydrochlorothiazide or equivalent) are a logical first step for pharmacologic therapy in elderly patients with ISH or diastolic hypertension. These agents are inexpensive, convenient to administer, well tolerated, and have been shown to prevent cardiovascular complications in controlled trials. It is prudent to monitor the patient's serum potassium level after the maximum diuretic dose is achieved, particularly for individuals with organic heart disease or patients receiving digitalis preparations. Although beta blockers tend to be less effective for older black patients than they are for younger hypertensive black patients, these agents may be useful in the treatment of individuals with coronary heart disease. This is particularly true in the first few years after an MI, provided that no contraindications to beta-blocker treatment exist.

Calcium antagonists are also effective antianginal agents and have become popular in the treatment of elderly individuals with high blood pressure. The ACE inhibitors can be used alone or in combination with diuretics, but acute renal failure can occur in patients with severe bilateral renal artery stenosis or severe stenosis of an artery to a solitary kidney. Centrally acting sympatholytic agents may also be useful but tend to produce sedation and dry mouth, particularly early in therapy. The alpha$_1$ receptor-blocking drugs and peripherally acting sympatholytic agents should be used with caution in elderly hypertensive patients because of the propensity to induce orthostatic hypotension.

For older individuals, antihypertensive drugs should be initiated at approximately one-half the usually recommended starting dose. Increments in doses should be smaller than those for younger patients and should be made at longer intervals. Patients' blood pressure should be monitored in both the erect and sitting or supine postures. Evidence from treatment trials clearly demonstrates that elderly individuals with diastolic hypertension (15) and ISH (14) benefit from a carefully monitored antihypertensive treatment regimen and that they tolerate antihypertensive drugs well without adverse effects on quality of life (43,69–71).

References

1. Fifth report of the Joint National Committee on Detection, Evaluation and Treatment of High Blood Pressure. Arch Intern Med 1993;153:154–183.

2. Report of the National High Blood Pressure Education Program Working Group on Hypertension in the Elderly. Hypertension 1994;23:275–285.

3. Centers for Disease Control and Prevention. Second National Health and Nutrition Examination Survey (NHANES II) 1976–1980, Hispanic HANES 1982–1984, and NHANES III 1988–1991. Hyattsville, MD: National Center for Health Statistics, 1992.

4. Hypertension prevalence and the status of awareness, treatment and control in the United States: final report of the subcommittee on Definition and Prevalence of the 1984 Joint National Committee. Hypertension 1985;7:457–468.

5. Kannel WB, Doyle JT, Ostfeld AM, et al. Optimal resources for primary prevention of atherosclerotic diseases: atherosclerosis study group. Circulation 1984;70:153A–205A.

6. Vokonas PS, Kannel WB, Cupples LA. Epidemiology and risk of hypertension in the elderly: the Framingham Study. J Hypertens 1988;6(suppl 1):S3–S9.

7. Kannel WB, Gordon T, Schwartz MJ. Systolic versus diastolic blood pressure and risk of coronary heart disease. Am J Cardiol 1971;27:335–346.

8. Kannel WB, Dawber TR, Sorlie P, Wolf PA. Components of blood pressure and risk of atherothrombotic brain infarction: the Framingham Study. Stroke 1976;7:327–331.

9. Kannel WB, Dawber TR. Hypertension as an ingredient of a cardiovascular risk profile. Br J Hosp Med 1974;11:508–523.

10. Society of Actuaries. Blood Pressure Study 1979. Chicago: Society of Actuaries and Association of Life Insurance Medical Directors of America, 1980.

11. Kannel WB. Implications of Framingham Study data for treatment of hypertension: impact of other risk factors. In: Laragh JH, Buhler FR, Seldin DW, eds. Frontiers in hypertension research. New York: Springer-Verlag, 1981:17.

12. Shekelle RB, Ostfeld AM, Klawans HL Jr. Hypertension and risk of stroke in an elderly population. Stroke 1973;5:71–75.

13. Colandrea MA, Friedman GD, Nichaman MZ, Lind CN. Systolic hypertension in the elderly: an epidemiologic assessment. Circulation 1970;41:239–245.

14. SHEP Cooperative Research Group. Prevention of stroke by antihypertensive drug treatment in older persons with isolated systolic hypertension. Final results of the Systolic Hypertension in the Elderly Program (SHEP). JAMA 1991;265:3255–3264.

15. Insua JT, Sacks HS, Tai-Shing T, et al. Drug treatment of hypertension in the elderly: a meta-analysis. Ann Intern Med 1994;121:355–362.

16. Gifford RW Jr, Borazanian RA. Treatment of hypertension in the elderly. In: Oreopoulos DG, Michelis MF, Herschorn S, eds. Nephrology and urology in the aged patient. The Netherlands: Kluwer, 1993:153–164.

17. Hypertension Detection and Follow-up Program Cooperative Group. Five-year findings of the Hypertension Detection and Follow-up Program, II. Reduction in stroke incidence among persons with high blood pressure. JAMA 1982; 247:633–638.

18. Hypertension Detection and Follow-up Program Cooperative Group. Five-year findings of the Hypertension Detection and Follow-up Program. II. Mortality by race, sex and age. JAMA 1979;242:2572–2577.

19. Borhani NO. Results of clinical trials regarding the efficacy of treating hypertension. Clin Geriatr Med 1989;5:675–690.

20. National Heart Foundation of Australia. Treatment of mild hypertension in the elderly: report by the management committee. Med J Aust 1981;2:398–402.

21. Amery A, Birkenhager W, Brixko P, et al. Mortality and morbidity results from the European Working Party on High Blood Pressure in the Elderly trial. Lancet 1985;1:1349–1354.

22. Amery A, Brixko R, Clement D, et al. Efficacy of antihypertensive drug treatment according to age, sex, blood pressure, and previous cardiovascular disease in patients over the age of 60. Lancet 1986;2:589–592.

23. Coope J, Warrender TS. Randomised trial of treatment in elderly patients in primary care. BMJ 1986;293:1145–1151.

24. Dalhöf B, Lindholm LH, Hansson L, et al. Morbidity and mortality in the Swedish Trial in Old Patients with Hypersion (STOP-Hypertension). Lancet 1991;338:1281–1285.

25. MRC Working Party. Medical Research Council trial of treatment of hypertension in older adults: principal results. BMJ 1992;304:405–412.

26. Hallock P, Benson IC. Studies on the elastic properties of human isolated aorta. J Clin Invest 1937;16:595–602.

27. Page LB. Hypertension and atherosclerosis in primitive and acculturating societies. In: Hunt JS, ed. Hypertension Update. Bloomfield, NJ: Health Learning Systems, 1980:1–12.

28. Tarazi RC, Gifford RW Jr. Clinical significance and mangement of systolic hypertension. In: Onesti G, Brest AN, eds. Hypertension: mechanisms, diagnosis, and treatment. Philadelphia: Davis, 1978:23–30.

29. Cressman MD, Gifford RW Jr. Clinicians' interpretation of the results and implications of the Hypertension Detection and Follow-up Program. Prog Cardiovasc Dis 1986;29(suppl 1):89–97.

30. Koch-Weser J. Correlation of pathophysiology and pharmacotherapy in primary hypertension. Am J Cardiol 1973;32:499–512.

31. Hricik DE, Browning PJ, Kopelman R, et al. Captopril-induced functional renal insufficiency in patients with bilateral renal artery stenoses or renal-artery stenoses in a solitary kidney. N Engl J Med 1983;308:373–376.

32. Messerli FH, Sundgaard-Riise K, Ventura HO, et al. Essential hypertension in the elderly: haemodynamics, intravascular volume, plasma renin activity, and circulating catecholamine levels. Lancet 1983;2:983–986.

33. Shimada K, Kitazumi T, Sadakane N, et al. Age-related changes of baroreflex function, plasma norepinephrine, and blood pressure. Hypertension 1985;7:113–117.

34. Rutan GH, Hermanson B, Bild DE, et al. Orthostatic hypotension in older adults. Hypertension 1992;19:508–519.

35. Peitzman SJ, Berger SR. Postprandial blood pressure decrease in well elderly persons. Arch Intern Med 1989;149:286–288.

36. Gifford RW Jr, Krikendall W, O'Connor DT, Weidman W. Office evaluation of hypertension: a statement for health professionals by a writing group of the Council for High Blood Pressure Research, American Heart Association. Circulation 1989;79:721–731.

37. Messerli FH, Ventura HO, Amadeo C. Osler's maneuver and pseudohypertension. N Engl J Med 1985;312:1548–1551.

38. O'Callaghan WG, Fitzgerald DJ, O'Malley K, et al. Accuracy of indirect blood pressure measurement in the elderly. BMJ 1983;286:1545–1546.

39. Vardan S, Moorkherjee S, Warner R, et al. Systolic hypertension. Direct and indirect BP measurements. Arch Intern Med 1983;143:935–938.

40. Luepker RV, Jacobs DR, Gillum RF, et al. Population risk of cardiovascular disease: the Minnesota heart survey. J Chronic Dis 1985;38:671–682.

41. Applegate WB, Miller ST, Elam JT, et al. Nonpharmacologic intervention to reduce blood pressure in older patients with mild hypertension. Arch Intern Med 1992;152:1162–1166.

42. Kaplan NM. Non-drug treatment of hypertension. Ann Intern Med 1985;102:359–373.

43. Curb JD, Borhani NO, Blaszkowski TP, et al. Long-term surveillance for adverse effects of antihypertensive drugs. JAMA 1985;253:3263–3268.

44. Martin BJ, Milligan K. Diuretic-associated hypomagnesemia in the elderly. Arch Intern Med 1987;147:1768–1771.

45. Whang R, Oei TO, Watanabe A. Frequency of hypomagnesemia in hospitalized patients receiving digitalis. Arch Intern Med 1985;145:655–656.

46. Carlsen JE, Køber L, Torp-Pederson C, Johansen P. Relation between dose of bendrofluazide, antihypertensive effect, and adverse biochemical effects. BMJ 1990;300:975–978.

47. Buhler FR, Hulthen UL, Kiowski W, et al. β-blockers and calcium antagonists: cornerstones of antihypertensive therapy in the 1980s. Drugs 1983;25(suppl 2):50–57.

48. Materson BJ, Reda DJ, Cushman WC, et al. Single-drug therapy for hypertension in men. A comparison of six antihypertensive agents with placebo. N Engl J Med 1993;328:914–921 [published correction, N Engl J Med 1994;330:1689].

49. Perry HM, Hall WD, Benz JR, et al. Efficacy and safety of atenolol, enalapril, and isradipine in elderly hypertensive women. Am J Med 1994;96:77–86.

50. Beta-Blocker Heart Attack Trial Research Group: a randomized trial of propranolol in patients with acute myocardial infarction. I. Mortality results. JAMA 1982;247:1707–1714.

51. Pederson TR, for the Norwegian Multicenter Study Group. Six-year follow-up of the Norwegian Multicenter Study on Timolol After Acute Myocardial Infarction. N Engl J Med 1985;313:1055–1058.

52. Yusuf S, Peto R, Lewis J, et al. Beta blockade during and after myocardial infarction: an overview of the randomized trials. Prog Cardiovasc Dis 1985;27:335–371.

53. Anderson MP, Beschgaard P, Frederiksen J, et al. Effect of alprenolol on mortality among patients with definite or suspected acute myocardial infarction: preliminary results. Lancet 1979;2:865–868.

54. Eisalo A, Virta P. Treatment of hypertension in the elderly with labetalol. Acta Med Scand 1982;665(suppl):129–133.

55. Weinberger MH. Influence of an angiotensin converting-enzyme inhibitor of diuretic-induced metabolic effects in hypertension. Hypertension 1983;5(suppl III):132–138.

56. Tuck ML, Katz LA, Kirkendall WM, et al. Low-dose captopril in mild to moderate geriatric hypertension. J Am Geriatr Soc 1986;34:693–696.

57. Forette F, Handfield-Jones R, Henry-Amar M, et al. Traitement de l'hypertension arterielle du suject âge par un inhibiteur de l'enzyme de conversion: enalapril. Presse Med 1985;14:2237–2247.

58. Lijnen P, Fagard R, Groeseneken D, et al. The hypertensive effect of captopril in hypertensive patients is age-related. Methods Find Exp Clin Pharmacol 1983;5:655–660.

59. Vidt DG. A controlled multiclinic study to compare the antihypertensive effects of MK 421, hydrochlorothiazide, and MK 412 combined with hydrochlorothiazide in patients with mild to moderate essential hypertension. J Hypertens 1984;2(suppl 2):81–88.

60. Corea L, Bentivoglio M, Verdecchia P, Providenza M. Converting enzyme inhibition vs diuretic therapy as first therapeutic approach to the elderly hypertensive patient. Curr Ther Res Clin Exp 1984;36:347–351.

61. The SOLVD Investigators. Effect of enalapril on survival in patients with reduced left ventricular ejection fractions and congestive heart failure. N Engl J Med 1991;325:293–302.

62. Pfeffer MA, Braunwald E, Moye LA, et al. Effect of captopril on mortality and morbidity in patients with left ventricular dysfunction after myocardial infarction. Results of the Survival and Ventricular Enlargement Trial. N Engl J Med 1992;327:669–677.

63. Pool PE, Massie BM, Venkataraman K, et al. Diltiazem as monotherapy for systemic hypertension: a multicenter, randomized, placebo-controlled trial. Am J Cardiol 1986;57:212–217.

64. Hallin L, Andren L, Hausson L. Controlled trial of nifedipine and bendroflumethiazide in hypertension. J Cardiovasc Pharmacol 1983;5:1083–1085.

65. Muiesan G, Agabiti-Rosei E, Castellano M, et al. Antihypertensive and humoral effects of verapamil and nifedipine in essential hypertension. J Cardiovasc Pharmacol 1982;4(suppl 3):325–329.

66. Aoki K, Kondo S, Mochizuki A, et al. Antihypertensive effect of cardiovascular Ca-antagonist in hypertensive patients in

the absence and presence of beta-adrenergic blockade. Am Heart J 1978;96:218–226.

67. Guazzi MD, Fiorentini C, Olivari MT, et al. Short- and long-term efficacy of a calcium antagonist agent (nifedipine) combined with methyldopa in treatment of severe hypertension. Circulation 1980;61:913–919.

68. Guazzi M, De Cesare N, Galli C, et al. Calcium channel blockade with nifedipine and angiotensin-converting enzyme inhibition with captopril in the therapy of patients with severe primary hypertension. Circulation 1984;70:279–284.

69. Goldstein G, Materson BJ, Cushman WC, et al. Treatment of hypertension in the elderly: II. Cognitive and behavioral function. Results of a Department of Veterans Affairs Cooperative Study. Hypertension 1990;15:361–369.

70. Applegate WB, Phillips HL, Schnaper H, et al. A randomized controlled trial of the effects of three antihypertensive agents on blood pressure control and quality of life in older women. Arch Intern Med 1991;151:1817–1823.

71. Gurland BJ, Teresi J, Smith WM, et al. Effects of treatment for isolated systolic hypertension on cognitive status and depression in the elderly. J Am Geriatr Soc 1988;36:1015–1022.

Chapter 37
Peripheral Arterial and Venous Disease

William R. Hiatt and Judith G. Regensteiner

dance mehitabel dance
caper and shake a leg
what little blood is left will fizz like wine in a keg.

Don Marquis
archy and mehitabel

Peripheral Arterial Disease

Peripheral arterial disease (PAD) affects a large number of individuals, with an age-adjusted prevalence of 12 percent (1,2). Approximately 50 percent of patients with PAD diagnosed by noninvasive studies are asymptomatic, 40 percent have intermittent claudication, and only a few percent have severe symptoms of ischemic rest pain, ulceration, or gangrene. Most symptoms of PAD occur with walking exercise when the limited arterial blood supply does not meet the metabolic demand of the muscles in the legs and results in muscle ischemia and the symptom of intermittent claudication. This symptom causes a walking impairment that may profoundly disrupt the activities of daily life. As much as 38 percent of patients younger than age 55 who seek treatment for claudication are disabled and require public assistance (3). In addition, the yearly health care costs of symptomatic PAD in a managed care environment averaged $3100 per patient in 1992 (4). If patients require interventional therapy (surgery, angioplasty, or amputation) the costs increase greatly, with an estimated 30.5 million dollars spent on these patients in 1989 in the state of Maryland alone (5).

Patients with PAD have a relatively stable natural history of their symptom of intermittent claudication (6–8). The history influences treatment decisions. For most patients with claudication as the primary symptom, the major goals are to modify the risk factors of the disease and to relieve the symptom of intermittent claudication and improve walking ability.

PAD Diagnosis

The diagnosis of PAD is often based on the clinical history of intermittent claudication (9) or the physical finding of an abnormal pedal pulse. However, these criteria significantly underestimate the true prevalence of PAD as defined by noninvasive measures of hemodynamics in the lower extremities (10,11). Noninvasive tests include recordings of systolic blood pressures, pulse volumes, and blood flow velocity in the lower extremity. Changes in distal blood pressure or flow occur only with a hemodynamically significant stenosis, and therefore these measures may miss lesser amounts of arterial disease. Newer, noninvasive methods employ duplex scanning of the arteries of the lower extremity in which real-time B-mode imaging provides visualization of the vessel, and Doppler ultrasound measures flow velocity.

Ankle-Brachial Systolic Pressure Index

The measurement of the ankle-brachial systolic pressure index (ABI) requires a Doppler ultrasonic instrument to detect reappearance of flow (systolic pressure) as a cuff is deflated. Systolic blood pressures are measured in each arm, and with a cuff on each ankle, pressures are also measured in the dorsalis pedis and posterior tibial arteries as well. In most patients with PAD, both ankle vessels in the same leg will have an abnormal pressure. Rarely, subjects will have an abnormal pressure in only one vessel of the leg. Causes of low pressures in only one ankle vessel include measurement error (Doppler probe not directly over the artery), vasoconstriction, or diabetes with occlusion of only one tibial artery. In this situation, confirmation of single vessel arterial disease may require more sophisticated testing by duplex ultrasonography. Once pressures are obtained, the ABI is formed from the average pressure in the arms (or the highest arm pressure if there is a greater than 10 mm Hg difference) and the pressure in each ankle vessel. Typically, an abnormal ABI is considered to be less than 0.90 (12).

Localization of arterial disease is determined by measuring Doppler systolic pressures in the thigh, calf, and ankle. In patients with isolated aortoiliac disease there is reduced thigh pressure; patients with isolated femoropopliteal disease have normal thigh pressures, but a pressure drop in the calf and ankle. Patients with disease below the popliteal artery (infrapopliteal) have normal thigh and calf pressures, with decreased ankle pressure. Examples of these patterns are shown in Table 37.1.

Because the ABI has a high sensitivity and specificity for angiographically defined PAD, it can be used in a variety of clinical settings (13,14). In epidemiologic studies, the ankle-arm ratio is an inexpensive and objective test for arterial occlusive disease (15). For example, in a large population-based study, the prevalence of the symptom of claudication (4.5%) underestimated the prevalence of PAD (18.2%) as estimated by the ABI (16). In patients with PAD, an abnormal ABI is a predictor of a markedly increased risk of cardiovascular mortality (17). In a 10-year study, individuals with an ABI less than 0.85 had a 2.36-fold increased risk of mortality, and if the ABI was less than 0.40, the mortality risk was increased 4.49-fold (18). In another long-term study, subjects with PAD (diagnosed by a variety of hemodynamic tests) had a relative risk of all-cause mortality of 3.1, and a risk of cardiovascular mortality of 5.9 (19). Patients with symptomatic or severe PAD were at the highest risk of mortality. Thus, the ABI is a simple and inexpensive measurement that identifies individuals with PAD who are at high risk of cardiovascular morbidity and mortality. Once identified, patients with PAD (whether symptomatic or asymptomatic) should be considered for aggressive treatment of cardiovascular risk factors.

PAD Risk Factors

Diabetes Mellitus

Patients with diabetes have a 2- to 4-fold increased risk of developing intermittent claudication as compared with risk for nondiabetics (20,21). In addition, diabetics tend to have a greater atherosclerotic disease burden, with a more distal distribution of peripheral arterial occlusions, and a worse natural history as compared with these factors for nondiabetics with PAD. Complicating the management of the diabetic with claudication is the associated peripheral neuropathy and a propensity for foot infections. Thus, a multifactorial approach must be taken with these patients.

Although diabetes is a major risk factor for PAD, at the time of presentation the degree of glycemic control as assessed by blood sugar level or glycosylated hemoglobin is not well correlated with the presence or severity of PAD (22). However in the diabetic, the associated risk factors of smoking and hyperlipidemia correlate strongly with disease severity (22,23). Unfortunately, no controlled clinical trials have been performed with diabetics to assess the effects of risk factor modification on the regression of vascular disease. The current available data suggest that excellent glycemic control may not be sufficient, and the clinician must also attempt to address the lipid status and

Table 37.1. Segmental Leg Pressures in the Diagnosis and Localization of PAD.*

	Normal		Aortoiliac		Fem-pop		Infra-pop		Aortoiliac + Fem-pop	
	BP	Ratio	BP	Ratio	BP	Ratio	BP	Ratio	BP	Ratio
Arm	130		130		130		130		130	
Thigh	130	1.00	100	0.77	130	1.00	130	1.00	100	0.77
Calf	130	1.00	100	0.77	90	0.69	130	1.00	70	0.54
Ankle	130	1.00	100	0.77	90	0.69	85	0.65	70	0.54

* Examples of pressure measurements and ankle-brachial systolic blood ratios are shown for different levels of arterial occlusive disease.
BP = blood pressure; fem-pop = femoropopliteal; infra-pop = infrapopliteal.

smoking behaviors of the patient (12). For diabetics, exercise training improves glycemic control and lipid profiles (24). Although exercise programs for diabetics with PAD have not been evaluated, exercise training for these patients may help to relieve claudication symptoms and improve glycemic control and other cardiovascular risk factors.

Hyperlipidemia

The major lipid risk factors for PAD are low high-density lipoprotein (HDL) cholesterol and elevated triglyceride levels (25,26). These findings are important in that a triglyceride elevation is not generally recognized as a cardiovascular risk factor. Several trials have been conducted evaluating the change in femoral atherosclerosis with the treatment of hyperlipidemia. In most studies, cholesterol lowering agents were used as the primary intervention, with niacin added to increase HDL cholesterol. Early studies suggested that lowering of triglycerides or increasing HDL cholesterol was associated with stabilization or regression of femoral atherosclerosis (27–29). More recent trials also support the observation that lipid modification is associated with stabilization or regression of femoral atherosclerosis (30,31). In a recent study, middle-aged men with coronary artery disease were randomized to diet and colestipol-niacin or diet and placebo (31). After 2 years of treatment, both groups had a lowering of low-density lipoprotein (LDL) cholesterol and triglycerides, but only the drug-treated group had an increase in HDL cholesterol. An increase in HDL cholesterol on drug therapy was associated with regression of moderately-diseased arterial segments or disease stabilization. In addition, these drugs may decrease cardiac morbidity and mortality (32).

Cigarette Smoking

In smokers, the risk of developing PAD is increased 2- to 3-fold, and smoking correlates more closely with development of intermittent claudication than any other cardiovascular risk factor (33,34). Patients with PAD who continue to smoke have a greater likelihood of vascular disease progression, myocardial infarction, stroke, and death than those who quit smoking (8). In contrast, smoking cessation is associated with improvement in the

symptoms of claudication and better surgical results (35). In patients with very severe PAD, smoking can cause cutaneous vasoconstriction, which aggravates the healing of ischemic ulcers. Therefore, smoking cessation is critical in the management of the patient with claudication.

Hypertension

Hypertension is an independent risk factor for claudication, raising the risk approximately 2-fold (33). The effects of the treatment of hypertension on the peripheral atherosclerotic disease process have not been evaluated. However, a clinical concern is that the lowering of blood pressure may also lower peripheral perfusion pressure and thereby worsen the symptoms of claudication. To address this question in patients with claudication, we previously conducted a randomized, double-blind trial of the effects of beta-adrenergic blockers on the peripheral circulation. The results demonstrated that both metoprolol and propranolol lowered resting and exercise blood pressure, but did not reduce peripheral blood flow or increase leg vascular resistance (36). Also, these patients did not have worsening symptoms of claudication during exercise. This study, and others, have concluded that patients with claudication may be safely treated with any class of drugs for hypertension. However, when drug therapy results in a large decrease in systemic blood pressure, some patients may experience a slight worsening of their claudication symptoms (37).

Homocysteine

Recently, several reports have shown a strong association between increases in plasma homocysteine concentration and PAD (38). This may be an important risk factor for patients younger than age 50 who present with claudication. However, screening for this disorder is not routinely available, and no therapeutic interventions have been evaluated.

Other Risk Factor Treatments

Other therapies have been targeted to slow the progression of peripheral atherosclerosis and to decrease cardiovascular mortality, such as the Physician's Health Study, in which low doses of aspirin were shown to reduce the relative risk of subsequent peripheral arterial surgery to

0.54 as compared with the effect of placebo (39). Aspirin combined with dipyridamole has also been shown to slow the progression of femoral atherosclerosis (40). Probucol is an antioxidant agent that is under investigation in the Probucol Quantitative Regression Swedish Trial (PQRST) as a means to treat femoral atherosclerosis, with the primary results still pending (41). These studies demonstrate that a multifactorial approach may be necessary to alter the natural history of peripheral atherosclerosis.

Drug Therapy for Claudication

Vasodilators
Arteriolar vasodilators were the first class of agents used to treat claudication. Examples include drugs that inhibit the sympathetic nervous system (alpha blockers), direct-acting vasodilators (papaverine), beta$_2$ agonists (nylidrine), and calcium channel blockers (nifedipine). These drugs have not been shown to have clinical efficacy in randomized, controlled trials (37,42). There are several theoretical reasons why vasodilators are not effective. In patients with PAD, the main determinant of arterial flow and oxygen delivery to skeletal muscle is the amount of large vessel arterial occlusive disease. Therefore, drugs that dilate arterioles distal to the large vessel occlusions do not augment blood flow. In addition, these drugs may create a steal phenomena by dilating vessels in normally perfused tissue and thus shunt blood away from the diseased circulation. Therefore, as a class of drugs, vasodilators are not recommended for claudication.

Anticoagulant and Antiplatelet Drugs
As discussed above, the use of aspirin and other antiplatelet agents may be important factors in the long-term treatment of peripheral atherosclerosis. Combinations of low-dose aspirin and low-dose warfarin are under investigation as agents to reduce cardiovascular mortality in patients with PAD. These drugs are also used in selected patients after bypass surgery to prevent graft thrombosis. However, studies that have evaluated the effects of aspirin or warfarin on the treatment of claudication have shown no benefit (43). Ticlopidine is a potent inhibitor of platelet aggregation that also has hemorrheologic effects. In one randomized, placebo-controlled trial, ticlopidine was shown to improve claudication symptoms and exercise performance (44).

Hemorrheologic Agents
Patients with PAD have been shown to have non-deformable red cells, elevated fibrinogen levels, and increased platelet aggregation, which leads to increased blood viscosity. The extent to which these phenomena reduce large vessel blood flow or flow in the microcirculation is unknown. Pentoxifylline improves red cell deformability, lowers fibrinogen levels, decreases platelet aggregation, and has been shown to increase walking distance in patients with PAD. In early controlled trials, the drug produced a 22 percent improvement over placebo in walking distance before the onset of claudication and a 12 percent improvement in the maximal walking distance (45). More recent studies have suggested that patients with symptoms for longer than 1 year and an ankle-arm systolic blood pressure ratio less than 0.80 comprise the subgroup most likely to respond to the drug (46).

Ketanserin is a selective serotonin (S$_2$) antagonist that lowers blood viscosity and also has vasodilator and antiplatelet properties. However, in controlled trials, this drug was not effective in treating claudication (47).

Metabolic Agents
Patients with PAD not only have a limited arterial blood flow, but also develop metabolic abnormalities in their skeletal muscle. Changes in carnitine metabolism are an example of the altered metabolic state observed in patients with PAD. Carnitine is an important cofactor for skeletal muscle intermediary metabolism during exercise. Carnitine is required for the mitochondrial oxidation of long-chain fatty acids and also helps to maintain normal cellular metabolism under conditions of metabolic or hypoxic stress (48). Patients with PAD have been shown to accumulate acylcarnitines (intermediates of oxidative metabolism) in their skeletal muscle (49). Abnormal accumulation of acylcarnitines is directly correlated with impaired exercise performance. Thus, it has been hypothesized that supplementation of patients with carnitine would improve ischemic muscle metabolism. Carnitine,

and an acyl form of carnitine (propionyl-L-carnitine), are experimental drugs that have been shown to increase exercise performance and improve claudication symptoms in patients with PAD (50,51). However, further investigation is necessary to fully establish the role of carnitine supplementation in treating patients with claudication.

Other metabolic factors that may be addressed in PAD include modification of the balance between fatty acids and carbohydrates as substrates for ischemic skeletal muscle. Although fatty acids are a plentiful source of energy, they require relatively more oxygen than carbohydrates for complete oxidation. The adenosine triphosphate (ATP)-oxygen ratio is 5.7 for fatty acids and 6.3 for glucose. Thus, when oxygen is limited as it is during claudication, a shift towards carbohydrate metabolism would be favorable in terms of ATP production. Several agents are now under investigation that modify substrate utilization in patients with claudication.

Other Claudication Drugs

Aminophylline inhibits adenosine receptors and thus may blunt the vasodilation response during exercise. This effect would theoretically limit the stealing of blood away from ischemic skeletal muscle. One study has shown that intravenous aminophylline improves treadmill exercise performance in patients with claudication (52).

Chelation therapy has been touted as a means to treat atherosclerosis and relieve symptoms of cardiovascular disease. However, there is no scientific basis to support these claims. One randomized, double-blind, multicenter trial has been conducted of edetic acid (EDTA) in patients with PAD (53). The drug was not shown to be effective in treating the symptoms of claudication or in improving the ABI.

Exercise Rehabilitation for Claudication

Exercise rehabilitation is an established and highly effective intervention for the treatment of claudication. Several controlled trials of exercise training have been conducted during the past 30 years. All studies of exercise treatment for claudication have reported an increase in treadmill exercise performance and a lessening of claudication pain severity during exercise (54–64). This consistent finding demonstrates that exercise training programs have a clinically important impact on functional capacity in patients

for whom other treatment options are limited and in whom spontaneous recovery does not occur. In addition, there is virtually no morbidity or mortality from exercise training.

A hospital-based, supervised treadmill exercise program is the most effective mode of exercise therapy for patients with claudication. The exercise sessions are typically held 3 times a week for approximately 1 hour each session, and 3-month periods of training are customary. Telemetry monitoring is not routinely used except for patients with clinical coronary disease or arrhythmias. A 5-minute warm-up period is used to increase the patient's heart rate slowly and promote flexibility, and should involve the use of large muscle groups, especially those muscles used for walking. At the end of the class there is a 5-minute cool-down period that involves stretching of the large muscle groups of the legs.

The beginning training workload is determined from the symptom-limited, maximal treadmill test on entry, such that the intensity of the treadmill exercise is set to the workload that initially brings on claudication pain in the patient. In subsequent visits, the speed or grade is increased if the patient is able to walk for 10 minutes or longer at the lower workload without reaching moderate claudication pain. Either speed or grade can be increased, but an increase in grade is recommended first if the patient can already walk at 2 miles per hour (mph). An additional goal of the program is to increase patient walking speed up to the normal 3.0 mph from the average PAD patient walking speed of 1.5 to 2.0 mph.

The initial training session is 35 minutes long with subsequent increases of 5 minutes each session until a 50-minute session is possible. During the exercise sessions, the patient walks on the treadmill until a mild or moderate level of pain is reached, and then has a rest period until the pain abates. After the pain is gone, the patient resumes walking until a moderate level of claudication pain is again reached, which is followed by another rest period. This process is repeated until the 50-minute exercise period has elapsed. In our experience, actual treadmill exercise comprises about 35 minutes, and rest periods total about 15 minutes of the 50-minute exercise time.

In previous trials of exercise training, the improvement in pain-free walking time on the treadmill ranged from 44 percent to 290 percent, with an average increase of 134 percent. The peak walking time increased from 25 percent to 183 percent, with an average increase of 96 percent. Thus, the ability to sustain walking exercise for longer durations with less claudication pain is improved by training. At the University of Colorado we have conducted a controlled trial of exercise conditioning for patients with claudication (65). Patients in the treated group were given a supervised, progressive treadmill walking program of 12 weeks' duration (36 1-hour sessions). Control subjects were asked to maintain their usual level of activity. Treated subjects increased their maximal walking time on a graded treadmill protocol by 123 percent and their peak oxygen consumption by 30 percent. Pain-free walking time on the treadmill increased by 165 percent. The control group had a 20 percent increase in peak walking time but no change in peak oxygen consumption or pain-free walking time.

The functional benefits of the training were further assessed by a walking impairment questionnaire (66). This analysis demonstrated that in the community, treated subjects could walk a greater distance, at a faster speed, and thus perform activities that had been considered difficult to impossible before the treatment (e.g., returning to work, dancing, doing outdoor activities, and shopping). Control subjects had no change in their level of disability (from questionnaire evaluations) during the course of the study. Thus, a progressive, walking-exercise program improved exercise performance, relieved the pain of intermittent claudication, and facilitated the ability to perform personal, social, and occupational activities.

Invasive Therapies for PAD

In patients with severe forms of PAD (ischemic pain at rest, nonhealing ulcers, and gangrene), peripheral bypass surgery is indicated to restore blood flow for tissue healing and limb salvage (67,68). In addition, bypass surgery or percutaneous transluminal angioplasty is recommended for patients with claudication if the symptoms limit occupational, social, or leisure-time activities (69–74). However, because most patients with claudication remain stable longer than 5 years (6,75), there are no uniform criteria defining when an invasive procedure is necessary in patients with claudication. Currently, practice standards vary widely, some institutions do not offer surgery for the treatment of claudication. In contrast, most reports indicate that 15 percent to 30 percent of peripheral bypass operations are for claudication (72,73,76,77), but this rate is as high as 70 percent to 80 percent in some institutions (78,79).

The most widely studied outcomes of invasive therapy have been long-term graft patency rates. In patients with aortoiliac disease, the 5-year graft patency is 89 percent, and the surgical mortality is 4.4 percent, with a morbidity of 11.4 percent (80). Patency rates for angioplasty are only 63 percent for a period of 5 years for aortoiliac disease, with a mortality of 0.2 percent and a morbidity of 2.3 percent (80). However, in other series, angioplasty had higher complication rates (79,81). For femoralpopliteal disease, surgery has a 5-year patency of 60 percent, mortality of 2.6 percent, and morbidity of 6.7 percent. With angioplasty for femoralpopliteal disease, the 5-year patency rate is only 40 percent to 60 percent, but morbidity and mortality rates are low and are similar to that described for aortoiliac angioplasty (81).

It is important to note that surgical graft patency rates do not necessarily translate into improved function. For patients in which functional evaluation has been performed, bypass surgery improved treadmill walking time and muscle function. However, the few studies that have been performed show that patients treated with surgery still have claudication and limited activity (57,63,82). The surgical risks and costs of a peripheral bypass operation for claudication may decrease the enthusiasm of the patient or referring physician to recommend surgery. It is estimated that the physician and facility fees for a peripheral bypass operation are $16,100 for the initial hospitalization alone (5).

Summary

Patients with intermittent claudication have cardiovascular risk factors that are distinct from those of patients with coronary and cerebrovascular disease. Recognition and modification of these risk factors are critical in the medical management of the patient with PAD. The medical treatments of claudication are limited to very few drugs, with pentoxifylline the only approved agent in the United States. However, an exercise rehabilitation program is a very effective means to treat claudication and should be recommended for all ambulatory patients.

Deep Vein Thrombophlebitis

Venous thromboembolism (DVT) is a major health problem in the United States. This is particularly true for patients undergoing surgery, in which the incidence of DVT is 25 percent to 50 percent and for fatal pulmonary emboli is 1 percent. Pulmonary emboli account for 12 percent of all deaths in acute care hospitals (83). Risk factors for DVT include age older than 40 years, malignant disease, congestive heart failure, obesity, acute paraplegia, trauma, varicose veins, and a history of thrombophlebitis, estrogens, hypercoagulable states, myocardial infarction, and immobilization.

Interventions to reduce the risk of DVT can be directed to intensive surveillance of high-risk groups with noninvasive techniques or prophylaxis. Prophylaxis is favored because surveillance is expensive, pulmonary emboli may not be effectively prevented by anticoagulants once venous thrombosis is present, and some cases may be missed by the noninvasive techniques.

DVT Prophylaxis

Mechanical

After patients have had surgical procedures, ambulation, leg elevation, and use of elastic stockings do not reliably reduce the risk of DVT. However, patients who are discharged from surgery within 4 days are at less risk of DVT than are those who remain 5 days or more. However, this may be a result of the nature of the underlying disease and the severity of illness rather than from the effects of early ambulation.

Use of external pneumatic compression stockings has been extensively studied and is of benefit in low-to-moderate-risk, general surgical, neurosurgical, urologic, and orthopedic patients. The results are similar to those for use of low-dose heparin, with a 3-fold reduction in the incidence of DVT in treated patients. Pneumatic compression decreases venous stasis and activates the fibrinolytic system.

Low-Dose Heparin

Heparin prophylaxis has been used for more than 20 years in both medical and surgical patients (84–86). In low doses, heparin prevents the coagulation cascade by enhancing the action of antithrombin III. The results of several controlled trials of low-dose heparin in surgical patients has shown a 3-fold reduction in DVT (from 25% to 7%) and a 10-fold reduction in pulmonary emboli (from 6.0% to 0.6%). The drug can be given as 5000 units every 8 to 12 hours. The two dosing schedules are equivalent, but more frequent dosing may result in increased bleeding complications. Low-dose heparin is ineffective for orthopedic and urologic surgery and should be avoided for neurosurgery.

Dihydroergotamine-Heparin

Dihydroergotamine (DHE) is an ergot derivative that, when given in low doses, is primarily a venoconstrictor. Administration of the drug is designed to prevent venous stasis, but when the drug is used alone, it is not an effective prophylactic agent. One large, controlled clinical trial in elective abdominal, pelvic, and thoracic surgery compared use of 5000 U heparin with 0.5 mg DHE with use of heparin alone or placebo (41). All drugs were given subcutaneously every 12 hours. The rates of DVT were 25 percent for placebo, 17 percent for heparin alone (not significant) and 9 percent for the combination of heparin and DHE ($p < 0.001$). It is therefore possible that the combination of drugs may be more effective than heparin alone, but more data are needed. Patients with angina, recent myocardial infarction, hypertension, peripheral vascular disease, or sepsis should not receive DHE. In these patients, heparin alone would be safer.

Low Molecular Weight Heparin

Low molecular weight heparin (LMWH) is derived from standard, unfractionated heparin. LMWH has a higher bioavailability, longer plasma half-life, and more consistent anticoagulant effect than standard heparin. These properties allow LMWH to be administered once or twice daily at a weight-adjusted dose, without need for laboratory monitoring or dose adjustment. LMWH may be associated with less bleeding and thrombocytopenia than standard heparin, but further investigation is needed to confirm these potential advantages.

As described above, standard low-dose heparin prophylaxis after general surgery is safe and effective. Because LMWH is more expensive than standard heparin, standard heparin is usually preferred for prophylaxis against DVT. However, several studies have compared

LMWH with standard heparin for patients at high risk for DVT. For patients undergoing abdominal or pelvic surgery for malignancy, LMWH and standard low-dose heparin are equally effective, but LMWH may have a reduced rate of bleeding (87). Further clinical trials are needed to address the safety and efficacy of LMWH prophylaxis for DVT in patients with malignancies. LMWH also prevents DVT in patients undergoing total hip replacement, with a risk reduction similar to that for warfarin therapy (88). For patients undergoing total knee replacement, LMWH is also effective when used with external pneumatic compression stockings (89,90).

Warfarin

Warfarin inhibits the synthesis of activated clotting factors II, VII, IX, and X. Although warfarin is effective for patients at very high risk for DVT, such as those undergoing hip surgery, the major complication is bleeding, which may occur as often as 20 percent of the time. When warfarin is used for prophylaxis, different strategies have been employed. The most aggressive approach is to start the drug preoperatively in therapeutic doses. Alternatively, warfarin may be given in low doses before surgery with an increased dose after surgery, or started only after surgery.

Dextran

Dextran decreases blood viscosity and platelet adhesiveness, and promotes fibrin degradation. Dextran 40 is given as a 500 to 1000 mL 10% solution during 6 hours starting on the day of surgery and then daily for as long as 5 days postoperatively. Dextran is used mainly for hip surgery, it is not as effective as warfarin, but is better than other agents. Serious side effects include volume expansion and anaphylactic reactions.

Acute Treatment of DVT

Thrombolytic Agents

Streptokinase and urokinase are plasminogen activators and induce a lytic state. They are most useful in extensive thrombotic disease, e.g., iliofemoral or subclavian vein thrombosis with extension into the vena cava. Studies have shown that these drugs are more effective than heparin in lysing clot and preserving venous valves.

The evidence that they prevent postphlebitic syndrome is not yet conclusive. These drugs are contraindicated for patients with recent surgery and intracranial neoplasms.

Heparin

Heparin remains the standard anticoagulant used in the initial treatment of acute, proximal DVT. Critical in the use of heparin is prompt and adequate anticoagulation of the patient presenting with DVT. In a recent study, 120 outpatients with proximal vein thrombosis were randomized to initial anticoagulation with acenocoumarol (a warfarin drug) alone and compared with patients receiving heparin followed by acenocoumarol (91). As expected, 40 percent of patients treated with acenocoumarol only had extension of clot during the first week of therapy as compared with 8 percent in the heparin-acenocoumarol group. The recurrence rate of DVT in the patients anticoagulated with acenocoumarol alone was also unacceptably high during 6 months of follow-up. This study has important implications for the initial treatment of DVT. In a recent survey of physician practices, 60 percent of patients presenting with DVT or pulmonary emboli were inadequately anticoagulated with heparin during the first 24 hours of hospitalization (92). Failure to adequately anticoagulate patients early in the course of the phlebitis may predispose them to clot extension and high rates of recurrence of DVT.

Once the patient is adequately anticoagulated on heparin, treatment needs to be continued for at least 5 days. In a recent study, 199 patients with DVT were randomized to 5 days compared with 10 days of heparin (93). The rates of bleeding complications and recurrent DVT during follow-up were the same for both groups, which suggests that 5 days of heparin is adequate and may also save hospital costs. When heparin is given for 5 days, it is important to begin warfarin immediately after the patient is adequately anticoagulated by heparin because it takes 4 to 5 days for warfarin to deplete activated clotting factors, particularly factor II.

A concern with the use of heparin is the development of thrombocytopenia. This complication usually occurs after 6 to 12 days of therapy and is reversible (94). Bovine heparin is more often associated with thrombocytopenia than is porcine heparin.

Chronic Management of DVT

Warfarin

Oral anticoagulants are usually given for 3 to 6 months after DVT. An important aspect of the monitoring of warfarin therapy is the use of the International Normalization Ratio (INR). The INR has been standard in Europe for many years, but its use has only recently become common practice in the United States. In a survey of coagulation laboratories, only 21 percent reported prothrombin times with the INR, but the INR is now more commonplace (95). For patients with DVT, recent work has shown that lower doses of warfarin are equally effective as the standard doses in preventing recurrent DVT, yet have a reduced risk of hemorrhage (96). Current recommendations are to maintain the INR at 2.0 to 3.0 with chronic warfarin therapy.

Heparin

For patients who cannot tolerate warfarin or who are in the first trimester of pregnancy, chronic treatment with heparin is acceptable. Patients are treated with a twice-a-day dose, adjusted so that the partial thromboplastin time is 1.5 times the control value (97). Under these conditions, heparin is as effective for DVT as full-dose warfarin.

Calf DVT

There remains a strong bias not to treat patients with isolated calf DVT with long-term anticoagulation because these patients have a low risk of embolization. However, choosing to not anticoagulate patients who have calf DVT may have serious consequences. In one study of patients with calf DVT, patients randomized to initial heparin therapy which was followed by 3 months of warfarin therapy had a 2 percent rate of DVT recurrence during a 12-month follow-up period (98). In contrast, those who received no therapy had a 29 percent rate of DVT recurrence and a 4 percent rate of pulmonary emboli. A review of the literature concluded that anticoagulation of symptomatic calf DVT prevents clot extension, embolization, and recurrence (99). Therefore, most patients with symptomatic calf vein DVT should be treated the same as patients with proximal vein DVT.

Summary

Venous thromboembolism is a common problem, particularly for hospitalized patients. The appropriate use of prophylactic agents designed to reduce the risk of DVT not only decreases morbidity and mortality, but also reduces health care costs. Prevention of DVT may be the only effective means to avert the development of the postphlebitic syndrome. Once a patient presents with DVT, prompt and adequate dosing with heparin remains the treatment of choice for most patients. Wafarin therapy should be monitored long-term with the INR.

References

1. Hiatt WR, Marshall JA, Baxter J, et al. Diagnostic methods for peripheral arterial disease in the San Luis Valley Diabetes Study. J Clin Epidemiol 1990;43:597–606.
2. Criqui MH, Fronek A, Barrett-Connor E, et al. The prevalence of peripheral arterial disease in a defined population. Circulation 1985;71:510–515.
3. Olsen PS, Gustafsen J, Rasmussen L, Lorentzen JE. Long-term results after arterial surgery for arteriosclerosis of the lower limbs in young adults. Eur J Vasc Surg 1988;2:15–18.
4. Stergachis A, Sheingold S, Luce BR, et al. Medical care and cost outcomes after pentoxifylline treatment for peripheral arterial disease. Arch Intern Med 1992;152:1220–1224.
5. Tunis SR, Bass EB, Steinberg EP. The use of angioplasty, bypass surgery, and amputation in the management of peripheral vascular disease. N Engl J Med 1991;325:556–562.
6. Jelnes R, Gaardsting O, Hougaard Jensen K, et al. Fate in intermittent claudication: outcome and risk factors. BMJ 1986;293:1137–1140.
7. Singer A, Rob C. The fate of the claudicator. BMJ 1960;633–636.
8. Juergens JL, Barker NW, Hines EA. Arteriosclerosis obliterans: a review of 520 cases with special reference to pathogenic and prognostic factors. Circulation 1960;21:188–195.
9. Rose GA, Blackburn H. Cardiovascular survey methods. Geneva: WHO monograph Series No. 56, 1968:172–175.
10. Criqui MH, Fronek A, Klauber MR, et al. The sensitivity, specificity, and predictive value of traditional clinical evaluation of peripheral arterial disease: results from noninvasive testing in a defined population. Circulation 1985;71:516–522.
11. Marinelli MR, Beach KW, Glass MJ, et al. Noninvasive testing vs clinical evaluation of arterial disease. A prospective study. JAMA 1979;241:2031–2034.
12. Orchard TJ, Strandness DE, Cavanagh PR, et al. Assessment of peripheral vascular disease in diabetes. Report and recommendations of an international workshop. Circulation 1993;88:819–828.
13. Carter SA. Indirect systolic pressures and pulse waves in arterial occlusive disease of the lower extremities. Circulation 1968;37:624–637.

14. Ouriel K, McDonnel AE, Metz AE, Zarins CK. A critical evaluation of stress testing in the diagnosis of peripheral vascular disease. Surgery 1982;91:686–693.

15. Fowkes FGR. The measurement of atherosclerotic peripheral arterial disease in epidemiological surveys. Int J Epidemiol 1988;17:248–254.

16. Fowkes FGR, Housley E, Cawood EHH, et al. Edinburgh Artery Study: prevalence of asymptomatic and symptomatic peripheral arterial disease in the general population. Int J Epidemiol 1991;20:384–392.

17. Dormandy JA, Murray GD. The fate of the claudicant–a prospective study of 1969 claudicants. Eur J Vasc Surg 1991;5:131–133.

18. McKenna M, Wolfson S, Kuller L. The ratio of ankle and arm arterial pressure as an independent predictor of mortality. Atherosclerosis 1991;87:119–128.

19. Criqui MH, Langer RD, Fronek A, et al. Mortality over a period of 10 years in patients with peripheral arterial disease. N Engl J Med 1992;326:381–386.

20. Kannel WB, McGee DL. Diabetes and cardiovascular disease: the Framingham Study. JAMA 1979;241:2035–2038.

21. Brand FN, Abbott RD, Kannel WB. Diabetes, intermittent claudication, and risk of cardiovascular events. Diabetes 1989;38:504–509.

22. Beach KW, Strandness DE. Arteriosclerosis obliterans and associated risk factors in insulin-dependent and non-insulin-dependent diabetes. Diabetes 1980;29:882–888.

23. Reunanen A, Takkunen H, Aromaa A. Prevalence of intermittent claudication and its effect on mortality. Acta Med Scand 1991;211:249–256.

24. Ronnemaa T, Mattila K, Lehtonen A, Kallio V. A controlled randomized study on the effect of long-term physical exercise on the metabolic control in type 2 diabetic patients. Acta Med Scand 1986;220:219–224.

25. Pomrehn P, Duncan B, Weissfeld L, et al. The association of dyslipoproteinemia with symptoms and signs of peripheral arterial disease. The lipids research clinics program prevalence study. Circulation 1986;73(suppl 1):1-100–1-107.

26. Montanari G, Vaccarino V, Franeschini G, et al. Metabolic approach to the diagnosis and treatment of atherosclerotic peripheral vascular disease. Int Angiol 1987;6:339–349.

27. Blankenhorn DH, Brooks SH, Selzer RH, Barndt R. The rate of atherosclerosis change during treatment of hyperlipoproteinemia. Circulation 1978;57:355–361.

28. Ost CR, Stenson S. Regression of peripheral atherosclerosis during therapy with high doses of nicotinic acid. Scand J Clin Lab Invest 1967;93(suppl):241–245.

29. Duffield RGM, Miller NE, Brunt JNH, et al. Treatment of hyperlipidaemia retards progression of symptomatic femoral atherosclerosis. A randomised controlled trial. Lancet 1983;2:639–642.

30. Olsson AG, Ruhn G, Erikson U. The effect of serum lipid regulation on the development of femoral atherosclerosis in hyperlipidaemia: A non-randomised controlled study. J Int Med 1990;227:381–390.

31. Blankenhorn DH, Azen SP, Crawford DW, et al. Effects of colestipol-niacin therapy on human femoral atherosclerosis. Circulation 1991;83:438–447.

32. Frick MH, Elo O, Haapa K, et al. Helsinki Heart Study: primary-prevention trial with gemfibrozil in middle-aged men with dyslipidemia. Safety of treatment, changes in risk factors, and incidence of coronary heart disease. N Engl J Med 1987;317:1237–1245.

33. Kannel WB, McGee DL. Update on some epidemiologic features of intermittent claudication: the Framingham study. J Am Geriatr Soc 1985;33:13–18.

34. Gofin R, Kark JD, Friedlander Y, et al. Peripheral vascular disease in a middle-aged population sample. The Jerusalem lipid research clinic prevalence study. Isr J Med Sci 1987; 23:157–167.

35. Krupski WC. The peripheral vascular consequences of smoking. Ann Vasc Surg 1991;5:291–304.

36. Hiatt WR, Stoll S, Nies AS. Effect of β-adrenergic blockers on the peripheral circulation in patients with peripheral vascular disease. Circulation 1985;72:1226–1231.

37. Solomon SA, Ramsay LE, Yeo WW. β-blockade and intermittent claudication: placebo-controlled trial of atenolol and nifedipine and their combination. BMJ 1991;303:1100–1104.

38. Clarke R, Daly L, Robinson K, et al. Hyperhomocysteinemia: an independent risk factor for vascular disease. N Engl J Med 1991;324:1149–1155.

39. Goldhaber SZ, Manson JE, Stampfer MJ, et al. Low-dose aspirin and subsequent peripheral arterial surgery in the physicians' health study. Lancet 1992;340:143–145.

40. Hess H, Deichsel G, Mietaschk A. Drug-induced inhibition of platelet function delays progression of peripheral occlusive arterial disease. A prospective double-blind arteriographically controlled trial. Lancet 1985;1:415–419.

41. Walldius G, Regnstrom J, Nilsson J, et al. The role of lipids and antioxidative factors for development of atherosclerosis. The Probucol Quantitative Regression Swedish Trial (PQRST). Am J Cardiol 1993;71:15B–19B.

42. Coffman JD. Vasodilator drugs in peripheral vascular disease. N Engl J Med 1979;300:713–717.

43. Deutschinoff A, Grozdinsky L. Rheological and anticoagulant therapy of patients with chronic peripheral occlusive arterial disease (COAD). Angiology 1987;38:351–357.

44. Balsano F, Coccheri S, Libretti A, et al. Ticlopidine in the treatment of intermittent claudication: a 21-month double-blind trial. J Lab Clin Med 1989;114:84–91.

45. Porter JM, Cutler BS, Lee BY, et al. Pentoxifylline efficacy in the treatment of intermittent claudication: multicenter controlled double-blind trial with objective assessment of chronic occlusive arterial disease patients. Am Heart J 1982;104:66–72.

46. Lindgarde F, Jelnes R, Bjorkman H, et al. Conservative drug treatment in patients with moderately severe chronic occlusive peripheral arterial disease. Circulation 1989;80:1549–1556.

47. PACK Claudication Substudy Investigators. Randomized, placebo-controlled, double-blind trial of ketanserin in claudi-

cants. Changes in claudication distance and ankle systolic pressure. Circulation 1989;80:1544–1548.

48. Bieber LL. Carnitine. Ann Rev Biochem 1988;57:261–283.

49. Hiatt WR, Wolfel EE, Regensteiner JG, Brass EP. Skeletal muscle carnitine metabolism in patients with unilateral peripheral arterial disease. J Appl Physiol 1992;73:346–353.

50. Brevetti G, Chiariello M, Ferulano G, et al. Increases in walking distance in patients with peripheral vascular disease treated with L-carnitine: a double-blind, cross-over study. Circulation 1988;77:767–773.

51. Brevetti G, Perna S, Sabba C, et al. Superiority of L-propionyl carnitine vs L-carnitine in improving walking capacity in patients with peripheral vascular disease: an acute, intravenous, double-blind, cross-over study. Eur Heart J 1992; 13:251–255.

52. Picano E, Testa R, Pogliani M, et al. Increase of walking capacity after acute aminophylline administration in intermittent claudication. Angiology 1989;40:1035–1039.

53. Guldager B, Jelnes R, Jorgensen SJ, et al. EDTA treatment of intermittent claudication–a double blind, placebo-controlled study. J Int Med 1992;231:261–267.

54. Lundgren F, Dahllof AG, Schersten T, Bylund-Fellenius AC. Muscle enzyme adaptation in patients with peripheral arterial insufficiency: spontaneous adaptation, effect of different treatments and consequences on walking performance. Clin Sci 1989;77:485–493.

55. Mannarino E, Pasqualini L, Menna M, et al. Effects of physical training on peripheral vascular disease: a controlled study. Angiology 1989;40:5–10.

56. Creasy TS, McMillan PJ, Fletcher EWL, et al. Is percutaneous transluminal angioplasty better than exercise for claudication? Preliminary results from a prospective randomised trial. Eur J Vasc Surg 1990:4:135–140.

57. Hedberg B, Langstrom M, Angquist KA, Fugl-Meyer AR. Isokinetic plantar flexor performance and fatigability in peripheral arterial insufficiency. Acta Chir Scand 1988;154:363–369.

58. Dahllof A, Holm J, Schersten T, Sivertsson R. Peripheral arterial insufficiency. Effect of physical training on walking tolerance, calf blood flow, and blood flow resistance. Scand J Rehab Med 1976;8:19–26.

59. Dahllof A, Bjorntorp P, Holm J, Schersten T. Metabolic activity of skeletal muscle in patients with peripheral arterial insufficiency. Effect of physical training. Eur J Clin Invest 1974;4:9–15.

60. Larsen OA, Lassen NA. Effect of daily muscular exercise in patients with intermittent claudication. Lancet 1966;2:1093–1096.

61. Ericsson B, Haeger K, Lindell SE. Effect of physical training on intermittent claudication. Angiology 1970;21:188–192.

62. Ernst EEW, Matrai A. Intermittent claudication, exercise, and blood rheology. Circulation 1987;76:1110–1114.

63. Lundgren F, Dahllof A, Lundholm K, et al. Intermittent claudication–surgical reconstruction or physical training? A prospective randomized trial of treatment efficiency. Ann Surg 1989;209:346–355.

64. Mannarino E, Pasqualini L, Innocente S, et al. Physical training and antiplatelet treatment in stage II peripheral arterial occlusive disease: alone or combined? Angiology 1991; 42:513–521.

65. Hiatt WR, Regensteiner JG, Hargarten ME, et al. Benefit of exercise conditioning for patients with peripheral arterial disease. Circulation 1990;81:602–609.

66. Regensteiner JG, Steiner JF, Panzer RJ, Hiatt WR. Evaluation of walking impairment by questionnaire in patients with peripheral arterial disease. J Vasc Med Biol 1990;2: 142–152.

67. Blair JM, Gewertz BL, Moosa H, et al. Percutaneous transluminal angioplasty versus surgery for limb-threatening ischemia. J Vasc Surg 1989;9:698–703.

68. Veith FJ, Gupta SK, Wengerter KR, et al. Changing arteriosclerotic disease patterns and management strategies in lower-limb-threatening ischemia. Ann Surg 1990;212:402–412.

69. Rutherford RB. Evaluation and selection of patients for vascular surgery. In: Rutherford RB, ed. Vascular surgery. Philadelphia: Saunders, 1984:11–18.

70. Health and Public Policy Committee American College of Physicians. Percutaneous transluminal angioplasty. Ann Intern Med 1983;99:864–869.

71. Wexler L. Percutaneous transluminal angioplasty of peripheral vascular occlusions: a clinical perspective. J Am Coll Cardiol 1989;13:1555–1557.

72. Donaldson MC, Mannick JA. Femoropopliteal bypass grafting for intermittent claudication. Arch Surg 1980;115:724–727.

73. Myhre HO. Is femoropopliteal bypass surgery indicated for the treatment of intermittent claudication? Acta Chir Scand Suppl 1990;555:39–42.

74. Jamieson C. The management of intermittent claudication. Practitioner 1988;232:613–616.

75. Imparato AM, Kim GE, Davidson T, Crowley JG. Intermittent claudication: its natural course. Surgery 1975;78:795–799.

76. Kent KC, Donaldson MC, Attinger CE, et al. Femoropopliteal reconstruction for claudication. Arch Surg 1988;123:1196–1198.

77. Brewster DC, Cambria RP, Darling RC, et al. Long-term results of combined iliac balloon angioplasty and distal surgical revascularization. Ann Surg 1989;210:324–331.

78. Spence RK, Freiman DB, Gatenby R, et al. Long-term results of transluminal angioplasty of the iliac and femoral arteries. Arch Surg 1981;116:1377–1386.

79. Wilson SE, Wolf GL, Cross AP. Percutaneous transluminal angioplasty versus operation for peripheral arteriosclerosis. J Vasc Surg 1989;9:1–8.

80. Doubilet P, Abrams HL. The cost of underutilization. Percutaneous transluminal angioplasty for peripheral vascular disease. N Engl J Med 1984;310:95–102.

81. Johnston KW, Rae M, Hogg-Johnston SA, et al. 5-year results of a prospective study of percutaneous transluminal angioplasty. Ann Surg 1987;206:403–413.

82. Strandness DE. Functional results after revascularization of the profunda femoris artery. Am J Surg 1970;119:240–245.

83. Anderson FA, Wheeler HB, Goldberg RJ, et al. A population-based perspective of the hospital incidence and case-fatality rates of deep vein thrombosis and pulmonary embolism. Arch Intern Med 1991;151:933–938.

84. Russell J. Prophylaxis of postoperative deep vein thrombosis and pulmonary embolism. Surg Gynecol Obstet 1983;157:89–104.

85. Hirsh J. Prophylaxis of venous thromboembolism. Mod Concepts Cardiovasc Dis 1984;53:25–29.

86. Gallus AS, Hirsh J, Tuttle RJ, et al. Small subcutaneous doses of heparin in prevention of venous thrombosis. N Engl J Med 1973;288:545–551.

87. Ficker JP, Vergnes Y, Schach R, et al. Low dose heparin versus low molecular weight heparin (Kabi 2165) in the prophylaxis of thromboembolic complications of abdominal oncological surgery. Eur J Clin Invest 1988;18:561–567.

88. Levine MN, Hirsh J, Gent M, et al. Prevention of deep vein thrombosis after elective hip surgery. A randomized trial comparing low molecular weight heparin with standard unfractionated heparin. Ann Intern Med 1991;114:545–551.

89. Hull RC, Raskob GE, Pineo GF, et al. Low-molecular-weight heparin (Logiparin) compared with less-intense warfarin prophylaxis against venous thromboembolism following total knee replacement. Blood 1992;1(suppl):167A.

90. Hull R, Delmore T, Hirsh J. Effectiveness of intermittent pulsatile elastic stockings for the prevention of calf and thigh vein thrombosis in patients undergoing elective knee surgery. Thromb Res 1979;16:37–45.

91. Brandjes DPM, Heijboer H, Buller HR, et al. Acenocoumarol and heparin compared with acenocoumarol alone in the initial treatment of proximal-vein thrombosis. N Engl J Med 1992;327:1485–1489.

92. Wheeler AP, Jaquiss RDB, Newman JH. Physician practices in the treatment of pulmonary embolism and deep venous thrombosis. Arch Intern Med 1988;148:1321–1325.

93. Hull RD, Raskob GE, Rosenbloom D, et al. Heparin for 5 days as compared with 10 days in the initial treatment of proximal venous thrombosis. N Engl J Med 1990;322:1260–1264.

94. King DJ, Kelton JG. Heparin-associated thrombocytopenia. Ann Intern Med 1984;100:535–540.

95. Bussey HI, Force RW, Bianco TM, Leonard AD. Reliance on prothrombin time ratios causes significant errors in anticoagulation therapy. Arch Intern Med 1992;152:278–282.

96. Hull R, Hirsh J, Jay R, et al. Different intensities of oral anticoagulant therapy in the treatment of proximal-vein thrombosis. N Engl J Med 1982;307:1676–1681.

97. Hull R, Delmore T, Carter C, et al. Adjusted subcutaneous heparin versus warfarin sodium in the long-term treatment of venous thrombosis. N Engl J Med 1982;306:189–194.

98. Lagerstedt CI, Olsson CG, Fagher BO, et al. Need for long-term anticoagulant treatment in symptomatic calf-vein thrombosis. Lancet 1985;2:515–518.

99. Philbrick JT, Becker DM. Calf deep venous thrombosis. A wolf in sheep's clothing? Arch Intern Med 1988;148:2131–2138.

Chapter 38
Cerebrovascular Diseases

Richard L. Hughes

I inhabit a weak, frail, decayed tenement; battered by the winds and broken in upon by the storms, and, from all I can learn, the landlord does not intend to repair.

John Quincy Adams
Old Age Is Not for Sissies

Cerebrovascular diseases continue to be the third leading cause of death among persons 65 years of age and older in the United States. Overall, stroke causes nearly 150,000 deaths each year (1). Stroke also is a major source of disability that leads to institutionalization. The American Heart Association estimates there are more than 2 million stroke survivors in the United States, many of whom require chronic nursing care or institutionalization (1).

The annual incidence and mortality rates for cerebrovascular diseases have been declining through recent decades (Figure 38.1), although a brief period of increased incidence attributed to the widespread use of computed tomography (CT) scanning with its improved sensitivity for stroke diagnosis occurred in the early 1980s (2). Reasons for the general trend toward decline are twofold. First, severity of stroke has steadily lessened, which has reduced death in the stroke population, and the 30-day mortality from stroke has decreased from more than 30 percent to less than 20 percent (2). Second, treatment of atherosclerotic and stroke risk factors, including lifestyle adjustments, have played a significant role in the decline.

The nomenclature for cerebrovascular disease is confusing and contains many archaic and imprecise terms, perhaps because of the evolution of knowledge in cerebrovascular disease and the use of similar terms for different conditions by clinicians, radiologists, and pathologists. *Stroke* is a general term that refers to any vascular injury to the brain. *Ischemic stroke* (often shortened to "stroke") is an ischemic injury to the brain that causes a persistent clinical deficit at 24 hours. Even mild, residual deficits are classified as strokes. The severity of the deficit is not the determinant, only that the deficit is present at 24 hours.

Transient ischemic attacks (TIAs) are ischemic neurological deficits that have *completely* resolved at 24 hours, regardless of their severity or relative duration (seconds or hours). Short TIAs that resolve within minutes do not cause permanent damage to the central nervous system, but a longer TIA that lasts for hours can be associated with cell death.

Hemorrhages in the central nervous system are classified by the anatomical area in which the hemorrhage occurs. For example, an epidural hemorrhage occurs between the skull and the dura; a subdural hemorrhage occurs between the dura and the thin arachnoid layer covering the brain. Subarachnoid hemorrhages occur next to the brain, underneath the arachnoid layer. Intraparenchymal hemorrhages include hematomas (formed blood clots that dissect into the brain) and hemorrhagic transformation of ischemic stroke (singular or multifocal regions of hemorrhage in an ischemic area). CT or magnetic resonance image (MRI) scanning can usually differentiate which type of hemorrhage has occurred.

Pathology

Ischemic Stroke

Many different types of vascular lesions cause stroke and TIA. Atherosclerotic lesions are by far the most common type, especially in the geriatric population. Hypertension-related vascular disease, primarily affecting the small arteries that penetrate the brain substance, commonly co-exists with atherosclerosis in the geriatric population. Less commonly, ischemic stroke can be caused by arteritis, fibromuscular dysplasia, arterial dissections, venous occlusions, and amyloid angiopathy. Although in-

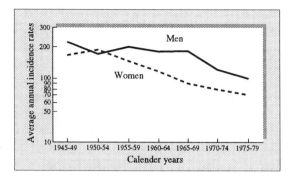

Fig. 38.1. Five-year average annual incidence rates per 100,000 population for all first episodes of stroke in Rochester, Minnesota. (Reproduced by permission from Whisnant JP. The decline of stroke. Stroke 1984;15:160.)

frequent because of the large number of strokes in this age range, these distinct processes often require different treatments, which makes diagnosis crucial.

Intracranial Hemorrhage

Intracranial hemorrhages are primarily caused by trauma, even in the older population. Typically, these hemorrhages include subdural hematomas, epidural hematomas, subarachnoid hemorrhages, and intra-parenchymal hemorrhages. Spontaneous hemorrhage (nontraumatic hemorrhage) is caused by rupture of a penetrating artery, which results in bleeding in or around the brain. Arteries rupture for different reasons, such as hypertensive degenerative disease, breakdown of a normal artery by amyloid (amyloid angiopathy), or rupture of a weakness, as occurs in arteriovenous malformation or aneurysmal subarachnoid hemorrhage. Spontaneous hemorrhage also can occur as a by-product of medical treatment or conditions such as use of anticoagulants and the broad number of bleeding disorders that are found in the elderly population.

Mechanisms of Ischemic Stroke

Once the diagnosis of ischemic stroke is made, it is necessary to determine the mechanism of the ischemic event (3). If the mechanism is known, appropriate intervention to prevent worsening or recurrent stroke is likely to be successful. Initial examination of the patient usually can determine whether the stroke is distributed in a large vessel or small vessel (3). Large vessel ischemia causes deficits in multiple systems. Typically, for example, a patient with a large vessel ischemic stroke has a hemiparesis, a hemisensory loss, and a homonymous hemianopsia contralateral to the ischemic side of the brain. A typical small vessel stroke produces an *isolated* motor (or isolated sensory) deficit on one side of the patient's body. The distinction between large vessel and small vessel stroke determines immediate care for the patient and directs a focused evaluation during the patient's hospital stay.

Large vessel strokes are generally caused by emboli from the heart, aorta, or carotid artery (4). Occasionally, a patient will have a paradoxical embolus that originates from the venous system and passes through a patent foramen ovale or other intracardiac defect. Focal thrombotic occlusion of an intracranial artery is an unusual cause of stroke but can occur in the very elderly population; it also is more common in Asian Americans and African Americans. Small vessel infarctions typically are caused by occlusion of the small penetrating vessels that course from large arteries deep into the brain. There occlusions produce "lacunar" infarctions and contribute to the process of multi-infarct dementia in the older population.

A third mechanism of stroke is hypoperfusion, which can occur with or without stenotic or diseased arteries. Profound systemic hypotension or inadequate perfusion during cardiopulmonary bypass can cause a multifocal ischemic injury in the end-arterial zones or arterial border zones. The elderly have a reduced ability to compensate for hypoperfusion, which makes them more at risk for such brain injury.

Other unusual mechanisms of stroke include arteritis, such as giant cell or temporal arteritis, traumatic or radiation injury to arteries, and vasospasm induced by drug, migraine, or idiopathic causes. Temporal arteritis, also called giant cell arteritis, produces inflammation and, eventually, occlusion of small to medium arteries. Typical symptoms include headache, scalp tenderness, and jaw claudication. The sedimentation rate is typically, but not always, elevated. Ischemia to the retina, optic nerve, or brain can be prevented by appropriate treatment with steroids. Primary injury to the arteries from trauma, radiation, or fibromuscular dysplasia results in stenosis or occlusion of the carotid or vertebral arteries and causes ischemia. Although a recent history of trauma or radiation (to the area of the neck) guides diagnosis in these patients, it is not unusual for patients to have little more than unexplained hypertension as a clue to fibromuscular dysplasia.

Venous infarctions typically cause hemorrhagic stroke in a brain distribution that is unusual for large vessel or embolic infarction. Often, there is an infectious or hematologic predisposition for venous occlusion.

Amyloid angiopathy is a poorly understood disorder of the small vessels in the central nervous system, and is distinct and unrelated to systemic amyloidosis, although the amyloid protein is found in both disorders. Typically occurring in the geriatric population, but occasionally in patients who are age 50 or so, this disorder causes a slow dementia, probably vascular, and is characterized by episodes of cerebral hemorrhage in a lobar or cortical pattern. These hemorrhages are remarkably well tolerated. Often, the diagnosis is made by CT scan in the outpatient setting many days after the hemorrhage. Unfortunately, no specific treatments are available for amyloid angiopathy except control of hypertension to reduce the risk of hemorrhage and antiplatelet agents to reduce the risk of ischemic injury. The characteristic nature of the lesions usually makes neurosurgical biopsy unnecessary.

Clinical Presentation

Infarction

The term "stroke" comes from the tendency of focal neurologic deficits to occur rapidly (within a few seconds) with no warning, headache, or change in consciousness. At onset, the deficit is usually most severe, with progressive improvement over seconds, minutes, hours, days, and weeks. Patients sometimes report severe deficit at onset but dramatic improvement when they are in the emergency department. The historic description given by the patient or patient's family, along with the neurologic examination, is usually sufficient to categorize the stroke as large vessel (perhaps with subsequent improvement) or small vessel ischemia.

Hemorrhage

Hemorrhages also present with sudden onset of neuro-logic deficit, but typically have associated headache, nausea, vomiting, and depressed level of consciousness. The onset of subarachnoid hemorrhage is cataclysmic and typically described as a "light switch" or "firecracker" in the head, which creates a severe headache. Sudden death occurs in about one-third of patients with hemorrhage. Intraparenchymal hematomas begin with a mild neuro-logic deficit and progress within a few minutes to include headache, nausea, and decreased level of consciousness. The patient's family often describes hemiparesis that steadily progresses to hemiplegia and a level of consciousness that steadily deteriorates to coma.

Localization

Crossed pathways from the brain to the body make possible clinical localization of a stroke to the right hemisphere, left hemisphere, brainstem, or cerebellum. The *left cerebral hemisphere*, if damaged, creates weakness in the right side of the body. Typically, the face and arm are affected more than the leg. Distal motor function and extensor arm function are more severely affected. Aphasia, which causes the patient to have difficulty with comprehension of words or difficulty expressing him- or herself in words, is common. Language localization to the left hemisphere is present in almost all right-handed individuals and in more than half of left-handed individuals. If visual function is involved, the patient is not able to see in the right visual field (right homonymous hemianopsia).

The *right hemisphere* controls the left side of the body and creates motor and sensory deficits to that side. Language function is not usually located in the right hemisphere, but large right hemisphere strokes often cause the patient to ignore the left part of the body and, sometimes, the left part of the room. Patients with right hemisphere stroke in its most severe form lie quietly in bed with their eyes closed. Although fully alert and able to speak, they may neglect their entire surroundings.

Localized *cerebellar injury* causes ipsilateral ataxia (incoordination). Many cerebellar ischemic strokes or hemorrhages also affect the brainstem. The *brainstem* contains cranial nerves, exiting to the *ipsilateral* side of the face, and long tracks from the brain to the body that control motor and sensory function to the *contralateral* body. Therefore, a brainstem infarction usually shows ipsilateral cranial nerve problems and contralateral deficits in the arm and leg. These crossed syndromes are typical of brainstem localization. Other clues for brainstem localization include any type of diplopia, dizziness, or dysphasia. Dysarthria, although a symptom of some brainstem problems, is a less useful diagnostic clue because it can be caused by cerebral injury or by local effects in the patient's face, mouth, and jaw.

Emergency Department Management

On the basis of the patient's history and physical examination in the emergency department, the identification of a cerebrovascular process is fairly straightforward. Often the nature of the process, such as ischemic or hemorrhage, is strongly suspected. Most emergency departments have CT scanning available to rapidly confirm or exclude the presence of hemorrhage (Figure 38.2) or, if the patient has a normal scan, to add strong radiographic confirmation that the diagnosis is ischemic stroke (5).

Without CT a sizable percentage of patients can receive only supportive care appropriate for either ischemic or hemorrhage events, and more specific therapies, such as anticoagulation or intracranial pressure monitoring, cannot be justified (5).

Emergency Management of Ischemic Stroke

The goal of ischemic stroke management is to preserve the noninfarcted areas of the patient's brain, prevent progression of infarction, avoid notorious complications of stroke (aspiration pneumonia, myocardial infarction, falls) and initiate a rational evaluation to guide long-term therapy. After stroke, most patients have relative hypertension that slowly improves during the next 7 to 10 days. There is little reason to initiate treatment unless the patient's blood pressure is elevated to very high levels (6) (Table 38.1). Because many stroke victims are dehydrated, fluids are often helpful. Rehydration tends to lower serum viscosity and may help prevent progression of stroke. The goal is to return the patient to a normal fluid state by replacing free water deficits, salt deficits, or both. Reluctance to use normal saline for fear of precipitating congestive heart failure is justified only when the patient has an appropriate history of severe heart failure or clinical signs of active heart failure at the time of the stroke. Free water (i.e., 5% dextrose water) may exacerbate cer-

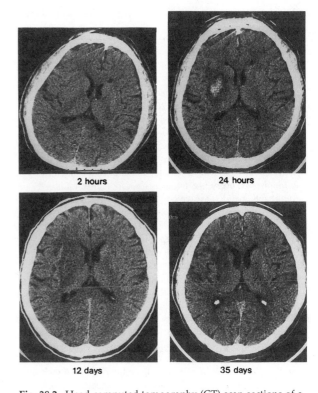

Fig. 38.2. Head computed tomography (CT) scan sections of a typical embolus to the brain demonstrating the evolution of an ischemic infarction. Clockwise from upper left: At two hours, there is no discernible change in CT scan. At 24 hours, the area of stroke is obvious as a low density (dark) region with a central area of hemorrhagic transformation (white). Hemorrhagic transformation of this type is seen in 30% to 40% of strokes at autopsy, but is usually not this apparent on scanning. At 12 days, the hemorrhagic area has decreased and the stroke has become almost "isodense" with surrounding normal brain. By 35 days the area of stroke is clearly seen as a low density (dark) area.

ebral edema in very extensive strokes but, in general, is appropriate for rehydration of any patient with an obvious free water deficit.

Considerable controversy exists regarding the use of glucose supplementation. Although glucose infusion is well described to abolish hemiplegic deficits in the rare hypoglycemic patient, increasing serum glucose levels correlate with more severe strokes in the typical atherosclerotic patient. The reason for this is acceleration of anaerobic glycolyses (and acidosis) or an increase in

Table 38.1. Algorithm for Emergency Antihypertensive Therapy for Acute Stroke.

1. If diastolic BP is >140 mm Hg on two readings 5 minutes apart, start infusion of sodium nitroprusside (0.5–10 mg/km/min).
2. If systolic BP is >230 mm Hg and/or diastolic BP is 121–140 mm Hg on two readings 20 minutes apart, give 20 mg labetalol IV for 1–2 minutes. The labetalol dose may be repeated or doubled every 10–20 minutes until a satisfactory BP reduction is achieved or until a cumulative dose of 300 mg has been administered via this minibolus technique. After the initial dosing schedule, labetalol doses may be administered every 6–8 hours as needed. (Labetalol is preferably avoided for patients with asthma, cardiac failure, or severe cardiac conduction abnormalities.)
3. If systolic BP is 180–230 mm Hg and/or diastolic BP is 105–120 mm Hg, emergency therapy should be deferred in the absence of documented intracerebral hemorrhage or left ventricular failure. If elevation persists with two readings 60 minutes apart, administer oral 200–300 mg labetalol 2–3 times daily as needed. Satisfactory alternative treatments to labetalol are 10 mg oral nifedipine every 6 hours or 6.25–25 mg captopril every 8 hours. If oral monotherapy is unsuccessful or if medications cannot be given orally, give labetalol IV as outlined above.
4. For acute stroke patients with systolic BP of <180 mm Hg and/or diastolic BP of <105 mm Hg, antihypertensive therapy is usually not indicated. Patients requiring heparin acutely should be anticoagulated after BP has been cautiously lowered to an acceptable range. A target BP range of 150/85–95 mm Hg for patients without previous hypertension or 160–170/90–100 mm Hg for patients with a history of hypertension is recommended. Because the benefits of heparin are modest even when indicated, rapid lowering of BP cannot be justified.

BP = blood pressure; IV = intravenously.
SOURCE: Reproduced by permission from Brott T, Reed RL. Intensive care for acute stroke in the community hospital setting. Stroke 1989;20:694–697.

viscosity that inhibits collateral circulation. The best approach is to check the patient's glucose level by finger stick in the ambulance or emergency room and treat hypoglycemia only when it exists. This prevents a worsening of the stroke through excess glucose administration.

A variety of unproven but compelling ways to resuscitate cerebral infarctions currently are being investigated. These methods include thrombolytic agents similar to those used for myocardial infarction within the first few hours after onset of ischemic stroke (7). Although there

are many anecdotal "successes" of use of these agents, their safety and efficacy remains to be determined. Hypervolemic hemodilution by use of albumen, dextrose, or other colloidal agents can increase the patient's intravascular fluid supply and improve collateral circulation. Although this treatment is effective for subarachnoid hemorrhage (SAH) vasospasm, results have been disappointing with its use for ischemic stroke.

Occasionally, infarctions worsen, not improve. This may be attributed to progressive arterial occlusion (stroke in progression), cerebral edema, secondary hemorrhagic transformation, or worsening of cardiopulmonary function. Unfortunately, none of these events has been definitively shown to respond to treatment. Hypotension and dehydration are the most important treatable problems that commonly prevent a stroke survivor from achieving the best outcome.

Emergency Management of Hemorrhage

The emergency management of intracranial hemorrhage is heavily dependent on rapid diagnosis to allow appropriate invasive intervention. Often, the placement of an intracranial pressure monitoring device or drainage device (ventriculostomy) is all that is necessary. Other types of hemorrhage require emergency surgery. The window of opportunity to intervene can be short; rapid diagnosis remains the crucial factor.

Intracranial hemorrhage causes damage to the brain by the mass effect of hemorrhage, focal and secondary ischemia, and the effects of irritating blood, which induce vasospasm. Intracranial pressure affects the patient's entire brain and can rapidly be fatal. General principles of management to support patients before a definitive procedure can be performed, or if a procedure is not necessary or helpful, include a reduction of intracranial pressure by a combination of diuresis and reduction of partial pressure of carbon dioxide (PCO_2) in the blood. Mannitol is traditionally the diuretic used, but other loop diuretics probably are as effective. Endotracheal intubation with hyperventilation is the only effective way to sufficiently reduce PCO_2 to about 25 mm Hg to reduce intracranial pressure.

Despite continuing controversy about efficacy, steroids are often used to minimize brain edema or an inflammatory component of the hemorrhage. Typically, dexamethasone is used in an intravenous 10-mg dose, followed by 4 to 10 mg every 6 hours. Other steroids are probably equally effective. Barbiturates, in doses sufficient to induce barbiturate coma, have also been used to manage chronic intracranial pressure elevations. Theoretically, barbiturates slow brain metabolism and allow the living cells to tolerate the hemorrhage with less morbidity.

The treatment of hypertension is difficult and controversial. Sufficient pressure is necessary to perfuse the brain and overcome elevations in intracranial pressure or venous pressure. In theory, pressure that is too high can worsen the hemorrhage or cause a recurrent hemorrhage. Ideally, the prehemorrhage blood pressure of the patient should guide therapy. The prehemorrhage pressure must be estimated in most cases. In general, systolic readings above 160 mm Hg probably are associated with higher risk of recurrent hemorrhage, but this level of pressure may be necessary for adequate brain perfusion.

Subarachnoid hemorrhage is a special case because the source of bleeding, usually an aneurysm or arteriovenous malformation (AVM), often requires surgery during the first few days of the patient's hospitalization. Patients with SAH benefit from sedation and relative hypotension because these conditions can reduce the risk of bleeding before surgical intervention. Treatment with nimodipine helps reduce the amount of ischemic damage from vasospasm, a process caused by irritation of blood vessels by the blood in the subarachnoid space.

Hospital Evaluation

Throughout the patient's hospitalization a number of goals should be addressed concurrently, even though the goals occasionally may conflict. First, emergency management is necessary to minimize any worsening of the initial event. Second, a sufficient understanding of the cerebrovascular event must be achieved to prevent further events. Third, the patient should be evaluated for rehabilitation, and, last, the important medical risk factors should be indentified and addressed.

In the case of ischemic stroke, the exact mechanism of stroke may require additional diagnostic testing. Usually after the emergency department evaluation, a history, examination, early hospital course, CT of the head, elec-

trocardiogram (ECG), and simple blood tests are available. These tests may define the mechanism of stroke without further testing. If there is uncertainty, carotid duplex ultrasound (ultrasound with Doppler velocity sampling of the arteries) and a transthoracic echocardiogram are often performed to look for the presence of a high-risk lesion, which may be the cause of the patient's stroke. Because these techniques are limited, conventional cerebral arteriography or transesophageal echocardiography occasionally are necessary if clinical suspicion of a carotid arterial lesion or a cardiac source of embolus is sufficiently high. For example, a patient with unexplained, recurrent TIAs that occur in the same carotid artery territory may require angiography of that carotid artery. Alternatively, a patient with a large embolus syndrome and unrevealing transthoracic echocardiogram often demonstrates abnormalities on transesophageal studies.

In contrast, a patient with a small vessel infarction determined on the basis of history, examination, and CT often needs no further testing to establish the mechanism of stroke. Similarly, a patient with a single event in a large vessel or embolic pattern and with atrial fibrillation seen on ECG needs no further testing to determine the mechanism of stroke, although cardiac considerations may require the performance of tests for separate indications.

Repeated CT scanning or MRI scanning of the patient a few days after a stroke to visualize the stroke is overrated and overused. A patient's clinical course usually predicts how large or small the stroke will appear on neuroimaging. However, repeated CT scanning is useful if a patient worsens, progresses, or has a change of level of alertness. In these cases, a CT scan may demonstrate secondary hemorrhage, hydrocephalus, a new stroke, or secondary cerebral edema.

Patients with brainstem strokes sometimes are difficult to image by CT, and MRI scanning may be necessary. Because MRI is costly, the usefulness of any information gained should be considered. A variety of other methodologies to measure cerebral blood flow are also available, such as positron emission tomography (PET), single photon emission computed tomography (SPECT), xenon enhanced computed tomography (Xe/CT), and additional MRI techniques. The application of cerebral blood flow testing is interesting in that it provides insight into the pathophysiology of stroke (8), but clear indications for use of these modalities are lacking.

Lumbar puncture is useful to determine neurosyphilis and vasculitis. Otherwise, it is not a routine part of evaluation of ischemic stroke. Perhaps the greatest use of lumbar puncture is to determine SAH, which may not show on CT scan in two situations. One, the SAH can occur days before the CT scan is performed, which gives the blood time to be diluted below the level of detection. Two, some patients have SAH from spinal or very low brainstem sources that are not within the region of CT scanning. Even if determination is delayed, SAH can be inferred by the presence of xanthochromia, which indicates that cerebrospinal fluid has been blood stained in the recent (weeks) past.

Prophylaxis

Ideally, the choice of an agent to prevent recurrent ischemic stroke is based on a clear understanding of the patient's medical risk factors and the mechanism of the initial ischemic stroke, TIA, or hemorrhage. Three agents effectively reduce risk of recurrent ischemic stroke—aspirin (9), ticlopidine (10), and warfarin (11) (Table 38.2). Aspirin has been established as the standard antiplatelet agent to prevent recurrent stroke (9). Most clinicians prescribe a single, coated aspirin once a day, but occasionally, a patient or subset of patients seems to respond better to larger doses. Although initially inexpensive, aspirin can cause gastrointestinal catastrophes, and the cost of aspirin therapy can be dramatically increased if an H_2 blocker is required on a regular basis.

Ticlopidine, a newer antiplatelet agent, appears to have some modest benefits over aspirin for certain subsets of patients (10), including patients in the first year after stroke, women, and patients with vertebral basilar ischemia. These are patient groups that have traditionally been considered to benefit also from anticoagulation. However, the modest benefit of ticlopidine is gained at the expense of both cost and the risk of neutropenia, which occurs in about 1 percent of patients. Nevertheless, ticlopidine offers a welcome alternative to patients who do not tolerate aspirin, fail with aspirin, or are perceived to be at higher risk. Ticlopidines require 5 to 7 days to achieve effective platelet effects. Diarrhea is a limiting effect in many patients but can be minimized by starting with single-day dosing that is increased to twice a day only as tolerated.

Anticoagulation has traditionally been used for higher risk patients, but the recent completion of five studies testing warfarin in primary prevention of stroke with atrial fibrillation has substantiated warfarin's role as a highly effective agent in the prevention of stroke (11). Most noticeably, the relative risk of stroke is reduced by about 70 percent, compared with 20 percent to 30 percent with antiplatelet agents. Furthermore, the use of lower international normalized ratio (INR) targets for anticoagulation has resulted in lower than expected bleeding complication rates. Factors that identify the highest risk patients are previous history of embolization, hypertension, and heart failure. Some factors, such as the type of atrial fibrillation (paroxysmal or prolonged) and the duration of atrial fibrillation, have no effect on risk.

There is some concern that patients older than age 75 accumulate higher risk of hemorrhage without a similar benefit of reduced stroke, which makes the choice of war-

Table 38.2. Agents to Reduce Risk of Recurrent Ischemic Stroke.

Agent	Type	Dose (mg)	Monitoring	Risk Reduction (%)*
Aspirin	Antiplatelet	325–1300/day	Gastrointestinal symptoms, bruising	20–25
Ticlopidine	Antiplatelet	250 twice a day	CBC, diarrhea	25–30
Warfarin	Anticoagulant	Adjust to INR	PT/INR, bleeding	70

*Risk reduction in secondary stroke prevention for aspirin and ticlopidine, and primary prevention in atrial fibrillation for warfarin.
INR = International Normalized Ratio; CBC = complete blood count; PT = prothrombin time.

farin less clear for elderly patients (11). Alternatives for elderly patients are use of aspirin or low-intensity warfarin therapy. Most clinicians also consider the apparent risk of embolization, on the basis of known factors (congestive heart failure, hypertension, previous embolization) to choose therapy, because the risks of serious hemorrhage seem to be distributed throughout all patients in this age group. Because a patient's compliance and tolerance of warfarin can only be estimated when therapy is initiated, 3 to 6 months of therapy may need to be completed before a patient's true risks are known.

For most patients, the choice of an antiplatelet or anticoagulant is simple. Anticoagulation is favored for patients with high risks of embolization or large vessel occlusion. For patients with small vessel infarctions, or with low risk of embolization and large vessel occlusion, antiplatelet agents are probably as useful as anticoagulation, but without the same risk. However, the data on these three agents were gathered from specific populations and require generalization to other patient groups that theoretically would respond in the same ways. Thus, there is considerable variability in practice, which prevents stricter guidelines from being used.

The use of intravenous heparin immediately after a stroke is highly controversial (12,13). Clearly, anticoagulation prevents recurrent embolization, which is at its highest risk in the first few days and weeks after an embolic event. Although there probably is some risk with heparinization, data are accumulating which indicate that heparin can be used safely even in strokes with hemorrhagic transformation (12). Furthermore, hemorrhagic transformation severe enough to harm or worsen the patient can occur with or without heparinization and may be related to factors other than anticoagulation (14). Given this incomplete knowledge, there are two general principles that help guide therapy. First, immediate heparinization is favored to prevent recurrent embolization or progression of large vessel syndromes. Other mechanisms of stroke probably are as well treated with an antiplatelet agent. Second, delaying the institution of anticoagulation for a few days and repeating the CT scan still reduces the bulk of the re-embolization risk for a few days to a week. Delay makes sense for very extensive strokes, which may be more susceptible to secondary hemorrhage.

Medical therapies to prevent intracranial hemorrhage are accomplished through two strategies. First, optimal control of blood pressure reduces the risk of virtually any intracranial hemorrhage. Second, some intracranial hemorrhages are caused by an initial ischemic event, followed by hemorrhagic transformation. If this is the mechanism, antiplatelet or anticoagulants paradoxically help prevent recurrent hemorrhage.

Surgical Management

Surgical therapy for cerebrovascular disease includes treatment for emergency management of intracranial hemorrhage, removal of intracranial aneurysms or AVMs, and revascularization procedures. In the emergency management of intracranial hemorrhage, occasional drainage of the hemorrhage, treatment of hydrocephalus, and placement of intracranial pressure monitoring routinely are performed (15). All these procedures are probably effective in some cases, but their use is still guided much more by experience than by outcome data. Especially lacking are good outcome data for the elderly population, in which the risks of surgery and prolonged stays in the intensive care unit are obviously greater. Fortunately, improved surgical techniques and improved neuroanesthesia are making intervention less risky for all patients, including the geriatric population.

The surgical removal of symptomatic (i.e., ruptured) and enlarging intracranial aneurysms and AVMs has long been effective in reducing the risk of recurrent catastrophic hemorrhage from these lesions (16,17). The case to intervene surgically in unruptured intracranial aneurysms and asymptomatic AVMs is much less clear, even in the younger population, in which benefits potentially could last for many decades. Risk is accumulated over years, so the *immediate* risk of surgical intervention must be weighed against the patient's long-term benefit, including life expectancy. The best markers of risk available include the size of an intracranial aneurysm: those larger than 10 mm have a significant risk for bleed; those under that size, provided they are not irregular or causing local compression of nervous structures, have less risk (17). AVMs probably bleed at a rate of 1 to 3 percent per year. The variable location, size, and resectability of AVM require their management to be individualized (16).

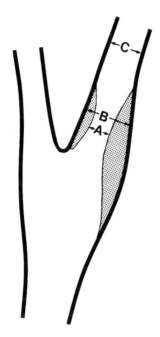

Fig. 38.3. Stenoses is calculated using the measurements A and C to apply the NASCET and ACAS criteria for carotid endarterectomy. Stenoses (%) = (C − A)/C × 100%. Using the measurement B will result in overestimation of the stenoses and cannot be accurately applied for selection of candidates for carotid endarterectomy.

In 1989, the North American Symptomatic Carotid Endarterectomy Trial (NASCET) demonstrated that endarterectomy was highly beneficial for symptomatic patients with high-grade stenosis (18). Further data have confirmed this procedure (19). The method used to establish a 70 percent stenosis is shown in Figure 38.3. Evidence to date suggests that geriatric candidates for asymptomatic carotid endarterectomy fare as well as younger patients (20).

In September 1994, the Asymptomatic Carotid Atherosclerosis Study (ACAS) demonstrated a 55 percent risk reduction for patients who underwent carotid endarterectomy in addition to receiving aspirin and other appropriate risk factor reduction methods. Patients with 60 percent or more stenosis benefitted (see Figure 38.3). This benefit is only for patients with a documented surgical risk of 3 percent or less (21). In this study, 37 percent of patients were from 70 to 79 years of age. Further analysis of subgroups is continuing.

References

1. American Heart Association. 1991 Heart and Stroke Facts. Dallas: American Heart Association, 1991.
2. Broderick JP, Phillips SJ, Whisnant JP, et al. Incidence rates of stroke in the eighties: the end of decline in stroke? Stroke 1989;20:577–582.
3. Caplan LR. Diagnosis and treatment of ischemic stroke. JAMA 1991;266:2413–2418.
4. Bozzao L, Fantozzi LM, Bastianello S, et al. Early collateral blood supply and late parenchymal brain damage in patients with middle cerebral artery occlusion. Stroke 1989;20:735–740.
5. Special resuscitation situations. JAMA 1992;268:2242–2250.
6. Brott T, Reed AL. Intensive care for acute stroke in the community hospital setting. Stroke 1989;20:694–697.
7. Wardlow JM, Warlow CP. Thrombolysis in acute ischemic stroke: does it work? Stroke 1992;23:1826–1839.
8. Hughes RL, Yonas H, Gur D, Latchaw RE. Cerebral blood flow determination within the first 8 hours of cerebral infarction using stable xenon-enhanced computed tomography. Stroke 1989;20:754–760.
9. Antiplatelet Trialists' Collaboration. Collaborative overview of randomized trials of antiplatelet therapy–I: prevention of death, myocardial infarction, and stroke by prolonged antiplatelet therapy in various categories of patients. BMJ 1994;308:87–106.
10. Hass WK, Easton JD, Adams HD, et al. A randomized trial comparing ticlopidine hydrochloride with aspirin for the prevention of stroke in high-risk patients. N Engl J Med 1989;321:501–507.
11. Atrial Fibrillation, Aspirin, Anticoagulation Study Group; Boston Area Anticoagulation Trial for Atrial Fibrillation Study Group; Canadian Atrial Fibrillation Anticoagulation Study Group; Stroke Prevention in Atrial Fibrillation Study Group; Veterans Affairs Stroke Prevention in Nonrheumatic Atrial Fibrillation Study Group. Risk factors for stroke and efficacy of antithrombotic therapy in atrial fibrillation. Arch Intern Med 1994;154:1449–1457.
12. Pessin MJ, Estol CJ, Lafranchire F, et al. Safety of anticoagulation after hemorrhagic infarction. Neurology 1993;43:1298–1303.
13. Ramirez-Lassepas M, Quinones MR. Heparin therapy for stroke: hemorrhagic complication and risk factors for intracerebral hemorrhage. Neurology 1984;34:114.
14. Lyden PD, Zivin JA. Hemorrhagic transformation after cerebral ischemia: mechanisms and incidence. Cerebrovasc Brain Metab Rev 1993;5:1–16.
15. Crowell RM, Ojemann RG, Ogilvy CS. Spontaneous brain hemorrhage. Surgical considerations. In: Barnett HJM, Mohn JP, Stein BM, Yatsu FM, eds. Stroke: pathophysiology, diagnosis, and management. 2nd ed. New York: Churchill Livingstone, 1992:1169–1188.
16. Stein BM. Surgical decisions in vascular malformations of the brain. In: Barnett HJM, Mohn JP, Stein BM, Yatsu FM,

eds. Stroke: pathophysiology, diagnosis, and management. 2nd ed. New York: Churchill Livingstone, 1992:1093–1133.

17. Wiebers DO, Whisnant JP, Sundt TM Jr, et al. The significance of unruptured intracranial saccular aneurysms. J Neurosurg 1987;66:23–35.

18. North American Symptomatic Carotid Endarterectomy Trial Collaborators. Beneficial effect of carotid endarterectomy in symptomatic patients with high-grade stenosis. N Engl J Med 1991;325:445–453.

19. Easton JD, Wilterdink JL. Carotid endarterectomy: trials and tribulations. Am Neurol 1994;35:5–17.

20. Loftus CM, Biller J, Godersky JC, et al. Carotid endarterectomy in symptomatic elderly patients. Neurosurgery 1988;22:676–680.

21. Clinical advisory: carotid endarterectomy for patients with asymptomatic internal carotid artery stenosis. Bethesda, MD: National Institute of Neurological Disorders and Stroke, 1994.

Chapter 39
Parkinson's Disease and Related Movement Disorders

Laurence J. Robbins

What can't be cured, must be endured.

Proverb

The neurodegenerative diseases include a wide array of illnesses afflicting victims of varying ages. Alzheimer's disease, Huntington's disease, amyotrophic lateral sclerosis (ALS), and Parkinson's disease (PD) are examples of neurodegenerative diseases preferentially affecting middle-aged to advanced-aged individuals (1). Early disease manifestations for each of these diseases reflect predilection for different parts of the central nervous system (CNS) or peripheral nervous system, e.g., early Alzheimer's disease causes memory loss and dysphasia, and early PD causes characteristic tremor and gait abnormalities. Although some neurodegenerative diseases remain confined to one part of the nervous system (e.g., ALS remains a "pure" motor neuron disease), other diseases may cause a broader range of neurologic symptoms as they progress over time (e.g., gait disorders in later stages of Alzheimer's disease and dementia in later stages of PD) (2,3). Alternatively, advancing age contributes substantially to the risk of developing a second neurodegenerative disease. The onset of a second disorder, rather than progression of a single neurodegenerative disease, may cause new neurologic symptoms. Because drug treatment for one neurodegenerative disease may worsen the symptoms of another, the physician must have the skills to distinguish between these diseases and recognize both the potential toxicity and the therapeutic benefit of pharmaceuticals used to treat these various disorders. This chapter focuses on the challenges of diagnosing and managing elderly patients with PD and related movement disorders.

Epidemiology

Although physicians diagnose only 50,000 new cases of PD annually, a long life expectancy (average 12.3 years) after diagnosis leaves from 500,000 to 1 million sufferers living with PD nationwide (4). As a neurodegenerative disease with onset typically occurring in the sixth decade or later, Parkinson's disease is more prevalent among the elderly. Indeed, the population older than 50 years of age has a tenfold increased prevalence of PD (1 in 100) compared with that for the general population (1 in 1000) (5). This disease is rarely familial and affects males and females equally. Although PD also affects every race and people from every region of the world, distribution data suggest some "environmental" factors (e.g., African Americans have a fivefold greater risk for PD than do blacks living in Nigeria) (4). Despite higher mortality rates among elderly patients with PD than rates for age-matched controls, life expectancy for PD has improved considerably during the past 30 years and is related to earlier diagnosis and to effective drug therapy. Most medications merely palliate symptoms in this relentlessly progressive disorder, but some controversial evidence suggests that the monoamine oxidase (MAO) inhibitor, selegiline, may briefly delay disease progression (see below) (6). The rate of clinical deterioration varies considerably among affected individuals and the etiology of this variable clinical course remains obscure (7).

Pathophysiology

The depletion of dopaminergic fibers in the basal ganglia, particularly the substantia nigra, is the pathological hallmark of idiopathic PD. Approximately 80 percent of dopaminergic neurons may be lost before clinical symptoms emerge and progression is relentless (8). Indeed, repleting dopamine relieves clinical symptoms but does not appear to arrest further loss of dopaminergic neurons. The etiology of the dopaminergic neuronal degeneration remains obscure. In addition, relative excess of other neurotransmitters such as acetylcholine and gamma aminobutyric acid (GABA) may also contribute to the clinical symptomatology, but medications aimed at blocking these neurotransmitters have produced only modest relief of motor symptoms in idiopathic PD (5).

Genetic factors, viruses, toxins, or other yet unidentified factors may contribute to dopaminergic neuronal loss. For example, excessive brain levels of copper in Wilson's disease may lead to destruction of dopaminergic neurons and the onset of parkinsonism in younger patients. This observation has led to a recommendation for routine screening for Wilson's disease among newly diagnosed parkinsonian patients, particularly patients younger than 40 years of age (9).

As another example of how neurotoxins may induce parkinsonism, a synthetic meperidine analogue, MPTP, led to an outbreak of parkinsonism in a group of young drug abusers (10). Among those who died, postmortem pathological findings in the substantia nigra were similar to those seen in idiopathic PD victims. Administration of MPTP to monkeys produces signs of parkinsonism and has served as a model for studying this disease and potential therapeutic interventions. For example, pretreatment with the MAO inhibitors appeared to prevent the signs of parkinsonism when MPTP was subsequently administered to monkeys (11). This and other research led to trials of antioxidants (vitamin E and selegiline) to retard progression of the disease in minimally symptomatic PD sufferers (6,12). Despite these advances, the etiology of idiopathic PD remains poorly understood and the disease progresses relentlessly in most patients.

Medications are a common cause of parkinsonism in the elderly (13). Most physicians are familiar with the propensity for antipsychotic medications like haloperidol (Haldol) to cause parkinsonism, but they may less readily recognize that the antihypertensive agent reserpine and antiemetics such as metoclopramide (Reglan) and prochlorperazine (Compazine) may also have extrapyramidal toxicity (9). Amoxapine (Asendin), an antidepressant, has some antidopaminergic properties and may induce parkinsonism (14). The pill-rolling resting tremor, a common early symptom of idiopathic PD, is said to be much less common in drug-induced parkinsonism, but this view remains controversial (13).

Clinical Features

In Dr. Parkinson's original description of the "Shaking Palsy" in 1817, three of his six cases were not patients but individuals he observed walking in his neighborhood (15). The now-characteristic appearance of the parkinsonian patient includes mask facies (hypomimia); pill-rolling resting tremor; stooped posture (i.e., universal flexion at the ankles, knees, hips, and elbows); impaired balance, and a festinating (propulsive) gait with loss of the normal arm swing. Patients or their families may also complain about deteriorating handwriting (micrographia) and decreased speech volume and clarity (hypophonia). These typical complaints belie the tetrad of clinical findings, namely, tremor, rigidity, bradykinesia, and postural instability (16,17). Autonomic dysfunction may provoke additional patient complaints of sialorrhea, orthostasis, constipation, and seborrhea. On physical examination, passive movement of affected limbs demonstrates rigidity, a uniform increase in tone throughout an extremity's range of motion. A tremor superimposed on the underlying rigidity gives the examiner a sense of "catch and release" or "cogwheel" rigidity. It is the rigidity rather than the cogwheeling, per se, that is most important in diagnosing PD.

Older patients with PD are more likely to complain initially about tremor (63%), bilateral signs (50%), and difficulty walking (33%); younger patients are more likely to complain of unilateral signs (>90%) and stiff muscles (43%) (18). Aged patients (>65 years) may suffer more rapid progression of their disease (19).

Tremor

Because tremor is a common and often isolated presenting complaint of elderly parkinsonian patients, distinguishing a parkinsonian tremor from other tremors is crucial to establishing the correct diagnosis. Cerebellar tremors are readily identified. Unlike the resting tremor of PD, which often improves with active movement of the affected limb, the cerebellar intention tremor worsens with movement, a side-to-side action that is most profound when a finger or toe approaches a fixed target (dysmetria) (20).

Distinguishing parkinsonian tremor from essential tremor (also referred to as "benign familial" or "senile" tremor) may be more challenging. Table 39.1 describes differences between these tremors. Parkinsonian tremors tend to be unilateral or asymmetric and predominantly affect the distal portion of the extremities. Conversely, essential tremor is typically bilaterally symmetric and is much more likely to extend to include the proximal extremities, the head (titubation), and even the larynx, which produces a vocal tremor. Beta blockers, particularly propranolol, are effective in alleviating essential tremor but have variable effect on parkinsonian tremors. Because essential tremor is also more common in patients with PD than it is with age-matched controls, co-existence of these diseases occurs frequently (21). Therefore, a therapeutic trial of beta blockers may help to distinguish an essential from a parkinsonian tremor. Doses of propranolol as low as 20 mg daily may control essential tremor but some patients may require as much as 320 mg or more for symptomatic relief (22,23).

Bradykinesia and Rigidity

Patients with advanced dementias may have significant poverty of movement and gait disorders that mimic PD. Subcortical dementias (e.g., multi-infarct dementia) may diminish facial expressiveness and thus mimic the masked facies of PD. The demented patient's flat affect, and halting, apractic, or magnetic gait (i.e., as if the patient's feet are stuck to the floor), and loss of gait-associated arm swing may be misdiagnosed as signs of PD. Similarly, patients with PD may develop memory impairment and other cognitive symptoms. To distinguish be-

tween PD and dementing disease, the patient's history is crucial. In most cases, gait abnormalities are a late manifestation of primary dementing illnesses. Patients with multi-infarct dementia or Alzheimer's disease typically have a long history of worsening cognitive impairment before the onset of parkinsonian-like expressionless facies and gait disturbances. In contrast, patients with PD usually suffer years of progressive motor problems before family or physician notice significant cognitive impairment (3). Because multi-infarct dementia, Alzheimer's disease and PD all occur more frequently with advancing age, these diseases may co-exist and clinical differentiation becomes difficult. Should all demented patients with movement disorders receive antiparkinsonian medication trials?

Unfortunately, little evidence exists to indicate that antiparkinson medications alleviate movement disorders caused by diseases other than idiopathic or drug-induced PD. In addition, virtually all medications prescribed to alleviate symptoms of PD may exacerbate cognitive impairment associated with dementing diseases (2,24). Therefore, patients with movement disorders and dementia require careful evaluation and, if antiparkinsonian medications are prescribed, the physician should monitor patients for adverse reactions, including worsening cognitive impairment.

Depression

The relationship between depression and PD is important for two reasons. First, depression may be mistaken for PD

Table 39.1. Comparison of Essential Tremor with Parkinson's Tremor.

Category	Essential Tremor	Parkinson's Tremor
Duration (before patient seeks medical attention)	Long, often >10 yr	Short, often <5 yrs
Distribution	Symmetric, distal and proximal (head involvement common)	Asymmetric, primarily distal limb involvement
Character	Fine; often worse with intentional movement	Coarse, pill-rolling; usually better with intentional movement
Associated finding	Usually none	Rigidity (often subtle)
Inheritance	Often familial	Usually sporadic
Medication		
Levodopa	No effect	Variable (may improve or worsen)
Beta blockers	Improves	Modest or no response

and second, depression is more common among patients with PD than it is among elderly persons without the disease (25). When flat affect and psychomotor retardation of depression mimic the masked facies and bradykinesia of PD, physicians may misdiagnose depression as PD. Interviews of patient and family usually reveal other symptoms of depression such as a history of depression, anhedonia (loss of pleasure in activities), sleep disturbances (e.g., early morning awakening), guilt, loss of energy, difficulty concentrating, poor appetite, and even suicidal ideation. While depressed nonparkinsonian patients appear immobile, their motor tone should be normal, and cogwheel rigidity and pill-rolling tremor are absent.

Depression is also more common among patients with PD than it is among elderly persons without PD. Nearly half of parkinsonian patients become significantly depressed during the course of their illness (26,27). Depression may explain why patients previously responsive to antiparkinsonian medications suddenly become less responsive. Treatment with traditional tricyclic antidepressants (e.g., nortriptyline) may relieve not only the patient's mood disorder but the mild anticholinergic effects may also relieve symptoms of the movement disorder, including sialorrhea, tremor, and rigidity (9). Similarly, electroconvulsive therapy may not only relieve symptoms in severely depressed patients but may also reduce rigidity and bradykinesia, independent of its mood elevating effects (28,29).

Autonomic Dysfunction and Other Symptoms

Although the classic tetrad of motor symptoms characterizes patients with PD, autonomic dysfunction frequently further compromises the functional status of PD sufferers (30). In particular, orthostatic hypotension is common in patients with PD and many antiparkinsonian medications exacerbate this problem. The Shy-Drager syndrome describes patients with both classic parkinsonian motor symptoms and severe orthostasis. The Shy-Drager syndrome along with olivopontocerebellar degeneration and supranuclear palsy form the Parkinson Plus syndromes, in which additional neurologic findings complicate the classic signs of PD. These patients often have a poor response to antiparkinsonian medication (9). Fortunately, these disorders are relatively uncommon.

Seborrheic dermatitis is extremely common among patients with PD and is often severe. The scaly rash not only involves the scalp but may also affect the ears, eyebrows, nasal folds, and chin (31). The etiology of the relationship between PD and seborrheic dermatitis is not well understood but some experts claim that levodopa treatment may alleviate the dermatitis (32).

Treatment

Three important caveats guide the approach to treatment of PD. First, pharmacologic treatment of PD is symptomatic; except for one controversial study of selegiline, medications do not alter the inevitable progression of the disease. Second, the available antiparkinsonian drugs have narrow therapeutic windows in elderly patients; relatively small differences separate the minimal effective dosage of a given medication and toxic dosage of the same medication. The symptoms of PD also fluctuate from one hour to the next and from day to day. Patients and their physicians should recognize this natural fluctuation and evaluate the impact of medication adjustments over days to weeks rather than changing the regimen daily. Table 39.2 includes some of the commonly prescribed medications, dosing recommendations, and costs.

Anticholinergics

Among the oldest class of drugs for treating parkinsonism, anticholinergic medications are modestly effective in reducing tremor and rigidity but only minimally effective in reducing bradykinesia (33). On occasion, patients with bother some sialorrhea may obtain relief from low doses of anticholinergic drugs. No specific anticholinergic agent is superior to others (34). Although most effective in treating drug-induced parkinsonism, these drugs have limited usefulness in the elderly with idiopathic PD because of significant side effects such as confusion, urinary retention, dry mouth, blurred vision, constipation, ataxia, and flushing.

Amantadine

Another of the older drugs used to treat PD, amantadine may provide modest relief for tremor, rigidity, and bradykinesia. Its mechanism of action remains obscure

Table 39.2. Dosage and Cost of Medications.

Drug	Starting Dose	Approximate Cost/Mo ($)	Avg Dose	Approximate Cost/Mo ($)
Trihexylphenidyl (Artance) (generic anticholinergic)	2 mg daily	2	2 mg 3–4 times/day	7–10
Amantadine (Symmetrel)	100 mg daily	10	100 mg 2–3 times/day	20–30
Carbidopa/levodopa	25/100 2–3 times/day	25–40	25:250 3–4 times/day	55–80
Sustained-release carbidopa/levodopa	25/100 2 times/day	40	50:200 2 times/day	160
Bromocriptine (Parlodel)	2.5 mg (1/2 tablet) 2 times/day	50	5 mg 3–4 times/day	225–300
Pergolide (Permax)	0.25 mg 2 times/day	50	1 mg 3 times/day	250
Selegiline (Eldepryl)	–	–	5 mg 2 times/day	120

(perhaps releasing endogenous dopamine or blocking reuptake of dopamine) (34). When amantadine was prescribed for influenza prophylaxis during influenza type A outbreaks in nursing homes, investigators reported that some bedridden or mute patients with unsuspected parkinsonism unexpectedly began walking or talking after receiving the drug (35). In addition to its use as a single agent, amantadine may be useful as an adjunct to levodopa therapy. Side effects of amantadine include confusion, edema, and livedo reticularis (a purplish mottling of the skin). Therapeutic response to amantadine usually wanes after a few weeks to a few months of therapy. Patients may again respond to the drug if it is reintroduced after it has been discontinued for weeks or months (34). The modest, short-lived efficacy of amantadine and its tendency to cause confusion in elderly patients often limits its usefulness for the geriatric population (36).

Dopamine Agonists

Dopamine agonists cross the blood-brain barrier and act directly on postsynaptic dopamine receptors. The older of the two available agents is bromocriptine. As a single agent, when given in doses of 15 to 30 mg daily, this D_2 receptor-agonist provides moderate relief of bradykinesia and rigidity but has variable effects on tremor (37). More often, bromocriptine is combined with carbidopa-levodopa to reduce a patient's requirement for the latter drugs as well as to improve symptom control. Gastrointestinal toxicity (nausea, vomiting) may limit tolerance of bromocriptine. Consequently, patients are begun on small doses (1.25 mg once or twice daily), which are gradually increased over several days or weeks. Other

dose-limiting side effects include dry mouth, orthostasis, erythromelalgia, confusion, delusions, hallucinations, and (rarely) pulmonary fibrosis (33).

Pergolide is a recently approved dopamine agonist with both D_1 and D_2 receptor activity. In clinical trials, pergolide may be effective alone or in combination with carbidopa-levodopa (38). Some patients who fail to respond to bromocriptine may respond to pergolide and vice versa (39). Pergolide and bromocriptine are expensive medications in therapeutic doses (see Table 39.2).

Levodopa

Levodopa has remained the most active agent in the treatment of rigidity and bradykinesia since its introduction in the late 1960s. Levodopa may ameliorate the pill-rolling tremor, but this effect on tremor is variable (40). Because dopamine does not cross the blood-brain barrier, levodopa is given because it crosses the blood-brain barrier and the remaining dopaminergic neurons in the basal ganglia convert it to dopamine. In the bloodstream, the enzyme dopa decarboxylase breaks down most of an administered dose of levodopa. Therefore, a dopa decarboxylase inhibitor, carbidopa, is administered in combination with levodopa to limit breakdown. To provide optimal blockade of dopa decarboxylase activity, patients should take at least 75 to 100 mg of carbidopa daily in divided doses (34). Combined carbidopa-levodopa tablets are available in 25/100, 10/100 and 25/250 formulations (carbidopa is always the first, smaller number). Patients may be started on as little as 300 mg of levodopa daily and still receive adequate amounts of carbidopa (i.e., 25:100 three times a day). Because total carbidopa should not exceed 200 mg daily, the 1:10 carbidopa-levodopa formulations (i.e., 10:100, 25:250) allow for larger doses of levodopa without excessive increases in carbidopa (e.g., average levodopa requirements for most patients is 500 to 1000 mg daily). Side effects of levodopa include confusion, anorexia, nausea, vomiting, orthostasis, dyskinesias, akathisia, hallucinations, arrhythmias, and flushing. Carbidopa has no significant toxicity of its own (34). Dietary proteins may interfere with absorption of standard preparations of levodopa and some patients may derive more therapeutic benefit if levodopa is taken on an empty stomach (41). Conversely, taking sustained-release carbidopa-levodopa (Sinemet CR) with food may increase bioavailability of the preparation (42).

Because patients may fail to respond to lower doses of carbidopa-levodopa, some experts suggest that the daily levodopa dose should approach 1500 mg before treatment-responsive PD can be ruled out (43). Unfortunately, elderly patients may develop toxicity from small doses of carbidopa-levodopa and thus cannot achieve optimal therapeutic trials.

Despite a drug half-life of only a few hours, carbidopa-levodopa may be given as infrequently as every 8 to 12 hours for early PD. This reflects the sustained benefit of the levodopa after its conversion to dopamine in the brain, although levodopa is undetectable in the serum a few hours after a dose. As PD progresses, the duration of the carbidopa-levodopa effect begins to parallel the serum concentration (44). Thus, the patient notes a shorter duration of response to carbidopa-levodopa and requires doses more frequently to avoid the "wearing off" effect. The sustained-release preparation of carbidopa-levodopa may reduce dosing frequency by approximately one-half to one-third but is less bioavailable than the standard preparation and total dose must be increased by 15 percent to 30 percent (33,42–47). The sustained-release preparation is also approximately twice as expensive as the standard preparation; therefore, patients may be reluctant to accept the greater cost in exchange for modest reduction in dosing frequency. In addition, the onset of action of the sustained-release preparation may be delayed for as long as 2 hours after a dose is taken and some patients prefer the swifter onset of action of the standard preparation (48,49). Although patients may notice an increase in "on" time with the sustained-release preparation, they often also notice an increase in dyskinesia (50). Some patients may prefer a regimen that includes both sustained-release and standard carbidopa-levodopa, the former to provide sustained control through the night and the letter to provide swifter relief of symptoms in the morning and during the day.

Many patients with PD notice a marked diminution in response to carbidopa-levodopa after as little as 5 years of treatment (32). The therapeutic window seems to narrow as patients require higher doses of levodopa to improve bradykinesia and rigidity, while toxicity such as dyskinesia, dystonia, and hallucinations seem to occur more frequently. Patients may suffer rapid swings in motor function (the "on-off" effect) (51). There is an ongoing study of the use of controlled-release carbidopa-levodopa alone in early PD to determine whether this preparation delays the onset of motor fluctuations as compared with the action of the standard preparation (42).

Various interventions may ameliorate motor fluctuations in later stages of PD. Prescribing smaller doses of carbidopa-levodopa more frequently may reduce fluctuations (e.g., 10:100 or 25:100 every $1\frac{1}{2}$–2 hours) (52). Sustained-release carbidopa-levodopa may improve "on" time and reduce dyskinesia, but many patients with motor fluctuation may not respond well to this preparation (49). Adding a dopamine agonist (e.g., bromocriptine or pergolide) may provide additional improvement in motor symptoms while permitting less frequent, or lower total doses, or both, of carbidopa-levodopa (39).

The MAO inhibitor selegiline in doses of 2.5 to 10 mg daily may block the metabolism of CNS dopamine and thus enhance the duration and effectiveness of carbidopa-levodopa (53,54). Maintaining serum levels of levodopa through continuous nasogastric tube infusion of carbidopa-levodopa has also been shown to reduce motor fluctuation but is impractical for chronic therapy of most elderly patients with PD (55). Recent reports suggests that a patient's entire daily carbidopa-levodopa requirement dissolved in tap water and stabilized by ascorbic acid may be continuously sipped throughout the day and produce a sharp reduction in motor fluctuation compared with conventional oral dosing with carbidopa-levodopa tablets (56). Patients should be reminded that taking standard carbidopa-levodopa with meals may result in lower absorption because levodopa competes with some dietary proteins for absorption. Taking the medication on an empty stomach or with low-protein meals may reduce motor fluctuation associated with reduced or delayed levodopa absorption (41).

Several investigational agents may become available to ameliorate levodopa-associated motor fluctuations. These include new dopamine agonists, additional MAO inhibitors, and a new class of compounds, the catecholomethyltransferase (COMT) inhibitors. Like the MAO inhibitors, the COMT inhibitors reduce dopamine breakdown in the CNS. Transdermal delivery systems for levodopa are also under investigation (33).

Muscular discomfort (cramping or aching) may become a disabling symptom of long-term carbidopa-levodopa therapy. These symptoms may occur at either peak dose effect or when patients are in an "off" period. The muscle relaxant orphenadrine (100 mg two or three times a day) may alleviate these symptoms and its mild anticholinergic effect may improve tremor and rigidity (57,58). However, orphenadrine may cause confusion and should be used cautiously in the elderly.

Sometimes, levodopa-induced delusions or hallucinations associated with peak serum drug levels may limit patient tolerance of escalating levodopa doses required by worsening bradykinesia and rigidity (33). Traditional major tranquilizers such as haloperidol often worsen parkinsonian symptoms and thus have limited usefulness in managing levodopa-induced psychotic symptoms. Preliminary evidence suggests that newer antipsychotic medications such as clozapine (Clozaril) have no extrapyramidal side effects and in low doses may alleviate drug-induced delusions and hallucinations and permit continued escalation of levodopa dosage (33,59). Unfortunately, clozapine may cause severe agranulocytosis in some patients and therefore requires frequent monitoring of patient's white blood cell count.

Selegiline

Selegiline, a monoamine oxidase (MAO) inhibitor, has been used not only as an adjuvant agent to reduce daily requirements for carbidopa-levodopa and ameliorate motor fluctuation (53,54) but also to prevent the progression of early PD (6,12). Older MAO inhibitors such as pargyline have both MAO-α and MAO-β blocking effects.

As a pure MAO-β inhibitor in doses of as much as 10 mg daily, selegiline is not associated with the adverse reactions seen when older MAO inhibitors are taken with tyramine-containing food such as cheddar cheese or chianti wine. Therefore, dietary restrictions are not necessary when selegiline is prescribed (9). Because MAO-β receptors predominate in the basal ganglia and substantia nigra, selegiline prevents oxidation of dopamine and thus may sustain levodopa's activity in this part of the CNS. Older MAO inhibitors' antidepressant activity depends on MAO-α receptors in higher CNS centers, but the MAO-β inhibitors such as selegiline appear to have no clinically significant antidepressant activity (38). Selegiline may increase the toxicity of concomitantly prescribed levodopa but has virtually no toxicity when administered alone.

In published reports of a double-blind, placebo-controlled study, the Deprenyl and Tocopherol Antioxidative Therapy of Parkinsonism trial (DATATOP), in patients with early PD, selegiline delayed the decision to begin carbidopa-levodopa therapy for progressive PD (6,12). Supporters argue that selegiline has no therapeutic benefit and consequently could only delay the need for carbidopa-levodopa by slowing disease progression. Critics argue that rather than preventing disease progression, selegiline has modest therapeutic effects on motor symptoms that delay the need for other symptomatic treatment such as carbidopa-levodopa. Because selegiline has virtually no adverse effects when administered alone, a major barrier to prescribing selegiline in early PD may be the substantial cost of the drug (see Table 39.2).

Surgery

Stereotactic thalamic surgery for PD has been used for many years and continues to have a role in therapy for younger patients with severe, refractory, unilateral tremors (60). Recently, pallidotomy has enjoyed renewed interest as a treatment for refractory bradykinesia and rigidity. However, the role of neurosurgical ablative procedures in the elderly patient with PD is extremely limited.

Promising recent research suggests that fetal cell transplantation in the brains of patients with PD may lead to amelioration of symptoms through the replenishing of dopaminergic neurons (61). Unfortunately, the procedure has benefited relatively few patients and, like ablative surgery, has been mostly limited to younger patients (<70 years old). In early transplant studies, persistent postoperative sleep disturbances and mental status changes were more common and more profound among older transplant recipients (62). Fetal cell transplantation is unlikely to become a significant alternative for elderly PD victims in the near future.

General Supportive Measures

Because average PD patients have a life expectancy similar to that of unaffected peers, they must face the challenge of maintaining their functional independence for many years. Support groups for PD (e.g., American Parkinson's Disease Association, 1-800-223-2732) often provide education, guidance, and emotional support for PD victims. Establishing predictable daily routines, reducing stress, and participating in regular exercise may improve a sense of well-being for patients with PD and facilitate better control of disease fluctuations (1). Physical and occupational therapy may help patients with PD maintain safe ambulation and facilitate self-sufficiency in activities of daily living. Speech therapy may help patients whose speech becomes inaudible as a result of decreased volume and increased speech velocity that accompany other PD motor symptoms.

Symptom control depends on accurate patient observation of disease activity, and patients must be encouraged to participate in assessing their response to medication. Because many patients may want to make suggestions for altering their medication regimen, physicians should solicit patient feedback and permit patients to share in treatment decisions. Depression is a frequent reversible cause of deterioration control, and physicians must remain vigilant in detecting early signs of depression and treating them appropriately. Like patients with brittle diabetes mellitus, patients with PD must have ready access to knowledgeable physicians so that unexpected fluctuations in disease control maybe addressed and corrected expediently.

Conclusion

PD is an aging-related, neurodegenerative disease that is becoming more common in our aging society. A careful medical history and physical examination will help to distinguish PD from other disorders that may mimic the motor symptoms and signs of PD. Patients with early signs of PD may be treated with selegiline to help delay disease progression, but this therapy remains controversial and expensive. Levodopa in combination with carbidopa is the single most effective agent in relieving the most disabling PD symptoms, namely, bradykinesia and rigidity. The dopamine agonists, bromocriptine and pergolide, may be effective as single agents or have additive benefits when combined with carbidopa-levodopa. Anticholinergic agents and amantadine have limited roles for elderly patients with PD because these drugs have only modest therapeutic benefit and significant toxicity (33). When added to a regimen of carbidopa-levodopa, selegiline may prolong the effect of levodopa and permit reduction in daily levodopa requirements. Neurosurgery presently has a very limited role in management of elderly patients with PD. Future management of PD will likely include additional choices within presently available drug classes (e.g., new MAO-β inhibitors and dopamine agonists) as well as new therapeutic approaches (e.g., COMT inhibitors). Successful care of aging PD patients requires the attention of physicians who are both accessible to the patients and knowledgeable about the rapidly changing pharmaceutical armamentarium available to treat this challenging disease.

References

1. Degenerative disease of the nervous system. In: Adams RD, Victor M, eds. Principles of neurology. New York: McGraw-Hill, 1993.
2. Mayeux R, Stern Y, Rosenstein R, et al. An estimate of the prevalence of dementia in idiopathic Parkinson's disease. Arch Neurol 1988;45:260.
3. Mortimer SA, Pirozzolo FJ, Hansch EC, Webster DD. Relationship of motor symptoms to intellectual deficits in Parkinson's disease. Neurology 1982;32:133.
4. Rajput AH. Frequency and cause of Parkinson's disease. Can J Neurol Sci 1992;19(suppl):103.
5. Pearce JMS. Aetiology and natural history of Parkinson's disease. BMJ 1978;277:1664.
6. The Parkinson Study Group. Effects of tocopherol and deprenyl on the progression of disability in early Parkinson's disease. N Engl J Med 1993;328:176–183.
7. Hoehn MM, Yahr MD. Parkinsonism: onset, progression and

mortality. Neurology 1967;17:427.

8. Hornykiewicz O, Kish SJ. Biochemical pathophysiology of Parkinson's disease. Adv Neurol 1986;45:19.

9. Standaert DG, Stern MB. Update on the management of Parkinson's disease. In: Biller J, ed. Contemporary clinical neurology. Med Clin North Am 1963;77:169.

10. Nutt JG. Parkinson's disease: evaluation and therapeutic strategy. Hosp Pract 1987;22:107.

11. Langston JW, Irwin I, Langston EB, Forno LS. Pargyline prevents MPTP-induced parkinsonism in primates. Science 1984;225:1480.

12. The Parkinson Study Group. Effect on deprenyl on the progression of disability in early Parkinson's disease. New Engl J Med 1989;321:1364.

13. Stephen PJ, Williamson J. Drug-induced parkinsonism in the elderly. Lancet 1984;2:1092.

14. Thorton JE, Stahl SM. Case report of tardive dyskinesia and parkinsonism associated with amoxapine. Am J Psychiatry 1984;141:704.

15. Parkinson J. An essay on the shaking palsy. London: Sherwood, Neely and Jones, 1817.

16. Calne DB, Snow BJ, Lee C. Criteria for diagnosing Parkinson's disease. Ann Neurol 1992;32:5125.

17. Zetusky WJ, Jankovic J, Pirozzolo FJ. The heterogeneity of Parkinson's disease: clinical and prognostic implications. Neurology 1985;35:522.

18. Gibb WRG, Lees AJ. A comparison of clinical and pathological features of young- and old-onset Parkinson's disease. Neurology 1988;38:1402.

19. Goetz CG, Tanner CM, Stebbins GT, Buchman AS. Risk factors for progression in Parkinson's disease. Neurology 1988;38:1841.

20. Dupont E. Parkinson's disease and essential tremor: a differential diagnostic and epidemiological aspects. In: Rinne UK, Klinger M, Stamm G, eds. Parkinson's disease: current progress, problems and management. New York: Elsevier/North-Holland, 1980.

21. Geraghty JJ, Jankovic J, Zetusky WJ. Association between essential tremor and Parkinson's disease. Ann Neurol 1985;17:329.

22. Koller WC. Dose-response relationship of propranolol in the treatment of essential tremor. Arch Neurol 1986;43:42.

23. Larsen TA, Calne DB. Essential tremor. Clin Neuropharmacol 1983;6:185.

24. Pederzoli M, Girotti F, Scigliano G, et al. L-dopa long-term treatment in Parkinson's disease: age-related side effects. Neurology 1983;33:1518.

25. Mayeux R, Stem Y, Rosen J, Levethal J. Depression, intellectual impairment and Parkinson's disease. Neurology 1981;31:645.

26. Gotham AM, Brown RG, Marsden CD. Depression in Parkinson's disease: a quantitative and qualitative analysis. J Neurol Neurosurg Psychiatry 1986;49:381.

27. Dooneie FG, Mirabello E, Bell K, et al. An estimate of the incidence of depression in idiopathic Parkinson's disease. Arch Neurol 1992;49:305.

28. Ward C, Stern GM, Pratt RTC, McKenna P. Electroconvulsive therapy in parkinsonian patients with the "on-off" syndrome. J Neural Transm 1980;49:133.

29. Balldin J, Granerus AK, Lindstedt G, et al. Neuroendocrine evidence for increased responsiveness of dopamine receptors in humans following electroconvulsive therapy. Psychopharmacology 1982;76:371.

30. Goetz CG, Lutge W, Tanner CM. Autonomic dysfunction in Parkinson's disease. Neurology 1986;36:73–75.

31. Moschella SL. Seborrheic dermatitis. In: Fitzpatrick TB, Arndt KA, Clark WH, et al. Dermatology in general medicine. New York: McGraw-Hill, 1971.

32. Barbeau A, Mars H, Gillo-Joffroy L. Adverse clinical side effects of levodopa therapy. In: McDowell FH, Markham CH, eds. Recent advances in Parkinson's disease. Contemporary Neurology Series. Philadelphia: Davis, 1971.

33. Calne DM. Treatment of Parkinson's disease. New Engl J Med 1993;329:1021–1027.

34. Berg MJ, Ebert B, Willis DK, et al. Parkinsonism-drug treatment: Part 1. Drug Intell Clin Pharm 1987;21:10.

35. Roca RP, Santmyer K, Gloth M, Denman S. Improved mental activity and appetite among long-term care patients treated with amantadine. J Am Geriatr Soc 1990;38:675.

36. Hunter KE, Stern GM, Laurence DR. Amantadine in parkinsonism. Lancet 1970;1:1127.

37. Goetz CG. Dopaminergic agonists in the treatment of Parkinson's disease. In: Colanow CW, Lieberman AN. The scientific basis for the treatment of Parkinson's disease. Park Ridge, NJ: Parthenon, 1992.

38. Abramowicz M, ed. Pergolide and selegiline for Parkinson's disease. Med Lett Drugs Ther 1989;31:82.

39. Lewitt PA, Ward CD, Larsen TA, et al. Comparison of pergolide and bromocriptine therapy in parkinsonism. Neurology 1983;33:1009.

40. Carlsson A. Basic concepts underlying recent developments in the field of Parkinson's disease. In: McDowell FH, Markham CH, eds. Recent advances in Parkinson's disease. Contemporary Neurology Series. Philadelphia: Davis, 1971.

41. Riley D, Lang AE. Practical application of a low-protein diet for Parkinson's disease. Neurology 1988;38:1026.

42. Gauthier S, Amyot D. Sustained release antiparkinson agents: controlled-release levodopa. Can J Neurol Sci 1992;19(suppl 1):153.

43. Calne DB, Snow BJ, Lel C. Criteria for diagnosing Parkinson's disease. Ann Nuerol 1992;32:S125.

44. Wooten GF. Progress in understanding the pathophysiology of treatment-related fluctuations in Parkinson's disease. Ann Neurol 1988;24:363.

45. Hutton JT, Morris JL, Roman GL, et al. Treatment of chronic Parkinson's disease with controlled-release carbidopa/levodopa. Arch Neurol 1988;45:861.

46. Hutton JT, Morris JL, Bush DF. Multicenter controlled study of Sinemet CR vs Sinemet (25/100) in advanced Parkinson's disease. Neurology 1989;39(suppl 2):S67.

47. Koller WC, Pahwa R. Treating motor fluctuations with

controlled-release levodopa preparations. Neurology 1994; 44(suppl 6):S23.

48. Abramowicz M, ed. Sinemet CR for Parkinson's disease. Med Lett Drugs Ther 1991;33:92.

49. Ahlskog JE, et al. Controlled-released Sinemet (CR-4): a double-blind crossover study in patients with fluctuating Parkinson's disease. Mayo Clin Proc 1988;63:876.

50. LeWitt PA, Nelson MV, Berchouc RC, et al. Controlled-release carbidopa/levodopa (Sinemet 50/200 Cr 4): Clinical and pharmacokinetic studies. Neurology 1989;39(suppl 2):S45.

51. Nutt JG, Woodward WR, Hammerstad JP, Carter JH, Anderson JL: The "on-off" phenomenon in Parkinson's disease. N Engl J Med 1984;310:483.

52. Cedarbaum JM, Olanow CW. Aspects of levodopa pharmacokinetics and pharmacodynamics: basis of the modification of drug response during chronic treatment of Parkinson's disease. In: Olanow CW, Lieberman AN. The scientific basis for the treatment of Parkinson's disease. Park Ridge, NJ: Parthenon, 1992.

53. Lieberman A. Experience with selegiline and levodopa in advanced Parkinson's disease. Acta Neurol Scand 1991; 136(suppl):66.

54. Golbe LI. Deprenyl as symptomatic therapy in Parkinson's disease. Clin Neuropharmacol 1988;11:387.

55. Sage JI, Troaskin S, Sonsalla PK, et al. Long-term duodenal infusion of levodopa for motor fluctuations in parkinsonism. Ann Neurol 1988;24:87.

56. Kurth MC, Tetrud JW, Irwin BA, et al. Oral levodopa/carbidopa solution versus tablets in Parkinson's patients with severe fluctuations: a pilot study. Neurology 1993;43:1036.

57. Drugs for Parkinson's disease. Lancet 1978;1:754.

58. Bassi S, Albizzati MG, Callari E, et al. Treatment of Parkinson's disease with orphenadrine alone and in combination with L-dopa. Br J Clin Pract 1986;40:273.

59. Abramowicz M, ed. Update on clozapine (use in levodopa-induced psychosis). Med Lett Drugs Ther 1993;35:16–18.

60. Abramowicz M, ed. Surgical treatment of Parkinson's disease. Med Lett Drugs Ther 1993;35:103.

61. Freed CR, Breeze RE, Rosenberg NL, et al. Survival of implanted fetal dopamine cells and neurologic improvement 12 to 46 months after transplantation for Parkinson's disease. N Engl J Med 1992;327:1549–1555.

62. Burns RS, Allen GS, Tulipan NB. The effects of adrenal medulla transplants in Parkinson's disease. Ann Neurol 1988;24:150.

Chapter 40
Osteoporosis in the Elderly

Paul D. Miller

Pain —has an Element of Blank—
It cannot recollect
When it begun —or if there were
A time when it was not.

Emily Dickinson

Osteoporosis is the most prevalent metabolic bone disease in the geriatric population, and its prevalence is increasing. By the year 2044 it is estimated that the prevalence of osteoporosis will double. It is also estimated that the number of worldwide hip fractures will increase fourfold by the year 2050.

Osteoporosis is a preventable and treatable disease that can be objectively diagnosed at an early stage, before fractures occur, by the measurement of bone mass. In addition, objective bone-mass measurement techniques can effectively monitor preventive programs to maintain bone mass. Bone-mass measurement(s) can also determine the efficacy of pharmacologic therapies designed to increase bone mass.

In general, the medical community's attitude toward osteoporosis, in the past, has been one of disinterest. The lack of interest in osteoporosis has been interpreted by the public to mean that osteoporosis is untreatable and, therefore, a normal, expected, process of aging. Thus, elderly women expect to lose height and to develop stooped posture as they get older. New generations of physicians need to accept responsibility for changing these attitudes. The expectations of the public need to be altered to increase the detection and diagnosis of osteoporosis before fractures occur. Physicians need to become aware that there are now methods of prevention and treatment of osteoporosis. A redefinition of the term osteoporosis is required.

Osteoporosis has previously been defined as a loss of bone calcium of sufficient magnitude to result in nontraumatic fractures of bone. Consequently, the osteoporotic process was in the advanced stages before the actual diagnosis was made. The new definition of osteoporosis includes criteria to diagnose osteoporosis *before* a fracture occurs. In this regard, analogies may be made between the processes of osteoporosis, hypertension, and elevated blood cholesterol levels. Each is a silent process, that, if left unrecognized and untreated, can result in a very serious clinical manifestation (i.e., fractured bones, cerebrovascular accident, or myocardial infarction). All these disease processes are quite prevalent and can be detected at an early asymptomatic stage.

The new definition of osteoporosis should be: a reduction in bone mass of sufficient magnitude associated with disordered microarchitectural changes in bone to render a patient *susceptible* to nontraumatic (i.e., fragility) fractures of bone. A fracture need not have occurred to define osteoporosis. Recently, both the World Health Organization and the Society for Clinical Densitometry established diagnostic thresholds (guidelines) to diagnose osteopenia (low bone mass) and osteoporosis in nonfractured individuals (1). *Osteopenia* is defined as a bone mineral density (BMD) that is 1.5 to 2.5 standard deviations (SD) below the mean peak bone mass of healthy young normal women. *Osteoporosis* is defined as a bone mineral density that is more than 2.5 SD below the mean peak bone mass of healthy young normal women, even in the absence of any fragility fractures. These diagnostic thresholds have been described because more than 95 percent of fragility fractures occur in women with more than 2.5 SD reduction in bone mass. Yet, it is important to identify women with lesser reductions in BMD because as bone mass declines, the risk of fragility fractures increases in an exponential manner. Detection of osteopenia or osteoporosis *before* a fracture occurs is important because the risk for a second fracture increases as much as 25-fold once the first fracture has occurred. Diagnosis of osteoporosis after the first fracture is analogous to diagnosing high blood pressure or high cholesterol after the stroke or heart attack has occurred.

Bone calcium loss is currently viewed as a universal aging process in both male and female human beings. Therefore, bone calcium loss could be viewed as a normal consequence of aging. However, this process of bone calcium loss results in fractures in nearly 50 percent of Caucasian or Oriental women older than age 50 (2). The physician should, therefore, no longer accept a substantial reduction in bone mass as "normal."

Epidemiology of Osteoporosis

Osteoporotic fractures currently affect 8 million Americans (2). This represents osteoporosis in its advanced stages, when fractures have already occurred.

The prevalence of osteoporosis in American women (defined as more than 2.5SD reduction in bone mass) across all ages is 30 percent of the population. However, for women older than 80 years of age, the prevalence doubles to include 60 percent of the population, 17 percent of whom will suffer a hip fracture and 30–40 percent of whom will develop vertebral fractures. Hence, in the lifetime of Caucasian women who receive no intervention for bone loss, fragility fractures develop in nearly 50 percent of the population. In the average life-span of Caucasian women, 1 of 6 will have hip fracture and 1 of 12 Caucasian men will do the same. If the criteria to define lesser reductions of low bone mass (osteopenia) in individuals who are also at higher fracture risk than someone with a normal bone mass are used, 50 percent of the Caucasian American population fulfill these criteria.

There is currently no certain method to predict which *individual* patient with low bone mass will ultimately develop fractures. Many cross-sectional and longitudinal studies have determined the relationship between low bone mass and future fracture risk, from which relative risks can be calculated on a population basis. However, it is still impossible to accurately predict future fractures in an individual patient with low bone mass. In addition, a physician cannot predict, on an individual basis, which asymptomatic, untreated, hypertensive patients will develop a high-blood-pressure-related complication. However, this does not negate the importance of detecting high blood pressure in the population because morbidity

and mortality caused by untreated hypertension can be reduced by identifying and intervening in those patients. Similarly, that all patients with significant low bone mass may not develop a fracture does not negate the importance of detecting all individuals with low bone mass to intervene and reduce future fracture risk for high-risk patients. Nontraumatic fractures do not occur without low bone mass and the risk of a fragility fracture has been shown to increase exponentially as bone mass declines (3).

It has been estimated that as much as 33 percent of women and more than 17 percent of men may experience a hip fracture by the age of 90 (4). When average life expectancy is considered, the lifetime risk of hip fracture is about 17 percent in women. Currently, 250,000 new hip fractures occur annually in the United States. The mortality rate of women with hip fractures is nearly 20 percent within the first 3 months after hip fracture. This mortality rate is nearly double for men, even when age-adjusted, after a hip fracture (5). Approximately 50 percent of the survivors of hip fractures require permanent nursing home or institutionalized care. Obviously, the magnitude of this problem is very great and is becoming greater.

Although a fracture of the distal forearm, the proximal humerus, or the vertebral body is ordinarily not fatal, the importance of these fractures on the morbidity and quality of life of patients, as well as the subsequent cost to society, cannot be minimized (6). Recently, it has also been recognized that mortality is also higher in women with vertebral compression fractures (7).

A study conducted in Rochester, Minnesota showed that approximately one-third of women older than age 65 had one or more vertebral compression fractures (7). The National Institutes of Health (NIH) Consensus Conference on Osteoporosis reported that as many as 50 percent of women older than age 65 in the United States have at least one nontraumatic vertebral compression fracture (2).

The problem of vertebral compression fractures has been minimized by many individuals in the medical community because of the assumed less dramatic morbidity and mortality consequences observed with these fractures as compared with consequences of hip fractures. Vertebral compression fractures, however, are quite significant and they may be very painful. The negative long-term effect of vertebral compression fractures is caused by the subsequent loss of height and resulting compromised multiple organ function in many individuals. Equally important, are the issues of the patients' perception of their quality of life. Their concerns include clothes that do not fit correctly and abdomens that protrude and cause personal and social embarrassment. Their individual self-esteem and body image deteriorate, and many aspects of their personal lives may be negatively affected (6). Hence, vertebral fractures, which often occur at an earlier age than do hip fractures, are a very important problem, both for the clinician and for the patient.

The total economic consequence of these various fractures is extremely large. It is estimated that the cost for acute and long-term care solely for patients with hip fractures now exceeds $10 billion annually in the United States. Although accurate estimates of the cost of other individual fractures have not yet been determined, it is estimated that more than $18 billion annually is spent on other osteoporotic fractures (2,7). Because the incidence of osteoporotic fractures is increasing, in part as a result of the aging population, these costs will also increase.

The prevalence of osteoporosis is also increasing as a result of factors *unrelated* to aging. The attainment of a normal peak bone mass, observed when a person is between 20 and 30 years of age, depends predominantly on genetic factors, which account for approximately 80 percent of peak bone development (8). However, dietary calcium intake and the amount of physical exercise during the building-block years of bone development, contribute the other 20 percent of peak bone mass development (9–11). More than 80 percent of the U.S. adolescent population does not consume as much as one-half the recommended dietary allowance (RDA) for calcium (1200 mg/day). It is estimated that only 60 percent of the U.S. adolescent population can pass standard physical fitness tests (12,13). These estimates raise concern that the current generation may never attain as high a peak bone mass as that of preceding generations. If this occurs, the prevalence of osteoporosis may increase from these factors, which blunt peak bone mass attainment and which are unrelated to aging. Because women who enter menopause with a lower peak bone mass may be at higher risk for future fracture than those whose peak bone mass is normal (14), attempts to influence the environmental factors that contribute to maximizing peak bone mass devel-

opment is vital. Therefore, to prevent a further increase in the prevalence of osteoporosis, attention must also be directed to the physical activity and the nutrition of adolescents.

Etiology of Low Bone Mass

There is not total agreement that bone loss occurs in premenopausal women or in men during the years immediately following the achievement of peak bone mass. In cross-sectional studies of men and women aged 30 to 50 years bone loss occurred at a rate of approximately 0.5 percent per year in predominantly cancellous bone of the axial skeleton. Cortical bone mass appeared to be well maintained until the time of menopause in women (15–18). Recently, however, four of the six longitudinal studies that examinined bone mass in various age groups have shown no bone loss at any skeletal site in premenopausal women (19).

However, there is universal agreement that at menopause bone loss occurs and may accelerate to average rates of 2 percent to 3 percent per year (18,20). In the center of the vertebrae (an area of nearly pure cancellous bone) this rate may increase to 6 percent to 8 percent per year during the first 5 to 10 years after menopause (21,22). In addition, during this period, cortical bone mass may also begin to decline. After approximately a decade of estrogen-dependent bone loss, the rates of loss at both skeletal sites decrease again to a slower rate but continue to decline throughout life, the so-called age-related bone loss. The cumulative effect, in a 65-year-old woman may be a 20 percent to 30 percent reduction in total skeletal mass over a period of approximately 20 years (21).

Prediction of Fracture

Although there is decline in bone mass after menopause as well as with aging, not all elderly women or men develop osteopenia to the degree that renders them susceptible to fractures. There is a large distribution of patients surrounding the mean bone mass for a given age in the population; therefore, certain elderly individuals may have relatively well-preserved bone mass and thus be less susceptible to fracture. However, decreased bone mass has been shown to be the most important predictor of future fractures caused by osteoporosis (3,23–25). Therefore, even for the elderly population, the objective measurement of the degree of osteopenia is valuable because it can define those individuals at little to high risk and assist clinical decision-making. Other factors, independent of bone mass, that are predictive of fragility fractures are 1) age, 2) the propensity to fall, 3) the presence of osteomalacia, 4) altered bone quality (26), and 5) the presence of existing fractures (25). Patients with osteoporotic fractures, on the average, demonstrate bone mass values that are more than 2.0 SD below the normal peak bone mass of young healthy individuals (27). The comparison of any patient's bone mass to young normals rather than the comparison to age-matched individuals defines osteoporosis and predicts future fracture risk. The future fracture risk, on the average, increases 2.5 times for each SD that a patient's bone mass is below normal peak bone mass. Over 90 percent of osteoporotic-related fractures occur in patients whose bone mass is at least 2 SD below normal. Therefore, the −2.0 SD level has often been referred to as the "fracture threshold" (27). However, there are patients with bone mass measurements above this level who will fracture and patients with bone mass measurements below this level who will never fracture (3,23–25,27). Thus, substantial overlap exists around this value. The curve relating declining bone mass to increasing fracture rate is exponential (Figure 40.1) (25). Therefore, it is important to identify patients early, when osteopenia is milder, to ensure that interventions to halt bone loss are effective and that bone mass is not continuing to decline, which would increase a patient's risk of future fracture. Objectively, insuring efficacy of interventions is vital to good patient care because future fracture risk becomes higher with each 1.0 SD decline in bone mass.

Bone mass measurements at various skeletal sites have been used for fracture prediction at any skeletal site (i.e., hip or vertebrae). Recent longitudinal data in patients with a mean age older than 60 years suggest that any skeletal site may be measured to predict future fracture risk at any other skeletal site (27). However, there is a trend toward better prediction of specific bone fractures with site-specific measurements (i.e., better prediction of spinal fractures measuring bone mass at the spine). This site-specific predictive relationship exists especially at the hip. Measuring BMD at the femoral neck predicts hip fracture better than measuring bone mass at the lumbar spine to predict hip fracture (28). The relative risk for hip

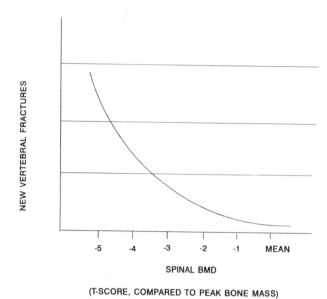

Fig. 40.1. The relationship between the incidence of new vertebral compression fractures and the number of standard deviations an individual patient's spinal bone mass is below the normal peak bone mass. (Reproduced by permission from Davis JW, Ross PD, Wasnich RD. Evidence for both generalized and regional low bone mass among elderly women. J Bone Miner Res 1994;9:305–309.)

fracture increased 2.6 times for each SD reduction in femoral neck BMD. In contrast, the relative risk of hip fracture increased 1.7 times for each SD reduction in lumbar spine BMD (28). Therefore, site-specific measurements of BMD may have advantages for the prediction of future fractures of a specific bone.

In all patients, both the lumbar spine and femoral neck sites may need to be measured. There may be justifiable reasons to measure *both* skeletal sites at baseline and, in some circumstances, longitudinally in patients. In individual perimenopausal patients with a mean age of 53 years, bone mass at various skeletal sites is not uniform (i.e., it is discordant) (29,30). Patients may have normal BMD of the spine but have low BMD at the hip or vice versa. In addition, patients may lose bone slowly at the spine but more rapidly at the hip or vice versa (29,30). A second important reason to consider measuring multiple skeletal sites in patients is that more patients with significant osteopenia may be detected by measuring multiple skeletal sites (27). If a community has access only to a device for wrist bone mass measurement and has no dual-photon x-ray absorptiometry (DXA) available, it is still valuable to use this equipment for patient care. Measuring any skeletal site is better than measuring no skeletal site, especially in the older population for fracture prediction. In perimenopausal women (aged 45–55), however, nearly 50 percent of those with low BMD may not be detected by wrist measurements alone (27). Wrist measurements measure predominantly cortical bone—cancellous bone is lost more rapidly after menopause.

Presently, there are no direct data relating BMD measurements to future fracture prediction for 50-year-old women or younger patients. Younger patients do not fracture enough to have longitudinal data. However, the long-term remaining lifetime fracture probability (RLFP) for a younger woman can be calculated on the basis of her current age and BMD with projected rates of bone loss and life expectancy (27,31,32). The RLFP for a younger woman is greater than it is for an older woman with comparable degrees of reduced bone mass because the younger woman has many more years of exposure to low bone mass in the future than does the older woman. In this regard, a young untreated woman with a femoral neck bone mass 3.0SD below the mean young normal value has a higher *lifetime* probability of hip fracture than does an 80-year-old woman with the same femoral neck bone density. However, the short-term (i.e., current) fracture risk is higher in the older woman because of the independent effect of age on fracture risk and the increased tendency to fall (28,33).

Although bone mass accounts for approximately 80 percent of bone strength and fracture susceptibility, qualitative defects in bone are also important to fracture risk (34). The latter qualitative factors have not been as well defined or as well quantitated using clinical measurements. Therefore, the current clinical practice is to use bone mass measurement as the clinical tool for the management of osteoporotic patients.

Bone mass of an individual at any age is related to peak bone mass attainment and subsequent rate of bone loss. There is a subset of women who lose trabecular bone, cortical bone, or both more rapidly than average. The rapid rates of bone loss may be related to hormonal, lifestyle, mechanical-loading, nutritional, genetic factors, or to all or combinations of these factors (14,35). Longitudinal direct measurement of bone mass is the only objective method to determine whether a patient is a fast or slow loser of bone mass. Rapid losers at menopause, particularly if they remain rapid losers, may have a higher risk of fracture 12 years later than will slow losers (14).

Biochemical markers of bone activity are also predictive of the rate of bone loss (36). However, there is sufficient individual biological variation in the ability of biochemical markers to define the rate of bone loss in individual patients not to warrant utilization of biochemical markers in lieu of direct bone mass measurement in individual subjects. In addition, the rate of bone loss may not be constant in an individual patient. Rapid bone losers may become slow losers and vice versa (37).

Data also indicate that the patient's initiation of osteoporotic preventive programs (including initiating estrogen replacement) may be enhanced by the objective measurement of BMD (38). Patients may be convinced they have a significant potential of developing osteoporosis when they are shown these objective BMD measurements; thus, they may realize that they may be at risk.

Another strong justification for bone mass measurements in the population is to detect osteoporosis *before* a fracture occurs. This recommendation is based on the independent relationship between low bone mass, existing fractures, and future fracture risk. Independent of bone mass, if one wedged vertebra exists, the relative risk for a second fracture in the subsequent 5 years is increased fourfold (3). However, the *combination* of low bone mass *and* one vertebral fracture increases the relative risk 25-fold (39). Hence, detection of a low bone mass to *prevent the first fracture* is vital. Therefore, clinicians can make a strong argument for more widespread use of bone mass measurement for detection of osteopenia to prevent the first fracture, particularly if the detection will influence a clinical decision.

Detection of Osteopenia

In any silent disease process, detection at a late stage is often not difficult, or ideal. Previously, physicians had to rely on plain x-rays, a very insensitive and subjective methodology, to detect significant osteopenia. Approximately 30 percent reduction in bone mass is required to detect significant osteopenia by plain lateral thoracic spine roentgenogram (40–43). Recently, more sensitive and objective radiological tests have been developed to detect osteopenia at much earlier stages. The first noninvasive radiological test developed was a single-photon densitometer (SPA) that measured bone mass at the wrist using a ^{125}I radioisotope source. This technique detected osteopenia when bone loss was only 2 percent to 3 percent below normal bone mass. Hence, SPA represented the first major breakthrough in early detection of osteoporosis (40–42).

The major disadvantage of SPA (or any cortical bone measurement) is that the wrist consists predominantly of cortical bone, a skeletal type that changes slowly over time without effect from pharmacologic intervention. Hence, cortical bone may not be the ideal bone structure to measure for the determination of longitudinal rates of bone loss or response to treatment. The newer modalities of measuring cortical bone mass at the wrist–single-photon x-ray (SPX), the new software available in DXA for wrist measurement, or quantitative computerized tomography (QCT) wrist measurements–are even more accurate and precise than SPA. Regardless of technological improvements, cortical bone is still by nature slow to change over time, with the exception of the effects of certain specific diseases (e.g., primary hyperparathyroidism) (41,44). The distal radius, which has substantial cancellous bone, is also more accurately measured by these newer techniques; thus, this site has been used to follow therapy in some studies (45,46). At this time, more data are needed before distal radius measurements can be advocated to monitor bone loss in place of axial skeletal measurements. For population studies, more perimenopausal women with substantial nonfractured osteopenia will be detected by measuring axial rather than wrist measurements (27).

Cancellous bone has a metabolic turnover rate higher than that of cortical bone and should, in most situations, reflect the impact of either preventive or active treatment programs more readily. This does not negate the possible importance of measuring cortical bone or monitoring bone mass at several sites in selected patients who have active disease or who are receiving active therapy.

The methods currently available for measuring cancellous bone mass of the axial skeleton are DXA and QCT (40–42,47). DXA has replaced the first-generation, dual-photon densitometer (DPA) because it has increased precision. Cancellous bone can also be measured by single-photon x-ray absorptiometry (SXA) at the calcaneus (heel) and is as accurate, precise, and predictive of fracture as is DXA (48).

Methods of measuring cancellous bone might be the preferred method for the earliest detection of osteopenia (49). Because cancellous bone often shows a response to pharmacologic intervention more rapidly than does cortical bone, cancellous bone techniques may be best suited for longitudinal follow-up of treated patients.

DXA and QCT for axial trabecular bone measurement are equally sensitive in detecting osteopenia (40,41). The advantages of DXA lie in its greater precision, lower radiation, and ability to measure the hip. The precision error of DXA, with good quality control, is approximately 1 percent (50). The precision error of single-energy QCT may be 4 percent to 5 percent (40,41). Hence, smaller longitudinal changes can often be detected by DXA. The recent development of the solid QCT phantom may improve the precision error of QCT in the future. However, the radiation exposure of QCT will always be much greater than DXA (1 mrem vs 100 mrem).

Vertebral DXA measurements in the anteroposterior (AP) plane measure the entire vertebral body, including the pedicles and the spinous processes. These processes are often affected by calcification and osteophyte formation, which are quite common in the elderly population and will often falsely elevate AP-DXA measurements. QCT, on the other hand, measures only the center of the vertebral body itself and is therefore not affected by osteophyte formation or sclerosis of the posterior elements. A careful review of the AP-spine DXA data is required to determine whether one or more vertebral bodies should be excluded from the analysis because of these artifacts. The recent development of lateral-spine DXA technology should eliminate the false elevation of AP-spine DXA because the posterior spinal elements may be eliminated from the results (51). Presently there is insufficient longitudinal data from DXA lateral spine scans across all age ranges for a basis for expected rates of change. In addition, patients with kyphosis may demonstrate overlap of the 12th rib on L-1, the iliac crest on L-4, or both. The effects of these overlaps on the interpretation of lateral scans has not yet been defined. Lateral-spine DXA will be an important addition to the clinical monitoring of patients as soon as these issues are clarified and normative data obtained.

Interpretation of Bone-Mass Measurements

A single low bone mass measurement in a nonfractured patient can indicate one of several things. First, the patient may never have achieved normal peak bone mass and the single, low bone-mass measurement may, therefore, not be indicative of previous decline in bone mass. However, because the normal distribution of peak bone mass in the population may not include individuals with more than 2.5 SD reductions in bone mass, patients below this value probably have lost bone. Second, the patient may have achieved normal peak bone mass, and the first low bone-mass measurement might, therefore, indicate that bone mass has been lost. A patient may also have attained relatively normal peak bone mass, had bone loss to a specific level, which is currently measured, and presently be stable with no further bone loss.

The distinction between these various possibilities can only be made with longitudinal measurements of bone mass over time. Correct interpretation of bone-mass measurement results is important in the care of patients with osteopenia. It is important to advise the nonfractured patient that, in many cases, annual measurements may be needed using the same technique (ideally, using the same machine) to define the potential significance of a single, low bone-mass measurement. It may be inappropriate to cause concern and alarm in a nonfractured patient, when the first low bone mass is detected, unless the bone mass is *very* low, because the low bone mass observed may have been present for a number of years. Appropriate clinical evaluation to assess the mechanism(s) of osteopenia is justified, and, in some cases, appropriate prevention interventions are indicated. However, exaggerated conclusions should be avoided.

The definition of "very low bone mass" in a nonfractured individual is currently a matter of debate. The World Health Organization (WHO) defines anyone with a bone mass lower than −1.0 SD below the mean peak bone mass of young individuals as osteopenia, and lower than −2.5 SD below this level as having osteoporosis, even in the absence of fractures. It is important to identify individuals with lesser degrees of low bone mass (between −1.0 and −2.5 SD) because their relative risk for future fracture is increased 2.5-fold for each 1.0 SD reduction. Over 95 percent of the osteoporotic-related fractures occur in individuals with a BMD that is at least 2.5 SD below normal mean peak bone mass. Therefore, this higher risk group is identified as having osteoporosis even if there is no fracture, because of their much greater fracture risk (52,53).

Another important issue in a patient with significant osteopenia is whether or not wedging of any vertebral body has occurred, because the future fracture risk increases dramatically when a patient has both low bone mass and a wedged vertebra. From a practical clinical standpoint, patients can be screened for height loss and potential wedged vertebrae by performing accurate annual height measurements. Annual measurements of a patient's height should be as routine as taking the patient's annual body weight. The clinician will often be surprised how frequently patients remark that they are actually taller than the physician has measured. If such a discrepancy (>1.5 in) is discovered, a lateral thoracic and lumbar spine x-ray is appropriate to determine whether vertebral compression or wedging has occurred. If none are seen, then height loss could easily represent intervertebral disk compression. Alternatively, if vertebral fractures or wedging are observed, the number and degree of deformities also has a gradient prognostic significance for future fracture risk independent of bone mass (3,25). Hence, the discovery of wedged vertebrae should be acted on, not ignored.

A patient with significant osteopenia of the axial skeleton without any loss of height usually does not have significant wedging of vertebrae. Significant wedging of the vertebrae generally requires 20 percent or more reduction in the anterior, posterior, or middle height of the vertebra, compared to its normal margins (54–57). If the vertebral margins are measured accurately with either precision calipers, a digitizer, or by DXA vertebral morphometry a 20 percent reduction in vertebral body height at the anterior or posterior border represents the generally accepted criteria for a vertebral fracture. A 20 percent reduction generally corresponds to a 3.0 SD reduction in vertebral height. This level is believed to be outside the range of nonsignificant vertebral deformity and is often associated with chronic pain syndromes. Ideally, vertebral wedging should be followed on an annual basis to correlate changes in BMD with any potential progression of compression fractures. Thus, in addition to monitoring bone mass, the other important aspect of osteoporosis therapy, the prevention of fractures, should also be monitored.

Use of Bone Densitometry

Risk factors alone cannot predict bone mass in individual patients (error range, >30%) (58). Therefore, a strong argument can be made for the widespread bone-mass testing of all women 50 years of age to identify high-risk individuals. Bone densitometry is the only objective method to diagnose osteoporosis in its early stage to aid women at menopause in making decisions about estrogen replacement therapy (38). Therefore, it is likely that widespread testing of the perimenopausal population will become a broadly accepted recommendation in the future. Epidemiological studies project significant reductions in medical costs related to a decrease in hip fractures and their related costs if more women receive estrogen replacement therapy (59,60).

Responsible guidelines for the use of bone-mass measurement were initially set forth by the National Osteoporosis Foundation (41,61,62):

1 To help in the decision-making process in women debating estrogen replacement therapy (ERT)

2 To assist in the decision for surgical intervention in individuals who have asymptomatic primary hyperparathyroidism

3 To monitor patients receiving chronic glucocorticoid therapy and determine intervention strategies

4 To confirm a diagnosis of osteoporosis in patients where plain x-rays show low bone mass

5 To monitor the efficacy of active treatment programs designed to pharmacologically increase bone mass in individual patients

The Society for Clinical Densitometry now recommends that bone-mass measurements be performed on any person of any age or sex if it will influence a clinical decision (63). Consideration should also be given to the measurement of bone mass even for women who begin ERT at menopause. Published data indicate that 70 percent of these individuals stop taking estrogen within 1 year, and most do not tell their doctor (64). Bone-mass measurements may be an excellent objective measure of compliance. Data also suggest that approximately 15 percent of women with adequate blood levels of estrogen may be estrogen nonresponders and continue to lose bone (65). Hence, women agreeing to begin ERT should be considered for a baseline bone-mass measurement and be followed up 1 year later with a second measurement. If the measurements are stable (indicating both compliance and responsiveness), a third measurement may not be required for many years.

The prevention of osteoporosis requires its detection. The efficacy of any preventive intervention requires proof, which is provided by the measurement of changes in bone mass. The efficacy of pharmacologic therapy to increase bone mass should be monitored by longitudinal bone-mass measurements. Bone-mass measurements are the only objective means available to provide data on prevention and treatment effectiveness.

Recently, biochemical methods have been developed to identify women who lose bone rapidly at menopause and thus predict more severe osteoporosis. These women may have normal bone mass at entry to menopause but lose bone rapidly for the first several years after menopause. Algorithms using a single bone-mass measurement at the time of menopause and several biochemical markers of bone remodeling suggest that this approach may help predict individuals who are at higher risk of developing more severe osteoporosis if they remain untreated (14). However, other investigators have suggested that rapid bone losers may not remain rapid losers and normal bone losers may become rapid bone losers. The only objective way to determine an individual's rate of bone loss is by direct bone-mass measurements (37). Once significant low bone mass is detected, each individual patient requires a differential diagnosis.

Differential Diagnosis of Low Bone Mass

A patient with low bone mass does not necessarily have osteoporosis. Although osteoporosis is the cause of low bone mass in most patients, some patients may have concomitant osteomalacia or other metabolic bone diseases. The prevalence of concomitant osteomalacia in patients who present with what appears to be pure osteoporosis is unknown. There is evidence, however, that the incidence of osteomalacia in the elderly population with femoral neck fractures is not insignificant (66–68). This may be related to the high prevalence, worldwide, of occult vitamin D deficiency. Nutritional vitamin D deficiency has been observed in ambulatory, as well as the institutionalized, elderly populations (69–74). In addition, data suggest that occult osteomalacia may also be present in a large number of individuals with axial low bone mass and vertebral compression fractures (75). This association might be related both to intestinal lactase deficiency, the prevalence of which increases in older age groups who avoid dairy products that provide the major source of dietary vitamin D and calcium (76), and to the seemingly high prevalence of asymptomatic celiac disease in this population. Celiac disease is presently underdiagnosed and should be considered in patients with osteomalacia (77,78) or osteoporosis (79). Celiac disease may lead to osteoporosis rather than to osteomalacia, possibly as a result of selective calcium malabsorption.

A number of items in the patient's history and biochemical profile should be considered when evaluating the differential diagnosis of an individual with osteopenia. Pertinent clinical factors or laboratory tests, if abnormal, increase the likelihood that osteomalacia may be present. They are listed in Table 40.1 and Table 40.2.

The biochemical testing of most osteopenic patients should include serum calcium, phosphorus, alkaline phosphatase and, in most cases, 25-hydroxyvitamin D_3 determinations. Serum calcium, phosphorus and 25-hydroxyvitamin D_3 levels are usually normal in patients with osteoporosis. Nutritional or sunlight exposure insufficiency can cause vitamin D deficiency in the elderly population. These conditions are usually associated with reductions (10–15 ng/mL) in plasma 25-hydroxyvitamin D_3. The abnormality can usually be corrected with 400 to 800 IU per day of vitamin D supplementation. If the serum 25-hydroxyvitamin D_3 level is markedly reduced (<10 ng/mL) or is not normalized by vitamin D supplementation, malabsorption is more likely.

Serum bone alkaline phosphatase is also normal in subjects with osteoporosis unless they have had a recent frac-

Table 40.1. Etiologies of Osteomalacia.

Vitamin D abnormalities
  Reduced 25-hydroxyvitamin D_3 levels
    Nutritional
    Malabsorption or hemigastrectomy
    Hepatic disease
    Phenobarbital or dilantin usage
  Reduced 1,25-dihydroxyvitamin D_3 levels despite normal 25-hydroxyvitamin D_3 levels and normal renal function
  Resistance to vitamin D
    Normal or elevated 1,25-dihydroxyvitamin D_3 levels
    Chronic renal failure
Calcium deficiency
Phosphorus deficiency
Drug-induced (aluminum, fluoride, lithium, diphosphonates, cadmium)
Hyperalimentation
Tumor-associated
Renal tubular acidosis
Primary hyperparathyroidism (after parathyroidectomy)
Beta-thalassemia

Table 40.2. Items in Patient History or Biochemical Profile That Increase Suspicion of Osteomalacia.

Hypocalcemia and/or hypophosphatemia
Low calcium-phosphorus product (<25 mg/de)
Renal disease or renal tubular acidosis
Malabsorption states
Hemigastrectomy
Chronic dilantin or phenobarbital use
Chronic antacid use
Osteopenia plus proximal muscle weakness
Osteopenia and/or bone pain with a sustained elevation of bone alkaline phosphatase
Constant bone pain, particularly at rest
Osteomalacia-associated fractures (Looser's transformation zones)

ture. Alkaline phosphatase increases in the serum during the repair phase of a bone fracture and then returns to normal. This usually occurs over a period of 6 to 8 weeks. An elevated bone alkaline phosphatase of more than 8 weeks' duration, in the absence of new fractures, is also a possible indication of osteomalacia. Bone alkaline phosphatase is also increased in metastatic disease, Paget's disease, and in some patients with primary hyperparathyroidism. Discrimination between bone alkaline phosphatase and alkaline phosphatase of other sources can be enhanced by the development of newer bone-specific alkaline phosphatase assays (80,81).

The only reliable method of confirming a diagnosis of osteomalacia is by quantitative histomorphological evaluation of a nondecalcified bone biopsy (82,83). Strict histologic criteria for the diagnosis of osteomalacia should be used to distinguish osteomalacia from subhistological varieties of osteoporosis and from the high-bone-remodeling states associated with osteoid accumulation (84,85). Double tetracycline labeling should also be performed before a bone biopsy to allow the assessment of the proper quantitative hallmarks distinguishing osteomalacia from osteoporosis (86,87).

The criteria for the diagnosis of osteomalacia are osteoid surface larger than 85 percent, osteoid thickness more than 12 microns, decreased mineral apposition rate, and prolonged mineralization lag time (88). Some preosteomalacia histomorphometric varieties have been described with lesser degrees of vitamin D deficiency (89). However, the previous nomenclature of "focal or localized" osteomalacia should not necessarily be accepted as representing a subvariety of osteomalacia, because it is recognized that these areas of bone often represent focal areas of active bone remodeling (90). The strict definition of osteomalacia allows the diagnosis of osteomalacia as a distinct metabolic bone disease whose etiology must be determined.

If a diagnosis of osteoporosis is confirmed, the etiology of this disease should also be determined. Elderly patients usually have one or both of the two most common forms of osteoporosis: type I (postmenopausal osteoporosis) and type II (age-related osteoporosis) (91).

Type I osteoporosis is related to estrogen deficiency and occurs in the early postmenopausal years. Other secondary consequences of estrogen deficiency are calcium malabsorption, hypercalciuria, elevated 1,25-dihydroxyvitamin D_3 levels, and normal parathyroid hormone levels. Increased bone resorption is related to estrogen deficiency and, when combined with a negative calcium balance, often leads to osteoporosis. Type II osteoporosis results from a reduction in 1,25-dihydroxyvitamin D_3 as the kidney ages and is followed by calcium malabsorption and elevated parathyroid hormone (PTH) levels. Elevated PTH levels have clinical implications because the predominant effect of PTH is a decrease in cortical bone mass, which may, in part, explain the increased hip fracture rate in type II osteoporosis. An inclusive list of possible etiologies of osteoporosis is shown in Table 40.3.

In the geriatric population, several secondary causes of osteoporosis are important, such as primary hyperparathyroidism, multiple myeloma, and hyper-

Table 40.3. Etiologies of Osteoporosis.

Primary osteoporosis
    Idiopathic juvenile osteoporosis (IJO)
    Idiopathic adult osteoporosis (premenopausal women; middle-aged or young men)
Secondary osteoporosis (partial list)
    Endocrine diseases
        Hypogonadism (including athletic amenorrhea)
        Ovarian agenesis
        Hyperadrenocorticism
        Hyperthyroidism
        Hyperparathyroidism
        Diabetes mellitus (?)
        Acromegaly
    Gastrointestinal diseases
        Subtotal gastrectomy
        Malabsorption syndromes (celiac disease)
        Chronic obstructive jaundice
        Primary biliary cirrhosis
        Severe malnutrition
        Anorexia nervosa
        Alactasia

Bone marrow diseases
    Multiple myeloma and related diseases
    Systemic mastocytosis
    Disseminated carcinoma
Connective tissue diseases
    Osteogenesis imperfecta
    Homocystinuria
    Ehlers-Danlos syndrome
    Marfan's syndrome
    Rheumatoid arthritis
Miscellaneous causes
    Immobilization
    Chronic obstructive
    pulmonary disease
    Chronic heparin therapy

thyroidism, which may also include the effects of excess thyroid hormone replacement therapy.

Primary hyperparathyroidism is a very prevalent disease, particularly in the postmenopausal population (92,93) (see also Chapter 33). Prevalence may reflect an actual increase in the prevalence of this disorder in this population or it may be the result of the enhanced biological expression of PTH in the estrogen-deficient state. Nevertheless, increased prevalence of primary hyperparathyroidism is observed in elderly, postmenopausal women—the same group of individuals with the highest prevalence of both postmenopausal and age-related osteoporosis. Therefore, primary hyperparathyroidism is an important disease to suspect even if an elderly patient is normocalcemic upon initial assessment.

The measurement of PTH is not appropriate as part of a routine biochemical assessment in postmenopausal or elderly osteoporotic patients unless some other biochemical marker suggests hyperparathyroidism. These biochemical abnormalities include hypercalcemia, an elevated chloride-phosphate ratio (>33), or persistent hypophosphatemia and renal phosphate wasting. If, however, additional data suggest hyperparathyroidism, then a serum PTH measurement is appropriate. The PTH level, measured by immunoradiometric (IRMA) assay (94), is often normal in cases of mild hypercalcemic hyperparathyroidism. In this situation, quantitative bone histology may provide valuable information to assist with the diagnosis (95–97). The treatment, for an elderly patient with normocalcemic or intermittent mild hypercalcemic primary hyperparathyroidism, is not always parathyroidectomy (98,99). Medical therapies for primary hyperparathyroidism should be considered (100–104) if parathyroidectomy is not performed. It is important to follow both cortical and cancellous bone by longitudinal bone-mass measurement in individuals who do not have surgery (105–107).

Multiple myeloma is more prevalent in the elderly population. Patients may have diffuse low bone mass with or without fractures. In the geriatric population, a sedimentation rate and a serum protein electrophoresis are justified in the initial medical assessment of a patient with osteoporosis. Table 40.4 lists the suggested laboratory tests.

Table 40.4. Laboratory Evaluation of the Elderly Patient with Low Bone Mass.

Routine tests
  CBC
  ESR
  TSH
  Biochemical profile (calcium, phosphorus, chloride, CO_2, creatinine, alkaline phosphatase)
  Protein electrophoresis
  25-hydroxyvitamin D_3 level
  24-hour urine (calcium, phosphorus, creatinine)
Selected tests
  Estradiol/FSH
  Free testosterone/LH
  Prolactin
  Plasma cortisol
  24-hour urine (free cortisol)
  1,25-dihydroxyvitamin D_3 level
  Parathyroid hormone level
  Osteocalcin/bone specific alkaline phosphatase
  Urinary hydroxyproline/creatinine
  Urinary pyridinoline, deoxypyridinoline/creatinine
  Urinary n-Telopeptide/creatinine
  Bone or skin biopsies

CBC = complete blood count; ESR = erythrocyte sedimentation rate; FSH = follicle-stimulating hormone; LH = luteinizing hormone; TSH = thyroid-stimulating hormone.

The biochemical markers of bone turnover have potential clinical value in the assessment and monitoring of patients with metabolic bone disease. Biochemical markers can often predict rapid bone losers, monitor the response to pharmacologic therapy, and follow the hyperparathyroid patient (36). It has been suggested that biochemical markers of bone turnover are predictive of, and are correlated to, bone histomorphometry (36). However, it is still unclear whether bone remodeling rates remain constant in a particular individual over time. The measurement of pyridinoline and deoxypyridinoline collagen crosslinks, formerly by high pressure liquid chromatography and now by radioimmunoassay, has advantages over urinary hydroxyproline because collagen crosslinks are not as dependent on dietary changes, and deoxypyridinoline appears to arise only from bone collagen. However, the usefulness of urinary collagen crosslinks in clinical medicine has yet to be well established and they are not yet routinely tested.

Serum osteocalcin, an osteoblast-derived biochemical marker, is also often elevated during high bone turnover. However, serum osteocalcin is often normal in Paget's disease. Osteocalcin levels may predict the clinical response to calcitonin therapy (108). It may also be valuable to measure noncarboxylated serum osteocalcin, the biologically inactive form of osteocalcin, the carboxylation of which is a vitamin K-dependent step. Noncarboxylated osteocalcin levels are elevated and positively correlated in elderly patients with hip fracture risk and may also suggest vitamin K deficiency.

A number of additional risk factors for hip fractures have been identified (Table 40.5) and these factors should be assessed in each elderly patient. Bone-mass measurement of the femoral neck is the most important predictor of hip fracture at the femoral neck. Although it has been suggested that trochanteric bone mass values best predict trochanteric fractures (109), other independent factors also contribute to hip fracture risk. Preventive interventions in these areas may reduce the risk of hip fracture. Prevention of falls, changing the direction in which falls occur, and the possible use of external hip padding may all reduce hip fractures (110,111).

A recent study described a significant relationship between hip axis length (HAL), the distance between the acetabulum and the lateral edge of the greater trochanter, and hip fracture (112). This predictor is independent of bone mass. Subjects with HAL more than 1 SD longer than the mean for the elderly population have a relative risk of hip fracture that is increased 1.7 times. The relative risk of hip fracture determined by HAL is less than that determined by bone-mass measurement of the femoral neck (1.7 vs 2.7 times the relative risk per 1.0 SD difference from the normal mean), but close to the predictive value of bone-mass measurement at other skeletal sites to predict hip fracture.

Hyperthyroidism has been shown to lead to accelerated bone loss. It has also been suggested that thyroid hormone replacement, in an otherwise euthyroid individual, may have a negative, although possibly reversible, effect on bone metabolism (113–115). Patients who receive thyroid hormone replacement but appear otherwise clinically euthyroid should have at least two measurements of bone mass, 1 year apart, to assess the potential bone loss caused by exogenous thyroid hormone replacement. This is particularly true for individuals with overly suppressed thyroid-stimulating hormone (TSH), especially if the thyroid replacement dose cannot be reduced. If none of these secondary causes of osteoporosis are present in the patient with osteoporosis, therapy for the maintenance of the existing bone mass should be considered.

Prevention of Osteoporosis and Augmentation of Bone Mass

The presence of low bone mass in a nonfractured individual should be followed by preservation of the existing amount of bone. In most instances, particularly for the elderly population with age-related bone mass loss, the longitudinal rate of change in bone mass is small. Even in the younger perimenopausal individual who may be a rapid bone loser, the rate of bone loss during a period of 12 months is usually about 4 percent to 5 percent per year. The significance of a 1-year loss of 5 percent of bone mass depends on the starting level of bone density. The lower the initial bone density, the more significant an additional loss of 5 percent of bone mass, because fracture risk is greater for individuals with the lowest bone mass. An unchecked 4 percent to 5 percent decrease per year in bone mass for several years may also result in severe consequences even if an individual enters menopause with normal bone mass.

Maintenance of bone mass depends on compliance of the patient with a preventive osteoporotic prescription:

1 Adequate exercise

2 Adequate calcium

Table 40.5. Risk Factors for Hip Fracture.

1. Low bone mineral density of the femoral neck or trochanter
2. Age
3. Increased hip axis length
4. Elevated noncarboxylated osteocalcin levels
5. Low vitamin D or vitamin K levels
6. Tendency to fall, characteristics of fall, and decreased standing/day
7. Maternal history of hip fracture
8. Previous fragility fracture of any type after 50 years of age
9. Low body weight after 25 years of age
10. Previous hyperthyroidism
11. Long-term treatment with drugs (e.g., prednisone, Dilantin)
12. Excess caffeine consumption

3 Adequate vitamin D

4 Appropriate estrogen replacement therapy

The effects of exercise on bone turnover are complex and poorly understood. However, there is a general consensus on some basic principles as they apply to the clinical aspects of exercise. Immobilization of an otherwise healthy individual results in excessive bone resorption, hypercalciuria, and loss of bone mass (116). Weightlessness, in space, also leads to accelerated loss of bone mass (117). Bone lost during these latter two situations may be recovered as soon as weight-bearing exercise or a return to an environment with gravity is accomplished. In addition, normal, menstruating women who exercise modestly, have a higher bone mass than their nonexercising, age-matched counterparts (118–120). Similarly, the bone mass of a person's dominant wrist is higher than that of the nondominant wrist (121), and bone mass of the nondominant femur is lower than that of the dominant femur in normal individuals (119).

Cross-sectional studies looking at the effect of exercise on bone mass in both pre- and postmenopausal women suggest a significant positive effect, even in the elderly (122,123). However, well-controlled longitudinal studies have shown only a small effect for aerobic or isometric exercise on bone mass in all adult age ranges (124,125). Immobility is detrimental to the skeleton, to muscle tone, and to balance maintenance, all of which may be important to the preservation of bone mass and the prevention of falls. Therefore, some exercise guidelines are important.

Patients should be encouraged to walk at least 1.5 miles three times per week. If this is not practical or safe for specific patients, simply standing with a walker or doing supervised water exercise may help the patient build muscle tone and provide useful emotional feedback to elderly patients. Retrospective studies suggest that there is a positive relationship between activity and hip fractures. The relative risk for hip fractures is lowest among elderly patients who have the highest degree of physical fitness (119,126).

There is a direct relationship between falls and hip fracture in the geriatric population (33,127). Therefore, it is important to prevent falls in this population because 90 percent of hip fractures occur after a fall (128) and 90 percent of falls occur in the bedroom or bathroom. In-creased activity should be accompanied by other preventive measures to decrease the probability of falls (129). Preventive measures include home protection assessments such as tacking down loose rugs, removing loose or unstable furniture, and providing good lighting in areas of the home used at night. Appropriate walking aids, canes, or walkers, and instructions on how to use them are also important. Central nervous system sedative medications should be used with caution, discontinued, or reduced to the lowest possible doses to avoid states of altered alertness that could cause falls (130). Many physical therapy departments provide home safety checks as a service to prevent falls at home.

Exercise may also help prevent osteoporosis in later life by increasing bone mass in adolescents to a degree higher than that predetermined by their genetic potential (131). Just as practitioners need to be alert to instructing patients about osteoporosis-preventive guidelines for the adult, the family practitioners and pediatricians need to educate parents and their younger patients about osteoporosis prevention.

Calcium is important for the attainment of a higher peak bone mass in adolescents (10), for the maintenance of a positive calcium balance, for the maintenance of bone mass in late postmenopausal osteoporosis (132,133), and, possibly, for the reduction of hip and vertebral fracture rates in late postmenopausal women (134–137).

The RDA of calcium for the adult, nonosteopenic population in the United States is currently 800 mg per day of elemental calcium (2,12). The NIH Consensus Conferences on Osteoporosis recommended that postmenopausal patients of any age with low bone mass consume 1500 mg per day of elemental calcium (2) and the most recent consensus conference suggested calcium intakes across a broad age range for women and men (138). Estrogen-deficient individuals require 2000 mg per day of elemental calcium to maintain positive calcium balance (76).

The loss of estrogen (type I osteoporosis) results in a negative calcium balance partly as a result of a decrease in gastrointestinal calcium absorption efficiency and, in part, to a decrease in renal conservation of calcium. In the early postmenopausal years, bone resorption increases and PTH levels fall, which causes the synthesis of 1,25-dihydroxyvitamin D_3 to decrease. This, in turn, causes renal tubular resorption and gastrointestinal calcium absorption to decrease. Patients older than age 65 have further impairment of calcium absorption from the gastrointestinal tract, particularly at lower dietary calcium intakes. In the elderly population with Type II osteoporosis, the normal gastrointestinal adaptation that increases the fractional absorption of calcium as calcium intakes become lower also declines with aging (139–141). In this situation, PTH levels are elevated because of a larger deficit in gastrointestinal calcium absorption and reduced levels of 1,25-dihydroxyvitamin D_3. Hence, it is important that patients with established osteoporosis receive higher daily intakes of elemental calcium (1500 mg/day).

The average American adult consumes only approximately 500 mg per day of elemental calcium (12). In much of the geriatric population, the average daily calcium consumption is probably lower, in part, from the higher incidence of intolerance to milk products in this population (142). Consequently, calcium supplements may need to be prescribed to make up the deficit. The form of calcium supplementation is important to consider for the elderly population. Calcium carbonate, the most prevalent and often the least expensive form of calcium supplementation, may not be bioavailable in the elderly or achlorhydric patient if taken without meals (140,143). However, most tested forms of calcium carbonate are well absorbed across all age ranges if taken with meals and in divided doses. Patients who have achlorhydria, a problem of increasing importance in the geriatric population, or individuals who cannot take their calcium carbonate with a meal, should be advised to use calcium citrate, which is well-absorbed independent of food consumption (144).

The effects of calcium on bone mass and fracture rate depends on the number of years a patient is beyond menopause and the skeletal site of interest. In *early* postmenopausal women (<7 years after menopause), calcium supplementation alone will not prevent estrogen-dependent bone loss, particularly from cancellous bone sites. However, calcium alone may have a positive effect on total body calcium and cortical bone in the wrist or hip in this population (142,145–147). Calcium alone is not as effective as the combination of calcium and ERT in preventing bone loss in early postmenopausal women. How-

ever, calcium alone seems to benefit cortical bone (145,148). Furthermore, there is reason to suspect that the integrity of the skeleton is worse in individuals who do not consume adequate amounts of calcium (12,21).

In studies of late postmenopausal women in which both calcium intake and the years postmenopause (>7 years) have been controlled, 12 of 12 studies demonstrated a positive skeletal effect of calcium *alone* at both axial and cortical sites (149). One study suggested that this effect was seen only in women whose baseline calcium intake was less than 400 mg per day and that calcium citrate malate was more effective in the prevention of bone loss than calcium carbonate (142). Investigators in New Zealand compared the skeletal effects of calcium supplementation to placebo in late postmenopausal women. These investigators found that calcium alone protected the axial skeleton over a 2-year period (133,136). The cortical bone mass (wrist and femoral neck) in this study was reduced by 35 percent.

Pharmacologic trials in the U.S. have most recently included groups treated with calcium and vitamin D alone as control (i.e., so-called placebo) groups because the Food and Drug Administration (FDA) will not allow pure, untreated, placebo controls in these trials. The trials have also shown positive effects on bone mass in the calcium-alone groups. These data, however, must be evaluated cautiously with regard to whether the positive effects were a result of calcium alone or because of other possible placebo effects of a clinical trial on patients' well-being (150).

The effect of calcium alone on hip fracture rates is unclear. Four retrospective studies suggest that populations with higher calcium intakes have fewer hip fractures than do populations with low calcium diets (134,151–153). This association may or may not be related to calcium alone, because these populations also consume varied amounts of protein, which may confound the results (149). Theoretically, however, calcium alone could have an effect on cortical bone loss of the hip if it lowers PTH in the elderly population, and thus lowers the rate of cortical bone turnover, which may in turn reduce hip fracture rates.

Vitamin D nutrition is as important as calcium nutrition for the elderly population. The current USA-RDA for vitamin D is 400 IU per day. Most adult Americans consume less than this amount. The only natural sources for vitamin D are sunlight activation of skin-stores of vitamin D-precursors and fortified dairy products. Many individuals receive their RDA for vitamin D from an over-the-counter multivitamin, most of which contain at least 400 IU. However, in the geriatric population, milk consumption and sunlight exposure is often limited. Hence, vitamin D deficiency may exist in the following groups of elderly patients: those who reside in institutionalized care centers, those who live alone and are more reclusive, or those ambulatory persons who live in regions of the country in which sunlight exposure is limited by the weather for much of the year (69–72,142).

Plasma levels of 25-hydroxyvitamin D_3, which is the best indicator of the nutritional intake and absorption status of vitamin D, are often low in the elderly American population. This biochemical abnormality is also associated with bone loss. Vitamin D supplementation to 800 IU per day, to ensure normal 25-hydroxyvitamin D_3 blood levels, is recommended for the geriatric population. An important study from France, where milk is not fortified with Vitamin D, showed that supplementing an elderly population with 800 IU per day of vitamin D reduced the incidence of hip fractures (154).

There are other important nutritional factors in the maintenance of normal bone mass. Excess dietary protein can lead to negative calcium balance and an increased urinary calcium excretion. Perhaps, in this case, the urinary calcium-nitrogen ratio is a better indicator of urinary calcium loss (21,149). In addition, a high caffeine intake, chronic cigarette smoking, and chronic excessive alcohol consumption have been shown to predispose a patient to bone loss (155). Consequently, patients need to be educated regarding the modification of these health factors to try to maintain bone mass.

Estrogen replacement in adequate doses prevents postmenopausal bone loss in most patients (156). The exact mechanism whereby bone resorption is inhibited with estrogen is unknown. Recent data suggest that estrogen binding to osteoblasts inhibits osteoblast production of interleukin-6 (IL-6) and other cytokines that mediate bone resorption (157). The sooner ERT is initiated after menopause, the better bone mass is maintained and the less likely a patient is to fracture. Most studies reporting fracture protection with estrogen are retrospective; however, they do suggest that ERT decreases fracture rates (158).

Currently, ERT is the only FDA-approved medication for the prevention of osteoporosis.

Despite the beneficial effects of ERT on osteoporosis prevention, ERT is not currently recommended for most postmenopausal individuals. There are some women for whom the use of ERT is absolutely contraindicated, such as women who have 1) known breast cancer, 2) unexplained vaginal bleeding, 3) pregnancy, 4) active unexplained thromboembolic disease or thrombosis occurring with ERT, and 5) active gallbladder disease. Women with any one or any combination of these contraindications should not be placed on ERT. Aside from this subset, other women refuse to take ERT for a variety of reasons. There is also a large group of women who begin ERT but stop the treatment when side effects or vaginal bleeding occur. Hence, the compliance with ERT is poor (159).

Estrogens increase the chance of endometrial cancer, although this increased risk can be effectively eliminated by the addition of appropriate doses of progesterone (160). The addition of progesterone, however, increases the incidence of vaginal bleeding and other side effects. Progesterone may also obliterate, at least in most of the doses recommended (10 mg), the favorable increase in high-density lipoprotein (HDL) that is observed with ERT alone. Preliminary evidence shows that low-dose, continual administration of progesterone (2.5 mg/d) in combination with proper ERT may also be protective against endometrial cancer with a lower incidence of vaginal bleeding, particularly in elderly women. This regimen does not negatively affect HDL (161). Alternatively, recent data suggest that the addition of various doses or types of progesterone does not affect the atherogenesis process (162,163). Therefore, a woman with an intact uterus should be advised either to take progesterone or to have an annual endometrial biopsy or transvaginal ultrasound to monitor potential endometrial changes as protection from the risk of endometrial cancer.

There is inadequate data regarding any potential beneficial effects of parenteral or vaginal estrogens. Parenteral estrogens expose women to unnecessary high and fluctuating estrogen levels; and, vaginal estrogens may only be beneficial locally. These local vaginal effects of topical estrogens may be quite important, however, to the postmenopausal woman's quality of life.

A woman who becomes aware of low bone mass after

measurement of bone density, may be more convinced of the need for ERT (164). In this situation, the physician has a stronger basis for recommending the initiation of ERT in a patient with low bone mass because the fracture risk is higher and continues to increase as bone mass declines. The measurement of bone mass at baseline and 1 year later, in those individuals who begin ERT, as well as those who have elected not to start ERT, is advisable to assess longitudinal changes. It is suspected that approximately 15 percent of women may not respond to adequate doses of estrogen even with good compliance (65).

How long a patient should remain on ERT is unknown. Withdrawal of ERT after 3 years of use results in the same rate of bone loss observed in untreated women immediately after menopause (165). It is broadly suggested that ERT be continued for a minimum of 15 years. This recommendation is based on meta-analysis data for breast cancer, which suggest that the detection of breast cancer increases 30 percent (relative risk, 1.3) after 15 years of ERT (166). However, the mortality from breast cancer was not greater in the meta-analysis study. It is possible that the subpopulation of patients who remain on long-term ERT are monitored more carefully, which may be the reason there is an increased detection of breast cancer in this subset and that the true breast cancer incidence is not increased. Data from a recent study suggest that women older than 75 years of age who previously received at least 10 years of ERT but discontinued the treatment at least 10 years before enrollment in the study had the same low bone mass as age-matched women who had never received ERT (167). It is therefore probable that ERT should be continued for the remainder of the patient's life. If ERT is discontinued, bone mass measurements can be used to objectively determine whether ERT should be re-initiated in patients who begin to lose bone mass.

The efficacy of beginning ERT in elderly (mean age 65 years), postmenopausal women who have severe osteoporosis and vertebral fractures and who have never previously received ERT, has recently been demonstrated (168). Within 1 year, bone mass of the axial skeleton increased significantly and the rate of new vertebral compression fractures declined. Estrogen, therefore, may be beneficial even for the elderly individual who has never received ERT. If fracture protection truly occurs after only 1 year of therapy with ERT in this population, ERT may be of value regardless of the patient's age or life expectancy.

Individuals with reduced bone mass, particularly if reduced to levels sufficient to result in bone fractures, who do not appear to respond to preventive interventions, may require additional pharmacologic therapy to increase bone mass to levels that reduce future fracture risk. At the very least, persons with low bone mass and existing fractures should receive pharmacologic therapy because their future fracture risk is very high.

Augmentation of bone mass through the pharmacologic manipulation of bone cells is difficult because of the inherent coupling of the cells responsible for bone resorption (osteoclasts) and the cells responsible for bone formation (osteoblasts) (169). Bone remodeling is a continuous process initiated by a number of local and systemic humoral factors. The most important systemic mediator of bone remodeling is PTH. Parathyroid hormone binds to osteoblastic receptors, which release cytokines that then initiate osteoclastic activity, which starts the remodeling process. The remodeling process begins with the formation of resorptive cavities at the bone surface. The stimulation of osteoclastic activity, in turn, also sends biochemical signals back to osteoblasts to stimulate osteoblastic activity (170–171). Hence, the initiation of bone remodeling by PTH and the subsequent resorption of bone creates resorptive cavities. After the osteoclasts have created resorption cavities, the osteoblasts begin forming new bone by first laying down nonmineralized bone matrix (osteoid), which is then mineralized with calcium and phosphorus. In normal biology, the amount of bone resorbed is replaced by an equal amount of bone formed.

Bone remodeling units (BMU) are always present along bone surfaces. At any given time, certain BMU's along the bone are undergoing active resorption, certain areas are undergoing active formation, and certain areas are quiescent (i.e., nonsynchronization exists). However, within any given BMU, the intimate coupling between osteoblasts and osteoclasts exists, and bone remodeling occurs in a very predictable, orderly cycle (172).

Pharmacologic manipulation of bone cells is conceptually difficult because of the possibility that whatever method is used to increase osteoblastic activity may also result in a subsequent increase in osteoclastic activity, and, therefore, in no net increase in bone mass. Alternatively, if the pharmacologic agent inhibits osteoclastic activity, there may also be an equivalent inhibition of osteoblastic activity. Again, the result could be no net increase in bone mass. The sustained uncoupling of the cell involved in the remodeling process to produce an increase in bone formation with a sustained decrease in bone resorption would be the ideal scenario to increase bone mass. To date, no single compound has this capability. There are drugs that inhibit bone resorption (Table 40.6) and other drugs that stimulate bone formation (Table 40.7). It is conceivable that a combination of compounds could achieve the end result.

Salmon calcitonin, in the parenteral form is the only compound, currently FDA-approved, for the treatment of postmenopausal osteoporosis in patients with established fractures. Salmon calcitonin inhibits bone resorption (173–175). It has been shown to increase bone mass in postmenopausal women with osteoporosis (176). The response may be dose-dependent (FDA approved dose: 100 MRC units/day). However, some patients respond to 100 MRC units, or even 25 MRC units every other day (175). The major side effect of parenteral calcitonin is nausea, which is also dose-dependent. Therefore, it may be more appropriate to begin treatment at a lower, less frequent dose and increase titration.

Longitudinal bone densitometry is the only certain method available to measure the response to therapy and

Table 40.6. Inhibitors of Bone Resorption.

1. Calcitonin
2. Estrogens
3. Bisphosphonates
4. Estrogen analogues (tamoxifen, raloxifene, tubulone)

Table 40.7. Stimulators of Bone Formation.

1. Fluoride
2. I-34 intermittent PTH
3. Zeolite
4. Cytokines (IGF$_2$, TGF$_\beta$)
5. Anabolic steroids

IGF = insulin-like growth factor; PTH = parathyroid hormone; TGF = T-cell growth factor.

should be performed annually even for patients who initially respond, because down-regulation of calcitonin receptors may occur and cause a decline in bone mass. Receptor down-regulation is a likely explanation for this observation because the development of calcitonin antibodies may not explain this decline in bone mass despite continued calcitonin administration (177). Properly designed studies to determine the effect of calcitonin on fracture rates have not yet been reported (178). Recent data claims a fracture reduction with nasal calcitonin. However, the small sample size and low fracture rates did not provide sufficient statistical power in this study for the results to be conclusive (179).

The potential of calcitonin to reduce pain in patients with acute vertebral compression fractures has been suggested by published studies (180). This potential analgesic effect can be valuable in preventing or shortening hospitalizations in these patients.

Nasal calcitonin, is approved and widely used in Europe and other areas of the world and was recently approved for use in the U.S. for the treatment of postmenopausal osteoporosis, on the basis of continued data from ongoing fracture studies. The more acceptable route of administration and decreased incidence of nausea are advantages of this formulation.

The *bisphosphonates* are also inhibitors of bone resorption. These compounds are biochemical analogues of naturally-occurring pyrophosphates that are not degraded in the body by pyrophosphatases. They have a high affinity for the skeleton, in which they inhibit bone resorption by impairing osteoclastic recruitment and function and by impairing mineral dissolution (181). As a class, they are poorly absorbed from the gastrointestinal tract and patients must not take these compounds with food or calcium-containing products.

The only published bisphosphonate clinical trial in the U.S. tested the first-generation bisphosphonate, etidronate. This drug has already been approved by the FDA for the treatment of Paget's disease, heterotopic ossification and, in the intravenous form, for hypercalcemia associated with malignancy. Cyclical etidronate increases bone mass and reduced vertebral fracture rate in patients after 2 years of therapy and bone mass is maintained at this higher level with longer use (7 yr) (182–185). In a higher-risk, lower bone mass subpopulation, cyclical etidronate has been shown to reduce vertebral fractures through 3 years of therapy (186). Osteomalacia, which has been observed only with long-term, daily, high-dose use of etidronate, has not been observed in bone biopsies, even after prolonged use of *cyclical* therapy (184,187). In fact, both the 4-year and 7-year bone biopsy data from the multicenter U.S. cyclical etidronate trial show that the initial decline in bone turnover seen after 2 years of cyclical etidronate returns toward baseline. Therefore, a fear of "frozen bone" is not seen with prolonged cyclical etidronate use.

Second- and third-generation bisphosphonates, which are more potent inhibitors of bone resorption, are currently being investigated in clinical trials. Preliminary reports on alendronate and tiludronate suggest that the observed rise in bone mass is approximately the same or slightly greater than that observed with cyclical etidronate (188). It has been suggested that even a 5 percent increase in bone mass may reduce fracture risk by approximately 30 percent to 40 percent (189), assuming bone quality is normal. Although bone mass contributes approximately 80 percent to the strength of bone, if bone quality is compromised, fracture protection may not be realized (190). *Sodium fluoride* (75 mg/day) has been shown to increase bone mass in a 4-year U.S. trial (191). However, this dose did not reduce vertebral fractures and may have increased appendicular fractures. This dose of sodium fluoride may impair bone mineralization; lower doses, used in European trials, did not. The European studies showed a reduced risk of fracture (192). Follow-up observations from the U.S. trial suggest that in a subgroup of patients with lower plasma fluoride levels, fracture rates were actually reduced (193). The toxic-therapeutic window for fluoride may be very narrow. Other fluoride preparations may ultimately prove to be beneficial (194,195).

Vitamin D analogues are proving to be increasingly useful for the treatment of postmenopausal osteoporosis (196). Careful monitoring of the serum calcium is required in patients receiving this therapy because hypercalcemia is a potential risk. In the elderly population, routine vitamin D replacement at doses slightly higher than those recommended in the U.S. may reduce hip fractures, especially for those patients with plasma vitamin D levels that are borderline-low (197). This safe approach may be a very cost-effective method of reducing the hip fracture rate worldwide.

Osteoporosis in Males

Osteoporosis in the male population is increasing as men live longer (5). Furthermore, age-adjusted mortality rates for hip fracture in males is higher than it is for females (5). The etiology of osteoporosis in males is shown in Table 40.8. It has been suggested that some cases of male idiopathic juvenile osteoporosis are really sporadic cases of osteogenesis imperfecta. Hence, skin biopsy for fibroblast culture to detect a defect in collagen synthesis is a consideration in such cases.

If male osteoporosis is hypogonadal, androgen replacement may augment bone mass. However, it is very important to determine the mechanism of the hypogonadism in all patients (198). Androgen replacement is difficult. Parenteral androgen is less toxic to the hepatic system, but liver function needs to be monitored. Androgens increase low-density lipoprotein (LDL)-cholesterol and increase the risk of prostate disease. Certainly, all men who receive androgens for the treatment of osteoporosis require careful monitoring of their prostate gland. If hypercalciuria is present, thiazide diuretics, to reduce urinary calcium excretion, may be beneficial (199).

There are no published data from well-designed clinical trials regarding the possible benefit of bisphosphonates or calcitonin in the treatment of male osteoporosis. However, in certain situations, these pharmacologic therapies are worthy of consideration (i.e., idiopathic osteoporosis seen in men, and osteoporosis in

Table 40.8. Etiology of Osteoporosis in Males.

1. Alcoholism
2. Hypogonadism
3. Myeloma
4. Hypercalciuria
5. Mastocytosis
6. Drug-induced
7. Acromegaly
8. Hyperparathyroidism
9. Hyperthyroidism
10. Gastrointestinal diseases
11. Idiopathic

young men with progressive fractures). Elderly men, like women, need couseling regarding proper calcium and vitamin D intake. Bone histology should be considered for young men with apparent aggressive idiopathic osteoporosis to exclude mastocytosis, a condition that may be more prevalent than previously recognized.

Conclusion

The prevalence of osteoporosis is increasing, but osteoporosis can be prevented and treated. It can be diagnosed before the first fracture occurs, an important intervention strategy to reduce the high risk for future fracture. Wider use of bone-mass measurements will allow greater detection of patients at high risk for future fracture. Appropriate intervention prevention strategies, including ERT, need to be more broadly employed in the elderly population. Newer pharmacology is also available to augment bone mass and reduce future fracture risk.

References

1. The WHO Study Group. Assessment of fracture risk and its application to screening for postmenopausal osteoporosis. Geneva: World Health Organization, 1994.
2. Consensus Conference: osteoporosis. JAMA 1984;799–802.
3. Ross PD, Davis JW, Epstein RS, Wasnich RD. Pre-existing fractures and bone mass predict vertebral fracture incidence in women. Ann Intern Med 1991;114:919–923.
4. Jacobson SJ, Goldberg J, Miles TP, et al. Hip fracture incidence among the old and very old: a population-based study of 745,435 cases. Am J Public Health 1990; 80:871–873.
5. Seeman E. Epidemiology and diagnosis of osteoporosis in men. In: Christiansen C, Riis B, eds. Fourth International Symposium on Osteoporosis. Hong Kong: Gardiner-Caldwell Communications Ltd; Hong Kong 1993.
6. Cook DJ, Guyatt GH, Adachi JD, et al. Quality of life issues in women with vertebral fractures due to osteoporosis. Arthritis Rheum 1993;36:750–756.
7. Melton LJ III, Riggs BL. Epidemiology of age-related factors. In: Avioli LV, ed. The osteoporotic syndrome. Orlando: Grune & Stratton, 1987:1–30.
8. Kelly PJ, Eisman JA, Sambrock PN. Interaction of genetic and environmental influences on peak bone density. Osteoporos Int 1990;1:56–60.
9. Kanders B, Dempster DW, Lindsay R. Interaction of calcium nutrition and physical activity on bone mass in young women. J Bone Miner Res 1988;3:145–149.
10. Johnston CC Jr, Miller JZ, Slemenda CW, et al. Calcium supplementation and increases in bone mineral density in children. N Engl J Med 1992;327:82–87.
11. Recker RR, Heaney RP. Peak bone density in young women. JAMA 1993;270:841–844.
12. Public Health Service Office of Disease Prevention and Health Promotion. The National Children and Youth Fitness Study: a summary of findings. JOPERD 1985:13–93.
13. Avioli LV. The calcium controversy and the recommended dietary allowance. In: Avioli LV, ed. The osteoporotic syndrome. Orlando: Grune & Stratton, 1987:57–66.
14. Christiansen C. Postmenopausal bone loss and the risk of osteoporosis. Osteoporos Int 1994;1(suppl):S47–S51.
15. Riggs BL, Wahner HW, Dunn WL, et al. Differential changes in bone mineral density of the appendicular and axial skeleton with aging; relationship to spinal osteoporosis. J Clin Invest 1981;67:328–335.
16. Riggs BL, Wahner HW, Seeman E, et al. Changes in bone mineral density of the proximal femur and spine with aging. J Clin Invest 1982;70:716–723.
17. Riggs BL, Melton LJ III. Involutional osteoporosis. N Engl J Med 1986;314:1676–1684.
18. Riggs BL, Wahner HW, Melton LJ III, et al. Rates of bone loss in the appendicular and axial skeletons of women. J Clin Invest 1986;77:1487–1491.
19. Recker RR, Lappe JM, Davies KM, Kimmel DB. Change in bone mass immediately before menopause. J Bone Miner Res 1992;7:857–862.
20. Nilas L, et al. Comparison of single- and dual-photon absorptiometry in postmenopausal bone mineral loss. J Nucl Med 1985;26:1257–1262.
21. Heaney RP. Prevention of osteoporotic fracture in women. In: Avioli LV, ed. The osteoporotic syndrome. Orlando: Grune & Stratton, 1987:67–90.
22. Genant HK, Ettinger B, Cann CE, et al. Osteoporosis: assessment by quantitative computed tomography. Orthop Clin North Am 1985;16:557–568.
23. Hui SL, Slemenda CW, Johnston CC Jr. Age and bone mass as predictors of fracture in a prospective study. J Clin Invest 1988;81:1804–1809.
24. Cummings SR, Black DM, Nevitt MC, et al. Appendicular bone density and age predict hip fracture in women. JAMA 1990;263:665–668.
25. Ross PD, Genant HK, Davis JW, et al. Predicting vertebral fracture from prevalent fractures and bone density among non-black, osteoporotic women. Osteoporos Int 1993;3:120–126.
26. Heaney RP. Osteoporotic fracture space: an hypothesis. Bone Miner 1989;6:1–13.
27. Melton LJ III, Alkinson EJ, O'Fallon WM, et al. Long-term fracture prediction by bone mineral assessed at different skeletal sites. J Bone Miner Res 1993;8:1227–1233.
28. Cummings SR, Black DM, Nevitt MC, et al. Bone density at various sites for prediction of hip fractures. Lancet 1993;341:72–75.
29. Pouilles JM, Tremollieres F, Ribot C. Spine and femur densitometry at the menopause: are both sites necessary in

the assessment of the risk of osteoporosis? Calcif Tissue Int 1993;52:344–347.

30. Davis JW, Ross PD, Wasnich RD. Evidence for both generalized and regional low bone mass among elderly women. J Bone Miner Res 1994;9:305–309.

31. Black DM, Cummings SR, Melton LJ III. Appendicular bone mineral and a women's lifetime risk of hip fracture. J Bone Miner Res 1992;7:639–646.

32. Wasnich RD. Fracture prediction with bone mass measurements. In: Genant HK, ed. Osteoporosis update. Berkeley: University Press, 1987:95–101.

33. Greenspan SL, Myers ER, Maitland LA, et al. Fall severity and bone mineral density as risk factors for hip fractures in ambulatory elderly. JAMA 1994;271:128–133.

34. Recker RR. Architecture and vertebral fracture. Calcif Tissue Int 1993;53(suppl 1):S139–S142.

35. Ott SM. When bone mass fails to predict bone failure. Calcif Tissue Int 1993;53(suppl 1):S7–S13.

36. Delmas PD. Biochemical markers of bone turnover for the clinical assessment of metabolic bone disease. Endocrin Metab Clin North Am 1990;19:1–18.

37. Hui SL, Slemenda CW, Johnston CC Jr. The contribution of rapid bone loss in postmenopausal osteoporosis. Osteoporos Int 1990;1:30–34.

38. Rubin SM, Cummings SR. Results of bone densitometry affect women's decisions about taking measures to prevent fractures. Ann Intern Med 1992;116:990–995.

39. Ross PD, Davis JW, Wasnich RD. Bone mass and beyond: risk factor for fractures. Calcif Tissue Int 1993;53(suppl 1):S134–S138.

40. Kimmel PL. Radiologic methods to evaluate bone mineral content. Ann Intern Med 1984;100:908–911.

41. Chesnut CH III. Noninvasive methods of measuring bone mass. In: Avioli LV, ed. The osteoporotic syndrome. Orlando: Grune & Stratton, 1987:31–43.

42. Cummings SR. Bone mineral density. Ann Intern Med 1987;107:932–936.

43. Wahner HW, Eastell R, Riggs BL. Bone mineral density of the radius: where do we stand? J Nucel Med 1985;26:1339–1341.

44. Riis BJ, Christiansen C. Measurement of spinal or peripheral bone mass to estimate early postmenopausal bone loss? Am J Med 1988;84:646–653.

45. Marslew U, Overgaard K, Riis BJ, Christiansen C. Two new combinations of estrogen and progestogen for prevention of postmenopausal bone loss: long-term effects on bone, calcium and lipid metabolism, climacteric symptoms and bleeding. Obstet Gynecol 1992;79:202–210.

46. Christiansen C. Use of nasally administered salmon calcitonin in preventing bone loss. Calcif Tissue Int 1991;49(suppl 2):S14–S15.

47. Mazess RB, et al. Performance of an x-ray dual-photon scanner. Second International Workshop on Non-Invasive Bone Measurements. Leuven, Belgium, 1987.

48. Ross P, Huang C, Davis J, et al. Predicting vertebral deformity using bone densitometry at various skeletal sites and calcaneous ultrasound. Bone 1995;16:325–332.

49. Melton LJ III, Chrischilles EA, Cooper C, et al. Perspective: how many women have osteoporosis? J Bone Miner Res 1992;7:1005–1009.

50. Faulkner KG, McClung MR. Quality control of DXA instruments in multicenter trials. Osteoporos Int 1995;5:218–227.

51. Finkelstein JS, et al. A comparison of lateral versus anterior-posterior spine dual energy X-ray absorptiometry for the diagnosis of osteopenia. J Clin Endocrinol Metab 1994;78:724–730.

52. Melton LJ III. How many women have osteoporosis now? J Bone Miner Res 1995;10:175–177.

53. Kanis J. World Health Organization–assessment of fracture risk and its application to screening for postmenopausal osteoporosis. Technical Report Series Geneva: World Health Organization, 1994.

54. Eastell R, Cedel SL, Wahner HW, et al. Classification of vertebral fractures. J Bone Miner Res 1991;6:207–215.

55. McCloskey EV, Spector TD, Eyres KS, et al. The assessment of vertebral deformity: a method for use in population studies and clinical trials. Osteoporos Int 1993;3:138–147.

56. Davies KM, Recker RR, Heaney RP. Revisable criteria for vertebral deformity. Osteoporos Int 1993;3:265–270.

57. Sauer P, Leidig G, Minne HW, et al. Spine deformity index (SDI) versus other objective procedures of vertebral fracture identification in patients with osteoporosis: a comparative study. J Bone Miner Res 1991;6:227–238.

58. Slemenda CW, Hui SL, Longcope C, et al. Predictors of bone mass in perimenopausal women. Ann Intern Med 1990;112:96–101.

59. Cheung AP, Wren BG. A cost-effectiveness analysis of hormone replacement therapy in the menopause. Med J Aust 1992;156:312–316.

60. Johsson B, Christiansen C, Johnell O, Hedbrandt J. Cost-effectiveness of fracture prevention in established osteoporosis. Osteoporos Int 1995;5:136–142.

61. Peck WA, et al. National Osteoporosis Foundation. Physician's resource manual on osteoporosis. Washington, DC: National Osteoporosis Foundation, 1987:14.

62. Johnston CC Jr, Slemenda CW, Melton LJ III. Clinical use of bone densitometry. N Engl J Med 1991;324:1105–1109.

63. Miller PD, Bonnick SL, Rosen C, for the International Panel of the Society for Clinical Densitometry. Consensus of an international panel on the clinical utility of bone mass measurements in the detection of low bone mass in the adult population. Calcified Tiss Int 1996.

64. Lindsay R. Criteria for successful estrogen therapy in osteoporosis. Osteoporos Int 1993;2(suppl):S9–S13.

65. Stevenson JC, Cust MP, Ganger KF, et al. Effects of transdermal versus oral hormone replacement therapy on bone density in spine and proximal femur in postmentopausal women. Lancet 1990;335:265–269.

66. Chalmers J, Edinburgh WD, Conacher WDH, et al. Osteomalacia – a common disease in elderly women. J Bone Joint Surg 1967;49:403–423.

67. Jenkins DHR, Roberts JG, Webster D, Williams EO.

Osteomalacia in elderly patients with fracture of the femoral neck. J Bone Joint Surg 1973;55:575–580.

68. Aaron JE, Gallagher JC, Anderson J. Frequency of osteomalacia and osteoporosis in fractures of the proximal femur. Lancet 1974;1:229–233.

69. Parfitt AM, Chir B, Gallagher JC, et al. Vitamin D and bone health in the elderly. Am J Clin Nutr 1982;36:1014–1031.

70. McKenna MJ, Freaney R, Meade A, Muldowney FP. Prevention of hypovitaminosis D in the elderly. Calcif Tissue Int 1985;37:112–116.

71. Clemens TL, Zhou X-Y, Myles M, et al. Serum vitamin D_2 and vitamin D_3 metabolite concentrations and absorption of vitamin D_2 in elderly subjects. J Clin Endocrinol Metab 1986;63:656–660.

72. Holick MF. Vitamin D requirements for the elderly. Clin Nutr 1986;5:121–129.

73. Salamone LM, Dallal GE, Zantos D, et al. Contributions of vitamin D intake and seasonal sunlight exposure to plasma 25-hydroxyvitamin D concentration in elderly women. Am J Clin Nutr 1994;59:80–86.

74. Chapuy MC, Arlot ME, Duboeuf F, et al. Vitamin D_3 and calcium to prevent hip fractures in the elderly women. N Engl J Med 1992;327:1637–1642.

75. Miller PD, Huffer WE, Krebs RA, et al. Axial osteopenia: the necessity of bone histology in distinguishing between osteoporosis and osteomalacia. First International Symposium on Osteoporosis. Copenhagen, Denmark, 1984.

76. Heaney RP. Calcium intake requirement and bone mass in the elderly. J Lab Clin Med 1982;100:309–312.

77. Hajjar ET, Vincenti F, Salti CS. Gluten-induced enteropathy: Osteomalacia as a principal manifestation. Arch Intern Med 1974;134:565–566.

78. Trier JS. Celiac sprue. N Engl J Med 1991;325:1709–1719.

79. Mazure R, Vazquez H, Gonzalez D, et al. Bone mineral affection in asymptomatic adult patient with celiac disease. Am J Gastroenterol 1994;89:2130–2134.

80. Panigrahi K, et al. Characteristics of a two-site immunoradiometric assay for measuring human skeletal alkaline phosphatase in serum. Clin Chem 1994;40:822–828.

81. Garnero P, Delmas PD. Assessment of the serum levels of bone alkaline phosphatase with a new immunoradiometric assay in patients with metabolic bone disease. J Clin Endocrinol Metab 1993;77:1046–1053.

82. Teitelbaum SL. Osteoporosis and the bone biopsy. In: Avioli LV, ed. The osteoporotic syndrome. Orlando: Grune & Stratton, 1987:45–55.

83. Hodgson SF, Johnson KA, Muhs JM, et al. Outpatient percutaneous biopsy of the iliac crest: methods, morbidity and patient acceptance. Mayo Clin Proc 1986;61:28–33.

84. Whyte MP, Bergfeld MA, Murphy WA, et al. Postmenopausal osteoporosis: a heterogenous disorder as assessed by histomorphometric analysis of iliac crest bone from untreated patients. Am J Med 1982;72:193–202.

85. Parfitt AM, Drezner MK, Glorieux FH, et al. Bone histomorphometry: standardization of nomenclature, symbols and units. J Bone Miner Res 1987;2:595–610.

86. Frost HM. Tetracycline-based histological analysis of bone remodeling. Calcif Tissue Res 1969;3:211–237.

87. Huffer WE, Leboff RB. An indirect method of measuring widths suitable for automated bone histomorphometry. J Bone Miner Res 1992;7:1417–1427.

88. Parfitt AM. Osteomalacia and related disorders. In: Krane SM, ed. Metabolic bone disease. 2nd ed. New York: Grune & Stratton, 1990:329–396.

89. Rao DS, Villanueva AR, Mathews M, et al. Histological evolution of vitamin-D depletion in patients with intestinal malabsorption or dietary deficiency. In: Frame B, Potts JT, eds. Clinical disorders of bone and mineral metabolism. Amsterdam: Excerpta Medica, 1983:224–226.

90. Parfitt AM. Osteomalacia and related disorders. In: Avioli LV, Krane SM, eds. Metabolic bone disease. Philadelphia: Saunders, 1990:329–396.

91. Riggs BL, Melton LJ III. Evidence for two distinct syndromes of involutional osteoporosis. Am J Med 1983;75:899–901.

92. Health H III, Hodgson SF, Kennedy MA. Primary hyperparathyroidism. N Engl J Med 1980;302:189–192.

93. Melton LJ III. Epidemiology of primary hyperparathyroidism. J Bone Miner Res 1990;6(suppl 2):S25–S29.

94. Nussbaum SR, Potts JT. Immunoassays for parathyroid hormone I-84 in the diagnosis of hyperparathyroidism. J Bone Miner Res 1991;6(suppl 2):S43–S50.

95. Christiansen P, Steiniche T, Vesterby A, et al. Primary hyperparathyroidism: iliac crest trabecular bone volume, structure, remodeling and balance evaluated by histomorphometric methods. Bone 1992;13:41–49.

96. Parisien M, Silverberg SJ, Shane E, et al. The histomorphometry of bone in primary hyperparathyroidism: preservation of cancellous bone structure. J Clin Endocrinol Metab 1990;70:930–938.

97. van Doorn L, Lips P, Netelenbos JC, Hackeng WHL. Bone histomorphometry and serum concentrations of intact parathyroid hormone (PTH(1-84)) in patients with primary hyperparathyroidism. Bone Miner 1993;23:233–242.

98. Coe FL, Favus MJ. Does mild, asymptomatic hyperparathyroidism require surgery? N Engl J Med 1980;302:224–225.

99. Bilezikian JP. Surgery or no surgery for primary hyperparathyroidism. Ann Intern Med 1985;102:402–403.

100. Medical management of primary hyperparathyroidism. Lancet 1984;1:727–729. Editorial.

101. Marcus R, Madvig P, Crim M. Conjugated estrogens in the treatment of postmenopausal women with hyperparathyroidism. Ann Intern Med 1984;100:633–640.

102. Selby PL, Peacock M. Ethinyl estradiol and norethindrone in the treatment of primary hyperparathyroidism in postmenopausal women. N Engl J Med 1986;314:1481–1485.

103. Coe FL, Favus MJ, Parks JH. Is estrogen preferable to surgery for postmenopausal women with primary hyperparathyroidism? N Engl J Med 1986;314:1508–1509.

104. McDermott, MT, Perloff JJ, Kidd GS. Effects of mild asymptomatic primary hyperparathyroidism on bone mass in women with and without estrogen replacement therapy. J Bone Miner Res 1994;9:509–514.

105. Marcus R, Madvig P, Young G. Age-related changes in parathyroid hormone and parathyroid hormone action in normal human. J Clin Endocrinol Metab 1984;58:223–230.

106. Martin P, Bergmann P, Gillet C, et al. Partially reversible osteopenia after surgery for primary hyperparathyroidism. Arch Intern Med 1986;146:689–691.

107. Kochersberger G, Buckley NJ, Leight GS, et al. What is the clinical significance of bone loss in primary hyperparathryroidism? Arch Intern Med 1987;147:1951–1953.

108. Civitelli R, Gonnelli S, Zacchei F, et al. Bone turnover in postmenopausal osteoporosis. J Clin Invest 1988;82:1268–1274.

109. Greenspan SL, Myers ER, Maitland LA, et al. Trochanteric bone mineral density is associated with type of hip fracture in the elderly. J Bone Miner Res 1994;9:1889–1894.

110. Hayes WC, Piazza SJ, Zysset DK. Biomechanics of fracture risk prediction of the hip and spine by QCT. Radiol Clin North Am 1991;29:1–18.

111. Lauritzen JB, Petersen MM, Lund B. Effect of external hip protectors on hip fractures. Lancet 1993;341:11–13.

112. Faulkner KG, Cummings SR, Black DM, et al. Simple measurement of femoral geometry predicts hip fracture: the study of osteoporotic fractures. J Bone Miner Res 1993;8:1211–1217.

113. Coindre JM, David JP, Riviere L, et al. Bone loss in hypothyroidism with hormone replacement. A histomorphometry study. Arch Intern Med 1986;146:48–53.

114. Stall GM, Harris S, Sokoll LJ, Dawson-Hughes B. Accelerated bone loss in hypothyroid patient overtreated with L-thyroxine. Ann Intern Med 1990;113:265–269.

115. Diamond T, Vine J, Smart R, Butler P. Thyrotoxic bone disease in women: A potentially reversible disorder. Ann Intern Med 1994;120:8–11.

116. Mazess RB, Whedon GD. Immobilization and bone. Calcif Tissue Int 1983;35:265–267.

117. Keller TS, Strauss AM, Szpalski M. Prevention of bone loss and muscle atrophy during manned space flight. Microgravity Q 1992;2:89–102.

118. Heath H III. Athletic women, amenorrhea, and skeletal integrity. Ann Intern Med 1985;102:258–259.

119. Pocock NA, Eisman J, Gwinn T, et al. Physical fitness is a major determinant of femoral neck and lumbar spine bone mineral density. J Clin Invest 1986;78:618–621.

120. Marcus R, Drinkwater B, Dalsky G, et al. Osteoporosis and exercise in women. Med Sci Sports Exerc 1992;24(suppl 6):S301–S307.

121. Huddleston AI, Rockwell D, Kulund DN. Bone mass in lifetime tennis players. JAMA 1980;244:1107–1109.

122. Krolner B, Toft B, Pors Nielson S, Tondevold E. Physical exercise as prophylaxis against involutional vertebral bone loss: A controlled trial. Clin Sci 1983;64:541–546.

123. Aloia JF, Cohn SH, Ostuni JA, et al. Prevention of involutional bone loss by exercise. Ann Intern Med 1978;89:356–358.

124. Dalsky G, Stocke KS, Ensoni AA. Weight-bearing exercise training and lumbar bone mineral content in postmenopausal women. Ann Intern Med 1988;108:824–828.

125. Pruitt LA, Jackson RD, Bartels RL, Lehnhard HJ. Weight-training effects on bone mineral density in early postmenopausal women. J Bone Miner Res 1992;7:179–185.

126. Kreiger N, Kelsey JL, Holford TR, O'Connor T. An epidemiologic study of hip fracture in postmenopausal women. Am J Epidemiol 1982;116:141–148.

127. Peck WA. Falls and hip fracture in the elderly. Hosp Pract 1986:72A–72L.

128. Tinetti ME, Speechley M. Prevention of falls among the elderly. N Engl J Med 1989;320:1055–1059.

129. Tinetti ME, et al. A multifactorial intervention to reduce the risk of falling among elderly people living in the community. N Engl J Med 1994;331:821–827.

130. Ray WA, Griffin MR, Schaffner W, et al. Psychotropic drug use and the risk of hip fracture. N Engl J Med 1987;316:363–369.

131. Slemenda CW, Miller JZ, Hui SL, et al. Role of physical activity in the development of skeletal mass in children. J Bone Miner Res 1991;6:1227–1233.

132. Heaney RP, Recker RR, Saville PD. Menopausal changes in calcium balance performance. J Lab Clin Med 1978;92:953–963.

133. Reid IR, Ames RW, Evans MC, et al. Effect of calcium supplementation on bone loss in postmenopausal women. N Engl J Med 1993;328:460–464.

134. Holbrook TL, Barrett-Conner E, Winegard DL. Dietary calcium and risk of hip fracture: 14-year prospective study. Lancet 1988;2:1046–1049.

135. Looker AC, Harris TB, Madans JH, Sempos CT. Dietary calcium and hip fracture risk: the NHANES I epidemiologic follow-up study. Osteoporos Int 1993;3:177-184.

136. Reid IR, Ames RW, Evans MC, et al. Long-term effects of calcium supplementation on bone loss and fracture in postmenopausal women: a randomized controlled trial. Am J Med 1995;98:331–335.

137. Recker RR, Kimmel DB, Hinders S, Davies KM. Anti-fracture efficacy of calcium in elderly women. J Bone Miner Res 1994;9(suppl 1):S154.

138. NIH Consensus Development Panel on Optimal Calcium Intake. Optimal calcium intake. JAMA 1994;272:1942–1948.

139. Gallagher JC, Riggs BL, Eisman J, et al. Intestinal calcium absorption and serum vitamin D metabolites in normal subjects and osteoporotic patients: effect of age and dietary calcium. J Clin Invest 1979;64:729–736.

140. Heaney RP, Recker RR. Estimation of true calcium absorption. Ann Intern Med 1985;130:516–521.

141. Heaney RP, Weaver CM, Fitzsimmons ML. The influence of

calcium load on absorption fraction. J Bone Miner Res 1990;11:1135–1138.

142. Dawson-Hughes B, Dallal GE, Krall EA, et al. A controlled trial of the effect of calcium supplementation on bone density in postmenopausal women. N Engl J Med 1990;323:878–883.

143. Recker RR. Calcium absorption and achlorhydria. N Engl J Med 1985;313:70–73.

144. Heaney RP. Calcium supplements: practical considerations. Osteoporos Int 1991;1:65–71.

145. Nilas L, Christiansen LN, Rodbro P. Calcium supplementation and postmenopausal bone loss. BMJ 1984;289:1103–1106.

146. Ettinger B, Genant HK, Cann CE. Postmenopausal bone loss is prevented by treatment with low-dosage estrogen with calcium. Ann Intern Med 1987;106:40–45.

147. Riis B, Thomsen K, Christiansen C. Does calcium supplementation prevent postmenopausal bone loss? A double-blind, controlled study. N Engl J Med 1987;316:173–177.

148. Aloia JF, Vaswani A, Yeh JK, et al. Calcium supplementation with and without hormone replacement therapy to prevent postmenopausal bone loss. Ann Intern Med 1994;120:97–103.

149. Heaney RP. Nutritional factors in osteoporosis. Ann Rev Nutr 1993;13:287–316.

150. Heaney RP. How do we know what we know? J Bone Miner Res 1991;6:103–105.

151. Matkovic V, Kostial K, Simonovic I, et al. Bone status and fracture rates in two regions of Yugoslavia. Am J Clin Nutr 1979;32:540–549.

152. Wickham CAC, Walsh K, Cooper C, et al. Dietary calcium, physical activity and risk of hip fracture: a prospective study. BMJ 1989;299:889–892.

153. Lau E, Donnan S, Barker DJP, Cooper C. Physical activity and calcium intake in fracture of the proximal femur in Hong Kong. BMJ 1988;297:1441–1443.

154. Meunier PJ. Prevention of hip fractures. Am J Med 1993;95:75S–78S.

155. Slemenda CW. Risk factors for low bone mass: Clinical implications. Ann Inter Med 1993;118:741–742.

156. Lindsay R. Estrogens in prevention and treatment of osteoporosis. In: Avioli LV, ed. The osteoporotic syndrome. Orlando: Grune & Stratton, 1987:91–107.

157. Jilka RL, Hangoc G, Girasole G, et al. Increased osteoclast development after estrogen loss: Mediation by interleukin-6. Science 1992;275:88–91.

158. Ettinger B, Genant HK, Cann CE. Long-term estrogen replacement therapy prevents bone loss and fractures. Ann Intern Med 1985;102:319–324.

159. Ryan PJ, Harrison R, Blake GM, Fogelman I. Compliance with hormone replacement therapy (HRT) after screening for post menopausal osteoporosis. Br J Obstet Gynecol 1992;99:325–328.

160. Persson I, Adami HO, Bergkvist L. Risk of endometrial cancer after treatment with oestrogens alone or in conjunction with progestogens: results of a prospective study. BMJ 1988;298:147–151.

161. Weinstein L. Efficacy of a continuous estrogen-progestin regimen in the menopausal patient. Obstet Gynecol 1987;69:929–932.

162. Wagner JD, Clarkson TB, St. Clair RW, et al. Estrogen and progesterone replacement therapy reduces low-density lipoprotein accumulation in the coronary arteries of surgically postmenopausal cynomolgus monkeys. J Clin Invest 1991;88:1995–2002.

163. Christiansen C, Riis B. Five years with continuous combined oestrogen/progestogen therapy. Effects on calcium metabolism, lipoproteins and bleeding pattern. Br J Obstet Gynecol 1990;97:1087–1092.

164. Rubin SM, Cummings SR. Results of bone density affects women's decisions about taking measures to prevent fractures. Ann Intern Med 1992;116:990–995.

165. Christiansen C, Christiansen MS, Transbol I. Bone mass in post-menopausal women after withdrawal of estrogen/gestagen replacement therapy. Lancet 1981;1:459–461.

166. Steinberg KK, Thacker SB, Smith SJ, et al. A meta-analysis of the effect of estrogen replacement therapy on the risk of breast cancer. JAMA 1991;265:1985–1990.

167. Ettinger B, Grady D. The waning effect of postmenopausal estrogen therapy on osteoporosis. N Engl J Med 1993;329:1192–1193.

168. Lufkin EG, Wahner HW, O'Fallon WM, et al. Treatment of postmenopausal osteoporosis with transdermal estrogen. Ann Intern Med 1992;117:1–9.

169. Raisz LG, Kream BE. Regulation of bone formation. N Engl J Med 1983;309:29–33, 83–89.

170. Slovik DM, Neer R, Potts JT Jr. Short-term effects of synthetic human parathyroid hormone-(I-34) administration on bone mineral metabolism in osteoporotic patients. J Clin Invest 1981;68:1261–1271.

171. Dewhirst FE, Ago JM, Peros WJ, Stashenko P. Synergism between parathyroid hormone and interleukin 1 in stimulating bone resorption in organ culture. J Bone Miner Res 1987;2:127–133.

172. Frost HM. The origin and nature of transients in human bone remodeling dynamics. In: Frame B, Parfitt AM, Duncan H, eds. Clinical aspects of metabolic bone disease. Amsterdam: Excerpta Medica, 1973:124–140.

173. Gennari C, Avioli LV. Calcitonin therapy in osteoporosis. In: Avioli LV, ed. The osteoporotic syndrome. Orlando: Grune & Stratton, 1987:121–142.

174. Fatourechi V, Heath H III. Salmon calcitonin in the treatment of postmenopausal osteoporosis. Ann Intern Med 1987;107:923–925.

175. Civitelli R, Gonnelli S, Zacchei F, et al. Bone turnover in postmenopausal osteoporosis: Effect of calcitonin treatment. J Clin Invest 1988;82:1268–1274.

176. Mazzuoli GF, Passeri M, Gennari C, et al. Effects of salmon calcitonin in postmenopausal osteoporosis: a controlled double-blind clinical study. Calcif Tissue Int 1986;38:3–8.

177. Reginster JY, Gaspar S, Deroisy R, et al. Prevention of osteoporosis with nasal calcitonin: effect of anti-salmon

calcitonin antibody formation. Osteoporos Int 1993;3:261–264.

178. Burckhardt P, Burnand B. The effect of treatment with calcitonin on vertebral fracture rate in osteoporosis. Osteoporos Int 1993;3:24–30.

179. Overgaard K, Hansen MA, Jensen SB, Christiansen C. Effect of salcalcitonin given intranasally on bone mass and fracture rates in established osteoporosis: a dose-response study. BMJ 1992;305:556–561.

180. Gennari C, Agnusdei D. Calcitonin in bone pain management. Curr Ther Res 1987;44:712–722.

181. Schenk R, Eggli P, Felix H, Rosini S. Quantitative morphometric evaluation of the inhibitory activity of new amino-phosphates on bone resorption in the rat. Calcif Tissue Int 1986;38:342–349.

182. Watts NB, Harris St, Genant HK, et al. Intermittent cyclic etidronate treatment of postmenopausal osteoporosis. N Engl J Med 1990;323:73–79.

183. Miller PD, Neal BJ, McIntyre DO. The effect of cyclical phosphorus-etidronate therapy (ADFR) on axial bone mass in postmenopausal osteoporosis. Osteoporos Int 1991;1:171–176.

184. Miller PD, Erickson AL. Long-term intermittent cyclical etidronate therapy for postmenopausal osteoporosis. Calcif Tissue Int 1995;56:493.

185. Chesnut C, et al. Bone marker changes in postmenopausal women on etidronate. J Bone Miner Res 1995;10(suppl 1):Calcified Tiss Int 1995;56:491.

186. Harris ST, Jackson RD, Genant HK, et al. Cyclical etidronate treatment of postmenopausal osteoporosis–4-year experience. Am J Med 1993;95:557–567.

187. Ott SM, Woodson GC, Huffer WE, et al. Bone histomorphometric changes following cyclic therapy with phosphate and etidronate disodium in women with postmenopausal osteoporosis. J Clin Endocrinol Metab 1994;78:968–972.

188. Fleisch H. Bisphosphonates and osteoporosis: future perspectives. In: Christiansen C, Riis B, eds. *Fourth International Symposium on Osteoporosis.* Hong Kong: Gardiner-Caldwell Communications 1993;23.

189. Riggs BL. A new option for treating osteoporosis. N Engl J Med 1990;323:124–125.

190. Riggs BL, Melton LJ, III. The prevention and treatment of osteoporosis. N Engl J Med 1992;327:620–627.

191. Riggs BL, Hodgson SF, O'Fallon WM, et al. Effect of fluoride treatment on the fracture rate in postmenopausal women with osteoporosis. N Engl J Med 1990;323:802–809.

192. Mamelle N, Meunier PJ, Dusan R, et al. Risk-benefit ratio of sodium fluoride treatment in primary vertebral osteoporosis. Lancet 1988;2:361–365.

193. Riggs B, O'Fallon W, Hodgson S, et al. Clinical trial of fluoride in osteoporotic women: Extended observation and additional analysis. Bone Miner 1992;17(suppl 1):74.

194. Antich PP, Boivin G, Meunier PJ, et al. Dependence of bone quality, mineral density and fluoride content on mode of fluoride administration. J Bone Miner Res 1992;7(suppl 1):S198.

195. Pak CY, Sakhaee K, Piaiak V, et al. Slow-release sodium fluoride in the management of postmenopausal osteoporosis. Ann Intern Med 1994;120:625–632.

196. Tilyard MW, Spears GFS, Com B, et al. Treatment of postmenopausal osteoporosis with calcitriol or calcium. N Engl J Med 1992;326:357–362.

197. Chapuy MC, Arlot ME, Duboeuf F, et al. Vitamin D_3 and calcium to prevent hip fractures in the elderly women. N Engl J Med 1992;327:1637–1642.

198. Jackson JA, Kleerekoper M. Osteoporosis in men: diagnosis, pathophysiology and prevention. Medicine 1990;69:137–152.

199. Middler S, Pak CY, Murad F, Bartter F. Thiazide diuretics and calcium metabolism. Metabolism 1973;22:139–146.

Chapter 41
Musculoskeletal Diseases

David H. Collier and William P. Arend

I am interested in physical medicine because my father was. I am interested in medical research because I believe in it. I am interested in arthritis because I have it.

Bernard Baruch
New York Post, 1959

Diseases involving the musculoskeletal system constitute the most common conditions affecting the elderly. It is important to realize, however, that most musculoskeletal symptoms do not signify underlying arthritis. Many aches and pains are due to self-limited problems such as bursitis, tendonitis, muscle sprain, and viral illnesses. In a random survey of 557 residents of Washtenaw County, Michigan, who were age 55 or older, 57 percent indicated the presence of arthritis (1). More significantly, 24 percent of these elderly individuals said that their arthritis interfered with daily activities in the home or at work. A study from the National Center of Health Statistics rating the frequency of the most common chronic conditions among persons aged 65 and older ranked arthritis first (prevalence of 470 per 1000) (2) over hypertension, hearing impairment, and heart conditions.

Precise prevalence figures for various forms of arthritis in the elderly are not available. A study from Goteborg, Sweden, categorized the types of arthritis found in 134 persons, 79 years of age. They found radiographic osteoarthritis (OA) of the wrist and fingers in 65 percent of the subjects and of the knees in 14 percent. Symptoms of osteoarthritis were reported by 6.2 percent of the subjects in the knee and by 4.5 percent in the hip. Rheumatoid arthritis (RA), as diagnosed by American College of Rheumatology (ACR) criteria, was noted in 10 percent. Calcium pyrophosphate dihydrate crystal deposition (CPPD) disease was present in 15 percent of the study subjects (23% of females, 6% of males), and hyperuricemia was found in 15 percent (6% of females, 29% of males).

Musculoskeletal diseases lead to a multitude of problems in the elderly. Not only can musculoskeletal diseases cause discomfort, weakness, and (at times) constitutional symptoms, but they can interfere with daily activities and threaten the individual's ability to live independently. Musculoskeletal disorders can decrease longevity; weakness and gait disturbances can cause falls and fractures that contribute to premature death. Patients with RA have been shown to have a decreased lifespan of 13 to 18 years (3).

Musculoskeletal symptoms in the elderly may indicate problems not directly related to rheumatic or autoimmune diseases. Metastatic malignancies, multiple myeloma, endocrine or metabolic disorders, and neurologic diseases all may have manifestations of joint or soft-tissue pain and disability. For example, diabetes mellitus can have manifestations of pain in the hands (with stiff fingers) and in the feet. The tendons of these patients may thicken and contract in the palmar surface of the hand and not allow full extension of the fingers. Elderly patients rarely present with their rheumatic illness as an isolated problem. More commonly they have multiple disorders and are taking one or more medicines. A recent study showed that 75 percent of patients with RA had at least one other illness (3). The diagnosis and management of arthritis is complicated by the presence of other medical conditions simultaneously treated with multiple drugs. For example, in a patient with RA who develops hypothyroidism, the stiffness, slowing down of function, and depression may all be falsely interpreted as a result of RA. Correction of the endocrine disorder may produce a dramatic benefit in the patient's symptoms and signs, whereas more aggressive treatment of RA would have been inappropriate.

The polypharmacy of elderly patients can cause two problems. First, there is an increased risk for drug interactions. Second, the treatment of one problem may exacerbate another. For example, the common use of nonsteroidal anti-inflammatory drugs (NSAIDs) can complicate renal disease, congestive heart failure, liver disease, hypertensive therapy or gastric ulcers. Thus, because of the multiple diseases, polypharmacy, and increased intolerance to many antirheumatic drugs, the diagnosis and management of rheumatic diseases in the elderly is more complex than in the young.

When a patient with a true arthritic condition is approached, it can be helpful to first categorize the patient by one of three conditions: inflammatory arthritis, degenerative arthritis, or metabolic arthritis. Inflammatory arthritis classically has symmetric distribution within an involved joint. Thus, for example, the medial and lateral compartment of the knee would have similar degrees of cartilage loss and destruction. Inflammatory arthritis usually demonstrates periarticular osteoporosis, cartilage loss, and erosions. Systemic manifestations of morning stiffness, easy stiffening of the joints at rest (gelling), and decreased energy in the evening are also common findings. Metabolic arthritis, such as gout, can lead to erosive changes in joints without much cartilage loss. Patients with metabolic forms of arthritis have fewer systemic symptoms. Degenerative joint disease (OA) commonly presents with an asymmetric distribution of involved joints and within joints. Thus, the usual

osteoarthritic knee has much greater loss of cartilage in the medial compartment than in the lateral compartment. Sclerotic bone, cartilage loss, and bony proliferation (osteophytosis) are classic x-ray findings of osteoarthritis. The end stage of all arthritis is a degenerative joint.

The specific diseases causing musculoskeletal complaints in the elderly can be divided into two groups: 1) those diseases seen primarily in the elderly, and 2) those diseases of which the elderly exhibit particular clinical characteristics (Table 41.1).

Osteoarthritis

OA, degenerative joint disease, is a heterogeneous clinical disorder representing a final common pathway of biochemical, metabolic, physiologic and pathologic changes characterized by loss of articular cartilage and remodeling of subchondral and marginal bone. It is the most common arthropathy. The frequency of diagnosis depends on which set of criteria are used: x-ray, symptoms, or pathologic specimens. The National Health and Nutrition Examination Survey (NHANES) estimated the incidence and prevalence of this disease (4). The U.S. population aged 25 to 74 years with *symptomatic* OA is estimated at 12.1 percent, about 15.8 million persons. The x-ray prevalence estimates for OA of the hands in adults aged 25 to 74 years are 32.5 percent, 42.4 million persons. Roentgenographic changes of OA are seen in 4 percent to 10 percent of people aged 15 to 24 years but are found in 80 percent of people older than age 55. In all studies, the relation of OA to aging is striking.

Not all patients with osteoarthritis seen by x-ray changes have associated symptoms. Symptomatic disease is seen in about 25 percent of individuals who have x-ray evidence of OA of the knees. There is better correlation of x-ray changes with OA of the hips. Similarly, not all pain in the knees of elderly patients should be attributed to arthritis. Bursitis, tendonitis, and other soft-tissue or muscle problems may be the cause of the pain.

Pathologic changes in weight-bearing joints at necropsy are found in almost all people by the time they are 40 years of age. Overall, the frequency of OA is equal in males and females. However, males younger than age 45 predominate; after age 45, women have an increased incidence of OA. Women tend to have more severe disease

Table 41.1. Musculoskeletal Diseases in the Elderly.

Diseases seen primarily in the elderly
  Osteoarthritis
  Calcium pyrophosphate dihydrate disease (pseudogout)
  Basic calcium phosphate disease (hydroxyapatite crystal deposition disease)
  Diffuse idiopathic skeletal hyperostosis
  Osteoporosis
  Paget's disease of bone
  Polymyalgia rheumatica, giant cell arteritis
Diseases with particular characteristics in the elderly
  Rheumatoid arthritis
  Systemic lupus erythematosus
  Sjögren's syndrome
  Polymyositis, dermatomyositis
  Systemic sclerosis
  Gout
  Septic arthritis
  Localized musculoskeletal disorders

with an increase in inflammatory or erosive osteoarthritis and in hereditary forms of OA.

Trauma is clearly associated with OA. Conflicting data exist regarding occupational risks (5). OA of the hips, knees, and shoulders is more frequent in miners. OA of the hands is more frequent in weavers. However, increased prevalence of OA was noted in pneumatic hammer drillers. Similarly, there is conflicting evidence whether playing sports can cause OA. If the presence of osteophytes is used as the primary criterion for the existence of OA, a number of studies demonstrate a correlation between athletic activity and OA. Some examples of the correlation of OA and athletics are shoulder and elbow involvement in baseball pitchers, the hands in boxing, the spine in weight lifting, and the knees in American and English football (soccer) (6). When strict x-ray criteria are used to diagnose OA, there is little evidence that exercise is deleterious to joints that have not been previously injured. One study of Finnish track record holders with an average age of 55 years demonstrated an incidence of OA of 4 percent as compared with an incidence of 8.7 percent in age- and sex-matched controls (7). A controlled prospective study of 498 long-distance runners aged 50 to 72 years compared with 365 controls found the runners to have less physical disability and no increased presence of OA (8). Obesity is associated with OA; in women, most commonly of the knees (9,10). However, obesity is also associated with OA of the hands, which promotes speculation that OA does not occur simply because of increased weight but possibly is secondary to some metabolic process.

Clinical Features

Certain clinical characteristics are common to most patients with OA. Significant symptoms are rarely present before age 40 unless the patient has had some trauma to the joint or possesses a congenital defect. The joints most commonly involved in OA are the distal interphalangeal (DIP), proximal interphalangeal (PIP), first carpometacarpal (CMC), hips, knees, first metatarsophalangeal (MTP), lumbosacral, and cervical spine. Early symptoms include joint pain with use and improvement with rest. There is relative preservation of function of the joint. Patients will complain of some stiffness, but it usually lasts less than 30 minutes and remains localized to involved joints. Systemic symptoms are distinctly unusual in OA.

Early in the course of OA, the first signs are localized tenderness, either of the joint or along periarticular ligaments and tendons. The joint may later develop secondary bony hypertrophy. Joint swelling is atypical in early OA but may develop later, especially in the knee. A joint with OA usually shows no signs of inflammation, such as erythema or warmth. Crepitance, a feeling of bone rubbing on bone when the joint is passively put through range of motion, can develop as a late finding.

Certain patterns of deformity are relatively specific for OA. Heberden's nodes, osteophytes around the DIP joints, or Bouchard's nodes, osteophytes around the PIP joints, may enlarge and deform the joints. Sometimes pseudocysts of the DIP joints may be prominent, representing outpouching of the synovium. Also the DIP and PIP joints may have erosions and other changes of inflammatory OA. The helpful signs that tell whether a patient has OA or RA are the DIP distribution, the lack of symmetry, and the involvement only of the fingers in the inflammatory process. Squaring of the first CMC, called the shelf sign, is characteristic of OA. An uneven loss of cartilage in the knees can lead to genu varus, a bow-legged appearance. The angulated knee then causes an added burden to the knee cartilage. A mild synovitis is often seen when the knee deformity is prominent. Hallux valgus, the big toe turning laterally, often with an associated bunion, is also a classic finding of OA, especially in women. If dorsal osteophytes form, the joint may demonstrate hallux rigidus. Isolated lumbar and cervical spine OA can commonly be seen on x-rays in the absence of pain. However, facet joint involvement or nerve root entrapment can cause localized or referred pain and stiffness. In the elderly, the combination of facet joint hypertrophy, bulging and degenerated discs, and thickened ligamentum flavum can contribute to spinal stenosis. In the lumbar spine, this manifests as pseudoclaudication, that is, radicular pain with walking, especially down a slope. In the cervical spine, OA may cause radicular pain and paresthesias down the arms or into the medial border of the scapula. Nerve root encroachment may lead to arm weakness and atrophy.

Clinical Syndromes

OA is often thought of as a single disorder, but actually has a variety of presentations and may represent the final common pathway of many pathological processes. OA may be classified into six different clinical syndromes (Table 41.2). *Primary generalized OA* is a common pattern of polyarticular joint disease most frequently seen in middle-aged and elderly women. This disease was first described by Kellgren and Moore in 1952 and commonly affects the DIPs, PIPs, first CMCs, knees, and spine (11). Patients with generalized OA exhibit a slow progression (occasionally acute) and usually have a good functional outcome. The incidence of hip involvement is low. *Inflammatory small joint (erosive) OA* is a separate clinical syndrome, is relatively uncommon, may be familial, and primarily affects postmenopausal women. The major joints involved are the DIP and PIP, and to a lesser extent the thumb, CMC, and scaphoid-trapezoid joints. The onset may be abrupt and appear to be gout, infection, or RA. Obvious inflammation and swelling may be present in erosive OA. The process leaves destructive and hypertrophic changes as it subsides over months or years. Although an inflammatory arthritis is present, patients with erosive OA characteristically have a negative rheumatoid factor, normal erythrocyte sedimentation rate, and no systemic symptoms. X-rays show erosions involving both sides of the joint, particularly the peripheral

subchondral region of the proximal joint surfaces which give the "gull wing" appearance. Joints outside the hand are not involved in erosive OA. *Isolated nodular OA* is another subgroup and includes the appearance of symmetrical Heberden's and Bouchard's nodes, usually in patients older than age 45. This disease is inherited and is autosomal dominant in women and recessive in men. Other joint involvement with nodular OA may be seen with time.

Unifocal large joint OA occurs commonly in the knees or hips, but an age-related increased incidence of shoulder involvement may occur. In these patients, causes of secondary OA should be considered, such as avascular necrosis of bone, acetabular dysplasia, slipped femoral epiphysis, leg-length discrepancy, congenital dysplasia, or Paget's disease. However, in many patients no apparent cause for unifocal large joint OA is found. Mechanical abnormalities with increased local shear stress on the cartilage are thought to be a major culprit. Many of these patients eventually require total joint replacement. Multifocal large joint OA usually involves bilateral hips, knees, or both, but may involve small joints and represent a form of secondary OA. In a patient presenting with shoulder, elbow, ankle, or wrist involvement, a careful assessment for an underlying cause of the OA should be pursued. These patients should be evaluated for crystal-associated arthropathies such as CPPD

Table 41.2. Clinical Patterns of Osteoarthritis.

Pattern	Site(s)	Special diagnostic features	Course
Generalized	DIP, PIP, CMC	–	Usually slowly progressive; often asymptomatic
Inflammatory, small joint	DIP, PIP; less often CMC, MTP, knee	Erosive x-ray changes; prominent signs of inflammation	Rapid course; early deformity
Isolated nodule	DIP, PIP	Prominent family history	Abrupt onset; rapid course
Unifocal, large joint	Knee, hip, shoulder	Mechanical or anatomic disturbance, osteonecrosis, Paget's disease	Slowly progressive; disabling
Multifocal, large joint	Shoulder, knees, hip wrist, MCP, ankle	Crystals–chondrocalcinosis on x-ray; rule out hemochromatosis, endocrine, neurologic cause	Variable–often progressive and disabling
Unifocal, small joint	DIP, PIP, MTP, CMC	Trauma or occupation; look for asymptomatic joints	Variable–often leads to chronic morbidity

CMC = carpometacarpal (joint); DIP = distal interphalangeal (joint); MTP = metatarsophalangeal (joint); PIP = proximal interphalangeal (joint).

(pseudogout), hypothyroidism, hyperparathyroidism, hemochromatosis, basic calcium phosphate (BCP) disease (Milwaukee shoulder, hydroxyapatite crystal disease), and acromegaly. *Unifocal small joint OA* is a related syndrome and may represent the result of local trauma from repetitive use of a particular joint or may be the presenting manifestation of more generalized OA. Two common examples of this syndrome are involvement of the first CMC joint and the first tarsometatarsal joint (the bunion deformity).

Laboratory Findings

Except for radiographic findings, laboratory data are generally not helpful in the evaluation of patients with any form of OA. The usual rheumatologic workup of a complete blood count (CBC), erythrocyte sedimentation rate (ESR), and rheumatoid factor are most likely to be found normal. The synovial fluid in OA patients is a nonspecific type I fluid with a white blood count of 200 to 1500 cells per µL and 20 percent to 50 percent polymorphonuclear leukocytes, normal viscosity, and normal glucose. If the patient has a secondary form of OA, crystals such as calcium pyrophosphate may be seen. Radiographic evaluation in OA can be diagnostic. Classic findings are the loss of cartilage space, especially in an asymmetric pattern, bony sclerosis of subchondral bone, cystic changes of subchondral bone, and osteophyte formation. Late findings may be the altered shape of bone and effusions of joints. There are specific patterns of x-ray changes in OA such as gull wing changes in interphalangeal joints, medial compartment disease of the knee, horizontal osteophytes of the spine, decreased joint space superiorly in the hip with relative medial preservation, and hallux valgus (bunion deformity) of the great toe without other metatarsophalangeal disease.

Pathophysiology

OA represents a failure of joint function resulting from many different disease mechanisms. Mechanical, environmental, and biochemical factors may all interact, possibly in a genetically predisposed individual, to produce the clinical syndrome called OA. The primary damage is to articular cartilage which is made up of collagen, giving tensile strength, and proteoglycans, which are large and highly hydrated molecules that contribute elasticity to cartilage. There are three major hypotheses regarding the pathogenesis of osteoarthritis: 1) OA is a degeneration of articular cartilage leading to denudation of a joint, 2) OA begins as a fibrillation of articular cartilage leading to secondary remodeling of bone, and 3) OA is a consequence of changes in the stiffness of subchondral bone.

Most researchers believe OA is a consequence of degeneration in the articular cartilage. In idiopathic or primary OA, early biochemical events in articular cartilage include changes in collagen structure that lead to an increase in water content. The collagen content of articular cartilage then decreases over time as disease progresses. The articular cartilage becomes less elastic and more prone to mechanical damage from normal or abnormal forces, with further destruction of collagen. Chondrocyte function in primary OA remains normal. The chondrocyte attempts to compensate by synthesizing more proteoglycans and collagen. Microfractures of subchondral bone then occur, and there is increased stiffness and change in the composition of proteoglycans. The late stage of OA occurs with chondrocyte failure and significant change in the amount and composition of proteoglycans and collagen. The gross and histologic changes of the cartilage show fissuring, fibrillation, and erosions. Radiologic changes of joint space narrowing, subchondral sclerosis, and hypertrophy of bone are evident. There may be an associated inflammatory reaction. Changes in subchondral bone may occur secondarily to abnormalities in the overlying articular cartilage.

There is some evidence for decreased hardness of subchondral bone in early OA. Multiple studies have demonstrated an inverse correlation between bone density and the prevalence of OA. In secondary forms, trauma, previous inflammatory joint disease, or the presence of metabolic disturbances damage the cartilage and lead to the same series of events. However, normal aging, in itself, does not lead to OA. The biochemical and structural changes in the joint that accompany aging are not the same. OA is more common in the elderly, not because of age-related changes, but because the involved pathophysiologic mechanisms require long periods of time to develop.

Moskowitz et al recently noted an abnormality in cartilage matrix structure in certain families with a hereditary form of OA that can affect patients at a relatively young age. A defect was described in the type II collagen gene, the major structural protein in cartilage, in which there is a substitution of the amino acid cysteine (not found normally in human type II collagen) for arginine (12–14). This single amino acid mutation was found in all affected members tested, but not in any of the unaffected members or in unrelated individuals.

Management

Therapy of osteoarthritis in the elderly should be conservative and influenced by the type, extent, and severity of joint disease. The physician should try to fit the treatment to the patient and to define whether treatment should be directed toward pain or limitation of motion. Even though a patient presents with knee pain with radiographic evidence of OA, pain may be due to a number of other causes such as crystalline disease, chronic ligament strain, anserine bursitis, popliteal or hamstring tenosynovitis, Baker's cyst, or referred pain from lumbosacral or sacroiliac disease. It is important to discuss a patient's concerns and what can or cannot be done. Monthly telephone calls from lay personnel to patients whose medical treatment regimens remain stable has recently been shown to reduce joint pain (15).

Physical modifications may also be very helpful in the treatment of OA. Obese patients should be encouraged to lose weight. Occupational therapists can help a patient to modify certain painful or harmful activities. They also can assess the need for assistive devices such as special door handles, toilet seat extenders, and special chairs. Canes, crutches, splints, and cervical pillows may ease pain and help with function. Physical therapy modalities such as the use of dry or wet heat, ice, massage, and exercise for range of motion and strengthening can be helpful in selected patients. Aerobic exercises have also been beneficial in patients with OA (16–18).

To assist with the selection of a treatment program for OA, a physician must decide whether pain or inflammation is the main problem. In one 4-week study, acetaminophen was shown to be as effective in treating OA of the knee as ibuprofen at low and high doses (20). NSAIDs have traditionally been the mainstay of treatment for OA. These drugs should be employed in the lowest effective dose by a physician who is aware of the possible complications of NSAIDs in the elderly. The

NSAID should be chosen on the basis of efficacy, safety, convenience of dosage, formulation, cost, concurrent diseases, and other drugs the patient may be taking. The patient is usually started on one-half the usual dose, which is increased cautiously as effectiveness and tolerability are assessed. Added analgesic therapy can be given with acetaminophen and, rarely, codeine. Topical agents are commonly used by patients and are mainly thought to have a counterirritative effect. Topical capsaicin applied at least four times a day over a joint has been shown to progressively decrease pain in the joint (21,22). The topical preparations work by decreasing neural transmitters in the main peripheral pain fibers, the polymodal nociceptors.

Intra-articular steroids may give great relief to OA patients but should not be administered more than three times a year to the same joint because successive injections may be increasingly less effective. Recent data suggest that corticosteroid injections can decrease osteophyte formation (23). Secondary fibromyalgia is a concomitant problem for many OA patients. Low doses of tricyclic antidepressants at night may help both sleep and pain. Presently, a number of agents are being studied to protect the cartilage or to actually cause new cartilage growth, which could dramatically alter future therapy.

When an osteoarthritic joint becomes so painful or nonfunctional that it greatly compromises lifestyle, surgical intervention should be considered. Arthroscopic examination with debridement of the knee to remove particles of cartilage and fibrous tissue can have a prolonged beneficial effect. Tidal joint irrigation, the washing out of the knee with normal saline using needles to enter the joint, has also been shown to produce pain relief (24). Patients with severe pain and destructive joint disease, especially of the hip and the knee, may benefit dramatically from total joint replacement. Age alone does not seem to be a factor in joint replacement. Hip replacements demonstrate a success rate of more than 95 percent in relieving pain.

Diffuse Idiopathic Skeletal Hyperostosis

Also known as ankylosing hyperostosis or Forestier's disease, diffuse idiopathic skeletal hyperostosis (DISH) is a radiographic diagnosis. Characteristics of DISH include

1) flowing ligamentous calcification and ossification along the anterolateral aspect of four or more contiguous vertebrae called syndesmophytes, 2) relative preservation of intervertebral disc height, 3) no significant apophyseal or sacroiliac involvement, 4) olecranon and calcaneal spurs, and 4) extraspinal ligamentous ossification. DISH is very common, with worldwide distribution. It is usually found incidentally in asymptomatic middle-aged to elderly men, but it may be the cause of spinal stiffness and low back pain. DISH also may accompany other rheumatic diseases such as RA (RADISH). Approximately 22 percent of DISH patients are diabetic. It should be emphasized that DISH is not a variant of osteoarthritis, but a separate entity that presents with ligamentous calcifications around the spine. The osteophytic spurs of OA differ radiographically as distinct bony outgrowths of the vertebrae usually with malalignment that results from loss of disc spaces.

Crystalline Arthritis

Calcium Pyrophosphate Dihydrate Deposition Disease (Pseudogout)

CPPD, osteoarthritis, and aging are interrelated. There is an increasing frequency with aging of asymptomatic deposition of CPPD crystals in articular cartilage, called chondrocalcinosis. CPPD disease is rare in persons younger than age 50, but increases to 10 percent to 15 percent in individuals aged 65 to 75 years and is present in more than 30 percent of those age 85 or older (25,26). CPPD exhibits a predominance in women of about 2 or 3:1 (26,27).

CPPD disease can be placed into three broad etiologic categories: sporadic, hereditary, and metabolic. The sporadic (idiopathic) form is found in 90 percent of the cases of CPPD disease and most elderly patients fit into this category. Multiple population groups in Czechoslovakia, Chile, the Netherlands, France, Spain, and other countries have reported a familial predisposition for CPPD disease (28). Genetically-influenced CPPD can be divided into two groups: early onset (3rd–4th decade) disease with severe, destructive, polyarticular disease, and late onset (6th–7th decade) disease that closely resembles the symptomatic sporadic form. A number of metabolic disorders are associated with CPPD disease, such

as hyperparathyroidism, hemochromatosis, hypophosphatasia, hypomagnesemia, and Wilson's disease, and there are possible associations of CPPD with gout, hypothyroidism, and ochronosis. Secondary CPPD disease should be considered when a patient has articular symptoms before age 50, has a florid polyarticular presentation, and when additional clues appear on the physical examination or on radiographs.

Six different clinical patterns of CPPD crystalline-induced arthropathy have been described (Table 41.3) (28). The classic presentation of CPPD disease is unilateral or bilateral knee pain with swelling, called pseudogout, or type A disease. Knee arthritis (gonagra) is to CPPD disease as first MTP joint arthritis (podagra) is to gout. Pseudogout is thought to occur from shedding of crystals from the articular cartilage. This shedding can occur from trauma, after surgery, or with other illnesses that cause prolonged immobilization. Pseudogout attacks can be acute or subacute and are usually self-limited. They can be as severe as a gout attack but are usually milder. The patient may be pain-free between attacks. Type B disease (pseudo-rheumatoid arthritis) is rare and occurs in about 5 percent of all patients with CPPD. Classically, type B presents with multiple joint involvement including wrists, elbows, metacarpophalangeals, knees, and shoulders. These patients may have systemic symptoms of morning stiffness, fatigue, and synovitis. The sedimentation rate may be elevated. The rheumatoid factor may be confusing in the pseudo-RA type of CPPD because 10 percent to 15 percent of elderly people are rheumatoid factor positive (29). Attacks may last weeks to several months.

Type C and type D CPPD disease consist of osteoarthritis associated with crystal disease, with type C also having an acute inflammatory or pseudogout presentation. Associated OA is very common. Helpful hints that indicate a patient may have CPPD disease accompanying OA are multiple atypical joint involvement (such as of the wrists, elbows, metacarpophalangeal (MCP) joints, shoulders, and knees), bilaterally symmetric involvement, and acute attacks on a background of chronic arthritis. With an inflammatory attack of CPPD disease, the elderly patient may appear ill, have fever, and be mildly confused. Type E, lanthanic (asymptomatic), CPPD is the most common type, representing about one-half of all patients

Table 41.3. Clinical Patterns of Calcium Pyrophosphate Dihydrate Deposition Disease.

Type	Prevalence of CPPD (%)	Sex ratio	Attack characteristics	Major joints	Miscellaneous features
A, pseudogout	25	M > F	Acute to subacute	50% knee cluster attacks	Chondrocalcinosis; 20% hyperuricemia; 5% gout
B, pseudo-RA	5	F > M	Subacute attacks; AM stiffness	MCPs, wrists	10% RF
C, pseudo-OA	25	F > M	Progressive DJD, inflammatory episodes	Knees, wrists, MCPs, hips, shoulders, elbows	Flexion contractures
D, pseudo-OA	25	F > M	Progressive DJD, noninflammatory	Knees, wrists, MCPs, hips, shoulders, elbows	Flexion contractures
E, lanthanic	4–25	F > M	Asymptomatic; chondrocalcinosis on X-ray	–	–
F, neuroarthropathic	Rare	–	CPPD crystals found in both neuropathic and pseudoneuropathic joints	–	–

CPPD = calcium pyrophosphate dihydrate; DJD = degenerative joint disease; MCP = metacarpophalangeal joint; OA = osteoarthritis; RA = rheumatoid arthritis; RF = rheumatoid factor.

with CPPD disease. The calcium deposition is usually present in both fibrocartilage and hyaline cartilage, but also can be seen in the synovial lining; tendon or ligament calcium deposition can even be present asymptomatically in the dura mater. Type F CPPD disease is the pseudoneuropathic type. A joint with this disease may resemble a Charcot joint with severe destruction, cartilage loss, debris and bony sclerosis, but the patient may exhibit no neurologic abnormalities.

The most helpful laboratory tests in the diagnosis of CPPD are synovial fluid analysis and plain radiographs. The practical, definitive diagnosis is made when synovial fluid is removed from the affected joint and positively birefringent intracellular rhomboid crystals from 2 to 10 μm in length are visualized. These are typically not as abundant as uric acid crystals in gout; the examiner must carefully look over the slide preparation of synovial fluid. The synovial fluid in CPPD usually has a white cell count in the range of 20,000 cells per μL but it can be much

higher. Polymorphonuclear cells usually constitute more than 90 percent of the total synovial fluid cells and the examiner must ensure that the patient does not have a septic joint by culture and Gram stain. The most common places to see chondrocalcinosis are in the 1) fibrocartilage in the symphysis pubis, wrist, knee meniscus, and annulus fibrosis; 2) hyaline cartilage in the knee, hip, shoulder, and elbow; and 3) spinal disc area along the outer margins. If the patient has CPPD, it is usually evident by taking x-rays of the knees, pelvis, and wrists. If the patient has indication of a metabolic problem, the physician may want to obtain serum calcium, magnesium, phosphorus, alkaline phosphatase, iron and total iron-binding capacity, ferritin, glucose, thyroid stimulating hormone, and uric acid. Further metabolic studies should be performed if abnormalities are found.

The aims of the management of CPPD should be to decrease symptoms, especially with an acute flare; identify and treat any underlying condition; and mobilize the patient as soon as possible. Acute attacks of CPPD can be treated with drainage of the affected joint. NSAIDs of the indole derivatives class such as indomethacin, tolmetin sodium, or sulindac are usually prescribed first. However, any NSAIDs may be used, and the newer agents such as nabumatone, oxaprozin, and etodolac may be safer. NSAIDs should always be used cautiously in the elderly and at the lowest effective dose. Colchicine has been shown to suppress acute synovitis caused by CPPD and can also be used chronically to prevent flares. The elderly are particularly sensitive to experiencing colchicine-induced diarrhea (30). If the patient clearly does not have a septic joint, aspiration followed by corticosteroid injection can stop an acute attack. NSAIDs, colchicine, and, in rare cases, low-dose corticosteroids have been used for long-term continuous treatment.

Apatite Deposition Disease (Basic Calcium Phosphate Deposition)

Apatite is a form of calcium phosphate. In the past, calcium phosphate-induced arthritis was called hydroxyapatite disease but it is now realized that the crystals found in tendons and joints represent a variety of apatite crystals. Apatite disease is now called basic calcium phosphate deposition disease. BCP has been associated with both an acute form of apatite deposition disease and with a destructive large joint arthropathy (chronic form) in elderly women. The study of BCP arthritis has been difficult because of the lack of a simple, reliable, diagnostic test.

The acute form of BCP deposition disease is associated with calcific tendonitis, calcific bursitis, and calcific periarthritis. Calcinosis of the skin and muscle is also seen with the acute form, and the calcific periarthritis can be unifocal or multifocal. The most common areas of involvement with acute BCP are the subdeltoid bursa and the trochanteric bursa, with occasional cases of periarthritis around the wrist, knee, or elbow. Attacks in most cases are of a single joint, abrupt in onset, and associated with intense local inflammatory signs that resemble an attack of gout. Familial forms of acute BCP deposition also occur, most often in middle-aged patients. Calcinosis also is found in a number of metabolic disturbances of calcium or phosphate, such as hyperparathyroidism, renal failure, metastatic neoplasms

affecting bone, and hypervitaminosis D. Calcinosis may also be seen in autoimmune diseases such as scleroderma or polymyositis.

The chronic form of BCP deposition is called Milwaukee shoulder or knee syndrome (31,32). This form of arthritis is usually found in elderly women and has a female-to-male ratio of 4:1 and occurs at a mean age of 72 years (range, 54–90 years) (33). The dominant shoulder is usually more affected but the disease often is bilateral. Glenohumeral joint degeneration with gross loss of the rotator cuff and instability are characteristically present. Chronic BCP disease can range from being asymptomatic to exhibiting severe pain after use or at night. Knee involvement is similar, with pain during and after ambulation; the knee may exhibit both lateral and medial instability. BCP deposition can overlap clinically with CPPD. No blood test can distinguish between the two diseases.

Radiographs of the chronic form of BCP deposition show glenohumeral joint degeneration with upward subluxation of the humeral head. Erosions of the coracoid process, of the under surface of the anterior third of the acromion, and of the acromioclavicular joint also are common. Erosions and roughening of the bony cortex over the greater tuberosity at the site of the insertion of the rotator cuff may be noted. The knee has atypical features of OA on x-ray showing lateral tibiofemoral and patellofemoral compartment narrowing.

The synovial fluid in BCP deposition disease characteristically has a low leukocyte count, usually less than 1000 cells per µL, with predominantly mononuclear cells. Apatite crystals are too small to be visualized by light microscopy but crystal aggregates that look like stacked coins may be seen. Calcium stains such as alizarin red S may stain apatite crystals but are of limited usefulness because of common false positives and false negatives. Electron microscopy, elemental analysis, or electron diffraction can establish the identity of the apatite crystals. Also, type II collagen particles are universally found in joints with BCP crystals. The BCP crystals are thought to be endocytosed by synovial cells and macrophages that, in turn, release collagenase, neutral proteases, and prostaglandins, all of which cause joint destruction and pain.

The treatment of chronic arthritis secondary to apatite

crystals is the same as that for severe OA. The joint should be rested and NSAIDs should be used carefully in this elderly population. Joint aspiration and corticosteroid injections are often employed, although some authors believe injections may promote further attacks and calcification of tissues. Patients with severe, unremitting pain may benefit from surgery. Acromioplasty with repair of the rotator cuff, subacromial spacers, or total joint replacement has been advocated for chronic BCP deposition disease with shoulder pain unresponsive to medications.

Gout

Gout is a metabolic disease with manifestations of an acute and chronic inflammatory arthritis caused by sodium urate crystals in synovial fluid. A gout attack is usually preceded by 20 to 30 years of asymptomatic hyperuricemia. Other manifestations of hyperuricemia include aggregated deposits of monosodium urate (MSU), called tophi, which occur chiefly in and around the joints of the extremities, urolithiasis, and renal disease involving inflammation and deposits of MSU in interstitial and tubular tissues. The prevalence of gout is 2 to 3 cases per 1000. Hyperuricemia in men usually starts after puberty; in females it begins in menopause. Thus, gout is more common in men by 2 to 7:1. Men develop gout at an average age of 50 years; women acquire gout later, usually after age 65.

A serum uric acid level more than 7.0 mg/dL is abnormal and supersaturates plasma and other body fluids. Hyperuricemia is caused either by an overproduction of uric acid (15–25% of the cases) or by an underexcretion of uric acid by the kidneys (75–85% of the cases). Urate is produced as a metabolic product of the purines, adenine and guanine. An overproduction of urate can be caused by rare genetic defects that promote either an increase in purine production, such as seen with enhanced phosphoribosylpyrophosphate synthetase activity, or a decrease in a salvage pathway, as occurs with hypoxanthine-guanine phosphoribosyltransferase deficiency. Although overproduction of urate usually is caused by a hereditary idiopathic process, other causes are myeloproliferative disorders, after chemotherapy with cytotoxic drugs, high purine intake, and alcohol consumption (34). Reduced renal elimination of urate is usu-

ally caused by intrinsic underexcretion that is genetically determined. Acquired causes of reduced renal elimination of urate include intrinsic renal disease, polycystic kidney disease, lead nephropathy, hypertension, and chronic use of drugs such as diuretics, low-dose aspirin, pyrazinamide, ethambutol, nicotinic acid, fructose, and levodopa. There is a well confirmed association of gout with obesity and hypertriglyceridemia.

Gout can evolve through four stages: asymptomatic hyperuricemia, acute gout, an intercritical period, and chronic tophaceous gout. The duration and degree of hyperuricemia increases the likelihood of a patient's developing a gouty attack or renal stones. As much as 50 percent of males with uric acid greater than 9 mg/dL eventually develop a gout attack. From 10 percent to 40 percent of patients with gout have experienced one or more attacks of renal colic before the first articular event. The first gout attack is monoarticular in 85 percent to 90 percent of patients. The first MTP joint is involved in 50 percent of initial gout attacks and eventually in 90 percent of all patients. Other joints frequently involved in acute gout are the instep, ankle, knee, wrist, finger, and elbow. Infrequent joints include the shoulder, hip, spine, sacroiliac, and temporomandibular. Tendonitis and bursitis also can be caused by deposition of urate crystals. The characteristic attack of gout is at night or in the early morning with an acute onset that reaches maximal pain in hours. Acute gout usually resolves in 3 to 7 days but, if untreated, attacks may become more frequent over time. About 10 percent of attacks are polyarticular, usually of a lower extremity, and asymmetric. This presentation is more common in women. Precipitating factors for acute attacks of gout are trauma, surgery, dietary excess, dehydration, hemorrhage, infections, and certain drugs.

Intercritical gout is the asymptomatic period between gout attacks. A patient has a 62 percent chance of developing a recurrent attack within 1 year, an additional 16 percent chance in the second year, 11 percent chance in 2 to 5 years, and 4 percent in 5 to 10 years. Seven percent of patients never experience another attack of gout. Later attacks are often polyarticular, more severe, last longer, and have more systemic signs. If acute gout is left untreated, it can progress to chronic tophaceous gout. The average time from the first gout attack to developing tophi is 11.6 years (range, 3 to 42 years). The longer the duration and the higher the level of hyperuricemia, the more likely tophi are to develop. In addition, tophi correlate with renal disease. Tophi can occur anywhere on the body–classic presentations are on the fingers, hands, knees, olecranon bursa, feet, and helix of the ear.

Gout in the elderly is of two types: early onset with inadequate treatment, or late in life onset. Early onset is basically the natural history of gout, but late onset may be a separate entity (35). Gouty arthritis in the elderly can be more indolent, which causes confusion when underlying OA is present. Hyperuricemia and pain in characteristic areas for gout does not mean the patient has gout. Similarly, OA in a joint that becomes worse may signify a gouty attack. It is much more common for multiple joints to be involved in the gouty attack of the elderly patient (36). Elderly women and men have similar incidences of new-onset gout. Medications that elderly patients take chronically are especially noted as predisposing factors. Diuretics cause hyperuricemia and are commonly associated with elderly onset gout. Another complication of gout in older age groups is the co-existence of other crystal diseases, such as CPPD, that can confuse diagnosis and treatment.

Laboratory evaluation of the patient with suspected gout should include CBC, serum uric acid, glucose, liver function tests, protein and albumin, calcium, creatinine, urinalysis, cholesterol, and triglycerides. Saturnine gout should be considered in a patient with hypertension and early-onset gout; a serum lead level may be helpful. The definitive diagnosis of gout is made by aspirating synovial fluid and looking for monosodium urate crystals under a polarizing microscope with a rose quartz filter. Monosodium urate crystals are needle-shaped and negatively birefringent. Because the definitive therapy for gout is distinctive from therapy for other forms of arthritis, diagnosis by arthrocentesis and crystal examination is essential. During an attack of gout, the patient's synovial fluid white cell count is usually high, with predominately polymorphonuclear leukocytes, and the fluid at times can appear pseudoseptic. During intercritical periods, synovial fluid may exhibit obvious monosodium urate crystals but demonstrate a normal white cell count. Radiographic findings of gout include sharply marginated lucent erosions with overhanging edges and sclerotic margins in such areas as the first MTP, fingers, and MCPs. There is a

relative preservation of joint space in spite of erosions. Osteoporosis is seen but generally is not prominent.

Asymptomatic hyperuricemia in the elderly is usually not treated except for prophylaxis in times of chemotherapy for certain malignancies. Treatment for gout is divided into therapy for acute attacks and therapy for chronic maintenance to suppress the serum urate level. NSAIDs are the usual first-line treatment for acute attacks, with the indole group of drugs used first, particularly indomethacin and, to a lesser extent, tolmetin sodium. Indomethacin (50 mg three to four times/day) is given for 2 days, then decreased to 25 mg four times/day. Most other NSAIDs are less effective but can be used. High-dose aspirin, because of its uricosuric effect and its theoretical ability to prolong an attack, should probably not be used. Chronic use of indomethacin in the elderly can cause central nervous system (CNS) problems such as hallucinations and depression.

Acute gout in the elderly can be treated with other approaches in patients in which NSAIDs cannot be used or are not well tolerated. Colchicine, 0.6 mg every hour to a maximum of 10 to 12 tablets or until diarrhea starts, can be used for an acute attack, but the elderly are more sensitive to the gastrointestinal and hematological toxicity of this drug. Aspiration of the affected joint followed by injection of corticosteroids can be particularly effective in the elderly patient, especially in the presence of systemic illness that precludes the use of other therapies. Oral corticosteroids are usually effective, but with a rapid taper, the patient typically experiences a flare of the acute attack. A slower taper of oral corticosteroids during a period of 6 weeks decreases the likelihood of a flare. Intramuscular injections of corticotropin (ACTH) have also been used to treat acute gout.

For long-term treatment of chronic gout, the patient should be educated to avoid alcohol, lose weight, and avoid trauma to susceptible joints. For the patient taking a medicine that causes hyperuricemia, simply discontinuing the offending drug can prevent future attacks. If the patient has had three attacks within 2 years, or has tophi, renal stones, or renal failure, chronic therapy to lower serum uric acid levels should be instituted. Maintenance therapy should be initiated only after an acute flare has subsided. The institution of maintenance drugs during an attack only prolongs and exacerbates the gouty attack.

Suppressive therapy is intended to lower levels of serum uric acid and consists of uricosuric agents or allopurinol. Uricosuric agents, probenecid or sulfinpyrazone, competitively inhibit uric acid resorption by the renal tubules. A 24-hour urine measurement for creatinine clearance and uric acid excretion should be taken. If the patient excretes more than 600 mg of uric acid on a purine-free diet or 800 mg on a regular diet, allopurinol should be used. If the patient has tophi or renal stones, allopurinol is also the drug of choice. The starting dosage for probenecid is 250 mg twice a day, increased to 500 mg twice a day. Serum uric acid level should be measured every 2 weeks with a goal of decreasing the level to below 5 mg/dL. Sulfinpyrazone dosage is 50 mg twice a day for 1 week, increased by 100 mg each week thereafter to a maximum dose of 800 mg, again with periodic titration of the patient's serum uric acid levels. Allopurinol is a competitive inhibitor of xanthine oxidase. The beginning dosage is 100 mg per day for 1 week, increased by 100 mg per day during each subsequent week. The usual maintenance dose of allopurinol is 300 mg/day but it can be increased to 600 mg/day in the presence of normal renal function. Drug interactions with azathioprine, thiazides, and ampicillin may occur with allopurinol and these combinations should be avoided.

Inflammatory Polyarthritis and Autoimmune Diseases

Multiple diseases can present as a polyarticular inflammatory arthritis in the elderly. RA, polymyalgia rheumatica, and a recently described arthritis called remitting seronegative symmetrical synovitis with pitting edema (RS₃PE) can all present in a similar fashion. Autoimmune diseases in the elderly can present differently than they do in a younger population.

Rheumatoid Arthritis

RA is an inflammatory polyarthritis that occurs in 1 percent to 2 percent of the adult population. Two percent to 33 percent of patients have onset of RA after age 60. In the elderly population, there is an equal frequency of RA in men and women. RA usually begins in the nonelderly population as a distal symmetric polyarthritis in the PIPs, MCPs, wrists, MTPs, and cervical spine. Over time, RA

progresses more proximally to include the knees, elbows, hips, and shoulders and actually can involve any joint.

Diagnostic Criteria

Revised criteria for the classification of RA have recently been drawn up by a committee of the American College of Rheumatology (Table 41.4). The clinical and laboratory manifestations of RA may develop over time, and thus not all be present initially. Therefore, these criteria are useful for classification of patients at any point but may have limited application as diagnostic criteria for any individual patient with disease of recent onset. If a patient fulfills four of the seven criteria, the diagnosis of RA has a sensitivity of 91 percent to 94 percent and a specificity of 89 percent. Criteria 1 through 4, that is, morning stiffness or clinical evidence of arthritis, must be present for at least 6 weeks, with joint findings observed by a physician.

Pathophysiology

The pathophysiology of RA is not known, but is believed to involve an abnormal or exaggerated immune response to an exogenous agent in a genetically predisposed host. More than 60 percent of white patients with RA are positive for human leukocyte antigen (HLA)-DR4 as compared with 30 percent or less of the normal population. How this genetic marker is related to the acquisition of RA has not been established. Although infectious agents are suspected to be involved in the induction of the disease, none has yet been proven.

RA begins as an inflammatory disease of the synovium, the lining layer of joints and tendon sheaths. The earliest histologic changes include an increase in the thickness of the synovial lining cells, which represents an infiltration from the blood of monocytes that develop into synovial macrophages, and a local proliferation of fibroblasts. The subsynovium exhibits an infiltration of monocytes and lymphocytes, as well as a new growth of blood vessels. The synovium becomes hyperproliferative and grows over the articular cartilage, called pannus, and destroys the cartilage. This synovial tissue also invades the adjacent bone and periarticular connective tissue. The cellular events in the synovium responsible for these events include activation of T cells, with release of factors that stimulate macrophages. These cells, in turn, release interleukin-1 and other mediators that induce fibroblasts

Table 41.4. 1987 Revised Criteria for Classification of Rheumatoid Arthritis*.

Criterion	Definition
Morning stiffness	Morning stiffness in and around joints, lasting at least 1 hour before maximal improvement.
Arthritis of 3 or more joint areas	At least 3 joints simultaneously with soft-tissue swelling or fluid (not bony overgrowth alone) observed by a physician; 14 possible areas are right or left PIP, MCP, wrist, elbow, knee, ankle, and MTP joints.
Arthritis of hand joints	At least 1 area swollen (as defined above) in a wrist, MCP, or PIP joint.
Symmetric arthritis	Simultaneous involvement of 3 or more joint areas (as defined above) on both sides of the body (bilateral involvement of PIPs, MCPs, or MTPs is acceptable without absolute symmetry)
Rheumatoid nodules	Subcutaneous nodules over bony prominences, extensor surfaces, or in juxtaarticular regions, observed by a physician.
Serum rheumatoid factor	Demonstration of abnormal amounts of serum rheumatoid factor by any method for which the result has been positive in <5% of normal control subjects.
Radiologic changes	Radiographic changes typical of rheumatoid arthritis on posteroanterior hand and wrist radiographs; must include erosions or unequivocal bony decalcification localized in or most marked adjacent to the involved joints (osteoarthritis changes alone do not qualify).

*For classification of purposes, a patient shall be said to have rheumatoid arthritis if he/she has satisfied at least 4 of these 7 criteria. Criteria 1 through 4 must have been present for at least 6 weeks. Patients with two clinical diagnoses are not excluded. Designation as classic, definite, or probable rheumatoid arthritis is *not* to be made.
SOURCE: Arnette FC, Edworthy SM, Bloch DA, et al. The American Rheumatism Association 1987 revised criteria for the classification of rheumatoid arthritis. Arthritis Rheum 1988;31:315–324.

in the synovium and chondrocytes in the cartilage to release enzymes. These enzymes degrade proteoglycans, collagen, and other connective tissue constituents and lead eventually to joint destruction.

Clinical Course

The clinical presentation and cause of RA are highly variable. Most patients present with insidious multiple joint involvement. However, a minority of patients may experience a rather abrupt onset of joint pain and swelling, representing the inflammatory synovitis. The course of RA is characterized by remissions and exacerbations with variable degrees of functional disability. As much as two-thirds of patients will maintain good joint function and be able to carry out near-normal activities of daily living. The remaining one-third or more of patients with RA, however, will experience sufficient joint destruction to impair function.

Serologic abnormalities in RA include a positive rheumatoid factor in 60 percent to 70 percent of patients. This factor is an antibody to the Fc portion of immunoglobulin G (IgG) and may be responsible for amplifying the inflammatory response in the synovium. Because the prevalence of rheumatoid factors increases with aging, a low titer in an older patient may not be significant. Although studies vary, about 10 percent to 15 percent of people older than 60 years of age have a positive rheumatoid factor. In addition, rheumatoid factors occur with other diseases such as systemic lupus erythematosus, subacute bacterial endocarditis, chronic lung disease, and chronic liver disease. Other serologic abnormalities found with RA include a positive test for antinuclear antibodies in as much as 50 percent of patients, usually in a low titer with a homogeneous pattern. The ESR may be elevated, and the patient may have an anemia secondary to chronic inflammation or blood loss. The synovial fluid in patients with RA is inflammatory, with 2000 to 75,000 cells per μL, greater than 50 percent neutrophils, negative cultures, and a glucose level less than 50 mg/dh, lower than normal blood levels.

In addition to joint disease, as much as one-half of patients with RA develop extra-articular manifestations. These are seen more often in patients with established destructive joint disease who have a high titer of rheumatoid factors. Extra-articular manifestations of RA include peripheral nodules, lung disease with interstitial fibrosis

(ILD) or pleural effusions, pericardial effusions, Sjögren's syndrome (dry eyes and mouth), neutropenia (Felty's syndrome), carpal tunnel syndrome, and vasculitis.

Rheumatoid Arthritis in the Elderly

Healey described three subsets of RA in the elderly (37) (Table 41.5). Subset one is the typical type of RA that would be seen in a younger patient. These patients have synovitis that starts in peripheral joints, is persistent, progressive, and usually leads to joint damage. There is radiographic evidence of joint erosions in patients with subset one of elderly-onset RA (EORA) and rheumatoid nodules are frequently found. Subset two of EORA exhibits features of Sjögren's syndrome. Sjögren's syndrome is an autoimmune disease associated with dry eyes and dry mouth (keratoconjunctivitis with xerostomia or sicca syndrome). Rheumatoid factor is commonly present. In this variant of RA in the elderly, synovitis is limited to a few joints, often the wrists and hands. Rheumatoid nodules are rare, and radiographic erosions are minimal. The third type of EORA resembles polymyalgia rheumatica. Rheu-

matoid factor is usually absent in these patients and there is a predilection for large joint involvement, characteristically shoulders, hips, and knees. Morning stiffness can be prominent. Rheumatoid nodules are typically not present, and radiographs do not show erosions. The joint disease does not progress and the mild synovitis is usually very responsive to low-dose corticosteroids.

Studies that have compared younger-onset RA (YORA) with EORA have emphasized that patients with EORA have a greater frequency of acute onset, systemic symptoms, and shoulder involvement (38–40). One of the more comprehensive studies (40) examined 78 patients with EORA and compared them with 134 patients with YORA. The results noted that an abrupt onset of RA with symptoms peaking in days to weeks occurred nearly twice as often in the EORA group than that in the YORA group (27% vs 14%). There was no difference in constitutional symptoms on presentation. The groups had similar amounts of extra-articular manifestations including dry eyes, dry mouth, and carpal tunnel syndrome. The joint scores at the first visit were nearly identical. The elderly patients had more arthritis in hips and knees; the younger patients had twice the amount of small joint disease. The EORA group had fewer subcutaneous nodules, a higher ESR, and fewer positive rheumatoid factors but similar values for hematocrit, white blood cell count, and antinuclear antibodies. A polymyalgia rheumatica-like presentation was seen in 23 percent of the patients with EORA. The outcome of patients with EORA at the last visit (4.8 years mean follow-up) was significantly better than that of the YORA group; the EORA group had less morning stiffness and fatigue, a lower total joint score, and one-half the number of subcutaneous nodules.

Therapeutic approaches are similar for patients with EORA and YORA, with some exceptions. NSAIDs are commonly used for both groups but cause more problems in the elderly. Recently, Healey suggested that low-dose corticosteroids (≤10 mg/day) are safer and more effective than NSAIDs (41). Second-line agents (formerly referred to as disease-modifying agents), such as gold, penicillamine, plaquenil, methotrexate, and azathioprine are used more frequently for patients with YORA. Methotrexate has become one of the most frequently used second-line agents for all RA patients. However, methotrexate is excreted by the kidneys and the elderly

Table 41.5. Subsets of Rheumatoid Arthritis in the Elderly.

Subset	Rheumatoid Factor	Manifestations
1	Present	Predilection for smaller joints (wrists, hands, feet)
		Synovitis likely persistent, progressive, leading to joint damage
		Frequent nodules
		Frequent radiographic erosion
2	Present	Sjögren's syndrome
		Synovitis limited to few joints (often wrists, hands)
		Responsive to anti-inflammatory drugs
		Rare nodules
		Minimal radiographic erosions
3	Absent	Predilection for large joints (shoulders, hips, knees)
		Marked stiffness
		Synovitis very responsive to low-dose steroid treatment
		Not progressive
		No nodules
		No radiographic erosions

with subtle chronic renal failure are particularly susceptible to the bone marrow suppression that can be induced by this drug. Similar incidences of oral ulcers, abnormal liver function tests, and pulmonary disease secondary to methotrexate have been seen in both young and old RA patients. Osteoporosis is associated with RA, with age, and with corticosteroids. Particular attention to this problem must be directed to the elderly; considerations for bone density studies and the therapeutic use of supplemental calcium, estrogens, calcitonin, or diphosphonates may be needed. Patients with RA who are scheduled for surgery should have x-rays of the cervical spine in flexion and extension views to look for C-1 or C-2 subluxation. If this is present, the anesthesiologist must take specific precautions to prevent spinal cord impingement.

In general, patients with RA have an increased mortality in comparison with aged-matched patients without RA. Prognostic factors that portend a worse prognosis in RA include extra-articular features of vasculitis, spine subluxation, pulmonary disease, infections, and sepsis. Laboratory tests that give a poor prognosis in RA include a high-titer rheumatoid factor, a persistently elevated ESR, and a low hemoglobulin level. A study by Pincus found that a lower level of education in RA patients was correlated with a worse prognosis (3), which may indicate the effects of multiple variables such as income, diet, access to care, general health habits, compliance, or overall lifestyle.

Polymyalgia Rheumatica and Giant Cell Arteritis
Polymyalgia rheumatica (PMR) is a disease of the elderly characterized by 1) onset above the age of 50 years; 2) pain and stiffness in the neck, shoulders, and pelvic girdle persisting for at least 1 month without significant weakness or atrophy; 3) elevated ESR; and 4) dramatic relief of symptoms by treatment with low-dose corticosteroids. The incidence of PMR in Olmstead County, Minnesota between 1970 and 1979 was 53.7 cases per 100,000 population older than 50 years of age (42). The incidence of RA was 77 cases per 100,000 in the same age group. A Swedish study suggested the incidence of PMR to be 20.4 per 100,000 in the age group older than 50 years. The female-to-male ratio of PMR is 2 to 2.5:1 and the age of patients is almost always greater than 50 years, with a mean of 65 to 70 years. Most reported cases of PMR have been in Caucasian individuals, but this may reflect an epidemiologic problem of ascertainment.

The presenting symptoms of PMR are stiffness in the morning and musculoskeletal pain most commonly localized to the shoulders and pelvic girdles. A 10-year epidemiologic study of 96 patients with PMR found complaints of pain in the shoulder (96%), hip (77%), upper arm (63%), neck (66%), thigh (54%), and torso (45%) (43). This study also noted that the patients' distal extremities were commonly painful; the lower extremities (knee to toe) exhibited pain 73 percent of the time and the upper extremities (elbow to fingers) 56 percent of the time. The onset of PMR may be gradual, but more often is abrupt, with symptoms developing as quickly as overnight. Weakness is not prominent, but musculoskeletal stiffness is characteristic. Patients with PMR often describe "rolling" out of bed in the morning, and gelling may make rising from a sitting position difficult. Many patients relate having had a viral illness 1 or 2 months before the onset of symptoms of PMR. Other systemic symptoms of patients with PMR include malaise and fatigue (30%), weight loss (15%), depression (15%), anorexia (14%), fever (13%), headache (13%), and blurred vision (3%) (43,44).

On physical examination about one-third of patients with PMR have tenderness in the shoulders, upper arms, and bicipital tendon groove. Concurrent synovitis has been noted in 12 percent to 32 percent of patients. Positive bone scans were found in 24 of 25 patients with PMR, the abnormal uptake most commonly being present in the shoulders (45). However, a more recent study examining 56 patients with PMR by isotope scans found peripheral synovitis in 5 (9%) and axial involvement in 7 (13%) (46). The synovitis is usually transient and mild, but may be prominent, and knee effusions can be quite large. The synovitis in PMR usually responds to treatment and leaves no residual damage.

Because of the close association of giant cell arteritis (GCA), or temporal arteritis, with PMR, it is important to look for symptoms and signs of GCA in patients presenting with PMR. Symptoms of GCA include headaches, visual changes, tender scalp, and jaw claudication manifest by pain in the jaw when the patient eats (Table 41.6) (47). Signs of temporal artery prominence and tenderness should be sought on physical examination. Eye findings in GCA may include diplopia or ptosis. Sudden blindness

Table 41.6. Initial Manifestations of Giant Cell Arteritis in 100 Mayo Clinic Patients.

Manifestations	No. of patients
Headache	32
Polymyalgia rheumatica	25
Fever	15
Visual symptoms without loss	7
Malaise/fatigue	5
Arterial tenderness	3
Myalgias	4
Weight loss/anorexia	2
Jaw claudication	2
Permanent visual loss	1
Tongue claudication	1
Sore throat	1
Arteritic angiogram	1
Hand/wrist stiffness	1

SOURCE: Calamia KT, Hunoler GG. Clin Rheum Dis 1980;6:389.

Table 41.7. Ischemic Syndromes in Giant Cell Arteritis.

Arteritic involvement	Manifestations
Temporal artery	Headache, scalp necrosis
Facial artery	Claudication of the jaw and/or tongue, odynophagia, gangrene of the tongue
Ocular arteries (ophthalmic, posterior ciliary, retinal)	Ptosis, diplopia, partial or complete loss of vision
Aorta and its major branches	Dissecting aortic aneurysm, aortic rupture, Raynaud's phenomenon, extremity claudication, bruits, absent pulses
Coronary artery	Angina, myocardial infarction
Renal artery	Glomerulitis, renal artery stenosis
Mesenteric arteries	Abdominal angina

may occur with funduscopic changes of ischemic optic neuritis including slight pallor, edema of the optic disc, scattered "cotton-wool" patches, and small hemorrhages. Optic atrophy may occur later. Spasm of jaw muscles may occasionally be a presenting manifestation of GCA. GCA is a vasculitis with invading macrophages and lymphocytes generally present in the entire circumference of the vessel wall. Langhans' giant cells are usually seen in the outer border of the internal elastic membrane. Because this form of vasculitis can affect large and medium-sized arteries, in severe or neglected cases the patient may complain of claudication and have unequal pulses or Raynaud's phenomenon, which can progress to gangrene of an extremity (Table 41.7). Occasionally, GCA may present as a fever of unknown origin with few physical findings (48).

The major laboratory abnormality in PMR is an elevated ESR that is greater than 45 mm/hr (Westergren) 90 percent of the time and is often more than 100 mm/hr (49). Case reports of normal ESR in patients with PMR and temporal arteritis exist, but are very rare. About one-half of patients with GCA have a mild to moderate normochromic anemia. Other less common findings include increases in serum levels of alpha$_2$-globulins and gamma globulins, abnormal liver function tests, and a decrease in albumin levels. Serum creatinine

phosphokinase levels, findings on electromyogram (EMG), and muscle biopsy test results are usually normal for patients with GCA. The muscle biopsy may occasionally show mild atrophy characteristic of disuse.

GCA is associated with PMR in 40 percent to 90 percent of cases (50,51). In a careful study by Nordborg, 7 of 27 patients with the clinical diagnosis of PMR had evidence of inflammation on temporal artery biopsies (52). Nordborg's hypothesis is that polymyalgia rheumatica and temporal arteritis (or GCA) represent different degrees or stages of the same disease process. Thus, should the temporal artery be biopsied in patients with PMR? Most patients with PMR have some symptom, other than blindness, to indicate whether temporal arteritis may be present.

Although controversial, recent evidence suggests that low-dose corticosteroid treatment may suppress PMR and possibly also temporal arteritis. However, most authors believe that prednisone needs to be given in doses larger than 40 mg per day to initially prevent blindness in patients with temporal arteritis. Most researchers recommend carefully following a patient with PMR for clinical symptoms of temporal arteritis and repeating the ESR. If there is any clinical suggestion of the presence of GCA, or if the ESR does not normalize with use of low-dose corticosteroids, the temporal artery should be biopsied.

Jaw claudication and clinically abnormal temporal arteries are the most suggestive symptoms of GCA. Temporal artery biopsies should be performed for every patient in whom high-dose corticosteroids are scheduled. Glucocorticosteroids are the only generally accepted treatment in GCA. To treat PMR, prednisone in a dose of 10 to 20 mg per day is the usual dose. The response is typically dramatic, often with overnight relief. However, some patients take 1 to 2 weeks or require a slightly higher dosage to see a good response. If no response is seen after 2 weeks, the diagnosis should be re-evaluated. To treat GCA, prednisone in a dose of 60 mg per day or larger is used. Symptoms and ESR should be followed closely in patients with either PMR or GCA. Steroids should be tapered slowly; a fast or sudden reduction may precipitate relapse of symptoms. In both PMR and GCA, corticosteroids should be continued at 7.5 to 10 mg per day for 12 to 24 months before a slow withdrawal of the medication is attempted.

Remitting, Seronegative, Symmetrical Synovitis with Pitting Edema

In 1985, McCarty (53) described a series of 10 patients with a peripheral seronegative polyarthritis and pitting edema of the hands and feet whose disease easily remitted with treatment and was not associated with joint destruction or deformity. It was proposed that this syndrome, RS3PE, represented a separate, benign form of polyarthritis in the elderly. Since McCarty's first description, an additional 22 cases have been reported in the literature (54,55). The mean age at onset is 69 years, the youngest patient age 45 and the oldest patient, age 82. All reported patients with RS3PE have been Caucasian. The male-to-female ratio is 2:1. The onset of RS3PE is frequently sudden, 1 to 7 days, and can be debilitating. Morning stiffness is a universal complaint and synovitis of the wrists and MCP joints is characteristic. Other joints frequently involved are PIPs, shoulders, knees, ankles, and elbows, with occasional involvement of the MTPs. Proximal myalgias have been described in several patients. Pitting edema of the distal extremities (of hands more often than of feet) is present. Flexor tenosynovitis is present in 65 percent of patients with RS3PE and clinical carpal tunnel syndrome is found in 30 percent. All patients achieved permanent remission with a variety of therapies.

Except for soft-tissue swelling, joint radiographs are normal in patients with RS3PE. Bone scans demonstrate uptake in involved joints. The patients do not possess rheumatoid factors, but 22 percent exhibit positive antinuclear antibodies (ANAs). The average ESR in RS3PE patients is 53 mm/hr, with a range of 5 to 104 mm/hr. Mild anemia is frequently noted. The synovial fluid is mildly inflammatory, with an average white cell count of 5077 cells per µL.

Symptoms in patients with RS3PE resolve most dramatically and rapidly with low-dose corticosteroid treatment. Other therapeutic agents are NSAIDs, hydroxychloroquine, gold, and intra-articular steroid injections. Remissions occur in about 5 months with corticosteroid treatment and in about 15 months with other agents.

Systemic Lupus Erythematosus

Systemic lupus erythematosus (SLE) is a multisystem autoimmune disease that occurs predominantly in women aged 20 to 40 years. The classification criteria for SLE are listed in Table 41.8 (56). Patients exhibiting 4 of 11 criteria, either serially or simultaneously, can be classified as having SLE with a sensitivity of 96 percent and a specificity of 96 percent. However, the full clinical picture of SLE may develop slowly over time and require an elapse of time before the diagnosis can be made with certainty.

SLE can involve most organs in the body, and its presenting clinical manifestations can vary widely. The cumulative clinical features of SLE are listed in Table 41.9 (56). Cutaneous manifestations are seen in 88 percent of patients, musculoskeletal in 83 percent, serositis in 63 percent, neuropsychiatric in 55 percent, Raynaud's phenomenon in 44 percent, vasculitis in 43 percent, and nephritis in 31 percent. The cumulative laboratory findings in SLE (Table 41.10) indicate that a positive test for ANA is found in 94 percent or more of patients. In the past, animal tissue substrates were used to screen for ANAs and these substrates did not detect anti-SSA/Ro antibodies. Now, human cell lines are used, and patients with SLE are virtually always ANA-positive.

In a compilation of seven selected studies of patients with SLE, 165 (12%) of 1426 patients had diagnosis of SLE made later than age 50 (58). After the age of 65, men and

Table 41.8. 1982 Revised Criteria for Classification of Systemic Lupus Erythematosus*.

Criterion	Definition
Malar rash	Fixed erythema, flat or raised, over the malar eminences, tending to spare the nasolabial folds.
Discoid rash	Erythematous raised patches with adherent keratotic sealing and follicular plugging; atrophic scarring may occur in older lesions.
Photo-sensitivity	Skin rash as a result of unusual reaction to sunlight, by patient history or physician observation.
Oral ulcers	Oral or nasopharyngeal ulceration, usually painless, observed by a physician.
Arthritis	Nonerosive arthritis involving 2 or more peripheral joints, characterized by tenderness, swelling or effusion.
Serositis	Pleuritis—convincing history of pleuritic pain or rub heard by a physician or evidence of pleural effusion. OR Pericarditis documented by electrocardiogram or rub or evidence of pericardial effusion.
Renal disorder	Persistent proteinuria greater than 0.5 grams per day or greater than 3+ if quantification not performed. OR Cellular casts—may be red cell, hemoglobin, granular, tubular, or mixed.
Neurologic disorder	Seizures in the absence of offending drugs or known metabolic derangements; e.g. uremia, ketoacidosis or electrolyte imbalance. OR Psychosis in the absence of offending or known metabolic derangements, e.g., uremia, ketoacidosis, or electrolyte imbalance.
Hematologic disorder	Hemolytic anemia with reticulocytosis OR Leukopenia less than 4,000/μL total on 2 or more occasions OR Lymphopenia less than 1,500/μL on 2 or more occasions OR Thrombocytopenia less than 100,000/μL in the absence of offending drugs
Immunologic disorder	Positive leukoerythrogenic cell preparation in abnormal titer OR Anti-DNA: antibody to native DNA in abnormal titer OR Anti-Sm: presence of antibody to SM nuclear antigen OR False positive serologic test for syphilis known to be positive for at least 6 months and confirmed by *Treponema pallidum* immobilization or fluorescent treponemal antibody absorption test.
Antinuclear antibody	An abnormal titer of antinuclear antibody by immunofluorescence or an equivalent assay at any point in time and in the absence of drug known to be associated with "drug-induced lupus" syndrome.

*The proposed classification is based on 11 criteria. For the purpose of identifying patients in clinical studies, a person shall be said to have systemic lupus erythematosus if any 4 or more of the 11 criteria are present, serially or simultaneously, during any interval of observation.

SOURCE: Tan EM, Cohen AS, Fries JF, et al. The 1982 revised criteria for the classification of systemic lupus erythematosus. Arthritis Rheum 1982;25:1271–1277.

women develop SLE with almost equal frequency. A meta-analysis of nine studies describing the clinical manifestations of older-onset SLE found the spectrum of SLE in the elderly to be different from that seen in a younger age group (59). Older-onset SLE patients were found to have an increased frequency of pleurisy, pericarditis, pulmonary fibrosis, and Sjögren's (sicca) syndrome. There were no differences between the two groups in the incidence of nephritis, photosensitivity, oral ulcers, and myalgias. Older patients with SLE exhibited a decreased incidence of neuropsychiatric illness, Raynaud's phenomenon, alopecia, fever, and lymphadenopathy than did

Table 41.9. Cumulative Clinical Features in 150 Patients with Systemic Lupus Erythematosus.

Manifestation	No. (%)	Manifestation	No. (%)
Cutaneous	132 (88)	Neuropsychiatric	83 (55)
Malar rash	91 (61)	Central nervous system	59 (39)
Alopecia	68 (45)	Peripheral neuropathy	32 (21)
Photosensitivity	68 (45)	Organic psychosis	24 (16)
Mucosal ulcers	35 (23)	Seizures	20 (13)
Discoid rash	22 (15)	Raynaud's phenomenon	66 (44)
Nodules	18 (12)	Vasculitis	65 (43)
Musculoskeletal	124 (83)	Cutaneous	40 (27)
Arthritis	114 (76)	Mesenteric	19 (13)
Ischemic necrosis	36 (24)	Digital ulcers	14 (9)
Myositis	7 (5)	Leg ulcers	9 (6)
Serositis	95 (63)	Nephritis	46 (31)
Pleurisy	85 (57)	Nephrotic syndrome	20 (13)
Pericarditis	35 (23)	Chronic renal failure	5 (3)
Peritonitis	12 (8)	Cardiopulmonary	8 (5)

Table 41.10. Cumulative Laboratory Features in 150 Patients with Systemic Lupus Erythematosus.

Manifestations	No. (%)
Hematologic	
Anemia	86 (57)
Leukopenia	62 (41)
Thrombocytopenia	45 (30)
Direct Coombs' positive	40 (27)
Immunologic	
Hypocomplementemia	89 (59)
Rheumatoid factor	45 (34)
Hyperglobulinemia	45 (30)
Chronic BFP-STS	34 (26)
Antinuclear antibodies	141 (94)
Anti-ssDNA	134 (89)
Leukoerythrogenic cells	67 (71)
Anti-nRNP	51 (34)
Anti-Sm	26 (17)
Anti-nDNA	42 (28)
Anti-Ro (SS-A)	48 (32)
Anti-La (SS-B)	18 (12)

younger patients (59). Although studies vary widely, older SLE patients probably develop less renal involvement and fewer hematologic manifestations (58–60). Serologically, older SLE patients demonstrate less frequent hypocomplementemia and possibly fewer anti-DS-DNA antibodies with about an equal incidence of rheumatoid factors in comparison with younger patients. Older patients with SLE display a higher incidence of anti-SSA/Ro and anti-SSB/La antibodies. In general, the prognosis for the older-onset SLE patient is good and probably better than it is for the younger-onset patient. Major organ system involvement influences prognosis; renal disease and thrombocytopenia in younger SLE patients decrease life expectancy (61), and possible lung involvement also decreases survival.

The modes of presentation of SLE in the elderly are diverse. The elderly can present with a single- or multiorgan involvement and usually manifest nonspecific constitutional symptoms such as weight loss, fever, fatigue, or malaise. The older SLE patient can present with polymyalgia rheumatica-type symptoms such as muscle stiffness, fatigue, high ESR, and anemia. The patient also may experience an isolated polyarthritis, skin rash, dyspnea, or neuropsychiatric problem. The neuropsychiatric symptoms may be depression, psychosis, or behavioral changes mimicking dementia. Late-onset Raynaud's phenomenon or peripheral neuropathy may be another sign of SLE in the elderly. The most prominent presentation of SLE in the elderly includes photosensitive dermatitis, pulmonary fibrosis, sicca syndrome, and peripheral neuropathy. Autoantibodies such as an ANA, anti-SSA/Ro, or anti-SSB/La along with anti-DS-DNA can be helpful in diagnosing SLE (58).

Drug-Induced Lupus

Drug-induced lupus is more common in the elderly. Over 50 drugs have been implicated in inducing a lupus-like illness (62). However, doubts exist with many of these drugs about their true association with lupus. Some of these drugs, such as anticonvulsants, may be used to treat early unrecognized signs of systemic lupus. Other drugs, such as oral contraceptives or sulfonamides, may have led to the unmasking of early subclinical SLE. Thus, drugs implicated in inducing a lupus-like syndrome have been divided into three groups (62): 1) drugs in which proof of the association is definite and for which appropriate, controlled prospective studies have been performed; 2) drugs that are possibly associated; and 3) drugs with somewhat unlikely associations or only a rare case report (Table 41.11). There are no definite criteria to distinguish idiopathic SLE from drug-induced SLE. The induction of

Table 41.11. Substances Associated with Drug-Related Lupus.

Group I	Group II	Group III
chlorpromazine	acebutolol	acecainide
methyldopa	captopril	p-aminosalicylic acid
hydralazine	hydrazine	chlorthalidone
procainamide	lithium carbonate	estrogens
isoniazid	methylthiouracil	gold salts
	oxyprenolol	methysergide
	phenytoin	nomifensine
	propylthiouracil	psoralen
	aromatic amines	sulfasalazine
	carbamazepine	thionamide
	labetalol	allopurinol
	mephytoin	benzylpenicillin
	metoprolol	chlorprothixene
	penicillamine	ethylphenacemide
	practolol	griseofulvin
	quinidine	metrizamide
	atenolol	oxyphisatin
	ethosuximide	reserpine
	levadopa	sulfonamides
	methimazole	tolazamide
	nitrofurantoin	aminoglutethimide
	phenylbutazone	1-canavanine
	primidone	domperidone
	trimethadione	isoquinazepon
		guanoxan
		minoxidil
		propafenone
		streptomycin
		tetracycline

SOURCE: From Solinger AM; Drug-related lupus: clinical and etiological considerations. Clin Rheum Dis 1988;14:187–202.

lupus-like symptoms and the development of a positive ANA after a patient begins a new drug, with resolution of the symptoms after withdrawal of the drug, are suggestive of drug-induced SLE.

The drugs most studied that induce ANAs and lupus-like symptoms are hydralazine and procainamide. Positive ANAs are induced in 24 percent to 75 percent of patients receiving these drugs, and lupus-like syndromes occur in 8 percent to 20 percent of these patients (63). Lupus symptoms usually occur within 2 years and can begin as early as 1 month after the patient begins these drugs. The most common symptoms are constitutional symptoms such as malaise, weakness, weight loss, and arthralgias. Arthritis is more common than it is in idiopathic SLE, but pleuropulmonary symptoms are simi-lar in occurrence. Skin rashes, adenopathy, myalgias, Raynaud's phenomenon, and renal involvement are more common in the idiopathic form of SLE. CNS involvement is extremely rare in drug-induced lupus.

Laboratory abnormalities of anemia and leukopenia or both occur in about 25 percent to 33 percent of patients with drug-induced SLE, and patients with drug-induced lupus exhibit positive ANAs. Elevated ESR and hypergammaglobulinemia are found relatively frequently in patients with drug-induced SLE. However, hypocomplementemia and anti-DS-DNA antibodies are not seen in these patients. Instead, drug-induced lupus is associated with antibodies to histone 1 and to the histone complexes H2A-H2B and H3-H4 (64).

One cannot predict who will develop a drug-induced lupus-like syndrome. However, a major predisposition is thought to be the genetically controlled hepatic acetylation of drugs by the acetyl transferase system. After taking hydralazine or procainamide, individuals who are slow acetylators develop positive ANAs much more rapidly than persons who are fast acetylators (62). Hydralazine, isoniazid, and procainamide share a common chemical structure, a primary aromatic amine or a hydrazine group, which causes the compound to be metabolized through acetylation. Slow acetylation of these drugs maintains the parent compound at a constant level, which implies that the lupus-like syndrome may be caused by the parent drug or a nonacetylated metabolite.

Treatment of Lupus

Drug-induced lupus is mainly treated by stopping the drug. For many patients, the symptoms abate within days or weeks. However, in some patients symptoms may persist for months or years. In this case, the patient is treated as if idiopathic SLE is present.

Management of idiopathic SLE in the elderly starts with education of the patient. First, the physician should explain to the SLE patient the nature of the illness and the approach to therapy. The clinician should allay anxiety and work toward building a relationship with the patient. The second step is therapy. Because SLE is varied and protean in nature, an organ system approach is advised. Some precautions may be taken to prevent flare-ups. Some patients are sun-sensitive and should use sunscreens and clothing that shades the skin when they go outside. Certain drugs such as sulfonamides and oral contraceptives, may induce exacerbations. However, there is no evidence that treatment with replacement estrogens exacerbates SLE. Patients with Raynaud's phenomenon should be cautioned to prepare for changes in weather and have clothing to keep their body and hands warm.

In the elderly with SLE, drug therapy should be used cautiously. Skin rashes can usually be treated with topical steroids, and arthralgias and arthritis can be treated with NSAIDs. If NSAIDs do not control the joint pain, if the patient develops discoid skin rashes, or if there is need to control fatigue and pleuritis, hydroxychloroquine at a dose of 200 mg once to twice a day should be used. At this low dose there is very little eye toxicity but patients should be advised to undergo routine eye examinations every 6 months. When potentially serious internal organ involvement of the muscles, heart, lungs, or CNS is present in idiopathic SLE, high doses of corticosteroids usually are given. Depending on the patient's response to corticosteroids and their side effects, azathioprine, methotrexate, and alkylating agents may be used in conjunction with, or as a means to decrease, the dose of steroids. Renal disease seems to respond best to cyclophosphamide, commonly administered at 1 to 2 g per meter^2 intravenously as a monthly pulse for 6 months, then every 3 months for another 18 to 24 months. Patients with late onset SLE tend to have relatively benign disease, and up to 40 percent of elderly patients will develop significant side effects to steroid treatment. Therefore, elderly patients with SLE should be treated in a conservative fashion with as little corticosteroid as possible. The clinical experience in elderly-onset SLE is quite limited and controlled studies of therapy are lacking.

Sjögren's Syndrome

Sjögren's syndrome (keratoconjunctivitis sicca and xerostomia) can occur as a primary disease or may be secondary to another autoimmune disease such as RA or SLE. The prevalence of this disorder in the general population has been estimated to be from 0.05 percent to 0.44 percent (65). However, screening of a female population with an average age of 81 years (range, age 63 to 92) indicated that complaints of dry eyes or dry mouth were present in 39 percent. Definite Sjögren's syndrome was present in only 2 percent, however, with a possible diagnosis made in 12 percent (65). The major cause of dry eyes and dry mouth in this elderly population was the use of medications that cause these side effects.

Primary Sjögren's syndrome is an autoimmune exocrinopathy that can affect saliva, tear formation, and pancreatic function (66). Patients with Sjögren's syndrome can experience extraglandular effects in the joints, lungs, kidneys, blood vessels, muscles, and CNS. In a typical presentation, the patient complains of dry eyes, including a sandy or foreign body sensation in the eyes, especially on awakening. The patient with Sjögren's syndrome may complain of itchiness or redness of the eyes and photosensitivity. Decreased production of saliva may cause a dry mouth and difficulty swallowing, changes in taste, and an increase in dental caries. Signs to look for in Sjögren's syndrome include pitting on the exposed cornea, a fissured, dry tongue, and parotid swelling. Standard tests to measure ocular dryness are corneal staining to detect pits and a Schirmer's tear test. A filter paper 30 mm long is placed on the inside of the lower eyelid with the remainder of the paper hanging down. The amount of tear formation in 5 minutes is measured and wetting of 5 mm or less is considered abnormal. Sometimes salivary flow rates or parotid scintigraphy are performed to document decreased salivary secretion. The definitive diagnosis of Sjögren's syndrome is made by a minor salivary gland biopsy. A focal collection of 50 or more lymphocytes in the gland is virtually diagnostic of Sjögren's syndrome. Other exocrine involvement in Sjögren's syndrome can include a dry upper respiratory tract, which causes recurrent bronchitis and pneumonitis. Also commonly found is loss of vaginal secretions and vaginal dryness. Rarely, acute or chronic pancreatitis with pancreatic insufficiency can develop.

Extraglandular involvement in Sjögren's syndrome can affect multiple organs. As much as 50 percent of patients with primary Sjögren's syndrome can have arthritis that mimics RA except for the absence over time of erosions. Raynaud's phenomenon can be seen in about one-third of patients. Pleuritis, interstitial lung disease, and, rarely, pulmonary hypertension have all been described in primary Sjögren's syndrome. Lymphocytic interstitial infiltration in the kidneys can cause a hypokalemic, hyperchloremic, distal renal tubular acidosis. About 5 percent of patients with Sjögren's syndrome can develop small to medium vessel vasculitis that can present with purpura, skin ulcers, urticaria and a mononeuritis multiplex. Sjögren's syndrome can overlap with polymyositis. Some observers have found a high incidence of CNS involvement with a wide spectrum of presentations in patients with Sjögren's syndrome (67). Focal CNS manifestations such as motor and sensory deficits, movement disorders, aphasia, seizures, and cerebellar syndromes have been described. Nonfocal deficits such as dementia, cognitive dysfunction, and psychiatric abnormalities also have been noted in these patients as well as spinal cord problems of transverse myelitis, neurogenic bladder, and chronic progressive myelitis. Other observers have not found such a high incidence or severity of CNS disorders in Sjögren's patients (68).

Primary Sjögren's syndrome in the elderly tends to be a more benign disease with fewer extraglandular features. Elderly patients with RA or SLE frequently develop secondary Sjögren's syndrome. Although the course is generally benign, there is also a higher incidence of pseudolymphoma and lymphoma in patients with Sjögren's syndrome.

Treatment for Sjögren's syndrome is aimed at protecting the mucous membranes and teeth in the mouth and the cornea of the eyes. The eyes are generally treated with artificial tear drops, such as carboxymethylcellulose, and ocular ointments or lubricants at night. If the eye dryness progresses, the tear ducts can be surgically occluded, which usually keeps the eyes moist. Hydroxypropyl cellulose opthalmic inserts also can be placed in the corner of the eye once a day for a continuous source of moisture. Oral hygiene is very important to protect the teeth from caries. Flossing the teeth and brushing frequently with a fluoride-based toothpaste are basic to saving the teeth. The teeth should be professionally cleaned two to three times a year. The patients should try to keep moisture in the mouth by using sugarless candies and gum, carrying water with them, or using an artificial saliva. The arthritis associated with Sjögren's syndrome is treated similarly to RA.

Polymyositis and Dermatomyositis
The inflammatory myopathies are systemic illnesses characterized by muscle weakness and the presence of lymphocytic infiltration on muscle biopsy. These myopathies are associated to a variable degree with vasculitis, dermatitis, malignancy, and other autoimmune diseases. In the past, inflammatory myopathies were divided into various subgroups according to their presentation and associations (69). The standard divisions were polymyositis (PM), dermatomyositis (DM), PM and DM with neoplasia, childhood DM with vasculitis, and overlap syndromes. In adults, the most frequent presentation is PM, followed by DM with associated neoplasms; overlap syndromes are less common. With advancements in histology and immunopathology, other categories of inflammatory myopathies have been noted, such as inclusion body myositis (IBM).

The incidence of the idiopathic inflammatory myopathies is about 5 to 10 cases per 1 million new cases per year (70). The age of presentation in adults is usually 40 or 50 years of age, with the cancer-associated group generally older. In a series with extensive literature review, the mean age of presentation of patients with PM was 50 years of age, for DM was 38.8 years of age, and for cancer-associated DM, 57.1 years of age (71). PM and DM occur more frequently in women (3:1) and blacks. IBM occurs more frequently in males older than age 50. The clinical onset of all types of inflammatory myopathies is more frequent in the winter and spring months.

The typical clinical presentation of PM and DM is an insidious, progressive, symmetric, proximal muscle weakness initially without pain but manifesting a variable amount of pain and tenderness over time. The more extensive the muscle involvement and the longer the condition goes untreated, the more likely that muscles will be tender and painful. IBM has a more insidious presentation and more diffuse muscle involvement than do DM and PM. Ocular and facial muscles are rarely involved. Pharyngeal and bulbar muscles may become weak over time and lead to aspiration pneumonia and dysphonia. Physical examination may show subtle to obvious weakness in specific muscle groups. The patient may exhibit a clumsy or waddling gait and may experience difficulty arising from a chair without the assistance of hands. Skin involvement seen in DM can include an erythematous or scaly rash over sun-exposed areas. Particularly characteristic is the heliotrope or lilac rash around the eyes and over the eyelids. Also characteristic of DM are flat plaques

579

over the PIP and MCP joints, called Gottron's papules. The fingers also may show dry and crackling skin over the finger pads, called "machinist" hands. Calcinosis may be seen on the extensor surfaces of the elbows and knees, in the fingers, or be sheet-like on the torso or in the muscles. Other extramusculoskeletal involvement in PM or DM includes esophageal dysmotility, seen in about one-third of patients. Primarily, the DM patients can exhibit cardiac involvement. Most frequently seen are arrhythmias followed by congestive heart failure and cardiomyopathies. Lung involvement can be one of the most serious consequences of PM and DM. The spectrum of pulmonary disease can range from an aggressive, diffuse alveolitis with rapidly progressive shortness of breath to more insidious but progressive ILD.

The major feature of DM that is relative to elderly patients is an association with malignancy. Although there is some controversy as to how significant this association is (72,73), most authors believe that malignancies increase in elderly patients with DM. In one study, the frequency of malignancy in DM was 8.5 percent in all patients, with figures of 19.2 percent and 17.9 percent in males and females, respectively, older than 50 years of age (74). In 70 percent of patients, the malignancy preceded the appearance of myositis by an average of 1.9 years. In the remaining 30 percent of patients, myositis preceded malignancy by an average of 2.8 years. The most common tumors are carcinomas of the breast, lung, stomach, or ovary (72). Thus, for the elderly patient who presents with DM, one should perform a thorough history and physical examination along with routine tests such as CBC, chemistries, liver function tests, urinalysis, and chest x-ray. Further consideration should be given to mammograms, gastrointestinal studies, and even computed tomography (CT) scans of the abdomen and pelvic area, as may seem appropriate for a particular patient. PM and DM can also overlap with scleroderma, SLE, RA, and Sjögren's syndrome.

Laboratory tests that are most helpful in diagnosing an inflammatory myopathy include creatine kinase (CK), which is invariably elevated; aldolase, which is elevated about 65 percent of the time; EMG, which typically demonstrates a myopathy; and muscle biopsy, which will not only confirm an inflammatory myopathy but can diagnose a specific subtype. In DM, the cellular infiltrates are

predominantly perivascular or in the interfascicular septa around the muscle fascicles. In PM, the infiltrate is mostly scattered in the muscle fibers. IBM looks like PM but demonstrates basophilic inclusions that rim vacuoles within individual muscle fibers. Tests for autoantibodies may be helpful in the diagnosis because 80 percent of PM and DM patients are ANA-positive. Anti-Jo-1 antibodies are particularly interesting. This is an antibody against histidyl-tRNA and is associated with fever, polyarthritis, Raynaud's phenomenon, and, most importantly, ILD. It is estimated that half the PM and DM patients that develop ILD will demonstrate anti-Jo-1 antibodies.

Prognosis and treatment depend on the form of inflammatory myositis. In one study, unfavorable prognostic signs were a failure to induce remission, leukocytosis, fever, older age, a shorter disease history, and dysphagia (75). IBM has a more insidious course with only moderately elevated CK and, in general, IBM is unresponsive to therapy. PM and DM are generally treated with high-dose corticosteroids, 1 to 2 mg/kg/day, until the CK and ESR normalize; the corticosteroids are then tapered slowly. A minority of patients may need to be maintained long-term on low-dose corticosteroids. Azathioprine and methotrexate are used when corticosteroids have failed or have caused serious side effects. Intravenous gamma globulin has been used with success when the above treatments have failed. Chlorambucil has been successful when azathioprine and methotrexate have failed. In patients with DM and malignancy, the muscle disease may regress once the tumor is treated successfully.

Scleroderma (Systemic Sclerosis)

Scleroderma is a heterogeneous set of diseases characterized by fibrosis of the skin and internal organs. There are localized forms of scleroderma that affect an extremity in a linear pattern (linear scleroderma) or in patches (morphea). These patients rarely have internal organ involvement. Patients with systemic sclerosis have tight skin and some internal organ involvement. Patients with systemic sclerosis are clinically divided into two groups, the limited form and the diffuse form. Patients with the limited form have tight skin evident distally to the elbows and knees and over the face and neck. In the past, this group was called the CREST (calcinosis, Raynaud's phenomenon, esophageal dysmotility, sclerodactyly, and *t*elangiectasias) subgroup. The diffuse form, by definition, demonstrates skin involvement proximal to the elbows and knees but excludes the head and neck. The distinctions between limited and diffuse forms of systemic sclerosis have prognostic significance.

Systemic sclerosis involves the skin and often multiple internal organs. Underlying this disease is a diffuse, noninflammatory vasculopathy with proliferation of endothelial cells in the intima of arterioles. More than 85 percent of patients have Raynaud's phenomenon and dysmotility of the lower two-thirds of the esophagus. The limited form of systemic sclerosis is more likely to exhibit telangiectasias and calcinosis than is the diffuse form, although both skin manifestations can be seen in the diffuse form. The lungs can be involved two ways, either with an interstitial fibrosing process or with pulmonary hypertension. The interstitial fibrosis can be of a limited form, primarily basilar fibrosis with no progression, or lung involvement can be progressive with potentially a more severe course. Patients with diffuse systemic sclerosis are at risk for developing serious ILD. Patients with the limited form of systemic sclerosis demonstrate a lower risk for developing serious ILD. However, a small subgroup of patients with the limited form of systemic sclerosis are at risk for developing pulmonary hypertension, which typically is unresponsive to traditional treatments used for idiopathic pulmonary hypertension. Almost all patients with diffuse systemic sclerosis develop esophageal dysmotility, and some patients exhibit fibrosis of the small and large bowel. Constipation with intermittent diarrhea from bacterial overgrowth can be a major problem in these patients. Malabsorption of calcium, iron, vitamin B_{12}, and, later, severe diffuse malabsorption with persistent weight loss can be seen. The heart commonly has patches of fibrosis noted on autopsy but significant arrhythmias, cardiomyopathy, or congestive heart failure are rarely noted, mainly in patients with diffuse systemic sclerosis.

Renal involvement is one of the most serious problems in diffuse systemic sclerosis and was a major cause of death in the past. With the advent of angiotensin-converting enzyme (ACE) inhibitors for the treatment of hypertension in scleroderma patients, the incidence of significant renal involvement has dramatically decreased.

Renal involvement is mainly a problem in patients with diffuse systemic sclerosis. Patients can exhibit some bone resorption, especially at the distal fingers, called acrosclerosis with osteolysis. Rarely do scleroderma patients develop a true arthritis, but tendon-sheath fibrosis with tendon rubbing is common. Patients with systemic sclerosis can demonstrate type 2 muscle fiber atrophy with mild weakness or can overlap with polymyositis and clinically display an inflammatory muscle disease treated similarly to polymyositis.

Laboratory tests can be helpful in distinguishing the limited and diffuse forms of systemic sclerosis. Almost all patients have a positive ANA. Most patients with the limited form also possess an anticentromere antibody. A subset of the diffuse form, probably less than 25 percent, has an antibody to topoisomerase 1, commonly referred to as anti-Scl-70. Anemia is common in all patients with systemic sclerosis. An elevated ESR can be seen with active disease but is not a consistent finding.

Systemic sclerosis typically affects women between 30 and 50 years of age with blacks exhibiting a higher incidence than whites. There is no clear consensus on whether patients with elderly-onset scleroderma have a different disease than do patients with younger-onset disease. An early report indicated that the elderly exhibited a higher prevalence of limited disease (76). However, this may represent the better prognosis of the limited form. Life-table analysis has demonstrated that elderly patients with scleroderma have poorer cumulative survival rates than do younger patients (77,78).

The approaches to treatment are similar for the two forms of systemic sclerosis. No well-accepted studies show that any treatment stops the fibrosis of the skin or internal organs. Standard therapy for the diffuse skin disease is as much as 1000 mg per day of D-penicillamine or 0.6 mg of colchicine twice a day. A number of experimental drugs are currently being evaluated. Patients with Raynaud's phenomenon should be told to keep their hands and body warm and to prepare for the worst possible weather when going outdoors. Calcium channel blockers are used to decrease attacks of Raynaud's phenomenon, with nifedipine the most thoroughly studied. All patients need to be placed on a regimen to prevent reflux esophagitis, including elevating the head of the bed higher than 2 inches, not eating for 3 hours before bedtime, and, usually, taking an antacid, H_2 blocker, or omeprazole at bedtime in standard doses. Patients who develop diarrhea are first treated with an antibiotic to decrease gut flora; if no response is seen, a diagnostic workup for diarrhea is performed. There is no known preventive measure for scleroderma lung disease, and it is typically unresponsive to any treatment. If the patient's diastolic blood pressure goes above 90 mm Hg, the patient should be treated with an ACE inhibitor because these drugs have been shown to decrease the incidence of renal failure.

Septic Arthritis

Infected joints once were considered a disease of children and adolescents but are now seen more often in adults, especially the elderly (79). In a review of infectious arthritis in 113 unselected patients, 27 percent were older than age 50 (80). If cases of gonorrhea are excluded, almost half the patients with septic joints are older than 50 years of age. Risk factors for the development of infected joints include immunosuppressive drugs such as corticosteroids, malignancies, diabetes, liver disease, underlying damaged joints such as those damaged by RA, and prosthetic joints. The elderly are more likely to possess these risk factors and thus exhibit an increased incidence of septic joints. Although Staphylococcus aureus is the most common organism cultured, there are increased incidences of β-hemolytic streptococcus and of gram-negative organisms in the elderly with septic arthritis in comparison with the adult population as a whole.

A septic joint is a medical emergency and one must have a high index of suspicion to make a proper diagnosis. The symptoms may at first be subtle, with fever present in only half the patients and rigors seen in less than one-fourth of patients. Typically, a septic joint is very painful with either active or passive movement and is usually warm, erythematous, and swollen. Septic arthritis is monarticular in about 85 percent of patients. The most common joints involved, in order of frequency, are the knee, hip, shoulder, ankle, wrist, and elbow, then all other joints. Blood leukocytosis is noted in 50 percent to 70 percent of patients and an elevated ESR is found in over 90 percent of patients. In nongonococcal arthritis, the synovial fluid Gram stain demonstrates organisms between 25 percent and 75 percent of the time, and synovial fluid cultures are positive in 60 percent to 100 percent. Blood cultures are important because in 10 percent of septic arthritis cases the organism is only grown from the blood. Although identification of crystals in a joint establishes the diagnosis of a crystal-induced arthropathy, crystals may be seen concomitantly with an infection. If there is any question concerning the diagnosis, the synovial fluid should be cultured and the patient treated for a septic joint. Radiographic studies in septic arthritis usually show soft-tissue swelling during the first week and within 10 days some osteoporosis may be visible with joint space narrowing. Subchondral bone destruction and periosteal elevation may develop rapidly thereafter. A bone scan can be used to assist in the early diagnosis of a septic joint, especially in areas difficult to aspirate, such as the sacroiliac joint or spine. A neglected septic joint may undergo rapid destruction and deterioration; thus, the more rapidly treatment is begun, the better the prognosis.

Treatment for septic arthritis usually includes antibiotics and drainage. Daily needle aspiration is performed until the synovial fluid normalizes or no synovial fluid is obtained. Needle drainage is used if the joint space is readily accessible and no loculations are suspected (81). This can be less traumatic for the patient and can more quickly lead to successful performance of range-of-motion exercises in comparison with surgical drainage. Certain joints, such as the hip, usually require surgical drainage. As the patient improves, physical therapy is started, first with passive range of motion, then with active motion as inflammation decreases. Poor prognostic signs in septic arthritis are a delay in instituting treatment of more than 7 days, hip involvement, prosthetic joint involvement, age older than 60 years, persistent synovial leukocyte count higher than 50,000 cells per μL after 5 days of therapy, and bacteremia (82).

An increasing number of joint replacements are being performed in elderly patients, and as much as 1 percent of arthroplasties become infected (83). Risk factors for infection include underlying RA, revision arthroplasties, and metal-to-metal prostheses. Infected prostheses may develop acutely in the immediate postoperative period or insidiously with indolent symptoms as long as 1 to 2 years after surgery. The major symptom suggesting developing infection of a prosthetic joint is pain on weight-bearing, which is often seen in the absence of any local or systemic evidence of infection. Radiographs may show loosening of the prosthesis, periosteal reaction, or both. Organisms most commonly cultured from infected prostheses are *S. epidermidis* and *S. aureus* with an increasing incidence of gram-negative and anaerobic organisms (83). Infected prostheses usually need to be removed before the infection will respond completely to appropriate antibiotics. However, there are some patients whose risk of surgery is so great that antibiotics are administered indefinitely.

Soft-Tissue Rheumatism

The geriatric population frequently experiences musculoskeletal problems related to the bursa, tendon, ligaments, and other soft tissue. In a recent study of 100 healthy subjects older than 65 years of age, 34 percent were found to possess a symptomatic shoulder disorder, with most having tendonitis (84). These soft-tissue problems can lead to varying degrees of pain and functional loss.

The most common diffuse soft-tissue syndrome is fibromyalgia. Although this was initially thought to occur primarily in a younger population, more recent demographic studies have placed the mean age at about 53 years, and about 73 percent of the patients are women (85). The age of onset may relate to other musculoskeletal disorders. Symptoms of fibromyalgia include moderate to severe generalized aches and pains most prominently in a proximal distribution described as "constant," "aching," or "dull." Stiffness is a common complaint but usually lasts less than 1 hour. Patients with fibromyalgia are easily fatigued. Weakness is claimed but is invariably a secondary response to pain. The duration of symptoms can be from months to 20 years or longer. Nonrheumatic symptoms commonly associated with fibromyalgia are sleep disturbance, headaches, anxiety or depression, and irritable bowel syndrome (86). Modulating factors that seem to exacerbate symptoms of fibromyalgia are weather changes (especially cold weather), sedentary states, unusual or excessive exercise, and emotional stress or anxiety. Factors that ameliorate symptoms include hot and dry weather, massage, vacation, and moderate exercise.

In general, patients with fibromyalgia display limited physical findings unless they posses a secondary disease. Secondary fibromyalgia is caused by a chronic pain process that may upset the patient's normal sleep cycle. In primary fibromyalgia, the patient's joints are not abnormal, and there is no demonstrated muscle weakness. Patients with primary or secondary fibromyalgia exhibit tender points. American College of Rheumatology criteria for the diagnosis of fibromyalgia suggest that the patient possess 11 of 18 possible tender points to establish the diagnosis (87). Tender points are discrete areas (2–3 cm in diameter) of normal appearing skin from which focal pain is elicited when pressure is applied to the underlying soft tissue and muscle. Adequate pressure should blanch the thumbnail. Frequently, palpation of these points will cause a sudden withdrawal, the "jump sign." The tender points are located at the lateral base of the occiput, anterior cervical muscles about midline of the sternocleidomastoid muscle, along the posterior lateral base of the neck, mid-trapezius, along the upper and lower area medial to the scapula in the paraspinous muscles, anterior pectoralis muscles, lateral to the lumbosacral joint, just distal to the lateral epicondyle, over the greater trochanteric bursa area, and medial to the mid-knee. Screening laboratory tests including CBC, ESR, creatine phosphokinase, serum calcium, and thyroid-stimulating hormone (TSH) should all be normal.

A major theory regarding the pathogenesis of fibromyalgia is that it is caused by a sleep disturbance. Patients experience interrupted stage 3 and stage 4 sleep, called an alpha-delta pattern (88). Interrupted sleep is hypothesized to induce an increased sensitivity to pain. The treatment for fibromyalgia is both nonpharmacologic and pharmacologic. First, the patient should be reassured that symptoms are not the result of a more serious disease. Local measures such as heat packs, gentle massage, and mild stretching exercises may provide temporary relief. The best therapeutic intervention may be the adoption of a graduated aerobic exercise program. Pharmacologic intervention is usually aimed at improving the quality of "restorative" sleep by using low doses of tricyclic antidepressants such as 10 to 50 mg of amitriptyline (89).

Bursitis and Tendonitis

Bursae are sacs filled with synovial fluid that act as cushions between tendons and bones. Trauma is the usual cause of bursitis but other causes include crystal precipitation and infection. A number of bursae can become inflamed. The subacromial bursa is under the acromial process and deltoid muscle over the shoulder capsule. Pain is usually elicited by abduction and flexion of the shoulder. The olecranon bursa is at the point of the elbow between the skin and the olecranon process. The patient with olecranon bursitis usually has mild pain with point tenderness but exhibits full range of motion of the elbow. The trochanteric bursa is directly over the greater trochanter of the femur, between the tendon of the gluteus maximus and the posterolateral aspect of the greater trochanter. Patients with trochanteric bursitis usually complain of a dull ache along the lateral aspect of the hip. Pain is usually worse with activity and crossing the legs. The patient may give a history of being unable to sleep on that side and point tenderness is present over the trochanteric bursa. The anserine bursa is about 5 cm below the joint margin of the medial aspect of the knee. Patients with anserine bursitis exhibit point tenderness and experience pain when they climb stairs. Osteoarthritis of the knee may confuse the presentation. The ischiogluteal bursa sits between the ischial tuberosity and the gluteus maximus muscle. Bursitis pain is noted in the buttock and posterior thigh area when the patient sits. The patient is tender locally over the ischial tuberosity and bending forward may result in severe buttock pain.

Therapy, in general, is similar for all inflamed bursae. First, the conservative approach of rest and NSAIDs should be tried. Adjunct therapy of ultrasound, heat, or cold may be used. If the patient does not improve, an intrabursal injection of corticosteroids should be performed. Infectious bursitis is treated with antibiotics and aspiration of the bursa.

Tendons attach muscle to bone. Tendons can become inflamed by trauma, by a degenerative process, as part of a systemic inflammatory disease, and by crystal deposition. The most common tendons to become inflamed are those involved in the rotator cuff of the shoulder. These tendons attach the supraspinatus, infraspinatus, and teres minor muscles into the greater tuberosity of the humerus. The patient with rotator cuff tendonitis complains of severe shoulder pain, and point tenderness over the greater tuberosity of the humerus usually is present. Abducting the arm 60 degrees to 120 degrees elicits pain. If the exam-

iner passively abducts the arm of the patient to 90 degrees and the patient cannot hold up the arm (the drop-arm sign), the patient may have a rotator cuff tear. Bicipital tendonitis presents with anterior shoulder pain and the examiner finds tenderness in the bicipital groove. Pain is elicited when the patient with a flexed elbow forcefully turns the palmar aspect of the hand upward (supination) against resistance (Yergason's sign). de Quervain's tenosynovitis is an inflammation of the abductor pollicis longus and the extensor pollicis brevis tendons as they traverse a thick fibrous sheath at the radial-styloid process. The patient notes pain on movement of the thumb or wrist with tenderness over the ulnar styloid. Characteristic of de Quervain's tenosynovitis is the Finkelstein sign – the patient folds the thumb into the palm and the fingers surround the thumb. Then the examiner grasps the folded hand and rotates the wrist ulnarly. This stretches the involved tendons eliciting pain.

The therapeutic approach is similar for all forms of tendonitis. The area is rested, the patient is given NSAIDs, and steroid injections can be administered into the tendon sheath. The patient is then given range-of-motion exercises to maintain mobility. If the above approach is unsuccessful, surgical intervention may be indicated for some forms of chronic tendonitis to relieve mechanical pressure.

Antiarthritic Therapy in the Elderly

All medications used to treat various forms of arthritis have side effects, and elderly patients are particularly susceptible to certain drug toxicities (90). NSAIDs are extensively used to treat a wide variety of symptoms. They are potent analgesic agents, have anti-inflammatory effects, inhibit platelet aggregation, and decrease fever. The elderly are particularly sensitive to NSAIDs (91). One of the major actions of NSAIDs is to inhibit production of prostaglandin. However, prostaglandins are generally made by a variety of cells and their therapeutic effect is to act locally to maintain homeostasis. Prostaglandins are involved in maintaining renal blood flow and sodium excretion by the kidneys, cytoprotection of the stomach mucosa, and dilatation of blood vessels. Prostaglandin E_1 is involved in the production of mucous, bicarbonate and in controlling blood flow to the stomach. NSAIDs can inhibit local prostaglandin production and lead to breakdown of the gastric mucosal barrier. The elderly are more likely to develop NSAID-induced gastric ulcers and major gastrointestinal bleeds than is a younger population. A synthetic prostaglandin E_1, misoprostol, can be administered with the NSAID to prevent the development of gastric ulcers. The main side effect of misoprostol is diarrhea.

In patients with compromised renal function, NSAIDs can cause a rise in creatinine or increased retention of sodium and precipitate congestive heart failure. All NSAIDs have the potential to cause hepatotoxicity, especially the indole derivatives such as indomethacin and sulindac. Diarrhea has been induced by some NSAIDs, most notably meclofenamate. Elderly patients may develop salicylate toxicity at lower drug doses than younger patients [92]. CNS side effects caused by salicylates are common in the elderly, particularly tinnitus, decreased hearing, or a depressed sensorium. The pharmacokinetics of NSAIDs are altered in elderly patients with decreased binding to serum proteins, decreased renal clearance, and altered distribution volumes [93]. Because many elderly patients take multiple drugs, NSAIDs are commonly involved in multiple drug interactions. NSAIDs may perturb warfarin, beta blockers, ACE inhibitors, diuretics, lithium, phenytoin, and digoxin. Thus, NSAIDs should be instituted judiciously in elderly patients and maintained at the lowest effective dose with careful monitoring.

Other antiarthritic medications also should be used cautiously in elderly patients. Disease-modifying drugs for RA can be used in older patients, but serious hematologic and renal toxicity from gold may occur, rashes and taste disturbance from penicillamine are more common, and retinal toxicity from hydroxychloroquine may be more prevalent [90]. Methotrexate is excreted renally. If an elderly patient has subtle renal compromise, methotrexate may remain in the blood at higher levels for a longer period of time and lead to additional bone marrow toxicity. Low serum albumin concentrations in elderly patients increase the risk of side effects from the therapeutic use of corticosteroids.

References

1. Barney JL, Neukom JE. Use of arthritis care by the elderly. Gerontologist 1979;19:548–554.

2. National Center for Health Statistics. Current estimates from the National Health Interview Survey: United States, 1986. Vital Health Statistics Series 1987;10:164.

3. Pincus T, Callahan F. Taking mortality in rheumatoid arthritis seriously – predictive markers, socioeconomic status and co-morbidity. J Rheumatol 1986;13:841–845. Editorial.

4. Lawrence RC, Hochberg MC, Kelsey JL, et al. Estimates of the prevalence of selected arthritis and musculoskeletal disease in the United States. J Rheumatol 1989;16:427–441.

5. Lee P, Rooney PJ, Sturrock RD, et al. The etiology and pathogenesis of osteoarthritis: a review. Semin Arthritis Rheum 1974;3:189–218.

6. Panush RS, Brown DG. Exercise and arthritis. Sports Med 1987;4:54–64.

7. Puranen J, Ala-Kebla L, Peltokallio P, Saarela J. Running and primary osteoarthritis of the hip. BMJ 1975;2:424–425.

8. Lane NE, Bloch DA, Wood PD, Fries JF. Aging, long-distance running, and the development of musculoskeletal disability. A controlled study. Am J Med 1987;82:772–780.

9. Felson DT, Anderson JJ, Naimark A, et al. Obesity and knee osteoarthritis. The Framingham study. Ann Intern Med 1988;109:18–24.

10. Felson DT, Zhang Y, Anthony JM, et al. Weight loss reduces the risk for symptomatic knee osteoarthritis in women: The Framingham study. Ann Intern Med 1992;116:535–539.

11. Kellgren JH, Moore R. Generalized osteoarthritis and Heberden's nodes. BMJ 1952;1:181–184.

12. Knowlton RG, Kalzenstein PL, Moskowitz RW, et al. Genetic linkage of a polymorphism in the type II procollagen gene (COL SA1) to primary osteoarthritis associated with mild chondrodysplasia. N Engl J Med 1990;322:526–530.

13. Eyre DR, Weis MA, Moskowitz RW. Cartilage expression of a type II collagen mutation in an inherited form of osteoarthritis associated with a mild chondrodysplasia. J Clin Invest 1991;87:357–361.

14. Moskowitz RW, Pun Y, Haggi TM. Genetics and osteoarthritis. Bull Rheum Dis 1992;41:4–6.

15. Rene J, Weinberger M, Mazzuca SA, et al. Reduction of joint pain in patients with knee osteoarthritis who have received monthly telephone calls from lay personnel and whose medical treatment regimens have remained stable. Arthritis Rheum 1992;35:511–515.

16. Bunning RD, Materson RS. A rational program of exercise for patients with osteoarthritis. Semin Arthritis Rheum 1989;21:33–43.

17. Kovar PA, Allegrante JP, MacKenzie R, et al. Supervised fitness walking in patients with osteoarthritis of the knee. A randomized controlled trial. Ann Intern Med 1992;116:529–534.

18. Gerber LH. Exercise and arthritis. Bull Rheum Dis 1990;39:1–9.

19. Minor MA, Hewell JE, Webel PR, et al. Efficacy of physical conditioning exercise in patients with rheumatoid arthritis and osteoarthritis. Arthritis Rheum 1989;32:1396–1405.

20. Bradley JD, Brandt KD, Katz BP, et al. Comparison of an anti-

inflammatory does of ibuprofen and acetaminophen in the treatment of patients with osteoarthritis of the knee. N Engl J Med 1991;325:87–91.

21. Deal CL, Schnitzer TJ, Lipstein E, et al. Treatment of arthritis with topical capsaicin: a double-blind trial. Clin Therapeutics 1991;13:363–395.

22. McCarthy GM, McCarty DJ. Effect of topical capsaicin in the therapy of painful osteoarthritis of the hands. J Rheumatol 1992;19:604–607.

23. Williams JM, Brandt KD. Triamcinolone hexacetonide protects against fibrillation and osteophyte formation following chemically induced articular cartilage damage. Arthritis Rheum 1985;28:1267–1274.

24. Ike RW, Arnold WJ, Rothschild EW, et al. Tidal irrigation versus conservative medical management in patients with osteoarthritis of the knee: a prospective randomized study. J Rheumatol 1992;19:772–779.

25. McCarty DJ. Calcium pyrophosphate dihydrate crystal deposition disease–1975. Arthritis Rheum 1976;19:275–285.

26. Doherty M, Dieppe PA. Clinical aspects of calcium pyrophosphate dihydrate crystal deposition. Rheum Dis Clin North Am 1988;14:395–414.

27. Dieppe PA, Jones HE, Scott DG, et al. Pyrophosphate arthropathy: a clinical and radiological study of 105 cases. Arthritis Rheum 1983;26:191–200.

28. McCarty DJ. Calcium pyrophosphate dihydrate crystal deposition disease (pseudogout syndrome)–clinical aspects. Clin Rheum Dis 1977;3:61–89.

29. Shmerling RH, Delbanco TL. The rheumatoid factor: an analysis of clinical utility. Am J Med 1991;91:528–534.

30. Brooks PM, Kean WF, Kassam Y, Buchanan WW. Problems of antiarthritis therapy in the elderly. J Am Geriatr Soc 1984;32:229–234.

31. McCarty DJ, Halverson PB, Carrera GF, et al. "Milwaukee shoulder"–association of microsplenoids containing hydroxyapatite crystals, active collagenase, and neutral protease with rotator cuff defects. I. Clinical aspects. Arthritis Rheum 1981;24:464–473.

32. Halverson PB, Cheung HS, McCarty DJ, et al. "Milwaukee shoulder"–association of microsplenoids containing hydroxyapatite crystals, active collagenase, and neutral protease with rotator cuff defects. II. Synovial fluid studies. Arthritis Rheum 1981;24:474–483.

33. Halverson PB, McCary DJ, Cheung HS, Ryan LM. Milwaukee shoulder syndrome: eleven additional cases with involvement of the knee in seven (basic calcium phosphate crystal deposition disease). Semin Arthritis Rheum 1984;14:36–44.

34. Toseland P. Beer drinking and gout. Br J Rheumatol 1984;23:203–209.

35. Borg EJT, Rasker JJ. Gout in the elderly, a separate entity? Ann Rheum Dis 1987;46:72–76.

36. Campbell SM. Gout: how presentation, diagnosis, and treatment differ in the elderly. Geriatrics 1988;43:17–77.

37. Healey LA. Rheumatoid arthritis in the elderly. Clin Rheum Dis 1986;12:173–179.

38. Terkeltaub R, Esdaile J, Décary F, Tannenbaum H. A clinical study of older age rheumatoid arthritis with comparison to a younger onset group. J Rheumatol 1983;10:418–424.

39. Inoue K, Shichikawa K, Nishioka J, Hirota S. Older age onset rheumatoid arthritis with or without osteoarthritis. Ann Rheum Dis 1987;46:908–911.

40. Deal CL, Meenan RF, Goldenberg DL, et al. The clinical features of elderly-onset rheumatoid arthritis. Arthritis Rheum 1985;28:987–994.

41. Caldwell JR, Furst DE. The efficacy and safety of low-dose corticosteroids for rheumatoid arthritis. Semin Arthritis Rheum 1991;21:1–11.

42. Hunder GG, Allen GL. Giant cell arteritis: a review. Bull Rheum Dis 1979;29:980–986.

43. Chuang TY, Hunder GG, Ilstrup DM, Kurland LT. Polymyalgia rheumatica. A 10-year epidemiologic and clinical study. Ann Intern Med 1982;97:672–680.

44. Jones JG, Hazelman BL. Prognosis and management of polymyalgia rheumatica/giant cell arteritis syndrome. Ann Rheum Dis 1983;42:168–170.

45. O'Duffy JD, Wahnmer HW, Hunder GG. Joint imaging in polymyalgia rheumatica. Mayo Clin Proc 1976;51:519–524.

46. Kyle V, Tudor J, Wraight EP, et al. Rarity of synovitis in polymyalgia rheumatica. Ann Rheum Dis 1990;49:155–157.

47. Calamia KT, Hunder GG. Giant cell arteritis (temporal arteritis) presenting as fever of undetermined origin. Arthritis Rheum 1981;24:1414–1418.

48. Petersdorf RG, Beeson PB. Fever of unexplained origin: report of 100 cases. Medicine 1961;40:1–30.

49. Ellis ME, Ralston S. The ESR in the diagnosis and management of the polymyalgia rheumatica/giant cell arteritis syndrome. Ann Rheum Dis 1983;42:168–170.

50. Huston KA, Hunder GG, Lie JT, et al. Temporal arteritis. A 25-year epidemiologic, clinical, and pathologic study. Ann Intern Med 1978;88:162–167.

51. Healey LA, Wilske KR. Polymyalgia rheumatica and giant cell arteritis. West J Med 1984;141:64–67.

52. Nordborg E, Bengtsson BA, Nordborg C. Temporal artery morphology and morphometry in giant cell arteritis. Acta Pathol Microbiol Immunol Scand 1991;99:1013–1023.

53. McCarty DJ, O'Duffy D, Pearson L, Hunter JB. Remitting seronegative symmetrical synovitis with pitting edema. RS₃PE syndrome. JAMA 1985;254:2763–2767.

54. Chaouat D, LeParc JM. The syndrome of seronegative symmetrical synovitis with pitting edema: a unique form of arthritis in the elderly? Report of 4 additional cases. J Rheumatol 1989;16:1211–1213.

55. Russel EB, Hunter JB, Pearson L, McCarty DJ. Remitting, seronegative, symmetrical synovitis with pitting edema–13 additional cases. J Rheumatol 1990;17:633–639.

56. Tan EM, Cohen AS, Fries JF, et al. The 1982 revised criteria for the classification of systemic lupus erythematosus. Arthritis Rheum 1982;25:1271–1277.

57. Hochberg MC, Boyd RE, Abram JM, et al. Systemic lupus erythematosus: a review of clinico-laboratory features and

immunogenetic markers in 150 patients with emphasis on demographic subsets. Medicine 1985;64:285–295.

58. Baker SB, Rovira JR, Campion EW, Mills JA. Late onset systemic lupus erythematosus. Am J Med 1979;66:727–732.

59. Ward MM, Polisson RP. A meta-analysis of the clinical manifestations of older-onset systemic lupus erythematosus. Arthritis Rheum 1989;32:1226–1232.

60. Wilson HA, Hamilton ME, Spyker DA, et al. Age influences the clinical and serologic expression of systemic lupus erythematosus. Arthritis Rheum 1981;24:1230–1235.

61. Reveille JD, Bartolucci A, Alarcon GS. Prognosis in systemic lupus erythematosus. Negative impact of increasing age at onset, black race, and thrombocytopenia, as well as causes of death. Arthritis Rheum 1990;33:37–48.

62. Solinger AM. Drug-related lupus: clinical and etiological considerations. Clin Rheum Dis 1988;14:187–202.

63. Harmon CE, Portanova JP. Drug-induced lupus: clinical and serological studies. Clin Rheum Dis 1982;8:121–135.

64. Monestier M, Kotzin BL. Antibodies to histones in systemic lupus erythematosus and drug-induced lupus syndromes. Rheumatic Dis Clin North Am 1992;18:415–436.

65. Strickland RW, Tesar JT, Berne BH, et al. The frequency of sicca syndrome in an elderly population. J Rheumatol 1987;14:766–771.

66. Fox RI, Howell FU, Bone RC, Michelson P. Primary Sjögren's syndrome: clinical and immunologic features. Semin Arthritis Rheum 1984;14:77–105.

67. Alexander E. Central nervous system disease in Sjögren's syndrome: new insights into immunopathogenesis. Rheumatic Dis Clin North Am 1992;18:637–672.

68. Binder A, Snaith ML, Isenberg D. Sjögren's syndrome: a study of its neurological complications. Br J Rheumatol 1988;27:275–280.

69. Bohan A, Peter JB. Polymyositis and dermatomyositis (first of two parts): N Engl J Med 1975;292:344–347.

70. Plotz PH, Dalakas M, Leff RL, et al. Current concepts in the idiopathic inflammatory myopathies: polymyositis, dermatomyositis, and related disorders. Ann Intern Med 1987;111:143–156.

71. Hochberg MC, Feldman D, Stevens MB. Adult onset polymyositis/dermatomyositis: an analysis of clinical and laboratory features and survival of 76 patients with a review of the literature. Semin Arthritis Rheum 1984;15:168–178.

72. Barnes BE. Dermatomyositis and malignancy: a review of the literature. Ann Intern Med 1976;84:68–76.

73. Lakhaupaul S, Bunch TW, Ilstrup DM, Melton LJ. Polymyositis-dermatomyositis and malignant lesions: does an association exist? Mayo Clin Proc 1986;61:645–653.

74. Bohan A, Peter JB, Bowman RL, Pearson CM. A computer-assisted analysis of 153 patients with polymyositis and dermatomyositis. Medicine 1977;56:255–286.

75. Benbassat J, Gefel D, Larhott K, et al. Prognostic factors in polymyositis/dermatomyositis: a computer-assisted analy-

sis of ninety-two cases. Arthritis Rheum 1985;28:249–255.

76. Hodkinson HM. Scleroderma in the elderly, with special reference to the CRST syndrome. J Am Geriatr Soc 1971;19:224–228.

77. Steen VD, Medsger TA. Epidemiology and natural history of systemic sclerosis. Rheum Dis Clin North Am 1990;16:1–10.

78. Masi AT. Clinical-epidemiological perspective of systemic sclerosis. In: Jayson MIV, Black CM, eds. Systemic sclerosis: scleroderma. Chichester: John Wiley, 1988:7–31.

79. Newman JH. The differential diagnosis of septic arthritis in the elderly. Compr Ther 1984;10:29–34.

80. Sharp JT, Lidsky MD, Duffy J, Duncan MW. Infectious arthritis. Arch Intern Med 1979;139:1125–1130.

81. Broy SB, Schmid FR. A comparison of medical drainage (needle aspiration) and surgical drainage (arthrotomy or arthroscopy) in the initial treatment of infected joints. Clin Rheum Dis 1986;12:501–522.

82. Goldenberg DL, Red JI. Bacterial arthritis. N Engl J Med 1985;312:764–771.

83. Harris JM. Orthopedic aspects of septic arthritis. In: Espinoza L, Goldenberg D, Arnett F, Alarson G, eds. Infections in the rheumatic diseases. New York: Grune & Stratton, 1988:65–75.

84. Chakravartz K, Webley M. Shoulder joint movement and its relationship to disability in the elderly. J Rheumatol 1993;20:1359–1361.

85. Wolf F. Fibromyalgia: the clinical syndrome. Rheum Dis Clin North Am 1987;15:1–18.

86. Yunus M, Masi AT, Calabro JT, et al. Primary fibromyalgia (fibrositis): clinical study of 50 patients with matched normal controls. Semin Arthritis Rheum 1981;11:151–171.

87. Wolfe E, Smythe HA, Yunus MB, et al. The American College of Rheumatology 1990 criteria for the classification of fibromyalgia: report of the multicenter criteria committee. Arthritis Rheum 1990;33:160–173.

88. Moldofsky H. Sleep-wake mechanisms in fibrositis. J Rheumatol 1989;16:47–48.

89. Goldenberg DL, Felson DT, Dinerman H. A randomized, controlled trial of amitriptyline and naproxen in the treatment of patients with fibromyalgia. Arthritis Rheum 1986;29:1371–1377.

90. Brooks PM, Kean WF, Kassom Y, Buchanan WW. Problems of anti-arthritic therapy in the elderly. J Am Geriatr Soc 1984;32:229–234.

91. Morgan J, Furst DE. Implications of drug therapy in the elderly. Clin Rheum Dis 1986;12:227–244.

92. Grigor RR, Spitz PW, Furst DE. Salicylate toxicity in elderly patients whth rheumatoid arthritis. J Rheumatol 1987;14:60–66.

93. Woodhouse KW, Wynne H. The pharmacokinetics of nonsteroidal anti-inflammatory drugs in the elderly. Clin Pharmacokinet 1987;12:111-122.

Chapter 42
Alzheimer's Disease and Other Dementias

David S. Geldmacher and Peter J. Whitehouse

Bodily decay is gloomy in prospect, but of all human contemplation the most abhorrent is body without mind.

Thomas Jefferson

Dementia will continue to grow in importance in geriatric medicine because of its overwhelming impact on patients and families, as well as society. Although cognitive decline in advanced age has been recognized throughout history, the understanding that it represents the result of specific disease states is more recent.

Dementia is an acquired loss of cognitive and intellectual functions severe enough to interfere with function at work or home, or in interpersonal interactions. It should be differentiated from the changes in cognition typical of healthy aging (*aging-associated cognitive decline*). Memory dysfunction is the typical early cognitive impairment. The term dementia, itself, is therefore a clinical description, not a pathologic diagnosis. It does not imply cause or progression because more than 55 illnesses that can lead to the diagnosis of dementia have been identified (1). These illnesses are collectively referred to as "dementing illnesses." Dementia has thus moved from being described as "senility," which implies that it is an obligate age-related state, to an illness state caused by many pathologic conditions. An important step in the growing understanding of dementia as an illness state was provided by Blessed et al (2) who reported that dementia severity was related to the amount of brain involved by specific pathologic changes.

The overall prevalence of dementia in the United States has been reported to be as high as 15 percent (3) and as much as 50 percent or higher for persons older than age 80 (4). One useful model for understanding the prevalence of dementia is to assume a doubling every 5 years beginning with 1 percent for persons age 60, doubling to 2 percent for those age 65, 4 percent for those age 70, 8 percent for

those age 75, 16 percent for those age 80, and 32 percent for persons age 85 (5). Incidence rates also increase with age. One estimate of overall estimates drawn from several populations around the world is 187.5 new cases per 100,000 population per year (6). When incidence is broken into age groups, dramatic increases occur among the older segments of the population. From 19.2 new cases per 100,000 population per year for the age group below 60 years, incidence increases to 130.0 for ages 60 to 69 years, to 740.8 for ages 70 to 79 years, and to 2175.1 for ages older than 80 years. The largest proportion of dementia results from primary degenerative diseases of the brain, such as Alzheimer's disease (AD). AD, alone or in combination with other illnesses, accounts for about 70 percent of dementia in most industrialized countries. In some circumscribed populations, such as African Americans or the Japanese, vascular dementia may be relatively more common possibly because of the frequency of hypertension in those populations.

Longer life spans and increasing knowledge of the causes of cognitive decline, particularly AD, has led to the prediction of dementia as an epidemic extending into the twenty-first century. The cost of caring for patients with dementia is already immense, over $90 billion annually in the U.S. Nonetheless, a major focus of current research is to slow the progression of dementing illnesses, which, if successfully applied to patients, may further increase the costs and burdens of care.

Alzheimer's Disease

In 1907, the German pathologist Alois Alzheimer reported the case of a 51-year-old woman with progressive cognitive decline and behavior change associated with distinctive neuropathologic features of senile plaques and neurofibrillary tangles. Although the senile plaques had been previously identified, the association of the clinical syndrome to specific pathologic findings was an important breakthrough in the understanding of dementia.

Clinical Features

Cognitive Decline

The primary cognitive feature of AD is usually progressive memory impairment. The memory dysfunction involves impairment of learning new information and is often characterized as short-term memory loss. In the early (mild) and moderate stages of the illness recall of remote well-learned material may appear to be preserved, but new information cannot be adequately incorporated into memory. Detailed evaluations show, however, that deficits in recall of remote events are also subtly present. Closely associated with the breakdown of learning is progressive disorientation in time and place. Finally, in the later stages, frank failure of recall of previously well-remembered information (i.e., names of the patient's own children) is observed.

Language impairments are also a prominent part of dementia of the Alzheimer type (DAT) (7). These are often manifest first as word-finding difficulty in spontaneous speech with compensatory circumlocutions. The language of the patient with AD is often vague, lacking in specifics, and may have increased automatic phrases and cliches. Impairment of object-naming ability, especially for parts of objects, is often prominent and is referred to as *anomia*. Subsequently, impaired comprehension of linguistic information becomes evident. Repetition is often preserved, even in more advanced cases. Communication patterns, or conversational *pragmatics*, become disrupted, and cause problems in the caregiving relationship (8). Progression to global aphasia or muteness (*aphemia*) is not uncommon.

Complex deficits in visual function are present in many patients with AD (9). These include many varieties of agnosia, such as the inability to recognize faces (*prosopagnosia*) and visual-object agnosia. Complex visual disturbances, such as Balint's syndrome may be observed. Deficits in visual attention probably contribute to many of the visual and memory disturbances in AD (10). There is also breakdown of elemental visual processing such as contrast and spatial frequency, perception, motion detection, and figure-ground discrimination, which may influence activities of daily living. Other focal cognitive deficits such as apraxia, acalculia, and left-right disorientation are also often present. Impairments of judgment and problem solving are frequently seen.

Noncognitive Symptoms

Noncognitive or behavioral symptoms are common in AD and may account for an even larger proportion of caregiver burden or stress than cognitive dysfunction. Personality changes are commonly reported (11), ranging from progressive passivity to marked agitation. Patients may exhibit changes such as decreased emotional expression, diminished initiative, and decreased expressions of affection (12). In some cases, personality change may predate cognitive abnormality.

Delusions are common in AD and affect as much as 50 percent of patients. The delusions are often paranoid in character and may lead to accusations of theft, infidelity, and persecution. A particular type of delusion common in AD is the reduplicative paramnesia known as *Capgras phenomenon*, in which patients believe that caregivers or family members are impostors or that their home is not their (real) home. The presence of delusions may be a poor prognostic sign, suggesting a faster rate of disease progression (13).

Hallucinations occur in as much as one-quarter of patients with AD. Hallucinations are typically visual but sometimes have auditory components. Frequent themes include seeing deceased parents or siblings, unknown intruders, and animals (12).

Depressive symptoms are very common and may be difficult to distinguish from an organic amotivational state or *abulia*. Estimates of the presence of depression in dementia range as high as 40 percent (12) with a similar rate for anxiety. Anxiety tends to be more prominent in the earlier phases of the illness and may be based on anticipation of potentially stressful circumstances or an adjustment reaction to the diagnosis of a dementing illness.

Changes in Neurologic Examination

Throughout most of the course, AD spares the patient's elemental neurologic examination. In later stages, extrapyramidal signs such as rigidity may become prominent. There is a significant overlap with Parkinson's disease, with as many as 20 percent to 30 percent of patients with AD demonstrating parkinsonian features including bradykinesia, rigidity, and tremor. Concomitantly, typical Alzheimer pathology can be frequently found in patients with Parkinson's disease and dementia (14). Seizures have been reported to occur in 10 percent to 20 percent of patients with AD, again often late in the disease. Myoclonus, brisk irregular muscle contractions, may occur in 5 percent to 10 percent of patients with AD. Multifocal myoclonus may be difficult to distinguish from seizures in later stage patients and may account for the apparent frequency of seizures.

Diagnostic Criteria

To bring uniformity to the diagnosis of such diverse symptoms, a working group composed of the National Institute of Neurologic and Communicative Disorders and Stroke, and the Alzheimer's Disease and Related Disorders Association (NINCDS-ADRDA), has developed criteria for the research diagnoses of definite, probable, and possible AD (15; Table 42.1). The diagnosis of AD is confirmed at autopsy in approximately 90 percent of individuals with probable AD by these criteria. In brief, the criteria require a 1-year course of decline in two or more areas of cognition such as memory, language, orientation, judgment, and problem solving. Onset should be between ages 40 to 90 and states of altered arousal, such as delirium, must be excluded as a cause. Treatable causes of dementia must also be excluded by structural imaging of the brain and laboratory evaluations to fully meet the criteria. By these criteria, the diagnosis of definite AD can be made only by biopsy or at autopsy with appropriate numbers of plaques and tangles determined from specific regions of the brain, in the presence of a clinical history consistent with dementia. No specific antemortem diagnostic tests for AD have been validated, which makes AD a clinical diagnosis made by exclusion of other causes of dementia.

Clinical Approach

The clinical approach to the patient presenting with memory problems is based on identifying the specific cognitive changes noted in the criteria and supportive laboratory testing. This approach involves careful physical and neurologic examination accompanied by mental status testing to identify the characteristic memory, language, other cognitive, and noncognitive symptoms (1).

The screening also involves laboratory testing with particular emphasis on tests to identify treatable sources of dementia, including thyroid function, vitamin B_{12} levels, and inflammatory or infectious states such as neurosyphilis (Table 42.2). Computed tomography (CT) or magnetic resonance imaging (MRI) are useful to exclude structural lesions that may contribute to dementia, such as cerebral infarctions, neoplasm, extracerebral fluid collections, and hydrocephalus.

Differential Diagnosis

Potentially treatable sources of dementia that may resemble AD include depression, hypothyroidism, vitamin B_{12} deficiency, cerebral vasculitis, neurosyphilis, AIDS and its complications, and strokes. It is fairly unusual that any of these would present with the characteristic pattern of multiple deficits in higher cortical function such as the subtle aphasia, apraxia, acalculia, and agnosias seen in typical AD. Patients with depression typically have psychomotor slowing and produce incomplete answers and poor effort on testing (e.g., "I don't know"), whereas patients with AD often give good effort but incorrect answers. The memory dysfunction in such conditions may, however, be indistinguishable on bedside evaluation.

Course

Average survival of patients diagnosed with AD is about 8 years, but is quite variable (16). Many patients require placement in nursing homes because of increasing dependence for personal care, such as total incontinence. Death most often results from secondary infections and complications of immobility, such as aspiration pneumonia, urosepsis, and decubitus ulcers.

Treatment Approaches

A multidisciplinary approach to care of the dementia patient is ideal. There are important roles for nursing and social work in the ongoing adaptation of patient and family to the disabling illnesses that typically cause dementia. Caregiver support and education are also of great value. Community support and advocacy groups, such as the Alzheimer's Association, can be a vital resource to caregivers. The Alzheimer's Association has many local chapters and offers a nationwide telephone help line (1-800-272-3900).

Table 42.1. NINCDS-ADRDA Criteria for the Diagnosis of Alzheimer's Disease.

I. The criteria for the clinical diagnoses of *probable* Alzheimer's disease include:
   1. Dementia established by clinical examination and documented by the Mini Mental State Test, Blessed Dementia Scale, or some similar examination, and confirmed by neuropsychological tests
   2. Deficit in two or more areas of cognition
   3. Progressive worsening of memory and other cognitive functions
   4. No disturbance of consciousness
   5. Onset between ages 40 and 90, most often after age 65
   6. Absence of systemic disorders or other brain diseases that in and of themselves could account for the progressive deficits in memory and cognition

II. The diagnosis of *probable* Alzheimer's disease is supported by:
   1. Progressive deterioration of specific cognitive functions such as language (aphasia), motor skills, apraxia, and perception (agnosia)
   2. Impaired activities of dally living and altered patterns of behavior.
   3. Family history of similar disorders particularly if confirmed neuropathologically
   4. Laboratory results of:
      a. Normal lumbar puncture as evaluated by standard techniques
      b. Normal pattern or nonspecific changes in EEG, such as increased slow wave activity
      c. Evidence of cerebral atrophy or CT with progression documented by serial observation

III. Other clinical features consistent with the diagnosis of probable Alzheimer's disease, after exclusion of causes of dementia other than Alzheimer's disease, include:
   1. Plateaus in the course of progression of the illness
   2. Associated symptoms of depression, insomnia, incontinence, delusions, illusions, hallucinations, catastrophic verbal, emotional, or physical outbursts, sexual disorders, and weight loss
   3. Other neurologic abnormalities in some patients, especially those with more advanced disease, including motor signs such as increased muscle tone, myoclonus, or gait disorder
   4. Seizures in advanced disease
   5. CT normal for age

IV. Features that make the diagnosis of *probable* Alzheimer's disease uncertain or unlikely include:
   1. Sudden apoplectic onset
   2. Focal neurologic findings such as hemipareses, sensory loss, visual field deficits, and incoordination early in the course of the Illness
   3. Seizures or gait disturbances at the onset or very early in the course of the illness

V. Clinical diagnosis of possible Alzheimer's disease:
   1. May be made on the basis of the dementia syndrome: in the absence of other necrologic, psychiatric, or systemic disorders sufficient to cause dementia; and in the presence of variations in the onset, presentation, or clinical course
   2. May be made in the presence of a second systemic or brain disorder sufficient to produce dementia, which is not considered to be the cause of the dementia
   3. Should be used in research studies when a single, gradually progressive, severe cognitive deficit is identified in the absence of other identifiable cause

VI. Criteria for diagnoses of *definite* Alzheimer's disease are:
   1. The clinical criteria for probable Alzheimer's disease
   2. Histopathologic evidence obtained from a biopsy or autopsy

VII. Classification of Alzheimer's disease for research purposes should specify features that may differentiate subtypes of the disorder, such as:
   1. Familial occurrence
   2. Onset before age 65
   3. Presence of trisomy-21
   4. Coexistence of other relevant conditions such as Parkinson's disease

CT = computed tomography; EEG = electroencephalogram.

SOURCE: Reproduced by permission from McKhann G, Drachman D, Folstein M, et al. Clinical diagnosis of Alzheimer's disease: report of the NINCDS-ADRDA work group under the auspices of the Department of Health and Human Services Task Force on Alzheimer's Disease. Neurology 1984:34:939–944.

Table 42.2. Screening Tests for Treatable Causes of Dementia*.

Test	Condition Evaluated
Complete blood count	Anemia (megaloblastic)
Chemistry panel	Metabolic disorders (i.e. delirium)
Liver function tests	
Thyroid function tests	Hypothyroidism
Vitamin B$_{12}$ test	B$_{12}$ deficiency
VDRL and FTA-ABS	Neurosyphilis
CT or MRI	Structural lesions

*Other tests, e.g., sedimentation rate, electroencephalogram, heavy metal screening, and cerebrospinal fluid examination may also be indicated in some patients, depending on the patient's history.

CT = computed tomography; FTA-ABS = fluorescent treponemal antibody absorption; MRI = magnetic resonance imaging; VDRL = venereal disease research laboratory test.

In 1993, the acetylcholinesterase inhibitor tacrine was approved in the U.S. for use as a cognitive enhancer in the treatment of AD. Tacrine may offer small, clinically observable, benefits to some patients (17). Its use is tempered by high rates (as high as 40%) of both symptomatic, dose-related gastrointestinal side effects such as nausea, vomiting, and diarrhea, and dose-independent hepatic toxicity, which requires frequent monitoring. High doses (e.g., 40 mg four times/day) appear to offer the maximum benefit, but many patients are unable to tolerate this level of cholinesterase inhibition (18,19). Other cholinesterase inhibitors with lower rates of adverse effects are being developed as are cholinergic agents with other means of action, such as direct-receptor agonists.

The noncognitive symptoms are often a greater source of caregiver difficulty than memory loss. Non-pharmacologic management of behavioral symptoms is desirable whenever possible. Increased socialization, through day-care programs and improved sleep hygiene, may minimize the need for pharmacologic intervention. When drugs are required for behavioral difficulties, conventional psychotropic agents such as neuroleptics, antidepressants, and anxiolytics are most often used, typically at doses lower than required for primary psychiatric indications. Low-dose neuroleptics are used by most clinicians to treat agitated symptoms. Antidepressants can have a beneficial effect on social withdrawal, depressed mood, and sleep disturbances. Benzodiazapine anxiolytics are often problematic in that they may cause increased cognitive impairments and paradoxical agitation. The atypical antidepressant trazodone has also been suggested as useful as a sedative treatment for agitation.

Neuropathology

On gross examination, the brain of a patient with AD often appears atrophic with enlarged ventricles and sulci. Overall brain weight is invariably reduced, but there is still significant overlap with the normal range. The distinguishing pathologic features of AD are *senile plaques* and *neurofibrillary tangles* (NFT) (Figure 42.1). These changes occur with normal aging but are seen at much higher densities in the brains of patients with AD. The contribution of these pathologic structures to the cause of cognitive decline is unclear because they may represent the result of another pathophysiologic process rather than being directly causally related. Neuronal and synaptic loss are a primary cause of intellectual and behavioral changes, regardless of the mechanism of cell death. Other pathologic findings include Hirano bodies, granulovacuolar degeneration, and intracerebral and intravascular deposition of amyloid protein. Senile or neuritic plaques are composed of glia, neuronal processes, and extracellular amyloid. They range in diameter from 15 μm to 100 μm and are distributed throughout the cortex and limbic nuclei such as the

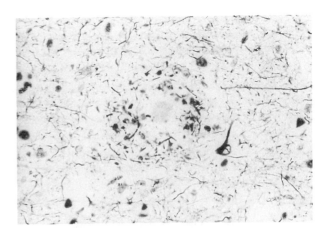

Fig. 42.1. Senile plaque (center) and neurofibrillary tangle (NFT) (right). The plaque consists of an amyloid core surrounded by dystrophic neural processes (neurites). The NFT is intracytoplasmic and consists of aberrantly arranged neurofilaments.

amygdala and hippocampus. Synaptic density, neuronal loss, and NFTs have also been found to correlate with declining mental ability.

Neurofibrillary tangles are collections of neurofilaments that have a distinctive, paired-helical, filamentous structure in AD. Other illnesses, such as progressive supranuclear palsy and dementia pugilistica, are also characterized by the presence of NFTs, but not all have the paired-helical structure. However, NFTs also appear in the brain as a result of healthy aging and may represent a nonspecific neuronal response. The protein components of NFTs have been identified as *tau* (a microtubular-associated protein) and *ubiquitin*. NFTs are also found throughout the neocortex and limbic nuclei and in the basal forebrain, locus ceruleus, substantia nigra, and raphe nuclei.

Widespread, cortical, neuronal loss is more obvious in younger patients. The deep layers of the temporal cortex appear most affected among cortical structures and the hippocampus is prominently involved. Neuronal loss also occurs in the cholinergic cells of the basal forebrain, the monoaminergic cells of the locus ceruleus (norepinephrine), and the raphe nuclei (serotonin). Neurotransmitter deficiencies as a result of cell death in these regions are important because they represent the target of symptomatic therapies for both cognitive and behavioral symptoms. The substantia nigra can also be affected, which may account for signs and symptoms of parkinsonism commonly observed late in the illness (20).

There are other nonspecific pathologic features found in AD. The pyramidal area of the hippocampus seems to be particularly prone to the development of *granulovacuolar degeneration*, which appears as clear zones 5 μm in diameter with an argyrophilic core. Hirano bodies are eosinophilic cellular inclusions that are also in the hippocampal pyramidal layer.

Neurotransmitters

Much attention has been paid to the neurotransmitter changes associated with AD, particularly changes in acetylcholine. Levels of cerebral cortical markers for acetylcholine metabolism, such as the synthetic enzyme choline acetyltransferase (CAT) and the degradative enzyme acetylcholinesterase (AChE), correlate with dementia severity. The degree of cholinergic reductions in cortex are closely associated with cellular loss in the basal forebrain nuclei that synthesize this neurotransmitter. Acetylcholine has been demonstrated to be important in memory and attentional function. There is a significant reduction in nicotinic cholinergic receptors in the cortex, but muscarinic receptors are more variably affected. DAT is not, however, the simple result of cholinergic deficits. Other ascending pathways, such as those for norepinepherine and serotonin, are also affected. Intrinsic classical neurotransmitters, such as gamma-amino butyric acid (GABA), are diminished, as are many cortically localized neuropeptides including corticotropin-releasing factor and, perhaps, somatostatin. Single-transmitter augmentation or replacement (such as dopaminergic therapy for Parkinson's disease) is therefore unlikely to be dramatically successful in AD.

Neurobiology

Although clear etiopathologic mechanisms for premature cell death in AD have not been established, the major clues come from genetics. Several kindreds of autosomal-dominant, familial AD have been identified. There are known linkages to chromosomes 21, 19, and 14. A genetic component has also been suggested in other, less obviously autosomal-dominant AD by Breitner and associates (21) who reported that the cumulative incidence of the illness among first-degree relatives of patients with AD approaches 50 percent in those surviving to age 87. Individuals with an affected first-degree relative have a four-fold increase in their age-adjusted risk for developing AD. Rates as high as 40 times normal have been suggested for individuals with two or more first-degree relatives with dementia (22). Thus far, twin studies have added little to clarify genetic risks. AD probably represents a final common pathway for several genetic abnormalities.

A peptide known as *beta amyloid protein*, *A4*, is deposited as a beta pleated sheet in the senile plaques of AD and in cerebral blood vessels. This is a hydrophobic portion of the senile plaques, and deposits are also found in normal aged brains. This peptide is a transmembrane portion of a larger, chromosome 21-encoded glycoprotein known as amyloid precursor protein. Proteolysis of the precursor protein is believed to be the source of the deposited amyloid, but what leads to pathologic accumulation in AD is unknown.

In 1993, the E4 allele of apolipoprotein E, a chromosome 19 gene, was reported to be linked with an increased risk for development of late-onset familial and sporadic AD (23,24). Preliminary reports suggest that the E4 allele is associated with abnormal phosphorylation and defective intracellular binding of tau proteins to microtubular structure. Evidence to date suggests that E4 is a marker for genetic susceptibility but has not established a causative role. Furthermore, the apparent greater risk associated with carriage of the E4 allele may represent a protective effect of the more common E2 and E3 alleles.

Pick's Disease

Pick's disease is another primary degenerative dementia seen in the elderly. It is much less common than AD, and occurs from 1 percent to 5 percent as often (25). Pick's disease was first described clinically by Arnold Pick in 1892. The histopathologic hallmark of the disease, the so-called Pick body, was reported by Alzheimer in 1911. More recently, the symptom complex attributed to Pick's disease has been recognized as not obligately associated with specific pathologic features. The term *dementia of the frontal lobe type* (DFT) has been offered as an alternative name for this clinical syndrome.

Clinical Features

Pick's original case had prominent aphasia, but current understanding suggests that changes in personality and behavioral regulation may predate language changes. Apathy is common, but some patients develop episodic disinhibition and socially inappropriate behaviors. Disorders of behavioral regulation, known as dysexecutive states, predominate in DFT. Initiation, goal setting, and planning are affected, are closely allied to attentional disorders, and can lead to disorientation in time, out of proportion to spatial disorientation (26). Language impairment is often characterized by abundant unfocused speech (*logorrhea*), echo-like spontaneous repetition (*echolalia*), and compulsively uttered repetitive phrases (*palilalia*), although anomia and dysfluency may evolve (27). Later in the course of the illness, muscle rigidity may be observed. The typical survival time is about 5 to 10 years (27).

Pathologic Features

There is a preponderance of atrophy in patients' frontal and anterior temporal lobes. The extreme atrophy results in a characteristic pattern of "knife-edged" gyri (Figure 42.2), generally sparing parietal and occipital cortices. Light microscopy reveals cortical neuronal loss and neuronal swellings (Figure 42.3). The classical Pick bodies can be seen on silver stains. On electron microscopy, Pick bodies are random accumulations of straight filaments 15 nm in diameter. They share antigenic characteristics with neurofibrillary tangles seen in AD, such as

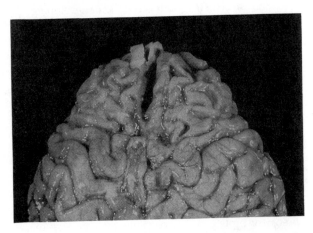

Fig. 42.2. Prominent frontal lobe atrophy demonstrating "knife edge" gyri in Pick's disease.

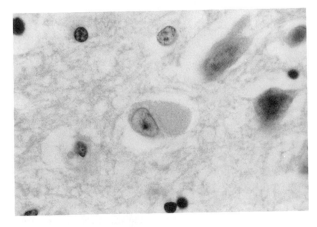

Fig. 42.3. Swollen or "ballooned" neuron with eccentrically displaced nucleus in Pick's disease.

immunocytochemical staining for ubiquitin and tau, but frequently lack the paired-helical configuration characteristic of AD.

Vascular Dementia

Cerebrovascular disease is a leading contributor to dementia worldwide. In most populations, only AD is a more common cause of dementia (28). In 1974, Hachinski et al popularized the phrase *multi-infarct dementia* (MID) to refer to the syndrome of dementia accompanied by focal neurologic signs or symptoms, characterized by stepwise deterioration, and frequently associated with hypertension (29). Recently, *vascular dementia* has emerged as a diagnostic category that includes not only the multiple discrete infarcts of MID, but other dementing syndromes attributed to cerebrovascular origins. Among these is dementia associated with diffuse, subcortical, white matter disease putatively attributed to chronic subcortical ischemia. This state is commonly, but controversially, known as *Binswanger's disease* or *subcortical arteriosclerotic encephalopathy*. Although there have been efforts to develop criteria for the diagnosis of vascular dementia (30,31), these remain controversial and no standard, such as the NINCDS-ADRDA criteria for AD, has arisen.

Given the high prevalence of cerebrovascular disease, strokes frequently contribute to the cognitive morbidity of individuals with dementia of all types, including AD. Although antemortem clinical evaluations and imaging may confirm the presence of multiple strokes, those techniques cannot exclude AD as a contributor to the overall condition. Consequently, the frequency of purely vascular changes in autopsy series of demented patients is 10 percent to 23 percent, comparable to that of "mixed dementia" with changes of both MID and AD (32).

Clinical Features

In about 90 percent of pathologically verified cases of MID, a history exists of acute unilateral motor or sensory dysfunction consistent with stroke (33). A history of acute impairment of cortical functions manifest as aphasia, apraxia, or agnosia may also exist. Urinary dysfunction and gait disturbance have been suggested as early mark-

ers for the development of MID (34). With accumulation of ischemic brain lesions, there is, typically, incremental impairment of memory and behavioral initiation, along with extrapyramidal features such as facial masking and rigidity. (More detailed discussion of the clinical and pathophysiologic features of cerebrovascular disease can be found in Chapter 38.)

An ischemic score (IS) was proposed by Hachinski and colleagues (35) as a means of distinguishing MID from primary degenerative dementia. A number of variants have been employed since the introduction of the original IS; a typical example is shown in Table 42.3. These scales are sensitive, but not specific, indicators of MID and do not address the presence or absence of AD pathology (28). In the clinical setting, an IS is most useful as an instrument for suggesting the presence of cerebrovascular contributors to a dementia syndrome. Imaging studies have an important role in the diagnosis of MID. In contrast to the diagnosis of AD, in which cerebral images are used to rule out structural changes contributing to the dementia, the CT or MRI scans in MID can clearly identify significant pathology. Interpretation of CT or MR imaging can be problematic because of their sensitivity to potentially age-related changes in the brain known as periventricular white matter hypodensities on CT. Hachinski and col-

Table 42.3. Hachinski Ischemia Score*.

Symptom-History	Score
Abrupt onset	2
Stepwise progression	1
Fluctuating course	2
Nocturnal confusion	1
Relative preservation of personality	1
Depression	1
Somatic complaints	1
Emotional incontinence	1
History of hypertension	1
History of strokes	2
History of associated atherosclerosis	1
Focal neurologic symptoms	2
Focal neurologic signs	2

* Scores of 5 or higher suggest that vascular disease may contribute to the dementia.

SOURCE: Reproduced by permission from Hachinski VC, Iliff LD, Zilhka E, et al. Cerebral blood flow in dementia. Arch Neurol 1975;32:632–637.

leagues introduced the term *leukoaraiosis* (literally, rarefaction of the white matter) to describe these changes, which are not obligately associated with cognitive decline (36). Nonetheless, in one neuropathologically verified series, 74 percent of patients with MID had cortical infarcts and 13 percent had deep infarcts on CT (33).

That treatment of vascular risk factors such as hypertension and smoking have been reported to improve cognition in patients with MID; similar treatments did not affect the cognition of AD patients in the same paradigm (37). With control of the risk factors, progression of the illness and, perhaps, current function are likely to be affected.

Degenerative Dementias with Prominent Motor Signs

Huntington's Disease

Huntington's disease (HD) is an autosomal, dominantly inherited, neurologic illness with clinical characteristics of dementia and abnormal movements. The dementia typically has prominent psychiatric characteristics including delusions, depression, and mania. Cognitive symptoms include problems with attention and concentration, memory, and executive function. Aphasic characteristics are uncommon, although dysarthria may result from the motor disabilities.

The classic motor characteristic of HD is chorea, more properly, choreoathetosis. This consists of involuntary twitching movements of the distal extremities (chorea) which progress to more writhing (athetoid) movements proximally. Onset is typically in the patient's fourth decade, although some cases have later onset and long duration of illness. Few new cases appear in persons older than age 70. The prevalence is about five per 100,000 in whites of European origin and lower among those of African or Asian ancestry. The genetic defect localizes to the short arm of chromosome 4, and reliable genetic testing is available; the ethical implications for presymptomatic diagnosis of this illness are complex.

Marked atrophy of the caudate nuclei, visible on cerebral imaging, is the characteristic gross pathological feature. There is extensive cell loss throughout the basal ganglia, but the cerebral cortex is relatively spared, at least until late in the illness. The characteristic neuro-

chemical change is a decrease in the major intrinsic inhibitory neurotransmitter of the basal ganglia, GABA. Neuronal excitotoxicity, mediated through glutamate neurotransmission has been suggested as the underlying cause for neuronal death in HD.

Parkinson's Disease

Although James Parkinson initially reported that intellect was spared during the course of "Paralysis agitans," cognitive changes can be detected in many patients. As discussed in Chapter 39, motor manifestations are the hallmark of the illness, but by age 85, more than 65 percent of patients with Parkinson's disease (PD) in one study had developed dementia (38). Older patients and those with a family history of dementia appear to have higher risk for the development of dementia with PD.

Visuospatial dysfunction is common and executive function abnormalities, similar to those reported for frontal lobe patients, have been identified. These cognitive changes occur even in testing paradigms that control for motor disability. Psychiatric changes also occur, particularly depression, which can occur in as much as 90 percent of patients with PD. Delusions and hallucinations also occur, and are often related to treatment with dopaminergic agents.

Progressive Supranuclear Palsy

Progressive supranuclear palsy (PSP) probably represents the second most common form of idiopathic parkinsonism (39) and was first described as a syndrome by Steele et al in 1964 (40). The initial symptoms most frequently appear in persons older than age 55 and include rigidity, particularly of the axial musculature, and gait dysfunction. Neuro-ophthalmologic features, typically beginning with impairment in downward gaze, are prominent. Along with ophthalmoparesis and parkinsonism, dementia has been considered a prototypical part of the syndrome. It now appears that dementia, although occurring in 60 percent to 80 percent of affected individuals, is not an obligate part of the syndrome (41). The dementia is usually characterized by bradyphrenia, dysexecutive states, and apathy or depression.

Other Degenerative Dementias

Other rare degenerative dementias can be identified by

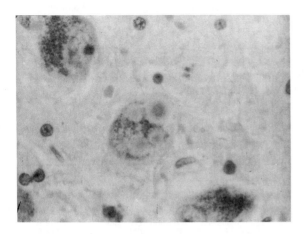

Fig. 42.4. Intraneuronal Lewy bodies, with eosinophilic core and clear halo.

Table 42.4. Major Clinical Characteristics of Dementia Syndromes.

Disease	Clinical Features
Alzheimer's disease	Amnesia, aphasia, agnosia, apraxia, personality and behavior changes
Pick's disease	Apathy or disinhibition, executive function impairment, speech/language abnormalities
Vascular dementia	Sensory/motor dysfunction on neurologic examination, gait disturbance, memory disturbance
Huntington's disease	Choreoathetosis, psychotic features, depression, impairments in memory, attention, and executive function
Parkinson's disease	Parkinsonism, bradyphrenia, executive function impairments, visuospatial dysfunction
Progressive supranuclear palsy	Parkinsonism, ophthalmoplegia, bradyphrenia
Lewy body disease	Parkinsonism, delusions, hallucinations
Corticobasal ganglionic degeneration	Parkinsonism, apraxia, "alien-hand" syndrome
Progressive subcortical gliosis	Personality change, innappropriate behaviors
Creutzfeld-Jakob disease	Myoclonus, irritability, visual disorders, rapid course

specific clinical or pathologic features. *Lewy body disease* is associated with Lewy bodies, identical to those found in Parkinson's disease (Figure 42.4), distributed throughout the cortex and subcortical nuclei. Behavioral changes, such as delusions and hallucinations, may be prominent early in the course and need not be associated with parkinsonian clinical features (42). *Corticobasal ganglionic degeneration*, another progressive dementia syndrome, has been increasingly recognized and is characterized by apraxia and prominent extrapyramidal signs (43). Some cases of *amyotrophic lateral sclerosis* (Lou Gehrig's disease) are also associated with dementia. *Progressive subcortical gliosis* is an unusual form of dementia with prominent personality change and inappropriate behaviors. Pathologic examination demonstrates extensive subcortical gliosis with relative sparing of the cortical ribbon (44). Some cases of progressive dementia lack any distinctive histopathology (45) and may be called "simple atrophy." Important clinical characteristics of these syndromes are presented in Table 42.4.

Creutzfeldt-Jakob Disease

Creutzfeldt-Jakob disease (CJD) is a rapidly progressive dementia, typically accompanied by myoclonus, although this cardinal feature may be absent early in the course. Other motor signs, such as parkinsonism, may also be prominent. The *Heidenhain variant* is characterized

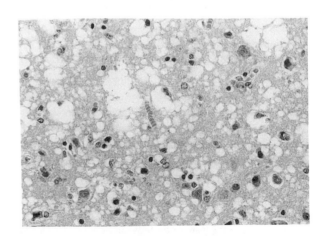

Fig. 42.5. Spongiform cerebral cortex degeneration in Creutzfeld-Jakob disease.

by early involvement and rapid decline of visual function. Onset is usually in patients in their sixth or seventh decade, with typical disease duration of 1 to 2 years. The onset can be difficult to determine because vague symptoms of irritability and unusual somatic sensations are common. These progress to more clear-cut disorders of memory and cognition and also to personality change in some cases. The patient's neurologic examination is characterized by myoclonus, but this may be absent in as much as one-fifth of cases. Electroencephalographic (EEG) changes of slowing and periodic complexes are essentially diagnostic when observed, but they are not obligate in the early stages of the illness. Pathologic changes include a spongiform degeneration of the cortex, which includes intraneuronal vacuoles as its distinctive feature (Figure 42.5).

Creutzfeldt-Jakob disease is a transmissible illness closely related to several animal diseases, such as scrapie. Although the illnesses are characterized by a distinctive infectious particle that has been called the *prion*, this agent is resistant to typical measures that inactivate nucleic acids, such as formaldehyde, heat, and radiation. The illness is not contagious in the conventional sense, but transmission has been reported in association with corneal transplant, intracranial electrodes, and cadaveric material. There is also a hereditary prion disease known as *Gerstmann-Straussler syndrome* with earlier onset and autosomal dominant transmission.

Acknowledgement. Supported by NIA Alzheimer's Disease Research Center Grant AG08012. The authors gratefully acknowledge Mark Cohen, MD, for providing the photomicrographs illustrating the chapter, and Ruth Archer for assistance in preparing the manuscript.

References

1. Mayeux R, Foster NL, Rossor M, Whitehouse PJ. The clinical evaluation of patients with dementia. In: Whitehouse PJ, ed. Dementia. 3rd ed. Philadelphia: Davis, 1993.
2. Blessed G, Tomlinson BE, Roth M. The association between quantitative measures of dementia and of senile change in the cerebral gray matter of elderly subjects. Br J Psychiatry 1968;114:797–811.
3. Jorm AF, Korten AE, Henderson AS. The prevalence of dementia: a quantitative integration of the literature. Acta Psychiatr Scand 1987;76:465–479.
4. Evans DA, Funkenstein HH, Albert MS, et al. Prevalence of Alzheimer's disease in a community population of older persons. Higher than previously reported. JAMA 1989;262:2551–2556.
5. White LR, Cartwright WS, Cornoni-Huntley J, Brock DB. Geriatric epidemiology. Ann Rev Gerontol Geriatr 1986;6:215–311.
6. Schoenberg BS, Kokmen E, Okazoki H. Alzheimer's disease and other dementing illnesses in a defined United States population: incidence rates and clinical features. Ann Neurol 1987;22:724–729.
7. Cummings JL, Benson DF, Hill MA, Read S. Aphasia in dementia of the Alzheimer type. Neurology 1985;35:394–397.
8. Ripich D, Vertes D, Whitehouse PJ, et al. Turntaking and speech act patterns in the discourse of senile dementia of the Alzheimer's type patient. Brain Lang 1991;40:330–343.
9. Mendez MF, Mendez MA, Martin R, et al. Complex visual disturbances in Alzheimer's disease. Neurology 1990;40:439–443.
10. Parasuraman R, Greenwood PM, Haxby JV, Grady CL. Visuospatial attention in dementia of the Alzheimer type. Brain 1992;115:711–733.
11. Patterson MB, Schnell A, Martin RJ, et al. Assessment of psychiatric symptoms in Alzheimer's disease. J Geriatr Psychiatry Neurol 1990;3:21–30.
12. Mendez MF, Martin R, Smyth KA, et al. Psychiatric symptoms associated with Alzheimer's disease. J Neuropsychiatry Clin Neurosci 1990;2:28–33.
13. Drevets WC, Rubin EH. Psychotic symptoms and the longitudinal course of senile dementia of the Alzheimer type. Biol Psychiatry 1989;25:39–48.
14. Boller F, Mizutani Y, Roessman U, Gambetti P. Parkinson disease, dementia and Alzheimer disease: clinicopathological correlates. Ann Neurol 1980;7:329–335.
15. McKhann G, Drachman D, Folstein M, et al. Clinical diagnosis of Alzheimer's disease: report of the NINCDS-ADRDA work group under the auspices of the Department of Health and Human Services Task Force on Alzheimer's Disease. Neurology 1984;34:939–944.
16. Barclay LL, Zemcov A, Blass JP, Sansone J. Survival in Alzheimer's disease and vascular dementias. Neurology 1985;834–840.
17. Davis KL, Thal LJ, Gamzu ER, et al. Tacrine in patients with Alzheimer's disease: a double-blind placebo-controlled multicenter study. N Engl J Med 1992;327:1253–1259.
18. Farlow M, Gracon SI, Hershey LA, et al. A controlled trial of tacrine in Alzheimer's disease. JAMA 1992;268:2523–2529.
19. Knapp MJ, Knopman DS, Solomon PR, et al. A 30-week randomized controlled trial of high-dose tacrine in patients with Alzheimer's disease. JAMA 1994;271:985–991.
20. Gibb WR, Mountjoy CQ, Mann DM, Lees AJ. A pathological study of the association of Lewy body disease and Alzheimer's disease. J Neurol Neurosurg Psychiatry 1989;52:701–708.

21. Breitner JCS, Silverman JM, Mahs RD, et al. Familial aggregation in Alzheimer's disease: comparison of risk among relatives of early- and late-onset cases, and among male and female relatives in subsequent generations. Neurology 1988;38:207–212.

22. Hoffman A, Schulte, Tanja TA, et al. History of dementia and Parkinson's disease in 1st-degree relatives of patients with Alzheimer's disease. Neurology 1989;39:1589–1592.

23. Saunders AM, Strittmatter WJ, Schmechel D, et al. Association of apolipoprotein E allele E4 with late-onset familial and sporadic Alzheimer's disease. Neurology 1993;43:1467–1472.

24. Strittmatter WJ, Saunders AM, Schmechel D, et al. Apolipoprotein E: high avidity binding to beta amyloid and increased frequency of type 4 allele in late onset familial Alzheimer disease. Proc Natl Acad Sci USA 1993;90:1977–1981.

25. Heston LL, Mastri AR, Anderson VE. Dementia of the Alzheimer type: clinical genetics, natural history, and associated conditions. Arch Gen Psychiatry 1981;38:1085–1090.

26. Tissot R, Constantinidis J, Richard J. Pick's disease. In: Frederiks JAM, ed. Handbook of clinical neurology. vol. 2. Neurobehavioral disorders. New York: Elsevier, 1985:233–246.

27. Mendez MF, Zander BA. Dementia presenting with aphasia: clinical characteristics. J Neurol Neurosurg Psychiatry 1991;54:542–545.

27. Heston LL, White JH, Mastri AR. Pick's disease: Clinical genetics and natural history. Arch Gen Psychiatr 1987;44:409–411.

28. Chui HC. Dementia: a review emphasizing clinicopathologic correlation and brain-behavior relationships. Arch Neurol 1989;46:806–814.

29. Hachinski VC, Lassen NA, Marshall J. Multi-infarct dementia: a cause of mental deterioration in the elderly. Lancet 1974;2:207–210.

30. Chui HC, Victoroff JI, Margolin D, et al. Criteria for the diagnosis of ischemic vascular dementia proposed by the State of California Alzheimer's Disease Diagnostic and Treatment Centers. Neurology 1992;42:473–480.

31. Roman GC, Tatemichi TK, Erkinjuntti T, et al. Vascular dementia: diagnostic criteria for research studies; report of the NINDS-AIREN International Workshop. Neurology 1993;43:250–260.

32. Katzman R, Lasker B, Bernstein N. Advances in the diagnosis of dementia: accuracy of diagnosis and consequence of misdiagnosis of disorders causing dementia. In: Terry RD, ed. Aging and the brain. New York: Raven, 1988:17–62.

32. Drachman DA. New criteria for the diagnosis of vascular dementia: do we know enough yet? Neurology 1993;43:243–245.

33. Erkinjuntti T, Haltia M, Palo J, et al. Accuracy of the clinical diagnosis of vascular dementia: a prospective clinical and post-mortem pathological study. J Neurol Neurosurg Psychiatry 1988;51:1037–1044.

34. Kotsoris H, Barclay LL, Kheyfets S, Hulyalkar A, Dougherty J. Urinary and gait disturbances as markers for early multi-infarct dementia. Stroke 1987;18:138–141.

35. Hachinski VC, Iliff LD, Zilhka E, et al. Cerebral blood flow in dementia. Arch Neurol 1975;32:632–637.

36. Hachinski VC, Potter P, Merskey H. Leuko-araiosis. Arch Neurol 1987;44:21–3.

37. Meyer JS, Judd BW, Tawaklna T, et al. Improved cognition after control of risk factors for multi-infarct dementia. JAMA 1986;256:2203–2209.

38. Mayeux R, Chen J, Mirabello E, et al. An estimate of the incidence of dementia in idiopathic Parkinson's disease. Neurology 1990;40:1513–1516.

39. Jankovic J. Parkinsonism-plus syndromes. Mov Disord 1989;4(suppl 1):S95–S119.

40. Steele JC, Richardson JC, Olszewski J. Progressive supranuclear palsy. Arch Neurol 1964;10:333–359.

41. Maher ER, Lees AJ. The clinical features of Steele-Richardson-Olszwewski syndrome (progressive supranuclear palsy). Neurology 1986;36:1005–1008.

42. Gibb WR, Luthert PJ, Janota I, Lantos PL. Cortical Lewy body dementia: clinical features and classification. J Neurol Neurosurg Psychiatry 1989;52:185–192.

43. Riley DE, Lang AE, Lewis A, et al. Cortico-basal ganglionic degeneration. Neurology 1990;40:1203–1212.

44. Neumann MA, Cohn R. Progressive subcortical gliosis, a rare form of presenile dementia. Brain 1967;90:405–407.

45. Knopman DS, Mastri AR, Frey WH, et al. Dementia lacking distinctive histologic features: a common non-Alzheimer degenerative dementia. Neurology 1990;40:251–256.

Chapter 43
Depression

Michael G. Moran, M.D.

Do not go gentle into that good night,
Old age should burn and rage at close of day;
Rage, rage, against the dying of the light.

Dylan Thomas, 1914–1953
Collected Poems, 1953

Because of its multiple causes, high prevalence, and significant morbidity and mortality, depression ranks as one of the most important clinical problems to confront the physician for the elderly patient. Depression is most appropriately considered a syndrome, not a specific disease, because many medical, pharmacologic, and psychiatric entities, either alone or in combination, can produce the clinical picture of depression (1). The importance of depression is underlined by its significant financial and prognostic impact on the medically ill patient (2).

This chapter explores the causes and differential diagnosis of depression in the elderly, the physiologic and cognitive aspects of depression, and the usefulness of special examinations such as computerized tomography (CT) and sleep studies. The chapter discusses unique problems in the institutionalized and medically ill patient and approaches to treatment, to suicidal ideation, and to the assessment of prognosis.

Myths and Facts

Ageism bias may be reflected in the assumptions made by the public in general and by physicians in particular regarding the mental health of the elderly. Because of fears of getting older, many young persons assume that all older persons are depressed, feel alone and abandoned, and hate their advanced age. In physicians, such prejudices may produce a simplistic approach to the diagnosis of depression, often manifest in a unitary concept of its origin. Although postmenopausal women have been traditionally seen as being at high risk for depression and

loss of sexual interest, contemporary epidemiologic studies fail to confirm this association (3). Loss and involutional changes with age account for some cases of depression, but multifactorial syndromes are understood to be quite common, and currently occupy the forefront of clinical and research attention (1,4). Some examples of the contributors to the clinical appearance and characteristics of affective disorders include genetics, medical illness, physiologic changes with aging, and social milieu.

Elderly persons with depression are less likely than their younger counterparts to have a family history of affective disorder (5). The earlier the onset of unipolar depression, the more likely the family history is positive. Among elderly who live *in the community*, depression is actually less common than it is among young persons. The homebound elderly and those living in nursing homes appear to be at greater risk. Other risk factors include smoking, lack of religious coping, female gender, and functional disability (6).

Only about 20 percent of elderly persons with depression are treated by mental health practitioners, which makes the detection of mood disorders by primary care and internal medicine physicians especially crucial. The masking of depression by somatic complaints or cognitive problems is common and may contribute to the underdiagnosis of depression (7).

Symptoms

There are few differences between the clinical presentations of depression in the elderly and in younger patients. However, older individuals with depression tend, as a group, to demonstrate more delusional thinking, more agitation, appetite loss, and psychotic thinking (8). They may be less likely to experience worthlessness or guilt. Although both young and old patients report about the same levels of depressive severity, clinicians rate the older patients as more depressed. Difficulty getting to sleep and preoccupation with somatic symptoms, considered characteristic of the elderly person with depression in earlier studies, were not found by Brodaty in 1991 (8). Compared with nondepressed older persons, the depressed patient may be more likely to "cocoon" – withdraw from the environment, confine himself to the bedroom with curtains drawn, and wrap up in a blanket (9).

If cognitive impairment is associated with the depressive syndrome (and is unrelated to another diagnosis such as Alzheimer's disease), the patient is also more likely to display manic symptoms and have a poorer prognosis. When severe, cognitive disturbances can resemble those of a dementia, and may even dominate the clinical picture (pseudodementia). This presentation may be caused by a subset of major depression that occurs late in life and may be related to occult brain pathology (4). Patients who go on to have overt manic episodes (late-life-onset mania) have a higher mortality rate than those who do not have these episodes (10).

Differential Diagnosis

Many nonpsychiatric medical disorders and several drugs can produce syndromes that mimic major depression. Because of this, *symptomatic evaluation in the physician's office is usually insufficient to complete the workup of the elderly patient with depression* (11).

A thorough history and physical examination form the cornerstone of the evaluation. A first depression in an elderly person for whom no psychosocial trigger (such as a major loss) can be found should prompt special consideration. The physician should review all medications the patient is taking, and ask about over-the-counter drug usage. Some elderly patients (and young ones) believe that, in the case of vitamins, "if a little is good, more is better." Such attitudes may result in excessive intake of vitamins poorly cleared, such as the fat-soluble group. These intoxications can look like depressive syndromes in the early stages, especially with excess vitamin D. Many centrally acting medications (including some antihypertensives) can produce or worsen depressive affect. Benzodiazepines and other sedating agents, including alcohol, can have a similar adverse effect on mood (Table 43.1).

Medical illness can also present with depressive symptoms *that are part of the illness itself, and not merely the result of the patient's emotional reaction to being sick*. Viral hepatitis, hypothyroidism, severe hyperglycemia, influenza, and metastatic and primary brain tumors are some of the many conditions to consider (Table 43.2) (12). Primary sleep disorders, such as obstructive sleep apnea (which increases in prevalence with a patient's age), often have mood disorders as part of the clinical picture, and the mood problem can be the presenting syndrome. Parkinson's disease (PD) is associated with a depression specific to that disease and is not a consequence of parkinsonian dementia or the patient's reaction to PD. Right hemispheric predominance in PD appears to be associated with more severe depressive symptoms (4).

Depression afflicts about 25 percent of patients who experience stroke, and comorbidity with anxiety disorders is also common. As in PD, these psychiatric problems result from the medical condition itself, not simply from the patient's reaction to having had the stroke. The severity of a comorbid medical condition is positively correlated with the occurrence and severity of a number of psychiatric conditions, including depression. Because medical illnesses increase in prevalence with age, one would expect the prevalence of depression to increase independent of other factors. But the level of health itself is less a factor in relapse or chronicity of depressive syndromes than *the direction of change of health*. Changes in

Table 43.1. Drugs That Cause Depressive Syndromes.

Sedative-Hypnotics	Antihypertensives	Narcotics	Others
Barbiturates	Reserpine	Oxycodone	Cimetidine
Benzodiazepines	α-methyldopa	Meperidine	Cycloserine
Alcohol	Propranolol		Corticosteroids
			Digitalis

Table 43.2. Medical Conditions That Cause Depressive Syndromes.

Neurologic	Neoplastic	Endocrine	Infectious
Stroke	Brain tumors	Hypothyroidism	Viral pneumonias
Parkinson's disease	Paraneoplastic syndrome	Diabetes mellitus	Viral hepatitis
Multiple sclerosis	Disseminated tumors	Cushing's disease	Infectious mononucleosis

independence seems most important in predicting re-lapse, independent of the baseline health status, number of medical conditions, or problems with activities of daily living (13).

Bereavement

Because acute and subacute grief share many symptoms with major depression, the physician must learn to distinguish between a normal period of bereavement and a pathological mood disorder *complicating* that grief (6,14). Ageism bias may obstruct the clinical vision of the doctor here: if all elderly are seen as being in "normal" states of grief because of their [actual] increased risk for loss, the physician may be less aggressive in diagnosing or treating a depressive mood disorder in a patient who has suffered a major loss.

Studies of the natural history of bereavement suggest that the persistence of depressive symptoms beyond 1 year after a spouse's death reflects a pathological condition (15). However, persistence of depressive symptoms for up to 6 months is not unusual (16). A woman at risk for depression after her husband's death is less likely to have worked outside the home and rates her support system as inadequate. She is likely to have had a previous psychiatric disorder. Initial depressive symptoms, while expectable may, if severe, predict pathologic reactions. A full depressive syndrome immediately after the loss may predict *persistence* of symptoms and the ultimate need for psychiatric intervention in the form of medication and psychotherapy. Young widows and widowers and those with a previous history of depressive disorders are also at greater risk for major depression. Widows tend to have more symptoms than widowers. At 13 months, 16 percent of widows meet criteria for a major depression, display suicidal ideation, and feelings of worthlessness. Intense

grief at 2 months after the loss predicted major depression at 1 year (17).

When the spouse's death is by suicide, bereavement tends to be prolonged and complicated. Surviving spouses demonstrate high levels of phobic behavior, hostility, and paranoid ideation (18). The picture may be worsened by the fact that these spouses usually receive less social support for their grief than do natural death survivors, and these spouses tend to avoid confiding in their friends (19).

Biologic and Physiologic Studies

Sleep studies among elderly persons with depression resemble those of younger patients—lower sleep efficiency, more early morning awakening, and shorter rapid eye movement (REM) latency. Because these findings are also present among acutely grieving older persons, the sleep electroencephalogram cannot distinguish these persons from those who do not have major depression (6). REM deprivation can be used, however, to distinguish between elderly persons with depression (who show no rebound after deprivation) and demented persons, who do rebound (20).

Magnetic resonance imaging demonstrates differences between depressed and nondepressed older patients. The patients with mood disorder have more subcortical atrophy, basal ganglia lesions, and subcortical hyperintensities (21,22). Positron emission tomography shows left prefrontal hypometabolism of glucose in depressed patients, an asymmetry that disappears after successful drug treatment (23).

Hormonal studies of depressed patients include elevated cerebrospinal fluid, corticotropin-releasing hormone, and decreased sleep-related growth hormone (GH) secretion. Sleep is a powerful stimulus for GH secretion;

secretion is unchanged on remission of the depression (6,24). Clinical diagnostic correlates of these findings have not yet been found. For instance, the dexamethasone suppression test may be positive in late-life depression, but tends to be so nonspecific as to be of little use (14).

Cognitive Disturbances

Cognitive disturbances may result from depressive disorders (pseudodementia of depression) or coexist with them (major depression *and* Alzheimer's disease, for example). As a result, the physician may fail to diagnose a treatable depression and write the patient off as having expectable memory problems associated with getting older. Thus, neither the patient's cognitive nor mood disturbance is evaluated. Physicians must familiarize themselves with the differential diagnosis of depression and dementia (7).

The depressed patient who is also cognitively impaired by the depression is likely to improve with conventional treatments (antidepressants or electroconvulsive therapy). Stoudemire and his co-workers found that depressed elderly patients *with cognitive disturbances* (from dementia or depression) may be at great risk for relapse, have more residual symptoms, and thus need closer follow-up than patients without cognitive symptoms (25,26). But Baldwin and colleagues found that the treatment of depression in patients *with dementia* was as successful as it was in those without dementia (27). Another group of investigators suggested that the "reversibly demented" depressed group may include some patients suffering from the early stages of irreversible dementing syndromes, and that early, thorough workup and consistent follow-up is necessary to detect treatable neurological disorders (28).

When the patient with Alzheimer's disease is depressed, the depression may be genetically related to the primary affective disorder, because dual-diagnosis patients have more first-degree relatives with depression (29). At variance with conventional wisdom is the finding that depression does not worsen the prognosis of the dementia (30). However, depression may be an acute *marker* for the stepwise progression of primary degenerative dementia (31).

Mildly demented patients report more mood distur-

bances than do severely demented patients. There could be several explanations, but these patients may be more alert to inner states and hence better able to report on (and react to) their cognitive losses. The *manifestation* of depression in more severely afflicted patients may simply be determined neurologically–patients who are more severely demented tend to show mood disturbance behaviorally, as decreased motivation (32).

Institutionalized or Hospitalized Patients

Studies conflict on whether depression contributes to morbidity or mortality in the nursing home patient. In a 30-month period, one group demonstrated variance in survival between depressed and nondepressed patients, but the differences were easily accounted for on the basis of differing severity of medical illness (33). Another investigator, looking at 454 nursing home admissions, found a 12.6 percent incidence of major depression, with an additional 18.1 percent of the patients showing some depressive symptoms. Major depression was *an independent risk factor* for mortality, increasing the risk by 59 percent in the first year (34). Federal regulations now mandate the assessment of depression in patients newly admitted to nursing homes.

There is less controversy surrounding the effects of depression in the medically ill, especially patients in hospitals. Comorbidity of medical and psychiatric illness is common. In fact, one study demonstrated a tendency for elderly medical patients to have more than one psychiatric diagnosis, with low rates of detection by physicians (35). The stress associated with medical illness appears to be a risk factor for both depressive symptoms and major depression (36). Depressed patients may refuse treatment of their medical condition, even when the prognosis is good (37). Comorbid patients have worse physical, social, and role functioning, and worse perceptions of their own health, as well as more complaints of pain (2). Among patients with coronary artery disease, for example, ventricular tachycardia occurs more frequently if the patient is depressed (38). Length of stay is greater for depressed medical inpatients, even if the patient has only depressive *symptoms* and not all the criteria for a depressive *disorder*. The successful treatment of depression may result in decreased overall health care resources (39). In general, the detection and treatment of depression, even the documentation of suicidal ideation, remains inadequate in the hospitalized elderly (40).

In both the nursing home and the hospital, the diagnosis of depression can be difficult to make because of the likely coexistence of confounding symptoms from a medical illness. Lethargy, decreased stamina and initiative, sleep disruptions, and anorexia may all be directly caused by chronic or acute medical conditions, and their presence may complicate the diagnosis of depression. In these situations, the physician should look for *intrapsychic* symptoms of depression. The presence of sustained hopelessness, a focus on guilt or worthlessness, suicidal ideation, or predictable diurnal mood variation point to a mood disorder. Medical illnesses may obviously be associated with these latter symptoms, and in those instances a psychiatric consultation may help distinguish expectable emotional reactions to disability, pain, and confinement from an autonomous depressive disorder (41).

Coping styles may be more or less adaptive for medically ill depressed patients. Male patients in this setting were studied for factors that protect against depression. Among the demographic and psychological variables studied, a religious coping style was found to be the single best protective mechanism (42).

Treatment

The treatment modalities available to physicians for treating the elderly are basically the same as those for treating younger patients. Special consideration lies not so much in the choice of modality as in attention to drug interactions, pharmacokinetic changes with age, target organ sensitivity, and the need for sustained follow-up. Although depression is probably the most common psychiatric disorder among the elderly (12), it may also be the most underrecognized (14,43). Primary care physicians tend to be unaware of the symptoms of depression, and few refer depressed elderly patients to specialists (44). The elderly tend to receive only symptomatic treatment with antianxiety agents and hypnotics, rather than definitive or therapeutic doses of antidepressants, and are likely to receive inadequate follow-up or maintenance therapy (11). Indeed, even patients with mild depression may benefit from antidepressant treatment, if they are appropriately screened (45).

Antidepressant medications (Table 43.3) have had few trials among the elderly, but they are believed to be equally effective. Response probably occurs later than it does in young patients, and compliance with medication is a significant problem (43). Medication should be continued for at least 9 to 12 months after the beginning of an acute episode, if not for life (46). When combined with interpersonal psychotherapy, nortriptyline was associated with remission in 79 percent of patients; 25 percent relapsed upon discontinuation of treatment.

One question asked by the National Institutes of Health (NIH) Consensus Conference regarding therapy was,

Table 43.3. Representative Antidepressants for Use in the Elderly.

Drug Class	Side Effects	Important Qualities
Sedating tricyclics (amitriptyline, imipramine)	Sedation, anticholinergic response	Metabolism affected by other drugs
Other tricyclics (nortriptyline, desipramine)	Mild sedation (NTP); activation (DSP)	Metabolism affected by other drugs
MAOIs inhibitors (phenelzine)	Agitation; weight gain	Tyramine-containing foods and sympathomimetic agents increase BP
Trazodone	Sedation; priapism	Does not affect metabolism of other drugs
SSRIs (fluoxetine, sertraline, paroxetine)	Sedation, anxiety, sexual dysfunction, GI distress	Interacts with MAOIs, serotonin, and dopamine (fluoxetine) agonists
Buproprion	Possible parkinsonian symptoms; seizures	Interacts with dopamine agonists and SSRIs (fluoxetine)

BP = blood pressure; DSP = desipramine; GI = gastrointestinal; MAOI = monoamine oxidase inhibitor; NTP = nortriptyline; SSRI = selective serotonin re-uptake inhibitor.
SOURCE: Preskorn SH. Recent pharmacologic advances in antidepressant therapy for the elderly. Am J Med 1993;94:2S–12S.

"What constitutes safe and effective treatment for late-life depression?" Several points arose in the answer. Traditional cyclic antidepressants are safe, but most clinicians choose either nortriptyline or desipramine, and *avoid amitriptyline and imipramine* because of their anticholinergic and orthostatic side effects. The newer-generation, selective serotonin re-uptake inhibitors (SSRIs) are also favored. Monoamine oxidase inhibitors (MAOIs) have been shown to be surprisingly safe, and are possibly underused. The patient factors that predict good or poor response are unknown, but considerable evidence documents that *treatment response depends on adequate length of treatment [it may not occur for up to 12 weeks], dosage and blood level of medication.* As much as 70 percent of patients fail to take 50 percent of their medication, and lack of compliance predicts poor outcome (14).

Many physicians reduce the dose of antidepressant after the patient has shown response. There are few trials testing this approach, but increasing data support continuation of medication at the dose that induced remission. The NIH Consensus Conference suggested maintaining patients for 6 months after remission from a first depressive episode, and *at least 12 months* after remission from a second or third episode (14).

The physician's choice of an antidepressant should be guided by the side effect profile of the agent because the drugs are equivalent in terms of efficacy. The beginning dose is often lower for the elderly than it is for a younger person (for example, 10 to 25 mg of nortriptyline, 25 mg of sertraline, or 10 mg of fluoxetine), and dosage advancement should occur at a slower pace. Decreased drug metabolism because of hepatic changes with aging and, probably, brain changes make the elderly more susceptible to drug side effects (47–50).

Sedating antidepressants and those that cause significant orthostasis may precipitate serious risk for falls and hip fractures (51). One report suggests that nortriptyline may adversely alter a patient's sensitivity to carbon dioxide and ability to compensate ventilatory load changes, even though the patient experiences less dyspnea and improved exercise tolerance (52). In this author's experience with a large number of depressed patients with pulmonary disease, nortryptyline has not been a problem. Further studies are needed, however, to clarify the effect of nortriptyline in the elderly population. Dry mouth, probably the most common troublesome side effect, may be controlled with judicious use of bethanecol (53).

The SSRIs offer the advantage of a very low incidence of severe side effects. Although they all block re-uptake of serotonin, the three drugs now on the market in this country are chemically quite different from each other, and have different pharmacokinetics. Of the three, the kinetics of sertraline change the least with age, which makes dosage and dosing interval adjustments less necessary, in theory. Sertraline also has less potential to inhibit the hepatic isoenzyme P450 IID6 than do the other two drugs. Theoretically, the plasma levels of many drugs (including cyclic antidepressants, carbamazepine, and neuroleptics) could increase if they are co-administered with fluoxetine or paroxetine (54). Use of the latter two drugs in the elderly is obviously not precluded by these differences, but should suggest appropriate attention to drug dosage, dosing intervals, and follow-up.

Several workers evaluated stimulant medications as alternatives to conventional antidepressants among the medically ill. Methylphenidate and dextroamphetamine are the most common choices, the former being somewhat better tolerated and requiring fewer daily doses. Any improvement in mood is likely to be shown within 48 hours of starting the medication. These drugs are probably underused because of physician reluctance. Delirious patients may not respond as well as others (55,56).

Psychosocial interventions hold an important place in the comprehensive therapeutic approach to the elderly patient. Combination therapy, in which the patient is treated with both antidepressant medication and psychotherapy, may be the most effective approach for a large group of patients (46).

Although there are no studies on the differential usefulness of psychosocial therapies in the comorbid elderly, or in the very old, several modalities show robust endurance of their efficacy in the older patient. These modalities include short-term psychotherapy, cognitive-behavioral therapy, and interpersonal psychotherapy (14). Such treatments are superior to placebo (11). Some authors suggest a greater acceptance of cognitive and behavioral approaches among these patients (12).

Freud was probably the first psychiatrist to suggest that older patients were too "unmalleable" for psychotherapeutic treatment. Few clinicians now agree with this bit of ageism bias. Many older patients are able to draw on their wide range of life experiences and their past adaptive approaches to crises and make good use of psychotherapy. This capacity may explain some findings of better outcome at 6 months for elderly patients, as compared with younger patients, even when the older patients have higher scales of medical illness symptoms (57).

In addition to psychotherapy with the individual patient, assessment and treatment of the marital couple and support system constitute essential ingredients in an overall approach. The caregivers of the frail elderly are themselves often under great burdens (14). This setting may contribute to physical abuse of the patient, with demented older patients at special risk (58).

Electroconvulsive therapy (ECT) is a safe and effective alternative or adjunctive approach for the depressed elderly patient. The patient who is so severely depressed as to be self-destructively withdrawn (not eating, virtually immobilized), who has persistent delusions, paranoia, or psychotic symptoms, and who is refractory to or not a candidate for other treatments, should be considered for ECT (12). Intuitively, ECT might seem to be dangerous for use in patients with cardiac conduction disorders, but in one study ECT was better tolerated by depressed patients with cardiac problems than were tricyclic antidepressants (59).

ECT can adversely affect memory, but newer techniques (unilateral, nondominant hemispheric administration) and equipment make it a safer modality than in the past. For patients whose depression included memory and concentration deficits, ECT may *improve* cognitive functioning (25).

Course and Outcome

Late-life depression has typically been regarded as refractory to usual treatments and particularly prone to relapse. However, the recent National Institute of Mental Health Collaborative Study of the Psychobiology of Depression suggests that treatment outcomes are similar in older patients compared with younger ones (60). After 1 year of study, 72 percent of older patients had improved; of that group, 19 percent had relapsed. No demographic characteristics of the *patients* predicted recovery or relapse, but three *family characteristics* predicted poor outcome: poor

spouse and adult children's health, their reports of difficulties in caring for the patient, and their psychiatric symptoms (61). Other investigators have also found that length of the depressive illness predicts lower recovery rates (62).

Alexopoulos and Chester found that active medical illness, high severity of depression, delusions, and morphologic brain abnormalities predicted chronicity, and chronicity may predict relapse (63). *Worsening* of a patient's health status is associated with persistent depressive symptoms (13).

Suicide

The elderly have the highest rates of suicide and completed suicide. Older white men are at greatest risk and generally have visited a primary care physician within the 6 months preceding their suicide. The patient at this typical presentation is suffering from a first major depression and has symptoms of moderate severity which were not recognized or treated (14). In another study of a similar population, the patients had never seen a mental health professional (64). *Expressed hopelessness* may be a particularly sensitive indicator of the likelihood of an attempt (65).

Patients with a history of suicide *attempts* tend to try suicide again. They generally have a high socioeconomic position and achieve only poor remission of index depressive episodes. Their spouses and children tend to have a number of psychiatric symptoms, perhaps associated with the detectable strain in their relationships with the patient (66).

For patients older than 80 years of age, *medical symptoms* play a central role in generating suicidal ideation and attempts. Men, more than women, seem to have economic stressors (67).

Conclusion

Depression among the elderly is a treatable illness with considerable morbidity and mortality, but it is underrecognized and often inadequately treated. Coexistent medical symptoms, ageism bias, and noncompliance make necessary a high index of suspicion for depression, with a thorough diagnostic workup and consistent aftercare. A variety of modalities demonstrate efficacy in treatment, but evidence suggests that few patients are referred to psychiatrists.

References

1. Small GW. Recognition and treatment of depression in the elderly. J Clin Psychiatry 1991;52:11–22.
2. Wells KB, Stewart A, Hays RD, et al. The functioning and well-being of depressed patients. Results from the Medical Outcomes Study. JAMA 1989;262:914–919.
3. Youngs DD. Some misconceptions concerning the menopause. Obstet Gynecol 1990;75:881–883.
4. McMahon FJ, DePaulo JR. Clinical features of affective disorders and bereavement. Curr Opin Psychiatry 1991;5:580–584.
5. Maier W, Lichtermann D, Minges J, et al. Unipolar depression in the aged: determinants of familial aggregation. J Affect Disord 1991;23:53–61.
6. Zisook S, Peterkin JJ. Mood disorders and bereavement in late life. Curr Opin Psychiatry 1993;6:568–573.
7. Yesavage J. Differential diagnosis between depression and dementia. Am J Med 1993;23S–28S.
8. Brodaty H, Peters K, Boyce P, et al. Age and depression. J Affect Disord 1991;23:137–149.
9. Baker FM, Miller CL. "Cocooning": a clinical sign of depression in geriatric patients. Hosp Community Psychiatry 1991;42:845–846.
10. Shulman KI, Tohen M, Satlin A, et al. Mania compared with unipolar depression in old age. Am J Psychiatry 1992;149:341–345.
11. Blazer D. Depression in the elderly. N Engl J Med 1989;320:164–166.
12. Mendels J. Clinical management of the depressed geriatric patient: current therapeutic options. Am J Med 1993;94:13S–18S.
13. Kennedy GJ, Kelman HR, Thomas C. Persistence and remission of depressive symptoms in late life. Am J Psychiatry 1991;148:174–178.
14. NIH concensus panel on depression in late life. Diagnosis and treatment of depression in late life. JAMA 1992;268:1018–1024.
15. Nuss WS, Zubenko GS. Correlates of persistent depressive symptoms in widows. Am J Psychiatry 1992;149(3):346–351.
16. Harlow SD, Goldberg EL, Comstock GW. A longitudinal study of the prevalence of depressive symptomatology in elderly widowed and married women. Arch Gen Psychiatry 1991;48:1065–1068.
17. Zisook S, Shuchter SR. Depression through the first year after the death of a spouse. Am J Psychiatry 1991;148:1346–1352.
18. Gilewski MJ, Fabernow NL, Gallagher DE, Thompson LW. Interaction of depression and bereavement on mental health in the elderly. Psychol Aging 1991;6:67–75.
19. Farberow NL, Gallagher-Thompson D, Gilewski M, Thompson L. The role of social supports in the bereavement process of surviving spouses of suicide and natural deaths. Suicide Life Threat Behav 1992;22:107–124.
20. Reynolds C, Buysse DJ, Kupfer DJ, et al. Rapid eye movement sleep deprivation as a probe in elderly subjects. Arch Gen Psychiatry 1990;47:1128–1136.
21. Coffey CE, Figiel GS, Djang WT, Weiner RD. Subcortical hyperintensity on magnetic resonance imaging: a comparison of normal and depressed elderly subjects. Am J Psychiatry 1990;147:187–189.
22. Rabins PV, Pearlson GD, Aylward E, et al. Cortical magnetic resonance imaging changes in elderly inpatients with major depression. Am J Psychiatry 1991;148:617–620.
23. Martinot JL, Hardy P, Feline A, et al. Left prefrontal glucose hypometabolism in the depressed state: a confirmation. Am J Psychiatry 1990;147:1313–1317.
24. Jarrett DB, Miewald JM, Kupfer DJ. Recurrent depression is associated with a persistent reduction in sleep-related growth hormone secretion. Arch Gen Psychiatry 1990;47:113–118.
25. Stoudemire A, Hill CD, Morris R, et al. Cognitive outcome following tricyclic and electroconvulsive treatment of major depression in the elderly. Am J Psychiatry 1991;148:1336–1340.
26. Stoudemire A, Hill CD, Morris R, et al. Long-term affective and cognitive outcome in depressed older adults. Am J Psychiatry 1993;150:896–900.
27. Baldwin RC, Benbow SM, Marriott A, Tomenson B. Depression in old age. A reconsideration of cerebral disease in relation to outcome. Br J Psychiatry 1993;163:82.
28. Alexopoulos GS, Meyers BS, Young RC, et al. The course of geriatric depression with "reversible dementia": a controlled study. Am J Psychiatry 1993;150:1693–1699.
29. Pearlson GD, Ross CA, Lohr WD, et al. Association between family history of affective disorder and the depressive syndrome of Alzheimer's disease. Am J Psychiatry 1990;147:452–456.
30. Lopez OL, Boller F, Becker JT, et al. Alzheimer's disease and depression: neuropsychological impairment and progression of the illness. Am J Psychiatry 1990;147:855–860.
31. Zubenko GS. Progression of illness in the differential diagnosis of primary dementia. Am J Psychiatry 1990;147:435–438.
32. Forsell Y, Jorm AF, Fratiglioni L, et al. Application of DSM-III-R criteria for major depressive episode to elderly subjects with and without dementia. Am J Psychiatry 1993;150:1199–1202.
33. Parmelee PA, Katz IR, Lawton MP. Depression and mortality among institutionalized aged. J Gerontol 1992;47:3–10.
34. Rovner BW. Depression and increased risk of mortality in the nursing home patient. Am J Med 1993;94:19S–22S.
35. Rapp SR, Parisi SA, Wallace CE. Comorbid psychiatric disorders in elderly medical patients: a 1-year prospective study. J Am Geriatr Soc 1991;39:124–131.
36. Turner RJ, Beiser M. Major depression and depressive symptomatology among the physically disabled. Assessing the role of chronic stress. J Nerv Ment Dis 1990;178:343–350.

37. Lee MA, Ganzini L. Depression in the elderly: effect on patient attitudes toward life- sustaining therapy [see comments]. J Am Geriatr Soc 1992;40:983–988.

38. Carney RM, Freedland KE, Rich MW, et al. Ventricular tachycardia and psychiatric depression in patients with coronary artery disease. Am J Med 1993;95:23–28.

39. Stewart JT. Diagnosing and treating depression in the hospitalized elderly. Geriatrics 1991;46:64–66.

40. Wells KB, Rogers WH, Davis LM, et al. Quality of care for hospitalized depressed elderly patients before and after implementation of the medicare prospective payment system. Am J Psychiatry 1993;150:1799–1805.

41. Koenig HG. Depressive disorders in older medical inpatients. Am Fam Physician 1991;44:1243–1250.

42. Koenig HG, Cohen HJ, Blazer DG, et al. Religious coping and depression among elderly, hospitalized medically ill men. Am J Psychiatry 1992;149:1693–1700.

43. Schneider LS. Treatment of depression, psychosis, and other conditions in geriatric patients. Curr Opin Psychiatry 1993;6:562–567.

44. Yesavage JA. Depression in the elderly: how to recognize masked symptoms and choose appropriate therapy. Postgrad Med 1992;91:255–261.

45. Stewart JW, McGrath PJ, Quitkin FM. Can mildly depressed outpatients with atypical depression benefit from antidepressants? Am J Psychiatry 1992;149(5):615–619.

46. Reynolds C, Frank E, Perel JM, et al. Combined pharmacotherapy and psychotherapy in the acute and continuation treatment of elderly patients with recurrent major depression: a preliminary report. Am J Psychiatry 1992;149:1687–1692.

47. Moran MG, Thompson TLI. Changes in the aging brain as they affect psychotropics: a review. Int J Psychiatry Med 1988;18:137–144.

48. Thompson TLI, Moran MG, Nies AS. Psychotropic drug use in the elderly, I. N Engl J Med 1983;308:134–138.

49. Thompson TLI, Moran MG, Nies AS. Psychotropic drug use in the elderly. II. N Eng J Med 1983;308:194–199.

50. Schiffer RB, Wineman NM. Antidepressant pharmacotherapy of depression associated with multiple sclerosis. Am J Psychiatry 1990;147:1493–1497.

51. Ray WA, Griffin MR, Schaffner W, Baugh DK, et al. Psychotropic drug use and the risk of hip fracture. N Engl J Med 1987;316:363–369.

52. Greenberg HE, Scharf SM, Green H. Nortriptyline-induced depression of ventilatory control in a patient with chronic obstructive pulmonary disease. Am Rev Respir Dis 1993;147:1303.

53. Rosen J, Pollock BG, Altieri LP, Jonas EA. Treatment of nortriptyline's side effects in elderly patients: a double-blind study of bethanechol. Am J Psychiatry 1993;150:1249–1251.

54. Preskorn SH. Recent pharmacologic advances in antidepressant therapy for the elderly. Am J Med 1993;94:2S–12S.

55. Rosenberg PB, Ahmed I, Hurwitz S. Methylphenidate in depressed medically ill patients. J Clin Psychiatry 1991;52:263–267.

56. Frierson RL, Wey JJ, Tabler JB. Psychostimulants for depression in the medically ill. Am Fam Physician 1991;43:163–170.

57. Hughes DC, DeMallie D, Blazer DG. Does age make a difference in the effects of physical health and social support on the outcome of a major depressive episode? Am J Psychiatry 1993;150:728–733.

58. Coyne AC, Reichmann WE, Berbig LJ. The relationship between dementia and elder abuse. Am J Psychiatry 1993;150:643–646.

59. Zielinski RJ, Roose SP, Devanand DP, et al. Cardiovascular complications of ECT in depressed patients with cardiac disease. Am J Psychiatry 1993;150:904–909.

60. Hinrichsen GA. Recovery and relapse from major depressive disorder in the elderly. Am J Psychiatry 1992;149:1575–1579.

61. Hinrichsen GA, Hernandez GA. Factors associated with recovery from and relapse into major depressive episode in the elderly. Am J Psychiatry 1993;150:1820–1825.

62. Keller MB, Lavori PW, Mueller TI, et al. Time to recovery, chronicity, and levels of psychopathology in major depression. A 5-year prospective follow-up of 431 subjects. Arch Gen Psychiatry 1992;49:809–816.

63. Alexopoulos GS, Chester JG. Outcomes of geriatric depression. Clin Geriatr Med 1992;8:363–376.

64. Horton-Deutsch SL, Clark DC, Farran CJ. Chronic dyspnea and suicide in elderly men. Hosp Community Psychiatry 1992;43:1198–1203.

65. Beck AT, Brown G, Berchick RJ, Stewart BL, Steer RA. Relationship between hopelessness and ultimate suicide: a replication with psychiatric outpatients. Am J Psychiatry 1990;147:190–195.

66. Zweig RA, Hinrichsen GA. Factors associated with suicide attempts by depressed older adults: a prospective study. Am J Psychiatry 1993;150:1687–1692.

67. Rich CL, Warstadt GM, Nemiroff RA, et al. Suicide, stressors, and the life cycle. Am J Psychiatry 1991;148:524–527. [Published erratum appears Am J Psychiatry 1991;148:960].

Chapter 44
Lung Disorders in the Elderly

Talmadge E. King, Jr.

It is not by muscle, speed, or physical dexterity that great things are achieved, but by reflection, force of character, and judgement; in these qualities old age is usually not only not poorer, but is even richer.

Cicero, 106–43 BC
On Old Age

Pneumonia

Lower respiratory tract infections are a major cause of morbidity among the elderly. In 1977, pneumonia (primarily bacterial) and influenza were the fourth leading causes of death in persons older than age 65. The prevalence of these infections is presumably caused by deterioration of the body's immunologic defenses and the presence of other chronic diseases that further impair immunity and allow colonization of the respiratory tract (1). Hospitalized geriatric patients are at increased risk because the use of respiratory therapy equipment, immunosuppressive drugs, and broad-spectrum antibiotics allows the entrance and proliferation of potential pathogens into the respiratory tract. Patients aged 65 and older account for nearly half of nosocomial pneumonias and more than half of the mortality from all types of nosocomial infections (2). In fact, increasing age is an independent risk factor for the development of nosocomial pneumonias. Other important risk factors include poor nutrition, neuromuscular disease, and tracheal intubation (2).

Clinical Picture

The presentation of pneumonia in the elderly patient may differ markedly from that seen in younger age groups. High spiking fevers, productive cough, and an elevated white cell count may not be seen. Instead, altered mental status, tachypnea, and evidence of dehydration may dominate the clinical picture. Although an alteration in mental status may be the result of hypoxia, septicemia, or volume depletion, meningitis must be excluded. Approximately 20 percent of elderly patients with community-acquired pneumonia may be afebrile on admission (3). The typical chest physical findings may not be heard because of an increase in the anteroposterior (AP) diameter. The characteristic radiographic appearance of lobar or segmental consolidation may be distorted by underlying emphysema, which produces a pattern of incomplete consolidation (Swiss cheese pattern). This pattern may be confused with tuberculosis or abscess formation.

Etiology

When considering the etiology of pneumonia in the elderly, it becomes important to determine whether the disease was acquired in the community or in an institution such as the nursing home or hospital. *Streptococcus pneumoniae*, respiratory viruses, *Hemophilus influenzae*, aerobic gram-negative bacilli, and *S. aureus* are the most frequent causes in outpatients with comorbidity, in patients 60 years of age or older, or both (4). *Moraxella catarrhalis*, *Legionella pneumophila*, *Mycobacterium tuberculosis*, endemic fungi, and enteric gram-negative bacteria are other causes in this setting. In one-third to one-half of cases, no etiology is identified (4). Hospitalization is required for 20 percent of patients initially treated as outpatients, and mortality in this setting is 5 percent to 25 percent. Most deaths occur during the first 7 days of hospitalization (4). Hospitalized and institutionalized persons are most commonly infected with *Klebsiella pneumoniae* and other enteric gram-negative bacilli; *L. pneumophila* and *S. pneumoniae* are also etiologic agents in this setting.

Diagnosis And Treatment

Standard posterioanterior and lateral chest radiographs should be performed on the patient when pneumonia is suspected. Attempts should be made to acquire the patient's sputum for Gram stain or other special stains and culture. A lack of sensitivity and specificity of sputum Gram stain significantly limits its usefulness. However, examination of the sputum may be diagnostic for some pulmonary infections (for example, *Legionella* sp., *Pneumocystis carinii, Mycobacteria*). Routine bacterial cultures also lack sensitivity and specificity, but recovery of organisms not found as part of the normal respiratory flora may be helpful (4). Viral cultures are rarely useful in the initial evaluation of a patient with community-acquired pneumonia (4).

If the patient is obtunded and unable to voluntarily expectorate, catheter suction and suction traps should be used. Other methods for obtaining uncontaminated specimens in patients with severe disease include transtracheal puncture and aspiration, fiberoptic bronchoscopy with a protected brush catheter, and bronchoalveolar lavage, with or without balloon protection. Blood cultures should be obtained from all hospitalized patients with pneumonia. Careful attention must be paid to gas exchange because many of these patients have underlying cardiopulmonary disease and the insult of a superimposed pneumonia can cause respiratory failure. The initial choice of antibiotic depends on the setting of the illness and on the Gram stain results. If indicated, initial therapy should be modified after culture results are available. Community-acquired pneumonia without comorbidity in a patient younger than 60 years of age can be treated initially with a macrolide or tetracycline (4). Patients with comorbidity, and patients who are older than 60 years of age (or both) should be initially treated with a second-generation cephalosporin, trimethoprim-sulfamethoxazole, or beta-lactam-beta-lactamase inhibitor (if *Legionella* sp. is suspected, erythromycin or other macrolide should be added) (4). Patients who are hospitalized with community-acquired pneumonia should have initial therapy started with a second- or third-generation cephalosporin or beta-lactam-beta-lactamase inhibitor, with or without a macrolide (4).

The decision to hospitalize a patient with community-acquired pneumonia is difficult. Several risk factors have been identified that increase the risk of a complicated clinical course or death. When these risk factors exist, especially if multiple, hospitalization is justified (4). Table

44.1 provides a summary of the specific risk factors for mortality or a complicated course of pneumonia. Severe community-acquired pneumonia has a distinctive pattern of etiologic agents: *S. pneumoniae* and *L. pneumophilia* are the most common causes; gram-negative bacilli is impor-

Table 44.1. Risk Factors for Mortality or Complicated Pneumonia That Support Hospitalization of a Patient with Community-Acquired Pneumonia.

Age older than 65 years
Presence of co-existing illnesses or other findings
   Chronic obstructive airway disease, including chronic structural disease of the lung (bronchiectasis, cystic fibrosis)
   Diabetes mellitus; chronic renal failure; congestive heart failure; chronic liver disease of any etiology; postsplenectomy state
   Previous hospitalization within 1 year of the onset of the current pneumonia
   Suspicion of aspiration (gastric or oropharyngeal secretions)
   Altered mental status
   Chronic alcohol abuse or malnutrition
Physical findings
   Respiratory rate in excess of 30 breaths/min
   Diastolic blood pressure ≤60 mm Hg or systolic blood pressure ≤90 mm Hg
   Temperature >38.3°C (101°F).
   Evidence of extrapulmonary sites of disease (e.g., presence of septic arthritis, meningitis)
   Confusion and/or decreased level of consciousness
Laboratory findings
   White blood count $<4 \times 10^9$/liter or $>30 \times 10^9$/liter or absolute neutrophil count below 1×10^9/liter
   PaO_2 >60 mm Hg or $PaCO_2$ >50 mm Hg while breathing room air
   Need for mechanical ventilation
   Evidence of abnormal renal function (serum creatinine >1.2 mg/dL, blood urea nitrogen >20 mg/dL or >7 mmol/liter)
   Presence of certain unfavorable chest radiographic findings, (>1 lobe involvement, presence of a cavity, rapid radiographic spreading, presence of pleural effusion)
   Hematocrit <30% or hemoglobin <9 gm/dL
   Other evidence of sepsis or organ dysfunction (metabolic acidosis, increased prothrombin time, increased partial thromboplastin time, decreased platelets, presence of fibrin split products >1 : 40)
Social circumstances that do not ensure adequate care and observation of the patient

SOURCE: American Thoracic Society. Guidelines for the initial management of adults with community-acquired pneumonia: diagnosis, assessment of severity, and initial antimicrobial therapy. Am Rev Respir Dis 1993;148:1418–1426.

tant in patients with co-existing illnesses; and *Pseudomonas aeruginosa* is rare, except in patients with bronchiectasis (4).

The assessment of the severity of illness is also difficult. The American Thoracic Society statement on community-acquired pneumonia (4) suggested the following criteria for defining severe community-acquired pneumonia and identifying increased likelihood of admission to an intensive care unit for management (especially if more than one of the following is present): 1) respiratory frequency more than 30 breaths per minute at admission; 2) severe respiratory failure defined by a partial pressure of arterial oxygen to fraction of inspired oxygen (PaO_2/FIO_2) ratio more than 250 mm Hg; 3) requirement for mechanical ventilation; 4) chest radiograph showing bilateral involvement or involvement of multiple lobes; 5) an increase in the size of the opacity by 50 percent or greater within 48 hours of admission; 6) shock (systolic blood pressure below 90 mm Hg or diastolic blood pressure below 60 mm Hg); 7) requirement for vasopressors for more than 4 hours; and 8) urine output lower than 20 mL/hr or total urine output lower than 80 mL in 4 hours (unless another explanation is available), or acute renal failure requiring dialysis.

The rate of resolution of the pneumonia in elderly patients may be atypical and thus present concern and a problem regarding management. Fein and colleagues (5)

have reviewed this issue and, as shown in Table 44.2, estimated the rate of resolution of pneumonia in the elderly, the likelihood of initial radiographic deterioration, and the likely presence of residual radiographic abnormalities.

Immunization

Vaccination against the influenza virus protects the high-risk elderly patient from influenza and its complicating pneumonia. Influenza immunization may also reduce mortality after an outbreak (6). The problem lies in the ability of the influenza A virus to antigenically shift about every 10 years. These shifts are often accompanied by a pandemic in a nonimmune population. The chronically debilitated elderly subject bears the brunt of this pandemic. Vaccines recommended for the particular year should be administered yearly to this high-risk population (7). Amantadine hydrochloride, an antiviral compound for the prevention of illness and treatment of symptoms of respiratory tract infections from influenza A viral strains, is a recommended (but not proven) treatment for older persons.

Pneumococcal pneumonia is still a major cause of death in the elderly population in spite of effective antibiotic treatment. A vaccine prepared from purified capsular polysaccharide material from 23 types of pneumococci theoretically should be protective against 85 percent of

Table 44.2. Resolution of Common Pneumonias in the Elderly.

Infection	Initial Radiographic Deterioration	Radiologic Clearing (mo)	Residual Radiologic Abnormalities (%)
S. pneumoniae			
Bacteremic	Majority	3–5	25–35
Nonbacteremic	Occasional	1–3	Rare
Group B *Streptococcus*	Common	1–3	Common
*S. aureus**	Majority	3–5	Common
*H. influenzae**	Occasional	1–5	Occasional
Legionella	Majority	3–5	25
TWAR (*chlamydia*)	Rare	1–3	Occasional
*B. catarrhalis**	Rare	1–3	Unusual, but confused by underlying cancer, COPD, CHF
Gram-negative*	Occasional	3–5	10–20
Viral	Variable depending on organism	Variable	Occasional fibrosis

*Data limited.
CHF = congestive heart failure; COPD = chronic obstructive pulmonary disease.
SOURCE: Fein AM, Feinsilver SH, Niederman MS. Nonresolving and slowly resolving pneumonia. Clin Chest Med 1993;14:555–569.

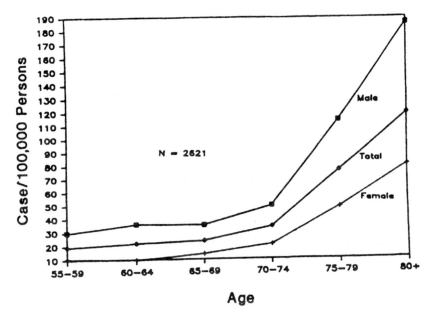

Fig. 44.1. Average age specific tuberculosis case rates (cases/100,000 persons per year) in Arkansas from 1979 through 1985. A sharp increase is apparent at about age 70. (Reproduced by permission from Stead WW, To T. The significance of the tuberculin skin test in elderly persons. Ann Intern Med, 1987;107:837–842.)

the bacterial pneumococcal pneumonias. After a single intramuscular dose, the resultant antibody responses are adequate enough to be 70 percent effective for persons older than 55 years of age (8). Unfortunately, this is not true for patients who are already immunosuppressed. Unlike influenza vaccine, pneumococcal vaccine is given once in a lifetime (9). Mass immunization is not necessary because pneumococcal pneumonia does not occur as pandemics; however, it is estimated that only 10 percent of persons for whom the vaccine is recommended have been vaccinated (9). Pneumococcal vaccine is recommended for asplenic patients with altered immunologic responses, all individuals aged 65 years and older, those with diabetes mellitus, chronic cardiorespiratory disease, or cirrhosis, and those living in special environments or social settings with an identified risk of pneumococcal disease (10).

Tuberculosis

Although tuberculosis is no longer a major health hazard in industrialized countries, it still occurs and is a serious problem among the elderly (11) (Figure 44.1). Unfortunately, the prevalence of tuberculosis is increasing in North America (12). The increase is related mainly to the increased risk that results from infection with the human immunodeficiency virus (HIV). Also, a number of outbreaks of multidrug resistant tuberculosis have been reported in a variety of settings, which highlights the need for renewed knowledge of the management of tuberculosis and an aggressive approach to tuberculosis control (12–14).

Because many geriatric patients have been exposed to tuberculosis infection (latent infection) as children, reactivation may occur during the adult years. It is estimated that in adults with negative chest films and positive tuberculin skin tests, the yearly infection rate will be 82 per 100,000 individuals (15). Among the elderly confined to nursing homes, the rate for active tuberculosis can be extremely high. This rate is enhanced by alcoholism, malnutrition, diabetes, immunosuppressive drugs, neoplasia, and renal dialysis. These data indicate that tuberculosis will continue to be a major health hazard in the geriatric population, and thus it has been recommended that a high index of suspicion for the disease should be maintained, especially for elderly patients who present with multiple medical problems and nonspecific complaints (16).

Clinical Picture

Tuberculosis is easily recognized in the patient who presents with fever, night sweats, weight loss, anorexia, and hemoptyses. Chest radiography demonstrates upper zone infiltrates, with or without cavitation, and a positive tuberculin skin test. Examination of the patient's sputum reveals acid-fast rods, which makes the diagnosis secure. Unfortunately, the typical clinical picture may not be seen in the elderly (17). In one study of 31 geriatric patients who died of tuberculosis, premortem diagnosis was made in only four (18). Rather than demonstrating a well-defined clinical illness, the geriatric patient may show only weight loss and anorexia or fever of unknown origin or may present as pneumonia, bronchitis, or even congestive heart failure with a pleural effusion (19,20). As much as 20 percent of patients with active tuberculosis have a negative tuberculin reaction (21). Instead of a typical chest radiograph demonstrating upper lobe infiltrative or cavitary disease, there may be single or multiple nodules, pleural effusion, miliary spread, or infiltrates in locations other than the upper lobes (22). Miliary tuberculosis can be very difficult to diagnose in the aged. As a result, more elderly individuals die of miliary tuberculosis without a diagnosis than do individuals in any other age group (23). The elderly patient may have a virtually negative chest radiograph with active extrapulmonary sites. It becomes imperative, therefore, to consider the diagnosis of tuberculosis for all geriatric patients with a wide variety of symptoms in whom diagnosis is not readily apparent.

Diagnosis

A high index of suspicion is key to the diagnosis of tuberculosis disease in the elderly (24). All patients suspected of having tuberculosis should have an intradermal skin test with 5U of purified protein derivative (PPD) (Table 44.3). A positive test (10mm or more of induration) indicates previous infection, but, as noted above, a negative test does not exclude the diagnosis (25). Skin test reactivity may be delayed, with a peak after 72 hours, in the elderly. Also, skin test reactivity appears to decline with

Table 44.3. Indications for Tuberculin Skin Testing.

Symptoms (cough, hemoptysis, weight loss) and/or laboratory abnormalities (e.g., radiographic abnormality) suggestive of clinically active TB

Recent contacts of persons known to have or suspected of having clinically active TB

HIV infection

Abnormal chest x-rays compatible with past TB

Other medical conditions that increase the risk of TB (silicosis, injecting drug use, diabetes mellitus, prolonged corticosteroid therapy, immunosuppressive therapy, hematologic and reticuloendothelial diseases, end-stage renal disease, clinical situations associated with rapid weight loss)

At high risk for recent infection with *M. tuberculosis* (immigrants from Asia, Africa, Latin America, and Oceania; medically underserved populations; personnel and long-term residents in hospitals, nursing homes, mental institutions, and correctional facilities)

HIV = human immunodeficiency virus; TB = tuberculosis.
SOURCE: American Thoracic Society. Control of tuberculosis in the United States. Am Rev Respir Dis 1992;146:1623–1633.

aging (26). Thus, a patient with a negative reaction should undergo a repeat test with the same dose after 1 week. A positive test at this time (booster or recall phenomenon) indicates a previously diminished skin hypersensitivity that has been activated by further exposure to tuberculous protein (27). Of importance, it has been shown that, in the elderly, the first significant reaction may not be elicited until the third test with the same dose of antigen. Tuberculosis disease (active tuberculosis in which an individual has an illness involving one or more organs) is diagnosed by positive bacteriologic studies (24).

Sputum, preferably an early-morning specimen, should be collected for 3 consecutive days. Induced sputums by the inhaled aerosol technique may be used for patients who are unable to voluntarily produce sputum. If these methods are ineffective, gastric aspiration or bronchoscopic specimens for culture may be obtained. If the patient has sterile pyuria, hematuria, proteinuria, or a combination of these conditions, the morning urine specimen should be cultured for tuberculosis. All positive cultures should be speciated to rule out atypical mycobacterial infections, and drug sensitivity studies should be performed because of the increased incidence of isoniazid (INH)-resistant strains, especially for both noncompliant patients and those who have received previous therapy. An intravenous pyelogram may further define the extent of renal tuberculosis. Specimen collection, smear examination, culture, methods for identification, and drug susceptibility testing for detection of initial and acquired drug resistance are important issues that have been recently reviewed (28). If the chest radiograph is not helpful, extrapulmonary tuberculosis should be considered. A miliary pattern may not be apparent on the chest radiograph until the disease is far advanced. Other sites that may be sampled, depending on symptoms, clinical findings, and laboratory results, include the bone marrow, spine (cold abscess), joints, meninges, liver, pericardium, and peritoneum.

Treatment

Modern chemotherapy is highly effective in treating tuberculosis. The major challenge in the elderly is to select a therapeutic regimen that produces minimal adverse reactions, is easily administered, and is acceptable to the patient (22). For most patients, a 6-month to 9-month regimen is recommended. Once active tuberculosis is diagnosed in a patient, therapy is often instituted in the hospital. After 2 to 4 weeks, the patient is considered noninfectious and may be discharged. Whether a patient should have normal activities restricted depends on the degree of infectiousness, the response to treatment, the nature of the activities, and who will be exposed in the course of those activities (12).

Short-course chemotherapy with isoniazid, rifampin, and pyrazinamide is currently recommended for pulmonary tuberculosis presumed to be caused by fully susceptible organisms. The 6-month regimen usually includes 2 months (induction phase) of INH (30 mg), rifampin (600 mg), and pyrazinamide (15 to 30 mg/kg, with a maximum dose of 2 gm/day). Then the patient is given 4 months (continuation phase) of daily INH (300 mg) and 600 mg of rifampin or a regimen of INH (15 mg/kg with maximum dose of 900 mg) and rifampin (10 mg/kg with a maximum dose of 2 gm/day) given twice weekly. There are also two protocols for the continuation phase of the 9-month regimen: INH (300 mg) and rifampin (600 mg) daily for the entire period or INH (300 mg) and rifampin (600 mg) daily for 1 to 2 months followed by INH (15 mg/kg with maximum dose of 900 mg) and rifampin (10 mg/kg with a maximum dose of 2 gm/day) given twice weekly. Pyridoxine (25 mg/day) should be given to pre-

vent the peripheral neuropathy associated with INH (24). If one is dealing with or suspects resistant organisms, second-line drugs (ethambutol or streptomycin) should be instituted after consultation with an expert in the treatment of tuberculosis (12). With resistant organisms, initial therapy for the 6-month treatment program includes INH, rifampin, pyrazinamide, and ethambutol (15–25 mg/kg daily, with maximum dose of 2.5 gm) until susceptibility testing is known and the regimen altered on the basis of the results. Streptomycin may be used instead

Table 44.4. High-Priority Candidates for Tuberculosis Preventive Therapy.

Preventive therapy recommended for the following persons with a positive tuberculin test, regardless of age:[a]
  Persons with known or suspected HIV infection[b]
  Close contacts of persons with infectious clinically active TB[b]
  Recent tuberculin skin text converters (≥10 mm increase within a 2-yr period for those <35 yr; ≥15 mm increase for those ≥35 yr). All children <2 yr old with a >10 mm skin test are included in this category
  Persons with medical conditions that have been reported to increase the risk of TB (e.g., diabetes mellitus, prolonged corticosteroid therapy, immunosuppressive therapy, some hematologic and reticuloendothelial diseases, injecting drug use, end-stage renal disease, and clinical situations associated with rapid weight loss)
Preventive therapy recommended for the following persons in high-incidence groups with a positive tuberculin test who are <35 yr and do not have additional risk factors:[c]
  Non-U.S.-born persons from high-prevalence countries (e.g., countries in Latin America, Asia, and Africa)
  Medically underserved low-income populations, including high-risk racial or ethnic populations, especially black, Hispanic, and Native American groups
  Residents of facilities for long-term care (e.g., correctional institutions, nursing homes, and mental institutions)

[a] Persons with fibrotic infiltrates on chest radiography thought to represent old, healed TB and those with silicosis, who were formerly considered candidates for preventive therapy, should receive 4-month multidrug chemotherapy (See ATS/CDC Treatment Statement).
[b] Persons in these categories may be given preventive therapy in the absence of a positive tuberculin test in some circumstances.
[c] Staff of facilities in which an individual with current TB would pose a risk to large numbers of susceptible persons (e.g., correctional institutions, nursing homes, mental institutions, other health-care facilities, schools, and child care facilities may also be considered for preventive therapy.
SOURCE: American Thoracic Society. Control of tuberculosis in the United States. Am Rev Respir Dis 1992;146:1623–1633.

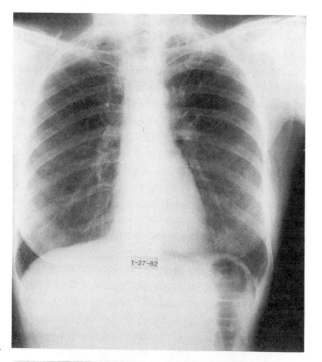

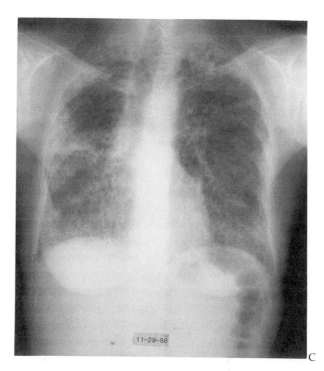

A

1-27-82

11-29-88

C

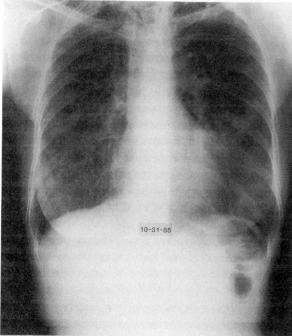

B

10-31-85

Fig. 44.2. Progressive pulmonary *Mycobacterium avium* complex tuberculosis. (*A*) Chest x-ray taken 6 years before diagnosis in a 70-year-old woman revealed ill-defined, patchy nodular opacities in lingula and right middle lobe areas. This chest x-ray was taken because of cough. (*B*) Chest x-ray taken 3 years before diagnosis revealed bilateral progressive nodular opacities in the mid lung zones. At this time, the woman complained of cough productive of scant sputum and breathlessness with exertion (climbing more than 2 flights of stairs). (*C*) Current chest x-ray revealed marked progression of disease with diffuse, bilateral reticular and irregular nodular opacities throughout all lung zones and evidence of volume loss with retraction of the hila upward. At this time, the woman complained of cough productive of scant sputum and breathlessness with exertion (walking 20–50 feet on level ground). Sputum cultures grew *Mycobacterium avium* and lung biopsy revealed necrotizing granulomas. (Reproduced by permission from Wade JF III, King TE Jr. Infiltrative and interstitial lung disease in the elderly. Clin Chest Med 1993;14:501–521.)

of ethambutol. For immunocompetent patients treated for the first time and who are fully compliant with the prescribed regimen, there is a better than 95 percent likelihood of a successful outcome of the treatment (12).

Isoniazid-induced hepatitis is a real problem in the elderly, particularly for those with active liver disease or impaired liver function. Because rifampin in combination with isoniazid increases the risk of further liver damage, streptomycin may be substituted for a total of 3 months. Streptomycin, however, should be avoided, if possible, because of its nephrotoxicity and ototoxicity, especially in elderly individuals. In low doses (15 mg/kg), the ocular complications of ethambutol are minimal (impairment of color vision and visual acuity). However, when ethambutol is used with isoniazid in a two-drug regimen, the recommended dosage is 25 mg/kg. At this dose, visual problems may occur, and the patient should receive monthly eye testing. Corticosteroids may occasionally be indicated in tuberculosis of the central nervous system (CNS), in tuberculous pericarditis, and in tuberculous peritonitis (29,30). Corticosteroids are thought to be effective in reducing fibrous adhesions.

Isoniazid prophylaxis for 6 months to 1 year is recommended for all high-risk patients, regardless of age, who have a positive skin test (induration of at least 12 mm) without culture evidence of active disease (31) (Table 44.4). Recent experience indicates that preventive treatment of elderly persons is effective in reducing the incidence of tuberculosis and that the incidence of toxicity from isoniazid is low (32). A year of preventive therapy is recommended if radiographic evidence of disease is present.

Mycobacterium Avium Complex

Pulmonary disease caused by nontuberculous mycobacteria (M. avium, M. intracellulare, M. scrofulaceum) are uncommon, but cases of M. avium complex appear to be rising (33–35). These opportunistic pathogens cause an estimated 2000 or more cases of infection annually in the United States (36). Despite intensive investigation, the exact transmission of M. avium complex remains an enigma. The organism is found in dust, soil, water, poultry, and other animals (35,36) Consequently, the prevailing assumption is that the disease is acquired directly from the environment by inhalation of ambient air.

The disease typically occurs in elderly men with underlying chronic lung disease, but increasingly, is being reported in patients without predisposing conditions and among elderly women (35,37–39). Most patients present with persistent cough and purulent sputum, usually without fever or weight loss (37). Radiographically, pulmonary disease caused by M. avium complex generally initially resembles reinfection tuberculosis and predominately involves the upper lobes (40). Two other patterns have recently been reported: progressive, multinodular opacities (37); and initial involvement of the periphery of the lingula or the right middle lobe (38,39). Hilar adenopathy, volume loss, and cavitary disease is not common (37,38). Iseman has noted that these apparently normal patients have a high prevalence of pectus excavatum (an abnormally narrow distance between the sternum and vertebrae), thoracic scoliosis, and mitral valve prolapse (35). He hypothesized that some patients with M. avium complex may have multisystem, connective-tissue disorder that renders them vulnerable to these environmental microbes (35). Reich and Johnson (39) suggested that habitual voluntary suppression of expectoration may account for the progression of this process in some women.

The natural history of the pulmonary infection with M. avium complex can be indolent. This often causes a delay in diagnosis and treatment. Progressive disease clearly occurs and can be the cause of death in these patients (Figure 44.2). Consequently, it is being increasingly recommended that patients be diagnosed and treated early in the course of their disease. Arresting this disabling and potentially lethal disease is believed to be worth a finite period of discomfort that may result from the therapy (35). Choosing the right medication to treat this disease is problematic. However, multidrug therapy may arrest or even cure the disease in some patients (35). In vitro susceptibility testing is strongly recommended as a method to select the drugs most likely to be successful in the treatment of M. avium complex because severe drug resistance is the rule. The possible benefits of resection of localized disease is unknown (41).

Pulmonary Aspiration

Aspiration of foreign material into the airways represents a debilitating and life-threatening problem for the elderly patient. Conditions predisposing to aspiration in this age group include altered level of consciousness, diminished or absent gag and cough reflexes, anesthesia, endotracheal intubation, the use of nasogastric tubes, tracheotomy during resuscitative attempts, and alcoholism (42). In a study of nursing home residents with the diagnosis of acute myocardial infarction (MI), autopsy revealed a 33 percent incidence of aspiration pneumonia (43). In these subjects, the aspiration was considered to be the cause of death. In general, aspiration has a high mortality (40% to 60%), which correlates with the amount of material aspirated and to the age and underlying general condition of the patient.

Types of Aspiration

Acid Aspiration (Mendelson's Syndrome)
The single most important factor in aspiration of gastric contents is the pH of the gastric juice. The pH of normal fasting gastric juice is between 1.5 and 2.4 (44). A pH below 2.5 appears to be critical in terms of resultant lung destruction (45). The pathologic picture is one of the adult respiratory distress syndrome (ARDS). There are areas of hemorrhage and atelectasis and an outpouring of protein-rich fluid. This progresses to destruction of the alveolar spaces, which become filled with necrotic debris and inflammatory cells (46). During the first 24 hours, the lung is sterile; however, if the patient survives several days, superinfection can occur (47).

Clinically, there is marked respiratory distress characterized by tachypnea, wheezing, cyanosis, and change in mental status. Hypoxemia is severe and unresponsive to high oxygen concentrations, indicating a large right-to-left shunt. Arterial hypotension is seen in 25 percent of cases. The chest radiograph demonstrates diffuse alveolar infiltrates with a normal cardiac silhouette (Figure 44.3). If aspiration of food particles accompanies the acid aspiration, bronchoscopy and removal are indicated, usually after endotracheal intubation. Corticosteroids and prophylactic administration of antibiotics are unproven modes of therapy and should not be begun empirically.

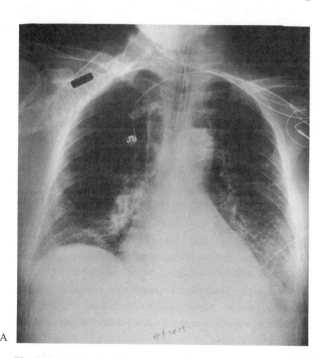
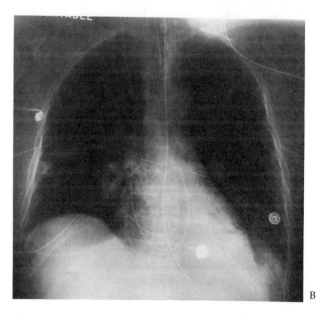

Fig. 44.3. Aspiration of gastric contents. (*A*) Chest x-ray taken several hours after the aspiration of gastric contents. (*B*) Chest x-ray taken of the same patient 24 hours after aspiration of gastric contents. Fiberoptic bronchoscopy revealed acute inflammation of the airways and food particles. Partial atelectasis of the left lower lobe persists although remarkable clearing of the infiltrate in the right lower lobe has occurred.

Superimposed bacterial pneumonia in patients with acid aspiration, however, carries considerable morbidity and mortality; therefore, recurrence of fever, purulent sputum, leukocytosis, new or expanding pulmonary infiltrates, unexplained clinical deterioration, increasing hypoxemia, and pathogens in sputum should prompt appropriate antimicrobial therapy. Positive end-expiratory pressure may be required to correct the hypoxemia. Because of the tremendous outpouring of plasma into the lung, hypoxemia results, and careful attention must be given to fluid replacement. Because there may be pre-existing cardiac disease in the elderly, large volume fluid replacement should be monitored with a Swan-Ganz catheter in place.

Aspiration of Solid Particles
The clinical manifestations that follow aspiration of solid particles are determined by the size of the particles. Occlusion of the large upper airways may cause acute suffocation and be immediately relieved by the Heimlich maneuver (a quick upward thrust over the abdomen causing a sudden elevation of the diaphragm that forces air through the trachea). Smaller objects reach and occlude more peripheral airways and result in eventual atelectasis and bacterial superinfection with abscess formation. Unexplained atelectasis is a definite indication for bronchoscopy (Figure 44.3). Failure to remove the obstructing object within 2 to 3 weeks may result in recurrent pneumonitis, bronchiectasis, lung abscesses, emphysema, or all of these conditions. Patients who aspirate large volumes of inert fluids such as barium, saline, and nasogastric feeding solutions, cause transient, self-limited hypoxemia and simple mechanical obstruction. Immediate tracheal suctioning usually results in immediate resolution, and further therapy should be aimed at prevention.

Chronic Aspiration of Gastric Contents
Chronic aspiration of gastric contents usually results from mechanical or neuromuscular problems. Disorders that interfere with the mechanical properties of swallowing include esophageal strictures, esophageal diverticula, hiatal hernias, nasogastric tubes, tracheostomy, and esophageal carcinoma. Neuromuscular problems include a myotonic esophagus and absent or poor gag reflex caused by a number of neurologic diseases. Recurrent aspiration often occurs at night, and the patient may report nocturnal dyspnea and wheezing. In most cases, the patient is seen for an infectious complication of chronic aspiration and presents with an infectious pneumonia, usually found in the dependent portions of the lung (i.e., the posterior segments of the upper lobes and the superior segments of the lower lobes). If the patient sleeps in the upright position, the basilar segments of the lower lobes are involved. The pneumonia may progress to lung abscess and emphysema. Occasionally, recurrent and small aspirations, particularly with hiatal hernia, can result in lower-zone pulmonary fibrosis without the history of recurrent pneumonia (48). Treatment consists of careful attention to oral hygiene because mouth flora, including anaerobes, are most often responsible for the infectious complications; proper use of antibiotics; and correction of the anatomic problem, if possible.

Mineral Oil Aspiration
Aspirations from the injudicious use of mineral oils may take several forms. There may be an acute pneumonitis with cough, sputum, and basilar infiltrates on chest radiographs and fat-filled macrophages present in the sputum. These patients may also be relatively asymptomatic except for progressive dyspnea and may develop lower-zone interstitial markings (lipoid pneumonia) or pulmonary nodules that pathologically are lipoid granuloma. In either case, history of the use of oily nose drops may be obtained, and discontinuing this practice may result in marked improvement (44).

Aspiration Causing Lung Abscess
Lung abscess frequently is one of the late complications of pulmonary aspiration. The presentation often is insidious, with weight loss, low-grade fever, and copious, foul-smelling sputum production as the prominent findings. Diagnosis requires appropriate identification of the infecting agent through cultures taken of the material obtained from transtracheal aspiration, blood, pleural fluid, bronchoalvolar lavage (BAL) and, occasionally, transthoracic needle aspiration. Exclusion of other causes of cavitary lung disease such as tuberculosis, fungal infection, carcinoma, cavitary infarction (i.e., bland or septic embolism or vasculitis), infected cyst, or bullae must be

determined. Fiberoptic bronchoscopy should be used to exclude an obstructing endobronchial lesion (tumor or foreign body).

Therapy demands drainage of the involved lung (postural drainage, steam inhalation, and, rarely, transthoracic needle aspiration or tube drainage) and antibiotic therapy. Antimicrobial therapy directed at anaerobes and the microaerophilic oral flora is important. Penicillin is usually adequate and has been the first choice of treatment. Recently, use of penicillin has been questioned because of the presence of beta-lactamase-producing organisms resistant to penicillin in as much as 60 percent of patients. Also, clinical trials have shown that clindamycin is superior to high-dose penicillin for the treatment of lung abscess (49). Consequently, clindamycin is thought to be the drug of choice by many authorities. Patients with mild symptoms and no major medical problems can be given parenteral penicillin (procaine penicillin, 600,000 U intramuscularly every 6 hr, or aqueous penicillin G, 5–20 million U/day intravenously in divided doses) or oral penicillin (500 mg, every 6 hr) and combined with 2 gm of metronidazole (an agent with activity against penicillin-resistant strains). Patients given parenteral penicillin can be switched to oral penicillin if clinical improvement occurs within several days and they can be continued on oral therapy until resolution of the cavity. In patients with severe symptomatic disease, therapy with intravenous aqueous penicillin (2 million U, every 4 hr) may be required for 5 to 10 days. If emphysema is present, chest tube drainage is required. Occasionally, thoracotomy with rib resection is necessary to drain loculated areas of pus. It should be noted that fever may persist for several days to 3 weeks despite adequate therapy, and it may take several more weeks for resolution of the cavity.

Pulmonary Embolism

Pulmonary embolism (PE) is responsible for approximately 50,000 deaths yearly, and about 300,000 to 600,000 patients suffer nonfatal PE, deep venous thrombosis (DVT), or both each year in the United States (50,51). In 60 percent of these patients, the diagnosis of PE is not suspected (52). A recent epidemiologic study found that the annual incidence rates per 1000 for persons age 65 to 69

years for PE and DVT were 1.3 and 1.8, respectively. Both rates increased steadily, to 2.8 and 3.1, respectively for persons aged 85 to 89 years (53). Pulmonary embolism results from venous thrombi that become lodged in the pulmonary arterial circulation. The elderly patient is at significant risk for the development of venous thrombosis because the patient is more likely to be inactive, at bed rest, and have concurrent clinical phlebitis, congestive heart failure, venous insufficiency, or carcinoma. The older patient is also at greater risk in the postoperative state (especially after pelvic or hip surgery) because of prolonged immobilization. In addition, because of already compromised cardiac and pulmonary function, PE represents a dangerous and often fatal event for the older patient (54). The diagnosis and management of DVT and PE has been recently reviewed (51,55).

Clinical Picture

The clinical picture of PE is dictated by both the size and extent of the embolic episode and the pre-existing cardiopulmonary reserve. Autopsy studies show that most cases of PE go unrecognized (Figure 44.4). A recent autopsy study of 3000 hospitalized geriatric patients determined that massive pulmonary thromboembolism in the main pulmonary trunk, branches, or both was the major cause of death in 21.2 percent of the patients (56). The diagnosis was not clinically suspected in 74.1 percent of these subjects (56). The missed diagnosis may result from failure of the medical profession to suspect the diagnosis or from the relative absence of symptoms in the patient. With massive PE, sudden syncope, chest pain, and acute dyspnea are common. Physical examination may reveal hypotension and signs of pulmonary hypertension, such as increased pulmonic component of second heart sound, tricuspid insufficiency, and distended neck veins.

With medium-sized PE, pleuritic chest pain, dyspnea, and hemoptyses are seen. Physical examination may be nonrevealing or demonstrate a pleural friction rub or findings of a pleural effusion. Mild temperature elevations may occur, but not higher than 39°C (57). In the hospitalized geriatric patient, symptoms may be limited to tachypnea, tachycardia, and a changing mental status. Diffuse wheezing is heard in a small percentage of patients and may be associated with pulmonary edema (58).

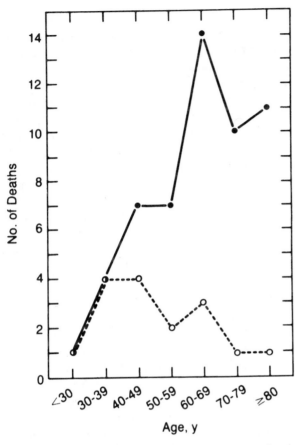

Fig. 44.4. Comparison of correct antemortem diagnosis of pulmonary embolism versus patient age. Solid line indicates all patients; broken line indicates patients with correct antemortem diagnosis. (Reproduced by permission from Gross JS, Neufeld RR, Libow LS, et al. Autopsy study of the elderly institutionalized patient: review of 234 autopsies. Arch Intern Med 1988;148:173–176.)

The third syndrome is insidious and is caused by recurrent episodes of small emboli that occlude the pulmonary arterial microvasculature and result in a picture of slowly progressive cor pulmonale. This syndrome is very difficult to differentiate from primary pulmonary hypertension, although the latter is more common in younger females with concomitant Raynaud's phenomenon and a familial predisposition (59). In all patients with suspected PE, a search for DVT must be undertaken. More often than not, signs of DVT including edema, unilateral calf enlargement, tenderness, positive Homan's sign, and palpable cord are absent.

Diagnosis

When PE is suspected, the diagnosis must be pursued in a logical sequence. Routine laboratory tests should be obtained to eliminate the many other possible diagnoses. Approximately 30 percent of patients with suspected PE on clinical grounds are actually proven positive. Although 60 percent have an abnormal ventilation-perfusion scan, only about 50 percent of patients have documented PE (i.e., 50 percent are false positive).

Arterial blood gases usually reveal mild to moderate hypoxemia, a widened $P(A-a)O_2$ gradient, and hypocarbia. A normal arterial blood gas, however, does not exclude the diagnosis of PE. The electrocardiogram (ECG) is usually normal, but an $S_1Q_3T_3$ pattern, evidence of right ventricular strain, right atrial abnormalities (P pulmonale), and supraventricular arrhythmias–particularly atrial fibrillation–may be present. However, tachycardia and nonspecific ST-T wave changes are most commonly present. In patients with a normal ECG at presentation, serial testing may reveal diagnostic features of embolism (60). The chest x-ray is usually normal or may have varying combinations of subtle or gross findings such as elevated hemidiaphragm, regional oligemia, pleural effusion, pleural-based infiltrate (Hampton's hump), subsegmental atelectasis, changes in the size of the pulmonary arteries, and right ventricular enlargement. Pneumothorax should be excluded. The principal value of the chest radiograph in the evaluation of acute PE is to exclude diagnoses that clinically mimic PE and to aid in the interpretation of the ventilation-perfusion scan (61).

The next diagnostic test is usually a perfusion lung scan with at least four views. A normal perfusion scan excludes the diagnosis of PE. If a perfusion defect is present, a ventilation scan should be performed, with particular attention given to the views that clearly show the perfusion defects. Matched ventilation-perfusion defects are characteristic of parenchymal diseases; mismatched defects, such as normal ventilation in zones of reduced perfusion, are characteristic of vascular obstruction. Therefore, a high-probability scan (i.e., greater than 87 percent frequency of PE) is characterized by perfusion defects substantially larger than the radiographic abnormalities, one or more large segmental defects, or two or more moderate-size ventilation-perfusion mismatches, without a corresponding radiographic abnormality. The clinical relevance of matched and mismatched subsegmental defects and multiple small perfusion defects is unknown. Many of these patients (as much as 40%) are found to have PE as confirmed by angiography.

If a high index of suspicion remains in the presence of a low-probability or indeterminate ventilation-perfusion scan, lower extremity venography, pulmonary angiography, or both should be performed. Venography has fewer complications than does angiography, but 20 percent to 30 percent of patients with documented PE have negative venograms. If the venogram reveals proximal DVT (above the knee), full anticoagulation is recommended. The venogram may be negative because the source of the thrombosis may be from the deep pelvic veins, the renal veins, the right atrium, or the vena cava.

Pulmonary angiography is considered the gold standard of tests and should be performed whenever doubt exists as to the correct diagnosis or when major therapy is contemplated (e.g., thrombolytic therapy, inferior vena caval ligation, or embolectomy). Approximately 50 percent of patients suspected of having PE require angiogram, of which only one-third are found to be positive. A normal angiogram excludes the diagnosis of PE. The combined morbidity and mortality from pulmonary angiography is 1 percent to 2 percent. Data from the Prospective Investigation of Pulmonary Embolism Diagnosis (PIOPED) study showed that major complications of pulmonary angiography among patients 70 years of age or older were not more frequent than complications among younger patients. However, renal failure (either major or minor) was more frequent in the elderly patients [62]. Dialysis was not required in these patients because the most frequent complication was either an elevation of the serum creatinine from previously normal levels to 2.1 mg/100 mL or more or an increase in a previously abnormal serum creatinine to 2.1 mg/100 mL or more [62].

Treatment

PE is a complication of DVT. Therefore, prevention is the key to successful management of PE. High-risk patients should be carefully monitored for the development of DVT, and a substantial number of patients with DVT may have asymptomatic PE [63]. Useful monitoring techniques are fibrinogen leg scanning, impedance plethysmography, Doppler flow studies with ultrasound (duplex ultrasound), and contrast venography.

Prophylactic therapy (e.g., 5000 U of low-dose heparin given subcutaneously every 12 hr) is effective in preventing DVT in selected high-risk patients. Treatment with aspirin and sulfinpyrazone appears to reduce the likelihood of DVT after hip replacement, especially among women. Early ambulation and elastic stockings are not protective in preventing DVT. Supportive care aimed at the treatment of hypoxemia (using oxygen therapy), hypotension, and reduced cardiac output is of first importance.

Heparin is the drug of choice for most patients with PE [64] and should be started as soon as the diagnosis is suspected on clinical grounds; the drug can be discontinued later if the workup is negative. Heparin prevents further clot formation, but it cannot prevent detachment of pre-existing venous thrombi. The ideal heparin regimen for PE is unknown. A useful regimen is to begin anticoagulation with a large intravenous bolus (5000 to 20,000 U), followed by a continuous infusion of 1000 to 1500 U/hr, or enough to prolong the whole-blood clotting time or the activated partial thromboplastin time (aPTT) 1.5 times control. Recent data suggest that use of weight-based nomograms for IV heparin result in significantly better early anticoagulation and fewer recurrences [65]. Starting with an initial heparin bolus of 80 U/kg followed by an intravenous infusion of 18 U/kg/hr, the subsequent dose of heparin is adjusted by the aPTT in the following way [65]:

aPTT <1.2 × control	80 U/kg bolus, then infusion of 4 U/kg/hr
aPTT 1.2–1.5 × control	40 U/kg bolus, then infusion of 2 U/kg/hr
aPTT 1.5–2.3 × control	no change
aPTT 2.3–3.0 × control	decrease infusion rate by 2 U/kg/hr
aPTT >3.0 × control	Hold infusion for 1 hr, then decrease infusion rate by 3 U/kg/hr

Full-dose heparin is usually maintained for at least 7 to 10 days. Most patients are maintained on anticoagulation therapy for at least 3 months, unless persistent risk factors are present that would prolong the therapy. Warfarin (adequate to prolong the prothrombin time 1.5 times the control value) or subcutaneous heparin (7500 U every 12 hr) are the two options for prolonged anticoagulation protection (64,66). Long-term heparin therapy represents a serious potential problem for the elderly (67), but older age is not a risk factor for bleeding with warfarin therapy (68). Complications with heparin therapy include bleeding in as much as 8 percent of patients, reversible thrombocytopenia, hyperkalemia, osteoporosis, and drug interactions (69,70). Increasingly, the International Normalized Ratio (INR) is used to monitor warfarin therapy (71). The INR corrects the plasma thromboplastin (PT) ratios obtained with thromboplastin reagents with different degrees of responsiveness to the warfarin-induced coagulation defect by standardizing the result against a common international reference preparation (71). The formula for calculation of INR is INR = (PT of patient/PT normal)^{ISI}, using the power representing the International Sensitivity Index (ISI) defined for the specific batch of thromboplastin used in the laboratory in which the test is performed. The goal for treatment of DVT and PE is to maintain the INR in the range of 2 to 3, with a target of 2.5.

In the presence of contraindications to anticoagulation, such as high risk of bleeding, recurrent emboli despite adequate anticoagulation, or severe embolization such that a recurrence may be fatal, surgical interruption of the inferior vena cava by vena caval plication, clipping, ligation, or insertion of a Mobin-Uddin umbrella or Greenfield filter is indicated. Documentation of proximal DVT should be obtained before surgical interruption is performed.

Thrombolytic therapy warrants consideration in patients with massive pulmonary emboli (i.e., involvement of more than two lobar arteries), pulmonary emboli accompanied by shock, submassive pulmonary emboli superimposed on underlying cardiopulmonary dysfunction leading to physiologic decompensation, and iliofemoral thrombosis to prevent chronic postphlebitic problems. Thrombolytic therapy does not replace heparin therapy but is instituted for 24 to 48 hours before heparin to accelerate clot resolution. Absolute contraindications include active internal bleeding and cerebrovascular disease or a surgical procedure performed within the previous 2 months. Thrombolytic therapy is administered by giving a loading dose, followed by a constant infusion

dose intravenously (a loading dose of 250,000 IU of streptokinase for 30 minutes, then 100,000 IU/hr for 24 hours; a loading bolus dose 4400 IU/kg of urokinase for 10 minutes, then 4400 IU/kg for 12 to 24 hours; or 100 mg of recombinant human tissue-type plasmogen activator for 2 hr). Therapeutic monitoring is performed by measurement of the whole blood euglobulin lysis time, the thrombin time, or the partial thromboplastin time (PTT) 4 to 6 hours after institution of the thrombolytic agent to identify and confirm activation of the fibrinolytic system. Further laboratory monitoring is not required after systemic fibrinolysis has been established. The PTT should be measured before anticoagulation therapy is started. These thrombolytic agents are extremely expensive and have not been proven to have a positive impact on morbidity, mortality, or recurrence. Complications include bleeding (severe in 5% to 25% of patients), urticaria (in approximately 5% to 15% of patients), and low grade fever (in approximately 25% of patients).

Acute embolectomy is indicated for patients with angiographically proven massive embolism and persistent shock despite medical therapy. Selected patients with chronic pulmonary emboli may benefit from thromboendarterectomy.

In the presence of antithrombin III deficiency, heparin therapy is ineffective, and oral anticoagulation is required. Some experts feel that antithrombin III levels should be determined as part of the initial evaluation of every patient in whom anticoagulation therapy is contemplated and should be followed in assessing the response to therapy. Patients with familial antithrombin III deficiency probably should be treated for life with anticoagulants.

Interstitial Lung Diseases

The interstitial lung diseases (ILD) are a heterogeneous group of diseases that are progressive, potentially fatal processes characterized by an interstitial and intra-alveolar inflammatory process, interstitial fibrosis, and revision of the distal lung architecture. Although these diseases are denoted as interstitial (i.e., involving that area bounded by the alveolar epithelial and endothelial basement membrane), the entire lung parenchyma can be involved. This heterogeneous group of disorders can be

Table 44.5. Etiologic Classification of Interstitial Lung Diseases.

Category	Examples
Idiopathic	Idiopathic pulmonary fibrosis
	BOOP
Connective tissue diseases*	Progressive systemic sclerosis
	Rheumatoid arthritis
	Polymyositis-dermatomyositis
	SLE
Occupational and environmental exposures	Inorganic dust diseases (silicosis, asbestosis, coal worker's dust)
	Hypersensitivity pneumonitis
	Farmer's lung
	Bird fancier's lung
Drug-induced	Drug-induced SLE
	Immunosuppressive and cytotoxic agents (bleomycin, methotrexate, busulfan, BCNU, radiation therapy, gold salts)
	Antimicrobial agents (nitrofurantoin, sulfonamides, penicillin)
	Vasoactive and neuroactive agents (heroin, methadone, barbiturates)
Primary diseases	Sarcoidosis (third stage)*
	Pulmonary histiocytosis X*
	Lymphangitic carcinomatosis
	Vasculitides
	Chronic infection, especially tuberculosis
	Chronic pulmonary edema
	Chronic gastric aspiration
	Pulmonary amyloidosis

*Rare for onset to occur in the elderly.
BCNU = carmustine; BOOP = bronchiolitis obliterans organizing pneumonia; SLE = systemic lupus erythematosus.
SOURCE: King TE Jr, Acute and chronic pulmonary disease in the elderly. In: Schrier R, ed. Geriatric medicine. The care of the elderly. Philadelphia: Saunders, 1990:273–323.

classified together because of common clinical, radiographic, physiologic, and pathologic features. Approximately two-thirds of these diseases have no known cause and are, therefore, classified by their clinical features, pathologic features, or both (72) (Table 44.5). The most common causes of ILDs are those related to occupational and environmental exposures, especially exposure to inorganic dust. Sarcoidosis is the most prevalent ILD of unknown etiology, but it occurs uncommonly in the elderly. Idiopathic pulmonary fibrosis (IPF), with or without associated connective-tissue disease, is also common, but most other conditions associated with ILD are rare.

Pathogenesis

A common pathogenetic sequence underlies most ILD regardless of etiology (Figure 44.5). The initial step appears to be injury to lung cells as a result of 1) direct toxicity to endothelial or epithelial cells from drugs or poisons; 2) generation of toxic oxygen radicals such as superoxide anion and hydrogen peroxide; 3) release of mediators and enzymes such as collagenase, elastase, beta glucuronidase from inflammatory cells (macrophages and neutrophils); and 4) alterations in the immune system, with deposition of immune complexes in the lung (vasculitic syndromes, IPF, some connective-tissue diseases, and histiocytosis X).

After injury to lung cells, several responses occur such as endothelial cell injury, resulting in the proliferation of neighboring cells; damage on the alveolar surface, causing type II epithelial cells to proliferate; and, in both instances, influx of inflammatory and immune effector cells, which results in alveolitis. The precise pathway leading from acute injury to fibrosis is not known. The major mechanism appears to be continued exposure to the inciting agent. In the presence of chronic alveolitis, derangement in the interstitium occurs and eventually leads to loss of alveolar gas exchanging units because of fibrosis and honeycombing.

UNKNOWN STIMULUS/INSULT

ACUTE ALVEOLITIS

EPITHELIAL INJURY & AIRSPACE EXUDATION

PERSISTENT ALVEOLITIS

PROGRESSIVE ALVEOLAR INJURY

FIBROBLAST PROLIFERATION & CONNECTIVE TISSUE SYNTHESIS

INTRAALVEOLAR & INTERSITIALFIBROSIS

END STAGE LUNG

("HONEYCOMB LUNG")

Fig. 44.5. Pathogenesis of interstitial lung disease. The specific stimulus and site of the initiating events remain unclear. An alveolitis occurs that can both damage the lung and initiate the complex process of repair. The extent of the alveolar epithelial and/or capillary endothelial injury appears to determine whether chronic inflammation and ultimately fibrosis develops. (Reproduced by permission from: Wade JF III, King TE Jr. Infiltrative and interstitial lung disease in the elderly. Clin Chest Med 1993;14:501–521.)

Clinical Picture

The typical patient with interstitial lung disease is 55 years of age or older and presents with the insidious onset of breathlessness with exercise and nonproductive cough (73). Other clinical manifestations depend on the underlying process, but include constitutional symptoms such as fever, weight loss, fatigue, and myalgias and arthralgias. Physical examination commonly reveals bibasilar and end-inspiratory dry rales ("velcro" rales). Clubbing of the fingers is common in some patients (those with IPF) and rare in others (those with sarcoidosis). Signs of pulmonary hypertension and cor pulmonale are generally seen only in advanced disease.

Diagnosis

The most important step in the evaluation of a patient with ILD is a carefully taken clinical history. Particular emphasis should be placed on possible occupational and environmental exposures. A strict chronologic listing of the patient's employment, including specific duties and known exposures to organic and inorganic dusts, gases, and chemicals, is important. Review of the home environment, especially as it relates to pets, air conditioners, and so forth, is valuable.

After the initial evaluation, the next most important issue is to confirm the diagnosis and determine the stage of disease so that decisions about prognosis and therapy can be made. Fiberoptic bronchoscopy with transbronchial lung biopsy may be the initial procedure of choice in many cases, especially when sarcoidosis, lymphangitic carcinomatosis, eosinophilic pneumonia, Goodpasture's syndrome, or infection is suspected. In many cases, open lung biopsy is required because a larger quantity of tissue, usually from two sites (i.e., an area of obvious abnormality and one that appears normal) is necessary to adequately define the process, especially in IPF. This approach decreases the sampling error that often occurs with transbronchial lung biopsy and allows the clinician to distinguish between active inflammation and end-stage fibrosis.

It is often difficult to decide whether to obtain a tissue diagnosis in elderly patients. Many clinicians opt for empiric treatment. Open lung biopsy is a low-morbidity procedure in experienced hands; therefore, tissue diagnosis is recommended if no other contraindications to anesthesia or surgery exist and if treatment with corticosteroids or cytotoxic agents is contemplated. The risks of open lung biopsy include persistent bronchopleural fistula, perioperative cardiac events, thoracic infection, postthoracotomy pain, and even death. Most of these problems occur in individuals with diseases other than ILD, for example, immunocompromised patients such as those with acquired immunodeficiency syndrome (AIDS) or cancer. Lung biopsy performed by stereoscopic thoracoscopy offers further reduction in morbidity, mortality, and hospital costs, especially for patients who are most ill, obese, or debilitated. In our experience, this method provides ample tissue, is very well tolerated, and offers advantages over traditional open lung biopsy procedures because of fewer days of hospitalization, a shorter period of thoracostomy tube drainage, and lower rates of postthoracotomy pain syndrome.

An elevated erythrocyte sedimentation rate (ESR) and hypergammaglobulinemia are commonly observed. Positive antinuclear antibodies (ANA), rheumatoid factors, and circulating immune complexes have been identified in many of these patients, even in the absence of a defined connective-tissue disorder, which may simply be a reflection of the higher incidence of ANA found in the elderly (74,75).

The chest x-ray is useful in suggesting the presence, but not the stage, of ILD and may be normal in as much 10 percent of these patients. The most common radiographic abnormalities are a reticular or a reticulonodular pattern. A coarse reticular pattern or multiple cystic areas (honeycombing) is a late radiographic finding and portends a poor prognosis. Radiographic evidence of pleural disease is uncommon in IPF, and its presence suggests a concomitant second process (e.g., a connective-tissue disease) as the underlying cause of the ILD. Increasingly, high-resolution computed tomography (HRCT) scanning (scans obtained with 1–2-mm collimation and reconstruction of the image with the use of a high-spatial-frequency algorithm) (76) is being used to diagnose and follow the course of ILD. HRCT scanning is more sensitive and specific than chest x-ray. HRCT is particularly helpful in symptomatic patients with a normal x-ray. Furthermore, HRCT scanning correlates better with measurements of disease activity and predicts the development of more severe disease better than routine chest x-ray. Also, HRCT evaluation is helpful in supporting the diagnosis when the patient cannot undergo lung biopsy because of relative contraindications–for example, the debilitated elderly patient, the patient with end-stage disease (honeycomb lung), or the patient with another major organ failure or systemic illness.

Pulmonary function abnormalities are common. The classic findings are consistent with a restrictive impairment (i.e., vital capacity and total lung capacity are reduced), and unless a complicating airway disease such as bronchiolitis obliterans, endobronchial sarcoidosis, or COPD exists, flow rates are well maintained. Occasionally, patients with associated obstructive airway disease or diffuse cystic disease have normal (in sarcoidosis and

rheumatoid disease) or increased total lung capacity (in advanced histiocytosis X or lymphangioleiomyomatosis). The diffusing capacity (corrected for alveolar volume and hemoglobin concentration) is reduced as a result of effacement of the alveolar capillary units and may precede or follow abnormalities in lung volumes. The resting arterial blood gas may be normal or reveal hypoxemia (secondary to a mismatching of ventilation to perfusion) and respiratory alkalosis. Commonly, blood gas abnormalities may only be elicited or accentuated by exercise. Despite the frequent presence of hypoxemia, erythrocytosis is uncommon. Serial lung function testing (especially exercise testing) is helpful in following the course and response to therapy.

Management of Interstitial Lung Diseases

Many ILDs are not responsive to therapy, therefore, it is extremely important that all treatable possibilities be given careful consideration. Because therapy does not reverse fibrosis, the major goals are 1) early identification and aggressive treatment directed at suppressing the acute and chronic inflammatory process to prevent further lung damage; 2) permanent removal of the offending agent, when known; and 3) palliation of complications. Unfortunately, no accurate or specific methods are available to stage the intensity of the alveolitis in a serial fashion. Open lung biopsy is both sensitive and specific for the evaluation of the alveolitis, but is generally used only once during the disease course. Symptoms, chest x-rays, pulmonary function tests, blood studies, gallium scanning, and BAL appear to reveal little information that is sensitive to or specific for the inflammatory process within the lung that actually defines disease activity (especially in an individual patient). In general, the responsive patient 1) reports a decrease in symptoms; 2) demonstrates radiographic improvement; 3) demonstrates physiologic improvement, such as increased total lung capacity (TLC) and diffusion capacity for carbon monoxide (D_LCO) or have an improvement in the exercise-induced oxygen desaturation; or 4) shows no further decline in lung function or other parameter of disease activity.

Corticosteroids remain the mainstay of therapy for suppression of the alveolitis present in these processes, but the success rate is low. In IPF, 40 percent to 50 percent of patients experience subjective improvement, but only 20 percent to 30 percent have objective improvement. Frequently, elderly patients with IPF are not treated, both because of their poor underlying condition and the hazards of corticosteroid therapy. When treated, only 32 percent of patients older than age 65 are likely to obtain a satisfactory response, with improvement in breathlessness and chest x-ray, compared with 95 percent of patients younger than 45 years of age, 62 percent of patients from 45 to 54 years of age, and 48 percent of patients from 55 to 64 years of age (77). High oral doses of prednisone (e.g., 80–100 mg/day for 6 to 12 weeks) followed by slow tapering (5–10 mg less every 2 to 3 weeks) is required to induce a response in most patients with IPF.

There is little evidence that corticosteroids influence the natural course of pulmonary manifestations in connective-tissue diseases except for patients with polymyositis-dermatomyositis, in whom approximately half have decreased dyspnea, clearing of the chest x-ray, and improved pulmonary function tests. Corticosteroid therapy, in addition to immediate removal from the etiologic agents in occupational and environmental processes, is generally recommended for symptomatic patients with acute inorganic dust exposure, acute radiation pneumonitis, and drug-induced disease. For organic dust disease (hypersensitivity pneumonitis), corticosteroids (60–80 mg/day of prednisone in tapering doses administered over 6 to 12 weeks) are recommended for both the acute and chronic stages. Cyclophosphamide (1–2 mg/kg/day), with or without corticosteroids, results in dramatic improvement in most patients with classic Wegener's granulomatosis. Cyclophosphamide, with or without prednisone, also appears to lead to improvement in selected patients with IPF. Objective response to prednisone and cytotoxic drugs commonly occurs in 6 to 12 weeks for most forms of ILD. Consequently, a treatment trial should not be less than this time period, unless complications or side effects occur. Most patients have relapses; thus, life-long treatment is frequently required. If patients demonstrate clinical and physiologic improvement, and the medication is discontinued, careful monitoring on a 6- or 12-month basis is essential to identify relapses.

Management Problems

Significant side effects can result from corticosteroid therapy such as increased appetite and weight gain; salt and water retention with exacerbation of cardiovascular disease, especially in elderly patients; hyperglycemia or overt diabetes mellitus (or both); depression, hyperexcitability, or frank psychosis, especially in elderly women; osteoporosis and joint destruction; peptic ulcer disease; and immunosuppression leading to opportunistic infections. Other side effects (e.g., hypokalemia, hypertension, renal lithiasis, poor healing, cataracts, ecchymosis, phlebitis, and hirsutism) may also occur. On the other hand, steroid withdrawal may result in serious symptoms and morbidity such as fatigue, weakness, arthralgia, anorexia, nausea, desquamation of skin, orthostatic dizziness and hypotension, fainting, and hypoglycemia.

Side effects of cyclophosphamide are bone marrow suppression, which requires that therapy be aimed at inducing a modest leukopenia with a total white cell count greater than $3000/\mu L$; hemorrhagic cystitis, which may be prevented with forced fluids and frequent bladder emptying; gastrointestinal symptoms such as anorexia, nausea or vomiting (or both); bone marrow suppression; azoospermia or amenorrhea; infection; development of hematologic malignancies; and ILD. Therapy should be altered if the patient has renal insufficiency. Consequently, if stabilization or clinical improvement cannot be documented, corticosteroid or cyclophosphamide therapy, or both, should be stopped because significant adverse reactions can occur.

Severe hypoxemia (PaO_2 less than 55 mm Hg) at rest, with exercise, or with both should be managed by supplemental oxygen. Patients with exercise-induced hypoxemia only should be given supplemental oxygen for use during exercise and possibly during sleep. If patients do not have supplemental oxygen, progressive reduction in the patient's level of activity may occur and the onset of right heart failure may be hastened. With the appearance of cor pulmonale, diuretic therapy and phlebotomy may occasionally be required. Pneumothorax, which is characteristic of eosinophilic granuloma of the lung, may also occur in other ILDs. This may be extremely difficult to treat because the lung is stiff and difficult to reexpand. Prolonged chest tube drainage, with high levels of negative pressure (20 to 40 mm Hg), may be necessary. Acute PE is an occasional cause of clinical deterioration in this group of patients. Sudden worsening of dyspnea, with unexplained deterioration in arterial blood gases and without evidence of superimposed infection, should prompt the clinician to consider lung scan, pulmonary angiography, or both procedures. Malignancy (particularly adenocarcinoma) develops in IPF and asbestosis with increased frequency (78).

Selected Interstitial Lung Diseases

Idiopathic Pulmonary Fibrosis

IPF, cryptogenic fibrosing alveolitis, is perhaps the most common ILD among the elderly (79). The mean onset is in a patient 55 years of age. Although the etiology is unknown, the clinicopathologic manifestations are specific. Careful evaluation of patients, often including lung biopsy, is needed before assigning this diagnosis. Patients generally present with gradually worsening dyspnea and cough with dry inspiratory rales on physical examination.

The duration of symptoms at the time of presentation is shorter for elderly subjects with IPF compared to that for younger patients (80). Digital clubbing is seen in 40 percent to 70 percent of patients and suggests late-stage disease. Laboratory findings are nonspecific and often include elevation in the ESR, low-titer positivity of ANA, immune complexes, and rheumatoid factor.

The chest radiograph usually shows reticular infiltrates in the mid and lower zones and small lung volumes, with or without honeycombing (Figure 44.6). Pleural disease and adenopathy are rare and should direct the clinician to an alternative diagnosis. High-resolution CT scan characteristically shows subpleural areas of reticulation and honeycombing (see Figure 44.6). Physiologic abnormalities include restrictive lung function with reduced D_LCO and lung compliance. Resting hypoxemia is common, but exercise-induced desaturation may be the only gas exchange abnormality early in the disease.

Although some authors feel that elderly patients with duration of symptoms for 2 years or longer, without fe-

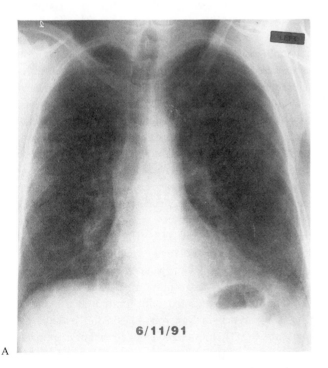
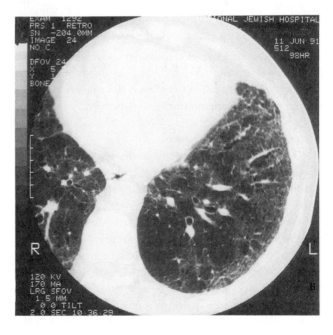

Fig. 44.6. Idiopathic pulmonary fibrosis. (*A*) Chest x-ray of a patient with long-standing idiopathic pulmonary fibrosis with diffuse, reticular opacities in the lower lung zones. (*B*) High resolution CT scan of the left lung from the same patient reveals the typical subpleural of usual interstitial pneumonia and honeycombing.

ver, and with compatible chest x-ray findings can be diagnosed clinically (81), it is important to rule out processes that closely mimic IPF, such as cryptogenic organizing pneumonitis (idiopathic bronchiolitis obliterans organizing pneumonia), chronic hypersensitivity pneumonitis, or respiratory bronchiolitis. Therefore, tissue diagnosis is warranted for many patients. Transbronchial biopsy is inadequate to make a definitive diagnosis of IPF. Open lung biopsy is generally required to obtain adequate tissue, but videothoracoscopic lung biopsy is likely to gain an increasing role in the diagnosis of IPF.

The natural history of IPF is generally one of steady progression. Consequently, for most patients a trial of immunosuppressive therapy with prednisone, cyclophosphamide, azathioprine or other experimental agents is recommended, although objective response rates are low (15%–20%). In a recent study, the median survival time for patients with IPF who were age 64 years or younger was 7.1 years; for elderly patients with IPF who were age 65 years or older, survival time was only 3.73 years (80). Age-related increased mortality has also been reported by others (73). In addition, patients with IPF have been shown to have a significant increase in the incidence of bronchogenic carcinoma (10%) (77,82) and an increased incidence of cardiovascular disease (ischemic heart disease and cerebrovascular accidents) (73,82). Infectious pneumonitis also occurs in IPF patients, probably as a result of immunosuppressive therapy.

Hypersensitivity Pneumonitis

The hypersensitivity pneumonitides are associated with repeated, intense inhalation of finely dispersed organic dusts, which produces diffuse, patchy, interstitial or alveolar infiltrates (or both) after the formation of antigen-antibody complexes (Arthus' reaction). Farmer's lung (exposure to moldy hay containing fungal spores) is the prototype, although air conditioner or humidifier lung disease (due to fungal overgrowth and aerosolization) and bird fancier's lung are more common in urban areas.

Disease can present in two forms. The first is an acute reaction after heavy exposure and is characterized by the abrupt onset (4–6 hours later) of fever, chills, malaise, nausea, cough, chest tightness, and dyspnea without wheezing, which subside over hours or days. Diffuse, fine rales throughout the chest, mild hypoxemia, and a restric-

tive ventilatory defect accompanies these symptomatic episodes. A fleeting, micronodular, interstitial pattern in the lower and mid-lower zone may be identified on chest x-ray. In the acute or subacute stage of hypersensitivity pneumonitis (HP), HRCT may be normal but most often reveals diffuse micronodules, ground-glass attenuation, focal air trapping or emphysema, and mild fibrotic changes, with relatively normal lung volumes (83). Hazy or ground-glass increase in lung density (that is, an increase in CT lung density that does not obscure the underlying lung parenchyma) or consolidation (a marked increase in attenuation with obliteration of underlying anatomic features) is observed in all stages of the process—acute, subacute and chronic disease—and appears to reflect the entire range of reversible interstitial processes—cellular interstitial infiltration, small granulomas within alveolar septa, and obstructive pneumonitis (83,84). Removal from exposure usually results in complete resolution. Pathologically, this stage is characterized by noncaseating, interstitial, granulomatous pneumonitis.

The second type is an insidious form that results if repeated acute episodes or continued low-level antigen exposure occur. A patient with chronic hypersensitivity pneumonitis may not have any acute episodes. This form of disease is particularly difficult to diagnose and manage. It appears to occur more commonly in middle-aged and elderly individuals, especially among bird fanciers. Disabling and frequently irreversible respiratory findings such as pulmonary fibrosis are characteristic. Hypoxemia, decreased diffusing capacity, and pulmonary function studies consistent with a combined obstructive and restrictive defect are frequently present. The chest film shows progressive fibrotic changes with fewer nodular densities and loss of lung volume, with shrinkage of the upper lobes. In chronic HP, two patterns of HRCT findings are identified: 1) honeycombing associated with ground-glass attenuation, parenchymal micronodules, emphysema, or all these conditions; 2) no honeycombing, but emphysema associated with ground-glass attenuation, and parenchymal micronodules. After cessation of exposure, the CT shows a return to normal or a dramatic improvement in patients with subacute disease and considerable reduction in ground-glass attenuation and micronodules in the chronic group. HRCT in patients with farmer's lung and persistent or progressive disease reveal centrilobular emphysema, focal fibrotic changes, and ground-glass opacities (85). In addition to granulomatous pneumonitis, biopsy specimens at this stage reveal bronchiolitis obliterans with destruction of alveoli (honeycombing) in association with densely fibrotic zones. The diagnosis of HP is important because HP is a reversible disease when diagnosed early. Intensive detective work is often required to uncover the source of the antigen. The serum can be tested against common antigens (the thermophilic actinomycetes, especially *Micropolyspora faeni* and *Thermoactinomyces vulgaris*), but the presence of precipitins does not make a definite diagnosis. Many chronic, progressive cases, particularly in patients who have died, show HP secondary to bird antigen exposure (83,84,86). Despite therapy, symptoms may persist for a prolonged time. High levels of bird antigen are detected for prolonged periods of time after bird removal and environmental cleanup (87). Continuous low-level exposure may explain the substantial mortality (29% at 5 yr) seen in chronic pigeon breeder's lung (86).

Drug-Induced Lung Disease

The elderly take more drugs per capita than does the population as a whole. The incidence of adverse drug reactions increases with age to the extent that patients in the eighth and ninth decades of life have three times the incidence of drug reactions than that observed in people younger than age 50.

Many elderly patients who present with dyspnea and cough may be taking one or more of the many drugs associated with drug-induced lung disease (Table 44.6). Consequently, drug-induced lung disease is an important consideration in the differential diagnosis of ILD in the elderly. Presentations of drug-related ILD are quite variable, ranging from acute fulminant deterioration to an insidious, progressive process mimicking IPF (88). The pathogenesis of drug-induced disease is poorly understood but may relate to direct toxic injury to pulmonary parenchyma or to indirect immune-mediated mechanisms, or to both, depending on the medication (89,90). While some forms of drug-induced ILD appear to be dose-related, others are clearly idiosyncratic. Discontinuation of the possible offending agent is always the first step in management of drug-related disease.

Table 44.6. Classification of Drug-Induced Interstitial Lung Disease.

Antibiotics
  Nitrofurantoin, acute and chronic
  Sulfasalazine
Anti-inflammatory agents
  Aspirin
  Gold
  Pencillamine
Antiarrhythmic agents
  Tocainide
  Amiodarone
Chemotherapeutic agents
  Antibiotics
    Bleomycin sulfate
    Mitomycin C
  Alkylating agents
    Busulfan
    Cyclophosphamide
    Chlorambucil
    Melphalan
  Antimetabolites
    Azathioprine
    Cytosine arabinoside
    Methotrexate
  Nitrosoureas
    BCNU (carmustine)
    CCNU (lomustine)
    Methyl-CCNU (semustine)
  Other
    Procarbazine hydrochloride
    Zinostatin
    Etoposide (VP-16)
Drug-induced systemic lupus erythematosus
  Procainamide hydrochloride
  Isoniazid
  Hydralazine hydrochloride
  Hydantoins
  Pencillamine
Illicit drugs
  Heroin
  Methadone hydrochloride
  Propoxyphene hydrochloride (Darvon)
  Talc
Miscellaneous
  O_2
  Drugs inducing pulmonary infiltrate and eosinophilia
  Radiation
  L-tryptophan

SOURCE: Reproduced by permission from Rosenow EC III, Martin WJ II. Drug-induced interstitial lung disease. In: Schwarz MI, King TE Jr, eds. Interstitial lung disease. St. Louis: Mosby Year Book, 1993:255–270.

Corticosteroids are occasionally helpful in some forms of disease, but they cannot be routinely recommended.

Chemotherapeutic agents are the most common culprits in drug-induced interstitial disorders. Unfortunately, the diagnosis is often missed or delayed because of the clinician's search for an opportunistic infection in immunocompromised patients. Bleomycin, busulfan, chlorambucil, cyclophosphamide, melphalan, and uracil mustard appear to cause fibrosis in a dose-dependent manner. The patient's age, number of cycles and cumulative dose, history of lung disease, hematologic abnormalities, combination chemotherapy, and most importantly, the concomitant use of radiation therapy or oxygen (FIO_2 greater than 40) appear to exert synergistic or additive effects. Nitrofurantoin is the most common of the antibiotics to produce lung disease and may cause either an acute, spontaneously resolving pneumonitis associated with peripheral eosinophilia or a chronic interstitial pneumonitis that is pathologically indistinguishable from IPF.

Coal Worker's Pneumoconiosis

Of the occupational lung diseases, coal worker's pneumoconiosis, silicosis, and asbestosis are the most common inhalation exposures that cause predominantly fibrosis and restrictive lung disease. Coal worker's pneumoconiosis usually occurs in association with silicosis. Two forms of disease predominate: simple pneumoconiosis, represented by small opacities (less than 1 cm in diameter) predominantly in the upper lung zones, and complicated pneumoconiosis or progressive massive fibrosis (opacity 1 cm or more in diameter). The prevalence rate among coal miners is approximately 10 percent, of whom 0.4 percent develop progressive massive fibrosis. Pulmonary function abnormalities occur in simple coal worker's pneumoconiosis, usually in the presence of a history of cigarette smoking, regardless of the extent of radiographic involvement.

Silicosis

Silicosis is found in miners, sandblasters, glass manufacturers, quarry workers, stone dressers, foundry workers, and boiler scalers. Silicosis has been regarded as a disease of the young that leads to disability and premature death. However, chronic cases are more commonly observed in

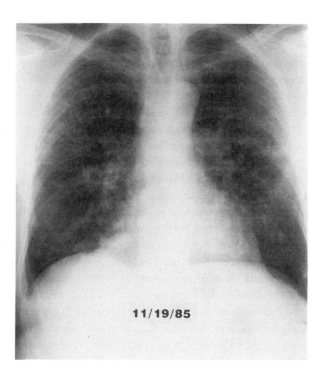

Fig. 44.7. Silicosis. Chest x-ray of a 62-year-old man with history of silicosis reveals diffuse nodular opacities in the mid to upper lung zones.

older individuals. Dyspnea and cough from chronic bronchitis is common, but patients are often asymptomatic. Inspiratory rales and clubbing are rare. Elevations in ESR with hypergammaglobulinemia, circulating immune complexes, and low titers of ANA are commonly found and perhaps explain progression of disease despite absence of continued exposure (91). Radiographically, silicosis appears as multinodular, rounded densities predominantly in both upper lung zones (Figure 44.7). The radiographic changes almost always occur before clinical and functional abnormalities. Progression from simple to progressive massive fibrosis occurs in a minority of patients. Patients with silicosis are highly susceptible to infection by *Mycobacterium tuberculosis* and other atypical mycobacteria. Furthermore, scleroderma and rheumatoid arthritis are unusually prevalent in patients with silicosis. There is no known treatment.

Asbestosis

Asbestos exposure is widespread because asbestos is used

extensively as an insulation material, a fire retardant, and a noise-reduction agent in many public facilities. Workers previously or currently employed in the shipyard, automotive, insulation, cement, textile, and asbestos mining industries are at greatest risk. There is a long latent period between exposure and the development of lung diseases; therefore, most of the cases occur in middle-aged or elderly persons. Paroxysmal, nonproductive cough is common and, unlike results for silicosis, inspiratory rales and clubbing are frequently found on physical examination. As with other ILD, restrictive pulmonary function tests with reduced D_LCO and abnormal gas exchange is common.

Smoking appears to facilitate the damaging effects of asbestos inhalation. Bilateral pleural thickening along the lower or mid-thoracic walls, calcified pleural plaques, and hazy infiltrates composed of irregular or linear small opacities, especially in the lower lung zones, are the most common changes seen on x-ray. Asbestos is also carcinogenic. Pleural and peritoneal mesotheliomas and bronchogenic carcinoma are recognized complications of asbestos exposure.

Connective-Tissue Diseases

The most common form of pulmonary involvement in the connective-tissue diseases is a chronic interstitial pattern that is indistinguishable from IPF. Pleuropulmonary disease may be the initial manifestation in patients with previously undiagnosed connective-tissue disease. Moreover, these findings may be a major cause of morbidity and mortality in these disorders. Connective-tissue disease is most prevalent in persons from 25 to 55 years of age. Although scleroderma, systemic lupus erythematosus, dermatomyositis-polymyositis, and Sjögren's syndrome can occur in the elderly, their respective prevalences in the aged is far less than the prevalence of rheumatoid arthritis. (Several comprehensive reviews of rheumatologically associated lung disease are recommended) (92,93). Rheumatoid arthritis is associated with 1) pleurisy, with or without effusion; 2) interstitial pneumonitis; 3) necrobiotic nodules (nonpneumoconiotic intrapulmonary rheumatoid nodules), with or without cavities; 4) Caplan's syndrome (rheumatoid pneumoconiosis); 5) pulmonary hypertension secondary to rheumatoid pulmonary vasculitis; 6) bronchiolitis

obliterans; and 7) upper airway obstruction caused by arytenoid arthritis.

Pulmonary lesions are commonly found in patients with progressive systemic sclerosis (scleroderma) and consist mainly of interstitial pneumonitis. Pulmonary function tests usually reveal a restrictive pattern, with reduced lung compliance and impaired diffusing capacity, often before any clinical or radiographic evidence of lung disease appears. Pulmonary vascular disease, alone or in association with pulmonary fibrosis, pleuritis, recurrent aspiration pneumonitis, and bronchiolar carcinoma, also occur. The ILD and pulmonary hypertension associated with scleroderma are strikingly resistant to current modes of therapy.

The pleuropulmonary manifestations of systemic lupus erythematosus are 1) pleurisy, with or without effusion; 2) atelectasis; 3) interstitial pneumonitis (less than 5% of patients), which exists in two forms – acute interstitial pneumonitis (tachypnea, dyspnea, high fever, cyanosis, and pulmonary hemorrhage that can be fatal) and chronic interstitial pneumonia (dyspnea, nonproductive cough, pleuritic chest pain, hypocapnia, impaired diffusing capacity and a restrictive ventilatory defect); 4) uremic pulmonary edema; 5) diaphragmatic dysfunction, with loss of lung volume; and 6) infectious pneumonia. Predominance in females is striking. Sjögren's syndrome (keratoconjunctivitis sicca, xerostomia, and recurrent swelling of the parotid gland), polymyositis and dermatomyositis may be associated with chronic diffuse interstitial pneumonitis and fibrosis.

Pulmonary Vasculitis

The pulmonary vasculitides are a heterogeneous group of disorders that have the common feature of necrotizing inflammation of blood vessels. The pathogenesis of pulmonary vasculitides is unknown. Most, if not all, are probably mediated by immune complex deposition in blood vessels, although cell-mediated immune processes may also be involved in some types. Wegener's granulomatosis (94,95) most commonly occurs in a patient's fifth decade of life and is characterized by the triad of 1) necrotizing granulomatous vasculitis of the upper respiratory tract (profuse rhinorrhea with sinus pain, epistaxis, and saddle nose deformity) and of the lower respiratory tract (cough, hemoptysis, and nodular, often cavitary, densities on chest x-ray); 2) disseminated vasculitis (leukocytoclastic vasculitis common); and 3) glomerulitis (azotemia, hypertension, and proteinuria).

Lymphomatoid granulomatosis, a disease that occurs in men in the fifth to sixth decade of life, is clinically similar to Wegener's granulomatosis. They differ, however, in that 1) involved organs are infiltrated by a pleomorphic mass of invasive atypical lymphocytes and plasmacytoid cells, which is accompanied by a granulomatous reaction in an angiocentric and angiodestructive pattern; 2) septal and palate perforations occur; 3) glomerulitis is rare; and 4) a tendency to progress to malignant lymphoma occurs in untreated patients.

The *hypersensitivity vasculitides* (Henoch-Schönlein purpura, cryoglobulinemia) are primarily systemic, with skin and visceral involvement. Although lung involvement is uncommon, it appears to occur more frequently in the elderly. Unlike the granulomatous vasculitides that involve the medium-sized vessels, these diseases primarily affect venules, arterioles, and capillaries.

Bronchogenic Carcinoma

For the past century, the incidence of bronchogenic carcinoma has been steadily increasing. It is responsible for an estimated 143,000 deaths a year in the United States and represents the most common cause of cancer deaths for both men and women (96). The age-specific incidence of bronchogenic carcinoma increases dramatically as a person ages. Persons older than 65 years of age, compared with those aged 45 to 64 years, have much higher incidence ratios (3.2 for men and 1.8 for women) (97). In fact, the group aged 65 and older constitutes roughly half all lung cancer cases (96). Lung cancer is associated with a number of carcinogenic pollutants. Although cigarette smoke is by far the most important, others are asbestos, uranium, nickel, chlormethyl ether, and chromium. Asbestos and uranium exposure seem to act synergistically with cigarette smoke and, thereby, increase the risk of a person to develop bronchogenic carcinoma more than that seen with cigarette smoking alone. In addition, scarring of the pulmonary parenchyma, secondary to diffuse interstitial fibrosis, or localized scarring after tuberculosis predisposes to the development of a scar carcinoma.

Clinical Picture

There are six major histologic subtypes of bronchogenic carcinoma: 1) squamous, 2) adenocarcinoma, 3) neuroendocrine (such as carcinoid tumor, small-cell, or oat cell), 4) mixed (adenosquamous or mixed small-cell and non-small-cell), 5) large cell undifferentiated, and bronchial gland (96). Most recent data suggest that adenocarcinoma and squamous carcinoma are the most common histologic types of lung cancer (98). Clinically, the patient is usually symptomatic or, rarely, has an asymptomatic lesion discovered on a chest radiograph performed for other reasons. Recent data suggest that lung cancer is initially seen at a less advanced stage as a person's age increases (98,99). If the tumor is endobronchial in location, an irritative cough may be present, which is difficult to distinguish from a cough associated with chronic airway obstruction (also likely to be present in this patient). Streaky hemoptysis, a new onset of localized wheezing, worsening dyspnea, and chest pain are all symptoms of endobronchial disease. An endobronchial lesion may be heralded by an obstructive infectious pneumonia. If the patient's chest wall is invaded, severe, deep, bone pain may be present. Pleural invasion may be associated with pleuritic pain and progressive dyspnea as a pleural effusion develops. Mediastinal spread is indicated by hoarseness (recurrent laryngeal nerve paralysis), raised diaphragm on chest radiograph (phrenic nerve paralysis), difficulty in swallowing (esophageal obstruction), pericardial tamponade, and headache and facial swelling (superior vena cava obstruction).

Extrathoracic metastatic manifestations are commonly the first signs of bronchogenic carcinoma. This is particularly true of the small or oat-cell variety. The most common sites of metastases are the CNS, bones, and liver. Symptoms may also be related to nonmetastatic extrathoracic manifestations, the paraneoplastic syndromes. The presence of a paraneoplastic syndrome indicates a poor prognosis. The endocrinopathies include inappropriate secretion of antidiuretic hormone (SIADH) seen with oat cell carcinoma, hypercalcemia secondary to parathyroid hormone-like material produced by squamous tumors, and adrenocorticotropic hormone (ACTH) production. Neuromuscular paraneoplastic syndromes include the Eaton-Lambert syndrome (reverse myasthenia gravis), peripheral neuropathy (sensory), and cerebellar degeneration. Patients with bronchogenic carcinoma may also present with dermatomyositis, pulmonary hypertrophic osteodystrophy (squamous cell), and acanthosis nigricans.

Diagnosis

Chest radiography can be highly suggestive of the diagnosis of bronchogenic carcinoma. A hilar mass may be represented by unilateral hilar enlargement or increase in hilar density. This may be associated with a homogenous parenchymal infiltrate, which may represent atelectasis or postobstructive pneumonia. Mediastinal enlargement may be present (metastatic lymph nodes) and may be associated with a paralyzed diaphragm (usually on the left) and an increase in size of the cardiac shadow, which represents pericardial metastases with effusion. Lytic rib lesions, pleural effusions and masses, and diffuse lymphangitic carcinomatosis may also be seen. A peripheral bronchogenic carcinoma may be associated with all of the above. If possible, it is important to obtain previous chest films to see whether a "coin" lesion is new. Cavitation in a peripheral bronchogenic carcinoma is most often seen with squamous cell carcinoma.

The staging of a potentially resectable bronchogenic carcinoma is still a matter of debate. To establish the diagnosis of central endobronchial lesions, sputum cytological examination is the initial step. If the cytology is positive for malignancy, and the patient demonstrates no evidence of local spread to the mediastinum or chest wall or no evidence of extrathoracic disease, fiberoptic bronchoscopy should be performed to determine the extent of the mucosal involvement. If cytology is negative, bronchoscopic examination is indicated, because it has been shown to be a well-tolerated, safe, and productive procedure, even for patients aged 70 years and older (100). Routine use of brain, bone, and liver-spleen scans has not been shown to be helpful unless there are symptoms that may indicate metastatic spread to these organ systems (101).

Intrathoracic spread of bronchogenic carcinoma may be easily determined by chest radiography if mediastinal, bone, or pleural disease is present, and these would be definite contraindications to surgical intervention. Mediastinoscopy is indicated for all central (endobronchial) lesions. The usefulness of mediastinoscopy for peripheral lesions is not certain. In one study, 9 of 46 patients with peripheral bronchogenic carcinoma had a positive mediastinal exploration. Seven of these, however, had positive chest radiographs for mediastinal enlargement. Compared with patients with central carcinomas, 50 percent of patients with peripheral bronchogenic carcinomas had negative chest radiographs and positive mediastinoscopy (102). Gallium-67 scanning and CT of the chest have also been recommended to evaluate mediastinal spread (103).

Treatment

Once all attempts have been made to detect metastatic disease, the decision of whether surgery is indicated must be made. This is particularly important for patients 70 years of age and older because the overall operative mortality (10%–14%) and morbidity is increased (104). Obviously, the mortality for pneumonectomy is greater than that for lobectomy or wedge resection. A diagnosis of oat cell carcinoma is a definite contraindication to surgery; these patients should be treated with chemotherapy and, depending on the extent of the disease (such as metastases to the CNS) with radiation therapy. The decision to operate on bronchogenic carcinoma in the elderly also depends on the patient's underlying cardiovascular and pulmonary status. In the older patient, this is often a matter of clinical exposure to the inciting agent. In the presence of chronic alveolitis, derangement in the interstitium occurs and eventually leads to loss of alveolar gas exchanging units because of fibrosis and honeycombing.

Carbon Monoxide Poisoning

Carbon monoxide is a colorless, odorless, highly toxic gas that binds avidly to hemoglobin (approximately 210 times greater than oxygen) so that oxygen transport in the body is markedly impaired and tissue hypoxia results. Acute exposure to high levels results in a well-documented clinical syndrome. On the other hand, the health effects of exposure to low levels is very controversial. One cannot help but wonder whether the elderly are not predisposed to potential problems because exposure in the home is increasing as a result of efforts to make buildings air tight, the use of gas stoves for heating (a common practice among the urban poor in northern climates), and the use of kerosene and gas space heaters and wood stoves. Furthermore, carbon monoxide levels may reach as much as twice the values identified in single-family residences. Although the health effects of low-level carbon monoxide exposure are controversial, it is nonetheless a syndrome that clinicians should recognize (105). This is especially relevant when one considers that carbon monoxide poisoning is frequently misdiagnosed as food poisoning, psychiatric disorders, cerebrovascular disease, intoxication, and heart disease.

Clinical Picture

The manifestations are related primarily to the level of carboxyhemoglobin present. Associated disease, especially cardiac disease and other factors that influence oxygen demand and delivery, also determine the severity of the clinical findings. Diagnosis depends on measurement of the patient's carboxyhemoglobin levels or oxygen content. Oxygen saturation should be measured directly and not calculated because the arterial PaO_2 usually is normal. At carboxyhemoglobin levels of 20 percent to 30 percent, headache, nausea, vomiting, weakness, dizziness, and diminished visual acuity are prominent symptoms. The finding of retinal hemorrhage on funduscopic examination should alert the clinician to possible carbon monoxide poisoning. At levels greater than 40 percent, little correlation exists between the symptoms and the blood carboxyhemoglobin level. Characteristically, manifestations are related to the brain, such as coma, seizures, ataxia, and diffuse and fluctuating neurologic deficits, and to the cardiac system, such as syncope, ECG abnormalities, and myocardial ischemia or infarction. A level greater than 60 percent is associated with coma and death.

Treatment

The half-life of carboxyhemoglobin is 4 to 6 hours, but increased alveolar ventilation and high inspired oxygen concentrations significantly alter the displacement of carbon monoxide. Therefore, the immediate institution of oxygen therapy (preferably 100 percent oxygen) is mandatory to improve tissue oxygen delivery and shorten the half-life of carboxyhemoglobin to 40 to 50 minutes. Intubation and mechanical ventilation may be required if the patient is hemodynamically unstable or if

hypoventilation (or both) is present. Hyperbaric oxygen hastens the removal of carbon monoxide and is recommended in the treatment of life-threatening cerebral or coronary hypoxia. Appropriate steps should be taken to manage any factor that reduces tissue oxygen delivery or increases tissue oxygen demand, such as anemia, hypothermia, hypotension, fever, or metabolic acidosis.

Sleep-Disordered Breathing

Age-related changes in sleep are common (Table 44.7). Of importance, apnea (cessation of breathing for 10 seconds or longer), underventilation, and oxygen desaturation (a decrease of 4% or more in oxygen saturation as measured by ear oximetry) occur commonly during sleep. These abnormalities may be responsible for potentially serious psychologic and physiologic consequences, especially in the elderly (Table 44.8). Disorders of sleep have been estimated to afflict approximately 50 percent of elderly per-

Table 44.7. Age-Related Changes in Sleep.

Variable	Change[a]
Time in bed	Increased
Total sleep time	None when nap time is included
Sleep efficiency (TST/TIB)	Decreased
Initial sleep latency	Small increase
Initial REM latency	Decreased secondary to advanced sleep phase
Sleep fragmentation	Increased secondary to transient arousals of less than 15 sec duration
NREM stage 1[b]	Small Increase
NREM stage 2[b]	Increased primarily due to decreased slow wave sleep delta waves
NREM stages 3–4[b]	No change in percent total sleep time but duration and timing of individual episodes are altered
Auditory awakening threshold	Decreased in NREM stages 2 and 4 and in REM sleep

[a] Compared with young adults.
[b] Measured as a percentage of total sleep time.
NREM = nonrapid eye movement; REM = rapid eye movement; TIB = time in bed; TST = total sleep time.
SOURCE: Reproduced by permission from Burger CD, Shepard JW Jr. Sleep-disordered breathing and aging. In: Mahler D, ed. Pulmonary disease in the elderly. New York: Marcel Dekker, 1993:61–80.

Table 44.8. Common Sleep-Related Complaints in the Elderly.

Difficulty initiating and maintaining sleep
Frequent arousals
Abnormalities in time spent asleep and excessive time spent in bed
Restless legs and periodic movements in sleep
Frequent use of sedative-hypnotics, including alcohol
Night wandering, frequent micturition

sons living at home and two-thirds of those living in long-term facilities (106). There is an increase in sleep fragmentation and a decrease in sleep quality (especially in women) in the elderly. This partially explains the frequent daytime complaints of the elderly: fatigue; frequent napping; excessive daytime sleepiness (especially while watching television, reading, driving, and eating) (106). Unfortunately, the clinical significance of the increased prevalence of sleep-related disorders of breathing in the elderly remains ill-defined. Further, the decision whether to treat the sleep-disorders found in a given patient is often difficult. Nonetheless, sleep-related disorders are a major factor in the poor quality of life and diminished sense of well-being of elderly patients. Consequently, the complaints must be evaluated and managed as best as possible without exacerbating frequent comorbid conditions, such as dementia, cardiac failure, and obesity. Detailed examination of sleep and breathing relationships has been extensively reviewed (106–110).

Sleep is divided into two broad phases, quiet and active sleep, primarily on the basis of electroencephalographic (EEG) wave changes that occur. Body functions also change during these phases. Quiet or nonrapid eye movement (non-REM) sleep is characterized by EEG wave slowing, with increased wave amplitude. Non-REM sleep (also called desynchronized or active sleep) is divided into *four stages*, representing progressively deeper stages of sleep. During stages 1 and 2 of non-REM sleep, the pattern is cyclical, with periods of Cheyne-Stokes breathing. As sleep becomes established, breathing stabilizes and is typically regular. In non-REM sleep, chemical control mechanisms determine ventilation. Periodic breathing during non-REM sleep increases as a person ages.

Active or rapid eye movement (REM) sleep is marked by EEG patterns of low-voltage, high-frequency waves indicative of intense cerebral activity. During REM sleep, heightened autonomic and metabolic activity occur, with increases in metabolic rate, body temperature, systolic blood pressure, and heart rate. Breathing becomes rapid and irregular, with periods of apnea as long as 15 to 20 seconds in normal adults. Similarly, airway smooth muscle tone fluctuates during REM sleep. Intercostal muscle activity is decreased and results in a paradoxical movement of the rib cage and decreased functional residual capacity. These findings indicate that mild degrees of hypercapnia and hypoxemia exist but are of little consequence in the healthy adult. In the presence of cardiac, neurologic, or pulmonary diseases, however, these episodes may be life-threatening. Many studies have now demonstrated that the presumably "normal" changes occur with greater frequency and severity in the elderly and in patients with chronic obstructive pulmonary disease (COPD). The clinical significance of oxygen desaturation is evident when one considers that nocturnal cardiac arrhythmias, pulmonary hypertension, and even sudden death are seen in these patients.

Sleep-Apnea Syndrome

Both sleep and respiration are disturbed during the sleep-apnea syndromes. Patients with this syndrome exhibit a constellation of clinical symptoms that resolve when the problem is appropriately treated (Table 44.9). Sleep apneas are classified, depending on the presence or absence of respiratory efforts, as central, obstructive, or mixed apneas (Figure 44.8). In each instance, air flow at the nose and mouth is absent, indicating apnea. In central

Table 44.9. Symptoms of Sleep Apnea Syndrome.

Noisy snoring (obstructive apnea)
Nocturnal insomnia (restless sleep or violent body movements)
Daytime somnolence
Intellectual and personality changes (depression)
Sexual dysfunction
Morning headache and/or nausea
Hallucinations, automatic behavior
Obesity
Systemic hypertension
Pulmonary hypertension, cor pulmonale, heart failure
Polycythemia
Edema
Cardiac arrhythmias
Unexplained nocturnal death

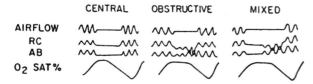

Fig. 44.8. Diagrammatic representation of the three patterns of apnea identified during sleep. In each, air flow at the nose and mouth is absent, indicating apnea. In central apneas, respiratory efforts, indicated in this instance by rib cage (RC) and abdominal (AB) displacement, are absent. During an obstructive apnea, efforts by the chest wall muscles are present throughout the entire episode of apnea. In mixed apneas, both central and obstructive patterns are present in the same apnea. Oxygen saturation (O_2 SAT%) falls according to the general degree of oxygen saturation and the length of the apnea. (Reproduced by permission from: Strohl KP, Cherniack NS, and Gothe B. Physiologic basis of therapy for sleep apnea. Am Rev Respir Dis 1986;134:791–802.)

apnea, respiratory efforts are not detected. In upper airway obstructive apnea, respiratory efforts are present but are not accompanied by airflow at the mouth or nose. Mixed, or complex, apnea resembles central apnea early in the episode and obstructive apnea as the episode progresses. All these situations result in alveolar hypoventilation, oxygen desaturation (decrease greater than 4 percent is considered abnormal), and sleep deprivation. Most often, obstructive or mixed apneas occur. Diagnosis of this syndrome frequently requires a searching inquiry when a patient presents with the symptoms outlined in Table 44.9. Snoring is increased in the elderly and appears to represent an intermediate stage in the transition from health to disease (111). Approximately 60 percent of men and 45 percent of women older than 60 years of age snore (111). Massively obese patients, those with COPD, stroke, and chronic heart disease, men, postmenopausal women, and patients with anatomic variations of the upper airway (e.g., hypognathia, nasal obstruction, and tongue or tonsillar enlargement) are others predisposed to the sleep-apnea syndrome.

The major pulmonary abnormalities occurring in sleep-apnea syndrome are 1) disordered breathing with oxygen desaturation, especially during naps and prolonged nocturnal sleep, usually of short duration (i.e., less than 60 seconds); 2) ventilation-perfusion mismatching that occurs during REM sleep, producing periods of oxygen desaturation that last for longer periods (i.e., longer than 5 minutes); 3) pulmonary hypertension; 4) decreased mucociliary clearance and cough depression, which may be particularly important in patients with COPD who have excess airway secretions; 5) decreased intercostal muscle contraction with resultant paradoxical movement of the chest wall; and 6) bronchoconstriction.

Other Sleep Disturbances

Before the clinician assumes that symptoms are related to sleep-apnea syndromes, the natural changes in sleep patterns that occur with aging must be carefully ruled out, especially that apparently healthy older individuals may require a longer time to fall asleep, may awaken more often during the night, and may need less sleep overall (112–115). Furthermore, sleep disturbances commonly occur in these patients as a result of concomitant illnesses such as depression, alcoholism, chronic use and dependence on sleeping pills, chronic pain syndrome, organic brain syndrome, and bereavement or situational insomnia. In the elderly, it is particularly difficult to distinguish between the normal variability of breathing during sleep and pathologic apnea (116). Aged men, especially those who are overweight, are more prone to impaired respiration during sleep than are aged women (117). The natural history and significance of the apneas found during sleep in the elderly is unclear (117,118).

Several additional points require emphasis. First, it is not always easy to predict the magnitude of the sleep disturbance on clinical grounds because clinical findings, blood gas analysis, and pulmonary function tests during wakefulness may be misleading. The important features that should alert the physician to examine the patient for the possibility of sleep-related disturbances are 1) pulmonary hypertension or cardiac failure in excess of that expected from the pulmonary function tests and arterial blood gases, and 2) a poor response to the standard measures of treatment and rehabilitation in COPD.

Second, the administration of nocturnal oxygen is a principal treatment modality for sleep hypoxemia. However, there is a subgroup of patients with predominantly obstructive apneas for whom low-flow oxygen results in a prolongation of the apneic periods, with a dramatic rise in $PaCO_2$ and resultant acidosis. Of importance, cardiac dysrhythmias occur more frequently in this setting (119).

How to determine which patients may suffer a deleterious effect from oxygen therapy is unclear. A further complicating factor in evaluating patients is the suggestion by Martin and coworkers that among this subset are patients who benefit from oxygen therapy with a reduced total amount of apneic time and the number of cardiac arrhythmias (120).

Third, not only does sleep aggravate gas exchange disturbances in patients with COPD, but COPD may aggravate sleep in ways that cause these elderly patients to develop changes in daytime behavior and performance, such as daytime somnolence, intellectual deterioration, impotence, depression, and essential hypertension (121).

Management

Management of sleep-apnea syndrome is important because many of the manifestations are reversible (108). Obstructive sleep apnea requires measures that will maintain the patency of the upper airway during sleep. Weight reduction is the primary mode of therapy in morbidly obese patients. Abstinence from alcohol and sedative-hypnotic agents, upright posture, and treatment of predisposing medical illnesses (e.g., hypothyroidism) are also very important aspects of treatment. Agents that enhance ventilatory responsiveness, such as medroxyprogesterone acetate (20 mg three times/day) or protriptyline (20 mg po at bedtime) have met with limited success in a few patients with obstructive sleep apnea. The application of nasal continuous positive pressure (CPAP) delivered by a device consisting of a small air blower attached by flexible tube to a snug-fitting nasal mask is the most commonly prescribed method to keep the upper airway open. Approximately 6 weeks of successful CPAP treatment is required for maximum improvement. When life-threatening cardiorespiratory events occur during sleep, tracheostomy is required. Surgical correction (i.e., removal of tonsillar and adenoid tissue) may also improve the syndrome.

In patients with central apneas, diaphragmatic pacing by way of the phrenic nerve or a rocking bed may be helpful. The long-term efficacy of this approach remains to be fully evaluated. Patients with primary alveolar hypoventilation occasionally respond to medroxyprogesterone. The role of nocturnal oxygen therapy has been discussed above. Sedatives and alcohol should be avoided in these patients.

Automobile accidents are more common in individuals with inattentiveness, fatigue, and sleepiness (as can occur in the elderly, especially those with sleep apnea) (110). Consequently, patients with sleep apnea should be cautioned about the potential risk of operating a motor vehicle. Some patients with sleepiness may have to stop driving because of the potential risk. These individuals should be referred to a pulmonary specialist familiar with sleep apnea who can assess the patient, begin treatment, ensure compliance, and offer advice regarding the potential risks to the patient and others. In addition, the American Thoracic Society has suggested that the physician has responsibility to report patients with sleep apnea to the licensing authority if 1) the patient has excessive daytime sleepiness and sleep apnea *and* a history of a motor vehicle accident or equivalent level of clinical concern; and 2) one of the following circumstances exists: the patient's condition is untreatable or is not amenable to expeditious treatment (within 2 months of diagnosis); or the patient is not willing to accept treatment or is unwilling to restrict driving until effective treatment has been instituted (110).

Cardiopulmonary Dysfunction and Critical Care

There has been a marked rise in the use of technologically sophisticated care in intensive care units during the past few decades. Although using approximately 7 percent of hospital beds in the United States, intensive care accounts for 20 to 30 percent of total hospital costs and represents 1 percent of the gross national product (122). The proportion of elderly patients treated in intensive care units approaches 50 percent (123). Cardiopulmonary dysfunction is a common feature of most patients cared for in intensive care units; however, there are little data concerning the actual incidence of ARDS or respiratory failure in the elderly. In addition, there is considerable debate regarding the value of using critical care resources for individuals who will benefit very little (124). A discussion of the intensive care management of acute and chronic respiratory failure and the important ethical issues has been published by several researchers (123,125–129).

Many of the basic principles of the management of respiratory failure are detailed in Chapter 45. Table 44.10

Table 44.10. Complications Associated with Acute Respiratory Failure and Its Management.

Complications associated with intubation and extubation
   Insertion trauma (laryngeal injury)
   Improper tube placement (esophagus or right mainstem)
   Cuff complications (tracheal stenosis, erosion or dilation, tracheoesophageal fistula, erosion of the innominate artery)
   Postextubation obstruction (supraglottic or subglottic edema)
   Gastric aspiration
   Airway obstruction (mucus, endotracheal tube)
   Endotracheal tube dislodgment (extubation)
Complications of ventilatory and monitoring procedures
   Pulmonary barotrauma (pneumothorax, pneumomediastinum, subcutaneous emphysema)
   Acid-base disturbances (alkalosis)
   Cardiovascular problems
   Arrhythmias (multifocal atrial tachycardia)
   Hypotension and low cardiac output
   Machine failure (patient disconnected, alarm malfunction)
   Flow-directed, balloon-tip catheterization
   Pulmonary infarction
   Pulmonary hemorrhage
   Arrhythmias
   Deconditioning (respiratory muscle failure)
Metabolic
   Syndrome of inappropriate antidiuretic hormone (SIADH)
   Electrolyte imbalances
   Hypokalemia and hypochloremia
   Severe hypophosphatemia and hypomagnesemia
Renal
   Fluid retention
   Renal failure
Gastrointestinal
   Gastrointestinal hemorrhage
   Ileus
   Gastric distention
   Pneumoperitoneum
Infection
   Sepsis
   Nosocomial pneumonia
Hematologic
   Anemia
   Thrombocytopenia
   Disseminated intravascular coagulation
Other problems
   Pulmonary embolism
   Drug toxicity (theophylline, digitalis)
   Oxygen toxicity
   Malnutrition
   Psychiatric disturbances ("intensive care unit psychosis," depression, agitation)

SOURCE: Reproduced by permission from King TE. Acute respiratory failure. In: Schrier RW, ed. Current medical therapy. New York: Raven Press, 1984:126–160.

outlines the many complications associated with respiratory failure and its management. It is important to understand that the aggressive management of respiratory failure in the elderly patient is justified. Although the long-term prognosis after respiratory failure is poor, the short-term prognosis in patients presenting with acute respiratory failure is better. In fact, studies of ventilatory management in the geriatric population emphasize an improved survival rate (130) and evaluation of long-term outcome of critically ill elderly patients requiring intensive care demonstrated that age alone was not an adequate predictor of long-term survival and quality of life (129,131).

ARDS and multiorgan dysfunction syndrome are catastrophic events, especially in the elderly (132,133). Severe pneumonia, sepsis syndrome, pulmonary aspiration, or multiple trauma are important risk factors for the development of ARDS, which is characterized by severe dyspnea, refractory hypoxemia (arterial PO_2 less than 150 mm Hg on an FIO_2 of 100 percent or PaO_2/FIO_2 less than 200 mg Hg regardless of positive end-expiratory pressure (PEEP) level) and diffuse bilateral pulmonary infiltrations, "stiff lung," right-to-left intrapulmonary shunting, usually normal or increased alveolar ventilation, increased physiologic dead space, and a pulmonary arterial wedge pressure of less than 18 mm Hg or no clinical evidence of left atrial hypertension. The mainstay of management is mechanical ventilation with PEEP and close hemodynamic monitoring of cardiac output and fluid balance. Despite appropriate and aggressive treatment, the mortality rate is extremely high (average, 65 percent) and can reach 90 percent to 100 percent in the presence of another organ failure (133–136).

Acknowledgment. I thank B.J. Burnett for excellent secretarial assistance.

References

1. Johanson WG, Pierce AK, Stanford JP. Changing pharyngeal bacterial flora of hospitalized patients: emergence of gram-negative bacilli. N Engl J Med 1969;281:1137–1140.
2. Hanson LC, Weber DJ, Rutala WA, Samsa GP. Risk factors for nosocomial pneumonia in the elderly. Am J Med 1991;92:161–166.

3. Gleckman RA, Bergman MM. Bacterial pneumonia: specific diagnosis and treatment of the elderly. Geriatrics 1987;42:29–41.

4. American Thoracic Society. Guidelines for the initial management of adults with community-acquired pneumonia: diagnosis, assessment of severity, and initial antimicrobial therapy. Am Rev Respir Dis 1993;148:1418–1426.

5. Fein AM, Feinsilver SH, Niederman MS. Nonresolving and slowly resolving pneumonia. Clin Chest Med 1993;14:555–569.

6. Gross PA, Quinnan GV, Rodstein M, et al. Association of influenza immunization with reduction in mortality in an elderly population. A prospective study. Arch Intern Med 1988;148:562–565.

7. Neiderman MS, Fein AM. Pneumonia in the elderly. Geriatr Clin North Am 1986;2:241–268.

8. Sims RV, Steinmann WC, McConville JH, et al. The clinical effectiveness of pneumococcal vaccine in the elderly. Ann Intern Med 1988;108:653–657.

9. Butler JC, Breiman RF, Campbell JF, et al. Pneumococcal polysaccharide vaccine efficacy. An evaluation of current recommendations. JAMA 1993;270:1826–1831.

10. Health and Public Policy Committee, American College of Physicians: Pneumococcal vaccine. Ann Intern Med 1986;104:118–120.

11. Stead WW, Lofgren JP. Does the risk of tuberculosis increase in old age? J Infect Dis 1983;147:951–955.

12. American Thoracic Society. Control of tuberculosis in the United States. Am Rev Respir Dis 1992;146:1623–1633.

13. Mahmoudi A, Iseman MD. Pitfalls in the care of patients with tuberculosis. Common errors and their association with the acquisition of drug resistance. JAMA 1993;270:65–68.

14. Iseman MD. Treatment of multidrug-resistant tuberculosis. N Engl J Med 1993;329:784–791.

15. Centers for Disease Control and Prevention. 1975 Tuberculosis Statistics. Washington, DC: Dept. of Health, Education, and Welfare (CDC)77-8249, 1976.

16. Alvarez S, Shell C, Berk SL. Pulmonary tuberculosis in elderly men. Am J Med 1987;82:602–606.

17. Korzeniewska-Kosela M, Krysl J, Muller N, et al. Tuberculosis in young adults and the elderly. Chest 1994;106:28–32.

18. Fullerton JM, Dyer J. Unsuspected tuberculosis in the aged. Tubercule 1965;46:193–198.

19. Stead WW. Raising physician awareness of tuberculosis in the elderly. Geriatr Focus Infect Dis 1991;1:1–3,10–11.

20. Van den Brande P, Vijgen J, Demedts M. Clinical spectrum of pulmonary tuberculosis in older patients: comparison with younger patients. J Gerontol 1991;46:M204–M209.

21. Holden M, Dubin MR, Diamond PH. Frequency of negative intermediate strength tuberculin sensitivity in patients with active tuberculosis. N Engl J Med 1971;285:1506–1509.

22. Chang SC, Lee PY, Perng RP. Lower lung field tuberculosis. Chest 1987;91:230–232.

23. Bradley SF. Tuberculosis in the elderly: forgotten but not gone. Geriatr Focus Infect Dis 1991;1:11, 16, 13–14.

24. Couser JI Jr, Glassroth J. Tuberculosis. An epidemic in older adults. Clin Chest Med 1993;14:491–499.

25. Rooney JJ, Crocco JA, Dramer S. Further observations on tuberculin reactions in active tuberculosis. Am J Med 1976;60:517–522.

26. Dorken E, Grzybowski S, Allen EA. Significance of the tuberculin test in the elderly. Chest 1987;92:237–246.

27. Thompson NJ, Glassroth JL, Snider DE Jr, Farer LS. The booster phenomenon in serial tuberculin testing. Am Rev Respir Dis 1979;119:587–597.

28. Heifets LB, Good RC. Current laboratory methods for the diagnosis of tuberculosis. In: Bloom BR, ed. Tuberculosis: pathogenesis, protection, and control. Washington, DC: American Society of Microbiology, 1994:85–110.

29. O'Toole RD, Thornton GF, Mukherjee MK. Dexamethasone in tuberculosis meningitis. Ann Intern Med 1969;70:39–49.

30. Kopanoff DE, Kilburn JO, Glassroth JL. A continuing survey of tuberculous primary drug resistance in the United States. March 1975 to November 1977. Am Rev Respir Dis 1978;118:835–842.

31. Stead WW, To T, Harrison RW, Abraham JH III. The significance of the tuberculin skin test in elderly persons. Ann Intern Med 1987;107:837–842.

32. Stead WW, To T, Harrison RW, Abraham JH III. Benefit-risk considerations in preventive treatment for tuberculosis in elderly persons. Ann Intern Med 1987;107:843–845.

33. Rosenzweig DY, Schlueter DP. Spectrum of clinical disease in pulmonary infection with Mycobacterium avium-intracellulare. Rev Infect Dis 1981;3:1046–1051.

34. O'Brien RJ, Geiter LJ, Snider DE Jr. The epidemiology of nontuberculous mycobacterial diseases in the United States. Results from a national survey. Am Rev Respir Dis 1987;135:1007–1014.

35. Iseman MD. Mycobacterium avium complex and the normal host. The other side of the coin. N Engl J Med 1989;321:896–898.

36. Kirschner RA Jr, Parker BC, Falkinham JO III. Epidemiology of infection by nontuberculous mycobacteria. Mycobacterium avium, Mycobacterium intracellulare, and Mycobacterium scrofulaceum in acid, brown-water swamps of the southeastern United States and their association with environmental variables. Am Rev Respir Dis 1992;145:271–275.

37. Prince DS, Peterson DD, Steiner RM, et al. Infection with Mycobacterium avium complex in patients without predisposing conditions. N Engl J Med 1989;321:863–868.

38. Reich JM, Johnson RE. Mycobacterium avium complex pulmonary disease. Incidence, presentation, and response to therapy in a community setting. Am Rev Respir Dis 1991;143:1381–1385.

39. Reich JM, Johnson RE. Mycobacterium avium complex pulmonary disease presenting as an isolated lingular or middle lobe pattern. The Lady Windermere syndrome. Chest 1992;101:1605–1609.

40. Christensen EE, Dietz GW, Ahn CH, et al. Pulmonary mani-

festations of *Mycobacterium intracellularis*. AJR 1979:133:59–66.

41. Corpe RF. Surgical management of pulmonary disease due to *Mycobacterium avium-intracellulare*. Rev Infect Dis 1981;3:1064–1067.

42. Zavala DC. The treatment of aspiration pneumonia in the aged. Geriatrics 1977;32:46–51.

43. Rossman I, Rodstein M, Bornstein A. Undiagnosed disease in the aging population. Arch Intern Med 1974;133:366–369.

44. Cameron JL, Mitchell WH, Zuidema GD. Aspiration pneumonia. Arch Surg 1973;106:49–52.

45. Ribano CA, Grace WJ. Pulmonary aspiration. Am J Med 1971;50:510–520.

46. Cameron JL, Anderson RP, Zuidema GD. Aspiration pneumonia: a clinical and experimental review. J Surg Res 1967;7:44–53.

47. Spencer H. Pathology of the lung. New York: Pergamon, 1962:122.

48. Mays EE, Dubois JJ, Hamilton GB. Pulmonary fibrosis associated with tracheobronchial aspiration. Chest 1976;69:512–515.

49. Levison ME, Mangura CT, Lorber B, et al. Clindamycin compared with penicillin for the treatment of anaerobic lung abscess. Ann Intern Med 1983;98:466–471.

50. Dalen JE, Alpert JS. Natural history of pulmonary emboli. Prog Cardiovasc Dis 1975;17:257–270.

51. Moser KM. Venous thromboembolism. Am Rev Respir Dis 1990;141:235–249.

52. Wilson JE. Pulmonary embolism diagnosis and treatment. Clin Notes Respir Dis 1986;19:13–15.

53. Kniffin WD Jr, Baron JA, Barrett J, et al. The epidemiology of diagnosed pulmonary embolism and deep venous thrombosis in the elderly. Arch Intern Med 1994;15:861–866.

54. Gross JS, Neufeld RR, Libow LS, et al. Autopsy study of the elderly institutionalized patient: review of 234 autopsies. Arch Intern Med 1988;148:173–176.

55. Hirsh J, ed. Venous thrombosis and pulmonary embolism: diagnostic methods. Edinburgh: Churchill Livingstone, 1987.

56. MacGee W. Causes of death in a hospitalized geriatric population: an autopsy study of 3000 patients. Virchows Arch A Pathol Anat 1993;423:343–349.

57. Murry HW, Ellis GC, Blumenthal DS, Sos TA. Fever and thromboembolism. Am J Med 1979;67:232–235.

58. Meth RF, Tashkin DP, Hansen KS. Pulmonary edema and wheezing after pulmonary embolism. Am Rev Respir Dis 1975;111:693–698.

59. Melmon KL, Braunwald E. Familial pulmonary hypertension. N Engl J Med 1963;269:770–775.

60. Sreeram N, Cheriex EC, Smeets JLRM, et al. Value of the 12-lead electrocardiogram at hospital admission in the diagnosis of pulmonary embolism. Am J Cardiol 1994;73:298–303.

61. Worsley DF, Alavi A, Aronchick JM, et al. Chest radiographic findings in patients with acute pulmonary embolism: observations from the PIOPED study. Radiology 1993;189:133–136.

62. Stein PD, Gottschalk A, Saltzman HA, Terrin ML. Diagnosis of acute pulmonary embolism in the elderly. J Am Coll Cardiol 1991;18:1452–1457.

63. Moser KM, Fedullo PF, LittleJohn JK, Crawford R. Frequent asymptomatic pulmonary embolism in patients with deep venous thrombosis. JAMA 1994;271:223–225.

64. Hirsh J. Heparin. N Egnl J Med 1991;324:1565–1574.

65. Raschke RA, Reilly BM, Guidry JR, et al. The weight-based heparin dosing nomogram compared with a "standard care" nomogram. Ann Intern Med 1993;119:874–881.

66. Hirsh J. Oral anticoagulant drugs. N Engl J Med 1991;324:1865–1875.

67. Vieweg WUR, Piscatelli RL, Houser JJ, Proulx RA. Complications of intravenous administration of heparin in elderly women. JAMA 1970;213:1303–1313.

68. Fihn SD, McDonell M, Martin D, et al. Risk factors for complications of chronic anticoagulation. A multicenter study. Ann Intern Med 1993;118:511–520.

69. Bell WR, Rayall RM. Heparin associated thrombocytopenia: a comparison of three heparin preparations. N Engl J Med 1980;303:902–906.

70. Glazier RL, Crowell EB. Randomized prospective trial of continuous vs intermittent heparin therapy. JAMA 1976;236:1365–1367.

71. Hirsh J, Poller L. The international normalized ratio. A guide to understanding and correcting its problems. Arch Intern Med 1994;154:282–288.

72. Schwarz MI, King TE Jr, ed. Interstitial lung disease. Philadelphia: Mosby-Year Book, 1993:1–22.

73. Turner-Warwick M, Burrows B, Johnson A. Cryptogenic fibrosing alveolitis: clinical features and their influence on survival. Thorax 1980;35:171–180.

74. Dreisin RB, Schwarz MI, Theofilopoulos AN, Stanford RE. Circulating immune complexes in the idiopathic interstitial pneumonias. N Engl J Med 1978;298:353–357.

75. Quaranta JF, Cassuto JJP, Giacobi R, Masseyeff R. Rheumatoid factor in the elderly. New methodology. New Methods Pathol Biol 1980;28:656–660.

76. Muller NL, Miller RR. Ground-glass attenuation, nodules, alveolitis, and sarcoid granulomas. Radiology 1993;189:31–32.

77. Turner-Warwick M, Burrows B, Johnson A. Cryptogenic fibrosing alveolitis: response to corticosteroid treatment and its effect on survival. Thorax 1980;35:593–599.

78. Turner-Warwick M, Lebowitz M, Burrows B, Johnson A. Cryptogenic fibrosing alveolitis and lung cancer. Thorax 1980;35:496–499.

79. King TE Jr. Idiopathic pulmonary fibrosis. In: Schwarz MI, King TE Jr, eds. Interstitial lung disease. 2nd ed. Philadelphia: Mosby-Year Book, 1993:367–403.

80. Schreiner R, Mortenson RL, Ikle D, King TE Jr. Interstitial lung disease in the elderly. In: Mahler D, ed. Pulmonary disease in the elderly. New York: Marcel Dekker, 1993:339–385.

81. Winterbauer RH. The treatment of idiopathic pulmonary fibrosis. Chest 1991;100:233–235.

82. Panos RJ, Mortenson R, Niccoli SA, King TE Jr. Clinical dete-

rioration in patients with idiopathic pulmonary fibrosis. Causes and assessment. Am J Med 1990;88:396–404.

83. Remy-Jardin M, Remy J, Wallaert B, Muller NL. Subacute and chronic bird breeder hypersensitivity pneumonitis: sequential evaluation with CT and correlation with lung function tests and bronchoalveolar lavage. Radiology 1993;189:111–118.

84. Buschman DL, Gamsu G, Waldron JA Jr, et al. Chronic hypersensitivity pneumonitis: use of CT in diagnosis. AJR 1992;159:957–960.

85. Lalancette M, Carrier G, Laviolette M, et al. Farmer's lung: Longterm outcome and lack of predictive value of bronchoalveolar lavage fibrosing factors. Am Rev Respir Dis 1993;148:216–221.

86. Perez PR, Salas J, Chapela R, et al. Mortality in Mexican patients with chronic pigeon breeder's lung compared with those with usual interstitial pneumonia. Am Rev Respir Dis 1993;148:49–53.

87. Craig TJ, Hershey J, Engler RJ, et al. Bird antigen persistence in the home environment after removal of the bird. Ann Allergy 1992;69:510–512.

88. Mahler DA, Rosiello RA, Loke J. The aging lung. Geriatr Clin Med North Am 1986;2:215–225.

89. Cooper JAD Jr. Drug-induced pulmonary disease. Clin Chest Med 1990;11:1–194.

90. Rosenow EC III, Martin WJ II. Drug-induced interstitial lung disease. In: Schwarz MI, King TE Jr, ed. Interstitial lung disease. 2nd ed. St. Louis: Mosby Year Book, 1993:255–270.

91. Doll NJ, Stankus RP, Hughes J, et al. Immune complexes and autoantibodies in silicosis. J Allergy Clin Immunol 1981;68:281–285.

92. Stokes LT, Turner-Warwick M. Lungs and connective tissue disease. In: Murray J, Nadel J, ed. Textbook of respiratory medicine. Philadelphia: Saunders, 1988:1462–1485.

93. King TE Jr. Connective tissue disease. In: Schwarz MI, King TE Jr, ed. Interstitial lung diseases. 2nd ed. Philadelphia: Mosby-Year Book, 1993:271–308.

94. Feigin DS. Vasculitis in the lung. J Thorac Imaging 1988;3:33–48.

95. Chakravarty K, Scott DGI, Blyth J, Courteney-Harris RG. Wegener's granulomatosis in the elderly–unusual presentations and misdiagnosis. J Rheumatol 1994;21:1157–1159.

96. Jett JM, Tazelaar HD. Lung cancer in the elderly. In: Mahler D, ed. Pulmonary disease in the elderly. New York: Marcel Dekker, 1993:239–277.

97. Levin DL. Cancer rates and risks, 2nd ed. Washington, DC: US Department HEW, 1974;3.

98. O'Rourke MA, Feussner JR, Feigl R, Laszlo J. Age trends of lung cancer stage at diagnosis: implications for lung cancer screening in the elderly. JAMA 1987;258:921–926.

99. DeMaria LC Jr, Cohen MJ. Characteristics of lung cancer in elderly patients. J Gerontol 1987;42:540–545.

100. Macfarlane JT, Storr A, Wart MJ. Safety usefulness and acceptability of fiberoptic bronchoscopy in the elderly. Age Ageing 1981;10:127–131.

101. Hooper RG, Beechler R, Johnson MC. Radioisotope scanning in the initial staging of bronchogenic carcinoma. Am Rev Respir Dis 1978;118:279–286.

102. Whitcomb ME, Barham E, Goldman AL. Indications for a mediastinoscopy in bronchogenic carcinoma. Am Rev Respir Dis 1976;113:189–195.

103. DeMeester TR, Golomb HM, Krichner P. The role of gallium 67 scanning in the clinical staging and preoperative evaluation of patients with carcinoma of the lung. Ann Thorac Surg 1979;28:451–464.

104. Kirsh MM, Rotman H, Bove E, et al. Major pulmonary resection for bronchogenic carcinoma in the elderly. Ann Thorac Surg 1976;22:369–373.

105. Samet JM, Marbury MC, Spengler JD. Health effects and sources of indoor air pollution. Am Rev Respir Dis 1987;136:1486–1508.

106. Burger CD, Shepard JW Jr. Sleep-disordered breathing and aging. In: Mahler D, ed. Pulmonary disease in the elderly. New York: Marcel Dekker, 1993:61–80.

107. Cherniack NS. Respiratory dysrhythmias during sleep. N Engl J Med 1981;305:325–330.

108. Strohl KP, Cherniack NS, Gothe B. Physiologic basis of therapy for sleep apnea. Am Rev Respir Dis 1986;134:791–802.

109. Feinsilver SH, Hertz G. Sleep in the elderly patient. Clin Chest Med 1993;14:405–411.

110. American Thoracic Society. Sleep apnea, sleepiness, and driving risk. Am J Respir Crit Care Med 1994;150:1463–1473.

111. Haponik EF. Obstructive sleep apnea in the elderly: more challenges for chest physicians. Pulm Perspect 1993;10:1–3.

112. Reynolds CF III, Coble PA, Black RS, et al. Sleep disturbances in a series of elderly patients: polysomnographic findings. J Am Geriatr Soc 1980;28:164–170.

113. Carskadon MA, Dement WC. Respiration during sleep in the aged human. J Gerontol 1981;36:420–423.

114. Bixler EO, Kales A, Cadieux RJ, et al. Sleep apneic activity in older healthy subjects. J Appl Physiol 1985;58:1597–1601.

115. Naifeh HK, Severinghaus JW, Kamiya J. Effect of aging on sleep-related changes in respiration variables. Sleep 1987;10:160–171.

116. Knight H, Millman RP, Gur RC, et al. Clinical significance of sleep apnea in the elderly. Am Rev Respir Dis 1987;136:845–850.

117. Bliwise DL, Feldman DE, Bliwise NG, et al. Risk factors for sleep disordered breathing in heterogeneous geriatric population. J Am Geriatr Soc 1987;35:132–141.

118. Bliwise DL, Pursley AM, Bliwise NG. Impaired respiration in sleep is associated with mortality in an ambulatory, non-institutionalized aged sample. Sleep RES 1986;15:104.

119. Guilleminault C, Commiskey J, Motta J. Chronic obstructive airflow disease and sleep studies. Am Rev Respir Dis 1980;122:397–406.

120. Martin RJ, Sander MH, Gray BA. Acute and long-term ventilatory effects of oxygen administration in adult sleep apnea syndrome. Am Rev Respir Dis 1982;125:175–180.

121. Phillipson EA. State of the art control of breathing during

sleep. Am Rev Respir Dis 1978;118:909–939.

122. National Heart, Lung, and Blood Institute. Report of the Task Force on Research in Cardiopulmonary Dysfunction in Critical Care Medicine. Washington, DC: Department of Health and Human Services, 1994:119.

123. Griffith D, Idell S. Approach to adult respiratory distress syndrome and respiratory failure in elderly patients. Clin Chest Med 1993;14:571–582.

124. Cohen IL, Lambrinos J, Fein IA. Mechanical ventilation for the elderly patient in intensive care: incremental charges and benefits. JAMA 1993;269:1025–1029.

125. King TE Jr. Acute respiratory failure. In: Schrier RW, ed. Current medical therapy. 2nd ed. New York: Raven, 1989:140–177.

126. Chin R, Pesce R. Practical aspects in management of respiratory failure in chronic obstructive pulmonary disease. Crit Care Crit Care Quarterly? 1983;6:1–21.

127. Carton RW, Brown MD. Ethical considerations and CPR in the elderly patient. Clin Chest Medicine 1993;14:591–599.

128. Chalfin DB. Outcome assessment in elderly patients with critical care illness and respiratory failure. Clin Chest Med 1993;14:583–589.

129. Chelluri L, Pinsky MR, Donahoe MP, Grenvik A. Long-term outcome of critically ill elderly patients requiring intensive care. JAMA 1993;269:3119–3123.

130. Pierson DJ, Neff TA, Petty TL. Ventilatory management of the elderly. Geriatrics 1973;28:86–95.

131. Pesau B, Falger S, Berger E, et al. Influence of age on outcome of mechanically ventilated patients in an intensive care unit. Crit Care Med 1992;20:489–492.

132. Fowler AA, Hamman RF, Zerbe GO. Adult respiratory distress syndrome: prognosis after onset. Am Rev Respir Dis 1985;132:472–478.

133. Bell RC, Coalson JJ, Smith JD. Multiple organ system failure and infection in adult respiratory distress syndrome. Ann Intern Med 1983;99:293–298.

134. Wade JF III, King TE Jr. Infiltrative and interstitial lung disease in the elderly. Clin Chest Med 1993;14:501–521.

135. King TE Jr. Acute and chronic pulmonary disease in the elderly. In: Schrier R, ed. Geriatric medicine. The care of the elderly. Philadelphia: Saunders, 1990:273–323.

136. King TE. Acute respiratory failure. In: Schrier RW, ed. Current medical therapy. New York: Raven, 1984:126–160.

Chapter 45

The Aging Lung, Chronic Obstructive Pulmonary Disease, Asthma, and Pulmonary Rehabilitation

Talmadge E. King, Jr. and Kenneth Newman

Keep breathing [key to longevity.]

Sophie Tucker
Newspaper Reports, Jan., 1964

Lung function declines with increasing age. This change occurs so gradually that in the absence of disease, breathing remains effortless. Throughout life, however, the respiratory system is continually exposed to factors such as pulmonary infection or environmental pollutants that may alter its function. Thus, in the elderly, it is often a major challenge to differentiate the normal decline in lung function (i.e., the changes attributed to the aging process itself) from the decline that results from disease or the external environment.

In general, there have been few longitudinal or cross-sectional studies of large numbers of elderly persons, either normal or those with specific pulmonary diseases. Consequently, a discussion of pulmonary diseases of the elderly is based on an impression of the important processes relative to the elderly rather than to that determined by firm scientific data. This chapter focuses on what is known regarding the effect of aging on the normal lung, and on asthma and chronic obstructive pulmonary disease (COPD).

Structure and Function of the Respiratory Tract

Morphologic Changes of Aging

Aging induces several changes in the respiratory system that collectively result in a decline in lung function (Table 45.1). The anteroposterior diameter of the chest increases, and skeletal deformities such as kyphoscoliosis frequently develop with age. Also, osteoporosis of the ribs and vertebrae, calcification of the costal cartilages, decreased respiratory muscle strength, progressive increase in chest wall stiffness, and progressive enlargement of the respiratory bronchioles and alveolar ducts, all contribute

to the reduced pulmonary function that underlies the increased susceptibility to cardiopulmonary diseases and diminishes the capacity for stress and exercise (1–3).

The chief physiologic manifestations of aging on lung functions, however, are related to the changes that occur in lung and chest wall compliance. The chest wall becomes stiffer with age, which results in a steady decline in chest wall compliance. In addition, the muscles of respiration (i.e., diaphragm, intercostal muscles, and accessory respiratory muscles), like other skeletal muscles, demonstrate a consistent decline in strength and endurance with age. This results in decreases in both maximal inspiratory and maximal expiratory pressures when the elderly are compared with a younger age group (2). In addition, respiratory muscle oxygen consumption (i.e., muscle energy use) for a given change in ventilation is increased in the healthy, elderly person (4). Conversely, as the chest wall stiffens and the muscles that move it weaken, an opposite and roughly equal process affects the lung parenchyma and conducting airways. There is a progressive loss of lung elastic recoil with age. The lung normally is able to collapse when the chest wall is opened (e.g., surgically or when a pneumothorax occurs) as a result of its elastic recoil. The diminution in static elastic recoil with senescence results in an increased expansibility. In other words, the compliance of the lung increases. (Compliance is defined as the change in volume per unit of change in pressure.) The decreased elastic recoil forces are believed to result from alterations in the connective tissue components of the lung. However, studies of age-related changes in collagen, elastin, and proteoglycans have yielded conflicting results. There is no evidence that the surface-active lining material of terminal respiratory units, a second determinant of elastic recoil, is altered with aging. One could expect, however, that the loss of alveolar surface area accompanying aging would result in a reduction of the surface tension forces normally present

Table 45.1. Effects of Aging On the Respiratory System.

Respiratory Abnormality	Physiologic Basis	Clinical Disorders
Decline in bellows function	Increased chest wall stiffness Loss of elastic recoil Decreased respiratory muscle strength Increased airway collapsibility	Aging lung
Abnormal gas exchange	Ventilation/perfusion mismatch Reduced diffusing capacity for carbon monoxide Increased alveolar-arterial oxygen gradient	Arterial hypoxemia
Abnormal breathing pattern	Diminished responsiveness to hypoxemia and hypercarbia Changing setpoint for ventilation caused by fluctuating level of wakefulness	Cheyne-Stokes breathing
Upper airway obstruction	Decreased airway muscle tone caused by loss of wakefulness stimulus, decreased metabolic respiratory drive	Snoring, sleep apnea, hypopnea, oxygen desaturation
Altered lung-host defense	Decreased ciliary action Impaired cough mechanisms Decreased IgA production Decreased phagocytic function of alveolar macrophages	Increased susceptibility to infection (pneumonia and chronic bronchitis)

and thereby result in some degree of loss of lung recoil. Consequently, the loss in elastic recoil of the lung, the stiffer chest wall, the weaker respiratory muscles, and the increased respiratory muscle oxygen consumption combine to make breathing more difficult for the elderly.

Changes in Dynamic Properties with Aging

Although the vital capacity (i.e., the amount of air that can be expelled from the lungs after a maximal inspiration) declines with age, total lung capacity remains constant. Although the elastic recoil of the lung decreases (i.e., the lung becomes more distensible), total lung capacity is not affected by aging because the concomitant reduced muscle strength and chest wall stiffness prohibit an increase in the maximum volume of the thorax. Therefore, the reduction in vital capacity results from an increase in the residual volume (i.e., the amount of air remaining in the lungs after a maximal expiration) (Figure 45.1). The increase in residual volume (and functional residual capacity) results from the collapse of small airways that occurs at higher lung volumes as age increases. Residual volume increases nearly 50 percent between early adulthood and 70 years of age.

In addition, standard spirometric measurements of lung function (i.e., forced expiratory volume in 1 second, peak expiratory flow rate, maximal midexpiratory flow

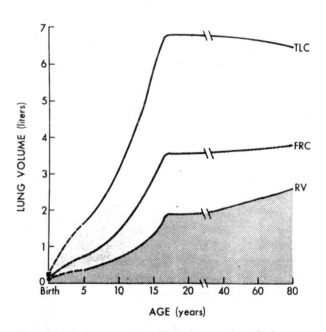

Fig. 45.1. Total lung capacity (TLC), functional residual capacity (FRC), and residual volume (RV) as a function of age from birth to 80 years of age for a male of average body build. (Reproduced by permission from Murray JF. The normal lung. Philadelphia; Saunders, 1976:312.)

rate, and maximal expiratory flow volume) have been demonstrated to decline with age (Figure 45.2). In fact, forced expiratory volume in 1 second (FEV$_1$) shows a steady decline of about 30 mL per year in healthy adult men, mainly from the diminished elastic recoil that occurs with aging (Figure 45.3). However, other nonage-related factors that affect airway geometry and resistance also play a role in this decline with age (5–8). In particular, cigarette smoking accelerates the age-related declines in flow rates.

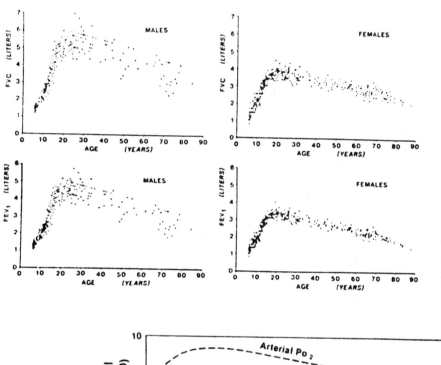

Fig. 45.2. Predicted values for forced vital capacity (FVC) (*A*) and forced expiratory volume in 1 second (FEV$_1$) (*B*) for males and females in the reference population. (Reproduced by permission from Knudson RJ, Lebowitz MD, Holberg CJ, Burrows B. Changes in the normal maximal expiratory flow volume curve with growth and aging. Am Rev Respir Dis 1983;127:725–734.)

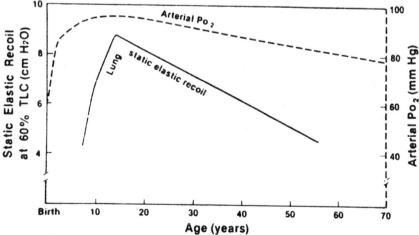

Fig. 45.3. Static elastic recoil at 60 percent TLC (solid line) and arterial PO$_2$ as a function of age (broken line). Both increase from birth to maturity followed by a gradual decline with advancing age. These two variables are believed to be related through the effects of elastic recoil on airway caliber and therefore the uniformity of ventilation. (Reproduced by permission from Young RC Jr, Borden DL, Rachal RE. Aging of the lung: pulmonary disease in the elderly. Age 1987;10:138–145.)

Alveolar Gas Exchange

The matching of ventilation and perfusion within the lung is critical for adequate gas exchange. Older persons have less uniform ventilation than young adults do when breathing at moderate tidal volumes. With deep breathing, however, the elderly have the ability to improve the uniformity of ventilation and, thereby, eliminate the difference between the two groups. The nonuniformity of ventilation at low lung volumes is believed to result from closure of the small airways in the dependent portions of the lung during tidal breathing, which results in a ventilation and perfusion mismatch throughout the lung.

In addition to the changes in ventilation that occur with age, there are also changes in the pulmonary circulation. Although pulmonary capillary blood volume and total lung perfusion remain normal, the alveolar capillary surface area progressively declines, which can be measured by a parallel decline in the single breath diffusing capacity for carbon monoxide (D_LCO). There is a progressive reduction in D_LCO ranging from 0.20 to 0.32 ml/min/mm Hg per year of adulthood for men and 0.06 to 0.18 ml/min/mm Hg per year for women (9). This change does not appear to be of clinical importance in an otherwise healthy individual.

The arterial oxygen tension slowly declines with age, at the rate of approximately 4 mm Hg per decade (see Fig. 45.3). This results predominantly from the imbalance in ventilation and perfusion caused by small airway closure in dependent lung zones that occurs during tidal breathing (10). The imbalance is particularly marked in the recumbent position. In addition, cardiac output and mixed venous oxygen (O_2) content also decline with aging, and therefore contribute to the fall in arterial partial pressure of oxygen (PO_2) seen in the elderly. In contrast, arterial partial pressure of carbon dioxide $PaCO_2$ and pH do not change with age. The $PaCO_2$ remains normal, despite an increase in the physiologic dead space, because minute ventilation increases with age.

Ventilatory Control

Normally, ventilation is regulated by a central controller in the brain that coordinates information fed to its various centers and modulates the activity of the respiratory muscles. There are two major sensors: the central chemoreceptors and the peripheral chemoreceptors. The central chemoreceptors are located in the medulla and have a slower response time than the peripheral chemoreceptors. The central receptors increase ventilation in response to acidosis, which causes a lowering of $PaCO_2$. They are responsible for three-fourths of the ventilatory response to CO_2. The peripheral chemoreceptors are located in the carotid bodies at the bifurcation of the common carotid arteries and in the aortic bodies above and below the aortic arch. The carotid body chemoreceptors are the most important in humans. The carotid body chemoreceptors respond to decreases in arterial PO_2 and pH by increasing alveolar ventilation. These receptors are solely responsible for the increase in ventilation that accompanies arterial hypoxemia (11). Although studies are limited, respiratory control appears to become less precise with age (1,12). Elderly subjects have a blunted response to hypoxemia and hypercapnia compared with that in young adults. The exact mechanism and the reason for these changes with aging are unknown.

Recently, considerable interest has been centered on sleep and the control of breathing. Numerous respiratory irregularities occur in adults during sleep, with apnea, hypopnea, and desaturation being common. These may occasionally be severe in the elderly (13–15).

Lung Host Defense

The lung also has important nonrespiratory functions, including purification of the inspired air and maintenance of an infection-free lung tissue (16). No systematic evaluation of host defenses has been reported in elderly persons. It appears likely, however, that the nonspecific components of lung defenses have an age-related decline similar to that of other organ systems (17).

Cell-mediated immunity and humoral antibody formation declines with age in some individuals; however, that this immune dysfunction is clearly involved in many disease processes in older adults has not been documented. The incidence of benign monoclonal gammopathies increases with age. Unfortunately, a subset of these individuals develop myeloma, macroglobulinemia, amyloidosis, or a malignant lymphoproliferative process (17). Autoantibody formation increases with age (i.e., antinuclear antibodies, antithyroglobulin antibodies, and rheumatoid factor). The importance of these types of changes remains to be clarified. These defects may reflect a loss of immune regulation (suppression) with "emergence of forbidden clones" (17). In addition, several defense mechanisms are altered in the aged and are thought to be responsible for the increased susceptibility of the elderly to chronic bronchitis, pulmonary infection, and autoimmune diseases. These alterations include 1) impaired cough mechanism; 2) ineffective ciliary action so that inhaled particles are not cleared readily from the tracheobronchial tree; 3) decreased immunoglobulin A (IgA), the secretory immunoglobulin of nasal and respiratory mucosal surfaces with neutralizing activity against viruses; 4) defective alveolar macrophages, or phagocytic cells, that ingest foreign material that reach the alveolar space, especially in smokers; 5) impaired T-cell proliferation, decreased cytokine-receptor expression (decreased interleukin-2 (IL-2) production and receptor expression, decreased production and response to T-cell growth factors) (17); and 6) diminished inflammatory response, as evidenced by decreased neutrophil-mediated killing and chemotaxis.

Manifestations of Pulmonary Disease

Cough, often associated with sputum production, and shortness of breath (dyspnea) are the most common manifestations of respiratory disorders. Hemoptysis, chest pain, cyanosis, and an abnormal breathing pattern are less common manifestations of chest disorders.

Cough

Cough plays a major role in host defense because of its ability to remove particles, such as bacteria, from the airways. In the elderly, the cough mechanism is frequently altered, in large part because of age-related changes in lung mechanics (e.g., decreased elastic recoil) and the decreased respiratory muscle strength. Chronic cough, with or without wheezing, should prompt careful attention to several important causes in the elderly.

Chronic bronchitis, acute respiratory tract infection, asthma, and postnasal drip are the most common causes of chronic cough. In this age group, it is very important to exclude other causes, such as gastroesophageal reflux or other mechanisms of aspiration, congestive heart failure, bronchogenic or metastatic carcinoma, interstitial lung disease, environmental irritant (e.g., tobacco smoke, noxious gases, dusts), foreign body in the airways, and pleural disease.

Because cough is an important protective reflex, its suppression should only be attempted when the underlying cause has been addressed or when it is important to prevent other complications of cough, such as rib fracture, muscle strain, significant sleep deprivation, urinary incontinence, or hernias. Codeine (10 to 30 mg orally every 4 to 6 hours, not to exceed 120 mg/day) is the most popular antitussive drug. In the elderly, cough suppression may result in the retention of respiratory secretions or lead to atelectasis, airway obstruction, or respiratory failure. Codeine may cause constipation, sedation, nausea, vomiting, dizziness, palpitation, pruritus, or agitation.

Dyspnea

Breathlessness, or dyspnea, is one of the most frequent complaints in the elderly patient and is commonly registered in patients with pulmonary, pleural, or cardiovascular processes. Unfortunately, dyspnea is a nonspecific sensation that may be extremely difficult for elderly patients to describe. Common expressions are an inability to get enough air, difficulty taking a deep breath or to breathe more rapidly, a smothering sensation, or a choking feeling. In a study of 70-year-old people, 45 percent of the study population had exertional dyspnea. In those who complained of exertional dyspnea, 64 percent of the men and 43 percent of the women suffered an identifiable illness of the cardiopulmonary system (18). In the pulmonary diseases, dyspnea results from the increased work of breathing that commonly occurs in the aged lung and is worsened by the disease process itself (19). In men 70 years of age or older, the presence of dyspnea is a risk factor for increased mortality (20). Many elderly persons suffer significant breathlessness as a result of inactivity and, thus, deconditioning. However, aging itself does not result in lung function changes that cause dyspnea at rest or with usual daily activity (21). Consequently, dyspnea is an important symptom that should be evaluated properly to rule out a specific cause (22).

Hemoptysis

The coughing up of blood, hemoptysis, varies from blood-tinged sputum to moderate or massive hemorrhage. It is sometimes difficult in the elderly to accurately determine where the blood being "coughed up" originates, such as from the nose or throat as a result of hematemesis (vomited blood) or from a portion of the bronchial tree. There are many causes of hemoptysis. Blood-streaked sputum is frequently seen with chronic bronchitis and upper respiratory infection and is an early finding of lung cancer. Massive hemoptysis (greater than 600mL in 48 hours) most commonly occurs with lung cancer, pulmonary tuberculosis (both active and inactive), bronchiectasis, and lung abscess. A general rule is that the occurrence of hemoptysis before a person is age 45 is most likely to result from mitral stenosis, tuberculosis, pneumonia, or bronchiectasis. After age 45, bronchogenic carcinoma, bronchitis, tuberculosis, and pulmonary embolus with infarction are more common causes of hemoptysis.

Massive hemoptysis is a medical emergency that can result in hypotension, anemia, cardiovascular collapse, and asphyxiation. Supportive measures to maintain vital functions are important (e.g., volume replacement, oxygenation, treatment with vasopressors). Control of the airway with endotracheal intubation should be carried out immediately, if required. The patient should be positioned with the bleeding side facing downward to prevent aspiration of blood into the contralateral lung. Localization of the bleeding site(s) by chest x-ray and fiberoptic bronchoscopy is an absolute preoperative requisite, and prompt surgical resection is the treatment of choice. Contraindications to surgery include diffuse lung disease that causes diffuse bleeding, coagulation abnormalities that may be associated with diffuse bleeding (e.g., anticoagulant therapy), inoperable lung cancer, and lung disease of such severity that the patient may not have adequate pulmonary reserve to survive resection of functioning lung tissue (i.e., a predicted $FEV_1 < 1.0$ liter after the procedure). In inoperable cases, bleeding can be controlled by tamponade of bronchial segment with a Fogarty balloon catheter or by embolization of the arterial supply to the bleeding segment. The latter technique is usually unsuccessful because the systemic bronchial circulation is the source of the bleeding. Recent data suggest that embolization of both the bronchial and pulmonary vessels is effective in controlling bleeding in some patients (23).

Chest Pain

Chest pain in the elderly patient is not always caused by myocardial ischemia. In fact, it may result from numerous causes and can present difficult differential diagnosis (24). Pleuritic pain caused by irritation of the parietal layer of the pleura complicates many pulmonary diseases. Pneumonia in a portion of the lung adjacent to the visceral pleural surface and pulmonary infarction are two important causes of pleurisy in the elderly. Rib fracture, costochondritis, pulmonary hypertension, postherpetic neuralgia, and muscle pain (after severe coughing) are other causes of chest pain in the geriatric population.

Breathing Pattern

The presence of an abnormal breathing pattern can be an important clue to the presence of disease in any patient, especially in the elderly. Considerable attention has been focused recently on sleep and the control of breathing (see Chapter 44). Normally, persons at rest breathe 8 to 16 times per minute, with a tidal volume of 400 to 800mL. Several abnormal patterns of breathing have been characterized and may provide helpful diagnostic clues.

1 *Kussmaul's breathing* is a form of hyperpnea characterized by a regular pattern, moderate rate, and large tidal volume, with little apparent effort and suggests metabolic acidosis.

2 *Obstructed breathing* is seen in patients with COPD and is characterized by a slow rate and increased tidal volume; wheezing is often present.

3 *Restricted breathing* is characterized by small tidal volume and rapid rate and is seen in patients with restrictive lung diseases, especially the interstitial lung diseases.

4 *Gasping respirations* consist of irregular, quick inspirations associated with extension of the neck and followed by a long expiratory pause. They are characteristic of severe cerebral hypoxia and are common in patients with severe cardiac failure.

5 *Cheyne-Stokes respiration* (an extreme form of periodic breathing) describes a cyclic pattern of alternating apnea and hyperpnea. It is sometimes seen in healthy, elderly persons but is generally found during sleep in patients with COPD, cardiac failure, or cerebrovascular insufficiency.

6 *Hypoventilation* is often difficult to identify and if not specifically sought, may be missed, often with grave conse-

quences for the elderly patient. It frequently results from severe obstructive lung disease, especially that associated with CO_2 narcosis, and from abnormalities in the control of breathing caused by cerebral vascular accidents, head trauma, oversedation, or administration of narcotics.

Chronic Obstructive Pulmonary Disease

Obstructive pulmonary diseases are characterized by alterations in ventilation that result from a limitation of expiratory flow. They are second only to heart disease as a cause of disability. Despite this frequency, the obstructive airways diseases are frequently overlooked and undertreated (25,26). The routine use of simple tests of lung function in clinical practice, office spirometry, or peak flow meter, is essential to improved identification and treatment of this common problem in the elderly (26) (Figure 45.4).

COPD includes localized disease of the upper airway, bronchiolitis, cystic fibrosis, bronchiectasis, asthma, bronchitis, and emphysema. Of these, bronchitis and emphysema are primarily diseases of later life, with peak incidence in a person's sixth and seventh decades. Bronchiolitis is seldom recognized after age 4; cystic fibrosis usually results in death by a person's second or third decade; and bronchiectasis, although seen at any age, is primarily a disease of middle age (27). Despite this broad range of causes of airway obstruction, COPD is most often applied to patients who have peripheral airway disease, emphysema, chronic bronchitis, or a mixture of the three, with or without airway hyperreactivity.

Emphysema

The indiscriminate use of the term *emphysema* when lower airway obstruction is referred to has resulted in considerable confusion about the exact definition. In addition, the separation of emphysema and bronchitis into two separate entities is occasionally misleading. The two diseases co-exist frequently; consequently, it is often difficult to differentiate them clinically. Emphysema is defined as "a condition of the lung characterized by abnormal, permanent enlargement of airspaces distal to the terminal bronchiole, accompanied by the destruction of their walls, and without obvious fibrosis" (28). Destruction in emphysema is further defined as nonuniformity in the pattern of respiratory airspace enlargement so that the orderly appearance of the acinus (the respiratory airspaces arising from a single terminal bronchiole) and its components are disturbed and may be lost. Consequently, only a presumptive diagnosis of emphysema can be made in the living patient. Obstruction to airflow is frequently present to some degree in emphysema and predominantly results from a decrease in the elastic recoil of the lungs and collapsible airways. The pathogenesis of emphysema remains unknown. The concept of protease-antiprotease imbalance remains the dominant hypothesis (29).

Three anatomic subtypes of emphysema are recognized on the basis of the portions of the acinus primarily involved (30). *Panacinar emphysema* is characterized by distention and destruction of all alveoli within the respiratory lobule. This type of emphysema has no definite regional preference, although the lower lobes may be more often affected. Interestingly, this form is associated with the primary emphysema seen in alpha$_1$-antiprotease deficiency (a familial disease with clinical manifestions that occur by the time a person who is homozygous for the Z gene is age 40).

Centriacinar emphysema is characterized by the destruction of the central part of the lobule; the proximal part of the acinus (respiratory bronchiole) is predominantly involved with the peripheral alveolar ducts and the alveoli unaffected. There are two subdivisions of this form of lesion. The first, known as *centrilobular emphysema*, is classically associated with cigarette smoking. Most of the lung changes with centrilobular emphysema occur in the apices of the upper lobe, but spread downward as the disease progresses. This type is rare before a person is 40 years of age and occurs without clinical manifestations in about one-fourth of those who die with no history of lung disease and a normal chest radiograph. In fact, half of individuals older than 70 years of age at autopsy have a mild form of centrilobular emphysema–the so-called aged lung–usually without disability. The second form is referred to as *focal emphysema* and occurs in individuals exposed to the inhalation of coal dust (i.e., coal pneumoconiosis) and other mineral dust. This lesion is relatively uniform in distribution in the lungs and is characterized by the dilation of respiratory bronchioles, with the intense accumulation of dust-laden macrophages in and around the respiratory bronchioles.

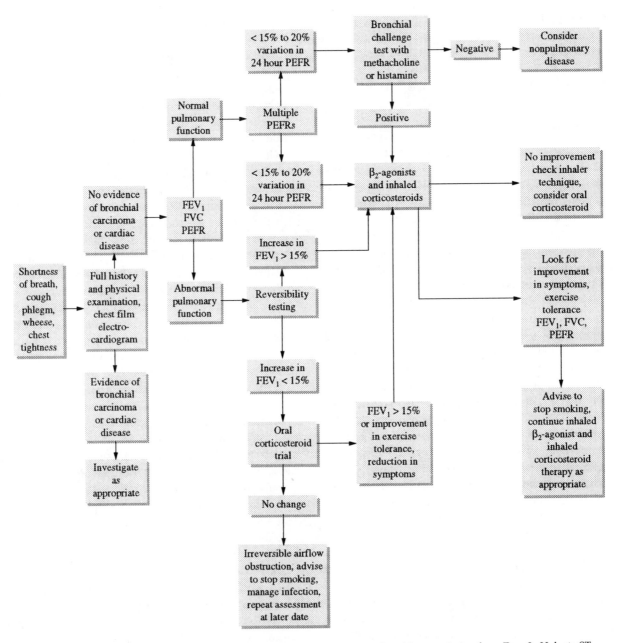

Fig. 45.4. Respiratory symptoms in the elderly: A management algorithm. (Reproduced by permission from Dow L, Holgate ST. Assessment and treatment of obstructive airways airways disease in the elderly. Br Med Bulletin 1990;46:230–245.)

Distal acinar emphysema involves the distal part of the acinus, alveolar ducts, and sacs that abut the pleura, vessel, and airways; thus, the emphysema is worse in these regions. Mild airflow obstruction, despite extensive

bullous emphysema, and the spontaneous pneumothorax of young adults are the clinical associations of this form of emphysema (28).

Clinical Picture

It is unusual to find a patient with pure emphysema. Although emphysema alone can result in a crippling and fatal disease, when hypoxemia and cor pulmonale supervene, it is almost invariably associated with chronic bronchitis. The diagnosis of emphysema in life is made indirectly by the collective changes found in the clinical, radiologic, and functional status. The clinical manifestations are predominantly breathlessness, with or without cough, that progresses to severe disability as a result of unrelenting dyspnea. Early in the disease, the clinical examination may be of little value. As the severity increases, the physician is confronted by an anxious, thin, and, occasionally, emaciated patient who demonstrates pursed-lip breathing with prominent use of accessory muscles of respiration because of the need to further inflate an already inflated chest. Breath sounds are markedly diminished, and heart sounds are faint.

Diagnosis

A combination of physiologic tests is necessary to indicate the presence of emphysema. The chest radiograph is suggestive but not specific for the diagnosis of emphysema (Figure 45.5). The presence of hyperinflation (low, flat diaphragm and large retrosternal air space); cardiovascular changes (a narrow vertical heart, prominent pulmonary trunk, and large hilar vessels with tapering peripheral vessels); and signs of local vessel loss (bullae that are demarcated by a thick, white line or with no definite margins) increases the diagnostic accuracy of the plain chest film. Few cases of mild emphysema can be recognized radiographically (31). Computerized tomography (CT) is suggested as a useful radiographic technique for detecting the morphologic changes of emphysema in life (32) (Figure 45.6). In general, when a patient has airway obstruction, increased total lung capacity, diminished elastic recoil, increased static compliance, and a decreased D_LCO, clinically significant emphysema is very likely to be present (33).

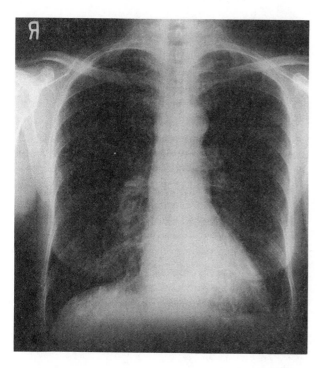

Fig. 45.5. Pulmonary emphysema, posteroanterior view. Both lungs are hyperradiolucent with classic appearance of arterial deficiency pattern in both upper lobes and associated with a flat diaphragm in a 70-year-old woman.

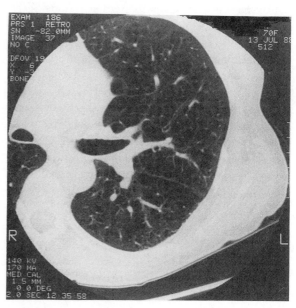

Fig. 45.6. Pulmonary emphysema, HRCT Scan. (Same patient as in Figure 45.5.) Retrospectively targeted 1.5-mm thick HRCT section through the left mid-lung shows characteristic pattern of emphysema, definable as well-defined zones of diminished lung density without definable walls.

Chronic Bronchitis

Chronic bronchitis is defined by the presence of sputum production and is characterized by cough, sputum production, airways obstruction, and chronic or recurrent bacterial infections. Simple chronic bronchitis is defined as mucous hypersecretion with resultant cough and expectoration on most days for at least 3 consecutive months during 2 successive years, with no other cause present. Morphologic changes are primarily hypertrophy of mucous glands in the large bronchi and evidence of chronic inflammatory changes in the small airways. Although multiple factors have been implicated in the etiology of chronic bronchitis, the most common association is cigarette smoking. Atmospheric pollution and occupational exposure have also been implicated.

Clinical Picture

A typical presentation of chronic bronchitis is that of a middle-aged or elderly man who has had a history of a productive cough for several years. The patient invariably is or was a cigarette smoker for many years. He usually has had a decline in exercise tolerance because progressive dyspnea severely limits his exertional efforts. Several factors are responsible for the exercise limitation seen in these patients (Table 45.2). Frequently, episodes of acute purulent bronchitis supervene; with time, these episodes become more frequent.

The clinical examination usually reveals a stocky or overweight man with a dusky complexion. Cyanosis may or may not be apparent at this time, but invariably these patients become "blue and bloated." Chest examination reveals mild to moderate diminution of breath sounds, with scattered rales and rhonchi. Evidence of right ventricular dysfunction with fluid retention (i.e., jugular venous distention and pedal edema) is usually present.

Diagnosis

The chest radiograph demonstrates a normal position of the diaphragm and lung fields that are normal or have increased bronchovascular marking. Cardiac enlargement may be present. Physiologic studies generally reveal airway obstruction with normal lung volumes and elastic recoil. The D_LCO is not diminished as it is in emphysema. The arterial blood gases are frequently abnormal, revealing hypercapnia and hypoxemia. With prolonged hypoxemia, erythrocytosis may be present, with hematocrits as high as 70 percent.

Complications of COPD

A number of complications may result from COPD. Table 45.3 lists several of the most common ones.

Cor Pulmonale

Cor pulmonale is defined by the World Health Organization as "hypertrophy of the right ventricle from diseases affecting the function and/or structure of the lung except when these pulmonary alterations are the result of diseases that primarily affect the left side of the heart, or of congenital heart disease" (34). The incidence of this form of heart disease is unknown. Although less than 50 percent of patients with COPD manifest right ventricular hypertrophy (RVH) at autopsy, chronic cor pulmonale most often results from COPD (35). Elevation of the pulmonary artery pressure is the prerequisite for the devel-

Table 45.2. Factors Leading to Exercise Limitation in Patients with COPD.

Abnormal pulmonary mechanics
Impairment of pulmonary gas exchange
Abnormal perception of breathlessness and ventilatory control
Presence of impaired cardiac performance resulting from cor pulmonale or occult coronary artery disease
Poor nutritional status
Development of respiratory muscle fatigue

SOURCE: Loke J, Mahler D, Man SFP, et al. Exercise impairment in chronic obstructive pulmonary disease. Clin Chest Med 1984;5:121–143.

Table 45.3. Complications of COPD.

Chronic hypercarbia
Chronic cor pulmonale, peripheral edema
Supraventricular and ventricular arrhythmias
Secondary erythrocytosis
Sleep disorders and hypoxemia, neuropsychological dysfunction
Pulmonary embolism
Spontaneous pneumothorax
Peptic ulcer disease
Acute respiratory failure
Side effects of adverse reaction to drug therapy
Malnutrition

opment of cor pulmonale. The significance of pulmonary hypertension in COPD cannot be overstated because its occurrence is clearly an important determinant of the quantity and quality of life in these patients (35). Patients with COPD frequently develop pulmonary arterial hypertension as a result of hypoxemia, hypercapneic acidosis, and an increased red cell mass (secondary polycythemia). Hypoxemia and acidosis induce hypertension by producing vasoconstriction of pulmonary vessels. In addition, irreversible anatomic destruction or restriction of pulmonary vessels occurs in patients with emphysema, thereby contributing to an increase in pulmonary vascular resistance. Polycythemia, usually seen in patients with hypoxemic bronchitis, increases pulmonary arteriole resistance as a result of increased blood viscosity. Also, the hypervolemia associated with polycythemia increases cardiac output, further complicating the pulmonary hypertension. Consequently, one or more of these factors set the stage for the development of cor pulmonale. Thus, longstanding, significant pulmonary hypertension produces right ventricular systolic and diastolic dysfunction by elevating afterload and reducing right ventricular myocardial oxygen supply relative to demand. This leads to subsequent dilation and hypertrophy and, finally, to cor pulmonale, with or without right ventricular failure (36).

Generally, the presentation of cor pulmonale is dominated by the manifestations of the underlying lung disease. In the elderly, co-existing coronary artery disease makes the distinction between right and left ventricular dysfunction important because therapeutic decisions depend on the accurate assessment of the relative role of each disease. In this regard, it is important to note that left ventricular dysfunction is rare in uncomplicated COPD (37).

Syncope and precordial pain are classic symptoms of pulmonary hypertension but are infrequent. Severe cyanosis, unexplained drowsiness, engorged neck veins, hepatomegaly, and fluid retention with dependent edema are often presenting findings. The presence of tachycardia, a right ventricular lift, a loud pulmonic component of the second heart sound, an atrial gallop, and a Graham Steell murmur (a soft, blowing, high-pitched diastolic murmur of pulmonic insufficiency) are extremely helpful in diagnosing pulmonary hypertension with cor

pulmonale. The chest radiograph usually demonstrates enlargement of the central pulmonary arteries. Two chest radiographic measurements–the diameter of the right descending pulmonary artery and the diameter of the left descending pulmonary artery–are sensitive indexes of pulmonary hypertension in patients with COPD. A right descending pulmonary artery greater than 16mm is a more specific and more accurate indicator than an enlarged left descending pulmonary artery greater than 18mm. If both arteries are enlarged, however, the combined sensitivity is 98 percent, and an accuracy of 90 percent for the presence of pulmonary artery hypertension is achieved (38).

RVH is difficult to diagnose by plain film of the chest. Measurements made from CT scanning are more helpful in identifying both pulmonary hypertension and RVH. Also, the sensitivity and specificity of the electrocardiogram (ECG) in the diagnosis of RVH is low. Autopsy studies reveal that 25 percent to 40 percent of patients with COPD and RVH have no associated ECG changes at the time of death (39). Nonetheless, it is extremely important that the presence or evolution of changes on the ECG consistent with right ventricular enlargement be identified because they signal the need for arterial blood gas analysis and the institution of supplemental oxygen therapy. The electrocardiographic findings of cor pulmonale may be present, including peaked P waves in leads II, III, and aVF, right axis deviation, RVH, and right bundle branch block. Continuous, long-term oxygen therapy helps ameliorate the effects of pulmonary hypertension and cor pulmonale in many patients with COPD and is discussed later in this chapter (40).

Arrhythmias

Supraventricular and ventricular arrhythmias are common complications of COPD, particularly during the stage of cor pulmonale and acute respiratory failure (41). Metabolic disturbances associated with respiratory failure are suspected as the cause of these arrhythmias. Consequently, arterial hypoxemia, hypercapnia, acidosis, and deficits in potassium, calcium, or magnesium must be treated aggressively. In addition, when these patients require mechanical ventilation, respiratory alkalosis secondary to overventilation occurs and may also trigger serious arrhythmias. Except in life-threatening situations, the use of antiarrhythmic drugs is appropriate only after all possible causes of the arrhythmias have been corrected.

Polycythemia

Secondary polycythemia, with hematocrits as high as 70 percent, occur because of the elevated renal erythropoietin that results from chronic hypoxemia. Polycythemia represents a mechanism that allows greater oxygen delivery to compensate for the chronically low arterial PO_2. The effectiveness of this response in COPD remains unclear. Supplemental oxygen to treat the hypoxemia present in these patients is the most important treatment modality. Occasionally, phlebotomy is indicated in patients who manifest congestive cor pulmonale with polycythemia.

Sleep Hypoxemia

It has been estimated that more than 80 percent of patients with COPD have serious nocturnal oxygen desaturation (42). Many of these patients, however, do not have classic features of sleep deprivation, such as daytime hypersomnolence or right heart failure. Obesity and increasing age, especially in men and postmenopausal women, are strongly associated with episodes of nocturnal desaturation (13,43,44). The causes of the hypoxemia noted during sleep are shown in Table 45.4.

The importance of identifying and managing the potentially severe nocturnal oxygen desaturation that occurs in patients with COPD cannot be overemphasized. Smolensky and coworkers reported several years ago that patients with chronic lung disease often die in the middle of the night (45). Furthermore, studies have demonstrated a relationship between nocturnal oxygen desaturation in the development of episodic pulmonary vasoconstriction

Table 45.4. Causes of Sleep Hypoxemia.

Alveolar hypoventilation
Ventilation-perfusion mismatch
Prolonged central apneas
Upper airway obstructive apnea
Mucus hypersecretion and accumulation
Disordered breathing and altered controls of ventilation
Nocturnal bronchoconstriction

and pulmonary hypertension and have suggested this as a possible mechanism for the progression to cor pulmonale and the blue and bloated syndrome (46,47). Equally important has been the demonstration that severe nocturnal oxygen desaturation in patients with COPD correlates with cardiac arrhythmias and other ECG evidence of myocardial hypoxia (48,49). The clinical manifestations and management of disordered respiratory function during sleep are discussed in Chapter 44.

Pulmonary Embolism

Pulmonary embolism (PE) is a significant complication of COPD; a 20 percent to 60 percent incidence has been reported (50). Inactivity and right heart failure are believed to be the primary risk factors. The clinical diagnosis of PE in patients with COPD is often difficult (51). Lippmann and Fein (50) and Fanta and colleagues (52) have suggested the following guidelines for the diagnosis of PE in patients with COPD.

1 Clinical manifestations are generally not helpful. However, any patient who develops severe tachypnea (more than 30 breaths per minute), the clinical manifestations of cor pulmonale in the absence of infection or other cause, and who is unresponsive to conventional bronchodilator therapy should be suspected of having PE. Typically, patients with COPD and cor pulmonale are not tachypneic to this degree because of their attempts to minimize the work of breathing.

2 As a corollary, an increase in alveolar ventilation (decreased $PaCO_2$) in a previously hypercapneic patient also suggests PE but is an uncommon finding (51). Patients who develop cor pulmonale on the basis of COPD alone typically present with both hypoxemia and carbon dioxide retention (mean $PaCO_2$ of 53 mm Hg). In patients with recurrent pulmonary emboli as the cause of their cor pulmonale, the mean $PaCO_2$ is 32 mm Hg (50,52).

3 Lung function tests in pulmonary emboli-induced cor pulmonale may not be impaired severely enough to explain the development of cor pulmonale in a patient with COPD. It is uncommon for patients with FEV_1 more than 1.5 liters to develop cor pulmonale solely on the basis of COPD.

4 Radioisotopic studies are not useful in differentiating PE from worsening obstruction. Often, the patient cannot hold a breath long enough for an adequate ventilation scan to be performed. Because the emboli are frequently small, the resolution of the scan cannot adequately distinguish between the changes caused by COPD from those caused by emboli.

5 When possible, angiography should be undertaken to confirm the diagnosis of PE.

6 Noninvasive tests for deep venous thrombosis (DVT) (Doppler ultrasound and impedance plethysmography) may be helpful in that a negative result has a high predictive value in excluding deep venous thrombi, particularly those that involve the proximal veins and are most likely to embolize (53).

Respiratory Failure

Respiratory failure is a common complication in patients with COPD. Respiratory failure often occurs in combination with or as a result of many of the problems just discussed. Acute respiratory failure is defined as arterial hypoxemia (PaO_2 less than 50 mm Hg). The precipitating causes of respiratory failure in this setting include 1) respiratory infection; 2) CO_2 narcosis secondary to respiratory depression caused by the administration of oxygen; 3) oversedation (sedatives, narcotics, tranquilizers), which causes a reduction in the cortical drive to breathe and, consequently, depresses respiration; 4) left ventricular dysfunction, primary or secondary to silent myocardial infarction; 5) thoracic cage abnormalities (e.g., flail chest); 6) pneumothorax; and 7) PE.

Other Complications

Spontaneous pneumothorax is a rare complication of COPD. However, it can have serious consequences when it occurs in the geriatric patient. Spontaneous pneumothorax, infection, and massive hemorrhage are important complications of bullous emphysema. Peptic ulcer disease occurs with greater frequency in patients with COPD (10% to 35%) than it does in the normal population (3%). Sexual dysfunction is relatively common in men with COPD and may be related to progression of the disease itself and not to associated illnesses (depression, cerebrovascular, cardiovascular, or peripheral vascular impairment) or to aging (54).

Management of the Elderly Patient with COPD

Although this group of diseases has been divided into chronic bronchitis and emphysema, most patients with COPD have a combination of both. In addition, many of these patients have wheezing (bronchospasm) as a prominent component and appear to be asthmatic.

Therapy of COPD is primarily directed at controlling the symptoms and complications (Table 45.5). Although both diseases can be treated with the same basic regimen, it is occasionally a grave error to oversimplify the management. Even the most precise and discriminating physician may lump these diseases and treat in a "cookbook" fashion. Consequently, patients with symptoms that are predominantly associated with emphysema, with no reversible bronchospasm, and with relative normoxia may be overmedicated with bronchodilators, corticosteroids, and antibiotics. On the other hand, the true bronchitic patient with significant bronchospasm may be undertreated and suffer needless morbidity. Therefore, every "chronic lunger" deserves a careful evaluation to determine as specifically as possible the predominant pathologic process, and careful attention must be paid to the components of the disease that are potentially reversible. This chapter emphasizes the key principles of treatment for the stable patient. Pulmonary rehabilitation is an extremely important adjunct in the management of the patient with COPD and is discussed in detail in the last section of this chapter (55). When to hospitalize a patient with COPD is often a difficult decision; some useful guidelines are provided in Table 45.6.

Table 45.5. Management of COPD.

Strongly urge smoking cessation
Patient and family education
Reduce work of breathing caused by airway obstruction
   Relieve bronchospasm (aerosol or oral sympathomimetic bronchodilators, with or without corticosteroids)
   Reduce secretions (remove all possible irritants, control infection, initiate appropriate antimicrobial therapy, administer influenza vaccine annually, pneumococcal vaccine once in a lifetime)
Chest physiotherapy
   Postural drainage and chest percussion
   Breathing retraining
   Exercise reconditioning
Low-flow oxygen therapy

Table 45.6. Principal Indications for Hospitalization of the Patient with COPD.

Acute exacerbation of symptoms unresponsive to outpatient treatment (e.g., markedly increased dyspnea, cough, sputum production) especially in presence of marked fatigue or exhaustion*

Acute respiratory failure characterized by respiratory distress, hypercarbia, worsening hypoxemia, or impaired mental status

Acute cor pulmonale with dependent edema, further impairment of exercise capacity, and hypoxemia

Complications of COPD, such as acute bronchitis or pneumonia

Performance of invasive diagnostic procedures on the lung, such as bronchoscopy, transbronchial biopsy, or needle aspiration of nodules

Need for surgery or other procedures that require significant amounts of analgesics or anesthesia

Diseases that may not require hospitalization in themselves but that in the presence of severe COPD, represent a significant risk to the patient

---

*When evaluating a patient during an acute exacerbation, the physician must obtain information from the family regarding the patient's baseline level of function (mental and physical). Previous arterial blood gas measurements (especially baseline, asymptomatic values), pulmonary function tests, and response to treatment should also be sought because they can often guide current management.

SOURCE: American Thoracic Society Statement. Standards for the diagnosis and care of patients with chronic obstructive pulmonary disease (COPD) and asthma. Am Rev Respir Dis 1987;136:225–244.

Patient Education

Patient education is unquestionably the most important aspect of a treatment program. Management of COPD requires patient and family cooperation and participation. The patient must be taught the basics of respiratory anatomy and physiology as well as how to deal with the psychological stresses of a chronic illness. The most important lesson must be smoking cessation. A steady stream of evidence clearly implicates COPD as a specific complication of smoking. In a 20-year follow-up of British physicians, it was demonstrated that a 15-year abstinence from cigarette smoking resulted in a reduction of the risk of dying of COPD from 36 times that of nonsmokers to 8 times (56). In addition, although low-tar, low-nicotine cigarettes may reduce the risk of lung cancer, there is no evidence that these cigarettes reduce the incidence of COPD. A common misconception is that once a patient presents with symptoms of COPD, it is too late to do any

good. Recent data, however, suggest that this attitude is not correct (57). Persons normally lose 20 to 30 mL per year in FEV_1. Patients susceptible to the effects of smoking have an annual FEV_1 decrement of 50 to 100 mL (58–60). In addition, it has been demonstrated that the cessation of smoking results in a definite, rapid beneficial response, especially the reduction of cough and sputum production. Therefore, every patient, regardless of age, should be encouraged to stop smoking (Figure 45.7).

Therapeutic Agents

Oxygen is the only medication shown to prolong life in patients with COPD (61,62). The criteria for the institution of oxygen therapy are given in Table 45.7. Oxygen should be prescribed to maintain oxygen saturations of more than 90 percent during rest, activity and sleep. The details of oxygen therapy and other important management modalities are discussed in the section on cardiopulmonary rehabilitation in this chapter.

Bronchodilator drugs are a mainstay in treatment of patients with COPD because they can improve airflow and reduce dyspnea. Many patients with COPD have some component of bronchospasm complicating their disease. Consequently, a defined trial of bronchodilator therapy is often recommended. Appropriate subjective and objective evaluation of the response and side effects is essential. It is important to note that a single pulmonary function test does not predict the response to chronic bronchodilator therapy. The drugs should be withdrawn if no improvement in dyspnea, cough, quantity of bronchopulmonary secretions, or lung function is achieved.

Anticholinergic agents, such as atropine or ipratropium bromide, have become a first-line therapy for patients with COPD (63) because ipratropium is very well tolerated, with a good margin of safety and excellent efficacy. However, it is not as useful for acute episodic periods of bronchospasm as are other bronchodilators. It has a slow onset of action with bronchodilator effect beginning about 15 minutes after use; the duration is about 3 to 5 hours. The recommended dose of ipratropium is 2 puffs four times daily, however, this produces less than maximal bronchodilatory effect. Therefore, this dose can be increased to three to six puffs given four times daily (64). For mild COPD it is reasonable to use ipratropium three

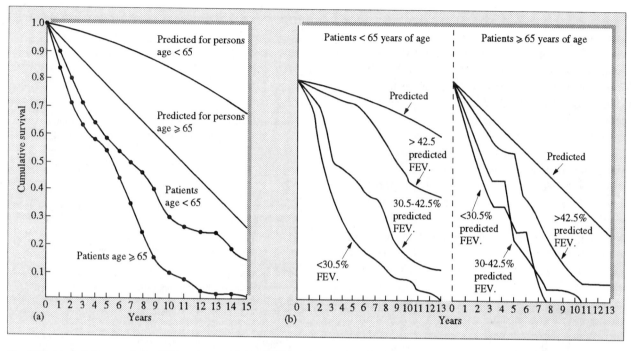

Fig. 45.7. Cumulative survival of 200 patients with chronic bronchitis and emphysema according to age (*A*) and according to age and pulmonary function (*B*) (Reproduced by permission from Dodge R, Burrows B. Chronic bronchitis and emphysema. In: Fries JF, Ehrich GE, eds. Prognosis. Contemporary outcomes of disease. Bowie, MD: Charles Press, 1981:228.)

Table 45.7. Criteria for the Institution of Home Oxygen Therapy.

Severe and persistent hypoxemia ($\leq PaO_2$ 55 mm Hg)[a]

Evidence of chronic hypoxemia ($\leq PaO_2$ 59 mm Hg) associated with mental impairment, markedly deteriorating exercise capacity, pulmonary hypertension, cor pulmonale, or right ventricular failure, polycythemia (hematocrit $\geq$55%)

Sleep hypoxemia (PaO_2 $\leq$55 mm Hg), especially if associated with above complications[b]

Selected patients with hypoxemia during exercise (PaO_2 $\leq$55 mm Hg) and exercise intolerance

---

[a] In patient receiving optimal medical management, measured at least two times, 3 weeks apart.

[b] After documented improvement during hospitalization.

to four times a day and beta agonists as "rescue" medications for bronchospasm. As the disease becomes more advanced, both should be used on a regular basis, three to four times daily. A theoretical reason for using the combination is that it may result in fewer side effects than high doses of either drug used alone. It produces rapid onset (beta agonist) and long duration (anticholinergic) of bronchodilation. In theory, the combination dilates both the large and the small airways, and does not significantly lower PO_2. Either agent probably does not result in greater airflow than either drug used alone in maximal doses.

Inhaled selective beta$_2$-stimulating agents (e.g., albuterol, bitolterol, or terbutaline) are very effective drugs to relieve bronchospasm. These drugs are best given via metered-dose inhalers (MDI). It is important that physicians and nurses properly instruct the patient in the use of MDIs. Unfortunately, many elderly patients have difficulty following the instructions and using the MDI properly (65). The most frequent problem for elderly patients is poor coordination of actuation of the MDI with inhalation. Use of a dry powder inhaler such as the "rotahaler" or use of a large volume reservoir improves the inhalation technique and enhances the likelihood that more of the drug will be deposited in the lungs and decrease the amount of oropharyngeal deposition. A few patients may require a powered nebulizer unit for best results. Patients with arthritic hands and wrists may benefit from devices that allow easier activation by the use of simple pincer movement or breath-activated MDIs (26). Oral beta$_2$ agonists are discouraged except for nocturnal use in patients who experience frequent awakenings because of cough, chest tightness, or wheeze despite inhaled therapy. Oral preparations require larger doses of the medication and can cause more side effects.

An area of ongoing debate is the role of theophylline for patients with COPD (66). Theophyllines produce little bronchodilator effect in addition to that of the inhaled agents. However, they have other actions that may be useful, such as respiratory stimulation, improvement of diaphragmatic strength, improvement in respiratory-muscle performance (67) and diuretic properties. The effects of theophylline and albuterol have been shown to be comparable, but additional benefits are obtained with the use of the two drugs in combination. Further, significant changes in functional status may occur despite relatively minor changes in spirometric indexes. In general, about 50 percent to 60 percent of patients with COPD respond to theophylline. The improvements may be considerable; therefore, as a second-line agent, it is reasonable to add theophylline compounds. Unfortunately, theophylline has a relatively narrow therapeutic range (10 to 20μg/mL).

A number of factors affect theophylline clearance including many drugs (e.g., erythromycin), environmental conditions (e.g., diet, illness), smoking, congestive heart failure, hypothyroidism, and liver disease. Many elderly patients are unable to tolerate theophylline even at therapeutic or subtherapeutic levels. Consequently, it is important to provide therapeutic drug monitoring in the elderly if dosage optimization is to be achieved. Generic, sustained-release theophylline preparations should be avoided because they have significant diurnal variability. Serum levels should be maintained in the low therapeutic range, titrating to therapeutic response but aiming for a level of 5 to 15μg/mL. This also allows for a certain amount of safety in dosing, especially in view of the potential for medication interactions with the theophyllines and the increased risk for toxicity in the elderly patient (see the section under asthma in this chapter).

Corticosteroids have also been used quite extensively in COPD, often accounting for much of the morbidity

Table 45.8. Potential Complications of Corticosteroid Therapy in the Elderly*.

Short term, high dose (may be of sudden onset)
  Mental and CNS disturbances—mood swings (euphoria to depression), jitteriness, severe psychosis (rare); pseudotumor cerebri (rare)
  Sodium and fluid retention
  Impaired glucose tolerance, hyperosmolar nonketotic coma (especially in presence of parenteral feedings)
  Hypokalemic alkalosis, systemic arterial hypertension, glaucoma, pancreatitis, peptic ulceration and gastrointestinal hemorrhage, proximal myopathy (rare)
Long term, daily steroids for months or years
  Suppression of the hypothalamic-pituitary-adrenal axis, with adrenal insufficiency
  Cushing's syndrome
  Osteoporosis with vertebral compression and multiple bone fractures, aseptic necrosis of bone
  Proximal myopathy
  Increased susceptibility to opportunistic infections
  Impaired wound healing, dermal atrophy
  CNS manifestations—depression, lability of mood, anxiety, seizures
  Posterior subcapsular cataract formation

*A number of the side effects are controversial and unproven.
CNS = central nervous system.
SOURCE: Chang SW, King TE. Corticosteroids. In: Cherniack RM, ed. Drugs for the respiratory system. Orlando: Grune & Stratton, 1986:77–138.

associated with this disease (Table 45.8). Some patients clearly benefit from long-term administration of steroids, either oral or inhaled, but it is not possible to predict who will benefit from these medications. Therefore, it is reasonable to give a closely monitored trial of therapy in patients who have continued symptoms despite maximum therapy with bronchodilators. Prednisone should be administered at 40mg a day for 14 days with pulmonary functions measured before and after administration. The spirometric response rate to this type of trial ranges in studies from 0 percent–44 percent. Corticosteroid responsiveness has been associated with acute bronchodilator response to beta agonists, and to sputum or blood eosinophilia, but there are no absolute predictors. In patients in whom there is no improvement in FEV$_1$ after a trial of steroids, the steroid should be discontinued. If there is significant improvement (>20% or more from the baseline value FEV_1), the oral corticosteroid dose should be reduced to the minimum possible, preferably on an alternate day schedule. At this stage, inhaled steroids can be added, but their role in the management of COPD remains unclear. In the absence of objective improvement, corticosteroid therapy should be discontinued because of the number and severity of potential side effects.

Adjunctive Therapy

Antibiotics are important agents in the treatment and prophylaxis of acute exacerbations of COPD (68). Exacerbation of COPD is commonly characterized by increases in breathlessness and cough and sputum production, with increased purulence in sputum. Respiratory infections are a primary cause of increased morbidity and mortality in patients with COPD. Most exacerbations appear to be initiated by viral infections (e.g., myxovirus, rhinovirus) or mycoplasma and then become secondarily infected by bacteria (most commonly *Hemophilus influenzae* or *Streptococcus pneumoniae*). Ampicillin, amoxicillin, tetracycline, erythromycin, and trimethoprim-sulfamethoxazole are the antibiotics currently prescribed. The duration of treatment must be individualized because recovery is usually prolonged. Most physicians treat patients with oral antibiotics for 7 to 14 days. Sputum cultures are not absolutely necessary for the institution of therapy in this setting because the so-called normal flora (i.e., normal oropharyngeal bacteria) are cultured, and there is little relationship between the organism identified and the response to antibiotics. Therefore, self-administration of antibiotics is desirable and safe in the properly instructed patient.

Repeated phlebotomy for the management of secondary polycythemia is not frequently indicated. The appropriate management of the hypoxemia with supplemental oxygen controls the hematocrit below 55 percent.

Annual prophylaxis against influenza and a single-dose pneumococcal vaccine are recommended, especially for the elderly, with or without chronic lung disease. Amantadine hydrochloride is a tricyclic amine that inhibits an early state of replication of the influenza A virus. In the event of an epidemic, prophylactic therapy should be seriously considered for elderly individuals who are unvaccinated, have serious co-existing medical illnesses, or are institutionalized. The recommended dosage is

100 mg twice daily and should be continued until the epidemic has passed or until 2 weeks after the patient has been vaccinated. For patients with suspected influenza, amantadine may reduce both the duration of the illness and the respiratory complications. In the elderly, the dose should be reduced to 100 mg daily after an initial loading dose of 200 mg because of the presence of renal insufficiency in this group. Furthermore, although side effects are not common (3% to 7% of treated individuals), they include confusion, disorientation, ataxia, tremors, and convulsions, especially in the elderly.

Air travel may be a stressful and difficult experience for elderly patients with COPD who are otherwise clinically stable on the ground. The prevalence of in-flight hypoxemia and related morbidity and mortality is unknown (69). The cabin of most commercial airlines is pressured to simulate an altitude of 5000 to 8000 feet. This results in a PO_2 of 106 to 130 mm Hg compared with 149 mm Hg at sea level (70). Patients with COPD may have difficulty adjusting to this degree of hypoxia and they may develop acute altitude stress because PaO_2 may fall to 40 mm Hg or lower in patients with severe COPD (71). It is important that the physician review the current status of any patient with COPD who wishes to fly. Gong (69) has reported that clinical stability, adequate exercise ability without significant dyspnea, and recent uncomplicated flights are favorable predictors of flying tolerance. Because these findings are unreliable and potentially misleading (69), it is important to determine the patient's likely PaO_2 at a reasonable altitude to be more certain of the safety and need for supplemental oxygen therapy. Two approaches are recommended to determine whether a patient will require oxygen therapy during air flight. First, ground-level PaO_2 and FEV_1 for stable, normocapnic patients with COPD to estimate the altitude PaO_2 the patient will likely experience may be calculated with use of the following formula (71,72):

$$PaO_2alt = 0.453 (PaO_2g) + 0.386 (FEV_1\% \text{ predicted}) + 2.440$$

where

PaO_2alt is the PaO_2 at altitude;
PaO_2g is the PaO_2 at ground level (71).

Second, an "altitude stress test" may be given, with use of

either hypoxic gas breathing (73–75) in a pulmonary function laboratory or monitoring in a hypobaric chamber (71) at an estimated altitude of 2438 meters (8000 feet) (69). In some patients, both approaches must be used to ascertain the potential risks. The minimal desired in-flight PaO_2 is 50 mm Hg or higher. If oxygen is found to be clinically indicated, the physician should prescribe supplemental oxygen and assist the patient in arranging in-flight oxygen with the commercial carrier at least 48 hours before the scheduled departure (69).

Bronchial Asthma

Epidemiology

Although asthma is a difficult disease to define, it is characterized by recurrent episodes of wheezing, coughing and shortness of breath, accompanied by a hyperresponsive airway with airflow obstruction and a bronchodilator response. The prevalence of asthma in the general population is approximately 3 percent (some estimates are as high as 8%) (76). Asthma prevalence rates increased 29 percent, and the death rate from asthma increased 31 percent from 1980 to 1987. National Asthma Education Program Expert Panel of the National Heart, Lung and Blood Institute (NHLBI) recently reported its *Guidelines for the Diagnosis and Management of Asthma* (Publication No. 91-3042). This report is available from the NHLBI and provides excellent guidelines for the management of asthma.

Asthma generally begins in childhood; that it may occur in the geriatric population is often not anticipated. It has been estimated that 85 percent of asthmatic patients have symptoms before they are 40 years of age (77). Only 3 percent of asthmatics present after age 40 and less than 1 percent after age 70 (78). Late-onset asthma can go undiagnosed for years, particularly if it is confused with other disorders in the elderly, such as heart failure, chronic bronchitis and emphysema (25). In addition, elderly people often rationalize increased age as the cause of decreased lung function. The prevalence of asthma in the elderly is unknown, but recent studies have suggested a prevalence of 3 percent to 9 percent. Burr and colleagues (79) using strict criteria (occurrence of wheezing and a 15% FEV_1 increased after bronchodilator use) to define asthma prevalence in a South Wales community found a

prevalence of asthma in the elderly of 6.5 percent. A difference in prevalence rate was noted with gender in the Tucson epidemiologic study in which the incidence of asthma in men older than 65 years of age was 3.8 percent compared with 7.1 percent in elderly women (80). The difference by gender may be caused by misdiagnosis—it is speculated that physicians are much more likely to diagnose men as having COPD instead of asthma.

Clinical Characteristics of Asthma in the Elderly

Most elderly patients with asthma have onset early in life. In the Tucson study, half the elderly asthmatics had a diagnosis before they were 40 years of age, (80). A common history relates that the patient had the onset of asthma in the first decade of life. The condition generally enters remission during the person's adolescence, but recurs during adulthood. Further, asthma is underdiagnosed in the geriatric population (Table 45.9). Most geriatric patients diagnosed with asthma have significant symptoms that appear at least 8 years before diagnosis (81). Usually no clear etiology is present, and elderly patients have no personal or family history of atopy. Suggested risk factors in the development of asthma include antibodies to chlamydia pneumonia, elevated immunoglobulin E (IgE) levels, blood eosinophilia, allergic rhinitis, and childhood asthma. However, patients who developed asthma at an early age tend to have a higher prevalence of having previous allergic disease. Wheezing (on most days) is the most common symptom but cough

Table 45.9. Possible Reasons for Misdiagnosis of Asthma in the Elderly.

Perception that asthma is a childhood disease
Common symptoms of asthma (wheezing, chest tightness, paroxysmal nocturnal dyspnea, and chest pain) are not distinctive and often are attributed to more common diseases of the elderly (congestive heart failure, ischemic heart disease, and chronic bronchitis)
Reduced perception of bronchoconstriction found in the elderly
Bronchodilators not appearing to be as effective in treatment, thus suggesting that the airway obstruction is not reversible because of decreased beta-adrenergic responsiveness; improper use of metered dose inhalers

SOURCE: Braman SS. Asthma in the elderly patient. Clin Chest Med 1993;14:413–422.

is also frequent. Studies of chronic cough show that cough-variant asthma is as common a cause of the persistent cough in the elderly population as it is in younger patients.

Spirometry consistently shows a greater obstructive component in older asthmatics than it does in younger asthmatics. Some nonsmoking patients with asthma develop severe, fixed airway obstruction. Bramen compared pulmonary function in a group of elderly nonsmoking asthmatics who developed asthma before or after age 65 (82). The patients with onset of asthma before age 65 (early onset) had a significantly lower postbronchodilator FEV_1 (59% predicted) than that in the late-onset group (75% predicted). This supported the clinical impression that long-standing asthma, usually of more than 20 years' duration, can lead to persistent airflow limitation, despite aggressive treatment with steroids and bronchodilators. The specific cause of the fixed obstruction is unknown. A recent autopsy study of six elderly patients with chronic asthma, who died of nonasthmatic causes, revealed no significant differences from controls (83). There is also some preliminary evidence that pulmonary function declines more rapidly in the asthmatic population than it does in the normal population. A study from Denmark showed that the drop in FEV_1 in nonatopic asthmatics was 50 mL per year, twice that of the control groups (84).

Treatment and Outcome

Treatment of asthma in the elderly patient tends to be more difficult than treatment for younger counterparts (76). The elderly tend to require more medications, and corticosteroid dependency is common. Often these patients are placed on multiple medications with complex schedules. Further, these patients have limited financial resources and decreasing cognitive function. Thus, compliance becomes a major problem. Education is a critical component to treating the disease. Education itself has been shown to increase compliance and improve asthma outcomes. Patients need to have a basic understanding of asthma and the medications used in treating it. They need to be instructed in the proper use of inhalers and in monitoring their own lung function with a peak flow meter. The elderly have been shown to have a much poorer perception of lung function than do younger patients. Consequently, a peak flow meter may become particu-

larly important as an early warning for asthma attacks for the elderly.

Older patients with asthma tend to deteriorate over longer periods of time than do their younger counterparts. Petheram and coworkers (85) found that more than half the patients had symptoms for longer than 2 weeks before admission for asthma flares. Spacers should be utilized in the geriatric population to increase pulmonary deposition of the medications and to decrease side effects. The elderly patient has difficulty coordinating the respiratory motions and hand action necessary to properly use a metered dose inhaler. There may also be a role for nebulizers in patients who are totally incapable of properly using an MDI despite a spacer device. It is also important for asthmatics to avoid the inciting factors that may set off their asthma, such as medications, irritants, or complicating medical conditions (Table 45.10).

Inhaled corticosteroids have assumed the place of first-line therapy for asthma because of recent understanding that asthma is a disease of inflammation and that inhaled steroids are the most effective medication for treating the inflammation for a prolonged period of time. Three inhaled steroids are available—beclomethasone, flunisolide, and triamcinolone. The major difference in these steroids is related to the output of medication per canister activation: 42 µg per puff of beclomethasone; 200 µg for triamcinolone; and 250 µg for flunisolide. In general, inhaled steroid use should be maximized to keep use or dosage of oral steroids to the minimum necessary. If

Table 45.10. Possible Precipitants of Asthma in the Elderly.

Chronic sinusitis
Aeroallergens
Gastroesophageal reflux
Respiratory infections, particularly viral infections
Irritants, such as smoke and strong smells (paints, varnish, household aerosols)
Medications used to treat other diseases
   Aspirin
   Nonsteroidal anti-inflammatory agents (NSAIDS) (ibuprofen, indomethacin, naproxen)
   Beta blockers (oral or ophthalmic)
Congestive heart failure
Metabisulfite ingestion (rare) (in wine, beer, and food preservatives)
Tartrazine allergies (rare)

prednisone is required chronically, an attempt should be made to taper the schedule to alternate days to decrease long-term side effects. Patients using inhaled steroids should be instructed to rinse their mouths with water immediately after use to prevent thrush. The use of spacer devices also significantly decreases the incidence of this complication. Recently, high-dose inhaled steroids have come into vogue as a treatment for severe asthmatics. Doses of steroids exceeding 1600 μg per day are available, but with the potential for adrenal suppression. However, the most common side effects of inhaled steroids are caused by local deposition in the upper airway and result in thrush, dysphonia, and dysgeusia.

The other part of pharmacologic management of asthma is bronchodilators. Beta agonists have been the mainstay of bronchodilator therapy and afford excellent and prompt relief of acute symptoms. Recent studies raise the concern that chronic use of beta agonists may actually intensify asthma. A study by Spitzer showed an increased risk of death for patients who regularly inhaled beta agonists (86). Although a great deal of debate exists about beta agonists, they are excellent bronchodilators, but they should not be relied on for chronic therapy of asthma, which is more appropriately controlled by steroid therapy. Furthermore, it is probably advantageous to use beta agonists on an as-needed basis if the patients can tolerate this approach.

Elderly patients tend to have a loss of beta receptors in the lung, however, and whether beta agonists are less effective in the elderly than they are in younger patients is controversial. The common side effects of inhaled and oral beta$_2$ agonists are tremor, tachycardia, hypokalemia (especially if the patient is taking diuretics), cardiac arrhythmias, or angina.

Ipratropium is an anticholinergic agent that is not as effective a bronchodilator as albuterol. However, it has an excellent safety profile and provides some additional bronchodilation to that offered by albuterol. Furthermore, response to ipratropium does not decline as a person ages and, therefore, for the elderly population it may be a better bronchodilator than it is for the younger asthmatic. Dryness of the mouth, bad taste, and throat irritation are side effects that the patient should be warned about. Ipratropium and theophylline may worsen urinary retention in older men with prostatism, but this is rare and is not a contraindication to use. Glaucoma is also not a contraindication to use.

In the past, theophylline was considered the first-line therapy for asthma, but it has been replaced by the inhaled steroids and by the beta agonist as the most important therapy for bronchospasm. However, theophylline still has a place in the treatment of moderate to severe asthma, particularly for patients who fail to respond to moderate doses of inhaled steroids. The narrow therapeutic ratio for theophylline makes careful monitoring of the theophylline level necessary because in the elderly population there is a significant increase in the rates of theophylline toxicity. Even with low or therapeutic blood levels, many patients develop side effects such as nausea, vomiting, insomnia, and tremulousness. The incidence of side effects can be decreased by starting the patient on a low dose of theophylline and slowly increasing the dose to a therapeutic response. Many patients do quite well with blood levels of 5 to 15 μg per mL instead of the generally accepted 10 to 20 μg per mL. Further, at comparable theophylline levels, elderly patients have more than a 16-fold increase in risk of significant toxicity as compared with that for patients younger than 25 years of age (87). The most important reason for theophylline toxicity is patient error—most commonly, patients take extra doses for relief of symptoms or are given more medication in error by the caretaker. Other important causes of theophylline toxicity include altered theophylline clearance because of concomitant disease (e.g., congestive heart failure, hepatic cirrhosis) or medication interactions with drugs such as erythromycin, cimetidine, ciprofloxacin, and allopurinol.

Elderly patients with moderate to severe asthma tend to have persistent symptoms and remain steroid-dependent (76,88). Most elderly patients with asthma die from causes common to the elderly population rather than from asthma—myocardial infarctions, stroke, or cancer (76,88). Nonetheless, the increased mortality from asthma throughtout the world is more marked in older patients (>55 years of age) for three major reasons: 1) diagnostic difficulties make a precise cause of the severe airflow obstruction sometimes difficult to identify in the elderly; 2) co-existing disease is relatively common and so asthma exacerbations can cause additional problems; 3) the medication employed to treat co-existent diseases may aggravate asthma. It must also be remembered that wheezing is not pathognomonic for asthma and that the differential diagnosis must consider congestive heart failure, chronic aspiration, pulmonary embolism, and lung or upper airway carcinomas (89).

Cardiopulmonary Rehabilitation

The capacity to perform physical tasks declines with age and the geriatric patient with chronic pulmonary disease is particularly likely to experience these effects of aging on cardiorespiratory performance during exercise. Thus, it is not surprising that the most common and distressing symptoms in such patients is dyspnea, especially with exertion and fatigue. Consequently, a comprehensive care program is required to allow elderly patients to lead as complete a life as possible despite their disease (Table 45.11) (55).

The American Thoracic Society (ATS) defines the objectives of pulmonary rehabilitation as methods to control and alleviate symptoms and pathophysiologic complications and to achieve optimal ability of the patient to carry out activities of daily living (30). The physician plays a central role in recognizing the need for a rehabilitation program and establishing the type of program required by the patient. Thus, it is extremely important that the physician not only prescribe the medications that may control and alleviate the patient's symptoms, but that the

Table 45.11. Benefits of Pulmonary Rehabilitation in the Elderly.

Improves quality of life, allows the patient to become more independent, improves the patient's chances of returning to work
Improves the patient's understanding of his/her disease
Enhances exercise capacity and improves the performance of activities of daily life
Improves psychosocial functioning (e.g., depression, fear)
Reduces respiratory symptoms (e.g., dyspnea)
Reduces the number of hospitalizations and use of medical resources
Possible improvement in survival

SOURCE: Rodrigues JC, Ilowite JS. Pulmonary rehabilitation in the elderly patient. Clin Chest Med 1993;14:429–436 and Ries AL. Pulmonary rehabilitation. In: Mahler D, ed. Pulmonary disease in the elderly. New York: Marcel Dekker, 1993:219–237.

physician pay particular attention to the physical and psychosocial factors that, when corrected or improved, will allow the elderly patient to re-establish an independent existence. The type of rehabilitation program must be individualized, but, in general, the key elements include those outlined below. Pulmonary rehabilitation is most beneficial for patients with COPD; however, certain aspects of the program are appropriate for most patients with any pulmonary disorder.

Education

Ongoing education of both the patient and family is one of the keys to successful management. Careful attention must be placed on making sure the patient and caretaker understand the principles of the treatment, the importance of compliance, the responses that are expected, when to contact the physician for advice, and the correct method for using the medication (particularly inhaler techniques). It is important that the cognitive ability of each patient be assessed and the program of education tailored to maximize understanding and allow for any difficulties the patient and spouse may have with memory, eyesight, or hearing. Care must be exercised in combining different drugs used to treat multiple diseases that may be present in an elderly individual. It is important that the patient and family know that they must tell all the physicians caring for the patient all the medications that have been given and that the patient is taking to avoid unwarranted drug interactions.

Smoking Cessation

Cigarette smoking remains the chief preventable cause of illness in the United States. As pointed out by Cox (90), older smokers pose a difficult problem for the physician: they have a higher nicotine addiction; they smoke more cigarettes; they have smoked longer; they have more social contacts who are also smokers; they have more smoking-related health problems; and many doubt their ability to quit smoking. Also, until recently, there were limited data on the value of smoking cessation in the elderly. However, it is now clear that quitting cigarette smoking at any age has positive consequences.

The physician and nurse are in unique positions to help

the elderly patient develop a strategy to increase the likelihood that he or she will quit smoking. Often the simple direct approach of advising the smoker to quit is effective. The benefits of quitting smoking should be stated: decreased cough, decreased dyspnea, increased stamina and energy (90). Frank discussion of the potential barriers to quitting should be held. Enrollment in a smoking cessation program and use of pharmacologic adjuncts to alleviate nicotine withdrawal symptoms are other useful approaches. Relapses are common, and the physician should be prepared to address this issue to reassure the patient that each attempt has a better chance of final long-term success (90).

Psychosocial Support

Psychosocial support is required for many patients with COPD and is an essential component of any rehabilitation program (30,91). Fear, anxiety, depression, and problems with cognitive, perceptual, and motor activity are common manifestations of chronic pulmonary diseases, especially COPD. Therefore, psychosocial intervention provides the patient with improved acceptance of the physiologic limitations, optimizes strength, and clarifies reasonable goals and priorities. Thus, effective psychosocial approaches provide the patient with a sense of control and mastery of his or her disease and enhances quality of life (30). Many options are available for psychosocial intervention, including education, counseling, individualized psychotherapy, group sessions, vocational counseling, and psychiatric consultation. Antidepressant medication should be used when indicated.

Nutritional Support

Nutritional support is important because poor nutrition is a major problem of the elderly and of patients with COPD, especially patients with severe emphysema, of whom approximately 30 percent have significant protein-calorie malnutrition (92,93). At present, the precise factors responsible for the malnutrition have not been identified, but elevated resting energy requirements appear to play a key role (Table 45.12). Insufficient protein-calorie intake may be responsible for the loss of weight and muscle mass (including that of the diaphragm and respiratory muscles) seen in patients with advanced COPD (Table

Table 45.12. Potential Factors Leading to Weight Loss in COPD.

Increased resting energy expenditure in malnourished patients with COPD
Increased diet-induced thermogenesis
Increased energy requirements for ventilation
Early satiety related to diaphragm flattening
Peptic ulcer disease
Abdominal symptoms related to air swallowing
Dyspnea with eating
Hypoxia during eating
Decreased appetite
Depression
Difficulty shopping and preparing food
Intake of foods low in calories
Dental problems

SOURCE: Fernandez E, Park S, Make BJ. Nutritional issues in pulmonary rehabilitation. Sem Respir Med 1993;14:482–495.

45.13). The methods of nutritional assessment and management of malnutrition in patients with COPD have been recently reviewed (94,95). The proper methods of nutritional assessment in this clinical setting and recommendations for nutritional support are described in Chaper 16.

Physical and Occupational Therapy

Physical and occupational therapy are essential components in a complete and effective pulmonary rehabilitation program (96). Specialists in these areas work together to determine the individual's potential and desire for improvement. They identify and develop goals that are mutually agreed on with the patient and family, and they implement a treatment plan and home care program designed to meet the short- and long-term functional goals established (Table 45.14).

Bronchial Hygiene

An attempt to maintain or improve airway clearance of bronchial secretions is important. Many patients with advanced disease have considerable difficulty mobilizing airway secretion. Consequently, adequate hydration, humidification of inspired gases, a regular program of postural drainage, breathing exercises, and assisted cough are felt to be useful adjuncts (30). Intermittent positive pressure ventilation (IPPB) has been demonstrated to have no benefit in hospitalized or ambulatory patients

Table 45.13. Nutritional Problems of Patients with COPD.

Nutritional Problem	Possible Causes
Weight gain	Excessive consumption of high caloric foods and beverages
	Decrease in activity level without appropriate decrease in food intake
	Increased appetite and food intake due to corticosteroid therapy
	Fluid retention
Loss of appetite	Shortness of breath
	Gastrointestinal symptoms such as nausea and vomiting
	Excessive sputum production
	Depression
Shortness of breath during or after meals, abdominal bloating	Eating too much at one time
	Eating too quickly
	Eating gas-forming foods
	Gulping air when eating or drinking
	Failure to relax before eating
	Failure to use supplemental oxygen
	Failure to use bronchodilator prior to mealtime
Nervousness, sleeplessness	Too much caffeine, especially in combination with theophylline
Thickened mucus or dehydration	Inadequate fluid intake
	Failure to increase fluid intake with fever, infection, increased ambient temperatures and exercise
	Fluid restriction due to cor pulmonale
Low serum albumin or muscle wasting	Inadequate protein intake
	Inadequate calorie intake leading to metabolism of dietary protein and breakdown of body tissues for energy
Low serum potassium	Inadequate intake of high potassium foods
	Thiazide diuretics
	Corticosteroid therapy
Fluid retention	Sodium retention due to corticosteroid therapy
	Cor pulmonale
	Congestive heart failure
	Excessive intake of high sodium foods

SOURCE: Reproduced by permission from Fernandez E, Park S, Make BJ. Nutritional issues in pulmonary rehabilitation. Sem Respir Med 1993;14:482–495.

with COPD and may be disadvantageous (97). The use of so-called expectorants has never been proven effective.

Chest Physiotherapy

Chest physiotherapy is frequently recommended for a patient with a variety of pulmonary problems. This encompasses the use of postural drainage, chest percussion and vibration administered by hand or mechanical means, and techniques of cough and deep breathing (30). Chest physiotherapy appears to benefit those patients with COPD who have excessive secretions (≥30 mL/day) that are difficult to expectorate. Despite widespread use at home and in most hospitals in the U.S., little objective evidence exists to indicate its efficacy in other situations.

Use of chest physiotherapy has not been shown to be effective for exacerbations of chronic bronchitis or for patients with pneumonia who do not have large volumes of sputum or who have status asthmaticus (28,98–100).

Results are optimized by giving bronchodilator therapy before chest physiotherapy. Complications are uncommon, but they include worsening hypoxemia (caused by positioning with the abnormal lung dependent) and bronchospasm. Even in the few situations in which chest physiotherapy is likely to be of benefit, it is difficult to establish in the home setting because it requires the patient and family members to undergo a complete educational program on the technique and goals. Trained

Table 45.14. Functional Problems Addressed by Physical and Occupational Therapy.

Functional Problem	Discipline
Decreased muscle strength and endurance	PT
Joint pain, limited range of motion, or both	PT
Lack of understanding of fitness and exercise	PT
Decreased cardiopulmonary endurance	PT
Dyspnea with activity	OT
Reduction in leisure and recreational activities	OT
Poor stress management and coping skills	OT
Decreased ambulation affecting performance of ADL	PT/OT
Inability to manage self-care	PT/OT
Vocational and work issues, including opportunities and skills evaluation	OT
Decreased work tolerance	PT/OT
Fear of exertion	PT/OT
Oxygen desaturation with activity	PT/OT

OT = occupational therapy; PT = physical therapy.
SOURCE: Reproduced by permission from Horne D, Corsello P. Physical and occupational therapy for patients with chronic lung disease. Sem Respir Med 1993;14:466–481.

respiratory care personnel, nurses, or physical therapists provide this instruction, and it usually requires several sessions and even home visit evaluations to ensure proper understanding and technique.

Physical Reconditioning

Most elderly people avoid regular exercise. Subsequently, they become deconditioned, which contributes to the exertional breathlessness and easy fatigue they experience. Age is not a deterrent to physical conditioning (101). Therefore, physical training should be encouraged. Before an elderly patient with COPD or other chronic pulmonary disease is enrolled in a physical reconditioning program, optimal medical management of the disease should be achieved. Motivation is the key factor in the selection of patients for this program. Several lines of reasoning can be used to help motivate the elderly to exercise: 1) quality-of-life issues such as the feeling of well-being, improvement in functional capacity, and performance of activities of daily living; 2) weight control, reduction of blood pressure, and probably reduced risk of coronary artery disease; and 3) reduction in medical care costs, chiefly from savings as a result of a decreased number of hospitalizations (91,102). Selection of patients for pulmonary reconditioning requires screening, which should in-

clude spirometry, studies of arterial blood gases at rest and during exercise (exercise oximetry may be used to determine the presence of exercise arterial desaturation), and cardiac stress testing.

Although difficult to assess, physical conditioning, inspiratory muscle training, breathing retraining, and energy conservation techniques are generally believed to be important modalities in the improvement of exercise performance that increases the dyspnea-limited level of activity or decreases the degree of dyspnea associated with the same level of activity (30).

Exercise reconditioning and inspiratory muscle training to improve performance and reduce the dyspnea experienced by patients with COPD have been shown to be beneficial in this setting. The accepted benefits of exercise reconditioning include increased endurance and exercise tolerance; increased maximal oxygen consumption (generally small); and increased skill in performance of a task, with decreased ventilation, oxygen consumption, and heart rate (30). The type of exercise (stair climbing, walking, treadmill walking, or stationary bicycling) appear unimportant; the type is best determined by the individual patient's physical ability, preference, and economic resources. Even arm and leg exercises in a chair or wheelchair are useful in more impaired patients. The minimal duration and frequency required to improve performance appears to be 20 to 30 minutes, three to five times per week. Unfortunately, the beneficial effects of exercise conditioning last only as long as the patient continues the exercise program. Isocapneic hyperventilation (the patient ventilates maximally while CO_2 is added to the breathing circuit to maintain a normal PCO_2 tension) and inspiratory resistance training (added resistance applied during inspiration for 15 minutes twice daily to train the inspiratory muscles) are the currently available methods for ventilatory muscle training. The efficacy of this therapy is unknown, but it appears to offer promise for selected patients, especially elderly patients who are unable to perform walking or bicycling exercise because of hip or knee problems that limit mobility.

Energy Conservation

Energy conservation is the planning and pacing of activities to improve performance. Instruction in work simplification and the use of energy conservation devices allow the patient more independence and greater participation in activities of daily living.

Breathing Retraining

Breathing retraining consists of teaching patients to use pursed-lip breathing, expiratory abdominal augmentation, synchronization of movement of abdomen and thorax, and relaxation techniques for the accessory respiratory muscles. Training appears to allow patients to increase tidal volume, decrease respiratory rate, and lower functional residual capacity, and thereby regain control of symptoms. It also seems to permit patients to overcome attacks of hyperventilation precipitated by fear and anxiety and to speed recovery from dyspnea induced by mild exercise.

Oxygen Therapy

Frequently, the institution of oxygen therapy is viewed as the "final insult" in an otherwise proud and independent life. The physician should be compassionate, and it should be suggested at a time when the pros and cons of its use can be fully discussed. It is important that the physician, patient, and family members understand the role of oxygen therapy in the management of hypoxemic patients with COPD. Long-term home oxygen use has been shown to improve exercise tolerance, alleviate pulmonary hypertension, reduce red cell mass, promote general well-being so that some patients return to work, markedly improve neuropsychiatric function, and reduce the number of hospitalizations (103).

Continuous oxygen therapy (at least 18 hr/day) is more efficacious than nocturnal therapy, especially for patients with severely altered pulmonary and cerebral function. Oxygen therapy is expensive; in the elderly in whom limitations of financial and social resources are commonplace, its use should be guided by careful monitoring and objective assessment because as much as 50 percent of patients meeting the criteria for the initiation of oxygen therapy (such as those with hypoxemia, with PaO_2 <55 mm Hg) have improvement in their hypoxemia after therapy directed at secretions, bronchospasm, and infection and further oxygen therapy becomes unnecessary.

Selection Criteria for Prescribing Home Oxygen

Oxygen therapy should be instituted only after the pa-tient has undergone at least a 3- to 4-week stabilization period during which aggressive management is employed to improve hypoxemia (e.g., secretion control, relief of bronchospasm, and control of infection). Room air arterial blood gases should be obtained on at least two separate occasions and reveal a PO_2 of 55 mm Hg or less or be consistently between 56 and 59 mm Hg in the presence of evidence of an adverse response to hypoxemia, such as cor pulmonale, impaired mental function, or erythrocytosis greater than 55 percent.

A minority of patients with COPD and interstitial lung diseases have only sleep hypoxemia (saturation less than 85 percent). Patients with COPD are usually obese or have CO_2 retention, unexplained erythrocytosis, or, rarely, cor pulmonale. Therefore, measurement of PaO_2 during sleep or continuous monitoring of oxygen saturation is required to identify nocturnal hypoxemia. Oxygen therapy that is adequate to produce a minimum nocturnal oxygen saturation of approximately 90 percent is a reasonable therapeutic goal (30). Patients with obstructive sleep apnea require additional treatment aimed at relieving nocturnal upper airway obstruction.

Other patients may have only significant exercise-induced hypoxemia. A treadmill, bicycle exercise study, or similar stress testing (walking in hall or up stairs) with use of oximetry to measure oxygen saturation will identify patients with this problem. If it is demonstrated that exercise is limited by exercise-induced hypoxemia, or if cardiac arrhythmias occur only during ambulation, prescribing oxygen with exercise appears warranted. It has not been clearly documented that the use of supplemental oxygen in this setting has long-term benefit. In the elderly, deciding to use oxygen for exercise-induced hypoxemia can be difficult because many of these patients spend very little time exercising. Thus, it is difficult to believe that exercise-induced hypoxemia plays a prominent role in survival or function at rest. Nonetheless, in selected patients, the institution of oxygen therapy in this setting can result in a remarkable increase in the level of activity and sense of well-being, especially if this therapy is combined with defined exercise reconditioning programs, breathing retraining, instructions in work simplification, the use of energy conservation devices, and adequate nutrition.

Methods of Oxygen Delivery and Types of Oxygen Systems
Nasal prongs are by far the most practical way to deliver home oxygen to patients. Recently, oxygen-conserving devices that supply oxygen only during inspiration have been developed (104). Also, a method of delivery of oxygen directly to the sublaryngeal trachea via a chronic transtracheal cannula has been developed (105). These systems require further study before they can be comfortably recommended for general use.

Compressed gas in cylinders or tanks has been the usual source of oxygen. Cylinders or tanks have several advantages, such as widespread availability and cost-efficiency, especially during intermittent use, and storage ability for long periods without loss of oxygen, which can decrease the frequency of oxygen deliveries. The disadvantages are that they are usually quite heavy and cannot be easily transported or moved; they require a pressure regulator; the high pressure presents a rare, but potential, explosive hazard; and they hold a limited supply of oxygen. This system is most convenient for patients who are house-bound. Small tanks on small carts are available for those who have limited ambulatory ability.

Liquid oxygen systems permit easy administration of oxygen during exercise and outside the home. Because of portability, liquid oxygen systems come closest to enabling the patient to be on oxygen 24 hours a day. The reservoirs are more attractive than the cylinders. The disadvantages are that these are the most expensive of the systems available; the oxygen is lost by venting when not used continuously; and the systems require frequent refilling. Nevertheless, liquid oxygen systems are preferred for patients who require the greatest range away from their stationary oxygen source. For example, the systems allow a patient to work several hours each day away from home.

Oxygen concentrators are stationary machines that concentrate oxygen by using a molecular sieve to impede nitrogen and create 90 percent to 100 percent oxygen from room air. The advantages of this system are that the concentrator provides a constant, inexhaustible home oxygen supply; it is more attractive equipment than the others; and it is very economical for long-term therapy. The disadvantages are that the concentrator requires electrical power and thus increases the patient's monthly electrical bill, it is somewhat noisy, and it requires periodic maintenance and a backup cylinder system in the event of a power failure or for travel.

Because ambulation is deemed extremely important for patients requiring oxygen therapy, the liquid system is preferred from an overall therapeutic point of view. The cost of oxygen, however, is expensive and varies between $250 and $500 per month, depending on location and the amount of oxygen used. The liquid system is the most expensive form of oxygen.

The oxygen prescription must provide the following documentation: 1) evidence that alternative therapies have been employed in an attempt to correct the hypoxemia (e.g., bronchodilators, corticosteroids, antimicrobials, physical therapy); 2) diagnosis (e.g., emphysema, chronic bronchitis, cor pulmonale, COPD, cystic fibrosis, interstitial lung disease, or bronchiectasis) for which home oxygen is appropriate therapy; 3) definite oxygen flow rate, (usually 1 to 2 liters/min via nasal cannula) and daily duration (usually continuously, 24 hours a day)–occasionally, documentation that hypoxemia drastically limits exercise or is accompanied by excessive tachycardia or cardiac arrhythmias or documentation of nocturnal hypoxemia must be provided; and 4) laboratory evidence of hypoxemia (PaO_2 <55 mm Hg or oximetry oxygen saturation <85 percent) while the patient is stable and breathing room air. Renewal of the oxygen prescription often requires documentation of the clinical benefit by an increase in exercise performance and performance of other activities of daily living.

Complications of Oxygen Therapy
There are few complications of low-flow oxygen therapy. On the other hand, the fear of significantly increasing hypercapnia and acidemia by oxygen administration in the acutely ill patient with COPD is well founded. Modest increases in $PaCO_2$ can be considered an expected adaptive response and are usually well tolerated. No good criteria exist to predict which patients will develop a rising $PaCO_2$ with oxygen therapy. The chance of a patient requiring intubation and mechanical ventilation is markedly reduced by avoiding uncontrolled or injudicious use of oxygen, avoiding sedatives or other medication that may lead to respiratory or cough suppression, and monitoring the effect of oxygen therapy on $PaCO_2$ by measur-

ing arterial blood gases. Severe hypoxemia causes death, but the disturbances associated with severe CO_2 retention are not usually lethal. Therefore, in an acutely ill and severely hypoxemic patient with COPD, once oxygen is started, it should not be discontinued, even in the event of hypercapnia (mechanical ventilation can be added). The lower the dose of oxygen (<40 percent O_2), the lower the risk of CO_2 retention. The use of humidified gas prevents drying of secretions and nasal irritation.

Summary

The aging lung is structurally and functionally different from the younger lung; however, the clinical significance of age-related changes in the lung is minor for an otherwise healthy older person. When lung disease supervenes, however, it may result in numerous problems, and in many instances, pulmonary diseases, especially respiratory failure and pneumonia, are terminal events. Nonetheless, the elderly patient with pulmonary disease can often lead a productive life if managed appropriately.

Patients require that the physician, nurse, and other allied health care professionals work collaboratively to develop a management plan that not only maximizes longevity but the quality of life. Through a comprehensive rehabilitation approach that is individualized for each patient, careful attention can be directed to the medical, physiologic, nutritional, and psychological problems that these patients face. The goal should be to provide a treatment program that allows these patients to remain in their own environment and to be with their family and friends.

References

1. Krumpe PE, Knudson RJ, Parson G, Reiser K. The aging respiratory system. Clin Geriatr Med 1985;1:143–175.
2. Mahler DA, Rosiello RA, Loke J. The aging lung. Geriatr Clin Med North Am 1986;2:215–225.
3. Crapo RO. The aging lung. In: Mahler D, ed. Pulmonary disease in the elderly. New York: Marcel Dekker, 1993;1–25.
4. Takishima T, Shindoh C, Kikuchi Y, et al. Aging effect on oxygen consumption of respiratory muscles in humans. J Appl Physiol 1990;69:14–20.
5. Knudson RJ, Clark DF, Kennedy TC, Knudson DE. Effect of aging alone on mechanical properties of the normal adult human lung. J Appl Physiol 1977;43:1054–1062.
6. Jones R, Overton T, Hammerlindl D, Sproule B. Effects of age on residual volume. J Appl Physiol 1978;44:195–199.
7. Knudson RJ, Lebowitz MD, Holberg CJ, Burrows B. Changes in the normal maximal expiratory flow volume curve with growth and aging. Am Rev Respir Dis 1983;127:725–734.
8. Fowler RW, Pluck RA, Hetzel MR. Maximal expiratory flow-volume curves in Londoners aged 65 and over. Thorax 1987;42:173–182.
9. Muiesan G, Sorbini CA, Grassi V. Respiratory function in the aged. Bull Physiopathol Respir 1971;7:973–1009.
10. Holland J, Milic-Emili J, Macklem PT, Bates DV. Regional distribution of pulmonary ventilation and perfusion in elderly subjects. J Clin Invest 1968;47:81–92.
11. Berger AJ, Mitchell RA, Severinghaus JW. Regulation of respiration. N Engl J Med 1977;297:92–97,138–143,194–201.
12. Kronenberg RS, Drage GW. Attenuation of the ventilatory and heart rate responses to hypoxia and hypercapnia with aging in normal men. J Clin Invest 1973;52:1812–1819.
13. Block AJ, Boysen PG, Wynne JW, Hunt LA. Sleep apnea, hypopnea, and oxygen desaturation in normal subjects: a strong male predominance. N Engl J Med 1979;300:513–517.
14. Naifeh KH, Severinghaus JW, Kamiya J. Effect of aging on sleep-related changes in respiration variables. Sleep 1987;10:160–171.
15. Smith PL, Bleecher ER. Ventilatory control during sleep in the elderly. Geriatr Clin North Am 1986;2:227–240.
16. Reynolds HY. Lung host defenses: a status report. Chest 1979;75:239–242.
17. Gyetko MR, Toews GB. Immunology of the aging lung. Clin Chest Med 1993;14:379–391.
18. Landahl S, Steen B, Svanborg A. Dyspnea in 70-year-old people. Acta Med Scand 1980;107:225–230.
19. Howell JBL, Campbell EJ. Breathlessness in pulmonary disease. Scand J Respir Dis 1967;48:321–329.
20. Sorlie PD, Kannel WB, O'Connor G. Mortality associated with respiratory function and symptoms in advanced age. Am Rev Respir Dis 1989;140:379–384.
21. Manning HL, Harver A, Mahler DA. Dyspnea in the elderly. In: Mahler D, ed. Pulmonary disease in the elderly. New York: Marcel Dekkeer, 1993;81–112.
22. Wade JF III, King TE Jr. Infiltrative and interstitial lung disease in the elderly. Clin Chest Med 1993;14:501–521.
23. Muthuswamy PP, Akbik F, Franklin C, Spigos D, Barker WL. Management of major or massive hemoptysis in active pulmonary tuberculosis by bronchial arterial embolization. Chest 1987;92:77–82.
24. Harris R. Evaluation of chest pain in the old patient. Intern Med 1980;10:65–69.
25. Banerjee DE, Lee GS, Malik SK, Daly S. Underdiagnosis of asthma in the elderly. Br J Dis Chest 1987;81:23–29.
26. Dow L, Holgate ST. Assessment and treatment of obstructive airways disease in the elderly. Br Med Bull 1990;46:230–

245.

27. Hogg JC, Williams J, Richardson JB, et al. Age as a factor in the distribution of lower-airway conductance and in the pathologic anatomy of obstructive lung disease. N Engl J Med 1970;282:1283–1287.

28. The definition of emphysema. Report of a National Heart, Lung, and Blood Institute, Division of Lung Diseases workshop. Am Rev Respir Dis 1985;132:182–185.

29. Snider GL. Emphysema: the first two centuries–and beyond. A historical overview, with suggestions for future research. Part 1 and Part 2. Am Rev Respir Dis 1992;146:1334–1344,1615–1622.

30. American Thoracic Society Statement. Standards for the diagnosis and care of patients with chronic obstructive pulmonary disease (COPD) and asthma. Am Rev Respir Dis 1987;136:225–244.

31. Thurlbeck WM, Simon G. Radiographic appearance of the chest in emphysema. AJR 1978;130:429–440.

32. Hruban RH, Meziane MA, Zerhouni EA, et al. High resolution computed tomography of inflation-fixed lungs: pathologic-radiographic correlation of centrilobular emphysema. Am Rev Respir Dis 1987;136:935–940.

33. Petty TL, Silvers GW, Stanford RE. Mild emphysema is associated with reduced elastic recoil and increased lung size but not with airflow limitation. Am Rev Respir Dis 1987;136:867–871.

34. World Health Organization. Chronic cor pulmonale. A report of an expert committee. Circulation 1963;27:594–615.

35. Stevens PM, Terplan M, Knowles J. Prognosis of cor pulmonale. N Engl J Med 1963;269:1289–1291.

36. Morrison DA. Pulmonary hypertension in chronic obstructive pulmonary disease: the right ventricular hypothesis. Chest 1987;92:387–388.

37. Kachel RG. Left ventricular function in chronic obstructive pulmonary disease. Chest 1978;74:286–290.

38. Matthay RA, Schwarz MI, Ellis JH Jr, et al. Pulmonary artery hypertension in chronic obstructive pulmonary disease: determination by chest radiography. Invest Radiol 1981;16:95–100.

39. Nicholas WJ, Liebson PR. ECG changes in COPD: what do they mean? Part 1, 2. J Respir Dis 1987;8:13–18,103–120.

40. Morrison DA, Henry R, Goldman S. Preliminary study of the effects of low flow oxygen on oxygen delivery and right ventricular dysfunction in chronic lung disease. Am Rev Respir Dis 1986;133:390–396.

41. Hudson LD, Kurt TL, Petty TL, Genton E. Arrhythmias associated with acute respiratory failure in patients with chronic airway obstruction. Chest 1973;63:661–666.

42. Wynne JW, Block AJ, Hemenway J, et al. Disordered breathing and oxygen desaturation during sleep in patients with chronic obstructive pulmonary disease (COPD). Am J Med 1979;66:573–579.

43. Block AJ, Wynne JW, Boysen PG. Sleep-disordered breathing and nocturnal oxygen desaturation in postmenopausal women. Am J Med 1980;69:75–79.

44. Bliwise DL, Feldman DE, Bliwise NG, et al. Risk factors for sleep disordered breathing in heterogeneous geriatric population. J Am Geriatr Soc 1987;35:132–141.

45. Smolensky M, Halbert F, Sargent F II. Advances in climatic physiology. New York: Springer-Verlag, 1972:281.

46. Boysen PG, Block AJ, Wynne JW, et al. Nocturnal pulmonary hypertension in patients with chronic obstructive pulmonary disease. Chest 1979;76:536–542.

47. Block AJ, Boysen PG, Wynne JW. The origins of cor pulmonale: a hypothesis. Chest 1979;75:109–110.

48. Tirlapur VG, Mir MA. Nocturnal hypoxemia and associated electrocardiographic changes in patients with chronic obstructive airways disease. N Engl J Med 1982;306:125–130.

49. Flick MR, Block AJ. Nocturnal vs diurnal cardiac arrhythmias in patients with chronic obstructive pulmonary disease. Chest 1979;75:8–11.

50. Lippmann M, Fein A. Pulmonary embolism in the patient with chronic obstructive pulmonary disease: a diagnostic dilemma. Chest 1981;79:39–42.

51. Lesser BA, Leeper KV, Stein PD, et al. The diagnosis of acute pulmonary embolism in patients with chronic obstructive pulmonary disease. Chest 1992;102:17–22.

52. Fanta CH, Wright TC, McFadden ER Jr. Differentiation of recurrent pulmonary emboli from chronic obstructive lung disease as a cause of cor pulmonale. Chest 1981;79:92–95.

53. Prescott SM, Richards KL, Tikoff G, et al. Venous thromboembolism in decompensated chronic obstructive pulmonary disease. Am Rev Respir Dis 1981;123:32–36.

54. Fletcher EC, Martin RJ. Sexual dysfunction and erectile impotence in chronic obstructive pulmonary disease. Chest 1982;81:413–421.

55. Rodrigues JC, Ilowite JS. Pulmonary rehabilitation in the elderly patient. Clin Chest Med 1993;14:429–436.

56. Doll R, Peto R. Mortality in relation to smoking: 20 years' observation on male British doctors. BMJ 1976;2:1525–1536.

57. Postma DS, Burema J, Gimeno F, et al. Prognosis of severe chronic obstructive pulmonary disease. Am Rev Respir Dis 1979;119:357–367.

58. Kanner RE, Renzetti AD Jr, Klauber MR, Smith CB, Golden CA. Variables associated with changes in spirometry in patients with obstructive lung disease. Am J Med 1979;67:44–50.

59. Bosse R, Sparrow D, Rose CL, Weiss ST. Longitudinal effect of age and smoking cessation on pulmonary function. Am Rev Respir Dis 1981;123:378–381.

60. Clement J, Van de Woestijne KP. Rapidly decreasing forced expiratory volume in one second or vital capacity and development of chronic airflow obstruction. Am Rev Respir Dis 1982;125:553–558.

61. Nocturnal Oxygen Therapy Trial Group. Continuous or nocturnal oxygen therapy in hypoxemic chronic obstructive lung disease: a clinical trial. Ann Intern Med 1980;93:391–398.

62. Timms RM, Kaule PA, Anthonisen NR, et al. Selection of patients with chronic obstructive pulmonary disease for long-term oxygen therapy. JAMA 1981;245:2512–2514.

63. Tashkin DP, Ashutosh K, Bleecker ER, et al. Comparison of

the anticholinergic bronchodilator iprotropium bromide with metaproterenol in chronic obstructive pulmonary disease. Am J Med 1986;81:81–89.

64. Ferguson GT, Cherniack RM. Management of chronic obstructive pulmonary disease. New Engl J Med 1993;328:1017–1022.

65. Allen SC, Prior A. What determines whether an elderly patient can use a metered dose inhaler correctly? Br J Dis Chest 1986;80:45–49.

66. Vaz Fragoso CA, Miller MA. Review of the clinical efficacy of theophylline in the treatment of chronic obstructive pulmonary disease. A Rev Respir Dis 1993;147:S40–S47.

67. Murciano D, Auclair MH, Pariente R, Aubier M. A randomized, controlled trial of theophylline in patients with severe chronic obstructive pulmonary disease. N Engl J Med 1989;320:1521–1525.

68. Anthonisen NR, Manfreda J, Warren CPW, et al. Antibiotic therapy in exacerbations of chronic obstructive pulmonary disease. Ann Intern Med 1987;106:196–204.

69. Gong H Jr. Advising patients with pulmonary diseases on air travel. Ann Intern Med 1989;111:349–351.

70. Cottrell JJ. Altitude exposures during aircraft flight. Flying higher. Chest 1988;93:81–84.

71. Dillard TA, Berg BW, Rajagopal KR, et al. Hypoxemia during air travel in patients with chronic obstructive pulmonary disease. Ann Intern Med 1989;111:362–367.

72. Dillard TA, Rosenberg AP, Berg BW. Hypoxemia during altitude exposure. A meta-analysis of chronic obstructive pulmonary disease. Chest 1993;103:422–425.

73. Schwartz JS, Bencowitz HZ, Moser KM. Air travel hypoxemia with chronic obstructive pulmonary disease. Ann Intern Med 1984;100:473–477.

74. Gong H Jr., Tashkin DP, Lee EY, Simmons MS. Hypoxia-altitude simulation test. Evaluation of patients with chronic airway obstruction. Am Rev Respir Dis 1984;130:980–986.

75. Vohra KP, Klocke RA. Detection and correction of hypoxemia associated with air travel. Am Rev Respir Dis 1993;148:1215–1219.

76. Brama SS. Asthma in the elderly patient. Clinics in Chest Med 1993;14:413–422.

77. Broder I. Barlow PP, Horton RJM. The epidemiology of asthma and hay fever in a total community, Tecumseh, Michigan. J Allergy 1962;33:513–523.

78. Derrick EH. The significance of age on the onset of asthma. Med J Aust 1971;1:1317–1319.

79. Burr ML, Charles TJ, Roy K, Seaton A. Asthma in the elderly: an epidemiological survey. BMJ 1979;1:1041–1044.

80. Dodge RR, Burrows B. The prevalence and incidence of asthma and asthma-like symptoms in a general population sample. Am Rev Respir Dis 1980;122:567–575.

81. Burrows B, Lebowitz MD, Barbee RA, Cline MG. Findings before diagnoses of asthma among the elderly in a longitudinal study of a general population sample. J Allergy Clin Immunol 1991;88:870–877.

81. Braman SS, Kaemmerlen JT, Davis SM. Asthma in the elderly: a comparison between patients with recently ac-

quired and long-standing disease. Am Rev Respir Dis 1991;143:336–340.

83. Sobonya RE. Quantitative structural alterations in long-standing allergic asthma. Am Rev Respir Dis 1984;130:289–292.

84. Peat JK, Woolcock AJ, Cullen K. Rate of decline of lung function in subjects with asthma. Eur J Respir Dis 1987;70:171–179.

85. Petheram IS, Jones DA, Collins JV. Assessment and management of acute asthma in the elderly. Postgrad Med J 1982;58:149–151.

86. Spitzer WO, Suissa S, Ernst P, et al. The use of β = agonists and the risk of death and near death from asthma. N Engl J Med 1992;326:501–506.

87. Shannon M, Lovejoy FH Jr. The influence of age vs. peak serum concentration on life-threatening events after chronic theophylline intoxication. Arch Intern Med 1990;150:2045–2048.

88. Braman SS, Corrao WM, Kaemmerlen JT. The clinical outcome of asthma in the elderly: a 7-year follow-up study. Ann NY Acad Sci 1991;629:449–450.

89. Braman SS, Davis SM. Wheezing in the elderly. Asthma and other causes. Geriatr Clin North Am 1986;2:269–283.

90. Cox JL. Smoking cessation in the elderly patient. Clin Chest Med 1993;14:423–428.

91. Paine R, Make BJ. Pulmonary rehabilitation for the elderly. Clin Geriatr Med 1986;2:313–337.

92. Hunter AM, Carey MA, Larsh HW. The nutritional status of patients with chronic obstructive pulmonary disease. Am Rev Respir Dis 1981;124:376–381.

93. Fernandez E, Park S, Make BJ. Nutritional issues in pulmonary rehabilitation. Sem Respir Med 1993;14:482–495.

94. Wilson DO, Rogers RM, Hoffman RM. Nutrition and chronic lung disease. Am Rev Respir Dis 1985;134:1347–1365.

95. NIH Workshop Summary. Nutrition and the respiratory system: chronic obstructive pulmonary disease (COPD). Am Rev Respir Dis 1986;134:347–352.

96. Horne D, Corsello P. Physical and occupational therapy for patients with chronic lung disease. Sem Respir Med 1993;14:466–481.

97. Intermittent Positive Pressure Breathing Trial Group. Intermittent positive pressure breathing therapy of chronic obstructive pulmonary disease: a clinical trial. Ann Intern Med 1983;99:612–620.

98. Kirilloff LH, Owens GR, Rogers RM, Mazzocco MC. Does chest physical therapy work? Chest 1985;88:436–444.

99. Mohsenifar Z, Rosenberg N, Goldberg HS, Koerner SK. Mechanical vibration and conventional chest physiotherapy in outpatients with stable chronic obstructive lung disease. Chest 1985;87:483–485.

100. Graham WGB, Bradley DA. Efficacy of chest physiotherapy and intermittent positive pressure breathing in the resolution of pneumonia. N Engl J Med 1978;299:624–627.

101. Fiatrone MA, O'Neill EF, Ryan ND, et al. Exercise training and nutritional supplementation for physical frailty in very

elderly people. N Engl J Med 1994;330:1769–1775.

102. Mahler DA, Cunningham LN, Curfman GD. Aging and exercise performance. Clin Geriatr Med 1986;2:433–452.

103. Petty TL, Neff TA, Creagh CE, et al. Outpatient oxygen therapy in chronic obstructive pulmonary disease: a review of 13 years' experience and an evaluation of modes of therapy. Arch Intern Med 1979;139:28–32.

104. Tiep BL, Lewis MI. Oxygen conservation and oxygen-conserving devices in chronic lung disease: a review. Chest 1987;92:263–272.

105. Christopher KL, Spofford BT, Petrun MD, et al. A program for transtracheal oxygen delivery: assessment of safety and efficiency. Ann Intern Med 1987;107:802–808.

106. Murray JF. The normal lung. Philadelphia: Saunders, 1976:334.

107. Young RC Jr, Borden DL, Rachal RE. Aging of the lung: pulmonary disease in the elderly. Age 1987;10:138–145.

108. Dodge R, Burrows B. chronic bronchitis and emphysema. In: Fries JF, Ehrich GE, ed. Prognosis. Contemporary outcomes of disease. Bowie, MD: Charles Press, 1981:228.

109. King TE Jr. Acute and chronic pulmonary disease in the elderly. In: Schrier R, ed. Geriatric medicine. The care of the elderly. Philadelphia: Saunders, 1990:273–323.

110. Loke J, Mahler D, Man SFP, et al. Exercise impairment in chronic obstructive pulmonary disease. Clin Chest Med 1984;5:121–143.

111. Chang SW, King TE. Corticosteroids. In: Cherniack RM, ed. Drugs for the respiratory system. Orlando: Grune & Stratton, 1986:77–138.

112. Ries AL. Pulmonary rehabilitation. In: Mahler D, ed. Pulmonary disease in the elderly. New York: Marcel Dekker, 1993:219–237.

Chapter 46
Diseases of the Prostate

Robert E. Donohue, E. David Crawford, and Marilyn Davis

The only two things we do with greater frequency in middle age are urinate and attend funerals.

Fred Shoenberg
Old Age is not for Sissies

Prostatitis

Prostatitis is a perplexing disease that requires very specific clinical and laboratory investigations to establish the diagnosis and to categorize properly the type of prostatitis present. Most patients believed to harbor bacterial prostatitis do not have a bacterial infection (1). Many health care resources are wasted on antibiotics to treat nonbacterial prostatitis and prostatodynia. It is important that the clinician be able to differentiate the types of prostatitis. Most cases are not due to bacterial infection, but are secondary to other pathogenic processes that cause inflammation of the prostate. In an elderly patient population, diagnosis and treatment require perseverance and precision. The proper classification system is based on a set of urine and prostatic cultures and the microscopic examination, known as the segmented urine culture technique, described by Meares and Stamey (2).

There are two types of bacterial prostatitis: acute bacterial prostatitis and chronic bacterial prostatitis. A patient with acute bacterial prostatitis is generally quite ill, experiencing systemic toxicity with fever, chills, lower back and sacral pain, perineal pain, and varying degrees of urinary obstruction. Rectal examination reveals an enlarged, tender, boggy prostate. Vigorous prostatic massage is not advisable because it may induce bacteremia. Acute bacterial prostatitis is relatively rare in young men; however, the elderly population has an increased incidence caused by the frequent use of indwelling urethral catheters.

Chronic prostatitis can be bacterial or nonbacterial and presents with varying degrees of dysuria, frequency, nocturia, or sharp, diffusely radiating perineal or lower back pain. The disease is characterized by periods of exacerbation and remission. Chronic bacterial prostatitis is the most common cause of recurrent urinary tract infections in men with a normal intravenous pyelogram (IVP) (3). Prostatodynia is another type of prostatitis and is, basically, pain in the prostate with no abnormal findings in the prostatic secretions or cultures.

Microorganisms most commonly gain access to the prostate gland in a retrograde fashion by ascending the urethral route. Theoretic seeding of the prostate with bacteria-laden urine is supported by the fact that prostatic calculi can contain extraneous constituents that originate in the urine. Rarely, hematogenous or lymphogenous routes are implicated in bacterial prostatic infection. There is some evidence that prostatitis may be sexually transmitted, in that partners of patients who have the disease often have positive vaginal introitus cultures for the same organism.

Nonbacterial prostatitis is believed to be inflammatory in nature, produced by irritants such as caffeine, alcohol, dietary factors, pharmacologic agents, and even physical activity. Increased intravesical pressure generated by heavy lifting or exercise against a closed external urethral sphincter can force urine into the prostatic ducts, creating a chemical prostatitis. Psychogenic factors such as stress and anxiety play an unquantifiable but demonstrable role in the promotion of prostatitis. Iatrogenic factors can also predispose patients to bacterial prostatitis, including, as noted, indwelling urethral catheters, surgical manipulation of the lower urinary tract, and transurethral resection of the prostate.

The most common organisms involved in bacterial prostatitis parallel those seen with urinary tract infections, including the enteric organisms *Escherichia coli*, *Pseudomonas*, *Enterobacter*, *Klebsiella*, and *Proteus* (4). Gram-positive pathogens are rarely cultured. Mixed cultures involving multiple organisms have been reported but are rare in the absence of indwelling foreign bodies such as a urethral catheter. Nonbacterial prostatitis is common and may be precipitated by agents such as *Trichomonas*, *Ureaplasma*, and *Chlamydia*.

Diagnosis

The proper method for diagnosing prostatitis is use of the segmented urine culture technique (5). With this method, it is possible to localize the infection to the prostatic substance. To perform these cultures, the physician requests that the patient report with a full bladder. The patient's external meatus is cleansed with soap and water. (Antiseptic solutions should be avoided because one drop in a collected specimen can inhibit growth.) The patient is asked to void 5 to 10 mL of urine in a container labeled VB1, and then to continue voiding to produce the classic midstream specimen, labeled VB2. At this point, a prostatic massage is carried out and the secretions are collected in a container labeled expressed prostatic secretion (EPS). The patient voids 10 more mL in another container labeled VB3. It is helpful to have the containers labeled and available at the time of collection of the specimens, and to inform patients, especially the elderly, in advance, of exactly what the procedure entails. The technique takes no longer than 5 minutes and is cost-effective, considering that many patients are needlessly placed on antimicrobial regimens when, in fact, they do not have bacterial prostatitis.

The same cultures and sensitivities, if performed in a hospital laboratory, can be quite expensive, exceeding $170. To reduce the cost of separate processing for cultures, a culture plate containing eosin methylene blue (EMB) or MacConkey's agar can be divided into four quadrants and each sample swabbed on a separate quadrant. The technique is not as precise as that performed in a commercial laboratory, but it is easy to visualize positive culture results and to determine whether there is a differential growth between the EPS or VB3 and VB1 or VB2.

To diagnose chronic bacterial prostatitis, there should be at least a 1 log difference in the growth between the EPS or VB3 and VB1 or VB2. However, any colony count is significant. For example, 1000 organisms in the EPS with 100 or less in VB1 and VB2 would indicate prostatitis. The next step is to examine the EPS for white

blood cells, oval fat bodies, and lecithin granules. Table 46.1 outlines the microscopic evaluation of the EPS and shows that in both chronic bacterial and nonbacterial prostatitis there are increased numbers of white cells and oval fat bodies and decreased numbers of lecithin granules. The culture establishes the presence of bacteria. Prostatodynia rarely produces any abnormalities of the EPS, and cultures are always negative.

Other urologic abnormalities, such as carcinoma in situ, stones, urethral diverticula, and strictures, may mimic the symptoms of prostatitis. Subtle urologic voiding dysfunctions, including detrusor sphincter dyssynergia, are known to precipitate nonbacterial prostatitis.

Treatment

Once the diagnosis of a bacterial prostatitis is made, the proper antibiotic must be chosen. The ideal antibiotic does not become ionized in the blood and is lipid soluble in its nonionized form; however, it ionizes at the pH of prostatic fluids. These characteristics cause the drug to diffuse into the gland, become ionized, and thus accumulate in prostatic tissue by a process known as iontrapping. The prostate possesses a barrier, analogous to the blood-brain barrier, which is breached in acute infection, allowing bacteria, as well as antibiotics, to diffuse freely into the gland. However, after resolution of the acute process, penetration of antimicrobial agents into the prostate depends on their lipid solubility and ionization potential.

In the patient acutely ill with prostatitis, therapy should be started with an aminoglycoside and ampicillin. These antibiotics are continued until the septic process abates; the patient is then given oral antimicrobial agents, chosen

Table 46.1. Microscopic Evaluation of Expressed Prostatic Secretions in the Diagnosis of Prostatitis*

	Chronic Bacterial Prostatitis	Nonbacterial Prostatitis	Prostatodynia
WEC	Increased	Increased	Normal
Oval fat bodies	Increased	Increased	Rare
Lecithin granules	Decreased	Decreased	Normal

*Prostatic massage is generally defined in an acute bacterial presentation.

on the basis of the sensitivity of the offending organism. In general, the antibiotic chosen has properties that allow it to penetrate into the prostate, such as carbenicillin and trimethoprim-sulfamethoxazole.

Data from clinical trials evaluating the efficacy of various antibiotics used to treat chronic prostatitis are limited. The ideal drug would be lipid soluble, thus promoting its passage into the prostate, and have a spectrum covering most common organisms associated with prostatitis. The first drug of choice is carbenicillin indanyl sodium (two 382-mg tablets four times a day for 1 month). Patients allergic to penicillin should be given trimethoprim-sulfamethoxazole (1 tablet twice a day for 1 month). Alternative drugs include the quinolones and tetracyclines. Although the data to support use of quinolones are not extensive, most urologists prescribe these drugs before carbenicillin.

Patients failing to respond to these regimens should be re-evaluated, and consideration given to a nonbacterial prostatitis. Urodynamic disorders may be effectively managed with short courses of anticholinergic agents such as oxybutynin. Patients with symptoms precipitated by infrequent voiding may benefit from timed voiding, such as trials every 2 hours. Approaches such as use of sitz baths and administration of anti-inflammatory agents and low-dose diazepam may be beneficial. For patients with prostatodynia, work and lifestyle patterns contributing to perineal, musculoskeletal dysfunction should be evaluated.

The diagnosis and treatment of prostatitis are clinically challenging. With our current understanding of the pathogenesis of the disease, prostatitis can now be more precisely defined and comprehensively managed. The segmented urine culture technique and microscopic examination of the EPS are of paramount importance in classifying the disease. The discovery of effective antibiotics that penetrate into the prostate now leads to cure of the disease in a substantial number of patients. For patients with nonbacterial prostatitis and prostatodynia, a careful, meticulous screening and diagnostic workup are indicated, followed by appropriate management strategies to alleviate the numerous etiologic causes. Establishing the proper diagnosis and implementing appropriate treatment can save the patient many visits to the clinician and eliminate inappropriate use of antibiotics in patients who may not benefit from such treatment. In our experience, less than 10 percent of patients have a bacterial prostatitis (6).

Benign Prostatic Hyperplasia

Etiology

The prostate gland, an accessory sexual gland located in front of the bladder, is responsible for 30 percent of the ejaculate in men. In the elderly man, growth of this gland causes elongation, tortuosity, and compression of the posterior urethra and leads to significant bladder outlet obstruction that often requires surgical correction. From a man's birth until puberty, the prostate grows slowly; with puberty, it begins a rapid increase in size, which continues until the person is approximately 20 years of age (7). The prostate remains constant at a weight of about 20 gm until the man is about age 45, when the onset of benign prostatic hyperplasia (BPH) commences, and the volume increases. In the person's fifth decade, the stroma undergoes a reawakening and stromal nodules are formed. They induce the proliferation and organization of the epithelial elements they support with new glandular elements.

The pathogenesis of BPH remains unclear and the etiology debatable (8). The role of the testis, intracellular dihydrotestosterone, and androgen-estrogen synergism are being researched. The normal size of the prostate before the onset of BPH is 20 gm. At 33 gm, the prostate becomes histologically identifiable but the usual size of the prostate in early studies of open surgical specimens was 52 gm. Current surgical specimens, most commonly secured by transurethral prostatectomy (TURP), are smaller. The early pathologic findings studied the pure leiomyoma nodule and the more common fibromyoadenomatous nodule. The latter is composed of varying proportions of glandular epithelium, smooth muscle, and fibrous tissue. The proportions vary with the patient's age and local growth factors.

The incidence of BPH in the United States detected at autopsy has been reported as 90 percent of men with microscopic nodular BPH; 50 percent of men with macroscopic nodular BPH, clinical BPH, or both; and 25 percent of men with symptomatic, clinical BPH.

Symptoms of prostatic disease can be obstructive or irritative. The obstructive manifestations of prostatic disease are hesitancy in initiating urination, weakened urinary stream, the inability to terminate urination abruptly without dribbling, incomplete emptying of the bladder at the time of voiding, the inability to void at all, acute urinary retention, and overflow incontinence (continuous leakage of a small volume of urine without bladder emptying). The irritative symptoms are nocturia, frequency, urgency, dysuria, and urge incontinence.

As the obstruction of the posterior urethra by elongation, tortuosity, and compression from prostatic tissues progresses, 50 percent to 80 percent of men develop an unstable bladder with frequency, urgency, and some urge incontinence (9). Residual urine increases and nocturia and daytime frequency occur. Often, a mass may appear in the lower abdomen, that is, distended bladder, and overflow incontinence ensues. At times, the patient may suffer from silent prostatism. The patient's symptoms do not represent the primary effects of urethral compression and tortuosity but the secondary system effects of bladder neck obstruction. The symptoms are 1) acute urinary retention, 2) overflow incontinence, 3) renal failure with blood urea nitrogen (BUN) and serum creatinine elevation, and 4) uremia. Acute retention, the final result of the progression of obstructive symptoms or silent prostatism, can be precipitated also by delay in voiding, by use of alcohol, or the use of anticholinergics, antidepressants, tranquilizers, and decongestants.

Diagnosis

The physical examination of the patient with BPH includes monitoring of vital signs and a generalized examination. Evaluation of the abdomen should include suprapubic percussion for a distended bladder and evaluation for the presence of inguinal hernia.

The rectal examination should not be considered only a prostate examination. A rectal examination yields information about the patient's anal sphincter tone, and about possible BPH, prostatic carcinoma, and rectal carcinoma. Fifty percent of rectal tumors (there is an expected incidence in men of 28,000 new cases in 1994) are accessible to the examiner's finger and are therefore detectable by a careful rectal examination. The examination is most easily and effectively completed with the patient on his knees and elbows on the examining table. This position allows the examiner to remain in a comfortable position during

the examination and facilitates examination of an obese male. The examination is also more comfortable for the patient when his legs are not supporting his body weight.

Rectal examination should include inspecting the patient's perineum and lower back, noting scars from previous laminectomies, detecting pilonidal sinus and sacral dimples, and assessing fissures, fistulae, and hemorrhoids. It should also evaluate the patient's anal sphincter tone and determine whether there is a narrowing just proximal to the anal sphincter muscle, which is suggestive of a previous aggressive hemorrhoidectomy and scar or, possibly, adenocarcinoma of the rectum.

The prostatic examination should include an evaluation for size, symmetry, nodularity, and hardness. The presence of nodules should be detected by use of two techniques. In the initial technique, to detect gross nodularity, the examiner's finger should traverse the patient's median sulcus and run superficially across the surface of each lateral lobe from the median sulcus to the lateral border of the gland. In the second technique, to detect nodules that are not obvious, each area of each lobe should be compressed individually and the prostatic tissue beneath the rectal wall evaluated. Any abnormality on either assessment should be diagrammed, highlighting the position of the abnormality for future comparison examination. The consistency of the prostate should be assessed and described as normal or hard, and hard areas should be diagrammed. Just above the prostate, the distal portion of the vas deferens may be palpated superiorly toward the midline and the seminal vesicles detected laterally. The rectal lumen should be palpated as far as possible to determine patency, and rectal wall palpated for abnormalities or growths.

The guaiac examination of stool removed at rectal examination is no longer recommended. The current view is that an atraumatically passed stool provides a better specimen to screen for blood than a digitally secured specimen because of the high incidence of false-positive tests on digitally obtained specimens.

Other laboratory evaluations, such as urinalysis for culture and sensitivity, should be made if appropriate. Assessment of residual urine and serum creatinine and electrolytes should also be done. A test to show the patient's level of prostatic specific antigen (PSA), the current serum protein under intense investigation as a screening tool for prostatic adenocarcinoma, may also be scheduled. PSA is a serine protease found in all prostatic tissue. PSA level is elevated in approximately 30 percent of men with BPH (see discussion of PSA in the section on prostate cancer).

Cystoscopy is the study of choice to anatomically evaluate outlet obstruction. By direct vision, the lumen and lining of the entire urethra are studied, and the anatomic relationship of the obstructing lobes (subtrigonal, subcervical, and lateral) of the prostate is visualized. The presence of bladder calculi, tumors, cystitis, and vesical hemorrhage can be easily detected. Changes in the bladder musculature (trabeculations, cellules, and diverticula) caused by the outlet obstruction can be seen directly. The sites in the trigone for the openings of the ureters can be seen, renal and ureteral hematuria diagnosed, and ureteral emptying recorded. The presence of a urethral stricture, a bladder neck contracture, or significant residual adenomatous prostatic tissue can be confirmed in patients who have recurrent outlet obstructive symptoms after previous TURP.

Uroflow studies yield the maximum information about the functional activity of the intact lower urinary tract. The generation of high pressure in the bladder but a low flow rate despite adequate urine volume in the bladder confirms functional obstruction.

Excretory urography yields excellent information about the anatomy of the urinary tract, renal anomalies, excretory capability of the kidneys, presence of renal masses, and filling defects of the collecting system. The anatomy, course, and caliber of the ureters are delineated; the presence of bladder wall trabeculations, cellules and diverticula, and effects of prostatic obstruction deter-

mined; and bladder filling evaluated. A postvoid film yields information about the degree of bladder emptying. The excretory urogram remains a controversial assessment study of the patient with BPH.

In the patient experiencing urgency and frequency, bladder pressure studies and cystometrography (either with water or with carbon dioxide) can be performed. Urgency and frequency also mandate a voided urine cytology to exclude transitional cell carcinoma in situ (CIS) in patients without obvious neurogenic disease. The direct observation of the urinary stream by the examining physician, a study that has fallen into disfavor recently, deserves to be used in selected cases.

The differential diagnoses of symptomatic BPH are 1) BPH, 2) uncontrolled diabetes mellitus, 3) transitional cell carcinoma of the bladder, 4) CIS, 5) uninhibited neurogenic bladder, 6) flaccid neurogenic bladder, 7) adenocarcinoma of the prostate, 8) bladder calculus, 9) prostatitis, 10) meatal stenosis, 11) urethral stricture disease, and 12) bladder neck contracture.

The American Urological Association symptom score is currently being used to quantify descriptions of symptoms and to compare therapeutic outcomes (10) (Table 46.2). Associated with a question of quality of life, it is serving as the benchmark for therapy assessment. Alterations of the symptom score are monitored sequentially to assess the success of the applied therapy.

Treatment
Medical Therapy
Historically, castration and steroidal antiandrogens have been tried, without success (11,12), as therapy for BPH. Intermittent self-catheterization is a nonsurgical therapy

Table 46.2. American Urologic Society Symptom Score

Frequency of Occurrence	0	<1 in 5	<50%	50%	>50%	always
OVER THE PAST HOW OFTEN HAVE YOU NOTED:						
Sensation of incomplete emptying	0	1	2	3	4	5
Had to urinate again in less than 2 hours	0	1	2	3	4	5
Stream stopped and started several times	0	1	2	3	4	5
Difficulty in postponing urination	0	1	2	3	4	5
A weak stream	0	1	2	3	4	5
Pushing or straining to begin urination	0	1	2	3	4	5
Need to get up from bed to urinate	0	1	2	3	4	5

TOTAL SCORE = •• MAXIMUM = 35

that has been employed successfully for generations. The patient catheterizes himself frequently enough in the day so that he never accumulates a volume of 500 mL at the time of any one catheterization. However, the risk of infection persists with this therapy.

Table 46.3 lists current methods of treating BPH (13). Modern medical therapies for BPH began in the mid-1970s with the work of Caine, who used dibenzyline, an alpha blocker, and flutamide, a nonsteroidal anti-androgen, in the treatment of BPH (12). Current medical therapies address the tone of the bladder neck, and provide hormonal control of the growth of the prostatic epithelial cell by decreasing testosterone in the cell, which interferes with the conversion of testosterone to its more active metabolite, dihydrotestosterone (DHT) by 5α-reductase inhibitors, interferes with the binding of the activated DHT to the receptor of nonsteroidal anti-androgens, and prevents transport of the DHT-receptor complex into the nucleus of the cell to stimulate protein synthesis. Luteinizing hormone-releasing hormone (LHRH) analogues are more than 100-fold more powerful than the hypothalamic hormone. They are used as a medical orchiectomy and achieve castrate levels of testosterone in the serum at 28 days after the initial injection. LHRH analogues, administered intramuscularly every 28 days, decreased the volume of the prostate by 31 percent in BPH and improved the symptom score and flow rate.

Alpha-adrenergic blockade with dibenzyline and prazosin have been most effective in relaxing the bladder neck to allow greater force to the urinary stream, higher flow rates, and more complete bladder emptying (14–16). Dibenzyline has significant side effects, such as fatigue, dizziness, nasal stuffiness, difficulty with ejaculation, difficulty with visual accommodation, and it is poorly tolerated in the elderly. Prazosin, in either single or double doses, also seems to work well but has similar side effects. Terazosin, a specific $alpha_1$ blocker that is administered once daily, is effective with few side effects. The required dose is determined by titration. Side effects include dizziness, lightheadedness, asthenia, and flulike symptoms. One distinct advantage of the alpha blockers is that the beneficial effects are noted almost immediately by the patient.

5α-reductase inhibitors have been studied for the treat-

Table 46.3. History of Treatment of Benign Prostatic Hyperplasia (BPH)

Treatment/Procedure	Date First Performed
Intermittent catheterization	?
Suprapubic transvesical prostatectomy	1880
Perineal prostatectomy	1894
Castration	1895
Transurethral prostatectomy (TURP)	1929
Edison 1879 lamp	
Hertz 1988 high-frequency current	
Young 1909 endoscopic instruments	
Retropubic prostatectomy	1947
Transurethral incision of the prostate	1951
Alpha adrenergic blockers (relaxants)	1976
Dibenzyline	
Prazosin	
Terazosin	
Antiandrogens	1976
Flutamide	1980s
Medical castration, LHRH analogues	1980s
Enzyme inhibitors – 5 α-reductase	1980s
Inhibitors	
Aromatase inhibitors	
Estrogen inhibitor	
Antiandrogens	
Steroidal	
Cyproterone acetate	
Megace	
Nonsteroidal	
Flutamide	
Nilutamide	
Casodex	
Balloon dilation	
Thermotherapy	
Permanent epithelial stent	
Laser prostatectomy	1990s

? = unknown

ment of BPH. The first-generation agent, which blocked the conversion of intracellular testosterone to DHT, was discontinued because of its side effects. The currently used inhibitor, finasteride, has much less toxicity and is tolerated well. Early studies show a reduction of prostate volume by 30 percent, an increase in the urine flow rate of 3 mL/sec, and an improvement in the patient's symptom score (17). These results have been sustained for at least 12 months. The side effects of decreased libido and ejaculatory disturbance occur in less than 5 percent of patients. An extensive study of the use of the combination of an alpha blocker and a 5α-reductase inhibitor is in progress.

Early studies of the nonsteroidal antiandrogen, flutamide, suggested potential usefulness of this drug as therapy for BPH, but it has recently been withdrawn as a treatment for this condition. Casodex, another nonsteroidal antiandrogen, was recently shown to decrease the prostate volume by 26 percent and increase urinary flow rate by 1.7 mL/sec. Breast tenderness was noted as a side effect, and impotence occurred in 50 percent of patients taking the drug.

Balloon dilation has been shown to be temporarily effective, but repeated dilations appear to be necessary to sustain benefit. Thermotherapy is coagulative necrosis by microwave therapy of periurethral BPH impinging on the urethra without injury to the urethra. This therapy appears to be beneficial, and further studies of its usefulness are under way. The insertion of a permanent indwelling urethral stent in the prostatic urethra is also undergoing investigation and early results appear promising.

Successful surgery for BPH dates to the 1880s, when the technique of suprapubic prostatectomy was introduced. Other successful surgical procedures were perineal prostatectomy in the 1890s, TURP in the 1920s, and simple retropubic enucleation of the prostate for benign disease in the 1940s. Better optics, better instrumentation, and more sophisticated application of electronic technology in the practice of urology, have made TURP the most popular method of prostatectomy, even for significantly enlarged glands. Spinal or continuous epidural anesthesia is the preferred method of anesthesia for the surgical procedure because a conscious patient allows the anesthesiologist to monitor the patient's mental status closely and alert the surgeon early to hypervolemic problems.

Intraoperative complications of TURP include bleeding, capsular perforation, bladder perforation, and urinary extravasation. Excessive absorption of irrigating fluid may result in hyponatremia, hypovolemia, restlessness, confusion, nausea, or vomiting. If the absorption is undetected, convulsions, coma, and death may occur. Postoperative complications include secondary hemorrhage, acute urinary retention, urinary retention caused by clot formation from secondary hemorrhage,

bladder neck contracture, and urethral stricture. Total urinary incontinence as a result of sphincteric injury occurs in about 1 percent of patients. More commonly, patients with preoperative urgency continue to have urgency and urge incontinence that will respond to anticholinergics.

Sexual function is also affected by TURP. The removal of the prostate gland and occlusion of the ejaculatory ducts that drain the seminal vesicles can eliminate ejaculation at orgasm. The seminal vesicles contribute 70 percent to the volume of ejaculate. If the ejaculatory ducts empty into the urethra with orgasm, loss of the bladder neck may lead to retrograde passage of the ejaculation into the bladder. Impotence also occurs, but the exact incidence remains to be determined. Not enough attention has been given to the objective preoperative assessment of erectile function, and therefore postoperative impotence is difficult to evaluate and interpret. Excessive periprostatic extravasation of irrigating fluid during TURP may contribute to impotence.

Recent studies show that in patients whose prostate weighs less than 30 to 35 gm (as estimated by rectal examination) unilateral or bilateral surgical incision of the prostate and bladder neck, beginning at the posterior trigone and ending near the apex of the prostate, allows adequate voiding and complete emptying of the bladder and has been accompanied by a significant reduction in morbidity and mortality, as compared with results of TURP (18,19). The incision is made deeply through the prostatic tissue from the posterior wall of the trigone, just medial to the ureteral orifice, down to and alongside the verumontanum in the distal prostatic urethra. With this incision, the bladder neck and prostatic urethra are widely opened. When this is accomplished unilaterally, approximately 40 percent of patients experience retrograde ejaculation. When the incision is performed bilaterally, approximately 70 percent of the patients experience retrograde ejaculation. Whether use of this type of transurethral incision of the prostate will continue to show beneficial results remains to be seen. Effective voiding can be restored, however, and except for retrograde ejaculation, sexual function remains unaffected.

BPH affects men older than 40 years of age. Symptoms may cause a significant alteration in lifestyle and necessitate therapy. Current therapy begins with medical attention to the symptoms and is followed by surgery only when medical therapy fails.

Cancer of the Prostate

Cancer originating in the prostate gland is the most commonly occurring tumor in men in the United States; the number of cases of prostate cancer has exceeded those of lung cancer since 1988 (20). Considered rare in the nineteenth century, prostate cancer presently is viewed as a morbid disease, with over 38,000 attributable deaths annually (21). Prostate cancer is a relatively uncommon disease in men younger than age 40; the mean age at presentation is 72 years of age.

No specific etiologic factors are known (22). Endogenous hormonal influences are implicated because DHT is essential to prostatic growth and metabolism. Geographic patterns show higher incidences of prostate cancer in northern and western European countries and lower incidences in eastern Europe and Japan (23). In the United States, incidence and mortality rates in black men are roughly twice those of white men. Rising disease rates in immigrants from countries considered low-risk areas for prostate cancer suggest environmental initiating or promoting factors. Dietary habits, specifically the high-fat North American diet, which alters hormone metabolism, are postulated as associative factors (24). Familial patterns are documented, which suggests genetic influences. Associative hormonal factors are implicated by the absence of prostatic cancer in androgen-deficient males (25) and the induction of prostate cancer in experimental animals by prolonged administration of male sex hormones (26).

As life expectancy increases, a corresponding increase in prostatic cancer has been demonstrated. Incidence data identifying latent (clinically unsuspected) carcinomas range from 0.85 percent in the large random series described by Alexejew and Dunajewski (27) to 66.7 percent per 100 men older than age 80 reported by Rullis and colleagues (28).

Diagnosis

Prostate cancer is curable if diagnosed while the cancer is localized to the prostate gland; however, detection while the cancer is confined within the prostate capsule is ac-

complished in only 10 to 15 percent of presentations. Before 1936, rectal examination was the only test to detect a suspicious prostatic lesion. With the description of serum acid phosphatase by Gutman in 1936, the field of biologic markers as potential indicators of the presence of tumors was introduced (29).

Evaluation

Since Gutman's report, numerous biologically active substances, including prostatic acid phosphatase (PAP) and PSA, have been examined. Radioimmunoassay of PAP is not entirely specific for prostate cancer; approximately 6 percent of patients with elevated PAP have BHP.

PSA, a glycoprotein serine protease discovered by Wang and associates in 1979, is found in the cytoplasm of prostatic epithelial cells and functions to liquefy the seminal coagulum in the adult man (30). At low concentrations, slightly above the upper limit of normal reference range of PSA, differentiation between benign prostatic conditions and cancer is mandated within the context of clinical and pathologic findings. PSA is currently the most useful marker for evaluating prostatic cancer and monitoring the presence or recurrence of disease after initial therapy. Because a rising PSA level may suggest disease progression, serial values may predict the clinical course of prostate cancer (31). The role of PSA as a screening modality is debated. In combination with other modalities, such as transurethral ultrasonography (TRUS) and digital rectal examination (DRE), PSA provided complementary evaluative data and exhibited the lowest error rate (the sum of the false-positive and false-negative rates) in contrast to TRUS and DRE (32). Levels of other markers such as carcinoembryonic antigen (CEA), lactic dehydrogenase (LDH), and urinary hydroxyproline may tend to rise with disease progression and fall with disease response, but the low percentage of efficiency does not justify their use as prostate cancer markers.

Newer modalities, specifically aspiration cytology and TRUS, have been promoted in the detection of prostate cancer. The technique of fine needle aspiration of sheets of cells for cytologic review, first reported by Esposti in 1956 and popularized in European centers, is now being applied in the United States (33). The spring-loaded bioptic needle technique with the ability to yield cores of tissue has been demonstrated to be a high-yield, cost-effective procedure with low morbidity. TRUS provides computerized images for viewing the entire prostatic structure and enhances the clinician's accuracy in guiding biopsy or aspiration needles to suspicious sites. However, TRUS alone is not a cost-effective, sensitive, or specific screening test. Cooner et al reported a positive predictive value of only 31 percent in individuals with a normal DRE and a PSA greater than 10ng/mL (34).

The DRE is a cost-efficient, readily performed test. Visualizing the prostate gland as having a central area or zone, a submucosal or transitional zone, and a horseshoe-shaped peripheral area may help with understanding disease distribution and the area accessible to digital rectal examination. Palpable areas include the posterior or posterolateral region of the peripheral zone with a midline furrow, which is felt as a shallow midline depression, and the two superiorly positioned seminal vesicles are identifiable landmarks on rectal palpation (35). Any change in glandular size, consistency, or contour may represent an inflammatory process, infarction, calculus, or tumor. As suggested by Guinan and associates, adherence to American Cancer Society guidelines for annual digital examination of the prostate gland for men over 40 years of age is recommended (36). Of the various test combinations (using PSA, DRE, and TRUS), PSA and DRE had the lowest prostate detection error rate (32). In support of the efficacy of this combined approach, the basic urologic recommendation for men at risk, as suggested by Oesterling, should be an annual DRE and PSA with further testing determined by an abnormality in one or both of these tests (37). The implications should be discussed with the patient.

Pathology

Histologic evaluation is needed to establish a definitive diagnosis; therefore, once the clinical suspicion of a prostatic cancer has arisen, the next step is biopsy. The common method used to confirm the diagnosis is needle biopsy of the prostate, performed either transperineally or transrectally. Needle biopsy may be done on an outpatient basis with ease, reliability, and safety. Needle tract tumor seeding is rarely reported. Other more invasive methods of prostatic biopsy are transurethral resection of the prostate and open perineal biopsy. Papanicolaou stain of prostatic fluid, obtained by prostatic massage, is positive in approximately 80 percent of patients with an established diagnosis of advanced prostate cancer.

The interpretation of prostatic biopsies by pathologists is often characterized by difficulty because of the similarity of a number of benign and malignant processes that can co-exist (38). Most prostatic carcinomas are adenocarcinomas, which are believed to arise from the epithelium lining the peripheral acini. In addition to the conventional carcinomas, a number of rare, unconventional ones also exist. Ductal carcinomas are often papillary or cribriform. Periurethral prostatic duct carcinomas arise at the junction of the large ducts with the prostatic urethra. Central, ductal tumors tend to be locally aggressive and metastasize later in their natural history. Endometrioid carcinomas, once thought to arise from the prostatic uricle, produce both PSA and PAP. They are, therefore, believed to be variants of ductal carcinoma. Mucinous carcinomas are uncommon (0.4 to 3.0 percent); however, as many as 20 percent to 20 percent of acinar carcinomas contain areas of mucin production. The possibility of invasive colorectal carcinoma should always be excluded in these cases. Other rare tumors, such as pure transitional cell carcinomas, small-cell (neuroendocrine) carcinomas, adenoid cystic carcinomas, and carcinosarcomas, have been reported.

Tumor Grade

Once the diagnosis of prostatic carcinoma has been established, a histologic grade is assigned in an attempt to predict prognosis. To date, over 40 prostatic cancer grading systems, which is reflective of the wide variety of histologic patterns admixed even for small biopsy fragments, have been described. Although a number of criteria have been examined for their prognostic significance, glandular architecture and nuclear anaplasia are the only two variables that have consistently been proven to be of value. The widely used Gleason system depends entirely on glandular architecture. In this systematic approach, the two most predominant patterns of carcinoma are assigned scores ranging from 1 to 5. The scores are then added to obtain a pattern sum for the individual's tumor. The sums have been shown to be predictive of stage and survival when used alone and when used in combination with clinical staging.

The system developed for use by the National Prostatic

Cancer Project (NPCP) uses both glandular architecture and nuclear detail (39). Numerous modifications to these systems have been presented with no universal acceptance. The Gleason system has served as the model to which other systems have been compared.

Recently, the definition of premalignant states, such as atypical hyperplasia and dysplasia, has raised a possibility of identifying patients at an earlier stage. These two lesions occur in both the presence and absence of BPH and seem, therefore, to be independent of BPH. Both these lesions have been shown to be present in small volume early tumors as well as in more advanced disease. With continued evaluation, atypical hyperplasia or dysplasia may be predictive, at a curable stage, of risk for development of significant disease.

Staging of Prostatic Carcinoma

After histologic confirmation, a staging workup is done to evalute localized extent and metastatic status, with awareness of the tumor's propensity to spread via blood vessels and lymphatics. Radiologic examinations include excretory urography, chest x-ray, bone scan, and bone survey or spot films of suspicious areas. Hepatomegaly or elevated liver enzyme studies require further evaluation. Pelvic and periaortic nodes are evaluated by computed tomography (CT). Because microscopic lymphatic metastases are not able to be imaged, pelvic lymphadenectomy remains the most accurate method for assessment of lymph node status. Transrectal ultrasonography may suggest size, shape, consistency, and border of the prostatic capsule. Magnetic resonance imaging (MRI), with its ability to illustrate the seminal vesicles and delineate the interface between the prostate gland and contiguous structures, may distinguish between BPH and cancer.

In 1956, Whitmore introduced a simple staging system ranging from A to D (40): stage A–tumor incidentally found upon prostatectomy; stage B–tumor confined to the prostate; stage C–tumor extended locally outside the prostate; and stage D–metastatic disease.

In 1975, another staging system, the Whitmore-Jewett modification, subdivided stage A disease into A1 and A2, reflective of tumor grade and quantity; stage B disease was classified as B1 and B2, indicative of palpable nodularity, size, and location; stage C disease was defined as C1 or C2, suggestive of degree of local invasion; and stage D disease was subdivided into D1 and D2, reflective of location of metastatic activity (41). Investigators have suggested two new categories of stage D disease: D0, reflective of an elevation in acid phosphatase in clinically determined, locally confined disease and D3, illustrative of disease recurrence after hormonal ablation for stage D1 or D2 prostate cancer (42).

The tumor, node, metastasis (TNM) system, a clinical and pathologic staging system for communication of assessment of primary tumor (T), presence and extent of nodal involvement (N), and distant metastasis (M), was adopted by the American Joint Committee for Cancer (AJCC) Staging and End Results Reporting in 1974. This system also recognized TX, NX and MX (X signifying factors that cannnot be assessed) and T0, N0, M0 (0 indicating that no tumor is detected; higher numerals [with letters for subdivisions] indicating increasing involvement). The AJCC system is contrasted to the Whitmore-Jewett system in Table 46.4.

Management of Disease

In developing an individual's treatment plan in the setting of viable alternative treatment options, key components in the person's data base should include age, family history of prostate cancer, occupational exposure, marital status, sexual activity pattern, dietary habits, urologic history, performance status, pain assessment, weight history, and other symptoms. These data complement the DRE, PSA, PAP, diagnostic imaging, histologic, and physical examination findings. All parameters viewed jointly provide landmarks for review and discussion of universal and individual concerns as well as establish the baseline on which to build a continuing therapeutic relationship.

Localized Prostate Cancer

Stage A1 (T1a) prostate cancer is managed by follow-up needle biopsies of the prostate gland 6 to 8 weeks after the initial prostatectomy. If no residual tumor is detected, routine prostate evaluation recommendations are instituted. Documentation of residual tumor results in reclassification of the patient to stage A2 (T1b).

Complete surgical removal of the prostate gland and seminal vesicles remains the optimal therapy for stage A2

Table 46.4. Comparison of Two Staging Systems for Prostate Cancer

Whitmore-Jewett System	Definition	AJCC System
A	No clinical neoplasm	T1
A1	Tumor <5% microscopic, well-differentiated foci	T1a
A2	Tumor >5% microscopic foci or moderately/poorly differentiated foci	T1b
B	Palpable intracapsular neoplasm	T2
B1	Focal <1.5 cm	T2a
B2	Diffuse >1.5 cm >2 foci	T2b
C	Locally advanced neoplasm	
C1	Bladder, seminal vesicles, prostatic capsule not fixed	T3
C2	Other sites, fixed	T4
D	Metastatic disease	N, M
D0	Elevated acid phosphatase with no clinical extraprostatic disease	NX, MX
D1	Regional lymph node involvement	
	1	N1
	2–5	N2
	>5	N3
D2	Distant nodes, bone, other organs	M
D3	Hormone-refractory disease	M

AJCC = American Joint Committee for Cancer.
SOURCE: Adapted from References 40–42.

(T1b) B1 and B2 (T2) lesions. Higher overall survival rates favor radical prostatectomy over radiotherapy at 10 and 15 years. A retropubic approach is preferred because the limited pelvic lymphadenectomy can be followed by radical prostatectomy if the nodal frozen section is negative for tumor. Although the perineal approach facilitates vesicourethral anastomosis and decreases blood loss, an additional surgical approach is necessary to adequately evaluate the pelvic lymphatics.

Rectal injuries, severe hemorrhage, infection, death are infrequent complications of radical prostatectomy. Postoperatively, urinary incontinence, bladder neck contracture, and urethral stricture may occur. Impotence has been universally experienced, although new nerve sparing surgical techniques preserve the pelvic nerve plexuses involved in penile erection and thus preserve potency.

The role of radiotherapy as a curative modality for early-stage prostate cancer has generated ongoing controversy. External-beam megavoltage radiotherapy has controlled disease limited to the prostate in an impressive number of patients. New implantation techniques for delivering radiation directly to target prostate tissue, used alone or with external-beam therapy, offer local control without loss of potency. Radiotherapy is clearly indicated for patients who are not good surgical candidates.

Stage C (T3) disease seems to be amenable to potentially curative therapy with LHRH analogue-antiandrogen "down-sizing" therapy. More than 50 percent of all prostate cancer lesions initially judged to be clinical stage C (T3 or T4) are actually stage D1 (N1–3) or even D2 (M) with micrometastatic foci of tumor to bone, distant nodes, or other organs. The curative potential of either radiotherapy or surgical intervention in advanced-stage lesions is slight.

Advanced Prostate Cancer

Since the Nobel Prize-winning demonstration of the androgen-dependent nature of prostate cancer by Huggins and Hodges in 1941, hormonal manipulation has been the cornerstone of therapy for advanced malignancy. Initially, Huggins thought that androgen deprivation had the potential to cure metastatic disease; however, continued evelution demonstrated recurrence in most patients between 12 and 24 months after bilateral orchiectomy.

The adult testicular Leydig cells produce 95 percent of all circulating androgens in the form of testosterone; the zona fasciculata and reticularis of the adrenal glands produce the remaining 5 percent in the form of dyhydroepiandrosterone (DHEA) and androstenedione. An intact hypothalamic-pituitary-adrenal-gonadal axis is required to maintain physiologic levels of testosterone. Interruption at any point in the axis circumvents the prostate supply of androgens, which deprives the gland of testosterone and produces objective improvement in disease control, subjective benefit, or both.

A number of pharmacologic agents and surgical interventions are designed to disrupt the axis. Pharmacologic agents include estrogenic compounds diethylstilbestrol (DES), chlorotrianisene (TACE), diethylstilbestrol diphosphate, progestational agents (megestrol acetate, medroxyprogesterone), LHRH analogues (leuprolide

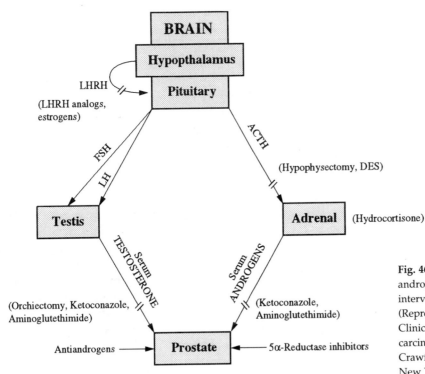

Fig. 46.1. Hormonal control of circulating androgens and pharmacologic and surgical interventions designed to disrupt the axis. (Reproduced by permission from Drago JR. Clinical presentation and diagnosis of carcinoma of the prostate. In: Das S, Crawford ED, eds. Cancer of the prostate. New York: Marcel Dekker, 1993.)

acetate, buserelin acetate), steroidal antiandrogens (cyproterone acetate and secondary action of megestrol acetate and medroxyprogesterone), nonsteroidal antiandrogens (flutamide, nilutamide, Casodex), androgen synthesis inhibitors (aminoglutethimide, ketoconazole, spironolactone), and a cytotoxic combination of nitrogen mustard linked to a phosphorylated estradiol (EMCYT). Surgical procedures include bilateral orchiectomy, hypophysectomy, and adrenalectomy. Figure 46.1 depicts the hypothalamic-pituitary-adrenal-gonadal axis and illustrates hormonal control of circulating androgens and various pharmacologic and surgical interventions designed to disrupt the axis (43).

Bilateral orchiectomy is the time-honored and cost-effective method for permanent disruption of the axis. It is a simple surgical procedure with minimal morbidity and continues to be effective as initial therapy for symptomatic advanced prostate cancer. Serum testosterone is permanently reduced to castrate levels, and impotence results. DES at an adequate suppression dosage (1 mg taken orally three times a day) binds the hypothalamic receptor for testosterone and thus decreases LHRH and LH release and increases levels of sex-steroid binding-globulin, which thereby reduces the amount of metabolically active testosterone. Remission rates approximating those of orchiectomy are achieved. Complications include sodium and water retention, embolic and thromboembolic episodes, cardiovascular compromise, testicular atrophy, and decreased libido. DES-associated gynecomastia can be prevented by delivery of 400 rad to each breast before initiation of the drug. Although DES continues to be widely used and is an effective, cost-efficient therapy, many clinicians consider the risk of cardiovascular side effects to be unacceptable in contrast to other therapeutic modalities.

LHRH is a naturally occurring decapeptide with a short half-life and was initially described in 1971 (44). Long-term supraphysiologic synthetic LHRH administration has been discovered to paradoxically cause androgen depletion, perhaps as a result of pituitary depletion or densensitization to the abundance of circulating LHRH. These agents are effective, although expensive, and have tolerable side effects including hot flashes, nausea and vomiting, edema, decreased libido, and impotence. The most common adverse event is associated with an initial surge in circulating testosterone, which can exacerbate bone pain, lymphadema, obstructive uropathy, and spinal cord compression.

A unique class of drugs known as nonsteroidal antiandrogens blocks the cellular action of androgens at the target organ by inhibiting the nuclear uptake of DHT. Rather than a lowering of serum androgens, a subtle rise may actually be seen. Side effects of the nonsteroidal antiandrogen, flutamide, include gynecomastia, diarrhea, elevated liver enzymes and, rarely, hepatic fatalities. This compound is used in conjunction with an LHRH analogue. Enthusiasm for combined androgen deprivation with an LHRH analogue and an antiandrogen has been generated by statistically significant progression-free survival and overall survival favoring the combined therapy in several series of large, randomized controlled trials conducted under the auspices of the National Cancer Institute (NCI) and the European Organization for Research and Treatment of Cancer (EORTC).

Surgical interventions, such as hypophysectomy for control of symptoms and adrenalectomy, have not affected objective or subjective parameters. Other agents, such as ketoconazole, a broad-spectrum antifungal, and aminoglutethimide, have been investigated for their ability to inhibit cytochrome p-450 enzyme-dependent steps and thus reduce adrenal androgen production but have no convincing efficacy.

In the continuing search for long-term control of the

heterogeneous prostate cancer cell lines, a number of chemotherapeutic agents have been evaluated in clinical trials as single agents, combination therapy, or adjuvant therapy. Complete responses to chemotherapy in stage D2 (M) disease have not been documented and partial responses have not been sustained. Disease stabilization and subjective responses have been achieved; the most effective chemotherapeutic agents have been cyclophosphamide, 5-fluorouracil, cisplatin, doxorubicin, and methotrexate (45). A role for nonhormonal chemotherapy has not been established for hormone refractory prostate cancer or for an initial therapy in stage D1 disease.

Current investigative approaches include testing drugs (e.g., somatostatin) that modulate the effects of growth factors, such as epidermal growth factor. These factors may be up-regulated through the action of an endogenous androgen, which stimulates the growth of both benign and malignant prostate cells. Suramin, a naphthylurea developed as a treatment for a protozoan parasitic infection, has been demonstrated to inhibit the binding of various tumor growth factors to their cell surface receptors, which affects their ability to stimulate tumor cells (46). Significant toxicity, including adrenal insufficiency, fatigue, peripheral neuropathy, and coagulopathy, has been observed. Clinical trials with suramin are under way.

Although no clear-cut pathway exists to facilitate prostate cancer prevention, interventions such as promotion of healthy dietary habits and chemopreventive agents, such as retinoids, offer compelling rationale. However, the design of a study to test such an intervention is impractical because of the number of subjects needed, the inability to blind the treatment arm, and difficulty in monitoring variables such as dietary compliance. A new class of compounds, 5α-reductase inhibitors, has been synthesized, of which the first agent to be approved was finasteride for the treatment of BPH. This compound's ability to result in intraprostatic androgen concentration similar to levels in castrate patients led to its selection as the agent to be tested in the large-scale Prostate Cancer Prevention Trial (PCPT) activated at 222 sites under NCI sponsorship.

The chemoprevention trial, which focuses new efforts on the prevention of prostate cancer, signals an exciting initiative in the field of prostate cancer research. By answering important questions posed by the PCPT, productive research opportunities will continue to be identified. Diagnosis of prostate cancer at an early stage, when cure is a likely outcome, is within the realm of current clinical reality. Advances in tumor markers, imaging techniques, and computerized tumor specimen visualization have greatly contributed to the clinician's ability to detect the disease early, determine its extent, and treat aggressively while predicting and monitoring response to therapy. New strategies in hormonal manipulation offer promise in contributing to progression-free and overall survival in advanced disease, and thus enhance the patient's quality of life. The continuing quest for unique agents has identified compounds that affect the elaboration of tumor growth factors. Traditional and new diagnostic, preventive, and therapeutic interventions offer promise, support the goals of prevention and early detection, and also suggest strategies to enhance the quality of life for patients living with advanced disease and the quality of life for their care providers.

References

1. Brunner H, Weidner W, Schiefer HG. Studies in the role of ureaplasma urealyticum and mycoplasma hominis in prostatitis. J Infect Dis 1983;147:807.
2. Meares EM Jr, Stamey TA. Bacteriologic localization patterns in bacterial prostatitis and urethritis. Invest Urol 1968;5:492.
3. Fair WR, Crane D, Schiller N, Heston WDW. A re-appraisal of treatment in chronic bacterial prostatitis. J Urol 1979;121:437.
4. Meares EM Jr. Acute and chronic prostatitis: diagnosis and treatment. Infect Dis Clin North Am 1987;1:855.
5. Stamey TA. Pathogenesis and treatment of urinary tract infections. Baltimore: Williams & Wilkins, 1980.
6. Crawford ED. Diagnosis and treatment of prostatitis. Hosp Pract 1985;20:77.
7. Berry SJ, Coffey DS, Walsh PC, et al. The development of human benign prostatic hyperplasia with age. J Urol 1984;132:474.
8. Wilson JD. The pathogenesis of benign prostatic hyperplasia. Am J Med 1980;68:745.
9. Turner-Warwick R. Clinical urodynamics. Urol Clin North Am 1979;6:171.
10. Lepor H, Machi G. Comparison of AUA symptom index in selected men between 55 and 79 years of age. Urology 1993;42:36.
11. Deming CL. The effect of castration on benign hypertrophy of the prostate in man. J Urol 1935;33:388.
12. Caine M, Perlberg S, Gordon R. The treatment of benign prostatic hypertrophy with flutamide (SCH 13521): a placebo-controlled study. J Urol 1975;114:564.
13. Lepor H. Medical therapy for benign prostatic hyperplasia. Urology 1993;42:483.
14. Caine M, Perlberg S, Shapiro A. Phenoxybenzamine for benign prostatic obstruction: review of 200 cases. Urology 1981;17:542.
15. Paulson DF, Kane RD. A prospective study in the pharmaceutical management of benign prostatic hyperplasia. J Urol 1975;113:811.
16. Caine M, Pfau A, Perlberg S. The use of alpha adrenergic blockers in benign prostatic hypertrophy. Urology 1976;48:255.
17. Stoner E, et al. Three-year safety and efficacy data on the use of finasteride in the treatment of benign prostatic hyperplasia. Urology 1994;43:284.
18. Orandi H. Transurethral incision of the prostate. Urology 1978;12:187.
19. Edwards L, Powell C. An objective comparison of transurethral resection and bladder neck incision in the treatment of prostatic hypertrophy. J Urol 1982;128:325.
20. American Cancer Society. 1986 cancer facts and figures. Cancer 1989;39:3.
21. Boring CC, Squires TS, Tong T, Montgomery S. Cancer statistics, 1994. Cancer 1994;4:19.
22. Murphy GP, et al. Prostate cancer. Part A. Research, endocrine treatment, and histopathology. New York: Alan R. Liss, 1987.
23. Jacobi GH, Hohenfellner RF. Prostate cancer. Baltimore: Williams & Wilkins, 1982:15.
24. Hill P, Wynder EL, Garnes H, Walker ARP. Environmental factor, hormone status, and prostatic cancer. Prev Med 1980;9:657.
25. Hovenanian MS, Deming CL. The heterologous growth of cancer of the prostate. In: Martin FH, ed. Surgery, gynecology and obstetrics. Chicago: The Franklin H. Martin Foundation, 1948:29–35.
26. Noble RL. The development of prostatic adenocarcinoma in the Nb rats following sex hormone administration. Cancer Res 1977;27:1929.
27. Alexejew M, Dunajewski L. Prostatakarzinom im kindesalter. Urol Chir 1930;1:64.
28. Rullis I, Schaeffer IA, Lilien OM. Incidence of prostatic carcinoma in the elderly. Urology 1975;4:295.
29. Gutman EB, Sproul EE, Autman AB. Significance of increased phosphatase activity of bone at the site of osteoblastic metastases secondary to carcinoma of the prostate gland. Am J Cancer 1946;28:485.
30. Wang MC, Valenzuela LA, Murphy GP, et al. Purification of a human prostate-specific antigen. Invest Urol 1979;17:159.
31. Chu TM, Murphy AP. What's new in tumor markers for prostate cancer? Urology 1986;27:487.

32. Catalona WJ, Smith DS, Ratliff TL, et al. Measurement of prostate specific antigen in serum as a screening test for prostate cancer. N Engl J Med 1991;325:1156.

33. Esposit PL. Cytologic diagnosis of prostatic tumors with the aid of transrectal aspiration biopsy: a critical review of 1,110 cases and a report of morphologic and cytochemical studies. Acta Cytol 1966;10:182.

34. Cooner WH, Mosley BR, Rutherford CL, et al. Prostate cancer detection in a clinical urologic practice by ultrasound, digital rectal exam, and prostate specific antigen. J Urol 1990;143:1146.

35. Walsh PC. Radical prostatectomy, preservation of sexual function, cancer control: the controversy. In: Donohue JP, ed. Controversies in urologic oncology. Urol Clin North Am 1987,14:663.

36. Guinan P, Bush I, Ray V, et al. The accuracy of the rectal examination in the diagnosis of prostate cancer. N Engl J Med 1980;303:499.

37. Oesterling JE. Prostate specific antigen: a critical assessment of the most useful tumor marker for adenocarcinoma of the prostate. J Urol 1991;145:907.

38. Miller GJL. An atlas of prostatic biopsies: dilemmas of morphologic variance. In: Fenoglip-Preiser CM, Wolff M, Rilke F, eds. Progress in surgical pathology, vol VIII. Philadelphia: Field and Wood, 1988:81.

39. Mostofi FK. Grading of prostatic carcinoma. Cancer Chemother Rep 1975;59:111.

40. Whitmore WJ Jr. Hormone therapy in prostate cancer. Am J Med 1956;21:697.

41. Jewett HJ. The present status of radical prostatectomy for stages A and B prostatic cancer. Urol Clin North Am 1975;2:105.

42. Whitesel JA, Donohue RE, Mani J, et al. Acid phosphatase–its influence on pelvic lymph node dissection. 1J Urol 984;131:70.

43. Drago, JR. Clinical presentation and diagnosis of carcinoma of the prostate. In: Das S, Crawford ED, eds. Cancer of the prostate. New York: Marcel Dekker, 1993.

44. Schally AV, et al. LH-RH agonists and antagonists. Int J Gynaecol Obstet 1980;18:318.

45. Scher HI, Sternberg CN. Chemotherapy of urologic malignancies. Semin Urol 1985;3:239.

46. Stein CA, LaRocca RV, Thomas R, et al. Suramin: an anticancer drug with a unique mechanism of action. J Clin Oncol 1989;7:499.

Chapter 47
Kidney Disease in the Elderly

Biff F. Palmer and Moshe Levi

Old age is like a plane flying through a storm. Once you're aboard, there is nothing you can do.

Golda Meir

Advancing age is associated with a number of structural and functional changes in the kidneys (Table 47.1). In spite of these changes, aging kidneys are remarkably capable of maintaining fluid and electrolyte balance within narrow limits. The adaptive capacity of aging kidneys to stress and disease is, however, quite restricted. As a result, elderly patients are predisposed to develop fluid and electrolyte disorders under conditions that would otherwise be well tolerated by younger individuals. Understanding of these alterations allows the clinician to anticipate and better treat many clinical conditions that occur in the elderly. This chapter reviews the normal, age-related changes that occur in renal anatomy and physiology. In addition, the chapter provides an overview of renal diseases that are most prevalent in the aged population.

Renal Anatomy

Advancing age is associated with progressive loss of renal mass in humans. Renal weight decreases from 250 to 270 gm in a young adult to 180 to 200 gm by a person's eighth decade (1). The loss of renal mass is primarily cortical, with relative sparing of the renal medulla. The total number of identifiable glomeruli falls with age, in accordance with the changes of renal weight (2–4). The number of hyalinized or sclerotic glomeruli identified on light microscopy increases from 1 percent to 2 percent during a person's third to fifth decade, to as high as 30 percent in some apparently healthy 80-year-olds, with a mean prevalence after age 70 of approximately 10 percent to 12 percent (5–7).

Changes also occur with age in the intrarenal vasculature, independent of hypertension or other renal disease. Normal aging is associated with variable sclerotic changes in the wall of the larger renal vessels, which are augmented in the presence of hypertension. Smaller vessels are spared, with less than 20 percent of senescent kidneys from nonhypertensive subjects displaying arteriolar changes (8–10).

Microangiographic and histologic studies have identified two very distinctive patterns of change in arteriolar-glomerular units with senescence (11,12). In one type, hyalinization and collapse of the glomerular tuft are associated with obliteration of the lumen of the preglomerular arteriole and a resultant loss in blood flow. This type of change is seen primarily in the cortical area. The second pattern, seen primarily in the juxtamedullary area, is characterized by the development of anatomic continuity between the afferent and efferent arterioles during glomerular sclerosis. As a result, there is loss of the glomerulus and direct shunting of blood flow from afferent to efferent arterioles. Blood flow is maintained to the arteriolar rectae verae, the primary vascular supply of the medulla, which are not decreased in number with age.

Renal Physiology and Pathophysiology

Renal Blood Flow

There is a progressive reduction in renal plasma flow (para-aminohippuric acid [PAH] clearance) of approximately 10 percent per decade, from 600 mL/min/1.73 m² in the 20 to 29-year-old age group to 300/mL/min/1.73 m² in the 80 to 89-year-old age group (13,14). The decrease in renal blood flow is associated with significant increases in both the afferent and efferent arteriolar resistance (14). The increase in the efferent arteriolar resistance may explain the age-related increase in filtration fraction (13,14). The exact relationship between renal plasma flow

Table 47.1. Renal Anatomic and Functional Changes with Aging

Decrease in total kidney mass: cortex > medulla
Decrease in renal blood flow
  Cortical flow > medullary flow
  Decreased response to vasodilators
Decrease in glomerular filtration rate
Altered tubular function
  Impaired Na conservation and excretion
  Impaired concentration/dilution of urine
  Impaired acidification of urine
  Impaired potassium metabolism

and cardiac output as a function of aging is not well established. Some studies have shown an age-related decrease in cardiac output, but others have shown no decrease in cardiac output with age (15–18). There is a small but definite decrease in the renal fraction of the cardiac output (renal blood flow/cardiac output [RBF/CO]) (19,20). The latter studies suggest that the major determinant of reduced renal blood flow with age is caused by functional or anatomic changes, or both, in the renal vasculature.

A study using the xenon washout technique to measure renal blood flow in 207 healthy potential renal donors who ranged in age from 17 to 76 years has shown that the age-related reduction in renal blood flow is not uniform within the kidneys (21). The investigators were able to demonstrate a preferential decrease in cortical blood flow. This finding is in accord with histologic studies showing a selective loss of cortical vasculature and preservation of medullary flow. The histologic and functional demonstration of a selective decrease in cortical blood flow may also explain the observation that filtration fraction actually increases with advancing age (13,14) because outer cortical nephrons have a lower filtration fraction than do juxtamedullary nephrons.

Whether the age-related decrease in renal blood flow is caused by anatomic or functional changes in the renal vasculature has been studied by two groups of investigators who have measured renal hemodynamics after intravenous administration of pyrogen (14), and intra-arterial administration of acetylcholine and angiotensin (21). During both pyrogen and acetylcholine administration, the vasodilator response was greater in the younger subjects than it was in the older subjects. However, the

vasoconstrictive response to angiotensin was identical in the young and old subjects.

More recently, renal hemodynamics were examined before and after an amino acid infusion in healthy, normotensive, young and elderly subjects without evidence of renal disease (22). At baseline, glomerular filtration rate (inulin clearance) and renal plasma flow (PAH clearance) were significantly lower and renal vascular resistance and filtration fraction significantly higher in the elderly as compared with those factors in the young subjects. After infusion of amino acids, effective renal plasma flow increased significantly in the young group but failed to do so in the elderly. By contrast, the glomerular filtration rate was found to increase to a similar extent in young and old subjects. The filtration fraction was found to increase in both groups but to a slightly greater extent in the elderly subjects (Figure 47.1). Renal vascular resistance fell in the young patients but did not change in the elderly. These data support the development of an age-related impairment in the vasodilatory response of the renal vasculature. Although an increase in renal blood flow was responsible for the rise in glomerular filtration rate in the young subjects, the lack of change in renal blood flow suggests an increase in intraglomerular pressure as the determinant responsible for the rise in glomerular filtration rate noted in the elderly subjects.

In summary, the bulk of data suggest that although the aging renal vasculature does respond to vasoconstriction and vasodilatation, the response to vasodilatation is markedly blunted. Anatomic changes as well as functional vasoconstriction mediate the age-related decrease in renal blood flow. Renal reserve, as defined by an increase in glomerular filtration rate in response to an amino acid infusion, remains preserved in elderly human subjects.

Glomerular Filtration Rate

Cross-sectional studies have shown a progressive, age-related decline in the glomerular filtration rate (GFR) in men and women older than 30 to 40 years of age (13,23). The results were confirmed by serial measurements of renal function in 548 healthy volunteers who participated in the Baltimore Longitudinal Study of Aging (24,25) (Figure 47.2). Creatinine clearance measurements showed a progressive linear decline from 140 mL/min/1.73 m^2 in

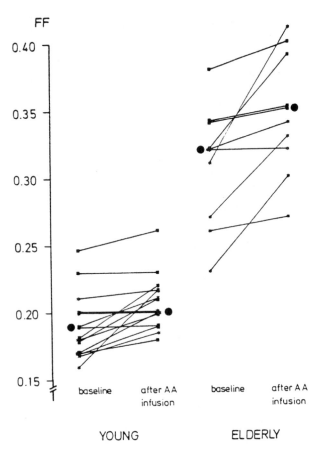

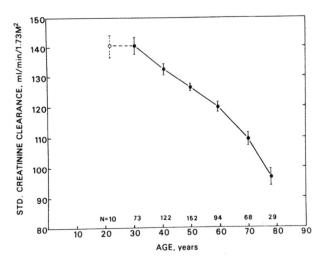

Fig. 47.2. Cross-sectional differences in standard creatinine clearance with age. The number of subjects in each age group is indicated above the abscissa. Values plotted indicate mean ± SEM. (Reproduced by permission from Rowe J, Andres R, Tobin J, et al. Age-adjusted standards for creatinine clearance. Ann Intern Med 1976;84:567–569.)

Fig. 47.1. Filtration fraction (FF) in young and elderly subjects at baseline and after amino acid infusion. Squares, men; asterisks, women; circles, median. (Reproduced by permission from Fliser D, Zeir M, Nowalk R, Ritz E. Renal functional reserve in healthy elderly subjects. J Am Soc Nephrol 1993;3:1371–1377.)

subjects 30 years of age to 97 mL/min/1.73 m² in subjects 80 years of age, at an approximate rate of 0.8 mL/min/1.73 m² per year (24,25). These results were reconfirmed in follow-up studies of 254 subjects in whom 5 to 14 serial creatinine clearance determinations were obtained between 1958 and 1981 (26). Of interest, 29 (36%) of the 254 subjects followed had no absolute decrease in creatinine clearance, and 7 of these subjects actually had a statistically significant increase in creatinine clearance over time.

In a similar study of 446 normal subjects, the age-related decline in creatinine clearance was found to be much steeper in blacks than in whites (27). In the setting of hypertension or diabetes mellitus, the decline in renal function is further magnified (28,29). An increased baseline renal vascular resistance and, possibly, a lower glomerular filtration surface area, fewer nephrons, or both, may underlie the accelerated decline in creatinine clearance noted in blacks (30). These factors may also account for the decrease in renal allograft survival noted when grafts are obtained from black or elderly donors (30,31). These data suggest that the age-related loss of glomerular function is not a universal phenomenon, and that racial, dietary, metabolic, hormonal, or hemodynamic factors may play a major role in modulating the age-related decrease in renal function.

The highly significant decrease in GFR that occurs with age is not usually accompanied with an elevation in serum creatinine concentration (24,25). Since muscle mass, from which creatinine is derived, falls with age at approximately the same rate as that of GFR, the rather striking age-related loss of renal function is not reflected by an increase in the serum creatinine concentration. Thus, the serum creatinine concentration usually underestimates the decline in GFR in the elderly.

The most important clinical implication for the age-

Table 47.2. Formulas Commonly Used to Estimate Glomerular Filtration Rate*

1. Creatinine clearance (mL/min/1.73 m²) = 133 − (0.64 × age)
2. Creatinine clearance (mL/min)

$$= \frac{(140 - age) \times weight (kg)}{72 \times serum\ creatinine\ (mg/dL)}$$

*Results are 15 percent less in females.

related decrease in GFR is the need for adjustment of the dosage of medications that are either directly excreted by the kidneys, by glomerular filtration, or by tubular secretion, or whose active metabolites, formed in the liver, are eliminated by the kidneys. When adjusting the dosage of such a medication, it is therefore very important to estimate GFR not only according to serum creatinine, but to measure or estimate it according to one of the formulas provided in Table 47.2. Either of these two formulas yields a reasonable estimation of the GFR. In fact, there is a very close correlation ($r = 0.85$) between calculated (formula 2) and measured creatinine clearance (32–34). In addition, it is also useful to monitor the serum levels of drugs that have a narrow therapeutic-to-toxic ratio.

Another important consequence of the age-related decrease in renal blood flow and GFR is potential predisposition to enhanced ischemic or toxic renal injury. An increase in baseline renal vascular resistance may explain why elderly patients are at high risk for acute cyclosporine nephrotoxicity (35). In addition to the absolute decrease in renal blood flow, the autoregulatory capacity of the renal vasculature is also impaired, which thus increases the risk of hemodynamically induced acute renal failure after severe volume depletion, septic shock, and major vascular surgery. Failure to properly adjust the dosage of renally excreted drugs, such as aminoglycoside antibiotics, nonsteroidal anti-inflammatory drugs (NSAIDs), and radiocontrast agents, may also increase the incidence of toxin-induced renal failure.

Fluid and Electrolyte Balance

Under normal circumstances, age has no effect on plasma sodium or potassium concentrations, on blood pH, or on the ability of the kidneys to maintain normal extracellular fluid volume. The adaptive reserve mechanisms

responsible for maintaining constancy of the extracellular fluid volume and composition in response to stress are, however, impaired in the elderly.

Sodium Conserving Ability

The ability of aged kidneys to conserve sodium in response to sodium deprivation is impaired (36) (Figure 47.3). Clearance studies in young and elderly subjects

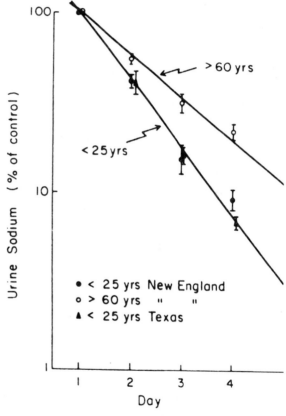

Fig. 47.3. Response of urinary sodium excretion to restriction of sodium intake in normal man. The mean halftime ($t_{1/2}$) for eight subjects older than 60 years of age was −30.9 ± 2.8 hours, exceeding the mean halftime of −17.6 ± 0.7 hours for subjects younger than 25 years of age ($p < 0.01$). When the subjects younger than 25 years of age were separated according to geographic area, the mean halftime for the Texas group (−17.9 ± 0.7) was similar to that of the New England group (−15.6 ± 1.4; $p < 0.3$). (Reproduced by permission from Epstein M, Hollenberg N. Age as a determinant of renal sodium conservation in normal man. J Lab Clin Med 1976;87:411–417.)

have shown a decreased distal tubular capacity for sodium reabsorption in the elderly (37). The distal tubular dysfunction could be caused by anatomic changes in aging kidneys, such as interstitial fibrosis. Alternatively, functional and hormonal changes, such as increased medullary blood flow or decreased renin-angiotensin-aldosterone activity, could also impair distal tubular reabsorption of sodium.

In this regard, there are important age-related alterations in the renin-angiotensin-aldosterone system. Basal plasma renin concentration or activity is decreased by 30 percent to 50 percent in elderly subjects, in spite of normal levels of renin substrate (38). During maneuvers designed to stimulate renin secretion (e.g., upright posture, 10 mEq/day sodium intake, and furosemide administration), the differences in plasma renin activity were further amplified (39–44) (Figure 47.4A). Although the precise mechanism is unknown, the age-related decrease in plasma renin activity has been attributed to 1) impaired renin secretion; 2) disturbances in the conversion of inactive to active renin; and 3) an enhanced tonic inhibitory effect of atrial natriuretic hormone on renin secretion. There is a similar 30 percent to 50 percent decrease in plasma aldosterone levels in elderly subjects during recumbency and normal sodium intake, which becomes more pronounced during upright posture, sodium restriction, and furosemide administration (40,44–47) (Figure 47.4B). The aldosterone deficiency appears to be related to the renin-angiotensin deficiency and not to intrinsic adrenal gland defects because both plasma aldosterone and cortisol responses to corticotropin (ACTH) infusion are normal in the elderly (44).

Thus, during sodium restriction, impaired angiotensin II, aldosterone response, or both may result in decreased renal tubular reabsorption in the elderly. In fact, clearance studies in young and elderly subjects have shown marked improvement in distal tubular sodium reabsorption in the elderly after treatment with aldosterone (48).

Sodium Excreting Ability

Excessive sodium retention and volume overload are commonly encountered problems in older patients. Short-term sodium loading studies (intravenous saline) show distinct, age-related differences in sodium excretion. Individuals older than 40 years of age excrete slightly less sodium per 24 hours after a 2-liter, normal saline load

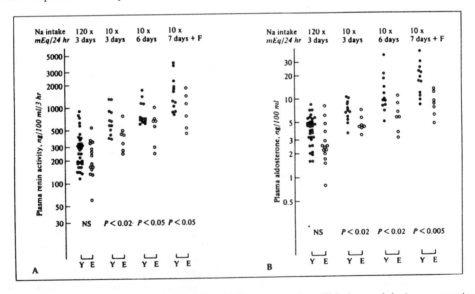

Fig. 47.4. Distribution of individual supine plasma renin (*A*) and aldosterone values (*B*) before and during progressive sodium depletion in young and elderly healthy subjects. Values indicating statistical significance refer to difference between young and elderly subjects. Plasma renin activity values are those obtained at incubation pH 5.7. Y, young subjects; E, elderly subjects. (Reproduced by permission from Weidmann P, De Myttenaere-Bursztein S, Maxwell M, De Lima J. Effect of aging on plasma renin and aldosterone in normal man. Kidney Int 1975;8:325–333.)

than do race-, sex-, and size-matched subjects younger than age 40 (27,48,49). In addition, the older subjects excrete a significantly greater portion of the sodium load at night than do their younger counterparts. Thus, both the excretory capacity for sodium and the circadian variation in excretion are influenced by age.

The age-related decrease in GFR is probably the major factor which limits the ability of aged kidneys to excrete an acute sodium load. Less well-studied are the roles of altered dopamine receptor activity and decreased renal sensitivity to circulating atrial natriuretic hormone in mediating the blunted natriuretic response (50–52).

Renal Concentrating Ability

Renal concentrating ability is well known to decline with age in humans (23,53,54). In one study, the concentrating ability of the kidneys, as measured by the urinary specific gravity, declined from 1.030 in 38 healthy men 40 years of age to 1.023 in men 89 years of age (23). In other studies, the maximal urine osmolality, measured after 12 to 24 hours of dehydration, was inversely related to age (53,54). The maximal urine osmolality was 1109 mOsm/kg in 31 subjects aged 20 to 39 years, compared with 1051 mOsm/kg in 48 subjects aged 40 to 59 years, and 882 mOsm/kg in 18 subjects aged 60 to 79 years. The age-related decline in the concentrating defect did not correlate with the age-related decline in GFR.

Studies in humans suggest that the concentrating defect is caused by an intrarenal defect rather than a failure in the osmotic release of arginine vasopressin (AVP) (55,56). After intravenous infusion of hypertonic saline (3% NaCl) in nine young (21–49 years of age) and three old (54–92 years of age) subjects, plasma AVP levels rose 4.5 times the baseline in the older men compared with 2.5 times the baseline in the younger group, despite similar free water clearances (55). The slope of the plasma AVP concentration (% baseline) compared with the serum osmolality, an index of the sensitivity of the osmoreceptor, was significantly increased in the older subjects. In addition, in the same study, intravenous infusion of ethanol caused a progressive decline in plasma AVP levels in the young subjects, but failed to have a similar effect in the older subjects. Plasma AVP levels have also been found to increase to a greater extent in elderly subjects as compared

with levels in younger controls in response to 24 hours of fluid restriction (57–58).

Evidence for an intrarenal defect comes from human studies demonstrating an age-related increase in solute excretion and osmolar clearance during dehydration (54). This phenomenon, which may be a reflection of an impaired solute transport by the ascending loop of Henle, may be responsible for the impairment in urine concentrating ability in elderly subjects. This possibility is supported by studies of clearance in water-diuresing subjects. The studies demonstrated a decrease in the sodium chloride transport in the ascending loop of Henle in elderly subjects (37,59). The defect in solute transport by the thick, ascending limb of Henle's loop could diminish inner medullary hypertonicity and thereby impair urinary concentrating ability. A relative increase in medullary blood flow, as suggested by the xenon washout studies (21), could also increase the removal of solutes from the medullary interstitium and thereby contribute to the decreased maximal urinary osmolality. Finally, a blunted responsiveness of the collecting duct to the hydroosmotic effect of AVP may also contribute to the impaired ability of the kidneys to maximally concentrate urine (60).

Age-related impairments in renal concentration and sodium conserving ability are associated with an increased incidence of volume depletion and hypernatremia in the elderly. Under normal physiologic conditions, increased thirst and fluid intake are natural defense mechanisms against volume depletion and hypernatremia. Elderly patients are particularly prone to develop hypernatremia because of an age-related impairment in the thirst mechanism (57,61). In comparison with young controls (aged 20–31 years), elderly patients (aged 67–75 years), after 24 hours of fluid restriction, have been shown to have a blunted sensation of thirst and mouth dryness, despite a higher serum sodium concentration and osmolality (57) (Figure 47.5). In addition, the hypertonic elderly subjects ingested less water after the period of fluid restriction in comparison with the young controls. Thus, an age-related impairment in the thirst mechanism renders the elderly patient particularly prone to the development of hypernatremia.

In practice, drugs that inhibit the thirst mechanism and the synthesis and release of AVP, including most of the sedatives and major tranquilizers, and drugs that inhibit

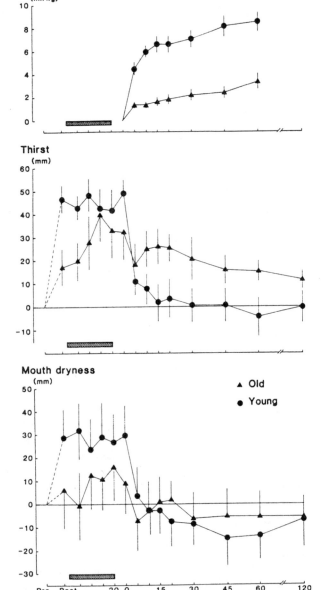

Fig. 47.5. Cumulative water intake, changes in thirst, and mouth dryness in old and young groups. Changes in thirst and mouth dryness were measured on a visual-analogue rating scale. (Reproduced by permission of the New England Journal of Medicine, from Phillips P, Phil D, Rolls B, et al. Reduced thirst after water deprivation in healthy elderly men. N Engl J Med 1984;311:753–759.)

the renal tubular action of AVP, especially lithium and demeclocycline, are best avoided (Table 47.3). The use of osmotic diuretics, enteral feeding containing high protein and glucose, and bowel cathartics should also be carefully monitored in the elderly. In addition, the complication of age-related decreases in thirst by systemic illness and dementia in many frail, elderly patients clearly places them at risk for the development of severe water deficiency.

The incidence of severe hypernatremia among the elderly exceeds one case per hospital per month (62). Hypernatremia in the elderly without underlying central nervous system disease may present with primary neurologic or psychiatric symptoms and delay the diagnosis. In subjects who are febrile and who have underlying neurologic disorders, AVP release may become impaired and thereby exacerbate the tendency toward hypernatremia (63,64). If not promptly diagnosed and treated, hypernatremia leads to coma, seizures, and death (65). In fact, in adults, acute elevation of serum sodium above 160 mEq per liter is associated with 75 percent mortality. Even in the absence of death, the neurologic sequelae can be severe in the elderly.

Renal Diluting Ability

Renal diluting ability is impaired as a function of aging (51,52,66,67). In water-diuresing subjects, minimal urine osmolality is significantly higher, 92 mOsm/kg in older

Table 47.3. Mechanism by Which Drugs Can Lead to Impaired Water Metabolism

Inhibit ADH Release	Inhibit Peripheral Action of ADH	Potentiate ADH Release	Potentiate Peripheral Action of ADH
Fluphenazine	Lithium	Nicotine	Tolbutamide
Haloperidol	Colchicine	Vincristine	Chlorpropamide
Promethazine	Vinblastine	Histamine	NSAIDs
Morphine (low doses)	Demeclocycline	Morphine (high doses)	
Alcohol	Glyburide	Epinephrine	
Carbamazepine	Methoxyflurane	Cyclophosphamide	
Norepinephrine	Acetohexamide	Angiotensin	
Cisplatinum	Propoxyphene	Bradykinin	
Clonidine	Loop diuretics	Clofibrate	
Glucocorticoids			

ADH = antidiuretic hormone; NSAIDs = nonsteroidal anti-inflammatory drugs.

subjects (ages 77–88) and 52 mOsm/kg in young subjects (ages 17–40). The solute-free water clearance (CH_2O) is also decreased: 5.9 mL/min in older subjects and 16.2 mL/min in young subjects. The impairment in CH_2O is mainly the result of the decrease in GFR. When CH_2O is factored for GFR, CH_2O/GFR is still decreased in the older subjects (52,67). Mechanisms of the impaired diluting ability of the kidneys in the elderly have not been well studied; in addition to the major role of impaired GFR, inadequate suppression of AVP release, or impaired solute transport in the ascending loop of Henle may also play a role.

The age-related impairment in maximal diluting ability and the enhanced osmotic release of AVP are associated with a high incidence of hyponatremia in the elderly. A random sampling of 160 patients in a chronic disease facility showed that 36 patients had hyponatremia, with a mean serum sodium of 120 mEq/liter, and 27 of these patients were symptomatic (68). In another study, a survey of hospitalized patients in a geriatric unit during a 10-month period revealed that 77 patients (11%) had plasma sodium concentration below 130 mEq/liter (69). Diuretics, especially the combination of hydrochlorothiazide and amiloride, and hypotonic intravenous fluid administration were determined to cause the hyponatremia in 56 of these patients. Forty-seven of the patients were symptomatic, and the mortality rate for the hyponatremic patients was twice the overall rate for the geriatric unit. Other reports also confirm that thiazide diuretics are a major cause of hyponatremia in the elderly (70). The well-known effect of thiazide diuretics to impair renal diluting ability under normal physiologic conditions seems to be compounded in the elderly who have a preexisting renal diluting defect (71). In addition, thiazide diuretics used in combination with the sulfonylurea chlorpropamide, which is known to potentiate the peripheral action of vasopressin, have synergistic effects in impairing renal diluting ability (72). In practice, drugs or agents that stimulate the nonosmotic release of AVP or drugs that potentiate the renal tubular action of AVP must be used with extreme caution in the elderly (73,74) (Table 47.3).

The symptoms of hyponatremia are most likely related to cellular swelling and cerebral edema caused by the water movement as a result of the lowering of extracellular fluid (ECF) osmolality. Patients may present with symptoms of lethargy, apathy, disorientation, muscle cramps, anorexia, nausea, or agitation, and with signs ranging from depressed deep tendon reflexes to pseudobulbar palsy and seizures. Differentiation of these symptoms from primary neurologic or psychiatric disease is important so that one can promptly institute appropriate therapy and avoid severe neurologic sequelae, such as central pontine myelinolysis.

Acid-Base Balance

Elderly subjects can maintain the pH and bicarbonate of blood within the normal range, and their basal acid excretion is not different from that of healthy younger volunteers (75). But when senescent kidneys are challenged with an acute acid load, they do not increase their acid excretion to the same degree as kidneys of young volunteers (76). In an earlier study, after a standard oral ammonium chloride acid load, older subjects (72–93 years) excreted only 19 percent of the acid load compared with 35 percent by the younger subjects (17–35 years) during an 8-hour period. Urinary ammonia accounted for less of the total acid excretion in the old subjects: 59 percent in the old subjects and 72 percent in the young subjects. In this study, the decrease in both these parameters was paralleled by a nearly equal drop in inulin clearance; thus, acid excretion per unit GFR was almost identical for both young and old subjects, which suggests that the decrease in acid excretion found in advancing age is caused by a decreased renal tubular mass rather than by a specific tubular defect (77).

A more recent study of elderly subjects with less impaired GFR, however, arrived at a different conclusion. In this study, the minimal urinary pH and net acid excretion, even when factored for GFR, were significantly decreased in the older subjects. There were no differences in the titratable acid excretion, but the older subjects showed a significant reduction in ammonium excretion even when it was factored for GFR: 34 mol/min in the elderly and 51 mol/min in the young subjects (76). Furthermore, a significant inverse correlation was found between the urinary pH and log ammonium excretion in young subjects, but the correlation was not significant in the elderly. However, for any given urinary pH, ammonium excretion in the elderly was less than that of younger subjects. The ammonium excretion depended on age rather than on pH of the urine. This study therefore suggests an intrinsic tubular defect in ammonium excretion as a function of aging. It is not known whether this defect is caused by anatomic changes or a result of functional defects, including the impairment in the renin-angiotensin-aldosterone axis that is frequently encountered in the aged.

Potassium Balance

Studies of the effects in humans of aging on renal and extrarenal adaptation to high potassium loads or dietary potassium deprivation are lacking. Two studies, however, have found that both total body potassium (78) and total exchangeable potassium (79) decrease with age in both sexes and that the decrease is more marked in women than in men. This decrease may relate to the decrease in muscle mass that occurs with advancing age. In response to exercise, the rate of increase in plasma potassium is higher in elderly subjects than it is in young subjects (80). The study also suggests that an age-related impairment may exist in the beta$_2$-adrenergic process that mediates potassium flux into skeletal muscle.

The presence of a renal acidification defect, and a decreased activity of the renin-angiotensin-aldosterone system may be the cause of the increased incidence of type 4 renal tubular acidosis (RTA), the syndrome of hyporeninemic hypoaldosteronism in the elderly. In fact, in a large clinical series, the mean age of the patients was 65 years (81). In addition, the elderly are also at increased risk for developing hyperkalemia from potassium-sparing diuretics, such as triamterene, aldactone, and amiloride and from drugs that inhibit the renin-angiotensin-aldosterone system, especially NSAIDs, beta blockers, converting enzyme inhibitors, heparin, and cyclosporine (Table 47.4).

Clinical Renal Diseases in the Aged

Renal Vascular Disorders

A major cause of vascular disease of the kidneys and renal insufficiency in the elderly is atheromatous renal disease. Atheromatous renal disease may present as 1) renal artery stenosis; 2) complex intrarenal lesions, with multiple stenoses of intrarenal vasculature; and 3) cholesterol embolism. In a recent report of 32 patients with various

Table 47.4. Drugs That May Predispose to Hyperkalemia

Potassium-sparing diuretics
Spironolactone
Triamterene
Amiloride
Beta blockers
Prostaglandin synthesis inhibitors
Converting enzyme inhibitors
Other
Heparin
Ketoconazole
Cyclosporine

forms of renal failure in patients with widespread atheroma, 22 patients had atheromatous stenosis of the renal arteries, 8 patients had renal artery lesions that coexisted with cholesterol emboli, and the remaining 2 patients had renal failure caused by cholesterol emboli alone (82). The natural history of atheromatous renal disease is progressive occlusion of the major renal arteries. In support, a recent review of 237 patients disclosed angiographic progression of renovascular disease in nearly 50 percent of patients (83). Most of these patients, if left untreated, develop progressive renal failure. In this regard, a prospective survey, conducted for 18 months, found that atheromatous renal disease was responsible for renal failure in 14 percent of patients older than 50 years of age who presented with end-stage renal disease (ESRD) (84). Thus, atheromatous renal disease may be an important cause of renal insufficiency in elderly patients who have generalized atherosclerosis and unexplained ESRD.

Because of the unique, intrarenal hemodynamic effects of angiotensin II, treatment of hypertension in patients with atheromatous renal disease by use of converting enzyme inhibitors may often result in a significant reduction in GFR (85). The diagnosis of renal artery stenosis should therefore be strongly considered for an elderly patient who presents with hypertension and renal failure. In accurately diagnosed patients, timely intervention, when technically possible, either in the form of percutaneous transluminal angioplasty or surgical revascularization, may result in significant improvement of the hypertension and may prevent further renal functional deterioration (83,86–88).

The most frequent triggering causes of cholesterol embolism are aortic surgery or abdominal, coronary, or carotid angiography (especially when performed via the femoral approach), and excess anticoagulation. This syndrome has also been reported to occur in patients with myocardial infarction for which thrombolytic therapy has been administered (89). Cholesterol embolism may also occur spontaneously (90). Patients may present with a combination of symptoms, such as purple discoloration of toes, which may progress to lower extremity focal digital necrosis, livedo reticularis of the abdominal or lumbar wall, gastrointestinal bleeding, pancreatitis, myocardial infarction, retinal ischemia, cerebral infarction, hypertension, and uremia (91). Cholesterol embolism may be associated with fever, increased erythrocyte sedimentation rate, eosinophilia, and hematuria without casts (92). Major differential diagnoses include contrast-induced acute renal failure, polyarteritis nodosa, allergic vasculitis, left atrial myxoma, and subacute bacterial endocarditis.

Episodic and labile hypertension caused by renal artery emboli is a common consequence of renal cholesterol emboli. Furthermore, there is a progressive decline in GFR within 1 to 4 weeks. This time course differentiates cholesterol emboli-induced acute renal failure from radiocontrast-induced acute renal failure, which usually occurs within 1 to 4 days after the angiographic procedure. The diagnosis of renal cholesterol emboli requires a high degree of suspicion and aggressive diagnostic workup. In addition to a careful funduscopic examination and skin and muscle biopsy, definitive diagnosis may require renal biopsy. Unfortunately, to date, no treatment modality has proved to be effective in reversing the disease process. At the present time, the recommendations are to avoid, if possible, excessive anticoagulation and invasive angiographic procedures in elderly patients with widespread atheromatous vascular disease, and when renal failure progresses, to provide supportive therapy, including dialysis.

Acute Glomerulonephritis

The most prevalent form of acute glomerulonephritis in the elderly is rapidly progressive glomerulonephritis. This is a clinical syndrome that describes the progressive loss of renal function during a period of weeks to months. The most common histologic lesion associated with this syndrome is the finding of glomerular crescents. An immunopathologic classification of rapidly progressive glomerulonephritis is given in Table 47.5. Approximately 20 percent of cases are mediated by antiglomerular basement antibodies and result in a linear staining of the glomerular basement membrane on immunofluorescent studies (type 1) (93). Forty percent of cases are thought to be immune complex-mediated and typically show a "lump-bumpy" pattern by immunofluorescence (type 2). The third major category, accounting for approximately 40 percent of cases, is characterized by the absence of immune deposits on immunofluorescent studies (type 3). The patients are often found to have circulating antineutrophil cytoplasmic antibodies (ANCA) (94).

Histologic studies of elderly patients with rapidly progressive glomerulonephritis have most commonly shown a type 2 or type 3 pattern (95). In a renal biopsy series of 115 patients aged 60 years and older who presented with glomerulonephritis, the nephrotic syndrome, or both, 19 patients were found to have idiopathic crescentic glomerulonephritis (96). In this series, antiglomerular basement membrane antibodies were detected in only 1 of 11 patients whose serum was checked. Linear deposition of immunoglobulin G (IgG) in the glomerular capillaries was observed only in two patients. Although granular deposits of IgG were observed in nine patients,

Table 47.5. Immunopathologic Classification of Crescentic Glomerulonephritis*

Type 1—Circulating antiglomerular basement antibody
  Without lung hemorrhage
  With lung hemorrhage (Goodpasteur's syndrome)

Type 2—Granular immune deposits
  Limited renal disease (IgA nephritis, membranoproliferative glomerulonephritis)
  Postinfectious disease (poststreptococcal, abscess, endocarditis)
  Systemic disease (systemic lupus erythematosus, cryoglobulinemia)

Type 3—No immune deposits (often associated with circulating antineutrophil cytoplasmic antibodies)
  Idiopathic glomerulonephritis
  Vasculitis
  Wegener's granulomatosis
  Microscopic polyarteritis nodosa

---

*Rapidly progressive glomerulonephritis is a clinical syndrome often associated with the histologic finding of glomerular crescents.

six other patients had no deposit disease. More recently, 8 of 10 patients older than age 65 who presented with rapidly progressive glomerulonephritis were found to have no immune deposits on immunofluorescent studies (97). Most of these patients tested positive for circulating ANCA. Similarly, 40 patients selected purely on the basis of renal histology that demonstrated findings of type 3 necrotizing crescentic glomerulonephritis were found to have an average age of 62 years (98). Circulating ANCA was present in most of these patients. Interestingly, extrarenal symptoms suggestive of vasculitis were commonly observed in these patients. In general, the prognosis for elderly patients with crescentic glomerulonephritis is poor. Use of pulse steroids, cyclophosphamide, plasmapheresis, or combinations of these therapies has been shown to be effective in small series of elderly patients (93,95,98). Because the side effects of these agents are increased in the elderly, careful consideration of the risk-benefit ratio must be undertaken for the individual patient.

Another prevalent form of acute glomerulonephritis in the elderly is diffuse proliferative glomerulonephritis, which commonly occurs in association with infection, especially poststreptococcal glomerulonephritis that is associated with streptococcal infections of the throat and the skin (99–101). Clinical features of poststreptococcal glomerulonephritis in the elderly are hypertension in 82 percent of patients, edema in 73 percent of patients, dyspnea and evidence of circulatory congestion in 41 percent of patients, and oliguria in 75 percent of patients. Although hypertension and edema are as frequently encountered in pediatric and young adult patients, circulatory congestion and renal insufficiency are most frequently encountered in the elderly, perhaps as a result of the age-related impairments in cardiopulmonary and renal reserve and function. Poststreptococcal glomerulonephritis may also present as crescentic glomerulonephritis and result in acute renal failure (see Table 47.5). Because of the overall favorable prognosis, maximal effort should be made for prompt diagnosis and appropriate therapy, including dialysis if indicated.

Nephrotic Syndrome

Nephrotic syndrome is a commonly diagnosed renal disease in the elderly. Review of nine international research studies, including those from the U.S., Japan, France, England, and Israel, that evaluated a total of 275 patients aged 60 years or older, revealed that the most common histopathologic lesions are membranous glomerulonephritis (123 patients, 45%), minimal change disease (52 patients, 19%), mesangial proliferative glomerulonephritis (32 patients, 12%), and membranoproliferative glomerulonephritis (32 patients, 12%) (102–110) (Table 47.6). Similar findings were reported in the Medical Research Council's glomerulonephritis registry consisting of 317 patients older than 60 years of age who presented with the nephrotic syndrome (111). The most frequent histologic findings were membranous nephropathy (36.6%) and minimal change disease (11.0%). Renal amyloidosis was found in 10.7 percent of patients. Other common causes of nephrotic syndrome in the elderly are diabetes mellitus and glomerulosclerosis.

In approximately 10 percent of elderly patients with the nephrotic syndrome, renal histopathology indicates glomerulosclerosis (see Table 47.6). This entity resembles the separate, well-known entity of focal segmental glomerulosclerosis, which is a common cause of the nephrotic syndrome in the younger patient population. Focal segmental (global) glomerulosclerosis especially affects the juxtamedullary glomeruli; immunofluorescence generally reveals granular deposits of immunoglobulin M (IgM) and serum protein C3. Although focal segmental glomerulosclerosis usually occurs as a separate and distinct entity, it may also occur as the end result of various other glomerulopathies or systemic diseases such as diabetes and hypertension. Hyperfiltration of the functioning glomeruli has been proposed to play an important role in the process of glomerulosclerosis (112,113). This process may be especially important for the juxtamedullary glomeruli because they have a significantly higher filtration fraction than do the superficial cortical glomeruli.

Renal biopsy is essential in establishing the correct histopathology because most often it is not possible to predict the histopathology solely from clinical data (114,115). Furthermore, in several of these series, elderly patients with minimal change disease responded to corticosteroid therapy, and complete remission was obtained without relapse. In addition, complete remission

Table 47.6. Histologic Lesions in 275 Elderly Patients with the Nephrotic Syndrome

Text Reference	Minimal Change	Membranous GN	Mesangial Proliferative GN	Membrano-proliferative GN	Glomerulo-sclerosis	Chronic GN
103	6	5	–	4	16	5
104	4	2	–	6	–	–
96	9	15	7	2	1	–
105	1	6	–	2	7	–
107	2	16	–	2	3	–
110	19	31	2	4	–	3
106	2	16	11	3	–	–
108	2	2	–	2	–	–
109	7	30	12	7	1	–
Total	52 (19%)	123 (45%)	32 (12%)	32 (12%)	28 (10%)	8 (3%)

GN = glomerulonephritis.

or partial remission was achieved in 50 percent to 70 percent of patients with membranous glomerulonephritis who were treated with corticosteroids and immuno-suppressants. On the other hand, the outcome of treatment of proliferative glomerulonephritis was highly variable. Thus, given the relatively high incidence of minimal change disease (19% of the nephrotic syndrome in the elderly), and the highly favorable response to therapy, it is recommended that the elderly patient with the nephrotic syndrome undergo a thorough workup that includes renal biopsy to establish the histopathology.

There is a known association between the presence of nephrotic syndrome and malignancy (116). The most common glomerular pathology in patients with malignancy is membranous glomerulopathy. In patients who present with the nephrotic syndrome, an associated malignancy has been reported in 7 percent to 20 percent of patients (110,117). The most common underlying tumors are cancer of the lung, colon, rectum, kidney, breast, and stomach. As a result, elderly patients with nephrotic syndrome should be screened for an underlying malignancy.

Renal Cysts

Simply renal cysts are commonly found in the aging adult population. More than 50 percent of people older than 50 years of age have at least one renal cyst on postmortem examination (118). Simple renal cysts are quite uncommon in children and are thus regarded as an acquired abnormality that is related to age.

With increased use of sonography and CT imaging of the abdomen, renal cysts are being recognized more frequently. In a recent sonographic study of 729 patients referred for reasons unrelated to the urinary tract, the prevalence of at least one renal cyst was found to progressively increase from 0 percent in those aged 15–29 years to 22.1 percent in the those aged 70 years and older (119). These findings confirmed earlier observations of an age-related increase in the development of simple renal cysts (120) (Figure 47.6). Simple cysts are usually unilocular, often cortical with some distortion of the renal contour, and increase in number with increasing age (121). Symptoms ascribed to renal cysts include abdominal or lumbar pain, hematuria, secondary infection, and renin-dependent hypertension. In most cases, however, simple cysts are asymptomatic and are discovered incidentally.

The major issue in the incidental discovery of a renal cyst is the differentiation between simple cyst and malignant mass. Sonographic criteria for a simple cyst are listed in Figure 47.7. If all three criteria are strictly satisfied, the cyst can be regarded as nonmalignant with virtually 100 percent accuracy (122). If the mass fails to satisfy these criteria, CT scanning is the next logical step. Strict criteria to identify simple cysts have also been established for this procedure, and if all CT diagnostic criteria are met, the cyst can be regarded as simple and no further evaluation is warranted (123). If the CT findings are intermediate, additional workup consisting of cyst puncture and aspiration for cytology is indicated. In selected patients,

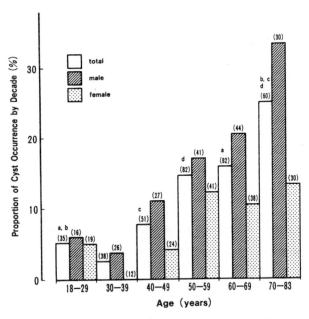

Fig. 47.6. Proportion of subjects with simple renal cysts by age decade. The number of subjects in each column is indicated in parentheses. Statistical analysis was performed between white columns (total of males and females): a versus a ($p < 0.05$), b versus b ($p < 0.01$), c versus c ($p < 0.25$), and d versus d ($p < 0.05$). (Reproduced by permission from Yamagishi F, Kitahara N, Mogi W, Itoh S. Age-related occurrence of simple cysts studied by ultrasonography. Klin Wochenschr 1988;66:385–387.)

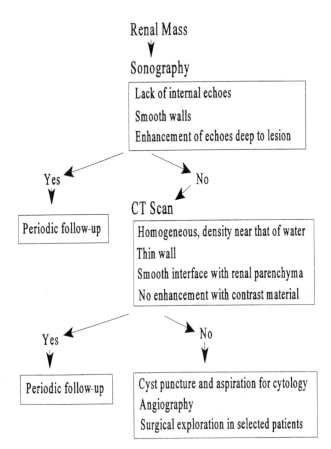

Fig. 47.7. Suggested workup of an asymptomatic renal cyst.

angiography or direct surgical exploration is required to fully exclude a malignant process.

Acute Renal Failure

A major cause of acute renal failure in the elderly is prerenal failure, i.e., decreased perfusion of the kidneys, which leads to a functional and potentially reversible type of acute renal failure. In addition to the age-related decreases in baseline renal blood flow and glomerular filtration rate, there is also evidence for age-related impairments in autoregulation of renal blood flow and renal functional reserve, which may render the aging kidneys more susceptible to prerenal failure. Even a modest contraction of blood volume induced by oral administration of a 120-mg dose of furosemide results in a larger decrease in GFR in subjects older than 40 years of age than that found in younger subjects (27).

In the elderly, a decrease in cardiac output secondary to an acute myocardial infarction or to congestive heart failure; a marked decrease in systemic vascular resistance secondary to sepsis; gastrointestinal losses caused by severe vomiting, diarrhea, bleeding, or third spacing; renal losses secondary to glycosuria or excessive use of diuretics; renal atheromatous disease; or use of converting enzyme inhibitors in the presence of bilateral renal artery stenosis can readily precipitate prerenal failure, which if not promptly recognized and reversed, may result in acute tubular necrosis. In fact, in several clinical series of acute renal failure in the elderly, the most frequently recognized cause of acute renal failure was hypovolemic or ischemic acute renal failure or both (124–128).

Complications of major surgery account for about 30 percent of cases of acute renal failure in the elderly. Hypotension during or after surgery, postoperative fluid loss from gastrointestinal or fistulous drainage, arrhythmias, and myocardial infarction are common postoperative complications in the elderly that may result in acute renal failure. Infection and especially gram-negative septicemia account for another 30 percent of cases of acute renal failure in the elderly. Gram-negative infections are frequently associated with endotoxin-induced renovascular vasoconstriction, which, in the susceptible individual, may result in acute tubular necrosis. In addition, most antibiotics used to treat serious infections, especially aminoglycoside antibiotics, are associated with a high incidence of acute tubular necrosis in the elderly. Age is a well-known risk factor for developing aminoglycoside nephrotoxicity (129). The reasons include possible overdosage as a result of inaccurate estimation of the GFR solely on the basis of serum creatinine concentration and age-related renal tubular functional and biochemical alterations (130), which may enhance the renal tubular toxic effects of aminoglycoside antibiotics.

Another major cause of acute renal failure in the elderly is use of NSAIDs (131–133). This is of special concern because several NSAIDs are now available as an over-the-counter medication. Inhibition of renal vasodilatory prostaglandin synthesis caused by NSAIDs can potentiate the renal vasoconstrictive effects of renal nerves, the alpha-adrenergic system, angiotensin II, and vasopressin (134). In the presence of an already reduced renal blood flow, acute renal failure may result in the elderly patient. This may be especially relevant in the hypertensive elderly subjects who have been found to have a significant reduction in urinary prostaglandin E_2 secretion (135). The elderly are also at increased risk for developing acute renal failure during converting enzyme inhibition therapy for left ventricular dysfunction or hypertension. This usually occurs in the presence of bilateral renal artery stenosis, or unilateral renal artery stenosis in the presence of a nonfunctioning or poorly functioning contralateral kidney. In view of increased recognition of atheromatous renal vascular disease in the elderly (82), elderly patients who are treated with any converting enzyme inhibitor need frequent determinations of GFR. The elderly are also at increased risk for radiocontrast-induced renal failure (90). The mechanisms of radiocontrast-induced renal injury are not completely understood, but include hemodynamic effects and direct tubular toxic effects that,

because of preexistent renal defects, may predispose the elderly to enhanced renal toxicity.

Another important cause of acute renal failure in the elderly is urinary tract obstruction, most frequently secondary to an enlarged prostate (136). Symptoms of prostatism, such as urinary frequency, difficulty in starting or stopping micturition, and nocturia, may not be apparent. A significant number of patients may therefore present with symptoms of ESRD rather than with prostatism. In addition, in clinically significant prostatism, residual urine is often infected, which may potentiate impairments in tubular function and reduction in renal blood flow and the GFR caused by the obstruction.

Most elderly patients respond well to treatment of acute renal failure with dialysis (126,128,137). Although the chances for survival or for recovery of renal function in the elderly with acute renal failure would seem to be markedly decreased, recent studies have found the mortality rate (50%–60%), and the recovery of renal function (50%–60%) not markedly worse than that for all adult patients who develop acute renal failure (126,128,137). It is therefore recommended that hemodialysis or peritoneal dialysis be initiated promply to alleviate uremic symptoms and to prevent uremic complications such as infection, myocardial infarction, congestive heart failure, and bleeding, which are the major causes of mortality in the elderly patient with acute renal failure.

Chronic Renal Failure

Many forms of chronic renal failure are commonly seen in older patients because the renal disease is secondary to other age-dependent medical diseases. Atherosclerotic disease of the renal vasculature causing renovascular hypertension and renal ischemia; diabetes, hypertension, or chronic glomerulonephritis causing glomerulosclerosis; and prostatic hypertrophy causing hydronephrosis are the most common causes of chronic renal failure in the elderly.

The clinical presentation of chronic renal failure in the elderly is often quite different than that seen in the general adult patient population. The elderly often present with decompensation of preexistent medical conditions, such as congestive heart failure, hypertension, peptic ulcer disease, or dementia, rather than with specific symptoms of

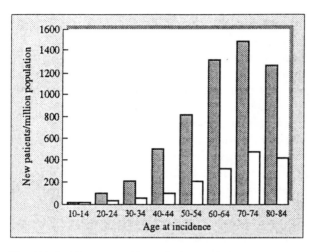

Fig. 47.8. Incidence per million population of ESRD by age and racial groups, 1987 to 1989 in the United States. (Adapted with permission from Nissenson A. Dialysis therapy in the elderly. Kidney Int 1993;43:S51–S57.)

uremia. In addition, the level of serum creatinine may underestimate actual renal reserve because, in the presence of decreased muscle mass, serum creatinine does not rise in direct proportion to the reduction in the GFR.

If the renal failure is advanced and no reversible causes can be identified, such as renal artery stenosis and urinary tract obstruction, early dialysis is advisable to prevent the disabling symptoms of uremia and organ dysfunction that may become irreversible. Age itself should not be the sole criterion to exclude dialysis. In fact, the number of elderly patients accepted for renal replacement therapy is increasing year by year (138) (Figure 47.8). In the absence of major extrarenal organ dysfunction, the elderly adjust to dialysis quite well, and their longevity rate, although not as favorable as that in younger patients, is not markedly reduced as a result of ESRD (139–141). In elderly patients who have cardiovascular disease and who may not tolerate hemodialysis, chronic ambulatory peritoneal dialysis (CAPD) has been successfully used (140–142). Age is also not an absolute contraindication for renal transplant; otherwise medically eligible elderly patients have undergone successful renal transplantation (143–144).

References

1. Tauchi H, Tsuboi K, Okutomi J. Age changes in the human kidney of the different races. Gerontologia 1971;17:87–97.
2. Dunnill MS, Halley W. Some observations on the quantitative anatomy of the kidney. J Pathol 1973;110:113–121.
3. McLachlan M, Guthrie J, Anderson C, Fulker M. Vascular and glomerular changes in the aging kidney. J Pathol 1977;121:65–78.
4. Moore RA. The total number of glomeruli in the normal human kidney. Anat Rec 1958;48:153–168.
5. Kaplan C, Pasternack B, Shah H, Gallo G. Age-related incidence of sclerotic glomeruli in human kidneys. Am J Pathol 1975;80:227–234.
6. Kappel B, Olsen S. Cortical interstitial tissue and sclerosed glomeruli in the normal human kidney, related to age and sex. A. Pathol Anat Histol 1980;387:271–277.
7. Sworn MJ, Path MRC, Fox M. Donor kidney selection for transplantation. Relationship between glomerular structure, vascular supply and age. Br J Urol 1972;44:377–383.
8. Moritz A, Oldt M. Arteriolar sclerosis in hypertensive and non-hypertensive individuals. Am J Pathol 1973;13:679–687.
9. Williams RH, Harrison TR. A study of the renal arteries in relation to age and to hypertension. Am Heart J 1937;14:645–658.
10. Yamaguchi T, Omae T, Katsuki S. Quantitative determination of renal vascular changes related to age and hypertension. Jpn Heart J 1969;10:248–258.
11. Takazakura E, Sawabu N, Handa A, et al. Intrarenal vascular changes with age and disease. Kidney Int 1972;2:224–230.
12. Ljungqvist A, Lagergren C. Normal intrarenal arterial pattern in adult and aging human kidney. A micro-angiographical and histological study. J Anat 1962;96:285–300.
13. Davies D, Shock N. Age changes in glomerular filtration rate, effective renal plasma flow, and tubular excretory capacity in adult males. J Clin Invest 1950;29:496–507.
14. McDonald R, Solomon D, Shock N. Aging as a factor in the renal hemodynamic changes induced by a standardized pyrogen. J Clin Invest 1951;30:457–462.
15. Brandfonbrener M, Landsdowne M, Shock NW. Changes in cardiac output with age. Circulation 1955;12:557–565.
16. Geokas MC, Lakatta E, Makinodan T, Timiras PS. The aging process. Ann Intern Med 1990;113:455–466.
17. Lammerant J, Veall N, DeVisscher M. Observations on cardiac output and "pulmonary blood volume" in normal man by internal recording of the intracardiac flows of ^{123}I-labelled albumin. Nucl Med 1961;1:353–359.
18. Strandell T. Circulatory studies on healthy old men. Acta Med Scand 1964;175:414–420.
19. Lee T, Lindeman R, Yiengst M, Shock N. Influence of age on the cardiovascular and renal responses to tilting. J Appl Physiol 1966;21:55–61.
20. Naeije R, Fiasse A, Carlier E, et al. Systemic and renal

haemodynamic effects of angiotensin converting enzyme inhibition by zabicipril in young and in old normal men. Eur J Clin Pharmacol 1993;44:35–39.

21. Hollenberg N, Adams D, Solomon H, et al. Senescence and the renal vasculature in normal man. Circ Res 1974;34:309–316.

22. Fliser D, Zeir M, Nowalk R, Ritz E. Renal functional reserve in healthy elderly subjects. J Am Soc Nephrol 1993;3:1371–1377.

23. Lewis W, Alving A. Changes with age in the renal function in adult men. Am J Physiol 1938;123:500–515.

24. Rowe J, Andres R, Tobin J, et al. The effect of age on creatinine clearance in men: a cross-sectional and longitudinal study. J Gerontol 1976;31:155–163.

25. Rowe J, Andres R, Tobin J, et al. Age-adjusted standards for creatinine clearance. Ann Intern Med 1976;84:567–569.

26. Lindeman R, Tobin J, Shock N. Longitudinal studies on the rate of decline in renal function with age. J Am Geriatr Soc 1985;33:278–285.

27. Luft F, Fineberg N, Miller J, et al. The effects of age, race, and heredity on glomerular filtration rate following volume expansion and contraction in normal man. Am J Med Sci 1980;279:15–24.

28. Retta T, Afre G, Randall O. Hypertensive renal disease in blacks. Transplant Proc 1993;25:2421–2422.

29. Cowie C. Diabetic renal disease: racial and ethnic differences from an epidemiologic perspective. Transplant Proc 1993;25:2426–2430.

30. Brenner B, Cohen R, Milford E. In renal transplantation, one size may not fit all. J Am Soc Nephrol 1993;3:162–169.

31. Kumar M, Stephan R, Chui J, et al. Effect of donor age on graft function and graft survival in cadaver renal transplantation. Transplant Proc 1993;25:2183–2184.

32. Luke DR, Halstenson CE, Opsahl JA, Matzke GR. Validity of creatinine clearance estimates in the assessment of renal function. Clin Pharmacol Ther 1990;48:503–508.

33. Gral T, Young M. Measured versus estimated creatinine clearance in the elderly as an index of renal function. J Am Geriatr Soc 1980;28:492–496.

34. Mcligeyo S. Calculation of creatinine clearance from plasma creatinine. East Afr Med J 1993;70:3–5.

35. Feutren G, Mihatsch M. Risk factors for cyclosporine nephropathy in patients with autoimmune diseases. N Engl J Med 1992;326:1654–1660.

36. Epstein M, Hollenberg N. Age as a determinant of renal sodium conservation in normal man. J Lab Clin Med 1976;87:411–417.

37. Macias Nunez J, Garcia Iglesias C, Bonda Roman A, et al. Renal handling of sodium in old people: a functional study. Age Ageing 1978;7:178–181.

38. Bauer J. Age-related changes in the renin-aldosterone system. Drugs Aging 1993;3:238–245.

39. Anderson GH, Springer J, Randall P, et al. Effect of age on diagnostic usefulness of stimulated plasma renin activity and saralasin test in detection of renovascular hypertension. Lancet 1980;2:821–824.

40. Crane M, Harris J. Effect of aging on renin activity and aldosterone excretion. J Lab Clin Med 1976;87:947.

41. Cugini P, Murano G, Lucia P, et al. The gerontological decline of the renin-aldosterone system: a chronobiological approach extended to essential hypertension. J Gerontol 1987;42:461–465.

42. Hall J, Coleman T, Guyton A. The renin-angiotensin system: normal physiology and changes in older hypertensives. J Am Geriatr Soc 1989;37:801–813.

43. Tsunoda K, Abe K, Goto T, et al. Effect of age on the renin-angiotensin-aldosterone system in normal subjects: simultaneous measurement of active and inactive renin, renin substrate, and aldosterone in plasma J Clin Endocrinol Metab 1986;62:384–389.

44. Weidmann P, de Chatel R, Schiffmann A, et al. Interrelations between age and plasma renin, aldosterone and cortisol, urinary catecholamines, and the body sodium/ volume state in normal man. Klin Wochenschr 1977;55: 725–733.

45. Weidmann P, De Myttenaere-Bursztein S, Maxwell M, De Lima J. Effect of aging on plasma renin and aldosterone in normal man. Kidney Int 1975;8:325–333.

46. Flood C, Gherondache C, Pincus G, et al. The metabolism and secretion of aldosterone in elderly subjects. J Clin Invest 1967;46:960–966.

47. Hegstad R, Brown R, Jiang N, et al. Aging and aldosterone. Am J Med 1983;74:442–448.

48. Luft F, Weinberger M, Grim C. Sodium sensitivity and resistance in normotensive humans. Am J Med 1982;72:726–736.

49. Luft F, Weinberger M, Fineberg M, et al. Effects of age on renal sodium homeostasis and its relevance to sodium sensitivity. Am J Med 1987;82(suppl 1B):9–15.

50. Brenner BM, Ballersmann BJ, Gunning ME, Zeidel ML. Diverse biological actions of atrial natriuretic peptide. Physiol Rev 1990;70:599–665.

51. Or K, Richards A, Espiner E, et al. Effect of low-dose infusions of ile-atrial natriuretic peptide in healthy elderly males: evidence for a postreceptor defect. J Clin Endocrinol Metab 1993;76:1271–1274.

52. Galbusera M, Garattini S, Remuzzi G, Menninit T. Catecholamine receptor binding in rat kidney: effect of aging. Kidney Int 1988;33:1073–1077.

53. Lindeman R, VanBuren H, Maisz L. Osmolar renal concentrating ability in healthy young men and hospitalized patients without renal disease. N Engl J Med 1960;262:1306–1309.

54. Rowe J, Shock N, DeFronzo R. The influence of age on the renal response to water deprivation in man. Nephron 1976;17:270–278.

55. Helderman J, Vestal R, Rowe J, et al. The response of arginine vasopressin to intravenous ethanol and hypertonic saline in man: the impact of aging. J Gerontol 1978;33:39–47.

56. Miller JH, Shock NW. Age differences in the renal tubular response to antidiuretic hormone. J Gerontol 1953;8:446–450.

57. Phillips P, Phil D, Rolls B, et al. Reduced thirst after water deprivation in healthy elderly men. N Engl J Med 1984;311:753–759.

58. Phillips P, Bretherton M, Risvanis J, et al. Effects of drinking on thirst and vasopressin in dehydration in elderly men. Am J Physiol 1993;264:R877–R881.

59. Macias Nunez J, Garcia Iglesias C, Tabernero Romo J, et al. Renal management of sodium under indomethacin and aldosterone in the elderly. Age Ageing 1980;9:165–172.

60. Bengele H, Mathias S, Perkins J, Alexander E. Urinary concentrating defect in the aged rat. Am J Physiol 1981;240:F147–F150.

61. Miller P, Krebs R, Neal B, McIntyre D. Hypodipsia in geriatric patients. Am J Med 1982;73:354–356.

62. Mahowald J, Himmelstein D. Hypernatremia in the elderly: relation to infection and mortality. J Am Geriatr Soc 1981;29:177–180.

63. Sonnenblick M, Algur N. Hypernatremia in the acutely ill elderly patient: role of impaired arginine vasopressin secretion. Miner Electrolyte Metab 1993;19:32–35.

64. Cooke C, Wall B, Jones G, et al. Reversible vasopressin deficiency in severe hypernatremia. Am J Kidney Dis 1993;22:44–52.

65. Arieff A, Guisado R. Effects on the central nervous system of hypernatremic and hyponatremic states. Kidney Int 1976;10:104–116.

66. Davis F, Van Son A, Davis P. Urinary diluting capacity in elderly diabetic subjects. Exp Gerontol 1986;21:407.

67. Crowe M, Forsling M, Rolls B, et al. Altered water excretion in healthy elderly man. Age Ageing 1987;16:285–293.

68. Kleinfeld J, Casimir M, Borra S. Hyponatremia as observed in a chronic disease facility. J Am Geriatr Soc 1979; 27:156–161.

69. Sunderam S, Mankikar G. Hyponatremia in the elderly. Age Ageing 1983;12:77–80.

70. Booker J. Severe symptomatic hyponatremia in elderly outpatients: the role of thiazide therapy and stress. J Am Geriatr Soc 1984;32:108–113.

71. Sonnenblick M, Friedlander Y, Rosin A. Diuretic-induced severe hyponatremia: review and analysis of 129 reported patients. Chest 1993;103:601–606.

72. Davis F, Boh D, Davis P. Factors modulating the effect of oral sulfonylureas on free water clearance. J Clin Pharmacol 1982;22:97.

73. Rault R. Case report: hyponatremia associated with nonsteroidal antiinflammatory drugs. Am J Med Sci 1993;305:318–320.

74. Crews J, Potts N, Schreiber J, Lipper S. Hyponatremia in a patient treated with sertraline. Am J Psychiatry 1993;150:1564.

75. Agarwal B, Cabebe F. Renal acidification in elderly subjects. Nephron 1980;26:291–295.

76. Hilton J, Goodboy M, Kruiesi O. The effect of prolonged administration of NH4CL on the blood acid-base equilibria of geriatric subjects. J Am Geriatr Soc 1955;3:697–703.

77. Adler S, Lindeman R, Yiengst M, et al. Effect of acute acid loading on urinary acid excretion by the aging human kidney. J Lab Clin Med 1968;72:278–289.

78. Allen TH, Anderson EC, Langham W. Total body potassium and gross body composition in relation to age. J Gerontol 1960;15:348–357.

79. Sagild U. Total exchangeable potassium in normal subjects with special reference to changes with age. Scand J Clin Lab Invest 1956;8:44–50.

80. Ford G, Blaschke T, Wiswell R, Hoffman B. Effect of aging on changes in plasma potassium during exercise. J Gerontol. 1993;48:M140–M145.

81. DeFronzo RA. Hyperkalemia and hyporeninemic hypoaldosteronism. Kidney Int 1980;17:118.

82. Meyrier A, Buchet P, Simon P, et al. Atheromatous renal disease. Am J Med 1988;85:139.

83. Rimmer J, Gennari F. Atherosclerotic renovascular disease and progressive renal failure. Ann Intern Med 1993; 118:712–719.

84. Scoble J, Haher E, Hamilton G, et al. Atherosclerotic renovascular disease causing renal impairment. A case for treatment. Clin Nephrol 1989;31:119–122.

85. Toto R. Angiotensin converting enzyme inhibitors and the kidney. Natl Kidney Found Letter 1993;10:41–52.

86. Zucchelli P, Zuccala A. Ischemic nephropathy in the elderly. Contrib Nephrol 1993;105:13–24.

87. Schlanger L, Haire H, Zuckerman A, et al. Reversible renal failure in an elderly woman wih renal artery stenosis. Am J Kidney Dis 1994;23:123–126.

88. Meier G, Sumpio B, Setaro J, et al. Captopril renal scintigraphy: a new standard for predicting outcome after renal revascularization. J Vasc Surg 1993;17:280–287.

89. Gupta B, Spinowitz B, Charytan C, Wahl S. Cholesterol crystal embolization-associated renal failure with recombinant tissue-type plasminogen activator. Am J Kidney Dis 1993;21:659–662.

90. Cronin RE. Southwestern internal medicine conference: renal failure following radiologic procedures. Am J Med Sci 1989;298:342–356.

91. Smith M, Ghose M, Henry A. The clinical spectrum of renal cholesterol embolization. Am J Med 1981;71:174.

92. Lye W, Cheah J, Sinniah R. Renal cholesterol embolic disease. Am J Nephrol 1993;13:489–493.

93. Donadio J. Treatment and clinical outcome of glomerulonephritis in the elderly. Contrib Nephrol 1993; 105:49–57.

94. Falk R, Jennette J. Anti-neutrophil cytoplasmic autoantibodies: a review and highlights of the third international ANCA workshop. Kidney 1991;24:1–10.

95. Furci L, Medici G, Baraldi G, et al. Rapidly progressive glomerulonephritis in the elderly. Contrib Nephrol 1993;105:98–101.

96. Moorthy AV, Zimmerman SW. Renal disease in the elderly: clinicopathologic analysis of renal disease in 115 elderly patients. Clin Nephrol 1980;14:223–229.

97. Bergesio F, Bertoni E, Bandini S, et al. Changing pattern

of glomerulonephritis in the elderly: a change of prevalence or a different approach? Contrib Nephrol 1993;105:75–80.

98. Bindi P, Mounenot B, Mentre F, et al. Necrotizing crescentic glomerulonephritis without significant immune deposits: a clinical and serologic study. Q J Med 1993;86:55–68.

99. Abrass C. Glomerulonephritis in the elderly. Am J Nephrol 1985;5:409–418.

100. Melby PC, Musick WD, Luger AM, Khanna R. Post-streptococcal glomerulonephritis in the elderly. Am J Nephrol 1987;7:235–240.

101. Volpi A, Meroni M, Battini G, et al. Postinfectious glomerulonephritis in the elderly. Am J Nephrol 1988;8:431–432.

102. Boner G, Lustig S, Ben-Bassat M, et al. Nephrotic syndrome in patients over 60 years of age. Seventh International Congress of Nephrology, Montreal, June 18–26, 1978:D3. Abstract.

103. Fawcett I, Hilton P, Jones N, Wing A. Nephrotic syndrome in the elderly. BMJ 1971;2:387–388.

104. Huriet C, Rauber G, Kessler Cuny G, Penin F. Le syndrome néphrétique après 60 ans, considérations étiologiques d'après une serie de 25 cas. Ann Med Nancy 1975;14:1021.

105. Ishimuto F, Shibasaki T, Nakano M, et al. Nephrotic syndrome in the elderly: a clinicopathological study. Jpn J Nephrol 1981;23:1321–1331.

106. Kingswood JC, Banks R, Tribe C, et al. Renal biopsy in the elderly: clinicopathological correlations in 143 patients. Clin Nephrol 1984;22:183–187.

107. Lustig S, Rosenfeld J, Ben-Bassat M, Boner G. Nephrotic syndrome in the elderly. Isr J Med Sci 1982;18:1010–1013.

108. Murphy P, Wright M, Rai G. Nephrotic syndrome in the elderly. J Am Geriatr Soc 1987;35:170–173.

109. Sato H, Saito T, Furuyama T, Yoshinaga K. Histologic studies on the nephrotic syndrome in the elderly. Tohoku J Exp Med 1987;153:259–264.

110. Zech P, Colon S, Pointet P, et al. The nephrotic syndrome in adults aged over 60: etiology, evolution and treatment of 76 cases. Clin Nephrol 1982;18:232–236.

111. Johnston P, Brown J, Davison A. The nephrotic syndrome in the elderly: clinico-pathologic correlations in 317 patients. Geriatr Nephrol Urol 1992;2:85–90.

112. Anderson S, Brenner BM. Effects of aging on the renal glomerulus. Am J Med 1986;80:435–442.

113. Hostetter TH, Rennke HG, Brenner BM. The case of intrarenal hypertension in the initiation and progression of diabetic and other glomerulopathies. Am J Med 1985;72:375–282.

114. Modesto A, Ah-Soune M, Durand D, Suc J. Renal biopsy in the elderly. Am J Nephrol 1993;13:27–34.

115. Moran D, Korzets Z, Bernheim J, et al. Is renal biopsy justified for the diagnosis and management of the nephrotic syndrome in the elderly? Gerontology 1993;39:49–54.

116. Eagan J, Lewis E. Glomerulopathies of neoplasia. Kidney Int 1977;11:297–306.

117. Donadio J. Treatment of glomerulonephritis in the elderly. Am J Kidney Dis 1990;16:307–311.

118. Kissane J. The morphology of renal cystic disease. Perspect Nephrol Hypertens 1976;4:31–63.

119. Ravine D, Gibson R, Donlan J, Sheffield L. An ultrasound renal cyst prevalence survey: specificity data for inherited renal cystic diseases. Am J Kidney Dis 1993;22:803–807.

120. Yamagishi F, Kitahara N, Mogi W, Itoh S. Age-related occurrence of simple cysts studied by ultrasonography. Klin Wochenschr 1988;66:385–387.

121. Dalton D, Neiman H, Grayhack J. The natural history of simple renal cysts: a preliminary study. J Urol 1986;135:905–908.

122. Pollack H, Banner M, Arger P, et al. The accuracy of gray-scale renal ultrasonography in differentiating cystic neoplasms from benign cysts. Radiology 1982;143:741–745.

123. McClennan B, Stanley R, Melson G, et al. CT of the renal cyst: is cyst aspiration necessary? Am J Radiol 1979;133:671–675.

124. Kumar R, Hill C, McGeown M. Acute renal failure in the elderly. Lancet 1973;1:90–91.

125. Lameire N, Matthys E, Vanholder R, et al. Causes and prognosis of acute renal failure in elderly patients. Nephrol Dial Transplant 1987;2:316–322.

126. McInnes EG, Levy EW, Chaudhuri M, Bhan G. Renal failure in the elderly. Q J Med 1987;243:583–588.

127. Rodgers H, Staniland J, Lipkin G, Turney J. Acute renal failure: a study of elderly patients. Age Ageing 1990;19:36–42.

128. Rosenfeld J, Shohat J, Grosskopf I. Acute renal failure: a disease of the elderly? Adv Nephrol 1987;6:159.

129. Moore R, Smith C, Lipsky J. Risk factor for nephrotoxicity in patients treated with aminoglycosides. Ann Intern Med 1984;100:352–358.

130. Levi M, Jameson D, Van Der Meer B. Role of BBM lipid composition and fluidity in impaired renal Pi transport in aged rat. Am J Physiol 1989;256:F85–F94.

131. Lamy P. Renal effects of nonsteroidal antiinflammatory drugs heighten risk to the elderly? J Am Geriatr Soc 1986;34:361–367.

132. Schwartz J, Altshuler E, Madjar J, Habot B. Acute renal failure associated with diclofenac treatment in an elderly woman. J Am Geriatr Soc 1988;36:482–483.

133. Gurwitz J, Avorn J, Ross-Degnan D, Lipsitz L. Nonsteroidal anti-inflammatory drug-associated azotemia in the very old. JAMA 1990;264:471–475.

134. Schlondorff D. Renal complications of nonsteroidal anti-inflammatory drugs. Kidney Int 1993;44:643–653.

135. MacKenzie T, Zawada E, Johnson M. The effect of age on urinary prostaglandin excretion in normal and hypertensive men. Nephron 1984;38:178–182.

136. Feest T, Round A, Hamad S. Incidence of severe acute renal failure in adults: results of a community based study. BMJ 1993;306:481–483.

137. Oliveira D. Acute renal failure in the elderly can have a

good prognosis. Age Ageing 1984;13:304–308.

138. Nissenson A. Dialysis therapy in the elderly. Kidney Int 1993;43:S51–S57.

139. Avram M, Pena C, Burrel D. Hemodialysis and the elderly patient: potential advantages as to quality of life, urea generation, serum creatinine, and less intradialytic weight gain. Am J Kidney Dis 1990;16:342–345.

140. Williams A, Nicholl J, El Nahas A, et al. Continous ambulatory peritoneal dialysis and haemodialysis in the elderly. Q J Med 1990;274:215–223.

141. Ismail N, Hakim R, Oreopoulos D, Patrikarea A. Renal replacement therapies in the elderly: Part 1. Hemodialy-sis and chronic peritoneal dialysis. Am J Kidney Dis 1993;22:759–782.

142. Gorban-Brennan N, Kliger A, Finkelstein F. CAPD therapy for patients over 80 years of age. Perit Dial Int 1993;13:140–141.

143. Ismail N, Hakim R, Helderman J. Renal replacement therapies in the elderly: Part 2. Renal transplantation. Am J Kidney Dis 1994;23:1–15.

144. Cantarovich D, Baranger T, Tirouvanziam A, et al. 155 cadavaric kidney transplants with cyclosporine in recipients more than 60 years of age. Transplant Proc 1993;25:1323.

Chapter 48
Geriatric Gynecology

Nora E. Morgenstern and Hugh R. K. Barber

It's wonderful to be married to an archaeologist—the older you get the more interested he is in you.

Agatha Christie in Jeffrey Feinman, The Mysterious World of Agatha Christie 1975

Geriatric gynecology is the prevention, diagnosis, care and treatment of illnesses and disability in the older woman (1). Because most women older than 65 years of age no longer see gynecologists for regular care (2), a thorough understanding of the postmenopausal state and the health care needs of the older woman is essential for the primary care provider.

A marked change in the average life expectancy of the population in the United States has occurred since the turn of the century. In the 1980s, more than 50 million women in the United States were older than age 50. Rapid increases in numbers of elderly women are expected as the "baby boomers" become menopausal. American women at the age of 50 years can expect to live another 30 years, on average, and therefore will live one-third of their lives in the postmenopausal state.

The percentage of the population that reaches 85 years of age and older is growing at a faster rate than is the population aged 65 to 84 years, and is the fastest growing population segment in the United States. As the phenomenon of aging of the population accelerates, the advantage in female survivorship will become more pronounced; in the next century, women will outlive men by 8.5 years.

Morbidity and Mortality

Women's advantage in mortality and life expectancy does not extend to morbidity. Women have more illnesses and disabilities than do men. They visit doctors more often and are hospitalized at a higher rate. Women also have a higher incidence of respiratory illnesses (except pneumo-

nia), digestive disorders, and infectious diseases than do men.

Cardiovascular disease is the leading cause of death in women aged 75 years and older, followed by cancer and cerebrovascular disease (3). Cardiovascular disease is the second cause of death (behind cancer) in women aged 55 to 74 years (3). Although women lag 10 years behind men in the onset of coronary artery disease and have a 20-year advantage for myocardial infarction and sudden death, within 10 years after menopause a woman's chance of sustaining a myocardial infarction or stroke equals that of men (4). Compared with men, women with coronary artery disease are more likely to die (5,6). Epidemiologic evidence supports estrogen deficiency and related lipid changes as major risk factors for coronary artery disease in women.

Evaluation of the Patient

History

The practitioner must be prepared to be unhurried when taking the medical history from an elderly woman. A significant number of elderly women may be unable to give a useful history of their obstetrical and gynecologic experience, or are uncertain whether they ever received hormone therapy. Although more than one-third of American women have had a hysterectomy by age 60 (7), many elderly women do not know why the procedure was performed. As much as one-third of elderly women who have had hysterectomies have a remnant cervix (8,9). This has important implications for cancer screening because these women are unlikely to have received adequate Papanicolaou (Pap) smears for cervical cancer screening.

The four most common genitourinary symptoms in older women are 1) stress urinary incontinence, 2) pruritus vulvae or pruritus anae, 3) vaginal discharge, and 4) dyspareunia. Some women are reluctant to volunteer these complaints, and need to be questioned directly. Another common symptom is so-called vaginal bleeding, but on close questioning, some elderly patients are uncertain whether the bleeding is coming from the urethra, vagina, or anal area.

Gynecologic Examination

The geriatric patient may be reluctant to have a gynecologic examination and must be educated about the importance of detecting common, treatable conditions. Fear of discomfort from the examination of atrophic vaginal and vulvar tissues is a barrier to regular screening. A successful examination requires proper positioning to ensure the patient's comfort. In the presence of severe osteoarthritis of the hips or knees or other musculoskeletal disorders, the patient may not be able to tolerate the lithotomy position. Examination of the external genitalia can be accomplished by the patient lying comfortably on her back, and drawing up her knees and dropping her legs to each side as much as she is able. Assistants then support the patient's legs to enable the clinician to perform the examination by speculum. Alternatively, the left lateral (Sims) position can be used. The upper leg should be flexed more than the lower leg to visualize the vaginal opening. It is important to explain each step of the examination to the patient and assure her that if there is any pain during the examination, the procedure will be stopped immediately.

The examination should start with careful observation and palpation of the vulva, urethra, and Bartholin's and Skene's glands. Next, a speculum should be carefully inserted, holding the blades parallel to the introitus and not rotating them until the speculum has been inserted to the depth of the vagina. The instrument should then be turned slowly so that the posterior blade rests against the posterior wall of the vagina. Gentle downward pressure on the instrument opens the vagina without disturbing the sensitive anterior organs. For patients with a stenotic vaginal introitus, a narrow (1 to 1.5cm) speculum is best tolerated. For patients in whom atrophic vaginitis causes the speculum examination to be painful, the physician must decide whether symptoms warrant speculum examination and whether a routine Pap smear is necessary in view of the low yield of cytologic abnormalities in the asymptomatic patient older than 60 years of age who has had previous Pap smear screening (10). Sometimes a visual examination alone can by accomplished by using a clear plastic anoscope.

The cervix is next identified. The practitioner should remember that with age and estrogen deficiency the cervix flattens and may be difficult to visualize. After any vaginal secretions have been removed, a Pap smear should be taken from the cervical canal. A small amount of lubrication on the speculum increases patient comfort and ease of sampling while maintaining adequate smear accuracy (11). The highest yield for sampling endocervical cells uses both the Ayre spatula and the saline-moistened cervical cytobrush (12,13). Using the brush after the spatula helps minimize bleeding from trauma to a friable atrophic cervix and results in a Pap smear that is easier to interpret. With age and genital atrophy, the cervical os may become stenotic and the squamocolumnar junction, or transformation zone, in which cervical cancers arise, moves back within the endocervical canal. Therefore, adequate sampling of endocervical cells for cervical cancer screening may be difficult in the elderly woman. In patients in whom a cervical Pap smear is impossible, some gynecologists suggest a vaginal pool smear, which occasionally detects occult gynecologic cancers (12).

A careful, one-finger examination of the entire length and breadth of the vagina, including the fornices, should be carried out before palpation of the uterus. Uterine size, shape, and mobility should be noted, and then the adnexal areas examined. A palpable ovary is unusual in elderly women and requires further investigation. After this, with the index finger in the vagina, the lubricated middle finger should be inserted into the patient's rectum for a rectovaginal exam that explores the rectovaginal septum, and cardinal and uterosacral ligaments. A careful rectal examination should be carried out, including a test for occult blood. Sometimes severe vaginal stenosis precludes a one- or two-finger vaginal examination, and bimanual palpation using the rectal approach is required.

Estrogen Deficiency

Menopause occurs, on average, when a woman is 51 years of age, or when ovarian production of estradiol ceases.

The most physiologically active estrogen, estradiol drops to 10 percent of its premenopausal level, with a small amount still produced in the adrenal glands. Estrone continues to exert mild estrogenic effects. Produced by peripheral conversion of adrenal androstenedione, estrone levels are increased in obese women because of increased conversion by adipose cells. Because adrenal androgen production is unchanged with menopause and testosterone continues to be produced by the ovaries, the postmenopausal years are characterized by a relative hyperandrogenicity.

The most noticeable immediate effect of the menopause is vasomotor instability, characterized by hot flashes or flushes, night sweats, and insomnia. Evidence is mixed regarding whether psychological symptoms, cognitive changes, and motor changes can also be attributed to estrogen deficiency. No consistent decrease in level of sexual interest or activity can be attributed to estrogen deficiency. Although for most women hot flashes resolve without treatment within 7 years of menopause, hot flashes persist into the sixth decade in 15 percent of women, and some women in their seventh and eighth decades continue to report hot flashes (14).

The effects of estrogen deficiency are manifested throughout the genitourinary tract and the body. The natural aging process of the skin is accelerated by estrogen deficiency, with thinning of the epidermis, decrease in collagen and elastic tissue in the dermis, reduction in the number of hair follicles on the scalp and extremities, and decreased activity of sebaceous glands. Hyperandrogenicity stimulates hair growth on the face, chest, axillae, and abdomen. In the breasts, glandular tissue atrophies and is replaced by fat, and the breasts become smaller. Fat and subcutaneous tissue is lost in the vulva, and pubic hair thins. Vaginal squamous epithelium thins, and submucosal elastic tissue, neural supply, and blood flow are reduced.

These physiologic changes contribute to the characteristic appearance of the atrophic vagina, in which the vagina is short and narrow, rugae are decreased, mucosa is thin, pale and friable, and tissues are dry. The cervix becomes smaller, paler and flatter, and the os may completely stenose. Mucosa of the urethra and bladder base exhibit changes similar to those of the vagina. Red urethral caruncles and symptoms of atrophic urethritis or the urethral syndrome (dysuria, urgency, frequency) may result. The endometrium becomes atrophic, shrinking from an average weight of 120 gm to 25 gm, and ovaries shrink to half of their premenopausal size.

Systemic effects of estrogen deficiency, such as osteoporosis, lipid abnormalities, and increased cardiovascular risk, are discussed extensively elsewhere in this text.

Diseases of the Vulva

The vulvar tissues of women in the geriatric age group who are not on estrogen replacement therapy are atrophic. The labia majora and minora and the clitoris become smaller. Shrinkage, loss of elasticity, and dryness of the vaginal introitus may make an examination uncomfortable. Lubrication from Bartholin's glands decreases, leading to painful penile intromission, and deflection of the penis anteriorly by rigid perineum may create pressure on the urethral meatus, causing urethritis, local inflammation, and dysuria.

In the geriatric population, there is an increase in the incidence of vulvar nonneoplastic epithelial disorders of the skin, formerly called vulvar dystrophies (Table 48.1). These include lichen sclerosus and squamous cell hyperplasia. Women with these lesions often present with burning, pruritus, or difficulty with coitus.

White lesions of the vulva traditionally have been treated as a group, and all thought to be premalignant.

Table 48.1 Classification of Vulvar Disease

Current Name		Former Name
Nonneoplastic epithelial disorders of skin and mucosa		
		Vulvar dystrophies
Squamous cell hyperplasia		Hyperplastic dystrophy
Lichen sclerosus		Lichen sclerosus et atrophicus
Other dermatoses		
Vulvar intraepithelial neoplasia		
VIN I	Mild dysplasia	Mild atypia
VIN II	Moderate dysplasia	Moderate atypia
VIN III	Severe dysplasia	Severe atypia
VIN IV	Carcinoma in situ	

SOURCE: Ridley CM, Frankman O, Jones I, et al. New nomenclature for vulvar disease: International Society for the Study of Vulvar Disease. Hum Pathol 1989;20:495–496.

However, lesions of the vulva can be either pigmented or white, depending upon local factors such as hygiene, excoriation, depigmentation, and vascularity. When a patient presents with a vulvar lesion that is white, gray, or simply pale, in which there is a change in skin surface and architecture and to which a specific cause cannot be ascribed, the clinician should biopsy the lesion for diagnosis. The outdated term leukoplakia should be discarded. On the basis of pathologic findings, a diagnosis is determined and appropriate treatment initiated. Overall, 2 percent to 5 percent of women with vulvar lesions have invasive carcinoma at the time of presentation, and 2 percent to 8 percent of dystrophic lesions demonstrate vulvar intraepitheliel neoplasia (VIN) when biopsied (15). Therefore, any suspicious or undiagnosed vulvar lesion must be biopsied.

Dystrophy is defined as defective or faulty nourishment or nutrition of the vulva and is associated with abnormal maturation of the squamous epithelium. The etiology of dystrophy is unknown, but recently an association between vulvar dystrophy and achlorhydria has been demonstrated, and papilloma viruses have been identified in a few patients (1).

Lichen sclerosus is the most common of the nonneoplastic epithelial disorders. Although it can affect patients of all ages, lichen sclerosus occurs most commonly in the postmenopausal woman. Its distribution is usually symmetric, involving the vulva and sometimes the thigh and perianal regions. Its appearance ranges from white or pale pink macules to thin pale plaques. Characteristically, it is described as "parchment" or "cigarette paper" because of its thin, dry, scaly, or finely wrinkled appearance. Pruritus is a common symptom of lichen sclerosus, and scratching can result in ecchymoses or ulcerations.

To be effective, treatment must interrupt the itch and scratch pattern. Any co-existing vaginitis must be treated, and the patient should be advised concerning vulvovaginal hygiene. The use of loose cotton underclothing and nonirritating soaps and detergents, as well as the avoidance of other possible irritants such as feminine hygiene sprays and scented powders and toilet tissue, are basic recommendations. It is important to instruct the patient to keep the area as dry as possible at all times, which may require temporarily minimizing physical activity. Use of a hairdryer set at low heat may be helpful in minimizing moisture.

In the acute phase, pruritus can be relieved by the use of cool, compresses wet with aluminum acetate (Burrough's solution). Once the acute phase is controlled, a short course of medium potency corticosteroid cream improves pruritus and edema. 2% testosterone proprionate ointment is helpful for patients whose primary symptom is burning. Daily use of this ointment for 2 or 3 weeks, followed by once or twice a week applications, can provide relief of symptoms and reduction of synechiae that may have developed between the labia and the clitoral prepuce. Topical testosterone can be absorbed and cause systemic side effects, which limits its usefulness in some patients.

Squamous cell hyperplasia has also been called hypertrophic dystrophy, hyperplastic dystrophy, hyperplastic vulvitis, neurodermatitis, and leukokeratosis. Most cases occur in the premenopausal woman. Distribution is patchy, with localized, thickened, raised, pink or white plaques. Unlike lichen sclerosus, the perineal and perianal areas are seldom involved. Pruritus is a universal symptom. Treatment is similar to that for lichen sclerosus and emphasizes vulvar hygiene and symptomatic use of topical corticosteroid cream. As the appearance of squamous cell hyperplasia can resemble carcinoma in situ or lichen sclerosus, multiple punch biopsies are necessary to establish the diagnosis. Dysplasia (atypia) is much more common in association with squamous cell hyperplasia than it is with lichen sclerosus.

Diseases of the skin found elsewhere on the body also occur in the vulvar region (16). Candidiasis and allergic vulvitis are common. Intertrigo is seen in obese older women who have difficulty with bathing and cleaning their perineum and vulva. The skin becomes superficially denuded, shiny, hyperemic, and moist, and may be covered by a scanty, malodorous discharge. Symptoms include itching and burning; treatment involves hygiene measures and keeping the area dry.

Clitoral phimosis may cause inspissated smegma to collect beneath the prepuce. The area is usually very red and uncomfortable, similar to balanitis in men.

Senile angiomas are small, usually multiple, red papules as large as 3 mm in diameter. Because they are a form of telangiectasia, senile angiomas bleed easily. If they are bothersome to the patient, they can be treated with cautery or laser.

Sebaceous cysts of the vulva are small, yellowish-gray nodules in the skin covering the labia and are rarely larger than 1 cm in diameter. Only very large cysts that become repeatedly infected need be excised. Cysts of the Bartholin's glands are distinctly unusual in the geriatric patient and require biopsy to exclude carcinoma.

Diseases of the Vagina

Estrogen deficiency contributes to a variety of symptoms in the postmenopausal woman, including leukorrhea, frequency and urgency of urination, dyspareunia, and itching. Atrophic vaginitis can produce either a scant alkaline discharge or bleeding. On wet prep, many white blood cells, red blood cells, and parabasal cells are seen. Decreased glycogen production by atrophic vaginal epithelium results in fewer lactobacilli; because the lactobacillus not only produces lactic acid, which maintains a protective acid vaginal pH, but also produces hydrogen peroxide, which is toxic to bacteria, the atrophic vagina is very susceptible to infection. Successful eradication of bacterial vaginitis in the postmenopausal woman may require both specific treatment of the pathogen and estrogen treatment of atrophic vaginitis. *Trichomonas vaginitis* thrives in an alkaline milieu, but *Candida albicans* is inhibited; recurrent candidiasis is suggestive of diabetes. The practitioner should also remember that all sexually transmitted diseases seen in younger persons can be contracted by the sexually active older woman.

Limited evidence suggests that sexual activity can help maintain a healthy vaginal epithelium. A study of 52 postmenopausal women, mean age 57 years, found that those engaging in sexual intercourse three or more times monthly exhibited significantly less vaginal atrophy than those who had intercourse less than 10 times a year (17).

Treatment of atrophic vaginitis can be accomplished by either topical or systemic estrogens. Topical estrogen cream should be applied a minimum of two or three times a week for 2 months, at a dose of 1/4 of an applicator (one gm or 0.625 mg of conjugated equine estrogen) inserted into the upper vagina. Because topical estrogens are absorbed systemically, women with an intact uterus who require prolonged estrogen treatment should receive con-current oral progesterone therapy to reduce the risk of carcinoma of the endometrium.

Estrogen Replacement

A variety of estrogen and progesterone regimens are efficacious for menopausal or symptoms of estrogen deficiency. In general, the lowest estrogen dose that alleviates symptoms should be used, with progesterone added for women who have an intact uterus. A dose-response relationship has been shown for transdermal estrogen, with a 53 percent reduction of hot flashes with a 0.05 mg twice weekly dose and an 83 percent reduction with 0.10 mg (18). Because the natural history of hot flashes is a gradual lessening over time, women requiring doses higher than the standard of 0.625 mg daily of conjugated equine estrogen (CEE) or 0.10 mg of 17-β-estradiol twice weekly for symptom control should receive regular attempts at dose reduction.

For women who cannot take estrogen, clonidine at an oral dose of 0.05 mg to 0.10 mg twice a day reduces hot flash frequency in as much as 40 percent of women (18). Although higher doses are more effective at suppressing hot flashes, side effects usually preclude their use. Progestins alone also decrease the rate of hot flashes in as much as 75 percent of women, with both 10 mg of medroxyprogesterone daily or 20 to 40 mg of megestrol acetate daily shown to be effective (18,19).

Estrogen replacement therapy (ERT) improves symptoms of both atrophic vaginitis and atrophic urethritis. Urgency, dysuria, and urge incontinence are improved with topical or systemic estrogens; estrogen may also prevent the development of urethral strictures related to atrophic urethritis (20). Estrogens are useful as adjunctive treatment for stress incontinence, but will not control symptoms completely if used alone. Topical estrogens (0.5 mg of estriol vaginal cream used nightly for 2 weeks followed by twice-weekly treatment for 8 months) have also been shown to help prevent recurrent urinary tract infections in postmenopausal women (21).

Another commonly accepted indication for ERT is prevention or treatment of osteoporosis. This indication requires a daily estrogen dose of 0.625 mg for at least 7 years after the menopause, as discussed in Chapter 40.

Estrogen and progesterone can be cycled or given continuously (Table 48.2). The most commonly used cyclic regimen is estrogen on days 1 to 25 and progesterone on days 13 to 25. The original recommendation of progesterone starting on day 16 was revised when it was learned that administration of progestins for at least 12 days per month prevents the development of endometrial hyperplasia or carcinoma (20). As this schedule commonly produces withdrawal bleeding, many older woman prefer a continuous regimen. A 40 percent incidence of breakthrough bleeding occurs with continuous combined therapy, especially for the first 6 months (20), but is unusual after 12 months of continuous therapy because the endometrium becomes atrophic.

Hormone replacement therapy for primary prevention of coronary heart disease is hypothesized, but not yet demonstrated to be effective in randomized, controlled trials. (The reader is referred to Chapter 33 for a more detailed discussion.) The most important lipid effects of ERT are a reduction in low-density lipoprotein (LDL) cholesterol and an increase in high-density lipoprotein (HDL) cholesterol; the effects are more pronounced with oral than with transdermal estrogen, by 10 percent to 15 percent (22,23). Oral estrogens also increase triglyceride (TG) levels; transdermal estrogen generally decreases TG levels. Progesterone therapy opposes the estrogen-induced rise in HDL, while eliminating the estrogen-induced rise in TG, or even lowering TG levels to below baseline (22). In general, neither estrogen alone nor combined estrogen

and progesterone therapy increases blood pressure, although a minority of women may experience blood pressure elevation after they begin taking estrogen (23).

The relationship of hormone replacement therapy to breast cancer risk is controversial. Several recent meta-analyses demonstrated a small, increased risk for the development of breast cancer associated with long-term use of estrogen in postmenopausal women (23–25). However, results are inconclusive because of the lack of prospective trials to follow a cohort of women after initiation of hormone replacement therapy.

Sampling of the endometrium of women receiving hormone replacement therapy is an unresolved issue. Endometrial biopsy at pretreatment and done annually is accepted procedure for women who are receiving only estrogen. On the other hand, standards for endometrial sampling for women taking continuous estrogen and progestin or sequential combination therapy are debatable. Pretreatment sampling in the absence of suspected pathology generally is not necessary. For women on a cyclic regimen, the pattern of withdrawal bleeding appears to correlate with endometrial histology, such that bleeding occurring before day 12 of estrogen therapy portends abnormal pathology and warrants endometrial sampling (26). For women taking continuous combined regimens, guidelines for when to sample are bleeding heavier than a normal menstrual period, bleeding lasting longer than 10 days, bleeding occurring more often than monthly, or bleeding persisting longer than 10 months after therapy was begun (27). Office sampling can be safely and effectively performed on most postmenopausal women. The endometrial Pipelle or similar technique is well tolerated, although cervical stenosis may preclude sampling and inpatient dilation and curettage (D&C) for endometrial sampling is required.

The relatively few absolute contraindications to ERT are current breast or endometrial cancer, active liver disease, active thrombophlebitis or thromboembolism, and vaginal bleeding of unknown cause.

Diseases of the Cervix

Atrophic cervicitis is associated with atrophic vaginitis and responds to estrogen therapy. Untreated atrophic cervicitis can lead to closure of the cervical os and mask

Table 48.2 Hormone Replacement Therapy

Therapy	Regimen
Estrogen (women without uterus)	
Conjugated equine estrogen (CEE)	0.3–0.625 mg daily
Micronized estradiol	1.0 mg daily
Estradiol valesate	0.10–2.0 mg daily
Transdermal estrogen (17-β-estradiol)	Patches of 0.05 or 1.0 mg twice weekly
Estrogen plus cyclic progesterone	
Conjugated estrogen	0.625 mg (days 1–25)
Medroxyprogesterone	5–10 mg (days 13, 14, 15, or 16–25)
Continuous estrogen plus progesterone	
Conjugated estrogen	0.625 mg daily
Medroxyprogesterone	2.5 or 5.0 mg daily

endometrial bleeding or cause late diagnosis of cancer of the cervix because an adequate Pap smear cannot be performed.

Chronic cervicitis may result from use of a pessary, poor hygiene, or chemical irritants such as douches. Sexual transmitted diseases affect the cervix of the postmenopausal woman, and the incidence of chlamydia, human papilloma virus, and herpes simplex virus in postmenopausal women is increasing.

With the exception of cervical polyps, benign tumors of the cervix are rare. Most cervical polyps arise from the endocervix, and are single and less than 2 or 3 cm in length. Although almost always benign, they should be removed for pathological examination. Abnormal-appearing tissue can be caused by cervical erosion, ulcers, or ectropion. Any suspicious lesion of the cervix should be investigated with biopsy, colposcopy, and possibly fractional curettage because of the possibility of invasive cervical cancer, even if the Pap smear results are normal.

Diseases of the Uterus

The uterus undergoes retrogressive changes with aging and becomes small and atrophic. Endometrial polyps, a common cause of postmenopausal bleeding, are usually benign, but occasionally develop malignant changes (28).

Leiomyomata also tend to atrophy. Found in 30 percent of white and 50 percent of black postmenopausal women, they are the most common cause of a pelvic mass (29). Because they require hormonal stimulation for growth, in the absence of hormone replacement therapy, a presumed uterine fibroid that is rapidly enlarging should be promptly evaluated to rule out malignancies such as sarcoma (29,30).

Endometrial ultrasound is a reliable means for excluding uterine pathology in postmenpausal women. Endometrial thickness of 5 mm or less throughout the cavity indicates an atrophic state, but pathology should be expected if there is focal or generalized endometrial thickness of more than 5 mm (31).

Atrophic changes render the postmenopausal uterus susceptible to infections. Pyometria has been reported in very elderly women with fever, and pelvic examination should be a routine component of the evaluation of fever of undetermined etiology.

Diseases of the Ovary and Adnexa

The postmenopausal ovary undergoes significant atrophy, shrinking from an average size of $3.5 \times 2 \times 1.5$ cm to as small as $1.5 \times 0.75 \times 0.5$ cm within 5 years of menopause (1). A postmenopausal palpable ovary (PMPO) that averages more than 1 cm in diameter is not a normal finding for the geriatric patient. Although an ovary this size usually does not signify cancer, the PMPO should be considered possibly malignant until proven otherwise (1,30). Physiologic cysts, a common cause of ovarian enlargement in premenopausal women, rarely occur in postmenopausal women (30).

Various strategies for evaluation of the PMPO and the adnexal mass have been proposed. Ultrasound and clinical characteristics can be helpful in differentiating benign from malignant disease. Benign tumors are more likely to be unilateral, cystic, mobile, and smooth. Malignant tumors tend to be solid, fixed, irregular, associated with ascites, and have a rapid growth rate (30). Malignancies are often bilateral because of the tendency of other carcinomas to metastasize to the ovaries.

Although size does not differentiate benign from malignant disease, cysts smaller than 5 cm in diameter are usually benign, and those 10 cm or larger are often malignant (32). In one series of 42 postmenopausal women with simple cysts that were unilocular, unilateral, not associated with ascites, and 5 cm or less in maximum diameter, serial ultrasound for as long as 73 months yielded no malignancies at subsequent surgery (33). On the basis of data from this and other small series, serial ultrasounds or diagnostic laparoscopy rather than laparotomy may be a reasonable option for postmenopausal women with asymptomatic simple cysts (32,33). Incidental scan-detected masses (SCAM) or a completely asymptomatic pelvic mass is likely to be benign (29,30) but should be followed closely. Abdominal computed tomography (CT) scan does not help differentiate benign from malignant disease and adds little diagnostic information to the ultrasound (29,30,33). Factors that increase the likelihood of malignancy are increasing age, positive family history of cancer (ovary, breast, colorectal), and an elevated CA-125 level (29,34–36). The CA-125 antigen is elevated in 60 percent to 90 percent of known ovarian tumors, but is often normal in small stage I ovarian cancer, and may be

Table 48.3 Differential Diagnosis of Adnexal Mass

Site	Cystic Mass	Solid Mass

Ovary	Neoplastic cyst
	  benign
	  malignant
	Endometriosis
		Neoplasm
		  benign
		  malignant

Fallopian tube	Tubo-ovarian abscess Hydrosalpinx	Tubo-ovarian abscess Neoplasm
Uterus	Pyometra Hematometra	Leiomyomata
Bowel	Palpable normal bowel	Diverticulitis, abscess Appendicitis Colon cancer Regional ileitis

Other	Distended bladder	Desmoid tumor
		Retroperitoneal tumor
		  (lymphoma,
		  sarcoma)

elevated secondary to other malignancies, such as adenocarcinoma of the colon, rectum, endometrium, and breast, or in cases of lymphoma. A myriad of nonmalignant conditions also are associated with increased CA-125 levels, including benign ovarian tumors and leiomyomata, as well as nongynecologic conditions such as pancreatitis and infections of the pelvis (35,37). However, despite its general lack of specificity, when used as a second diagnostic test in postmenopausal women with an ultrasound-confirmed adnexal mass, the positive predictive value for malignancy of an elevated CA-125 (>35 U/mL) approaches 100 percent (35).

Nongynecologic conditions causing a pelvic mass are not uncommon at exploratory laparatomy, even with negative presurgical radiographic evaluations (Table 48.3). Diagnoses include carcinoma of the colon and rectum, other carcinomas metastatic to the ovary, and diverticular disease. Although tubo-ovarian abscess is usually a disease of young sexually active women, it can occur in older women secondary to acute diverticulitis or bowel perforation, or be related to concurrent genital tract pathology such as malignancy or large leiomyomata (38).

Disorders of Pelvic Support

Support of pelvic structures depends on the endopelvic fascia, the uterosacral and cardinal ligaments, and the levator ani muscles. An intact fascial system with its attachments to the vaginal fornices and upper two-thirds of the lateral vagina provides a well-supported vaginal tube, which in turn is the most important supporting structure of the uterus and vaginal vault. A variety of circumstances lead to postmenopausal weakness and pelvic relaxation syndromes (39). Pelvic prolapses are seen in most multiparous elderly women and are very common in women with four or more childbirths and age 72 years or older; both these factors result in stretching and laxity of the pelvic floor fascia and musculature (40).

Cystocele

Descent of a portion of the posterior bladder wall and trigon into the vagina is usually caused by trauma during childbirth. Urethrocele (sagging of the urethra) is commonly associated with cystocele and frequently occurs in women who have urinary stress incontinence. However, urethrocele alone is not a cause of incontinence, nor do large cystoceles invariably cause stress incontinence. Patients with a large cystocele may have repeated bouts of cystitis and symptoms of incomplete emptying of the bladder, urinary frequency, and vaginal fullness or pressure. On examination, a soft, reducible mass bulging into the anterior vagina and sometimes distending the vaginal introitus is found; straining or coughing increases the bulging.

A cystocele requires surgical repair if there are recurrent urinary tract infections, significant postvoid residual, or protrusion into the vaginal introitus causing ulceration of the vaginal wall.

Uterine Prolapse

Uterine prolapse occurs either into the upper vagina, from weakness of the cardinal and uterosacral ligament complex, or as eversion of the lower vagina, caused by damage to the pelvic floor and urogenital diaphragms. Occasionally, both conditions occur together. The etiology usually is childbirth trauma, with contributing factors including atrophy of the vaginal epithelium, vascular insufficiency, and chronically increased intraabdominal pressure, as in obesity.

Prolapse is classified as 1) first degree if the cervix appears at the vaginal introitus; 2) second degree if the cervix and half the uterus appear at the vaginal orifice; and 3) third degree if the entire uterus protrudes through the orifice and the vaginal walls are completely everted. Third degree is also known as procidentia; it is often associated with cystocele and rectocele and can occur after hysterectomy (vaginal prolapse). Complications of procidentia include trophic ulceration of exposed vagina, decubitus ulcer of the uterus, and ureteral obstruction, usually bilateral, which causes hydroureteronephrosis and risk of renal failure. Urinary tract infection is seen in 50 percent to 100 percent of women with severe prolapse (40).

Evaluation should include a pelvic examination in the standing position, with straining; urinalysis; postvoid residual; assessment of renal function; and consideration of renal ultrasound or intravenous or retrograde pyelography in second- or third-degree prolapse (40). Ureteral obstruction or other severe complications are best treated surgically, even in the very elderly woman. An alternative to vaginal hysterectomy in the frail elderly woman is partial colpocleisis (the Le Fort procedure), in which obliteration of the vagina by suturing the bladder to the rectum is performed under local anesthesia. Either hysterectomy or partial colpocleisis can be complicated by cystocele or stress urinary incontinence.

Pessaries are a reasonable alternative to surgery for some women. Indications for pessary use include symptomatic uterine prolapse after failed surgery; as an interim measure for symptom relief while awaiting surgery; and for long-term supervised use in women who are at increased risk for surgical intervention (41). Pessaries are unlikely to be successful with marked outlet relaxation and associated cystocele and rectocele, and they are usually contraindicated with uterine displacement by a mass such as a leiomyoma, previous pelvic surgery, or pelvic radiotherapy with significant fibrosis. Successful use of a pessary also requires adequate estrogenization of the vaginal mucosa; hormone replacement therapy should be initiated before a pessary trial.

Several pessary models are now commonly available, including the ring, which is similar to a diaphragm, the Gellhorn disc, and the doughnut. The patient must be advised that pessary use sometimes causes urinary incontinence. After initial successful fitting, follow-up examinations must be performed at least every 6 months. Daily topical estrogen therapy (0.3 mg) is suggested, and the pessary must be removed and cleaned weekly. Because of a slightly increased risk of cervical and vaginal cancer, Pap smears should be obtained annually. Complications include vaginitis or cervicitis from inadequate hygiene, actinomycosis infections with secondary abscess or fistula formation, impactions from a forgotten pessary, vaginal erosions, bleeding, urethral obstruction, and (rarely) vaginal or cervical cancer (41).

Rectocele

Bulging of the posterior vaginal wall by the underlying rectum through the rectovaginal septum results in a rectocele. A mild degree of rectocele, which is usually asymptomatic, is a common finding in multiparous elderly women. A large rectocele may produce a sense of pelvic pressure, rectal fullness, constipation, or incomplete evacuation of stool. Occasionally, a patient may find it necessary to push the posterior vaginal wall manually in a backward direction to effectively evacuate stool. A bowel program should be initiated to avoid hard stools and straining at the stool. Pessaries are not helpful for this condition, and surgical repair should be considered if the rectocele significantly affects the patient's quality of life.

Enterocele

An enterocele results from the small bowel pushing into the peritoneum between the rectum and the vagina. Although usually asymptomatic, an enterocele occasionally pulls on the mesentery of the bowel and causes upper abdominal discomfort. Enteroceles, similar to other hernias, can be complicated by bowel obstruction.

Examination shows a bulge in the upper part of the vagina in the posterior fornix. The diagnosis is made by asking the patient to stand and strain or cough while the examiner places the index finger in the rectum and the thumb in the vagina. The small intestine will produce an impulse which is easily felt. Because an enterocele is a true hernia, surgical repair is indicated. This process entails high ligation of the hernia sac and closure of the fascia, either by sewing together of the uterosacral ligaments or by obliterating the cul-de-sac to prevent recurrences.

Postmenopausal Bleeding

Although postmenopausal bleeding is usually caused by benign causes, most studies show that the older the woman and further she is past menopause, the higher the probability that bleeding is caused by malignancy (42,43). Because bleeding is the most common symptom of endometrial cancer, which causes 15 percent to 20 percent of cases of postmenopausal bleeding (42–45), this and other cancers must always be looked for.

A variety of conditions can cause postmenopausal bleeding (Table 48.4). Of benign etiologies, atrophic vaginitis, cervical or endometrial polyps, atrophic endometrium, and endometrial hyperplasia are the most common. Although atrophic vaginitis is the most common etiology found in some research series (46,47), it is a diagnosis of exclusion. Merely finding atrophic vaginitis on pelvic examination does not confirm that it is the cause of bleeding. Evaluation of bleeding thought to be caused by atrophic vaginitis requires vaginal cytology and endometrial biopsy if the woman's uterus is intact. If daily application of topical estrogen cream does not eradicate the bleeding within 2 weeks, other etiologies must be considered. Similarly, although cervical polyps can also

Table 48.4 Causes of Postmenopausal Bleeding

Gynecologic	Nongynecologic
Benign	
Vulvar lesion	Gastrointestinal
Vaginitis	Urinary tract
Atrophic*	Caruncle
Infectious	Urethral prolapse
Cervicitis	Hematuria
Cervical polyps*	
Endometrial atrophy*	
Endometrial hyperplasia*	
Leimyomata	
Endometritis	
Erosion of prolapsed vagina, cervix, uterus	
Malignant	
Vulvar carcinoma	
Vaginal carcinoma	
Cervical carcinoma*	
Uterine adenocarcinoma*	
Uterine sarcoma	
Tubal carcinoma	
Ovarian carcinoma	

*Most common etiology.

bleed, as can uterine fibroids on rare occasions, their presence does not obviate the need for more thorough assessment, including Pap smear and endometrial sampling. The practitioner should also remember that endometrial polyps are associated with cancer, usually of the endometrium, in as much as 15 percent of cases (48).

It can be difficult to ascertain solely from the patient's history whether bleeding is vaginal or from other sites; therefore, initial evaluation always requires a careful pelvic examination, a rectal examination including test for fecal occult blood, and urinalysis. Sometimes examination of undergarments is useful. The possibility of coagulapathies also should be considered.

Careful visual inspection of the vulva, vagina, and cervix is the first step in evaluation of postmenopausal bleeding, along with biopsy of suspicious lesions. A Pap smear of the cervix, or in absence of a cervix, of the vaginal wall, should be performed. Appropriate cultures for sexually transmitted diseases should be obtained, and vaginal discharge evaluated for infections such as trichomonas, which can cause a bloody discharge.

Evaluation of the endometrium should be done for all cases of postmenopausal vaginal bleeding in which the patient's uterus is intact. A Pap smear alone is not sufficient because the sensitivity of the Pap smear for detecting endometrial cancer is only 18 percent to 66 percent (26,44,45). Several devices are available for outpatient endometrial biopsy, such as the Vabra aspirator and the endometrial Pipelle, both of which have a sensitivity rate of 89 percent to 95 percent for detection of endometrial pathology (26,45,49). A pelvic ultrasound should be obtained if any pelvic masses are palpated, or if the endometrium cannot be sampled because of cervical stenosis. Transvaginal ultrasonography findings of a uniform endometrial thickness of 5 mm or less is considered an appropriate cutoff for conservative management of postmenopausal bleeding (31,49).

D&C should be reserved for the following indications: 1) nondiagnostic office endometrial sampling; 2) technical barriers to office sampling, such as cervical stenosis; and 3) patients requiring examination under anesthesia for diagnosis and management of the problem, including women with heavy uterine bleeding (26,45). Unfortunately, the sensitivity of D&C for diagnosis of endometrial cancer is not 100 percent. Although hysteroscopy, in which the endometrial cavity is visualized directly to guide biopsies, is a promising procedure, randomized trials are needed to demonstrate its superiority to D&C (26,50).

Gynecologic Malignancies

Persons older than 65 years of age have a one in five chance of developing cancer, and 50 percent of all cancer deaths occur in persons older than age 65. Moreover, the death rate from cancer in persons older than age 65 is increasing, with those 85 years and older at highest risk of death from cancer.

As a person ages, not only does the incidence of gynecologic cancers rise, but also cancers of the endometrium, cervix, ovary and vulva are diagnosed at a more advanced stage (2,51). Epidemiologic data suggest that at least some of the delay in diagnosis is related to lack of gynecologic examinations (2).

One study of gynecologic cancer in women age 75 years and older found the following diagnoses: cancer of the endometrium, 36 percent, invasive cervical cancer, 25 percent, cancer of the vulva, 19 percent, ovarian cancer, 12 percent, and vaginal cancer, 7 percent (51). 1992 data showed ovarian cancer to be the leading cause of death from gynecologic cancer in women age 75 years and older, following deaths from carcinoma of the colon or rectum, lung, breast and pancreas (3). A key health promotion goal for the year 2000 identified by the U.S. Department of Health and Human Services (52) is:

> Increase to at least 95 percent the proportion of women aged 70 and older with uterine cervix who have ever received a Pap test, and to at least 70 percent those who received a Pap test within the preceding 1 to 3 years (Baseline: 76 percent "ever" and 44 percent "within the preceding 3 years" in 1987).

Endometrial Cancer

Three-quarters of cases of endometrial cancer occur in postmenopausal women, with peak incidence in the sixth and seventh decades. It is the most common gynecologic cancer in the United States. The lifetime probability of a 50-year old woman developing it is 2.6 percent (23). Although most cases are diagnosed at stage I and are well differentiated or moderately well differentiated in grade, endometrial cancer is not a benign disease. Five-year survival is 75 percent overall, with black women having only a 53 percent 5-year survival rate (53); and mortality increases with advancing age (54).

Identified risk factors for endometrial cancer are primarily chronic, unopposed estrogen stimulation and associated conditions, such as early menarche, nulliparity, or late menopause. Estrogen can either be endogenous, as in obesity, in which adipose tissue conversion of ovarian and adrenal androgen increases estrone levels, or exogenous, as in ERT or use of digoxin or spironolactone, which can exert estrogenic effects. Other risks are history of pelvic radiation therapy, family history of endometrial cancer, and personal history of cancer of the ovary or breast.

The relative risk for endometrial cancer in women who have ever received estrogen compared with those who have never used it is 2.31 (23). The risk increases with dose and duration of use, with relative risk increasing to 4.5 after 5 or more years of unopposed estrogen at a daily dose of 0.625 mg (23). However, the addition of progestins for 12 to 13 days monthly eradicates the increased risk. Tamoxifen, possessing both estrogen-agonist and estrogen-antagonist effects, also has been shown to be a risk factor for endometrial cancer when used as adjunctive treatment for breast cancer (55,56).

Endometrial hyperplasia results from chronic, unopposed estrogen stimulation and develops in as much as 40 percent of women who take unopposed estrogen (23). Adenomatous hyperplasia with atypia is a premalignant state, with 25 percent to 30 percent progression to carcinoma within 10 years (57). Adenomatous hyperplasia with atypia may regress with progesterone therapy, but progestin-treated women, especially if obese, warrant close follow-up for development of endometrial cancer. Although approximately 30 percent of endometrial cancers can be attributed to hyperplasia and estrogen use, most endometrial cancers are found in an atrophic endometrium (57).

Bleeding or spotting is the most common symptom of endometrial cancer and is seen in 90 percent of cases (54). A purulent vaginal discharge from pyometra is occasionally a presenting symptom. Although Pap smears are an insensitive screening technique, presence of endometrial cells on cervical cytology in the postmenopausal woman is suspicious for uterine carcinoma. Studies have found from 1 percent to 11 percent incidence of carcinoma in women with typical endometrial cells on Pap smear, a 16 percent incidence with presence of atypical cells, and a 63 percent incidence with presence of suspicious cells (58,59).

In the asymptomatic woman, no screening approaches have been shown to be cost-effective for detection of endometrial cancer. However, annual endometrial sampling should be considered for high-risk patients, including postmenopausal women receiving unopposed exogenous estrogen, obese women (particularly those with a family history of endometrial cancer), and women receiving tamoxifen prophylaxis. In elderly women with a stenosed cervix, office endometrial sampling may be technically difficult and require a D&C.

Ovarian Cancer

Ovarian cancer has the highest fatality rate of all gynecologic cancers. Data from the Surveillance, Epidemiology, and End Results Program of the National Cancer Institute (SEER) show that peak incidence rates occur between the ages of 60 and 85 years, with maximum rate of 54 per 100,000 population in the group 75 to 79 years of age (60). Age is adversely associated with stage, with a disproportionate number of advanced stage cases diagnosed in women older than age 65 (60,61). Overall, the 5-year survival rate is 40 percent, with survival approaching 90 percent for women whose disease is confined to the ovary at diagnosis but dropping to 28 percent to 33 percent for the two-thirds of women whose disease is diagnosed at an advanced stage (62).

Over 95 percent of ovarian malignancies diagnosed after the patient is age 65 are epithelial tumors (61). Risk factors for ovarian cancer are advanced age; nulliparity; a personal history of endometrial, colon, or breast cancer; and a family history of ovarian cancer. Although the most important risk for ovarian cancer is family history in a first-degree relative, only 7 percent of ovarian cancers are familial (62). Pregnancy, any use and duration of use of oral contraceptives, and tubal ligation are associated with a decreased risk for developing this malignancy (62,63). In addition to early-stage diagnosis, independent prognostic factors are age, functional status, postoperative tumor burden, tumor grade, and histologic type (64).

Because ovarian cancer is often minimally symptomatic in its early stages, most patients have widespread disease at time of diagnosis. It is unusual, however, for ovarian cancer to be completely asymptomatic. Many women have had vague abdominal complaints for long periods of time before the diagnosis is made. Other presenting symptoms are nonspecific, such as fatigue, anorexia, and weight loss. Paraneoplastic syndromes are rarely the presenting symptom. They include a syndrome of cerebellar degeneration (65). The ovary is the recipient of metastases from a variety of malignancies. Breast and colon cancers are most likely to spread to the ovary.

Currently, there is no evidence to support mass screening for ovarian cancer, nor is there data demonstrating that screening reduces mortality in high-risk women, such as those with two or more afflicted first-degree relatives (62,66). CA-125 and transvaginal ultrasound are the most effective screening methods currently available (62,67). Pelvic examination is a poor screening test because ovarian malignancies usually have disseminated by the time they are palpable. Transvaginal ultrasound, using pooled data, has a sensitivity of 85 percent and a specificity of 93.8 percent for detection of cancer, with specificity likely to improve with addition of the color-flow Doppler technique (62,67). The specificity of the CA-125 radioimmunoassay for detecting ovarian cancer in postmenopausal women is better than 99 percent if the cutoff value of more than 35 U/mL is used, but the sensitivity for detecting stage I disease ranges from 25 percent to 75 percent (62). Prospective studies for mass screening using combined modalities are in progress.

Numerous studies have demonstrated a treatment bias toward elderly patients, who are less likely to receive optimal treatment than are their younger counterparts. In part this discrepancy can be explained by the presence of comorbid conditions, but bias against use of more aggressive therapy in older patients with ovarian cancer also appears to be a factor (64). Several studies, however, have shown that most elderly patients can tolerate both aggressive chemotherapeutic regimens and surgery (64,68,69).

Cervical Cancer

Invasive cervical cancer is a disease of older women, with 27 percent of new cases diagnosed after the patient is age 65 and 44 percent of deaths occurring after the woman is

60 years of age. The mean age at diagnosis is 52.2 years, with a bimodal distribution peaking at both 35 to 39 years of age and 60 to 64 years of age. Although the 5-year survival rate is 90 percent for women with localized cervical cancer, the rate drops to about 40 percent for women with advanced disease. Increased mortality for older women is thought to be a result of the disease being diagnosed at a more advanced stage in older women.

The high incidence of invasive cervical cancer in older women is clearly associated with lack of regular cytologic screening, and the decline in age-adjusted cancer deaths in the past 30 years is largely attributable to the use of the Pap test (8,61,70–72). More than half of women diagnosed with invasive cervical cancer have not received a Pap test within the previous 3 years (73). Those at highest risk for lack of Pap smear screening are the elderly and persons of low socioeconomic status. In addition to lack of screening, risk factors for invasive disease include early sexual activity, multiple sexual partners, lack of use of barrier contraception, genital infections (in particular, certain oncogenic types of the human papilloma virus), acquired immunodeficiency syndrome (AIDS), and cigarette smoking (carcinogenic by-products of cigarette smoking can be found in cervical mucus) (11,72,74–77). Hispanic, African American, and Native American women have higher incidence of invasive cervical cancer than do other nationalities, in part because of inadequate screening (9,72,74,78,79). Chronic pessary use is rarely a cause of cervical cancer in elderly women, but can occur after prolonged use (80).

Women with preinvasive disease are usually asymptomatic, but those with invasive cancer may have symptoms of bleeding or persistent vaginal discharge. Use of Pap smears for screening can detect early cancers, but unfortunately, the Pap smear becomes a less reliable test for older women. Although the prevalence of abnormal Pap smears increases with age, both the number of abnormal Pap smears that indicate invasive carcinoma and the number of false-positives rises (53,61).

Abnormal nonneoplastic Pap smears in the postmenopausal woman can be classified in two etiologic groups: infectious, and reactive or reparative. The former manifests as atypical squamous cells on Pap smear and is usually caused by organisms such as candidiasis or trichomonas. With appropriate treatment, the smear should normalize by 3 or 4 months. The latter causes atypical or dysplastic cells on Pap smear, and is associated with such conditions as inflammation, atrophy, chemotherapy, or radiation changes. Because atrophy is such a common condition in the elderly woman, the initial approach to a Pap smear demonstrating atypia in a woman with atrophic vaginitis and no obvious pathologic lesions is treatment with topical estrogen cream for 3 or 4 weeks and repeating the smear. If atypia or dysplasia persists with treatment, colposcopy is necessary because atypical squamous cells are associated with cervical intraepithelial neoplasia (CIN) in 19 percent to 30 percent of cases, and CIN is found with dysplasia in as much as 90 percent of cases (81).

A less common finding is endocervical glandular atypia, intermediate between reactive changes and CIN. Endocervical atypia requires colposcopic assessment because dysplasia, CIN, or invasive malignancy is found in as much as 50 percent of cases (81). Endometrial cells found on Pap smear, even if not atypical, require assessment of the uterus because of the likelihood of underlying endometrial hyperplasia or cancer (58).

False-negative Pap smears also become increasingly common with age, in part because of errors in Pap smear technique (such as inability to sample endocervical cells in the geriatric patient), and in part because of laboratory error. Even in the best of laboratories and with a correctly obtained sample, the false-negative rate for cervical pathology is about 5 percent (82).

Cytologic screening is less accurate for invasive disease than it is for premalignant conditions or carcinoma in situ because of the presence of associated conditions such as inflammation, necrosis, and bleeding. 20% to 50% of patients with invasive disease have negative Pap smears (82). Therefore, suspicious lesions of the cervix require biopsy, even if the Pap smear is normal. Colposcopic evaluation of the cervix should be performed for 1) preinvasive changes on Pap smear, such as dysplasia or low-grade CIN; and 2) two Pap smears taken 3 to 6 months apart that show inflammatory or atypical changes after appropriate management. Multiple colposcopically directed biopsies of abnormal areas should be taken, along with a curetting of the endocervical canal (ECC). Aging changes may prevent adequate colposcopy in elderly women and require careful ECC by surgical technique or by loop electrosurgical excision procedure (LEEP) (76).

The consensus of current cervical cancer screening recommendations is that all women, regardless of age, who have not had previous Pap smears undergo Pap smears every 1 to 3 years. An analysis of the efficacy of Pap smears in elderly women concluded that triennial screening reduced mortality at a cost of $2254 per year of life saved, which is comparable to the cost of influenza and pneumococcal vaccination programs in persons aged 65 and older (73). Medicare added a triennial screening Pap smear benefit in 1990 (72).

Women aged 65 to 70 years who have had normal Pap smears every 1 to 3 years, and within the past 10 years, develop cervical cancer very rarely; Pap smears may be discontinued for this group (83,84). Some advocate discontinuing screening at an earlier age. A recent Scottish retrospective case analysis of women with CIN, microinvasive, or invasive cancer of the cervix found no cases of CIN in women older than age 50 who had received triennial Pap smears since early adulthood (10). Disadvantaged groups that have had little access to health care services need special targeting efforts. An analysis of the cost-effectiveness of cervical cancer screening for low-income, elderly urban women found a single Pap smear to be cost-effective in terms of saving lives (85).

It is important to remember that women with a cervical stump after hysterectomy must follow the same Pap smear schedule guidelines. In one research series, more than 5 percent of cervical cancer cases, most of which were invasive, were found in the cervical stump (86).

Cancer of the Vulva

Invasive cancer of the vulva accounts for 4 percent of gynecologic cancers. More than 95 percent of vulvar cancer is the squamous cell type; more unusual malignancies of the vulva include malignant melanoma. Invasive squamous cell carcinoma is a disease primarily of older women, with mean age at diagnosis for stage I and stage III at 65 and 71 years of age, respectively. A secondary primary malignancy affecting the cervix, breast, or uterus is found in about 15 percent of the cases.

VIN is usually a disease of younger women. It is diagnosed on biopsy by the presence of definite mitoses seen above the basal cellular layer. The natural history of VIN has been regression in most patients (87); however, an association of VIN with smoking, presence of human papilloma virus (HPV), and sexual history has been described in women with invasive vulvar squamous cell cancer (88). The association of VIN, HPV, and invasive vulvar squamous carcinomas also confers risk for other genital primary neoplasms (89).

Additional risks for invasive vulvar squamous cancer pertinent to the elderly woman are vulvar epithelial hyperplasia or atrophy, with or without cellular atypia (88). Symptoms of pruritus, a lump or ulcer, or dysuria usually herald the diagnosis.

Treatment for invasive carcinoma of the vulva in the past was radical vulvectomy, with distressingly negative psychosexual consequences. Since the 1980s, good results for early-stage invasive disease have been achieved with radical local excision (87,90). Size of the lesion and lymph node status are independent prognostic variables, with excellent prognosis when groin nodes are uninvolved and lesion diameter is 2 cm or less (91). Combined modality approaches using chemotherapy and radiotherapy are being studied for patients with more advanced disease, with the goal of achieving good survival rates and avoiding extensive radical surgery (87). The overall 5-year survival rate for operable cases is 70 percent, with the rate falling to 50 percent or less if the patient has two or more positive nodes (87).

Paget's disease of the vulva is seen in patients aged 60 years and older. The lesion characteristically presents as white islands of hyperkeratosis over a bright red base. Often there is a history of pruritus vulvae. Because the patient may have an underlying invasive cancer, the lesion must be biopsied down to the fascia. Ten percent to 25 percent of these lesions are associated with current or previous adenocarcinoma elsewhere, most commonly in the breast.

Vaginal Cancer

Invasive carcinoma of the vagina is very rare, comprising 1 percent to 3.6 percent of gynecologic malignancies. Vaginal intraepithelial neoplasia (VaIN), although even less common, is being diagnosed more frequently because of more widespread use of cytological screening and vaginal colposcopy. Mean age of patients at diagnosis is

50 years of age, but cases have been seen in very elderly women. Lesions may be unifocal or multifocal and may occur at the same time on the cervix and vulva. Both invasive vaginal cancer and VaIN are associated with hysterectomy performed for benign conditions or for neoplastic disease, particularly CIN (92,93). Abnormal vaginal cytology may be seen within 1 year of hysterectomy for CIN; with no history of CIN, the average time in which the patient develops an abnormal Pap smear is 11 years (93). Most cases of VaIN are silent and require cytologic screening for diagnosis. In one study of 32 patients with VaIN, 28 percent were subsequently diagnosed with invasive vaginal cancer (93).

Treatment for VaIN can be carried out by excisional biopsy, CO_2 laser, cryotherapy, or intravaginal 5-fluorouracil (5-FU) cream. The latter is indicated for treatment of extensive lesions that involve much of the vaginal epithelium or for multifocal lesions such as those seen with HPV infection (92). It is important to protect the vulva during this treatment, because leakage of topical 5-FU onto the vulva can cause ulceration. Vaginectomy and radiotherapy are treatment options for invasive cancer.

Major Gynecologic Surgical Procedures

Disorders of the female genital organs are certainly not among the major causes of death, but they give rise to important illnesses that produce discomfort and disability, and they therefore warrant treatment.

Medical advances in diagnosis and treatment and better understanding of physiologic and pathophysiologic processes in the elderly now justify the performance of major operations in this age group. Numerous reports have shown that age alone does not contraindicate surgery. Both vaginal hysterectomy for benign conditions and major gynecological cancer surgery can often be successfully performed in very elderly women (68,69,94). The physician should remember that sexual activity in some women continues into very old age; therefore, surgery should be performed with this factor in mind, particularly gynecologic cancer surgery, which is often followed by sexual dysfunction (53).

As the population ages, women who no longer accept age alone as a barrier to active life will request more elective surgery. Contraindications to surgical intervention should not include chronologic age as the sole basis for exclusion of surgery.

References

1. Barber HRK. Perimenopausal and geriatric gynecology. New York: Macmillan, 1988.
2. Grover SA, Cook EF, Adam J, et al. Delayed diagnosis of gynecologic tumors in elderly women: relation to national medical practice patterns. Am J Med 1989;86:151–157.
3. Boring CC, Squires TS, Tong T. Cancer statistics, 1992. Cancer 1992;42:19–38.
4. Byyny RL, Speroff L, eds. A clinical guide for the care of older women. Baltimore: Williams & Wilkins, 1990.
5. Lerner DJ, Kannel WB. Patterns of coronary heart disease morbidity and mortality in the sexes: a 26-year follow-up of the Framingham population. Am Heart J 1986;11:383–390.
6. McGovern PG, Folsom AR, Sprafka JM, et al. Trends in survival of hospitalized myocardial infarction patients between 1970 and 1985: the Minnesota Heart Survey. Circulation 1992; 85:172–179.
7. Carlson KJ, Nichols DH, Schiff I. Indications for hysterectomy. N Engl J Med 1993;328:856–860.
8. Mandelblatt J, Gopaul I, Wistreich M. Gynecological care of elderly women: another look at Papanicolaou testing. JAMA 1986;256:367–71.
9. Mandelblatt J, Traxler M, Lakin P, et al. Breast and cervical cancer screening of poor, elderly, black women: clinical results and implications. Harlem Study Team. Am J Prev Med 1993;9:133–138.
10. Wijngaarden WJ, Duncan ID. Rationale for stopping cervical screening in women over 50. BMJ 1993;306:967–971.
11. Mandelblatt J. Cervical cancer screening in primary care: issues and recommendations. Prim Care 1989;16:133–150.
12. Koss LG. The Papanicolaou test for cervical cancer detection: a triumph and a tragedy. JAMA 1989;261:737–743.
13. King A, Clay K, Felmar E, et al. The Papanicolaou smear. West J Med 1992;156:202–204.
14. Kronenberg F. Hot flashes: epidemiology and physiology. Ann NY Acad Sci 1990;592:52–86.
15. Ridley CM, Frankman O, Jones I, et al. New nomenclature for vulvar disease: International Society for the Study of Vulvar Disease. Hum Pathol 1989;20:495–496.
16. Soper JT, Creasman WT. Vulvar dystrophies. Clin Obstet Gynecol 1986;29:431–439.
17. Leiblum S, Bachmann G, Kemmann E, et al. Vaginal atrophy in the postmenopausal woman. JAMA 1983;249:2195–2198.
18. Walsh B, Schiff I. Vasomotor flushes. Ann NY Acad Sci 1990;592:346–355.
19. Loprinzi CL, Michalak JC, Quella SK, et al. Megestrol acetate for the prevention of hot flashes. N Engl J Med 1994;331:347–352
20. Belchetz P. Hormonal treatment of postmenopausal women. N Engl J Med 1994;330:1062–1071.

21. Raz R, Stamm W. A controlled trial of intravaginal estriol in postmenopausal women with recurrent urinary tract infections. N Engl J Med 1993;329:753–756.

22. Lobo RA, Speroff L. International consensus conference on postmenopausal hormone therapy and the cardiovascular system. Fertil Steril 1994;61:592–595.

23. Grady D, Rubin SM, Petitti DB, et al. Hormone therapy to prevent disease and prolong life in postmenopausal women. Ann Intern Med 1992;117:1016–1037.

24. Dupont WD, Page DL. Estrogen therapy and breast cancer. Arch Intern Med 1991;151:67–72.

25. Steinberg KK, Thacker SB, Smith SJ, et al. A meta-analysis of the effect of estrogen replacement therapy on the risk of breast cancer. JAMA 1991;265:1985–1990.

26. Chambers JT, Chambers SK. Endometrial sampling: when? where? why? with what? Clin Obstet Gynecol 1992;35:28–39.

27. American College of Physicians. Guidelines for counseling postmenopausal women about preventive hormone therapy. Ann Intern Med 1992;117:1038–1041.

28. VanBogaert L-J. Clinicopathologic findings in endometrial polyps. Obstet Gynecol 1988;71:771–773.

29. Soper DE. Pelvic masses. In: Shingleton HM, Hutt WG, eds. Postreproductive gynecology. New York: Churchill Livingstone, 1990:259–275.

30. Creasman WT, Soper JT. The undiagnosed adnexal mass after the menopause. Clin Obstet Gynecol 1986;29:446–452.

31. Nasri MN, Coast GJ. Correlation of ultrasound findings and endometrial histopathology in postmenopausal women. Br J Obstet Gynecol 1989;96:1333–1338.

32. Rulin MC, Preston AL. Adnexal masses in postmenopausal women. Obstet Gynecol 1987;70:578–581.

33. Goldstein SR, Subramanyam B, Snyder JR, et al. The postmenopausal cystic adnexal mass: the potential role of ultrasound in conservative management. Obstet Gynecol 1989;73:8–10.

34. Lin JY, Angel C, DuBeshter B, Walsh CJ. Diagnosis after laparotomy for a mass in the pelvic area in women. Surg Gynecol Obstet 1993;176:333–338.

35. Finkler NJ, Benacerraf B, Lavin PT, et al. Comparison of serum CA 125, clinical impression, and ultrasound in the preoperative evaluation of ovarian masses. Obstet Gynecol 1988;72:659–663.

36. Killackey MA, Neuwirth RS. Evaluation and management of the pelvic mass: a review of 540 cases. Obstet Gynecol 1988;71:319–322.

37. Van Nagell JR, DePriest PD, Gallion HH, Pavlick EJ. Ovarian cancer screening. Cancer 1993;71:1523–1528.

38. Hoffman M, Molpus K, Roberts WS, et al. Tuboovarian abscess in postmenopausal women. J Repro Med 1990;35:525–528.

39. Adkins RB Jr, Scott HW, eds. Surgical care for the elderly. Baltimore: Williams & Wilkins, 1988.

40. Jay GD, Kinkead T, Hopkins T, Wollin M. Obstructive uropathy from uterine prolapse: a preventable problem in the elderly. J Am Geriatr Soc 1992;40:1156–1160.

41. Zeitlin MP, Lebherz TB. Pessaries in the geriatric patient. J Am Geriatr Soc 1992;40:635–639.

42. Schindler AE, Schmidt G. Post-menopausal bleeding: a study of more than 1000 cases. Maturitas 1980;2:269–274.

43. Pacheco JC, Kempers RD. Etiology of postmenopausal bleeding. Obstet Gynecol 1968;32:40–46.

44. Fortier KJ. Postmenopausal bleeding and the endometrium. Clin Obstet Gynecol 1986;29:440–445.

45. Merrill JA. Management of postmenopausal bleeding. Clin Obstet Gynecol 1981;24:285–299.

46. Dewhurst J. Postmenopausal bleeding from benign causes. Clin Obstet Gynecol 1983;26:769–776.

47. Gambrell RD. Postmenopausal bleeding. J Am Geriatr Soc 1974;22:337–343.

48. Peterson WF, Novak ER. Endometrial polyps. Obstet Gynecol 1956;6:40–49.

49. Deppe G, Malviya VK. Uterine neoplasms. In: Hajj SN, Evans WJ, eds. Clinical postreproductive gynecology. Norwalk, CT: Appleton & Lange, 1993:189–199.

50. Downes E, Al-Azzawi F. The predictive value of outpatient hysteroscopy in a menopause clinic. Br J Obstet Gyn 1993;100:1148–1149.

51. Kennedy AE, Flagg JS, Webster KD. Gynecologic cancer in the very elderly. Gynecol Oncol 1989;32:49–54.

52. Department of Health and Human Services. Healthy People 2000: National Health Promotion and Disease Prevention Objectives. DHHS Publ. No. (PHS)91-50212. Washington, DC: U.S. Government Printing Office, 1991.

53. Shingleton HM, Alvarez RD. The role of the general gynecologist in cancer care. In: Shingleton HM, Hurt WG, eds. Postreproductive gynecology. New York: Churchill Livingstone, 1990:277–299.

54. McGonigle KF, Lagasse LD, Karlan BY. Ovarian, uterine and cervical cancer in the elderly woman. Clin Geriatr Med 1993;9:115–130.

55. Van Leeuwen FE, Benraadt J, Coebergh JWW, et al. Risk of endometrial cancer after tamoxifen treatment of breast cancer. Lancet 1994;343:448–452.

56. Fornander T, Rutqvist LE, Cedermark B, et al. Adjuvant tamoxifen in early breast cancers: occurrence of new primary cancers. Lancet 1989;1:117–120.

57. Richards-Kustan CJ, Kase NG. Diagnosis and management of perimenopausal and postmenopausal bleeding. Obstet Gynecol Clin North Am 1987;14:169–189.

58. Yancey M, Magelssen D, Demaurez A, Lee RB. Classification of endometrial cells on cervical cytology. Obstet Gynecol 1990;76:1000–1005.

59. Cherkis RC, Patten SF, Andrews TJ, et al. Significance of normal endometrial cells detected by cervical cytology. Obstet Gynecol 1988;71:242–244.

60. Yancik R, Ries LG, Yates JW. Ovarian cancer in the elderly: an analysis of Surveillance, Epidemiology, and End Results Program data. Am J Obstet Gynecol 1986;154:639–647.

61. Weintraub NT, Freedman ML. Gynecologic malignancies of the elderly. Clin Geriatr Med 1987;3:669–692.

62. Carlson KJ, Skates SJ, Singer DE. Screening for ovarian cancer. Ann Intern Med 1994;121:124–132.
63. Hankinson SE, Hunter DJ, Colditz GA, et al. Tubal ligation, hysterectomy, and risk of ovarian cancer: a prospective study. JAMA 1993;270:2813–2818.
64. Marchetti DL, Hreshchyshyn MM. Is ovarian cancer undertreated in older women? Drugs Aging 1994;5:81–84.
65. Scully RE, Mark EJ, McNeely WF, NcNeely BU, eds. Case records of the Massachusetts General Hospital: Case 34–1989. N Engl J Med 1989;321:524–534.
66. American College of Physicians. Screening for ovarian cancer: recommendations and rationale. Ann Intern Med 1994;121:141–142.
67. Van Nagell JR, DePriest PD, Gallion HH, Pavlik EJ. Ovarian cancer screening. Cancer 1993;71:1523–1528.
68. Kirschner CV, DeSerto TM, Isaacs JH. Surgical treatment of the elderly patient with gynecologic cancer. Surg Gynecol Obstet 1990;170:379–384.
69. Lawton FG, Hacker NF. Surgery for invasive gynecologic cancer in the elderly female population. Obstet Gynecol 1990;76:287–289.
70. Fletcher A. Screening for cancer of the cervix in elderly women. Lancet 1990;335:95–99.
71. Power EJ. Pap smears, elderly women, and Medicare. Cancer Invest 1993;11:164–168.
72. Fahs MC, Mandelblatt J, Schechter C, Muller C. Cost effectiveness of cervical cancer screening for the elderly. Ann Intern Med 1992;117:520–527.
73. Nasca PC, Ellish N, Caputo TA, et al. An epidemiologic study of Pap screening histories in women with invasive carcinomas of the uterine cervix. NY State J Med 1991;91:152–156.
74. Devesa SS, Young JL, Brinton LA, Fraumeni JF. Recent trends in cervix uteri cancer. Cancer 1989;64:2184–2190.
75. El-Sadr W, Oleske JM, Agins BD, et al. Clinical practice guideline: Evaluation and management of early HIV infection. AHCPR Publ. No. 94-0572. Washington, DC: U.S. Department of Health and Human Services Agency for Health Care Policy and Research, 1994.
76. Ferenczy A. Management of the patient with an abnormal Papanicoloaou test. Obstet Gynecol Clin North Am 1993;20:189–202.
77. Peters RK, Thomas D, Hagan DG, et al. Risk factors for invasive cervical cancer among Latinos and non-Latinos in Los Angeles County. J Natl Cancer Inst 1986;77:1063–1077.
78. Becker TM, Wheeler CM, Key CR, Samet JM. Cervical cancer incidence and mortality in New Mexico's Hispanics, American Indians, and non-Hispanic whites. West J Med 1992;156:376–379.
79. Trapido EJ, Chen F, Davis K, et al. Cancer in South Florida Hispanic women. Arch Intern Med 1994;154:1083–1088.
80. Schraub S, Sun XS, Maingon PH, et al. Cervical and vaginal cancer associated with pessary use. Cancer 1992;69:2505–2509.
81. Goff BA, Atanasoff P, Brown E, et al. Endocervical glandular atypia in Papanicoloaou smears. Obstet Gynecol 1992;79:101–104.
82. Koss LG. Cervical (Pap) smear: new directions. Cancer 1993;71:1406–1412.
83. Clinical Practice Committee. Screening for cervical carcinoma in elderly women. J Am Geriatr Soc 1989;37:885–887.
84. Miller AB, Anderson G, Brisson J, et al. Report of a national workshop on screening for cancer of the cervix. Can Med Assoc J 1991;145:1301–1325.
85. Mandelblatt JS, Fahs MC. The cost-effectiveness of cervical cancer screening for low-income elderly women. JAMA 1988;259:2409–2413.
86. Barillot I, Horiot JC, Cuisenier J, et al. Carcinoma of the cervical stump: a review of 213 cases. Eur J Cancer 1993;29A:1231–1236.
87. Farias-Eisner R, Berek JS. Current management of invasive squamous carcinoma of the vulva. Clin Geriatr Med 1993;9:131–143.
88. Anderson WA, Franquemont DW, William J, et al. Vulvar squamous cell carcinoma and papillomaviruses: two separate entities? Am J Obstet Gynecol 1991;165:329–336.
89. Mitchell MF, Prasad CJ, Silva EG, et al. Second genital primary squamous neoplasms in vulvar carcinoma: viral and histopathologic correlates. Obstet Gynecol 1993;81:13–18.
90. Hacker NF, Van der Velden J. Conservative management of early vulvar cancer. Cancer 1993;71:1673–1677.
91. Homesley HD, Bundy BN, Sedlis A, et al. Assessment of current International Federation of Gynecology and Obstetrics staging of vulvar carcinoma relative to prognostic factors for survival. Am J Obstet Gynecol 1991;164:997–1004.
92. Audet-LaPointe, Body G, Vauclair R, et al. Vaginal intraepithelial neoplasia. Gynecol Surg 1990;36:232–239.
93. Ireland D, Monaghan JM. The management of the patient with abnormal vaginal cytology following hysterectomy. Br J Obstet Gynecol 1988;95:973–975.
94. Nahhas WA, Brown M. Gynecologic surgery in the aged. J Repro Med 1990;35:550–554.

Chapter 49
Common Gastrointestinal Diseases

Randall E. Lee and William R. Brown

Avoid fried meats which angry up the blood. If your stomach disputes you, lie down and pacify it with cool thoughts. Keep the juices flowing by jangling around gently as you move. Go very light on the vices, such as carrying on in society. The social ramble ain't restful. Avoid running at all times. Don't look back. Someone might be gaining on you.

Leroy (Satchel) Paige
Prescription for staying young
Collier's, June 13, 1953

Diseases of the digestive system are among the most common diseases of the elderly. According to one study 27 percent of elderly patients admitted to hospitals as medical emergencies had major diseases of the digestive system, and 42 percent of those with chronic illness had important digestive disorders. Although no digestive disease is unique to the elderly, several have more severe consequences for this age group or their frequency increases in persons with advancing age.

Advancing age may bring changes in all major functions of the digestive tract, but elderly patients' abdominal symptoms ordinarily should not be ascribed to age alone. In particular, symptoms that suggest the irritable bowel syndrome occurring for the first time in advanced age or changes in the pattern of bowel movements should not be dismissed as functional or psychosomatic in origin before a thorough search for organic illness has been conducted.

The dramatic improvements in the capabilities and safety of gastrointestinal endoscopy now allow physicians to provide elderly patients with endoscopic therapy for diseases that previously required more expensive and dangerous surgical procedures. For example, endoscopic hemostasis therapy for severe upper gastrointestinal bleeding does not have an increased complication rate when performed in the elderly and is considered to be first-line therapy in many hospitals (1). Similarly, endoscopic laser therapy or placement of a stent is now an accepted nonsurgical alternative for the palliation of an obstructing esophageal, biliary, or colonic malignancy in high-surgical-risk patients. Nevertheless, because procedure-related complications may have more serious consequences in the elderly, the risks and benefits of an endoscopic procedure should always be assessed before performing the procedure.

Dysphagia

The symptom of dysphagia, difficulty with swallowing, should never be dismissed as a functional consequence of aging until organic pathology has been excluded from diagnostic consideration. Indeed, *presbyesophagus*, a term describing a complex that includes increased frequency of nonpropulsive esophageal tertiary contractions and decreased peristaltic contraction amplitudes, is now believed to have little clinical significance (2).

In general, dysphagia may be divided into two subtypes: oropharyngeal (transfer) dysphagia and esophageal dysphagia. Oropharyngeal dysphagia results from a mechanical obstruction in the oropharynx or from a disruption in the complex neuromuscular pathways linking the brain, tongue, pharynx, and upper esophageal sphincter. It is typically manifest by an inability to transfer the food bolus from the oropharynx into the proximal esophagus. Attempts to initiate a swallow result in aspiration, coughing, or regurgitation through the nose. Thin liquids may be more troublesome than soft solids. Clinical conditions that commonly are associated with mechanical oropharyngeal dysphagia in the elderly are reduced compliance of the upper esophageal sphincter (cricopharyngeal achalasia), hypopharyngeal (Zenker's) diverticulum, and cancers of the head and neck. Clinical conditions that commonly are associated with neuromuscular oropharyngeal dysphagia in the elderly are stroke, amyotrophic lateral sclerosis, myasthenia gravis, and Parkinson's disease. A videofluoroscopic, barium-swallowing study usually will provide sufficient evidence to confirm clinical diagnosis of oropharyngeal dysphagia. Consultation with a speech therapist often is helpful for the palliation of early symptoms of oropharyngeal dysphagia. The progression of dysphagia symptoms may warrant consideration of a gastrostomy tube.

The causes of esophageal dysphagia can usually be categorized as those that impair the propulsive motility of the esophageal body or those that produce a mechanical obstruction. Patients with impaired esophageal motility, such as that caused by achalasia, may provide a history of dysphagia for both solids and liquids without a clear sequence of progression. On the other hand, patients with a mechanical obstruction, such as that caused by a peptic stricture or by an esophageal carcinoma, almost always relate a progression of solid to liquid dysphagia.

The evaluation of a patient with symptoms of esophageal dysphagia generally includes a barium swallow or an esophagogastroduodenoscopy (EGD) as the initial diagnostic test. The advantage of the EGD is that biopsies and cytologic brushings of lesions that are suspicious for cancer can be obtained and immediate dilation of a symptomatic stenosis can be performed. Elderly patients who present with symptoms suggestive of a mechanical esophageal obstruction should be presumed to have esophageal carcinoma until proven otherwise.

Esophageal Food Impaction

The initial approach to food impacted in the esophagus should begin with a rapid assessment of the patient's ability to breathe, because aspiration of food or secretions may cause the situation to deteriorate rapidly. Commonly, the patient reports a story of food suddenly becoming stuck and of failed attempts to wash it down with liquids. Pharmacologic techniques to relax the esophagus include the intravenous administration of glucagon or the sublingual administration of nitroglycerin. Even if the food bolus passes spontaneously, the patient should undergo endoscopic evaluation to determine whether there is underlying esophageal pathology, such as esophageal

carcinoma or a peptic stricture. Meat tenderizer should not be used because of the risk of digesting the esophagus. Contrast radiography should not be performed; water-soluble contrast agents cause an intense pneumonitis if aspirated, and barium sulfate interferes with endoscopy (3).

Gastroesophageal Reflux Disease

The symptoms of gastroesophageal reflux disease (GERD) are very common, with some estimates indicating that more than one-third of the population of the United States regularly has "heartburn" symptoms (4). Although the prevalence of GERD in the elderly is not precisely known, the elderly may have a higher prevalence of conditions that contribute to the pathogenesis of reflux and may have a higher prevalence of GERD complications as a result of longer duration of the disease.

Conditions that predispose to reflux symptoms include inappropriate relaxation of the lower esophageal sphincter (LES), decreased saliva production, delayed gastric emptying, and the presence of a hiatal hernia. Other factors that may contribute to the severity and frequency of esophageal reflux include the use of medications such as nitrates and calcium channel blockers that lower the LES pressure, overeating, obesity, and cigarette smoking. The predominant symptom of esophageal reflux is heartburn, a burning retrosternal pain, which may be relieved by the ingestion of an antacid. Some special features of esophageal reflux in the elderly may include 1) very subtle symptoms; 2) dysphagia, secondary to an inflammatory stricture in the distal esophagus, as the predominant symptom; 3) aspiration of gastric contents, which causes coughing, wheezing, morning hoarseness, sore throat, or pulmonary infection; and 4) frequent misinterpretation of the esophageal symptoms as pain of cardiac origin.

Distinguishing between noncardiac chest pain of esophageal origin and that of ischemic heart disease origin may be as difficult as it is important (5). Classically, pain caused by esophageal reflux may be made worse by drinking coffee, tea, or acidic juices; it may be relieved by taking antacids or assuming an upright position; it usually is not exacerbated by exertion. In contrast, the typical pain caused by ischemic heart disease usually is unaffected by the composition of foods swallowed or by a change in position and is worsened by exertion. Nevertheless, the clinical history often is confusing, and both esophageal and cardiac disease may co-exist in the same patient. Therefore, a patient who complains of chest pain should first undergo an evaluation for ischemic heart disease. Making a definitive diagnosis of esophageal noncardiac chest pain may require an esophageal manometric study with acid perfusion (Bernstein test) or, if available, an ambulatory esophageal pH monitoring study (6). Esophageal abnormalities, other than GERD, that may cause angina-like chest pain include diffuse esophageal spasm (repetitive, simultaneous, nonperistaltic esophageal contractions of prolonged duration interspersed with normal contractions), and "nutcracker" esophagus (peristaltic but high-amplitude contractions and no or incomplete relaxation of the lower esophageal sphincter).

Patients who have a brief and uncomplicated history of esophageal reflux may be treated symptomatically for a period of 2 to 4 weeks without previous diagnostic study. However, a more complicated history or an inadequate response to the therapeutic trial should prompt further evaluation.

Because the barium esophagogram is not sensitive in detecting mucosal abnormalities, esophagoscopy with biopsy of the mucosa is usually the most effective study in suspected reflux esophagitis. The patient's symptoms of reflux may be more severe than visual inspection of the esophagus would suggest, so the biopsy may be necessary to establish the presence of esophagitis.

The initial treatment for GERD symptoms should consist of changes in the patient's eating habits and lifestyle patterns combined with the use of nonsystemic antacids. The basic therapy involves advising the patient to

• Eat three small meals a day and avoid between-meal snacks
• Avoid foods that decrease LES pressure (alcohol, fats, chocolate, peppermint)
• Take nothing by mouth for 3 to 4 hours before bedtime
• Elevate the head of the bed 3 to 6 inches with bricks or blocks
• Stop smoking
• Decrease dietary intake of fat and lose weight if obese.
• Avoid drugs that decrease LES pressure (progesterones, methylxanthines, anticholinergics, benzo-

diazepines, beta-adrenergic agonists, calcium channel blockers)
• Take a liquid antacid 1 and 3 hours after meals and at bedtime

Patients who do not respond to basic medical therapy should begin systemic pharmacologic therapy with an H_2 receptor antagonist (H_2RA). Many clinical trials have demonstrated that successful treatment of GERD symptoms may require a much higher dose and more frequent administration of the H_2RA than that used for treatment of peptic ulcers. For example, although 20 mg of famotidine once daily may be used to heal peptic ulcers, 20 to 40 mg of famotidine twice daily may be required to treat GERD.

The use of older prokinetic agents such as metoclopramide to treat GERD has generally fallen out of favor because of the relatively high incidence of associated side effects of these agents as well as their relatively low clinical efficacy as compared with that of H_2RAs. A newer prokinetic agent, cisapride, has a much lower incidence of central nervous system (CNS) side effects compared with metoclopramide and is more effective than placebo in healing GERD. The role of cisapride in the overall treatment of GERD remains to be determined pending the results of large randomized controlled clinical trials (7).

Severe GERD may require therapy with H^+/K^+-ATPase inhibitors, such as omeprazole. These drugs, also known as proton-pump inhibitors, irreversibly block secretion of acid by the gastric parietal cell. Proton-pump inhibitors heal erosive and ulcerative reflux esophagitis faster than do other drugs and often provide patients with GERD with the first symptomatic relief they have had in years.

GERD is considered to be a chronic disease that, if responsive to medical therapy, usually requires lifelong treatment for continued suppression of symptoms. Although the safety profile of the proton-pump inhibitors and of the H_2RAs is excellent, concerns remain about the theoretical risks to humans during long-term treatment (8,9). Antireflux surgery performed by experienced surgeons remains a useful and effective therapeutic option for patients with intractable GERD and for those who face long-term treatment with high-dose H_2RAs or proton-pump inhibitors (10). Antireflux surgery should be approached with caution in the elderly; the real risks of surgery should be weighed against the theoretical risks of continued medical therapy (11).

Peptic Ulcer Disease

Peptic ulcer disease (PUD) of the stomach and duodenum is a serious health problem for the elderly. More than half of patients hospitalized for complications from PUD are older than 60 years of age, and most deaths from PUD occur in persons older than age 65 (12). PUD in the elderly is more likely to present either with atypical or nonspecific symptoms or as a major complication, such as perforation or bleeding, without antecedent symptoms. Although the overall incidence of PUD is decreasing, the incidence of PUD in the elderly is increasing. Some factors believed to be responsible for this trend are the increased use by the elderly of nonsteroidal anti-inflammatory drugs (NSAIDs) and the increased prevalence in the elderly of gastric mucosal infection by *Helicobacter pylori*.

Use of NSAIDs is recognized as a major risk factor for the development of PUD in all age groups, but the elderly appear to be at higher risk for developing ulcers from NSAIDs. Part of this higher risk may be explained by the fact that about one-half of all NSAID prescriptions are written for patients over the age of 65 years. Other factors that may contribute to the increased risk in the elderly are the different metabolic actions of NSAIDs and the reduced amounts of mucosal prostaglandins in the elderly population. The concurrent use of NSAIDs impairs the healing of peptic ulcers by H$_2$RAs. The prostaglandin analogue, misoprostol, at a dose of 200μg four times a day, has been demonstrated to significantly reduce the 3-month incidence of both gastric and duodenal ulcers in patients who take NSAIDs for arthritis (13).

The prevalence of *H. pylori* infection of the gastric mucosa clearly increases in persons as age advances. Some studies report 80 percent to 90 percent of their study population who are older than 70 years of age as *H. pylori* seropositive. Because of the strong evidence that associates *H. pylori* infection with peptic ulcer disease, a recent National Institutes of Health consensus panel concluded that patients with duodenal or gastric ulcers, who also are infected by *H. pylori*, should undergo antimicrobial therapy (14). There are at present many different protocols for the treatment of *H. pylori*, most of which

consist of an antibiotic combined with an H$_2$RA or with a proton-pump inhibitor. The best protocol remains to be determined by comparative randomized clinical trials. The question of whether all patients with PUD should be empirically treated for *H. pylori* without a confirmed diagnosis by endoscopic biopsy, *H. pylori* antibody serology, or breath tests is the subject of intense debate at the present time.

Peptic ulcer disease may be diagnosed by barium contrast radiography or by endoscopy. The sensitivities of each technique for the detection of ulcers are both operator dependent, but endoscopy clearly is superior for the detection of ulcers smaller than 0.5cm; endoscopy also permits immediate biopsies.

Special Considerations

Several studies have confirmed that neither the radiologist nor the endoscopist can reliably exclude malignancy in a gastric ulcer solely on the basis of visual clues. In addition, the healing of a gastric ulcer does not exclude malignancy. Therefore, unless a patient has contraindications to surgical resection of a gastric carcinoma, an individual with a gastric ulcer must undergo thorough endoscopic biopsy to exclude malignancy. Most benign gastric ulcers heal after 12 weeks of standard-dose H$_2$RA, proton-pump inhibitor, or sucralfate therapy. Patients whose gastric ulcers fail to heal within this time period may require high-dose omeprazole therapy (40mg daily). Surgical resection should be considered for gastric ulcers that are refractory to intensive medical therapy.

Severe Ulcer Bleeding

Severe upper gastrointestinal (UGI) bleeding is one of the most common complications of peptic ulcer disease in the elderly. The higher incidence of concurrent medical illnesses in the elderly places this patient population at a much higher risk for morbidity and mortality. Bleeding peptic ulcers in the elderly have been associated with mortality rates ranging from 25 percent to 60 percent (15).

The initial management of the elderly patient with UGI bleeding should include a rapid evaluation of the patient's overall clinical condition and comorbid problems, with special attention given to the intravascular volume status. When confounding factors such as renal insufficiency or congestive heart failure are present, the physician should consider inserting a right heart catheter. An EGD should be performed to determine the cause of the bleeding and to provide immediate endoscopic hemostasis with injection, electrocautery, or thermocautery. Endoscopic therapy for active ulcer bleeding is about 90 percent effective in stopping active ulcer bleeding, and when compared with conventional medical therapy, it significantly reduces the rates of rebleeding, the amount of blood products transfused, the need for emergency surgery, and mortality (16). If emergency endoscopic therapy fails to provide hemostasis, or is unavailable, alternative treatments such as angiographic embolization or surgery should be considered.

Elderly patients who have bled from peptic ulcers belong to a high-risk subset of all patients with peptic ulcer disease. In spite of previous successful therapy for *H. pylori*, these high-risk patients should be maintained on chronic acid-suppression therapy to reduce the chance of ulcer recurrence (14).

The side effects of medications used in ulcer therapy deserve special consideration in the elderly. Calcium-containing antacids may exacerbate constipation, magnesium-containing antacids may cause diarrhea, and aluminum-containing antacids must be used with caution if the patient has poor renal function. Generally, the complications caused by H$_2$RAs are few. CNS symptoms such as agitation and confusion have been associated with H$_2$RA administration, but controlled trials demonstrating a causal relationship are lacking. Similarly, H$_2$RAs have been reported to affect the metabolism of other drugs such as warfarin and phenytoin. In certain individuals this effect may be clinically significant. Sucralfate may cause constipation. Misoprostol may produce a dose-dependent diarrhea. The following are general recommendations for management of peptic ulcers:

• An H$_2$RA is generally the first-line medication. When given at equivalent doses, cimetidine, ranitidine, famotidine, and nizatidine heal 70 percent to 80 percent of duodenal ulcers at 4 weeks, and about 90 percent of duodenal ulcers at 8 weeks. H$_2$RAs are also effective for gastric ulcers.

• Sucralfate, given as 1 gm four times a day, has efficacy comparable to that of H$_2$RAs.

• Omeprazole, given at 40 mg per day heals duodenal

ulcers more rapidly than do standard doses of H$_2$RAs at 2 and 4 weeks.

• High-dose antacid therapy is effective, but should be prescribed rarely because of poor patient compliance and diarrhea.

• Anticholinergics are not recommended for initial treatment of duodenal ulcer because of the frequency of untoward side effects, especially in the elderly.

• NSAIDs should be avoided when possible, and alternate therapies such as acetaminophen or gold should be used.

• Misoprostol should be co-administered if NSAIDs must be used.

• *H. pylori* infections should be treated.

• Gastric ulcers and refractory duodenal ulcers should undergo endoscopic biopsy.

• Patients should be stopped from smoking because smoking impedes healing and promotes recurrence of peptic ulcers.

• Chronic maintenance therapy with half-standard doses of H$_2$RAs or sucralfate significantly reduces duodenal ulcer recurrence rates and is indicated for patients who have frequent recurrences, complicated ulcers, or medical problems requiring the use of ulcerogenic drugs.

• Unresponsiveness of duodenal ulcers to routine medical treatment should prompt an evaluation for a gastric hypersecretory state (Zollinger-Ellison syndrome).

• Surgery for duodenal ulcer disease should be reserved for complications of the ulcer (major hemorrhage, perforation, gastric outlet obstruction).

Diverticular Disease

Diagnostic Considerations

The prevalence of colonic diverticulosis increases with age and is estimated to be about 25 percent to 40 percent in people aged 65 to 74 years. Diverticular disease predominantly affects people in the Western world and has been attributed to the low fiber content of the usual Western diet. Most diverticula are diffusely distributed in the sigmoid colon, but they may be present anywhere in the colon and can vary in number from single to many in an individual patient. As the number of diverticula increases, the frequency of symptoms attributed to them also increases, but many symptoms, such as nonspecific abdominal pain, diarrhea, and constipation, that may be associated with the diverticulosis may be caused by other conditions. About 80 percent of persons with colonic diverticula seem to remain symptom-free throughout life. The most common symptom that seems reliably correlated with the presence of diverticula is colicky or gripping pain in the left lower quadrant of the abdomen, which is worse after meals. A cord-like loop of colon may be palpable in the left side of the false pelvis. The diverticula may be demonstrated by barium enema or by an endoscopic examination.

Treatment of Uncomplicated Diverticulosis

The treatment of uncomplicated diverticulosis usually includes an increased dietary intake of vegetable fiber, especially of cereal grains. The effectiveness of bran in the relief of symptoms of diverticular disease has been reported in most of the relevant controlled trials (17). The rationale for using a high-fiber diet in the treatment of diverticular disease is based on observations that increased volume and weight of stool in the sigmoid colon increase the radius of the bowel and concurrently decrease intraluminal pressure. Anticholinergic drugs often are tried in the treatment of diverticulosis, but their efficacy is unestablished, and their use may be a factor in inducing pseudo-obstruction of the colon (Ogilvie's syndrome), which can be a serious complication in the elderly, as well as the more common side effects of dry mouth, blurred vision, and urinary retention.

Complications of Diverticulosis

The principal complications of diverticulosis are diverticulitis and hemorrhage.

Diverticulitis

In most persons, the course of diverticulitis consists of self-limited episodes, but in others, the disease may be severe and may even require surgical intervention. Patients with diverticulitis typically complain of pain of increasing severity in the left lower quadrant of the abdomen and have associated signs of abdominal infection (fever, leukocytosis, and peritoneal signs). In the aged, however, the signs of an acute inflammatory process may be muted, and the severity of the patient's condition underestimated. Diagnostic evaluation of suspected diverticulitis should include supine and erect plain radiographs of the abdomen for the presence of free air. The use of invasive tests such as sigmoidoscopy and barium enema in the workup of suspected diverticulitis remains controversial. Sigmoidoscopy is useful primarily for detecting other conditions such as rectal carcinoma, rather than for establishing the diagnosis of diverticulosis, and some believe this procedure should be deferred until the acute attack has subsided. Similarly, some believe that barium enema should be deferred during the acute inflammatory process because of the risk of "blowing out" an infected diverticulum. A computed tomography (CT) scan may be very useful for noninvasively establishing the diagnosis by demonstrating the diverticula and pericolic inflammation.

The treatment of diverticulitis usually includes broad-spectrum antibiotics and careful management of fluid requirements by intravenous infusion. Antibiotic coverage should include gram-negative aerobes such as *Escherichia coli*, as well as anaerobic organisms. Antibiotic treatment, once started, should be continued for 7 to 10 days. An urgent resection of the colon (usually a staged operation requiring a temporary colostomy) is indicated if generalized peritonitis, persistent colonic obstruction, or signs of pericolic abscess are present.

Hemorrhage

Rectal bleeding in some form occurs in 10 percent to 25 percent of patients with known diverticular disease, and severe hemorrhage occurs in 3 percent to 5 percent of patients, but the bleeding does not always originate in the diverticula. When bleeding is from a diverticulum, it is located in the right colon in about two-thirds of cases. Typically, the bleeding is brisk and painless.

As in all patients who present with severe hematochezia, the initial diagnostic evaluation of the patient with severe bleeding presumed to be from colonic diverticulosis must include efforts to exclude bleeding from an upper gastrointestinal source. Initially this is accomplished by placement of a nasogastric tube, but if there is any doubt about the interpretation of the nasogastric aspirate, an EGD should follow. The initial treatment of hemorrhage from colonic diverticular disease involves the usual measures of fluid and blood replacement, with special attention to the decreased tolerance for hypovolemia in the elderly and the associated diseases and medication use that often characterize this age group.

Several tests are available to search for and treat the cause of a lower GI bleed. The order in which these tests are performed depends on local availability and expertise. Radionuclide imaging after injection of ^{99m}Tc-labeled autologous erythrocytes may give the approximate location of the bleeding site. The more invasive selective mesenteric angiography is useful for the purposes of both diagnosis and therapy. If the bleeding diverticulum is identified by contrast extravasation, the bleeding artery may then be selectively infused with vasopressin or embolized with metal coils or absorbable gelatin sponge. Urgent colonoscopy, preceded by a rapid bowel purge with polyethylene glycol solution, may provide a diagnostic accuracy similar to that of angiography. Colonoscopy also is a sensitive means of identifying angiodysplastic lesions, which in the elderly may be an even more common cause of massive colonic bleeding than are diverticula. A bleeding site identified by colonoscopy may be injected with epinephrine to achieve acute hemostasis. A barium enema should not be performed in any patient with severe lower GI bleeding because it has no therapeutic potential and because the barium interferes with the more appropriate tests discussed above. Surgical excision of the affected segment of colon sometimes must be undertaken if hemorrhage continues despite these measures.

Colorectal Cancer

Colorectal cancer is one of the leading causes of cancer-related deaths in the United States, especially in the elderly. In 1990, colorectal cancer ranked third as a cause of cancer-related deaths in men older than age 75 and first for women of that same age group. The incidence of colorectal cancer increases dramatically after a person is 40 years of age until its peak in persons about 75 years of age (18).

Colorectal cancer should be regarded as a preventable disease. Strong evidence supports the hypothesis that most colorectal carcinomas arise from adenomatous polyps, and that removal of these polyps results in a dramatic reduction in the incidence of colorectal cancer. For instance, the data from the National Polyp Study indicate that colonoscopic polypectomy reduced the incidence of colorectal cancer by a statistically significant 76 percent to 90 percent (19). It is estimated that approximately 5 to 12 years elapse from the time a benign adenoma appears until the subsequent development of a malignant focus. Hence, one method for preventing colorectal cancer is to screen patients for premalignant adenomatous polyps and to remove such polyps before they become carcinomas. Unfortunately, at present there is no ideal test that screens for colorectal neoplasms. The fecal occult blood test (FOBT) is easy to perform and initially is inexpensive; however, it is criticized for being insensitive for the early detection of adenomas and for being susceptible to multiple factors that cause false-positive results. In addition, the initial low cost of the FOBT must be balanced against the total expense of investigating the significant number of false-positive findings. Flexible sigmoidoscopy has gained increased popularity as a screening tool for colorectal cancer, and training in its use is now recommended by the American Board of Internal Medicine for residents in internal medicine. This test has a high sensitivity and specificity for lesions within its 60-cm reach, but recent clinical trials have demonstrated that only about 50 percent of patients with adenomatous polyps had adenomas in the distal colon; the remainder of the patients had adenomatous polyps beyond the reach of the flexible sigmoidoscope. Colonoscopy is also increasingly advocated as a method for colorectal cancer screening. The advantages of colonoscopy include examination of the entire colon and the chance to remove all polyps with a single test. The potential disadvantages include the current cost to perform a colonoscopy in the United States, as well as the risk of the procedure itself. Final recommendations for colorectal cancer screening await the results of ongoing research trials.

Other important considerations in the management of colorectal adenomas are the relationship between the size of the polyps and the likelihood of cancer being associated with them, and the duration required for progression of an adenoma to a carcinoma. In large series, the malignancy rate for adenomas less than 1 cm in diameter has been about 1 percent; for adenomas larger than 2 cm the malignancy rate is nearly 50 percent (20). Data on the interval between the detection of an adenoma and its progression to a carcinoma are fragmentary, but the interval is estimated at 5 to 15 years (20). Investigators from the National Polyp Study Workgroup recently advised that most patients who have undergone an initial colonoscopic removal of all adenomatous polyps can wait at least 3 years before subsequent follow-up colonoscopy without incurring an increased risk of developing colorectal cancer (21).

Balanced judgment is necessary in screening for colonic adenomas and for their removal in the elderly. Although surveillance for colonic neoplasms is generally favored, the risk of performing a sigmoidoscopic or colonoscopic polypectomy may outweigh the risk of cancer developing from an adenoma, especially a small one, within the expected lifetime of a patient. Some aspects of colorectal cancer are also discussed in Chapters 11–54.

Hemorrhoids

Hemorrhoids usually present with the symptom of painless hematochezia or as an anal mass that protrudes when the patient defecates. Although hemorrhoids are very common, the diagnosis of hemorrhoidal bleeding is one of exclusion; both hematochezia and occult blood loss should be investigated by a full examination of the colon to exclude neoplasms, inflammatory bowel disease, or other sources of bleeding. Hemorrhoids are not painful unless they have become thrombosed.

The initial treatment of nonthrombosed hemorrhoids usually includes the use of stool softeners and suppositories and a dietary change to a high-fiber diet. Persistently symptomatic internal hemorrhoids may respond to treatments designed to fibrose the hemorrhoids to the underlying tissue. These treatments include rubber-band ligation, direct current cauterization, bipolar electrocauterization, sclerotherapy, and photocoagulation with an infrared probe. The choice of treatment frequently depends on local expertise and the availability of equipment. Several clinical trials have documented the effectiveness of all these treatments, although some may be more effective than others (22). Hemorrhoids that remain unresponsive to these treatments or that are complicated by thrombosis or prolapse may require surgical excision (23).

Gallstone Disease and Associated Complications

Gallstones are common in the elderly; many studies suggest a prevalence of about 20 percent to 30 percent in persons older than 70 years of age (24). Nonetheless, most elderly patients with gallstones remain asymptomatic, and the risk of therapy is greater than the risk of developing gallstone-associated complications. On the other hand, if symptoms do develop, the risk of recurrent symptoms and subsequent complications is more than 50 percent. Therefore, therapy for gallstones usually is reserved for patients who develop symptoms of biliary pain or complications of cholelithiasis such as acute cholecystitis, choledocholithiasis, cholangitis, or biliary pancreatitis (25).

Diagnostic Considerations

Making the diagnosis of symptomatic gallstone disease in elderly patients can be challenging because they may not present with classic manifestations. Biliary pain usually is described as a gradually increasing, upper abdominal pain that reaches a plateau and then diminishes over several hours. The presence of fever, leukocytosis, jaundice, or severe pain lasting more than several hours typically suggests the development of a complication, such as acute cholecystitis. However, elderly patients with acute cholecystitis may have only minimal abdominal tenderness and no fever. Similarly, elderly patients with cholangitis may initially present with mental obtundation, rather than the more common manifestations of Charcot's triad (abdominal pain, fever, and jaundice). Atypical clinical presentations may impede the timely diagnosis and treatment of symptomatic gallstone disease and contribute to increased morbidity in elderly patients.

Generally, transcutaneous abdominal ultrasonography is the preferred initial imaging test to confirm gallstone disease because this test has a sensitivity for gallbladder stones of about 90 percent to 95 percent. The presence of localized gallbladder tenderness under pressure from the ultrasound transducer (Murphy's sign) is about 90 percent accurate in confirming acute cholecystitis. Ultrasonography also is useful for detecting the presence of dilated bile ducts, a finding that should raise the suspicion for choledocholithiasis or a malignant bile duct stenosis.

Treatment of Uncomplicated Gallstone Disease

The usual treatment for uncomplicated *symptomatic* cholelithiasis in the elderly is the same as that for younger patients: cholecystectomy, either by the traditional open method or by the laparoscopic method. Cholecystectomy effectively prevents the recurrence of symptoms and the development of complications from cholelithiasis. The mortality rate for elective open cholecystectomy increases with advancing age and is estimated to be between 1 percent and 3 percent for persons 70 years of age. Laparoscopic cholecystectomy offers the advantage of reduced postoperative recovery time. The operative risks of laparoscopic cholecystectomy performed by an experienced surgeon may approach that of open cholecystectomy (25). Advanced age alone should not preclude surgery, but concurrent illnesses, such as obstructive lung disease or congestive heart failure, elevate the surgical risk and should prompt consideration of nonsurgical treatment options.

The most widely available nonsurgical treatment option for uncomplicated gallstone disease is oral bile acid therapy. Candidates for this therapy have gallstones that are not calcified and are less than 1.5 cm in diameter. The treatment must be sustained for as long as 2 years, and the best reported rates of complete gallstone disappearance are about 60 percent (26). A disadvantage of oral bile acid therapy is its recurrence rate of about 50 percent after therapy is discontinued.

Other nonsurgical treatment options for uncomplicated gallstone disease include extracorporeal shock wave lithotripsy (ESWL) and direct-contact dissolution by a solvent infused through a catheter directly into the gallbladder. These treatments are available only at specialized centers, and at the time of this writing are considered investigational by the Food and Drug Administration.

Treatment of Complicated Gallstone Disease

The most common complications of gallstone disease are acute cholecystitis, choledocholithiasis, cholangitis, and acute biliary pancreatitis. The usual treatment for acute cholecystitis in the elderly is clinical stabilization by the prompt administration of intravenous fluids and broad-spectrum antibiotics, followed shortly thereafter by cholecystectomy. Early cholecystectomy is associated

with less morbidity and a more rapid postsurgical recovery compared with cholecystectomy that is delayed several weeks after the initial episode of acute cholecystitis.

Elderly patients with acute cholecystitis who are high-surgical-risk candidates and whose clinical status is deteriorating may benefit from emergency gallbladder drainge by surgical cholecystostomy, percutaneous cholecystostomy performed under local anesthesia, or by endoscopic retrograde cholangiopancreatography (ERCP) and insertion of a transpapillary gallbladder catheter. All these methods were reported effective in various small clinical series, but no large randomized trial has demonstrated the superiority of one of these methods. The selection of a particular method should mainly depend on local expertise (27).

Common bile duct stones may cause severe complications such as acute cholangitis or biliary pancreatitis more often than do stones confined to the gallbladder. These complications can be particularly devastating in the elderly, and the removal of common bile duct stones is

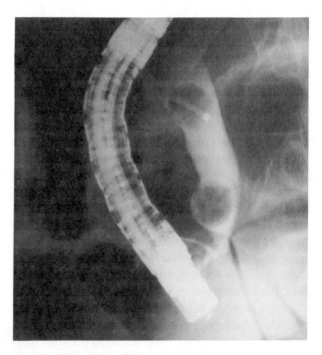

Fig. 49.1. ERCP reveals a stone obstructing the distal end of a dilated common bile duct. A 1.5-cm diameter, balloon-tipped catheter is poised proximal to the stone in preparation to sweeping the stone out through an endoscopic sphincterotomy.

recommended even for patients who are asymptomatic at the time of diagnosis. The stones may be removed either by ERCP, percutaneous transhepatic cholangiography (PTC), or surgery. Again, local expertise may favor one method to another, and at times, the clinical situation may require combining some or all of the above techniques (Figures 49.1 and 49.2).

Acute cholangitis usually is a complication of choledocholithiasis. The most common offending bacteria are gram-negative aerobes such as *E. coli*, *Klebsiella*, or *Pseudomonas*. Most patients with acute cholangitis dem-

onstrate clinical improvement after intravenous fluids and broad-spectrum antibiotics are administered. Patients who do not improve should undergo ERCP with biliary drainage. Emergency endoscopic biliary drainage may be performed without fluoroscopic guidance at the patient's bedside. Several large series have favored endoscopic biliary drainage to surgical decompression (28). One randomized controlled trial showed that patients with severe acute cholangitis who were treated by ERCP had a significantly lower mortality rate compared with that for patients who were treated by surgery (29). If endoscopic drainage is not successful, the biliary system should be drained by urgent PTC.

The usual follow-up to nonsurgical intervention for choledocholithiasis is cholecystectomy. However, endoscopic sphincterotomy and removal of the common bile duct stones without subsequent cholecystectomy may be appropriate in the high-risk elderly patient. Several studies suggest that the need for subsequent cholecystectomy in patients with cholelithiasis who have undergone endoscopic sphincterotomy is only about 2 percent to 3 percent per year (30).

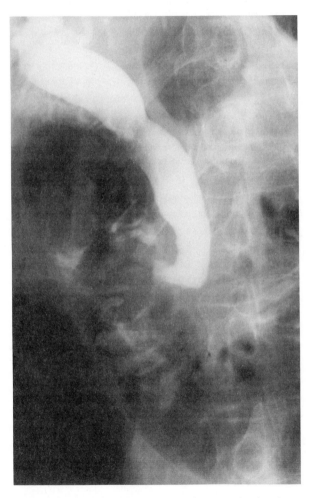

Fig. 49.2. A cholangiogram obtained a few seconds after the stone was swept out and the endoscope was removed demonstrates free flow of contrast into the duodenum and absence of the obstructing stone.

References

1. Gilbert DA, Silverstein FE, Tedesco FJ, et al. The national ASGE survey on upper gastrointestinal bleeding. III. Endoscopy in upper gastrointestinal bleeding. Gastrointest Endosc 1981;27:94.
2. Dantas RO, Cook IJ, Dodds WJ, et al. Biomechanics of cricopharyngeal bars. Gastroenterology 1990;99:1269–1274.
3. Brady PG. Management of esophageal and gastric foreign bodies. Clin Update Am Soc Gastrointest Endosc 1994;2:1–4.
4. Nebble OT, Fornes MF, Castell DO. Symptomatic gastroesophageal reflux: incidence and precipitating factors. Am J Dig Dis 1976;21:953.
5. Benjamin SB, Castell DO. Chest pain of esophageal origin. Arch Intern Med 1983;143:772.
6. Richter JE, Bradley LA, Castell DO. Esophageal chest pain: current controversies in pathogenesis, diagnosis, and therapy. Ann Intern Med 1989;110:66–78.
7. McCallum RW. ACG Committee on FDA-related matters. Cisapride: a new class of prokinetic agent. Am J Gastroenterol 1991;86:135–149.
8. Klinkenberg-Knol EC, Festen HPM, Jansen JBMJ, et al. Long-term treatment with omeprazole for refractory reflux esophagitis: efficacy and safety. Ann Intern Med 1994;121:161–167.

9. Freston JW. Omeprazole, hypergastrinemia, and gastric carcinoid tumors. Ann Intern Med 1994;121:232–233. Editorial.

10. Spechler SJ, Department of Veterans Affairs Gastroesophageal Reflux Disease Study Group. Comparison of medical and surgical therapy for complicated gastroesophageal reflux disease in veterans. N Engl J Med 1992;326:786–792.

11. Richter JE. Surgery for reflux disease – reflections of a gastroenterologist. N Engl J Med 1992;326:825–827. Editorial.

12. World Health Organization. World health statistics annual of 1986. Geneva: World Health Organization, 1987.

13. Graham DY, White RH, Moreland LW, et al. Duodenal and gastric ulcer prevention with misoprostol in arthritis patients taking NSAIDs. Ann Intern Med 1993;119:257–262.

14. NIH Consensus Development Panel on *Helicobacter pylori* in Peptic Ulcer Disease. *Helicobacter pylori* in peptic ulcer disease. JAMA 1994;272:65–69.

15. Silverstein FE, Gilbert DA, Tedesco FJ, et al. The national ASGE survey on upper gastrointestinal bleeding. II. Clinical prognostic factors. Gastrointest Endosc 1981;27:80.

16. Cook DJ, Guyatt GH, Salena BJ, Laine LA. Endoscopic therapy for acute nonvariceal upper gastrointestinal hemorrhage: a meta-analysis. Gastroenterology 1992;102:139–148.

17. Almy TP. Some disorders of the alimentary tract. In: Andorran R, Bierman EL, Hazzard WR, eds. Principles of geriatric medicine. New York: McGraw-Hill, 1985:662–681.

18. Boring CC, Squires TS, Tong T, Montgomery S. Cancer statistics, 1994. CA Cancer J Clin 1994;44:7–26.

19. Winawer SJ, Zauber AG, Ho MN, et al. Prevention of colorectal cancer by colonoscopic polypectomy. N Engl J Med 1993;329:1977–1981.

20. Day DW, Morson BC. The adenoma-carcinoma sequence. Major Probl Pathol 1978;10:58.

21. Winawer SJ, Zauber AG, O'Brien MJ, et al. Randomized comparison of surveillance intervals after colonoscopic removal of newly diagnosed adenomatous polyps. N Engl J Med 1993;328:901–906.

22. Randall GM, Jensen DM, Machicado GA, et al. Prospective randomized comparative study of bipolar versus direct current electrocoagulation for treatment of bleeding internal hemorrhoids. Gastrointest Endosc 1994;40:403–410.

23. Abcarian H, Alexander-Williams J, Christiansen J, et al. Benign anorectal disease: definition, characterization and analysis of treatment. Am J Gastroenterol 1994;89:S182–S193.

24. Mendez-Sanchez N, Jessurun J, Ponciano-Rodriquez G, et al. Prevalence of gallstone disease in Mexico: a necropsy study. Dig Dis Sci 1993;38:680–683.

25. Ransohoff DF, Gracie WA. Treatment of gallstones. Ann Intern Med 1993;119:606–619.

26. Plaisier PW, van der Hul RL, Terpstra OT, Bruining HA. Current treatment modalities for symptomatic gallstones. Am J Gastroenterol 1993;88:633–638.

27. Van Dam J. Endoscopic treatment of acute cholecystitis: all your troubles down the drain? Gastroenterology 1994;107:311–312.

28. Siegel JH, Rodriquez R, Cohen SA, et al. Endoscopic management of cholangitis: crital review of an alternative technique and report of a large series. Am J Gastroenterol 1994;89:1142–1146.

29. Lai ECS, Mok FPT, Tan ESY, et al. Endoscopic biliary drainage for severe acute cholangitis. N Engl J Med 1992;326:1582–1586.

30. Silvis SE. Endoscopic sphincterotomy with an intact gallbladder. Gastrointest Endosc Clin North Am 1991;1:65–77.

Chapter 50
Infections

F. Marc LaForce

One evil in old age is that, as your time is come, you think every little illness the beginning of the end. When a man expects to be arrested, every knock at the door is an alarm.

Sydney Smith, 1771–1845

Infectious diseases cause 30 percent of geriatric deaths and are the most frequent cause of hospitalization for the elderly (1). For the most part, infections in the elderly are similar to those of younger patients except for two key factors: 1) the prevalence of associated cardiopulmonary, neurologic and genitourinary illnesses that interfere with normal host defenses, and 2) the failure of normal homeostatic responses to infectious challenges. These two characteristics ensure that geriatric infections are likely to result in death, disability, or prolonged hospitalization. This chapter reviews common geriatric infections and emphasizes treatment and preventive strategies. Because of the importance of respiratory and urinary infections in the elderly, these illnesses are discussed in detail.

With the continued expansion of the geriatric population, particularly of the very old, both generalists and subspecialists must be knowledgeable in the diagnosis and management of infections in the elderly. This is not an easy task because serious infections in the elderly present subtly. For example, elderly patients with pneumococcal bacteremia are less likely to be febrile than are younger bacteremic patients (2). A high index of suspicion of infection is a usual hypothesis when an older patient deteriorates clinically.

Aging and Host Defenses

Alterations in host defenses associated with aging are summarized in Table 50.1. Organ-specific defenses usually deteriorate because of the effects of a chronic illness. Cigarette smoking causes chronic bronchitis, ciliostasis, squamous metaplasia, and depressed mucociliary clearance. Dyspepsia, a frequent condition in the elderly, is treated with antacids and H_2 blockers that can effectively control gastric acid secretion, but do so at the cost of decreasing acid-mediated destruction of potential gastrointestinal pathogens. Foreign bodies facilitate certain infections and indwelling intravenous lines can serve as conduits for cutaneous bacteria and are clearly associated with an increased risk of bacteremia. All prostheses are associated, to a greater or lesser extent, with an increased risk for local infection.

Nonspecific cellular and humoral defense mechanisms, such as macrophages, polymorphonuclear leukocytes, and complement, are largely unaffected by age (3). Antibody response is somewhat depressed with age but probably not to a clinically relevant degree. Poor antibody response to influenza and pneumococcal vaccines are usually associated with co-existing diseases or use of immunosuppressive drugs. In contrast, cell-mediated immune responses do become depressed with age. Thompson and colleagues evaluated the immune response of 17 centenarians (4). These studies showed that serum immunoglobulin levels, total white cell counts, differential counts, natural killer cell activity, and the number of circulating monocytes were normal. The most striking abnormality was in the population of T4-positive helper T lymphocytes, which were decreased more than twofold when compared to those of controls. Because the number of OKT8 cells was normal, the T4/T8 ratio was decreased from the normal of 1.7 to a level of 0.7. The decrease in T4 cells was reflected in poor responses to the mitogen phytohemagglutinin. Such changes are consistent with earlier human and murine experimental studies that have shown that the aging immune system is generally intact except for a significant decrease in OKT4 cells (5). These changes appear to be closely related to thymic involution (5).

Table 50.1. Effect of Aging on Susceptibility to Infection

Deterioration of organ-specific defenses
Decline in cell-mediated immunity
Presence of indwelling devices
Prevalence of underlying diseases

Table 50.2. Factors that Can Modify Use of Antibiotics in the Elderly

Subtle early manifestations of infection
Advanced infection when diagnosed
Presence of prosthetic devices
Drug interactions
Drug compliance (particularly in the ambulatory setting)

Murasko and colleagues evaluated immune function in 260 patients who were 70 to 106 years of age (6). They also noted a decrease in lymphocyte phytohemagglutinin response but were unable to demonstrate clear-cut deterioration of cell-mediated immunity with increased age. For example, persons older than 90 years of age had the least reduction in immune function, an observation that prompted investigators to propose that great age may be a selective factor that favors those with intact immune systems, a hypothesis for which there is some supportive evidence (7).

Other factors, such as malnutrition, may worsen the decline in cellular immunity. Overt and subclinical malnutrition is common in the elderly, and nutritional repletion has been shown to enhance delayed hypersensitivity and antibody response in adults (8).

Use of Antibiotics in the Elderly

In Table 50.2 several clinical and pharmacologic factors that can influence the selection and dosing of antibiotics in the elderly are summarized. The subtlety of clinical findings associated with serious infection in the elderly has been well described; confusion, incontinence and anorexia are often the only manifestations of serious infection. Elderly persons generally have lower temperatures with infections and more than 10 percent of older patients with bacteremia are afebrile (9). Since the elderly have basal body temperatures that are about 0.3 to 0.5°C lower than temperatures of young persons, clinicians should suspect infection as a possible explanation of minimal elevations in temperature in the elderly.

Difficulty in making an early diagnosis of infection in the elderly, plus their poor response to sepsis, have led to some general assumptions that influence the treatment of suspected infections in the elderly (10). Empiric therapy is often the rule, and the choice of an antibiotic tends to be different for older patients than for younger patients. In general, the variety of organisms that can cause infections in the elderly is broader than that seen with similar infections in younger patients. In addition, many older patients have compromised host defenses and live in institutionalized settings in which the resident bacterial flora are more resistant to treatment than those seen in the community setting. The physiologic decline in renal function with aging favors the selection of less toxic antibiotics that are renally excreted. Thus, beta lactam antibiotics, particularly the second- and third-generation cephalosporins, ampicillin/sulbactam, ticarcillin/clavulanate are attractive agents because of their broad spectrum of activity and low toxicity. Of course, the usual caveats associated with prudent antimicrobial therapy, such as obtaining smears of potentially infectious material, prompt Gram stain interpretation of such smears, taking proper cultures, knowing local bacterial sensitivity patterns, and antibiotic costs, must always be considered whenever an antimicrobial regimen is being decided.

There are now more than 70 licensed cephalosporin products. No practitioner can be expected to be completely knowledgeable about all these agents. Most of the newer antibiotics, particularly the cephalosporins, fall into the "me too" category—despite being more expensive, they offer little therapeutic advantage to less expensive alternatives. Most clinicians become familiar with a panel of antibiotics that they prescribe regularly. Objective reviews, particularly those published in *Medical Letter on Drugs and Therapeutics*, are reliable sources of useful information about new antibiotics.

The likelihood or severity of infection can be expressed as being directly proportional to inoculum size and the virulence of the organism and inversely proportional to the integrity of host defenses (Figure 50.1). Antibiotics can play a crucial role in reducing or eliminating viable organisms while allowing time for host defenses to completely eliminate infecting pathogens. During the process

$$\text{Severity of infection} = \frac{\text{Inoculum size} \times \text{Virulence}}{\text{Integrity of host defenses}}$$

Fig. 50.1. Determinants of infection. Antibiotics can play a key role in decreasing or eliminating the inoculum size.

of inactivating pathogens, specific immune mechanisms are stimulated such that a second challenge with the same pathogen results in a vigorous and specific response that rapidly destroys the organism.

A seductive tendency that should be resisted is one whereby antimicrobial coverage is progressively broadened when a patient with a suspected infection is not progressing as well as might be hoped. There are several reasons for apparent antibiotic failure, not the least of which is the presence of an undrained focus of infection or that the presumption of infection is incorrect. In such circumstances, it is usually safe to discontinue antimicrobial therapy to re-evaluate a patient. These patients are under observation and antimicrobial therapy can be promptly restarted, if necessary. All too frequently, broadening antimicrobial coverage serves to comfort the physician; additional antibiotic may delay the performance of diagnostic tests.

In a person's seventh decade, renal tubular secretory capacity and glomerular filtration rate are about half the values noted in a person's second decade of life (11). The physiologic deterioration of renal function results in higher blood levels of penicillins and cephalosporins, agents that are normally filtered and secreted. Fortunately, cephalosporins and penicillins have such a high therapeutic-toxic ratio that their use in the setting of moderate renal insufficiencies poses no great risk. Aminoglycosides are primarily excreted by glomerular filtration and will achieve higher than expected levels in the elderly. Even with careful use of published nomograms, dosing is difficult and becomes problematic because of the large number of serious gram-negative infections that occur in these patients. Blood levels must be used to follow therapies because underdosing of aminoglycosides is as big a problem as are toxic levels (9). The introduction of third-generation cephalosporins and the monobactam, aztreonam, represents a major advance

because of the relative safety and extended spectrum against gram-negative rods of these drugs.

Use of vancomycin has increased in recent years because of reports of patients' increased hypersensitivity to penicillin, the increase in methicillin-resistant organisms, staphylococcal infections, and the convenience of twice-daily parenteral outpatient therapy for vancomycin. The most important and serious adverse reaction to vancomycin is auditory nerve toxicity. This complication occurs most frequently in the elderly because of their age-related decrease in renal function, which limits renal clearance of this agent. Blood levels should be checked to maintain peak and trough levels of 30 and 8 µg/mL, respectively. Infusions should be given during a period of 60 minutes to reduce the incidence of histamine flushing.

Third-generation cephalosporins have good antibacterial activity against most aerobic gram-negative bacilli, including *Pseudomonas aeruginosa*, and have good activity against staphylococci. These agents are relatively non-toxic, which makes them useful for treating complicated infections in the elderly. Quinolones have a broad spectrum of activity against many aerobic gram-negative rods but do not have sufficient activity against *Streptococcus pneumoniae* and cannot be considered first-line empiric therapy for pneumonia in the elderly. Because ciprofloxacin can be given orally, use of this agent has simplified home-based therapy for a wide variety of infections. Nitrofurantoins frequently cause adverse drug reactions in the elderly and because of the availability of alternative drugs, their use should be limited.

Home intravenous antibiotic therapy has been shown to decrease the cost of extended antibiotic therapy with little or no difference in clinical outcome. Published studies have emphasized acceptability to patients and good clinical outcomes, as long as patients or their families are capable of providing good intravenous care (12). Medicare reimbursement has limited the use of home antibiotic therapy in the elderly because Medicare reimbursement for outpatient intravenous therapy requires a physician to directly administer or supervise the administration of intravenous antibiotics (13). However, since 1990, some intravenous therapy has been covered by Medicare, which may stimulate the Health Care Financing Administration (HCFA) to seriously evaluate home antibiotic therapy.

Clinicians should be on the alert for drug interactions

because of the concurrent use of many drugs in elderly patients—the average patient in the United States who is older than 65 years receives 10.7 new and refilled prescriptions annually (14). For example, ciprofloxacin can increase serum theophylline concentrations. Rifampin is a potent inducer of the hepatic microsomal enzyme system, which can result in accelerated breakdown of a wide variety of drugs including warfarin, digoxin and phenytoin (10,15). Conversely, metronidazole and sulfonamides potentiate the action of anticoagulants (10,15). The possibility of drug interactions helps validate the decision by most physicians to limit the antibiotics prescribed to a group of compounds with toxicities and interactions that are well known to them.

Respiratory Tract Infections

Pneumonia is characterized clinically by fever, cough, chest pain, chills, increased sputum production, and a new infiltrate on chest x-ray. The disease follows unrestrained multiplication of a virulent pulmonary pathogen such as *S. pneumoniae* or a less aggressive organism such as *Escherichia coli* that grows because of a defect in pulmonary defenses. Pathogens that can cause pneumonia are aspirated from colonized upper airways, and the efficiency with which these aspirated bacterial challenges are cleared depends on the patient's cough reflex, mucociliary escalator system, or phagocytosis by alveolar macrophages and polymorphonuclear leukocytes (16). Older persons are at significant risk from acute lower respiratory tract infections; pneumonia is the fifth leading cause of death and accounts for about 4 percent of all deaths. Pneumonias in the elderly are best described in the context of four descriptive categories: 1) community-acquired pneumonia, 2) nursing home pneumonia, 3) nosocomial pneumonia, and 4) aspiration pneumonia.

Community-Acquired Pneumonia

Bennett et al have published the results of the largest community-based study of pneumococcal bacteremia and noted an annual rate of 56.3 cases per 100,000 population for persons 65 years of age and older (17). Assuming that there are, on average, four nonbacteremic pneumococcal infections for each bacteremic one, the elderly can be assumed to have, at a minimum, an annual incidence rate of

pneumococcal infection of about two cases per 1000 population. These data are consistent with published hospitalization rates for pneumonia of 5.3 per 1000 reported for Halifax County, Nova Scotia (18). Mortality rates for community-acquired pneumonia are also age-related, with an overall mortality of about 20 percent in the elderly (18).

Co-existing chronic obstructive lung disease, congestive heart failure or recent viral infection, particularly with influenza virus, are important predisposing factors. Determining a specific etiology for cases of community-acquired pneumonia continues to be an unsolved problem. Sputum samples are often hard to obtain and in only about one-half of cases of community-acquired pneumonia can a specific agent be identified (19). *S. pneumoniae* and *Haemophilus influenzae* continue to be the most common bacterial isolates and, because of their frequency, all empiric regimens used to treat community-acquired pneumonia in the elderly must cover these two pathogens (19).

Evaluation of elderly patients with community-acquired pneumonia is straightforward. Blood cultures should always be drawn before initiation of therapy. Patients who are producing phlegm should have their sputum examined microscopically and cultured if Gram stain shows a predominance of polymorphonuclear leukocytes. Therapy should be tailored according to the Gram-stain findings. About half of elderly patients with community-acquired pneumonia are unable to produce a sputum sample, and these patients should be treated empirically. If chest x-rays show an effusion associated with the infiltrate, the effusion should be tapped to determine whether empyema or a complicated effusion is present.

Treatment guidelines are given in Table 50.3. Patients with sputum Gram stains consistent with pneumococcal pneumonia can be safely treated with penicillin. Patients with mixed flora, suggestive of *H. influenzae* and pneumococci should be treated with ampicillin/sulbactam or a third-generation cephalosporin. Therapy should be continued for 10 days. Nonresolving community-acquired pneumonias in the elderly can be problematic (20). These patients usually require fiberoptic bronchoscopy with lung lavage and chest computerized tomography (CT) studies. Confounding diagnoses are the

Table 50.3. Treatment Guidelines for Empiric Antibiotic Therapy for Elderly Patients with Pneumonia[a]

Type of Pneumonia	Usual Pathogens	Suggested Antibiotic
Community-acquired	Pneumococcus	IV-administered Ceftriaxone
	H. influenzae	Ampicillin/sulbactam TMP-SMX
		PO-administered TMP-SMX Amoxicillin or amoxicillin/clavulanate
Nursing home	Pneumococcus	IV-administered Ceftriaxone
	H. influenzae	Ampicillin/sulbactam
	Aerobic gram-negatives	Ampicillin and gentamicin[b]
		PO-administered Amoxicillin plus ciprofloxacin Amoxicillin/clavulanate
Nosocomial	Aerobic gram-negatives	IV-administered[c] Piperacillin and gentamicin[b]
	(special attention to Pseudomonas)	Ceftazidime and gentamicin[b]
	Staph. aureus	Vancomycin and gentamicin[b] Imipenem IV-administered
Aspiration	Pneumococcus	Ceftriaxone
	H. influenzae	Ampicillin/sulbactam
	Aerobic gram-negatives	Ampicillin and gentamicin
		PO-administered Amoxicillin plus ciprofloxacin Amoxicillin/clavulanate

[a] Empiric therapy presupposes that sputum Gram stain information or culture data are not available.
[b] Aztreonam can be substituted for gentamicin in patients with azotemia.
[c] Recommendations should take into account local sensitivity patterns.
IV-intravenously; PO = orally; TMP-SMX = trimethoprim-sulfamethoxazole.

Table 50.4. Strategies to Prevent Community-Acquired Pneumonias

Improvement of host defenses
  Control underlying medical conditions
  Adequate nutrition
  Counseling about tobacco and alcohol use
  Enhance host immune system
    Yearly influenza vaccines
    Pneumococcal vaccine
Nonhost factors
  Limit exposure to crowds during influenza epidemics
  Immunize caregivers with influenza vaccine
  Limit risk factors leading to aspiration (e.g., avoid over sedation)
Chemoprophylaxis against influenza type A
  Amantadine
  Rimantadine for high-risk groups

medical management of these medical conditions is a necessary first step to prevent community-acquired pneumonia. For example, pulmonary congestion and edema, conditions associated with high rates of pulmonary infection, have been shown to impair intrapulmonary bacterial clearance in experimental animals (16). Similarly, cigarette smoking has been shown to impair both ciliary activity and intrapulmonary antibacterial activity (16). The treatment of pulmonary congestion and smoking cessation then become high priorities to prevent community-acquired pneumonia. Acute alcohol intoxication depresses pulmonary antibacteria activity in experimental animals, promotes aspiration, facilitates gram-negative colonization of the oropharynx and has clearly been identified as a risk factor for community-acquired pneumonia. Counseling patients about the dangers of alcohol use, particularly in the setting of chronic pulmonary and cardiac disease, is an important but often underused preventive strategy. Comprehensive immunization with influenza and pneumococcal vaccines is always a high priority.

Nursing Home Pneumonia

Pneumonia is a common infection among nursing home residents. These infections are the second most common cause of bacteremia in nursing home residents and account for about one-quarter of transfers to acute hospitals (21). The etiologic agents associated with these infections tend to be a mixture of the pathogens seen with commu-

commonest cause of nonresponse and include chronic aspiration secondary to oropharyngeal dysphagia, congestive heart failure, lung cancer, and malnutrition. Occasionally, lung lavage specimens grow unusual organisms like *Mycobacterium tuberculosis*, *Aspergillus* species, or *Nocardia*, all pathogens that can be treated.

Steps that can be taken to prevent community-acquired pneumonia are summarized in Table 50.4. Because of the prevalence of cardiopulmonary diseases in the elderly and their deleterious effect on host defenses, aggressive nity-acquired pneumonia and nosocomial pneumonia. The increased incidence of gram-negative rod pneumonias in these patients reflects the increased use of antibiotics in the nursing home setting and progressive disability, two factors associated with increased rates of oropharyngeal colonization with gram-negative rods. In one study, 40 percent of nursing home patients had *Klebsiella* isolated from their sputum as compared with 8 percent for patients with community-acquired pneumonia (22). The clinical presentation of pneumonia in these patients can be subtle: confusion and disorientation are described as common symptoms; as much as one-third of patients are afebrile. Most of these patients have physical findings consistent with pneumonia on chest examination. The frequency of these findings underscores the importance of percussing and auscultating lungs in elderly patients with confusion (23). Some can be treated in the nursing home, but more often these patients are referred to hospitals. Empiric therapy (see Table 50.3) should cover *S. pneumoniae*, *H. influenzae*, and the more common enterobacteriaceae such as *E. coli* and *Klebsiella*. Nursing home patients are at particular risk from influenza, and all residents should receive annual influenza immunizations.

Nosocomial Pneumonia

The elderly, once hospitalized, are at increased risk for developing nosocomial pneumonia. These infections are frequently associated with three risk factors: 1) superinfection complicating recovery from a community-acquired pneumonia, 2) ventilator-associated pneumonia, and 3) abdominal or thoracic surgery (24). The oropharyx of hospitalized elderly patients rapidly becomes colonized with aerobic gram-negative rods that can be aspirated. *E. coli*, *Klebsiella*, *Enterobacter*, *Proteus* and *Pseudomonas* are the most common pathogens isolated from these infections. Because these organisms originate from the hospital flora, they are frequently resistant to multiple antibiotics. Antimicrobial therapy should be tailored to the local sensitivity patterns; common regimens are given in Table 50.3. Mortality rates for these infections are high, and recovery, when it occurs, is often agonizingly slow. Because of the extended convalescence associated with these infections, it is important to maintain proper nutrition in these patients.

Aspiration Pneumonia

Skilled nursing facilities often accrue a group of patients who are highly susceptible to chronic aspiration. These patients have severe oropharyngeal dysphagia secondary to chronic neurologic diseases such as multi-infarct dementia, Parkinson's disease, or Alzheimer's disease. These patients are at high risk for nosocomial pneumonia. McDonald and coworkers documented an attack rate for nosocomial pneumonia of 1.9 per 1000 days in a high-risk, institutionalized population in Veterans Administration (VA) hospitals (25). As in other studies of pneumonia in the elderly, lethargy was a common symptom in these high-risk patients. The infections were serious and the mortality rate was about 20 percent per episode; however, all patients with more than two episodes of nosocomial pneumonia died within 2 years of the first infectious event. A follow-up, prospective study in the same population used multivariate analysis to evaluate risk factors associated with aspiration in high-risk patients and showed that presence of a feeding tube, having a hyperextended fixed neck position, and receiving benzodiazepenes or anticholinergics were independent risk factors for aspiration. More comprehensive preventive strategies to prevent aspiration in these patients should be studied. The respiratory pathogens isolated from these patients and treatment guidelines are similar to those seen in patients with nursing home pneumonia (see Table 50.3).

Urinary Tract Infections

Importance of Residual Volume as a Risk Factor

The volume of residual bladder urine plays a key role in determining whether bacteriuria remains constant and helps predict whether a short course of antibiotics is likely to be successful in patients with urinary tract infections. This phenomenon is of greater importance when the physician manages urinary tract infections in the elderly because of increased prevalence of age-related diseases characterized by incomplete emptying of the bladder. Bladder bacterial counts are largely determined by the number of bacteria in the postvoid residual urine (Figure 50.2). These organisms serve as a reservoir and, in the absence of antimicrobial therapy, significant postvoid residual urine guarantees that significant bacteriuria will be

$$\text{Bladder bacteria at time t} = \frac{\text{Urine bact. cts. x resid. vol. x multiplication rate of bact. through time t}}{\text{Residual volume + new urine volume over time t}}$$

Fig. 50.2. Factors determining bladder bacterial counts.

constant. Normally, postvoid residual urine is about 0.5 mL and in a state of water diuresis, significant bacteriuria (greater than 10^5 bacteria/mL) will be rapidly cleared. However, presence of a residual volume as small as 3 mL, allows for continued reseeding of bacteria in the bladder. For example, a bacterial doubling time of 20 minutes, a bladder volume of 300 mL, and a residual volume of 3 mL results in the return of bladder bacterial population to its prevoid level in about 2.5 hours (26,27). Single or short-course antibiotic therapy is highly effective in persons without postvoid residual urine.

Urinary Tract Infections in Uninstrumented Patients

Asymptomatic bacteriuria is a frequent finding in the elderly (Table 50.5) and, although this laboratory test is associated with a significant reduction in survival, it is not related to an increased incidence of fatal genitourinary infections (28). Controlled studies have shown that routine bacteriologic screening of asymptomatic elderly with treatment of bacteriuric episodes has not decreased morbidity or mortality, and routine culturing of urine is not recommended (29).

The prevalence of bacteriuria is also related to the level of functional disability. Forty percent of elderly, noninstrumented, institutionalized male veterans are bacteriuric at any given time and Nicolle and coworkers noted an acquisition rate of bacteriuria of about 40 percent per year (30). Once bacteriuria developed in these veterans, it persisted or, if it cleared, tended to recur.

E. coli is the most common uropathogen in the elderly; however, geriatric patients are more likely to suffer from infection with *Klebsiella, Enterobacter, Serratia, Pseudomonas* and *Proteus* (31). Enterococcal infections occur more frequently in elderly men. In a study of asymptomatic bacteriuria in the elderly, Kaye et al noted that 93 percent of the isolates in women were *Enterobacteriaceae*, but 56 percent of the isolates in men were gram-positive

cocci. Polymicrobial bacteriuria is more common in the elderly institutionalized patients (31). The increased variety of organisms isolated from the urine in older patients has been ascribed to their increased exposure to hospital flora (31).

After middle age, urinary tract infections in men increase progressively because of prostatic enlargement and the development of obstructive uropathy with residual urine after voiding. Symptoms of prostatism are usually evaluated by instrumentation of the urinary tract, which often results in bacterial colonization of the bladder. Bladder bacteria may also invade the prostate and cause chronic bacterial prostatitis, a condition not only difficult to treat, but which can also seed the bladder and cause relapsing infections of the urinary tract (32).

Elderly patients can present with typical symptoms of urinary tract infection such as increased frequency, dysuria, fever, and flank pain. However, symptoms such as nausea, vomiting, confusion and respiratory distress often dominate the clinical picture. Lack of fever does not rule out the presence of an invasive urinary tract infection (33). Flank pain, even in the presence of active

Table 50.5. Prevalence of Bacteriuria in Various Populations

Population	Sex	
	Male (%)	Female (%)
Community-based		
65–85 years of age	5	15
85+ years of age	15	25
Adult inpatients		
<70 years of age	7.5	30
≥70 years of age	25	30
Institutionalized elderly	>30	>30

SOURCE: Lipsky BA. Urinary tract infections in men. Ann Intern Med 1989;110:138–150.

pyelonephritis may be absent (33). In Gleckman's study of acute pyelonephritis in the elderly, the diagnosis was missed in 21 percent of patients because of the presence of gastrointestinal symptoms, pulmonary symptoms, or both (34). Urinary tract infections are the most common cause of community-acquired bacteremia in the elderly. A change in clinical status, particularly one associated with fever, should always include a search for urosepsis.

Treatment of urinary tract infections is straightforward, and a wide variety of antimicrobial agents have been used to treat these infections. One frequently neglected but helpful step in determining therapy for patients with suspected urosepsis is a urine Gram stain on the unspun urine sediment. When only gram-positive cocci in chains are seen, which suggests an enterococcal infection, therapy with parenteral ampicillin (6–12 gm/day) is appropriate. Presence of gram-negative bacteria requires therapy with one of several possible agents, the choice of which should depend on where the patient acquired the infection. Community-acquired infections in the absence of previous instrumentation or evidence of obstruction can be treated with trimethoprim-sulfamethoxazole, ampicillin/sulbactam, an aminoglycoside, a fluoroquinolone, a third-generation cephalosporin, or aztreonam. Urinary infections in patients who have been recently hospitalized or who come from nursing homes are more likely to be caused by multi-resistant bacteria. Many infectious disease clinicians favor a combination of piperacillin and gentamicin or imipenem or piperacillin/clavulanate as initial therapy for these patients. Follow-up therapy should be dictated by antimicrobial susceptibility tests. Whenever possible, antibiotics should be changed to less expensive single-agent therapy. Continuation of broad-spectrum antibiotics instead of narrower, more specific therapy, just because the patient is doing well, is financially and microbiologically inappropriate.

In uninstrumented elderly patients without postvoid residual urine, a short, three-day course of antibiotics usually suffices to treat lower urinary tract infection. All elderly patients with suspected pyelonephritis should be treated for at least 2 weeks. Patients should be carefully followed and those who relapse should be retreated for 6 weeks. A major problem, particularly in elderly men, is recurrent urinary tract infection, usually occurring within a month after completion of apparently successful treatment. Relapses are alleged to reflect chronic prostatic infection. In two studies of patients with recurrent urinary tract infections, cure rates were better after 6 to 12 weeks of therapy. This may be a reflection of the difficulty of treating chronic prostatic infections and the poor penetration of beta lactams and aminoglycosides into noninflamed prostate (35). Trimethoprim, erythromycin, quinolones, and doxycycline achieve adequate prostatic levels, and many urologists and infectious disease specialists recommend from 6 to 12 weeks of therapy with one of these agents. Even after extended therapy, relapse rates of 30 percent to 40 percent have been reported (35,36).

Urinary Tract Infections in Persons with Indwelling Catheters

The use of indwelling bladder catheters is far more common in the elderly. After an indwelling catheter is in place, bacterial colonization occurs in about one-half of patients within 2 weeks and virtually all of the patients show bacterial colonization within 6 weeks (37,38). Enteric gram-negative rods are the common colonizing bacteria and their antibiograms reflect local resistance patterns. Attempts at eradicating bladder bacteria in the presence of a catheter are futile and result in colonization with resistant organisms.

Table 50.6 summarizes important guidelines for the prevention of urinary tract infections in persons who have been catheterized. Both the presence of a foreign body in the bladder and the manipulation of the indwelling catheter cause local damage to the bladder. Superimposed bladder distension favors the dissemination of bacteria into submucosal layers and bacteremia. Attempts to eradicate bladder colonization with prophy-

Table 50.6. Guidelines to Prevent Urinary Infections in the Elderly with Indwelling Catheters

Maintain fluid intake at 1.5 liter/day.
Avoid unnecessary catheter manipulations (e.g., routine
  changing of catheter or routine bladder irrigation)
Change catheter when urine flow has ceased for 4 h

SOURCE: Seiler WD, Stahelin HB. Practical management of catheter-associated UTIs. Geriatrics 1988;43:43–49.

lactic antibiotics, special meatal care, bladder irrigation, bladder lavage, or use of antiseptic additives into the drainage bag have all failed (37,39). The single most important step to minimize the threat of systemic infection in the catheterized elderly is to ensure constant urine flow and to minimize bladder distension. Catheters should be minimally manipulated and drainage bags ought never to be placed above the level of the bladder to prevent retrograde filling of the bladder with heavily contaminated urine. A significant decrease in urine flow should result in prompt changing of the urinary catheter.

Elderly patients with indwelling Foley catheters and who develop systemic signs of infection, and those who have no other identifiable source of infection should be presumed to have urosepsis and be treated accordingly. Blood and urine cultures should be taken, if possible, and therapy directed at aerobic gram-negative rods. Antibiotic recommendations depend on local susceptibility patterns; aminoglycosides, ampicillin/sulbactam, fluoroquinolones, and third-generation cephalosporins have all been shown to be effective (37,39,40,41). Perhaps the most important step is a careful evaluation of the status of the urinary catheter. If there is no evidence for catheter obstruction, the catheter may be safely left in place. If there is bladder distension, leakage of urine around the catheter or palpable encrustations in the catheter, the catheter should be replaced. Catheter replacement should *follow* initiation of systemic antibiotic therapy, if possible.

A rectal examination should be done in all men to ensure that active prostatitis is not present. If a boggy prostate is noted, the indwelling catheter should be removed and the bladder drained suprapubically. There are no absolute rules governing the length of antibiotic therapy. In general, a 10-day course is prescribed and most patients respond well. Broad-spectrum empiric therapy can be individualized after the results of the urine cultures are available. In most circumstances, oral antibiotics are used to complete therapy. Antibiotics should not be continued longer than 10 days in patients who have responded because of the risk of increasing the rate of colonization with resistant organisms. Most patients who are being treated appropriately clear the bacteriuria for several days but become recolonized quickly when antibiotics are stopped. Recolonization is the norm and should be expected.

Bacteremia and Endocarditis

Bacteremia

Bacteremia in the elderly has been reviewed by Richardson, who analyzed eight clinical studies done from 1980 to 1989 and which included data for more than 1000 patients (42). Clinical findings of bacteremia in the elderly were consistent in all studies, with confusion and delirium in the patients listed as common findings at the time of evaluation. Predicting bacteremia in the elderly is difficult. Fontanarosa, working in a community hospital emergency room, compared clinical and laboratory parameters of 750 elderly patients who had blood cultures drawn (43). Seventy-nine bacteremic patients were compared with a random sample of 136 patients who were not bacteremic. Logistic regression analysis showed that altered mental status, vomiting, and band forms more than 6 percent were the only characteristics that were independent predictors of bacteremia. The presence of one of these three characteristics had a sensitivity of 0.85 and a specificity of 0.45 for predicting bacteremia. Not unexpectedly, specificity increased when more predictive criteria were included but at the cost of a marked decrease in sensitivity. The authors concluded that their best statistical model was not sufficiently accurate to be clinically useful and that the diagnosis of bacteremia in the elderly remains an unresolved clinical problem.

All studies showed that the urinary tract was the most common source of bacteremia (from 24%–56%); other common sites included lungs and the biliary tree (42). Aerobic gram-negative rods accounted for more than 60 percent of blood isolates and included E. *coli, Klebsiella, Providentia*, and *Proteus* as the most common strains. *Staphylococcus aureus* was the most common gram-positive isolate but *S. pneumoniae*, enterococcus, and *S. viridans* were not unusual isolates. Mortality was highly dependent on the functional status of the patient; case fatality rates ranged from 9 percent for community-dwelling patients with more than 5 years' life expectancy to 47 percent for patients with nosocomial bacteremia. Co-existing disease was believed to account for the differences in mortality rates.

Muder and coworkers published a prospective, 5-year study of 163 episodes of bacteremia in a long-term care VA facility (44). They noted an increase in the nosocomial bacteremia rate from 0.2 per 1000 patient-days in 1985 to 0.4 per 1000 patient-days in 1989. They isolated 205 bacteria and two yeasts from blood cultures; 22 of the bacteremic episodes were polymicrobial. The overall mortality was 21.5 percent, with major differences depending on the site of primary infection; urinary tract infections had a mortality rate of 15 percent in comparison to the 50 percent mortality rate among patients with bacteremic pneumonia. There was a strong association between bacteremic urinary tract infection and the presence of an indwelling catheter (44).

These data are consistent with the observation that bacteremia in the elderly is difficult to diagnose and likely to be particularly serious under two circumstances: 1) acquisition of bacteremia as a nosocomial infection, and 2) a site of primary infection outside the urinary tract.

Endocarditis

Steckelberg and coworkers published an important population-based study of infective endocarditis in Olmstead County, Minnesota (45). All patients with infective endocarditis, who lived in the county, were part of a single data base; thus, for the first time, the true impact of age on the incidence of endocarditis could be calculated. From 1970 to 1987, there were 68 episodes of endocarditis, with 32 occurring in the elderly. The incidence rate in the population 65 years of age or older was almost nine times that seen in the group younger than 65 years of age. There was an equal number of mitral valve and aortic valve sites. About one-third of infections were caused by *Staph. aureus* and a second third caused by *S. viridans*; 8 percent of cases were caused by enterococci. No cases were caused by enterobacteriaceae or fungi. Twenty-eight percent of these patients died, and about one-third suffered major embolic events. The authors concluded that the risk for endocarditis increases with age and that clinicians should vigorously adhere to recommendations for prophylaxis in this age group.

Previous dental work, genitourinary tract instrumentation, and prolonged intravenous lines are three predisposing factors for endocarditis in the elderly, although in about one-half of patients no specific predisposing event is identified (46). Gram-positive organisms account for most of the cases of endocarditis in the elderly. Enterococci are usually related to a urinary tract source

and dental sources are believed to be responsible for *S. viridans* infections. *S. bovis* endocarditis is commonly associated with gastrointestinal disease, particularly colon carcinoma (47).

The clinical manifestations of endocarditis in the elderly can be subtle because systolic murmurs are common in the elderly. Any illness with fever and a possible embolic event should prompt the clinician to obtain at least two blood cultures. The key to making the diagnosis is a positive blood culture, and multiple positive blood cultures of any of these organisms provides strong presumptive evidence for infective endocarditis. Particular attention should be paid to the extent of valvular damage, particularly of the aortic valve, because of the possible need for valvar replacement to manage congestive heart failure. Elderly patients should be treated according to standard regimens with a prolonged course of intravenous antibiotics depending on the isolate (35). Prognosis of infective endocarditis is poorest in the elderly, with a mortality rate of about 45 percent (46,47).

Because of the high case fatality rate of endocarditis in the elderly, there has been renewed interest in encouraging the use of prophylactic regimens that might decrease the incidence of these infections. Use of these regimens is based on the hypothesis that the initial step in infective endocarditis is a transient bacteremia that allows for the implantation of bacteria to damaged valves (48). The American Heart Association has identified certain high-risk procedures for which prophylaxis should be offered

Table 50.7. High-Risk Procedures in the Elderly for Chemoprophylaxis for Infective Endocarditis

---

Dental work producing gingival bleeding or performed in an infected mouth (e.g., tooth abscess)

Surgical intervention or biopsy of respiratory mucosa

Incision and drainage of infected tissue

Genitourinary procedures (cystoscopy, prostatic surgery, urethral dilatation, urinary tract surgery, vaginal hysterectomy)

GI procedures (gallbladder and colon surgeries, esophageal dilatation, scleral therapy for esophageal varices, colonoscopy, upper GI endoscopy with biopsy, or proctosigmoidoscopy with biopsy)

GI = gastrointestinal.
SOURCE: Dajani AS, Bisno AL, Chung KJ, et al. Prevention of bacterial endocarditis. Recommendations by the American Heart Association. JAMA 1990;264:2919.

Table 50.8. Infective Endocarditis Chemoprophylaxis for Oral and Respiratory Tract Procedures

Standard regimen*
  Amoxicillin, 3 gm PO, given 1 h before procedure; follow with 1.5 gm PO, 6 h after initial dose.
  For penicillin-allergic patients, give erythromycin ethylsuccinate, 800 mg, or erythromycin stearate, 1 gm PO, 2 h before procedure; repeat with 1/2 dose 6 h later. Alternatively, give clindamycin, 300 mg PO, 1 h before procedure and repeat with 150 mg 6 h later.
Alternate regimens
Ampicillin, 2 gm IV or IM, 30 min before procedure; repeat in 6 h with ampicillin 1 gm IV or IM, or with ampicillin, 1.5 gm PO.
Clindamycin, 300 mg IV, 30 min before procedure; repeat with clindamycin, 150 mg IV or PO, 6 h later.
Vancomycin, 1 gm IV, infused during 60 min, beginning 1 h before procedure; no repeat dose necessary.

*Includes patients with prosthetic heart valves and high-risk patients.
IM = intramuscularly; IV = intravenously; PO = orally.
SOURCE: Dajani AS, Bisno AL, Chung KJ, et al. Prevention of bacterial endocarditis. Recommendations by the American Heart Association. JAMA 1990;264:2919.

Table 50.9. Chemoprophylaxis for Infective Endocarditis for Gastrointestinal and Genitourinary Procedures

Ampicillin, 2 gm IV or IM and gentamicin* 1.5 mg/kg of body weight (not to exceed 80 mg) IV or IM 30 min before procedure; repeat both drugs at the same dose 8 h later (adjust dose and interval for gentamicin in patients with renal dysfunction). Amoxicillin, 1.5 gm PO 6 h after initial dose may replace parenteral ampicillin.
In penicillin-allergic patients, ampicillin is replaced by vancomycin; 1 gm IV (infused during 60 min) before procedure; repeat dose of vancomycin is administered 8 h later (or adjusted for renal dysfunction). Gentamicin is administered as described above.

*Equivalent aminoglycoside may be substituted.
IM = intramuscularly; IV = intravenously; PO = orally.
SOURCE: Dajani AS, Bisno AL, Chung KJ, et al. Prevention of bacterial endocarditis. Recommendations by the American Heart Association. JAMA 1990;264:2919.

to persons with prosthetic valves or who have evidence of valvular disease (Table 50.7). Chemoprophylactic regimens for oral and respiratory tract procedures and for gastrointestinal and genitourinary procedures are reproduced in Tables 50.8 and 50.9, respectively. As a practical rule, any older patient, with either a prosthetic valve, a cardiac murmur, or a history of endocarditis, should be a candidate for prophylaxis.

Other Infections

Bacterial Meningitis

Central nervous system (CNS) infections are unusual in the elderly but are important because of their high mortality rate. Community-based studies from Rhode Island have documented an average annual incidence rate of bacterial meningitis of 9.4 per 100,000 population (49). Cases occurred predominantly in women (59 cases versus 25 cases in men). Cases of meningitis in the elderly constituted only about 15 percent of the total number of cases, but they accounted for 67 percent of the total mortality for all age groups. There were 46 deaths among the 84 cases reported (54.8% case fatality ratio) in persons aged 65 years or older.

The typical clinical presentation of bacterial meningitis in the elderly includes fever, change in mental status, and a stiff neck. Poor outcome is related to the degree of obtundation on admission (50). Occasionally in the elderly, the important physical finding of nuchal rigidity may be difficult to evaluate because of co-existing cervical spondylosis. When nuchal rigidity is a result of meningeal irritation, the neck resists flexion but can be passively rotated from side to side. With cervical spine disease lateral rotation, flexion and extension of the neck are associated with resistance.

When meningitis is suspected, prompt examination of the cerebrospinal fluid is critical. It has become a routine practice to delay a lumbar puncture until a CT scan is done to ensure that a focal intracranial mass is not present. However, a lumbar puncture can be safely performed without CT in the absence of focal neurologic deficits disclosed by the patient's history or physical examination. If CT is necessary, and if meningitis is part of the differential diagnosis, the patient should be given a dose of a third-generation cephalosporin such as ceftriaxone while waiting for the test. A preferred approach is to perform the lumbar puncture expeditiously and to begin antibiotic therapy while the laboratory work is being done on the spinal fluid. White blood cell counts in spinal fluid from patients with bacterial meningitis are usually larger than 1000 cell/µL. Polymorphonuclear leukocytes predominate, and in about 60 percent of cases, a positive diagnosis can be made from a study of the spinal fluid Gram stain. The most common organisms causing meningitis in the elderly are *S. pneumoniae* and enteric gram-negative bacilli. *Listeria monocytogenes* can be isolated from immunosuppressed patients (49–51).

Empiric therapy should always be directed against *S. pneumoniae* and aerobic gram-negative rods. Immunosuppressed patients should be covered for listeriosis. In the absence of a specific pathogen by Gram stain, a third-generation cephalosporin should be given and ampicillin added to cover *Listeria* if the patient is immunosuppressed. Patients with a positive spinal fluid Gram stain consistent with pneumococci can be treated with penicillin. There are good data to suggest that the use of dexamethasone decreases postmeningitic sequelae in patients with meningitis, and all elderly with bacterial meningitis should receive 10 to 20 mg per day of dexamethasone for the first 4 days (52).

Diarrhea

Deaths from diarrhea in the elderly are probably more important than has been realized. Lew et al reviewed U.S. mortality data collected from 1979 to 1987 and found that for that 9-year period, more than 28,000 persons died of diarrhea, and more than half the deaths were in persons 75 years of age or older (53). The diarrheal deaths in the elderly had a clear, winter seasonality, a trend that was not corrected when concurrent diagnoses of pneumonia, influenza, or both were removed. About 70 percent of the deaths from diarrhea in older persons had their onset in nursing care facilities. Gastrointestinal infections are not unusual in long-term care facilities, and associated deaths, as uncovered in this epidemiologic analysis, are often unnoticed.

Antibiotic-associated diarrhea is a major problem in hospitalized elderly. *Clostridium difficile* spores have colonized many of our hospitals and are frequently spread to patients during hospitalization (54). Systemic antibiotics can perturb normal gut flora, allowing the proliferation of *C. difficile* and the production of powerful exotoxins, which can cause a severe enterocolitis. Patients usually present with diarrhea, but soon develop abdominal pain, cramps, and diarrhea. The diarrhea frequently has red cells, mucus, and almost invariably, polymorphonuclear

leukocytes. Stool toxin assays are positive for *C. difficile* toxin. Patients with known or suspected *C. difficile* enterocolitis should be treated with oral metronidazole (250 mg four times/day) or oral vancomycin (125 mg four times/day). Because of the cost, metronidazole is the preferred therapy. Patients usually respond with a decrease in symptoms within 48 hours after therapy is initiated, and diarrhea and colitis resolve after 10 days of therapy. Patients can usually also be continued on their original course of antibiotics. Relapses occur in about 20 percent of patients and these relapses, if severe enough, are treated no differently than are first episodes. There has been a significant increase in cases of *C. difficile* enterocolitis, and virtually any antibiotic has been shown to be capable of disrupting normal gut flora sufficiently so that *C. difficile* spores can vegetate, proliferate, and produce toxin. These iatrogenic infections emphasize the principle that antibiotic therapy in the elderly should not be prescribed without a good reason.

Somewhat analogously, gastroenterologists have described antibiotic-associated diarrhea caused by overgrowth of *Candida* species. The character of the diarrhea is different from that seen in *C. difficile* enterocolitis in that no white blood cells are seen. All patients have negative *C. difficile* toxin assays and have more than 10^4/mL of *Candida* in the stool; fecal Gram stain reveal many yeast forms. Of interest, all patients described to date have responded to oral nystatin therapy with a decreases in stool *Candida* colony counts and the disappearance of diarrheal symptoms (55,56).

Tuberculosis

The elderly are an important reservoir of tuberculous infection because they may have been infected decades earlier at a time when tuberculous infection was more common than it is today. Cellular immunity wanes with age and it is not surprising that some latent infections become active as persons become older. Recent epidemiologic studies of outbreaks of tuberculosis in nursing homes have suggested that the elderly are also susceptible to reinfection (57).

Tuberculosis in the elderly is a less dramatic illness compared with that in younger patients. In a recent series, only one-third of elderly patients with active pulmonary tuberculosis complained of fever or weight loss, whereas

62 percent of younger men with pulmonary tuberculosis were febrile (58). Chest x-rays often suggest the diagnosis and positive acid-fast smears are diagnostic in the appropriate setting. Occasionally, the diagnosis is delayed when infiltrates on radiographs are misdiagnosed as being a result of old disease. The most important step in the diagnosis of tuberculosis is suspecting its presence.

Elderly persons in long-term care facilities both pose a risk and can be at risk from tuberculosis. All nursing homes and other long-term care facilities should have an organized tuberculin screening program. Patients should undergo two-step testing on admission to the facility in order to identify patients who are negative and to offer isoniazid chemoprophylaxis to those with positive skin tests, when indicated. All persons with negative skin tests should be tested annually to identify recent converters. The identification of recent tuberculin converters should prompt an immediate search for an active case of tuberculosis within the facility and the initiation of isoniazid chemoprophylaxis for the converters (59).

Herpes Zoster

Herpes zoster is an important disease in the elderly because its incidence increases with each decade of life and because the frequency of postherpetic pain is more troublesome with advancing age. The disease is caused by varicella zoster virus (VZV) and represents a reactivation of a latent virus acquired in childhood. The virus resides in sensory neurons, most often in the thoracolumbar area of the cord or in the fifth nerve, particularly the ophthalmic branch. The disease is characterized by a vesicular rash in a dermatomal distribution. The rash is often preceded by a burning or painful sensation. The rash usually appears 2 to 5 days after the beginning of pain and is unilateral. It does not cross the midline. The lesions resemble those of chicken pox and go through a rapid evolution from papules to vesicles to crusted lesions over a period of approximately a week. Pain in the affected dermatome often persists for 1 to 6 months, longer in more elderly individuals. A number of varicelliform lesions may be seen on other parts of the patient's body and, occasionally, a full-blown rash resembling varicella may be seen.

Before the appearance of the rash, the diagnosis of herpes zoster may be confused with many other causes of pain, such as pleurisy, appendicitis, or a collapsed intervertebral disc, and occasionally results in unnecessary surgery. After the rash appears, the diagnosis is almost always obvious. Confirmations of the diagnosis may be made by Tzanck smear, virus isolation, or one of a number of serologic tests for VZV.

At the present time, acyclovir is the preferred treatment for herpes zoster (800 mg five times daily PO for 7 to 10 days, or 5 mg/kg of body weight IV every 8 hours for five days). Steroids were once considered to reduce the incidence of post herpetic neuralgia but more recent data do not support this approach. Patients with VZV infection of the eye should be seen by an ophthalmologist.

Zoster in adults is thought to occur because of waning, age-related immunity. Levine and coworkers studied the immune response of live attenuated varicella-zoster virus vaccine in the elderly (60). The vaccine was well tolerated and 6 to 245 injections resulted in systemic spread of vaccine virus as manifested by a minimal skin rash. Antibody levels against VZV were increased at 12 but not at 24 months, and VZV-specific, proliferating T cells in peripheral blood monocytes were increased in vaccinees. These data are encouraging and suggest that immunization of adults may stimulate immune responses and might prevent episodes of zoster. However, a recommendation to use VZV vaccine in adults must await the results of vaccine trials that are underway in adults (61).

Infectious Hazards of Travel

Travelers' diarrhea affects about one-third of travelers going to tropical areas, and enterotoxigenic E. coli account for most of these infections (62). Although these infections are self-limited, they are disruptive and may precipitate dehydration in the elderly traveler. The best way to prevent travelers' diarrhea is to avoid contaminated food and water. Food served hot and fruits that can be peeled are considered safe. Bottled water and beverages are considered safe; ice is not and should be avoided. Trimethoprim-sulfamethoxazole (TMP-SMX) (800 mg TMP/160 mg SMX orally, twice daily for three days) is effective empiric therapy for travelers' diarrhea and, when combined with the anti-motility agent loperamide, can effectively control symptoms (63). Antibiotic resistance to TMP-SMX has been reported, and some infectious diseases specialists recommend fluoroquinolones because of their activity against TMP-SMX-resistant *Salmonella* and *Campylobacter* (64). Elderly patients with diarrhea should be careful about ensuring that they remain properly hydrated. Oral rehydration packets are readily available and they should be used.

Vaccine requirements for each country are listed in *Health Information for International Travel*, which is published annually by the Centers for Disease Control and Prevention (CDC). The need for special vaccines, such as yellow fever, Japanese B encephalitis, and rabies, are updated annually. In addition to these special needs, all persons older than 65 years of age should receive one dose of pneumococcal vaccine and a diphtheria-tetanus (DT) booster, if indicated. The risk for poliomyelitis to an international traveler is very small. Because the elderly are likely to have come into contact with wild polio virus at a time before the introduction of poliomyelitis vaccine, routine vaccination is not recommended. Under special circumstances in which extensive exposure to unsanitary conditions is likely to occur, two doses of enhanced potency inactivated poliomyelitis vaccine given 1 month apart are recommended (65).

Influenza epidemics occur from December to April in the northern hemisphere and from May through September in the southern hemisphere. The seasonality of influenza is less dramatic in tropical countries, but outbreaks are more common during the rainy seasons. The elderly are at increased risk from respiratory infections, and influenza immunization should be given to the elderly person planning winter travel in northern and southern latitudes (66). Chemoprophylaxis with rimantadine is a less attractive alternative strategy to prevent influenza A (66).

Hepatitis A occurs from one to ten times per 1000 travelers to developing countries who stay for 2 to 3 weeks and who have not received immune globulin (65). Visitors to rural areas should be given immune globulin.

All travelers should be aware of the risk of malaria. Chloroquine-resistance is now widespread, and it is important to tailor a chemoprophylactic regimen accordingly (67). For travel to malaria endemic areas with chloroquine-resistant malaria, mefloquine chemoprophylaxis is recommended (three tablets: 75 mg pyrimethamine plus 1500 mg sulfadoxine). Mefloquine prophylaxis should begin 1 to 2 weeks before travel and

be continued for 4 weeks after leaving the malarious area. Malaria recommendations may change, and it is important that up-to-date reviews be consulted. Many clinicians, in addition to prescribing prophylactic regimens, also provide travelers with a single therapeutic dose of combination pyrimethamine-sulfadoxine (250 mg salt PO once a week) to be taken if the traveler experiences a febrile illness and professional medical care is not available.

Immunizations and Chemoprophylaxis

Routine immunizations which are recommended for all elderly patients are summarized in Table 50.10.

Tetanus Toxoid

Tetanus in the United States is now a geriatric disease (68). Of 114 tetanus cases reported to the CDC in 1989 and 1990, 58 percent of cases were in persons 60 years of age or older. Prevention of tetanus in the adult population has relied on proper wound care and routine decennial boosters with tetanus toxoid (Td). However, more than two-thirds of reported tetanus cases are related to wounds not considered serious enough to need medical attention (68). Errors are also made during wound care. In a study of six emergency rooms, Brand and coworkers found that patients at highest risk for tetanus were least likely to receive correct treatment (69).

The recommendation for routine booster doses of Td in adults has been poorly followed. Mullooly reviewed 1900 randomly selected adult members of a health maintenance organization (HMO) who were eligible to receive Td boosters at no cost out-of-pocket and reported that only 39 percent received one or more Td injections during a 10-year period (70). Furthermore, immunization rates were inversely related to age – 47 percent for persons aged

Table 50.10. Routine Immunizations Recommended for Adults Older Than 65 Years

Vaccine	Frequency
Tetanus/diphtheria	Primary series, then every 10 yr or single booster at age 60 yr
Pneumococcal	Single dose
Influenza	Yearly in fall

20 to 39 years and 28 percent for those older than age 70 years. Several serosurveys done in the U.S. since 1977 have shown consistently that at least half of Americans aged 65 years or older have unprotective tetanus antitoxin levels (71,72). Failure to immunize adults has left older Americans, particularly women who were not vaccinated as part of military service, unprotected.

Balestra and Littenberg have compared the cost-effectiveness of various adult tetanus immunization schedules (73). The authors compared three antitetanus strategies: 1) a booster of Td every 10 years, 2) a single booster for persons aged 65 years, and 3) no intervention for persons older than age 6 except for wound prophylaxis. The decennial strategy was marginally more effective in preventing cases but was far more expensive than the single-booster strategy (discounted cost-effectiveness ratio of about $140,000 per year of life saved with the decennial strategy, compared with $4,500 for the single booster at 65 years of age).

If a change in strategy to a single-booster dose of Td is considered, a key question pertains to the durability of protective antibody titers in persons who have received a primary series. The answers are encouraging: all studies measured protective tetanus antitoxin levels in 87 percent to 100 percent of patients as long as 15 to 25 years after these persons had completed a primary series, and all study subjects had prompt and vigorous anamnestic responses after revaccination (74,75). Perhaps the most relevant serologic data are those from Sweden, which has had a national immunization schedule since the 1950s of three doses of diphtheria-tetanus-pertussis (DTP) or diphtheria-tetanus (DT) at intervals of 4 to 6 weeks starting in a person's second or third month of life, followed by a booster dose when the person is 8 to 10 years of age. No further doses of Td are given to women, but men receive another booster dose in their late teens as part of military service. Christenson and Bottiger measured tetanus antitoxin levels in all age groups, which provided information on the comparability of protective antitoxin levels after four- and five-dose schedules (76). All men and 94 percent of women aged 21 to 30 years had protective levels; between 31 and 50 years of age, 94 percent of men and 73 percent of women had protection. In the age group 60 years and older, 80 percent of men and 56 percent of women had protective levels. These data are consistent with the premise that a Td booster given during the teenage years to persons who received primary immunization results in protection from tetanus for decades.

These data suggest that an appropriate alternative to a decennial tetanus immunization strategy in the U.S. would be a single DT booster to persons aged 60 years who have received the primary DTP immunization series and a DT booster in their teens (77). Linking pneumococcal vaccine to the DT booster dose given to persons aged 60 years is an attractive option.

Pneumococcal Vaccine

Pneumococcal vaccine, licensed since 1977 and reformulated in 1983, contains the capsular polysaccharides of the 23 pneumococcal types responsible for 85 percent to 90 percent of bacteremic infections in the U.S. These antigens induce type-specific antibodies that enhance the opsonization, phagocytosis, and killing of pneumococci by leukocytes and other phagocytic cells. The 23-valent vaccine contains 25 μg of each capsular antigen. After vaccination, more than 80 percent of healthy, young adults develop a twofold or more rise in antibody titer against each antigen. Elderly patients, diabetics, and patients with chronic obstructive lung diseases or alcoholic cirrhosis may develop lower antibody titers than those of normal, young adults, but these levels are still considered adequate for protection.

Pneumococcal vaccine was shown to be protective against pneumococcal pneumonia and bacteremia in healthy, young adults in the setting of high rates of the disease in early randomized controlled studies done among South African gold miners (78). More variable results have been found in studies of the elderly. Pneumococcal vaccination has not been demonstrated to prevent pneumococcal pneumonia in randomized controlled studies that have been criticized methodologically (78). Further case-control studies based on pneumococcal vaccine immunization rates in persons with pneumococcal bacteremia and their controls have demonstrated efficacy in the 60 percent range (79). In 1991, Shapiro and colleagues published the largest and most comprehensive case-control study to study the efficacy of pneumococcal vaccine (80). The vaccine had an efficacy of 61 percent (95% confidence interval, 47%–72%) in immunocompetent recipients. As part of this study, pneumococcal isolates were collected from patients. There were 170 pairs of case patients and controls in which the case patient was infected with a pneumococcal serotype not present in the 23-valent vaccine. Vaccine No efficacy was reported in this group, important confirmational data that the vaccine was effective only against the serotypes found in the vaccine.

Pneumococcal vaccine should be given as a single intramuscular or subcutaneous dose (0.5 mL). Both pneumococcal and influenza vaccines can be given at the same time at different sites without an increase in side effects or a loss of antibody response (68). Serious adverse reactions are relatively few. Minor local side effects such as local pain or redness are common and occur in as much as 50 percent of persons given the vaccine (81). Local Arthus-like reactions have been reported occasionally after the second dose of the 14-valent vaccine but are infrequent with revaccination with the 23-valent vaccine.

Influenza Vaccine

Influenza virus infections remain a significant cause of mortality and morbidity in the U.S. (82). During influenza epidemics, hospitalization among elderly patients with chronic lung and heart diseases may increase two- to fivefold compared with rates of hospitalization during nonepidemic periods. Mortality from pneumonia and general cardiopulmonary diseases is also increased during epidemics of influenza (83,84). Ten thousand or more excess deaths have been documented in each of seven different epidemics in the U.S. during the years 1977 to 1988.

Influenza viruses are single-stranded RNA viruses that are transmitted person-to-person by aerosols or droplets from the respiratory tracts of infected persons. The virus attaches, penetrates, and multiplies in the ciliated columnar epitheliums of a person's upper and lower respiratory tract and leads to cell necrosis and sloughing. This insult markedly impairs the airway's defense system and predisposes to bacterial colonization and local infection in the bronchiopulmonary tree. Secondary bacterial pneumonia is usually due to *S. pneumoniae, H. influenzae* and *Staph. aureus.* Primary influenza viral pneumonia, which often ends fatally, occurs less frequently.

The most effective way of preventing influenza infection is through annual immunization with killed influenza virus trivalent vaccine. Since 1977, influenza vaccine has contained one virus from one of the three major categories of currently circulating influenza viruses; usually a B-type virus and one of A(H1N1) and another of A(H3N2) type. Selection of candidate strains is made after reviewing data on the prevailing strains from the previous season in the U.S. and worldwide isolates. The vaccine contains 15 µg of each antigen per 0.5 mL dose. The vaccine contains only thimerosal as a preservative and minute amounts of egg protein. Because of continued changes in the virus, so-called antigenic drift, immunizations must be given annually. In the U.S., influenza vaccine is usually offered during the months of September through November.

The effectiveness of influenza vaccine in preventing or attenuating illness depends primarily on the age and immunocompetence of the vaccine recipient and the similarity between the virus strains included in the vaccine and those that are circulating during the influenza season. When there is a good match, the vaccine has been shown to prevent illness in 70 percent of healthy children and younger adults (85). Similar results are seen among elderly persons living in the community in the prevention of hospitalization for community-acquired pneumonia.

Among the nursing home elderly, influenza vaccine is most effective in preventing severe illness, secondary complications, and death. In this population, the vaccine has been shown to be about 50 percent effective in preventing hospitalization and pneumonia and about 80 percent effective in preventing death, despite a vaccine efficacy of only about 30 percent among frail, elderly persons (85,86). Thus, yearly influenza vaccination is the single most important measure for reducing the impact of influenza in frail, institutionalized elderly. Results of a 10-state, 4-year influenza immunization demonstration with Medicare recipients sponsored by the CDC and the HCFA showed that the vaccine was cost effective (87). As a result of this trial, Medicare now fully covers influenza vaccine for Part B beneficiaries. A second, important outcome of this study was the realization that high influenza immunization rates could be reached in the community; coverage rates in the ten intervention sites averaged 59 percent compared with rates of 46 percent in the nonintervention sites. Four of the 10 study sites reached much higher levels and, in 1991, the last year of the study, Monroe

County, New York immunized 74 percent of its population aged 65 years or older.

Influenza vaccine can cause minor local reactions (88). Malaise and myalgia may occur in recipients not previously exposed to vaccine antigens; these reactions begin about 6 to 12 hours after vaccination and subside within 48 hours. Recipients of the 1976 swine influenza vaccine developed Guillain-Barré syndrome at a rate of about one case per 100,000 persons vaccinated. Neurologic complications have not been reported in subsequent influenza vaccines (85). Individuals with hypersensitivity to eggs should not receive influenza vaccine but are candidates for chemoprophylaxis.

Chemoprophylaxis Against Influenza

Two antiviral drugs have specific activity against influenza A viruses: amantadine hydrochloride and rimantadine hydrochloride (89). Both agents are now available in the U.S. Amantadine and rimantadine interfere with the replication cycle of type A influenza viruses, although specific mechanisms of their antiviral activity are not completely understood. Both drugs are 70 percent to 90 percent effective in preventing illnesses caused by

Table 50.11. Indications for Anti-Influenza Type A Agents

Chemoprophylaxis
As adjunct to late vaccination of high-risk persons during 2 wk to develop antibodies
In unvaccinated persons, to reduce spread of infection and maintain care for high-risk persons
For immunodeficient persons who may have poor antibody response
For persons for whom influenza vaccine is contraindicated
Amantadine, 200 mg, daily for adults <65 years old; 100 mg daily for those ≥65.
Rimantadine, 100 mg twice a day; for persons with severe hepatic dysfunction or renal impairment (creatinine clearance <10 mL/min) and for elderly nursing home patients, 100 mg daily
Amantadine or rimantadine for duration of influenza type A outbreak, usually 5–7 wk

Therapeutic regimen
Any symptomatic persons, especially those at high risk, during an ongoing influenza type A outbreak
Dose schedule similar to that for chemoprophylaxis except duration of 5–7 days after onset of symptoms

naturally occurring strains of influenza A (89,90). They are not effective against type B influenza. Table 50.11 summarizes the indications for the use and dosage schedule of antiviral agents for influenza type A viruses.

In addition to prophylactic efficacy, both drugs have therapeutic benefit if started within 48 hours of symptoms. Amantadine and rimantadine differ phamacokinetically (89). Both have rapid gastrointestinal absorption, but amantadine is excreted unmetabolized in the urine. The plasma half-life for amantadine is 12 to 18 hours in normal volunteers, but in the elderly and in patients with impaired renal function, the half-life is markedly prolonged. Amantadine should be used in lower doses in these groups (90).

Rimantadine has a much larger volume of distribution and at least 90 percent of the drug is metabolized after oral administration. The plasma half-life is about twice that of amantadine (24 to 36 hours). In clinical trials, both amantadine and rimantadine have been proven to be effective chemoprophylactic agents (89,90). However, amantadine use is associated with a higher incidence of CNS side effects such as lightheadedness, difficulty in concentrating, insomnia, loss of appetite, and nausea (90). These side effects are dose related and, not unexpectedly, occur with increased frequency in patients with impaired renal excretion. Rimantadine should now be the preferred agent for the elderly, for patients with renal impairment, and for children, especially those with a history of seizures.

References

1. Infectious disease in the elderly. Cuhna BA, ed. Chicago: Year Book, 1988.
2. Esposito AL, Gleckman RA, Cram S, et al. Community-acquired bacteremia in the elderly: analysis of one hundred consecutive episodes. J Am Geriatr Soc 1980;28:315–319.
3. Gardner ID. The effect of aging on susceptibility to infection. Rev Infect Dis 1980;2:801–810.
4. Thompson JS, Wekstein DR, Rhoades JL, et al. The immunity status of healthy centenarians. J Am Geriatr Soc 1984;32:274–281.
5. Hirokawa K, Utsuyama M, Kasai M, Kurashima C. Aging and immunity. Acta Pathol Jpn 1992;42:537–548.
6. Murasko DM, Nelson BJ, Silver R, et al. Immunologic response in an elderly population with a mean age of 85. Am J Med 1986;81:612–618.

7. Roberts-Thomson IC, Whittingham S, Youngchaiyud U, Mackay IR. Aging, immune response and mortality. Lancet 1974;2:368–370.

8. Law DK, Dudrick SJ, Abdou NI. Immunocompetence of patients with protein-calorie malnutrition: the effects of nutritional repletion. Ann Intern Med 1973;79:545.

9. Richardson JP. Bacteremia in the elderly. J Gen Intern Med 1993;8:89–92.

10. Yoshikawa TT. Antimicrobial therapy for the elderly patient. J Am Geriatr Soc 1990;38:1353–1372.

11. Ljungberg B, Nilsson-Ehle I. Pharmacokinetics of antimicrobial agents in the elderly. Rev Infect Dis 1987;9:250–264.

12. Poretz DM. Home intravenous antibiotic therapy. Clin Geriatr Med 1991;7:749–763.

13. Balinsky W, Nesbitt S. Cost-effectiveness of outpatient parenteral antibiotics: a review of the literature. Am J Med 1989;87:301–305.

14. Kasper JA. Prescribed medicines: uses, expenditures and source of payment. Preview 9, National Health Care Expenditure Study. Washington, DC: Department of Health and Human Services, DHHS Publ No. (PHS)82-3320, 1982.

15. Gleckman RA. Antibiotic use in the elderly. Infect Dis North Am 1989;3:507–516.

16. Reynolds HY. Host defenses impairment that may lead to respiratory infections. Clin Chest Med 1987;8:339–358.

17. Bennett NM, Buffington J, LaForce FM. Pneumococcal bacteremia in Monroe County, New York. Am J Public Health 1992;82:1513–1516.

18. Marrie TJ. Epidemiology of community-acquired pneumonia in the elderly. Semin Respir Infect 1990;5:260–268.

19. LaForce FM. Antibacterial therapy for lower respiratory tract infections in adults: a review. Clin Infect Dis 1992;15(suppl 2):S233–S237.

20. Fein AM, Feinsilver SH. The approach to nonresolving pneumonia in the elderly. Semin Respir Infect 1993;8:59–72.

21. Crossley KB, Thurn JR. Nursing home-acquired pneumonia. Semin Respir Infect 1989;4:64–72.

22. Garb JL, Brown RB, Garb JR, et al. Differences in etiology of pneumonias in nursing home and community patients. JAMA 1978;240:2169–2172.

23. Musgrave T, Verghese A. Clinical features of pneumonia in the elderly. Semin Respir Infect 1990;5:269–275.

24. Hanson LC, Weber DJ, Rutala WA, Samsa GP. Risk factors for nosocomial pneumonia in the elderly. Am J Med 1992;92:161–166.

25. McDonald AM, Dietsche L, Litsche M, et al. A retrospective study of nosocomial pneumonia at a long-term care facility. Am J Infect Control 1992;20:234–238.

26. Kunin CM. Role of the host defense. In: Kunin CM, ed. Detection, prevention, and management of urinary tract infections. Philadelphia: Lea & Febiger. 1987:299–323.

27. O'Grady F, Cattell WR. Kinetics of urinary tract infection. II. The bladder. Br J Urol 1966;38:156–162.

28. Nicolle LE, Henderson E, Bjornson J, et al. The association of bacteriuria with resident characteristics and survival in elderly institutionalized men. Ann Intern Med 1987;106:682–686.

29. Boscia JA, Abrutyn E, Kaye D. Asymptomatic bacteriuria in elderly persons: treat or do not treat? Ann Intern Med 1987;106:764–766.

30. Nicolle LE, Bjornson J, Harding GKM, MacDonnel JA. Bacteriuria in elderly institutionalized men. N Engl J Med 1983;208:1420–1425.

31. Baldassarre JS, Kaye D. Special problems of urinary tract infection in the elderly. Med Clin North Am 1991;75:375–390.

32. Gleckman R, Crowley M, Natsios GA. Therapy of recurrent invasive urinary tract infections of men. N Engl J Med 1979;301:878–880.

33. File TM, Tan JS. Urinary tract infections in the elderly. Geriatrics 1989;44:15–19.

34. Gleckman R, Blagg N, Hibert D, et al. Acute pyelonephritis in the elderly. South Med J 1982;75:551–554.

35. Pfau A. Prostatitis: a continuing enigma. Urol Clin North Am 1986;13:695–715.

36. Krieger JN. Prostatitis syndromes: pathophysiology, differential diagnosis, and treatment. Sex Transm Dis 1984;11:100–112.

37. Kunin CM. Care of the urinary catheter. In: Kunin CM, ed. Detection, prevention, and management of urinary tract infections. Philadelphia: Lea & Febiger. 1987;245–288.

38. Warren JW, et al. A prospective microbiologic study of bacteriuria in patients with chronic indwelling urethral catheters. J Infect Dis 1982;146:719–723.

39. Seiler WD, Stahelin HB. Practical management of catheter-associated UTIs. Geriatrics 1988;43:43–49.

40. Lipsky BA. Urinary tract infections in men. Ann Intern Med 1989;110:138–150.

41. Nickel JC, Pidutti R. A rational approach to urinary tract infections in older patients. Geriatrics 1992;47:49–55.

42. Richardson JP. Bacteremia in the elderly. J Gen Intern Med 1993;8:89–92.

43. Fontanarosa PB, Kaeberlein FJ, Gerson LW, Thomson RB. Difficulty in predicting bacteremia in elderly emergency patients. Ann Emerg Med 1992;21:842–848.

44. Muder RR, Brennen C, Wagener MM, Goetz AM. Bacteremia in a long-term-care facility: a five-year prospective study of 163 consecutive episodes. Clin Infect Dis 1992;14:647–654.

45. Steckelberg JM, Melton LJ, Ilstrup DM, et al. Influence of referral bias on the apparent clinical spectrum of infective endocarditis. Am J Med 1990;88:582–588.

46. Terpenning MS. Infective endocarditis. Clin Geriatr Med 1992;8:903–912.

47. Gantz NM. Geriatric endocarditis: avoiding the trend toward mismanagement. Geriatrics 1991;46:66–68.

48. Dajani AS, Bisno AL, Chung KJ, et al. Prevention of bacterial endocarditis. Recommendations by the American Heart Association. JAMA 1990;264:2919.

49. Aronson SM, DeBuono BA, Buechner JS. Acute bacterial meningitis in Rhode Island: a survey of the years 1976 to 1985. RI Med J 1991;74:33–36.

50. Behrman RE, Meyers BR, Mendelson MH, et al. Central ner-

vous system infections in the elderly. Arch Intern Med 1989;149:1596–1599.

51. Roos KL. Meningitis as it presents in the elderly: diagnosis and care. Geriatrics 1990;45:63–75.

52. McGowan JE, Chesney PJ, Crossley KB, LaForce FM. Guidelines for the use of systemic glucocorticosteroids in the management of selected infections. J Infect Dis 1992;165:1–13.

53. Lew JF, Glass RI, Gangarosa RE, et al. Diarrheal deaths in the United States, 1979 through 1987. JAMA 1991;265:3280–3284.

54. Kelly CP, Pothoulakis C, LaMont JT. *Clostridium difficile* colitis. Current concepts. 1994;330:257–262.

55. Danna PL, Urban C, Bellin E, Rahal JJ. Role of *Candida* in pathogenesis of antibiotic-associated diarrhoea in elderly inpatients. Lancet 1991;337:511–514.

56. Gupta TP, Ehrinpreis MN. Candida-associated diarrhea in hospitalized patients. Gastroenterology 1990;98:780–785.

57. Stead WW. Tuberculosis among elderly persons: an outbreak in a nursing home. Ann Intern Med 1981;94:606–610.

58. Alvarez S, Shell C, Berk SL. Pulmonary tuberculosis in elderly men. Am J Med 1987;82:602–606.

59. Bailey WC, Albert RK, Davidson PT, et al. Treatment of tuberculosis and other mycobacterial diseases. Am Rev Respir Dis 1983;127:790–796.

60. Levin MJ, Murray M, Rotbart HA, et al. Immune response of elderly individuals to a live attenuated varicella vaccine. J Infect Dis 1992;166:253–259.

61. Takahashi M. Current status and prospects of live varicella vaccine. Vaccine 1992;10:1007–1014.

62. Patterson JE. The pre-travel medical evaluation: the traveler with chronic illness and the geriatric traveler. Yale J Biol Med 1992;65:317–327.

63. Ericsson CD, DuPont HL, Mathewson JJ, et al. Treatment of travelers' diarrhea with sulfamethoxazole and trimethoprim and loperamide. JAMA 1990;263:257–261.

64. Taylor DN, Sanchez JL, Candler W, et al. Treatment of travelers' diarrhea: ciprofloxacin plus loperamide compared with ciprofloxacin alone. A placebo-controlled, randomized trial. Ann Intern Med 1991;114:731–734.

65. Hill DR. Immunizations. Infect Dis Clin North Am 1992;6:291–312.

66. Pomilla PV, LaForce FM. Evaluation of respiratory problems. Infect Dis Clin North Am 1992;6:473–487.

67. Schwartz IK. Prevention of malaria. Infect Dis Clin North Am 1992;6:313–331.

68. Prevots R, Sutter RW, Strebel PM, et al. Tetanus surveillance–United States, 1989–1990. MMWR 1992;41:1–9.

69. Brand DA, Acampora D, Gottlieb LD, et al. Adequacy of tetanus prophylaxis in six hospital emergency rooms. N Engl J Med 1983;309:636–640.

70. Mullooly JP. Tetanus immunization of adult members of an HMO. Am J Public Health 1984;74:841–842.

71. Weiss BP, Strassburg MA, Feeley JC. Tetanus and diphtheria immunity in an elderly population in Los Angeles. Am J Public Health 1983;73:802–804.

72. Crossley K, Irvine P, Warren JB, et al. Tetanus and diphtheria immunity in urban Minnesota adults. JAMA 1979;242:2298–3000.

73. Balestra DJ, Littenberg B. Should adult tetanus immunization be given as a single vaccination at age 65? A cost-effectiveness analysis. J Gen Intern Med 1993;8:405–412.

74. Gottlieb S, McLaughlin FX, Levine L, et al. Long term immunity to tetanus: a statistical evaluation and its clinical implications. Am J Public Health 1964;54:961–971.

75. McCarroll JR, Abrahams I, Skudder PA. Antibody response to tetanus toxoid 15 years after initial immunization. Am J Public Health 1962;52:1669–1675.

76. Christenson B, Bottiger M. Epidemiology and immunity to tetanus in Sweden. Scand J Infect Dis 1987;19:429–435.

77. LaForce FM. Routine tetanus immunizations for adults: once is enough. J Gen Intern Med 1993;459–460.

78. Austrian R, Douglas RM, Schiffman G, et al. Prevention of pneumococcal pneumonia by vaccination. Trans Assoc Am Physicians 1976;89:184.

79. Buter JC, Breiman RF, Campbell JF, et al. Pneumococcal polysaccharide vaccine efficacy: an evaluation of current recommendations. JAMA 1993;270:1826–1831.

80. Shapiro ED, Berg AT, Austrian R, et al. The protective efficacy of polyvalent pneumococcal polysaccharide vaccine. N Engl J Med 1991;325:1453.

81. DeStefano F, Goodman RA, Noble GR, et al. Simultaneous administration of influenza and pneumococcal vaccines. JAMA 1982;247:2551.

82. Glezen WP. Serious morbidity and mortality associated with influenza epidemics. Epidemiol Rev 1982;4:25.

83. Barker WH. Excess pneumonia and influenza-associated hospitalizations during influenza epidemics in the United States, 1970–1978. Am J Public Health 1986;76:761.

84. Lui KJ, Kendal AP. Impact of influenza epidemics on mortality in the United States from October 1972 to May 1985. Am J Public Health 1987;77:712.

85. Recommendations of the Advisory Committee on Immunization. Prevention and control of influenza. Part 1. Vaccines. MMWR 1993;42:1.

86. Gross PA, Quinnan GV, Rodstein M, et al. Association of influenza immunization with reduction in mortality in an elderly population: a prospective study. Arch Intern Med 1988;148:562.

87. Centers for Disease Control and Prevention. Final Results. Medicare influenza vaccine demonstration–selected states, 1988–1992. MMWR 1993;42:601–610.

88. Margolis KL, Poland GA, Nichol KL, et al. Frequency of adverse reactions after influenza vaccination. Am J Med 1990;88:27.

89. Douglas RG. Prophylaxis and treatment of influenza. N Engl J Med 1990;322:443.

90. Dolin R, Reichman RC, Madore HP, et al. A controlled trial of amantadine and rimantadine in the prophylaxis of influenza A infection. N Engl J Med 1982;307:580.

Chapter 51
Endocrine Disorders in the Elderly

Thomas Hornick and Jerome Kowal

What we think and feel and are is to a great extent determined by the state of our ductless glands and our viscera.

Aldous Huxley
Meditation on El Greco

The process of aging has been defined as a genetically programmed, slowly progressive, irreversible change that involves cell loss and replacement events and the adaptation to these changes. Age-related development starts at birth, peaks during and after puberty, and declines steadily thereafter. Primary aging, the process that results from inherent changes in cells with age, needs to be differentiated from changes caused by the effects of disease. In the endocrine system, there is sufficient redundancy in most organs to tolerate substantial loss before abnormalities appear. Characteristically, function may be normal unless the organ is stressed. This becomes increasingly important in very old persons, those 80 years of age and older, when homeostatic reserve becomes more limiting. Although the neuroendocrine theory of aging has its proponents, aging is not generally believed to be merely a decline in hormone or neurotransmitter function.

Most endocrine studies in human subjects have been cross-sectional (subjects of all ages are measured at the same time or different age groups are compared). This methodology provides ease of application and speed of assessment of a potential effect of age on the variable being studied. However, cross-sectional studies cannot measure the rate of change of a variable in an individual, and only measure different age groups at a single point in time without regard for differences in cohorts. Longitudinal studies have shown that, although progression of aging in individual subjects does reflect age-related changes observed from cross-sectional data, the rate of change with age differs greatly in individual subjects. Separating the effects of senescence from those of progressively more sedentary behavior presents a major challenge.

The advent of more sensitive assays for circulating hormones in humans has not eased the difficulty in delineating the relationship between hormone levels and biologic response. Hormone level at a given point in time is a result of a complex interplay of secretion and metabolic clearance. The complexities of the endocrine system indicate that aging effects may occur at a number of points. These include the central nervous system (CNS), and hypothalamic control of the pituitary, pituitary control of target endocrine glands, hormone secretion by the endocrine glands, binding of hormones in the circulation, hormone degradation rate, receptor levels, and postreceptor phenomena.

Thus, endocrine function in the aging patient should be considered in terms of homeostatic adjustments to changes in physiologic function. Basal hormonal levels in humans reflect changes in glandular aging, hormone metabolism, feedback regulation, and other age-related changes (Table 51.1). Renin, aldosterone, triiodothyronine (T_3) in men, and dehydroepiandrosterone (DHEA) are reduced. With advancing age, there appears to be a general decline in secretion rate and metabolic clearance of some hormones, such as testosterone, insulin, adrenal androgens, aldosterone, and thyroid. Normal regulatory mechanisms are generally still present, but for some hormones there is a decrease in feedback, which leads to increased secretion. This is reflected in the elevated secretion of follicle-stimulating hormone (FSH) and luteinizing hormone (LH) as a result of gonadal involution. Antidiuretic hormone (ADH) responses are exaggerated in response to increased serum osmolality in older individuals. There is a decrease in metabolic clearance of cortisol and thyroxine, with diminished production rate to maintain the hormone at normal levels. In contrast, epinephrine clearance rate increases. Some classes of receptors, such as intracellular steroid receptors, appear to decline with age, but insulin receptors and other mem-

Table 51.1. Effect of Age on Circulating Hormone Levels

Definite increase with age
    FSH
    LH
    Norepinephrine
    Insulin
    PTH
    ANP
Probable increase with age
    ADH (with stimulation)
    Prolactin
Definite decrease with age
    Renin
    Aldosterone
    DHEA and DHEA-S
    Estrone and estradiol
    (women)
    Testosterone
    Androstendione
    Progesterone
Probable decrease with age
    GH and IGF-1
    T_3 (men)
Unchanged with age
    T_4
    TSH
    ACTH
    Cortisol

ACTH = corticotropin; ADH = antidiuretic hormone; ANP = atrial natriuretic protein; DHEA = dihydroepiandrosterone; DHEA-S = dihydroepiandrosterone-sulfate; FSH = follicle-stimulating hormone; GH = growth hormone; IGF-1 = insulin-like growth factor (somatomedin-C); LH = luteinizing hormone; PTH = parathyroid hormone; T_3 = triiodothyronine; T_4 = levothyroxine; TSH = thyroid-stimulating hormone.

brane associated receptors do not. Postreceptor age-related alterations occur with somatomedin action, insulin-induced glucose metabolism, catecholamine, and steroid hormone responsiveness.

Comparable normative anatomic changes occur with aging in all endocrine glands. Each gland appears to decrease in weight and to develop a patchy, atrophic appearance accompanied by vascular change and fibrosis. Thyroid, prostate, and adrenal glands have a tendency to form adenomas. The prevalence of certain endocrine diseases, such as diabetes mellitus and hypothyroidism, increases in elderly populations. Endocrine disease in advanced age groups may occur without classic signs and symptoms and present as chronic symptoms of syn-dromes generally associated with elderly patients: fatigue, loss of motivation, anorexia, weight loss, failure to rehabilitate, failure to thrive, and difficulty concentrating. The challenge to the physician is to be aware that some of these symptoms and syndromes may be aggravated or caused by disordered endocrine function.

Thyroid

Thyroid function is a balance between hypothalamic thyrotropin-releasing hormone (TRH), pituitary thyrotropin (TSH) stimulation of the thyroid, and feedback regulation of TRH and TSH by thyroid secretion of thyroxine (T_4) and T_3. TSH increases thyroglobulin content, increases iodide uptake and organification to form mono- and diiodotyrosines, with subsequent synthesis of T_4 and conversion to T_3, and secretion of T_4 and T_3. With aging (Table 51.2), there is a progressive decrease in the metabolic clearance rate of T_4, which reaches levels in patients older than 80 years to less than half that of younger patients, with a concomitant decrease in thyroid hormone production. Although the basal metabolic rate (BMR) decreases with age, oxygen consumption as a function of lean body mass shows no change. Radioactive iodine uptake (RAIU) by the thyroid decreases in the elderly, consistent with the decrease in T_4 production. Plasma thyroid-binding globulins are also unchanged in healthy individuals. As a result, T_4 in the plasma is unaffected.

Serum T_3 tends to decline to levels that are lower than the mean level found in younger subjects but are within a broader normal range in well, elderly persons. The de-

Table 51.2. Alterations in Thyroid Physiology in the Elderly

Test	Result
Basal metabolic rate	Normal
Radioactive iodine uptake	Decreased
T_4 and T_3 production	Decreased
Serum T_4 and T_3 concentration	Normal
T_4 and T_3 degradation	Decreased
TSH concentrations	Normal to decreased
TSH response to TRH	Decreased in men
TSH suppression by T_4	Decreased

T_3 = triiodothyronine; T_4 = levothyroxine; TRH = thyrotropin-releasing hormone; TSH = thyroid-stimulating hormone.

crease in T_3 is presumably caused by a decline in peripheral conversion of T_4 to T_3. This is partially offset by an increased conversion of T_4 to T_3 within the thyroid. Concomitant with the decrease in T_3 levels, there is an increase in the inactive metabolite of T_4 metabolism evolving from proximal ring deiodination (rT_3). T_3 levels may be markedly decreased in individuals with debilitating nonthyroidal disease.

Studies of octogenarians reflect either no change or a slight overall decrease of 24-hour basal TSH secretion, with normal diurnal variation. However, serum TSH may be mildly elevated even in healthy older individuals. TRH stimulation of TSH production is blunted, especially in elderly men, reducing its diagnostic value in the evaluation of hyperthyroidism.

The major clinical conditions encountered in older individuals are apathetic thyrotoxicosis and unsuspected hypothyroidism. Routine screening for thyroid disease has become an essential aspect of assessment of frail, elderly patients. With appropriate blood tests, these disorders can be generally distinguished from normal function at a reasonable cost. For screening purposes, there is no need to draw a battery of thyroid tests (Table 51.3). A single high-sensitivity serum TSH level is generally all that is required. This includes the evaluation of suspected hypo- and hyperthyroidism in the presence and absence

Table 51.3. Patients Who Can Be Assessed by TSH Measurement Alone

No previous thyroid disease
New hypothyroidism
Hyperthyroidism (previous treatment)
T_4 replacement therapy
T_4 suppression therapy (TSH >0.05 mU/liter)

T_4 = levothyroxine; TSH = thyroid-stimulating hormone.

Table 51.4. Patients for Whom Clinical Decisions Cannot Be Made by TSH Alone

T_4 suppression therapy (TSH <0.05 mU/liter)
New goitrous disease
New hyperthyroidism
Hyperthyroidism (current treatment)
Pituitary/hypothalamic disease
Secondary hypothyroidism treated with T_4

T_4 = levothyroxine; TSH = thyroid-stimulating hormone.

of nodules, and of patients taking thyroid hormones. However, if the serum TSH is less than 0.1 mU/liter, additional testing for T_4 or T_3 levels may be warranted, particularly to monitor the progress of patients who have thyrotoxicosis and who are undergoing therapy, individuals who are receiving thyroid replacement therapy, and patients with nodular disease without clinical signs of hyperthyroidism (Table 51.4). Although the combination of low serum TSH and elevated serum T_4 captures 100 percent of thyrotoxic patients, as much as one-third of elderly patients with these results may not be clinically thyrotoxic. Additional confirmation of thyrotoxicosis, in the presence of a low TSH and normal or marginally elevated T_4 or T_3, can be attempted with a 24-hour RAIU.

Hypothyroidism

Clinical manifestations of hypothyroidism do not occur unless there is reduced delivery of thyroid hormones to peripheral tissues. Epidemiologic studies of the prevalence of hypothyroidism have been highly variable, ranging from 0.9 percent to 17.5 percent. In the Framingham study the prevalence of TSH greater than 10 mU/liter was 5.9 percent; with TSH at 5 to 10 mU/liter, the prevalence was 14.4 percent.

The concurrence of the clinical features of hypothyroidism with decreased serum T_4 to less than 4.5 µg/dL and TSH in excess of 10 mU/liter is diagnostic of hypothyroidism. A serum TSH level in excess of 20 mU/liter is also considered to be diagnostic of hypothyroidism and merits initiation of treatment. The natural history of the development of hypothyroidism is depicted in Figure 51.1. Serum TSH rises above the normal range before the fall in total or free T_4. Therefore, reliance on the laboratory for screening is mandatory to avoid the cardiac and neurologic consequences of early myxedema.

Hypothyroidism in the elderly is most commonly associated with autoimmune thyroiditis or previous treatment for Graves' disease (Table 51.5). The pathogenetic role of thyroid autoantibodies in the development of hypothyroidism is unclear. In one study, 80 percent of patients with elevated TSH, normal T_4, and antibody (microsomal) titers more than 1:1600 went on to develop overt hypothyroidism within 4 years. However, antithy-

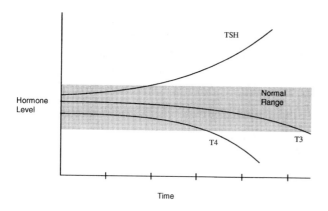

Fig. 51.1. TSH elevation occurs before an appreciable decline in T_4 levels. T_3 levels are preserved until late in the disease.

Table 51.5. Causes of Hypothyroidism in the Elderly

Autoimmune thyroiditis
Late consequences of treated Graves' disease
Previous head and neck surgery or radiation
Iodine deficiency
Amiodarone
Lithium
Pituitary failure

poglobulin and antimicrosomal titers were elevated in only two-thirds of proven cases of hypothyroidism. They were not specific for the development of hypothyroidism because their prevalence was higher (30% in women, 15% in men) than the prevalence of hypothyroidism.

Patients who have had RAIU for Graves' disease should be monitored at least yearly. Head and neck surgery or remote irradiation of the neck may cause thyroid damage that leads to failure years after the initial insult. Iodine deficiency, although not a problem in the United States, is a leading cause of hypothyroidism in many parts of the world and is associated with goiter formation. Iodine excess can lead to hypothyroidism in patients with previous autoimmune thyroiditis by blocking iodide oxidation and organification. Amiodarone, an antiarrhythmic agent, and radiocontrast agents are iodinated compounds that can cause hypothyroidism by this mechanism. Lithium impairs the formation and release of T_4, but rarely causes hypothyroidism. Hypo-

pituitarism is rare and can cause hypothyroidism from a central TSH deficiency. The clinical features of myxedema are absent.

The symptoms of early hypothyroidism in the elderly population are often subtle and are difficult to distinguish from common complaints (Table 51.6). Patients frequently consider them as a normal part of aging. In one study, only 10 percent of individuals with laboratory-determined hypothyroidism were recognized solely by clinical examination. Low recognition is generally ascribed to the fact that hypothyroidism is a great masquerader and frequently appears along with other problems. It is not uncommon to find elderly patients who complain of fatigue, intolerance to cold, weight gain, arthralgias, dry skin, or constipation. However, hoarseness, physical or mental slowing, excessive sleepiness, and paresthesias are not as common in the general population and require evaluation of thyroid status.

Thyroid failure can have a global effect on the frail elderly and should also be considered in patients with carpal tunnel syndrome, myopathy, cerebellar ataxia, ileus, fecal impaction, ischemic heart disease, congestive heart failure (CHF), obstructive sleep apnea, reduced ventilatory drive, and pericardial or pleural effusions. In advanced hypothyroidism, bradycardia is common but not universal.

The presence of delayed relaxation time of the knee or ankle reflex is frequently hard to elicit in an elderly patient with decreased reflexes. Checking radial and biceps reflexes is preferable and more effective. Puffy, nonpitting edema from myxedema may appear in the subcutaneous tissue, especially in the face and around the eyes; dry thickened skin, particularly of the fore-

Table 51.6. Common Symptoms of Hypothyroidism in the Elderly

Fatigue, weakness, lack of energy, excessive sleepiness
Intolerance to cold
Anorexia with weight gain or weight loss
Arthralgias, muscle cramps, paresthesias
Dry skin, coarse skin
Constipation
Hoarseness, coarsening of the voice
Decreased memory, mental slowing
Swelling of hands, face, or extremities

arms and hands, thinning of the outer third of the eyebrows, and coarsening of hair are present in advanced cases. Other suggestive evidence includes low voltage and bradycardia on electrocardiogram (ECG), hypercholesterolemia, macrocytic or normocytic anemia, elevated serum creatinine phosphokinase (CPK), aspartate aminotransferase (SGOT), and lactate dehydrogenase (LDH), and hyponatremia.

Neurologic symptoms in patients with hypothyroidism include difficulty concentrating, psychomotor slowing, and diminished cognitive function. A recent study using neuropsychologic testing on nondemented hypothyroid patients demonstrated impaired learning, word fluency, visual-spatial abilities, attention, motor speed, and visual scanning as compared with nonhypothyroid controls. There was some improvement in these measures after treatment (see Osterweil et al, 1992). Progressive disease in the elderly may lead to social withdrawal and paranoia. Thyroid function tests should be routinely included in the evaluation of dementia. However, "myxedema madness" is a rare cause of the dementia syndrome.

As previously described, hypothyroidism is confirmed by elevated serum TSH with depressed free T_4. Even in patients with severe nonthyroidal illness, the presence of a low free T_4 and elevated TSH indicates primary hypothyroidism. Patients with TSH between 10 and 20 mU/liter and normal serum T_4 without overt symptoms of hypothyroidism are regarded as having subclinical hypothyroidism. There is no clear consensus on treatment for this population. Although many consider this to be an early stage of hypothyroidism and recommend treatment, others suggest close follow-up of thyroid function with treatment only if overt hypothyroidism occurs. In patients who have mildly elevated TSH, a trial of thyroxine may be both therapeutic and prophylactic: 1) left ventricular function measurably improves after T_4 replacement in patients with mild TSH elevation, and 2) after normalization of serum TSH with therapy, some patients note improvement in nonspecific symptoms not originally attributable to hypothyroidism.

T_4 is the treatment of choice for hypothyroidism and should be given once daily. Other preparations of thyroid hormones are not recommended because hormone preparations containing T_3 may cause side effects from the rapid absorption of T_3. The initial recommended dose is 0.025 mg/day with gradual increases every 4 to 6 weeks until the TSH is normal. T_4 has a half life in plasma longer than 7 days in older hypothyroid patients; thus it is not useful to check serum TSH levels more frequently than every 3 to 4 weeks. Because T_4 is cleared less rapidly in the elderly, the full replacement dose required is less than that for younger patients. The effective dose is generally between .075 and 0.125 mg/day and should be individualized using the serum TSH level as a guide.

Thyroid replacement has to be advanced slowly to avoid aggravating co-existing myocardial ischemia, CHF, or arrhythmias. Patients with known coronary artery disease should be followed closely as L-thyroxine therapy progresses. If symptoms increase, treatment should be reduced to a level at which the symptoms are not aggravated and antianginal therapy maximized before the dose is increased. Therapy with a beta blocker can be helpful to protect against cardiac overload.

Decreased bone mass has been documented in patients with chronic thyroid suppression, but the incidence of fractures has not been shown to be increased. Because patients may receive thyroid replacement therapy for decades, cumulative bone loss may be significant; thus, it is important to titrate the dose to the serum TSH in patients receiving chronic thyroid replacement.

Myxedema coma is a medical emergency requiring immediate intervention. Myxedema coma generally occurs in association with acute stress such as severe infection. Hypothermia and respiratory depression are frequent and intensive care management is required. Thyroid replacement is given intravenously along with stress doses of glucocorticoids to treat coincident adrenal insufficiency. Treatment should begin before laboratory confirmation if the diagnosis is suspected. Supportive care and successful treatment of complicating infections are important for survival. Mortality remains high.

Hyperthyroidism

Various surveys put the prevalence of thyrotoxicosis in the elderly population at 0.5 percent to 2.3 percent. Hyperthyroidism can be difficult to diagnose in an elderly person. Only 25 percent of patients older than 65 years of age present with typical symptoms of hyperthyroidism such as weight loss, palpitations, weakness, nervousness, and heat intolerance, which are seen in 70 percent to 90 percent of young patients. In contrast, in patients older than 75 years, only 44 percent have weight loss, 36 percent have palpitations, and 32 percent have weakness. Significantly, Tibaldi found that the average number of symptoms per patient was two, and 2 of the 25 patients in his series had no symptoms (see Tibaldi et al, 1986).

Physical findings of tachycardia, lid lag, fine skin, tremor, and goiter are also less common in the elderly than they are in younger persons. Tachycardia, an almost universal finding in younger patients, was present in 28 percent of Tibaldi's series. Fine skin and tremor were recognized in roughly 40 percent, and 68 percent did not have a goiter. Ophthalmopathy is rare. Atypical presentations include change in bowel habits, depression, chronic fatigue, emotional lability, or muscle weakness and wasting (particularly in proximal upper and lower limbs). In the elderly population, hyperthyroidism can present as generalized wasting and failure to thrive, which mimics patients with occult malignancies (Table 51.7). This was recognized as early as 1931, when Lahey reported a series of patients with "apathetic hyperthyroidism". He noted that these patients presented with fatigue and apathy and without eye findings, goiters, or tachycardia.

Any patient who presents with atrial fibrillation or refractory CHF should be screened for thyroid disease. Studies reported from England and the United States

have revealed that as many as 25 percent of nursing home residents older than age 75 with atrial fibrillation have masked thyrotoxicosis. Conversely, the prevalence of atrial fibrillation in older patients with hyperthyroidism is 32 percent to 39 percent.

Hyperthyroidism in the elderly is most frequently caused by toxic multinodular goiter. The incidence of Graves' disease tends to decline sharply in persons older than 60 years of age. In toxic multinodular goiter, one or more nodules autonomously secrete excessive T_4, with suppression of TSH. In Graves' disease, an autoantibody directed at the TSH receptor on the thyroid cell surface stimulates the gland to produce thyroxine. In contrast, the mechanism of hormone overproduction in thyroid nodules has not been elucidated. Self-limited, iodine-induced hyperthyroidism (Jod-Basedow phenomenon) is occasionally seen in patients with nontoxic multinodular goiter after excessive intake of iodine. Thyrotoxicosis from factitious administration or inadvertent ingestion of thyroid hormone can be strongly considered if RAIU is suppressed. Thyrotoxicosis can appear insidiously in a patient who has been on the same dose of thyroid for many years because of an age-associated decrease in metabolic clearance of thyroid hormone.

Diagnosis has been aided by the advent of high-sensitivity TSH assays. Suppression of serum TSH levels below 0.5 mU/liter associated with elevated serum T_3 or T_4 levels is diagnostic of thyrotoxicosis. In 4 percent to 12 percent of cases, only serum T_3 is elevated; total or free serum T_3 should be measured when T_4 is normal and clinical suspicion remains high. In the setting of debilitating nonthyroidal illness, a serum T_3 more than 100 ng/dL should prompt investigation for hyperthyroidism. Other common but nondiagnostic laboratory test results include decreased serum cholesterol, elevated alkaline phosphatase and mildly increased serum calcium, the latter two presumably caused by increased bone turnover.

TRH stimulation of TSH is marginally useful to diagnose hyperthyroidism in the presence of a low serum TSH. In several series of normal older individuals, TRH responses have been shown to be suppressed in the absence of thyroid disease. RAIU and scan can confirm Graves' disease or toxic multinodular goiter. In Graves' disease, the uptake is diffuse, but there is focal uptake in "hot" nodules in toxic multinodular goiter, or in a single

Table 51.7. Symptoms of Apathetic Hyperthyroidism

Cardiovascular
  Chronic or paroxysmal atrial fibrillation
  Congestive cardiac failure (usually resistant to therapy)
  Paroxysmal atrial tachycardia
Gastrointestinal
  Anorexia, nausea
  Weight loss
  Constipation
  Chronic diarrhea (rarely)
Musculoskeletal
  Generalized asthenia
  Proximal muscle weakness
  Temporal muscle wasting
Mental state
  Depression
  Apathy, lethargy

nodule in Plummer's disease. Very rarely, TSH- or TRH-secreting adenomas can be diagnosed by an elevated serum TSH associated with elevated serum T$_4$.

The treatment of choice in the elderly is thyroid ablation with ^{131}I. A single course of radioiodine therapy is usually successful in most patients with Graves' disease. However, for toxic multinodular goiter, repeat treatment may be required at 6-month intervals if normalization does not occur. In the presence of ischemic heart disease, achieving a euthyroid state before thyroid ablation is recommended to prevent transient release of thyroid hormone and exacerbation of cardiac symptoms. Oral administration of propylthiouracil (PTU) (100–150 mg every 8 hr) or methimazole (10 mg every 6 hr) interferes with the organification step in the formation of thyroxine and induces a euthyroid state within 2 to 4 weeks. In patients with a symptomatic tremor, atrial fibrillation, or tachycardia, propranolol can be used for symptomatic relief until thyroid function is normalized. Unfortunately, some of the contraindications for propranolol, such as bronchospasm, CHF and insulin usage, occur commonly in elderly persons.

In general, in this population, radioactive iodine sufficient to produce hypothyroidism is warranted to achieve a rapid cure. Thyroid replacement for life is required. The use of suppressive drugs has been associated with remission in some cases in younger patients with Graves' disease, but, in general, the frequent dosage interval and toxicity of the drugs (agranulocytosis) make this a less attractive choice for the older patient unless the patient refuses thyroid ablation. Surgical resection of the gland is generally not recommended because of the operative risks in this age group.

Nontoxic Nodular Goiter

Autopsy data reveal that the prevalence of thyroid nodules increases with increasing age. By the age of 70 years, 90 percent of women and 70 percent of men have clinically undetectable thyroid nodules. Ultrasound studies show an incidence of 50 percent in patients who are screened when they are older than 50 years of age. In contrast, nodules were found on physical examination in only 4.2 percent of Framingham study patients, with a greater incidence in women. The differential diagnosis of a new palpable thyroid nodule includes Hashimoto's thyroiditis, follicular and papillary adenoma, nontoxic multinodular goiter, thyroid cyst, and carcinoma.

Single nodules are more commonly associated with cancer than are multiple nodules. Radioisotope imaging of the thyroid determines whether a nodule actively takes up iodine (hot) or does not (cold). As much as 10 percent of single, cold nodules are malignant. Factors that increase the likelihood of a nodule being malignant are a history of radiation to the head and neck, hoarseness, rapid growth of the mass, tracheal compression, and hard consistency of the mass. The evaluation of a nodule requires assessment of the thyroid status of the patient and fine needle aspiration (FNA) of the nodule for histologic diagnosis. FNA is a reliable, safe way to determine the presence or absence of malignancy in a cold nodule.

Neoplasms commonly found in the elderly are papillary carcinoma (35%), follicular carcinoma (20%), medullary carcinoma (15%), anaplastic carcinoma (20%), and lymphoma, sarcoma, and metastatic cancer. The incidence of death from thyroid cancer is low (<1% all cancer deaths). The 10-year survival rate of patients with papillary and papillary-follicular cancers is greater than 90 percent. The prognosis of anaplastic cancers is poor.

If the patient's thyroid function is normal, and there is no impairment of breathing or swallowing, observation is the best management. Thyroid suppression therapy generally sufficiently shrinks the gland, but carries the risk of transient hyperthyroidism if autonomously functioning nodules are present in the gland. Long-term suppression therapy with thyroid hormone also carries the risk of decreasing bone mass and altering cardiac function. Patients with a rapidly growing malignancy should have surgical removal of the tumor. If a patient is placed on thyroid suppression, it must be maintained continuously. A "breakthrough" nodule deserves re-evaluation.

Syndrome of Inappropriate Secretion of Antidiuretic Hormone

The syndrome of inappropriate secretion of antidiuretic hormone (SIADH) is defined by 1) hyponatremia, with normal or low serum potassium; 2) inappropriate elevation of urine osmolality and sodium; 3) elevated plasma volume, which is frequently not clinically evident but suggested by low blood urea nitrogen (BUN) or creatinine; and 4) absence of edema, hypertension, CHF.

Two-thirds of all cases of SIADH occur in the elderly. Table 51.8 lists some of the more common etiologies in an elderly population. Acute respiratory infections, such as pneumonia, lung abscess, and tuberculosis, are among the most common causes. Acute stress from surgery, severe infection, and, occasionally, psychological crisis can produce hyponatremia. Intracranial events such as brain tumor, stroke, and brain surgery cause transient hyponatremia. Medications that are frequently implicated are listed in the Table 51.8. SIADH may not be initially apparent because of a patient's reduced fluid intake. However, on hospital admission or during an illness in which fluids are managed, the patient's increased fluid intake leads to hyponatremia. This hyponatremia is generally mild, self-limited, and requires no treatment.

Symptoms relate to the severity of the hyponatremia and the rapidity of change. When the patient's serum sodium levels fall below 125 mEq/liter, fatigue, lethargy,

Table 51.8. Common Causes of SIADH

Pulmonary infections
Acute stress from surgery
Intracranial disease
    Stroke
    Brain tumor
    Meningitis/encephalitis
Malignant tumors with ectopic ADH secretion
    Bronchial
    Pancreatic cancer
    Thymoma
Drugs
    Chlorpropamide
    Tolbutamide
    Thiazide diuretics
    Narcotics
    Tricyclic antidepressants
    Barbiturates
    Carbamazepine
    Indomethacin, other NSAIDs

ADH = antidiuretic hormone; NSAID = nonsteroidal anti-inflammatory drug; SIADH = syndrome of inappropriate secretion of antidiuretic hormone.

and muscle cramping may occur. CNS manifestations indicate severe hyponatremia and should be an indication for rapid correction. Seizures, delirium, and coma can result from severe hyponatremia and it is potentially fatal.

Management of hyponatremia depends on its severity. Rapid correction to near normal levels has been associated with central pontine myelinosis. Correction in severe symptomatic cases aims for restoration of serum sodium to 120 mEq/liter, a level at which the risk of seizures decreases and other neurologic symptoms should clear. The rate of correction in severe cases should be about 2 mEq/liter/hr, accomplished by fluid restriction and administration of 3% saline (200–300 mL during 3–4 hr). Fluid restriction to 800 to 1000 mL/day is the treatment of choice for mildly symptomatic cases. For patients with no symptoms and mild hyponatremia, close monitoring is all that is generally required. In refractory cases, demeclocycline, 600 to 1200 mg/day, induces a mild nephrogenic diabetes insipidus and can maintain normal sodium levels secondary to polyuria. Unfortunately, the risk of dehydration is high with this agent. Orally active antidiuretic hormone (ADH) antagonists are now under clinical investigation.

Anterior Pituitary

In general, hypothalamic-pituitary axis function is intact in persons of older age. Circadian rhythms are unaffected. However, evidence suggests that sensitivity to feedback is diminished, which results in a higher baseline level of pituitary hormone secretion. Corticotropin (ACTH) and TSH feedback loops remain responsive to cortisol and to T_4/T_3, respectively, but at serum hormone levels that may be normal or slightly elevated. LH and FSH are increased in postmenopausal women as a result of loss of ovarian function. LH and FSH may be normal or slightly elevated in males. Hypogonadism in older males may be caused by inadequate pituitary responses to diminished testosterone production. Serum prolactin levels increase with age in men and women. Elevated prolactin levels may be a result of other causes such as drugs (phenothiazines, butyrophenones), renal failure, hypothyroidism, cirrhosis, and prolactinoma of the pituitary.

Growth hormone (GH) and insulin-like growth factor-1 (IGF-1) levels both decrease with aging in men and women, but GH secretion is greater in women than in men. The number of growth hormone-producing cells (somatotrophs) declines in the absence of pituitary pathology; however, the GH content of the pituitary is normal. With aging, there is a decrease in the frequency and amplitude of the nocturnal pulses of GH. Secretory responses to direct growth hormone-releasing hormone (GHRH) and indirect (e.g., exercise, hypoglycemia, arginine) stimulation of the pituitary have been reported to be decreased or unaffected.

Deficiency of GH in young adults with panhypopituitarism is associated with decreased protein synthesis, decreased lean body mass, decreased bone mass, and an increase in body fat, all of which are reversed with administration of recombinant GH. Because similar changes in body habitus occur with advancing age, the lower secretion of GH in older individuals has been implicated in these changes. Administration of human recombinant GH to malnourished elderly men for 3 weeks resulted in increased body weight, mid-arm circumference and urinary nitrogen retention (see Kaiser et al, 1991). Longer periods of administration in men resulted in increased lean body mass, increased skin thickness, and decreased adiposity (see Rudman et al, 1990). The incidence of side effects was low in these trials. GH administration appears to be safe for short periods of administration, with reversal of some of the effects of aging on body habitus. Other trials of the effect of GH on bone density have found that there is appendicular loss of density with relative sparing of axial bone. Therefore, in patients with osteoporosis, GH may have deleterious effects. The long term effect of GH administration on frail, elderly persons is not known.

Potential side effects of GH therapy include edema, arthralgias, carpal tunnel syndrome, hypertension, fasting hyperglycemia, and increased alkaline phosphatase, which are present to varying degrees depending on the dose administered. The possible risk of accelerating atherosclerotic vascular disease (as seen in acromegaly) has not been fully dispelled, even in short courses of therapy. In addition, GH therapy is costly and requires systemic administration. The efficacy of alternative approaches using pulsatile GHRH therapy have yet to be proven. However, GH may have a useful role in short-term therapy of catabolic disease producing cachexia or burns.

Hypopituitarism is rare, but its symptoms can be easily confused with nonspecific complaints of an aging patient. Symptoms include impotence, tiredness, lethargy, pallor, and intolerance of cold. The evaluation of pituitary insufficiency is similar to that for younger patients. The most sensitive parameter of pituitary secretion is secretion of GH; GH is absent in 90 percent of these patients, TSH in 60 percent. A reduced adrenal response to hypoglycemia occurs in 50 percent of these patients and adrenal insufficiency in 30 percent of patients with large pituitary adenomas. Initial serum testing should include assays for GH, TSH, cortisol, LH, and FSH. Decreased TSH in the setting of decreased thyroxine or low ACTH coincident with low cortisol strongly suggests hypopituitarism. Insulin-induced hypoglycemia to elicit GH response is not recommended because of risk to the elderly patient. Radiographic workup for a pituitary adenoma should include computed tomography (CT) or magnetic resonance imaging (MRI) scan of the sella. Therapy is aimed at replacement of deficient thyroid and cortisol, or gonadal steroids and GH, as indicated.

Adrenocortical System

Aldosterone, DHEA, DHEA-sulfate (DHEA-S), androstendione, and cortisol are the major hormones secreted by the adrenal gland. Basal, circadian, and ACTH-stimulated secretion of cortisol is normal in older individuals. Metabolic clearance of cortisol decreases with age, but is compensated by a decrease in production. Serum levels of corticosteroid-binding globulin (CBG) are unchanged with age. Although elderly patients with acute myocardial infarction have basal and stimulated cortisol output similar to that of younger patients, a delay in recovery from stress levels has been described in elderly patients undergoing surgical procedures, which implies an impairment in the hypothalamic feedback response. Patients with diabetes mellitus or hypertension have a greater stimulated cortisol peak and prolonged return to baseline than that in matched, healthy elders. The clinical significance of this delayed return is unclear.

Adrenal reserve is not impaired under normal conditions, but in chronically ill patients, severe stress can produce transient hypocortisolism and steroid and ACTH-responsive hypotension. The pituitary-adrenal glucocorticoid response is altered by gender and disease. Women may have increased responses to corticotropin-releasing hormone. In some patients with Alzheimer's disease, stroke, or affective disorders, overnight suppression with dexamethasone does not suppress ACTH, and basal cortisol levels may be high.

DHEA and DHEA-S, the principal products of the zona reticularis of the adrenal gland, have the closest association with aging of any hormone system. In the fetal adrenal gland DHEA serves as a precursor for gestational estrogens. Shortly after the infant is born, the fetal zone shrinks dramatically and DHEA production drops to unmeasurable levels. DHEA remains at low levels until a person is 5 to 6 years of age, at which time it increases in an accelerating fashion and reaches a peak when a person is approximately 18 to 20 years of age. This surge is called adrenarche and occurs concomitantly with, or may precede, puberty.

After peaking at adrenarche, DHEA levels gradually decline at a rate of approximately 0.10 to 0.18 μmol/liter/year of age. Both the basal level of DHEA production and ACTH-stimulated DHEA production decline in parallel. The increase in adrenal androgen levels observed before and during adrenarche and puberty is associated with increasing width of the adrenal zona reticularis. There is a correlation between zona reticularis involution and diminished adrenal androgen production in humans during aging. Because of the dissociation of DHEA production from other ACTH-dependent adrenal steroid function, a putative androgen-stimulating peptide has been hypothesized.

Recent studies have suggested that elderly individuals who retain higher plasma DHEA levels have a lower incidence of cardiovascular disease and greater life expectancy than persons with lower levels. No difference in serum DHEA-S levels has been observed between normal individuals and those with Alzheimer's disease. Although DHEA therapy has been recommended in parts of the world to deter aging, its efficacy remains highly conjectural.

Metabolic clearance of aldosterone, volume of distribution and plasma half-life of aldosterone are unchanged with age. Renin production is decreased in many older individuals; in patients who have low levels of renin, there is correspondingly low output of aldosterone.

Adrenal Insufficiency

Although adrenal insufficiency is relatively rare in the elderly, it is reversible, and must be considered for patients with unexplained hypotension or shocklike conditions. Antecedent symptoms can include weight loss, failure to thrive, weakness, change of mental status, arthralgias, diffuse or patchy hyperpigmentation, nausea, and abdominal pain. The principal cause of primary adrenal insufficiency (Addison's disease) in the elderly is autoimmune disease. However, tuberculosis, and, more rarely, bilateral metastatic disease or amyloidosis have to be considered. Atrophic adrenals on CT scan of the abdomen are most consistent with autoimmune disease. Enlarged adrenals should raise suspicion of an infiltrative process and warrant evaluation for tuberculosis. Significant laboratory findings include hyperkalemia, hyponatremia, and hypoglycemia, with or without azotemia.

Adrenal suppression by prolonged steroid administration is not uncommon for patients taking chronic steroids for rheumatoid arthritis or bronchospastic disease. Sudden withdrawal of steroids can lead to adrenal insufficiency, with fever, abdominal pain, and hypotension. If a patient's initial AM serum cortisol level is low, the diagnosis of adrenal insufficiency can be confirmed with a cosyntropin stimulation test. In a patient who has been receiving steroids, repetitive stimulation with ACTH to increase adrenal function may be warranted. Treatment involves replacement with cortisol; care should be taken not to exceed 37.5 mg of cortisol per day to avoid complications of hypercortisolism. If the patient remains weak or hypotensive, addition of fludrocortisone is warranted. The principal differences in the presentation of secondary and primary adrenal insufficiency are the absence of hyperpigmentation and electrolyte abnormalities in secondary insufficiency. Hyperpigmentation and electrolyte abnormalities are associated with excess production of ACTH and diminished aldosterone, respectively.

Cushing's Syndrome

Cushing's syndrome is rare in elderly persons. The disease primarily occurs in middle-aged women, with a lower incidence in men. The presence of centripetal obesity, striae, buffalo hump, glucose intolerance, and hypertension warrants a diagnostic screen. Cushing's syndrome can be caused by an adrenal tumor or pituitary or ectopic ACTH-secreting tumors; the incidence of malignant adrenal tumors increases in older women. Workup includes analysis of cortisol and adrenal androgen production, followed by serum ACTH, dexamethasone suppression test, and CT scan of the abdomen if there is chemical evidence for hypercortisolism. High adrenal androgen levels suggest an adrenal tumor. Severe metabolic alkalosis and rapid onset suggests an ectopic ACTH-secreting tumor. On CT scan, bilateral adrenal enlargement suggests pituitary Cushing's disease or an ACTH-secreting tumor. Unilateral enlargement with contralateral suppression suggests an adrenal tumor. Therapy is primarily surgical. The reader is referred to standard textbooks of medicine for a more complete treatment of the features of this disease.

Adrenal Masses

Adrenal masses are discovered incidentally in 1 percent to 10 percent of high-resolution abdominal CT scans. This incidence is similar to autopsy series, which show a 2 percent to 9 percent incidence of unsuspected adrenal micro- and macroadenomas. The problem presented to the clinician is to distinguish clinically important masses from benign disease. Most adrenal masses are benign, nonsecretory adenomas. The risk of malignancy increases with larger masses. The differential diagnosis of an adrenal mass is broad and includes adrenal carcinoma, adrenal adenoma, pheochromocytoma, metastatic malignancy, tuberculosis, ganglioneuroma, or other rarer causes.

Laboratory workup is aimed at the relatively more common pheochromocytoma and aldosteronomas and should include an AM serum cortisol, plasma catecholamines, plasma renin activity, and aldosterone. Pheochromocytoma would be unlikely in a patient without episodic or sustained hypertension. Aldosteronomas generally cause hypertension and hypokalemia. Hypertension and obesity are seen in glucocorticoid excess, and their absence decreases the likelihood of a glucocorticoid-secreting adenoma. Metastatic disease to the adrenal is generally not an isolated phenomenon. The patient with an incidental adrenal mass can be followed clinically with repeat CT scanning to follow growth of the mass. If the mass is larger than 5 cm, the incidence of malignancy is high enough to warrant CT-guided biopsy or removal of the mass.

Parathyroid

The major physiologic role of parathyroid hormone (PTH) is the regulation of free serum calcium. PTH increases the calcium level by increasing intestinal calcium absorption, activating osteoclastic resorption of bone, and increasing tubular reabsorption of calcium in the kidney. The serum free calcium does not change with age, but PTH has been shown to increase with age in men and women and has been implicated as a factor in bone loss in the elderly. Several age-related changes can account for the rise in PTH: 1) decreased sensitivity of the intestine to vitamin D, which leads to decreased calcium absorption; 2) decreased phosphate reabsorption in the kidney; and 3) decreased renal responsiveness to PTH. In addition, decreased dietary intake of calcium and vitamin D (and/or synthesis of vitamin D), necessary for adequate calcium absorption from the intestine, results in increased PTH-mediated bone resorption to maintain the calcium pool.

The incidence of primary hyperparathyroidism is increased in the elderly, with approximately 188.5 cases/100,000/year in women and 92.2 cases/100,000/year in men. Many cases are discovered serendipitously by routine calcium measurement. As a result, most cases of hyperparathyroidism are asymptomatic at the time of discovery. Symptoms attributable to hyperparathyroidism are usually related to the elevated calcium level or to the effect of PTH on the skeleton and kidneys. Elevated calcium causes lethargy, fatigue, depression, "restless legs," arthralgias and chondrocalcinosis, hypertension, polydipsia and polyuria; gastrointestinal symptoms include anorexia, nausea, vomiting, and constipation. Cognitive deficits and behavioral disorders are commonly seen, particularly at markedly increased serum calcium levels. Depression is the most frequent psychiatric symptom and improves after surgery in 30 percent to 100 percent of patients.

Bone loss may appear as generalized osteopenia. Subperiosteal absorption of the radial aspect of the phalanges is a classic radiologic finding signifying osteitis fibrosa cystica in later stages of the disease. Despite the absence of radiologically apparent bone loss, significant cortical, and to some extent, trabecular bone loss occurs and can lead to osteoporotic fractures or exacerbate osteoporosis. After parathyroidectomy, there is partial recovery of bone mass, associated with accelerated absorption of the circulating calcium.

Nephrolithiasis, hypercalciuria, and renal insufficiency can occur with long-standing, otherwise asymptomatic, hyperparathyroidism and are an indication for evaluation and treatment.

The differential diagnosis of hypercalcemia is listed in Table 51.9. Malignancy and primary hyperparathyroidism account for 90 percent of the cases of hypercalcemia. Hypercalcemia increasing over a short period of time strongly suggests an underlying malignancy. Elevated serum calcium and decreased serum phosphorus in association with normal or elevated PTH (by N-terminal PTH or intact PTH specific assay) is definitively diagnostic of hyperparathyroidism. If PTH is suppressed in association with hypercalcemia, hypercalcemia of malignancy should be strongly considered, and a search for a primary tumor should be undertaken. Abnormalities that suggest hyperparathyroidism in the absence of a PTH assay include hypophosphatemia, hyperchloremic acidosis, hypomagnesemia, hyperuricemia, increased alkaline phosphatase, anemia, and elevated sedimentation rate.

Serum albumin greatly influences total calcium concentration. Most circulating calcium is bound to albumin. This is generally corrected by adding 0.8 mg/dL calcium for each mg/dL albumin less than 4 mg/dL. Thus, a serum calcium of 10 mg/dL in a chronically ill patient with an albumin of 2.5 mg/dL suggests that the true measurement of calcium may be 11.2 mg/dL. If there is doubt, an ionized calcium level should be ordered.

Not all patients with asymptomatic primary hyperparathyroidism progress to symptomatic disease. A 10-year prospective study of 142 patients with asymptomatic hyperparathyroidism found that 23 percent (33 patients) underwent surgery, most in the first 5 years (Scholz and Purnell, 1981). Patients should be considered for surgical resection of the parathyroids if they are 1) symptomatic, including having a recent history of nephrolithiasis, refractory peptic ulcer disease, or pancreatitis; 2) have evidence of osteitis fibrosa cystica or osteopenia by bone density measurement; 3) have a serum calcium level in excess of 12 mg/dL; or 4) have mental status changes associated with elevated calcium.

The decision for surgery should be determined by the patient's life expectancy and quality of life. At present, no data support parathyroidectomy for asymptomatic older individuals. Surgical cure rates are generally higher than 95 percent. Postoperatively, there is frequently rapid improvement in mental symptoms and cessation of rapid bone resorption. The major complications of the surgery include recurrent laryngeal nerve injury and hypoparathyroidism in less than 5 percent of patients. In advanced cases, rapid repletion of calcium in bone can produce severe, life-threatening hypocalcemia.

A trial of medical therapy may be warranted for patients with only vague symptoms, such as lethargy, fatigue, and weakness. No agents counteract the effects of PTH. Estrogen therapy has been shown to be effective in reducing the effect of PTH on bone loss in women. The primary focus of nonsurgical management is control of hypercalcemia. Adequate fluid intake should be ensured and thiazide diuretics should be avoided. Other diuretics should be used cautiously because dehydration exacerbates hypercalcemia. Patients with asymptomatic hyperparathyroidism should be followed with periodic measurement of calcium, PTH, bone density, renal function, and checks for the presence of symptoms.

Hypoparathyroidism in the elderly is most frequently

Table 51.9. Causes of Hypercalcemia

Primary hyperparathyroidism
Hypercalcemia of malignancy
Drug-induced (thiazides, lithium, hypervitaminosis D, "milk alkali" syndrome)
Familial hypocalciuric hypercalcemia
Immobilization in patients with high bone turnover (Paget's disease)
Granulomatous disease (tuberculosis, sarcoidosis)

iatrogenic, either from previous surgery for hyperparathyroidism or from thyroidectomy. Idiopathic forms exist but rarely appear in later life. Functional hypoparathyroidism accompanies hypomagnesemia. An increase in blood pH from respiratory alkalosis increases the amount of bound serum calcium, which reduces free serum calcium and produces symptoms related to hypocalcemia. In unsuspected cases of hypocalcemia, stress may precipitate muscle spasms.

Symptoms range from perioral paresthesias in mild cases, to spasm, tetany, and seizures. Mental depression, seizures, and dementing syndromes have been noted in hypoparathyroidism. Neuromuscular hyperexcitability is the hallmark of hypocalcemia and can be elicited by Trousseau's or Chvostek's test. The presence of hyperphosphatemia and hypocalcemia strongly suggests hypoparathyroidism. The diagnosis is confirmed by low or absent serum PTH. However, PTH can be suppressed to undetectable levels by hypomagnesemia, and restoration of magnesium in cases of functional hypoparathyroidism restores normal calcium and PTH levels.

Treatment is directed at increasing serum calcium levels. In the absence of PTH and with hyperphosphatemia, conversion of 25(OH)D to 1,25(OH)2D is poor. Therefore, treatment is undertaken with 1-alpha hydroxylated vitamin D or its analogues. The danger of this therapy is hypercalcemia, which can occur without symptoms and result in significant renal impairment. Thus, calcium levels must be monitored closely, at least every 1 to 2 months.

Further Reading

General Aging

Kowal J, Cheng B. General principles of endocrine function after the sixth decade. In: Bardin CW, ed. Current therapy in endocrinology and metabolism. Philadelphia: Decker, 1993.

Tietz NW, Shuey DF, Wekstein DR. Laboratory values in fit aging individuals—sexagenarians through centenarians. Clin Chem 1992;38:1167–1185.

Thyroid

Davis P, Davis F. Hyperthyroidism in patients over the age of 60 years. Medicine (Baltimore) 1974;53:161–181.

Drinka PJ, Nolten WE. Review: subclinical hypothyroidism in the elderly: to treat or not to treat? Am J Med Sci 1988;295:125–128.

Griffin MA, Solomon DH. Hyperthyroidism in the elderly. J Am Geriatr Soc 1986;34:887–892.

Leger A, Massin J, Laurent M, et al. Iodine-induced thyrotoxicosis: an analysis of eighty-five consecutive cases. Eur J Clin Invest 1984;14:449–455.

Levy EG. Thyroid disease in the elderly. Med Clin North Am 1991;75:151–167.

Olsen T, Laurberg P, Weeke J. Low serum triiodothyronine and high reverse triiodothyronine in old age: an effect of disease not age. J Clin Endocrinol Metab 1978;47:1111–1115.

Osterweil D, Syndulko K, Cohen S, et al. Cognitive function in non-demented older adults with hypothyroidism. J Am Geriatr Soc 1992;40:325–335.

Rosenthal MJ, Hunt WC, Garry PJ, Goodwin JS. Thyroid failure in the elderly. JAMA 1987;258:209–213.

Ross DS, Daniels GH, Gouvea D. The use and limitations of a chemiluminescent thyrotropin assay as a single thyroid function test in an outpatient endocrine clinic. J Clin Endocrinol Metab 1990;71:764–769.

Sawin CT, Castelli WP, Hershman JM, et al. The aging thyroid: thyroid deficiency in the Framingham study. Arch Intern Med 1985;145:1386–1388.

Tibaldi JM, Barzel US, Albin J, Surks M. Thyrotoxicosis in the very old. Am J Med 1986;81:619–622.

Pituitary

Blackman MR. Pituitary hormones and aging. Endocrinol Metab Clin North Am 1987;16:981–994.

Corpas E, Harman SM, Blackman MR. Human growth hormone and human aging. Endocrin Rev 1993;14:20–39.

Impallomeni M, Yeo T, Rudd A, et al. Investigations of the anterior pituitary functions in elderly patients over the age of 75. Q J Med 1987;64:505–515.

Kaiser FE, Silver AJ, Morley JE. The effect of recombinant human growth hormone on malnourished older individuals. J Am Geriatr Soc 1991;39:235–240.

Mannakkara JV, Datta-Chaudhure M. Recognizing pituitary insufficiency in the elderly. J Am Geriatr Soc 1991;39:273–276.

Rudman D, Feller AG, Nagraj HS, et al. Effect of human growth in men over 60 years old. N Engl J Med 1990;323:1–6.

Urban RJ. Neuroendocrinology of aging in the male and female. Endocrinol Metab Clin North Am 1992;21:921–931.

Adrenal

Dedon JF, Courtney DL, Holmes FF. Addison's disease from tuberculosis in a centenarian. J Am Geriatr Soc 1992;40:618–619.

Greenspan S, Rowe J, Maitland L, et al. The pituitary-adrenal glucocorticoid response is altered by gender and disease. J Gerontol 1993;48:M72–M77.

Gross MD, Shapiro B. Clinically silent adrenal masses. J Clin Endocrinol Metab 1993;77:885–888.

Mason AS, Meade TW, Lee AJ, Morris JN. Epidemiological and clinical picture of Addison's disease. Lancet 1968;2:744–747.

Neurup J. Addison's disease: clinical studies. A report of 108 cases. Acta Endocrinol (Copenh) 1974;76:126–141.

Parathyroid

Potts JT. Management of asymptomatic hyperparathyroidism. J Clin Endocrinol Metab 1990;70:1489–1493.

Scholz D, Purnell D. Asymptomatic primary hyperparathyroidism: 10-year prospective study. Mayo Clin Proc 1981;56:473–478.

Sier HC, Hartnell J, Morley JE, Giuliano AE, Kaiser FE, Frankl D. Primary hyperparathyroidism and delirium in the elderly. J Am Geriatr Soc 1988;36:157–170.

Chapter 52

Thermoregulatory Disorders

Nora E. Morgenstern

We grow with years more fragile in body, but morally stouter,
and we can throw off the chill of a bad conscience almost at once.
Logan Pearsall Smith
Afterthoughts, 1931

Elderly persons are particularly vulnerable to disorders of thermoregulation, presenting as hypothermia or hyperthermia. Because humans are endothermic, as are all vertebrates, they must maintain body temperature within a narrow temperature range, independent of ambient temperature, for survival. Older persons are less able to withstand extremes of heat and cold because of reduction of homeostatic ability, presence of other diseases and syndromes (such as malnutrition), and effects of some medications. Older persons with hypothermia and hyperthermia have higher morbidity and mortality than do younger persons and have increased death rates from cardiovascular and respiratory disease. As seen with other geriatric syndromes, manifestations can be subtle or confusing, which can contribute to delayed diagnosis and poorer outcome.

Pathophysiology of Temperature Regulation

The usual, normal, human body temperature ranges from approximately 97°F to 99°F (36°C to 37.5°C) rectal temperature, with oral temperatures ranging 0.3° to 0.6°C lower (Table 52.1) (1,2). Circadian rhythms create modest diurnal variations, with lowest temperatures in the early morning hours during deep sleep and highest temperatures between 4 P.M. and 10 P.M. Diurnal variation is preserved with aging and with Alzheimer's disease (3); however, elderly persons reach their highest body temperature earlier in the evening (4). Basal temperatures of healthy older persons do not differ significantly from those of young adults, but frail, elderly, nursing home residents may have slightly lower core temperatures (5).

Oral temperatures depend on ambient temperature, and breathing patterns and may be misleadingly low in elderly persons with conditions such as stroke, Parkinson's disease, and delirium. Esophageal and rectal temperatures are therefore considered the most reliable measurement of core body temperature (1,6). Infrared tympanic membrane thermometry correlates fairly well with rectal temperatures in frail elderly persons (7).

The *thermoneutral zone* is the environmental temperature range at which minimal activation of metabolic, evaporative, and thermoregulatory processes maintain normal body temperature. In unclothed adults, the thermoneutral zone is 27°C to 33°C (6,8).

The regulation of normal temperature is achieved by balancing heat production with heat loss. The preoptic region of the anterior hypothalamus and the posterior hypothalamus are the feedback centers responsible for integration of thermoregulatory responses and receive both neural inputs from peripheral skin heat and cold receptors and temperature inputs from surrounding blood. The preoptic anterior hypothalamus is bathed by a specialized vascular network, through which the anterior hypothalamus responds to core blood temperatures by activating mechanisms in the autonomic nervous system and the endocrine system for heat production, conservation, or dissipation. With increases in body temperature, heat-sensitive neurons in the anterior hypothalamus increase their firing rate two- to tenfold for every increase of 10°C (9). Heat-dissipating responses mediated by the anterior hypothalamus include cutaneous vasodilatation and increased activity of sweat glands (10). Cold-sensitive neurons increase their firing rate as body temperature decreases, which stimulates sympathetic outflow tracks to cause peripheral vasoconstriction and shivering. The hypothalamus also has linkages to the cerebral cortex, which leads to behavioral changes such as putting on more clothes in response to cold.

Table 52.1. Normal Body Temperatures

Type of Measurement	Elderly Subjects (≥70 yr)		Young Adults (18–40 yr)	
	Range (°C)	Mean (°C)	Range	Mean
Rectal	36.7–37.5	37.2		
Auditory canal	36.4–37.2	36.8		
Sublingual	36.2–37.0	36.6	35.6–37.7(°C)	36.8°C (±0.4°)
Axillary	35.5–37.0	36.3	96.0–99.9(°F)	98.2°F (±0.7°)

SOURCE: Darowski A, Weinberg JR, Guz A. Normal rectal, auditory canal, sublingual, and axillary temperatures in elderly afebrile patients in a warm environment. Age Ageing 1991;20:113–119 and Mackowiac PA, Wasserman SS, Levine MM. A critical appraisal of 98.6°F, the upper limit of normal body temperature, and other legacies of Carl Reinhold August Wunderlich. JAMA 1992;268:1578–1580.

The thermoregulatory center may be damaged by a range of metabolic or structural insults to the brain. Destruction of the posterior hypothalamus results in hypothermia or poikilothermia, a condition in which body temperature is highly dependent on external temperature (11). Structural damage from infarction, hemorrhage into the third ventricle, Parkinson's disease, or other degenerative central nervous system (CNS) diseases can destroy enough of the anterior hypothalamus to result in hypothermia, as can metabolic processes such as uremia and infections such as encephalitis. The hypothermia seen in septic shock is caused in part by a change in the hypothalamic set point.

Normal body temperature requires a balance between heat production, heat maintenance (insulation), and heat loss. Thermogenesis (heat production) is a product of basal metabolic rate (BMR), muscle activity, thyroid hormones and catecholamines, the sympathetic nervous system, and availability of nutrients.

In healthy young persons, basal metabolic processes significantly affect thermogenesis. At rest, BMR generates 55 to 75 kcal/hr, with kcal production increasing four- to sixfold with moderate physical activity (9). Aging diminishes the efficacy of these processes. A healthy, 30-year-old man has a BMR, on average, of 37 kcal/m²/hr, but an 80-year-old man has a BMR of 33 kcal/m²/hr. Similarly, BMR drops from 36 kcal/m²/hr in a healthy, 30-year-old woman to 32 kcal/m²/hr in an 80-year-old woman (9,12). The decrease in average BMR with age is caused in part by a decrease in lean body (muscle) mass (13,14), and in part by a decrease in muscular activity as a result of a

sedentary lifestyle (13). In humans, as in other endotherms, about 80 percent of calories derived from food is employed in temperature maintenance (15). The thermic response to eating is blunted in healthy older persons (16,17). Malnutrition also reduces heat production because of reduced glucose stores and impaired gluconeogenesis.

Thyroid hormone thermogenesis is a significant source of basal heat production. Both thyroxine and thyrotropin-releasing hormone generate heat (15). The ability of thyroxine levels to alter metabolism does not appear to change with age (15). Although catecholamines are known to stimulate thermogenesis, and beta-adrenergic responsiveness decreases with age, it is unclear to what extent the decrease in thermogenesis seen in old age can be attributed to changes in action of catecholamines.

Heat maintenance is controlled by the insulating properties of skin and subcutaneous tissue, especially subcutaneous fat. Loss of subcutaneous fat with aging, as well as decreased total adipose tissue mass in persons with weight loss and malnutrition, predispose to hypothermia. On the other hand, obese elderly persons show decreased tolerance to environmental heat, in part because fat provides excess insulation (10).

Heat loss occurs by radiation, conduction, convection, and evaporation. Radiation losses, as in heat loss from a person's uncovered head, may account for as much as half of the body's heat loss in moderate temperatures (18). The most potent mechanism of heat loss from conduction is immersion in cold water, in which the thermal conductivity is 32 times that of air; wet clothes also increase heat loss twentyfold. Merely lying immobilized on a cold surface can be a clinically significant cause of conductive heat loss and hypothermia. Convection losses are exemplified by wind disrupting the layer of warm air surrounding the body (windchill). Evaporative heat losses occur in the lungs and from skin. Evaporation of sweat becomes the critical mechanism for maintaining the body's core temperature in hot environments and when a person exercises vigorously.

Mechanisms that control body temperature appear to be less effective with advancing age, particularly in frail, elderly persons. Peripheral vasoconstriction or vasodilation are the first lines of defense against cold or hot temperatures. Blood flow to the skin depends on both a normally functioning autonomic nervous system, and the ability of the cardiovascular system to change cardiac output to shift blood flow to and from the periphery. Both longitudinal and cross-sectional studies have demonstrated impairment in blood flow responses to variations in the external temperature with advancing age (12,19–21). A minority of apparently healthy elderly do not experience peripheral vasoconstrictor response to cold (13). Forearm vasodilation response to heat is also impaired and occurs with a lesser magnitude in some healthy elders (22) and at higher core temperatures than that seen in younger persons (23). Likewise, motor response changes with aging, with onset delayed in older persons (21,24,25). Together with a blunted perception of thirst (25,26), these changes increase an elderly person's

risk of significant dehydration and hyperthermia.

Shivering is an important defense against drops in core temperature and can increase heat production two- to fivefold (8). The shivering response becomes less efficient as persons age, with increased latency of onset and smaller muscle contractions (13). Shivering is also reduced in persons with hypoglycemia (27). But, once an older person (even a person age 80 years or older) generates a shivering response, the person is able to effectively increase heat production (13).

Physiologic studies suggest that persons aged 60 years and older are less able to maintain normal temperatures in response to hypothermic stimuli such as drinking ice water than are younger persons (28). Some studies also indicate reduced perception of cold, impaired sensitivity to temperature changes, and lessened behavioral responses to cold in healthy elders (29). However, no conclusive evidence exists to substantiate the assertion that healthy older persons are more subject to clinically important hypothermia than are younger persons solely on the basis of exposure to low environmental temperatures (29–31).

Many medications impair thermoregulatory function (Table 52.2). Phenothiazines can precipitate hyperthermia or hypothermia, as well as the neuroleptic malignant syndrome. Ethanol predisposes to hypothermia because it is a CNS depressant, an anesthetic, a vasodilator, and a risk for hypoglycemia, trauma, and environmental exposure (see Table 52.2) (32–34).

Table 52.2. Medications Associated with Hyperthermia and Hypothermia

Medical Condition	Medication	Effect
Hyperthermia	Thyroid hormone	Increased metabolic rate
	Anticholinergics	Decreased sweating
	Phenothiazines	Block neurotransmission in central hypothalamic thermoregulatory paths; decreased sweating
	Tricyclic antidepressants	Anticholinergic action; muscular hyperactivity
	Lithium	Muscular hyperactivity
	Monoamine oxidase inhibitors	Cutaneous vasoconstriction; muscular hyperactivity
	Diuretics	Decreased sweating
Hypothermia	Ethanol	Peripheral vasodilatation; inhibition of shivering; impaired environmental perception
	Reserpine, clonidine	Peripheral vasodilatation
	Sedative-hypnotics	Impaired environmental perception; reduced muscular activity
	Phenothiazines	Variable peripheral alpha blockade causing vasodilatation
	Hypoglycemic agents	Insufficient fuel

Hypothermia

Hypothermia is defined as core body temperature of 35°C (95°F) or lower (35).

Epidemiology

Accidental hypothermia results from exposure to sudden or prolonged drops in environmental temperature. Typically, the victim has suffered overwhelming cold stress, such as in cold-water immersion or winter outdoor injuries. Hypothermia develops at milder temperatures in persons whose underlying diseases, or use of alcohol or various medications, predispose them to low body temperatures. Elderly persons who fall and lie on the ground, even indoors, for a period of time are at risk to develop accidental hypothermia. Although most cases occur in winter months, hypothermia is a year-round disease and may occur in all climates, including the tropics. Immersion hypothermia and frostbite confer high risks of mortality, but mortality is also significant in elderly persons found indoors with hypothermia (36). Indoor cases of hypothermia are associated with low socioeconomic status and inadequate heating (29,37).

A myriad of conditions render the older person vulnerable to hypothermia (Table 52.3). Myxedema coma presents with low body temperature in 80 percent of patients (38). Diabetes, with and without complications such as ketoacidosis and hypoglycemia, predisposes to hypothermia (27,39). Stroke, head trauma, degenerative CNS diseases, alcoholism, Wernicke's encephalopathy, cirrhosis, malnutrition, and cachexia all are risk factors for hypothermia. In an Israeli series of older persons hospitalized with hypothermia, hypoproteinemia was the most common associated condition. It was found in 50 percent of patients in association with cachexia (30%) and neuroleptic use (21%) (40). Also, although most persons with sepsis develop fever, 20 percent to 25 percent of elderly persons with sepsis present with hypothermia, and infections of various types, including bacteremia, soft tissue, respiratory, and urinary tract infections are found in 41 percent to 78 percent of elderly hypothermic patients (35–37,40).

Drugs also place older persons at risk of developing hypothermia. Alcohol is the most common cause of drug-induced hypothermia at all ages, but other categories of

Table 52.3. Conditions Predisposing to Hypothermia

Endocrine abnormalities
  Hypothyroidism
  Diabetes
  Diabetic ketoacidosis
  Hypoglycemia
  Adrenal insufficiency
  Hypopituitarism
CNS abnormalities
  Stroke
  CNS tumor, CNS trauma
  Parkinson's disease, other degenerative CNS diseases
  Hypothalamic dysfunction
  Dementia
Other neurologic conditions
  Spinal cord injury
  Autonomic insufficiency
  Peripheral neuropathy
  Wernicke's encephalopathy
Skin conditions
  Burns
  Psoriasis
  Exfoliative dermatitis
Other conditions
  Malnutrition and cachexia
  Hypoproteinemia
  Alcoholism
  Sepsis, other serious infections
  Uremia
  Mobility disorders

CNS = central nervous system.

pharmaceuticals also are associated with hypothermia in elderly persons. Depression of central thermoregulatory function can be seen with phenothiazines, tricyclic antidepressants, benzodiazepines, narcotics, and reserpine. Phenothiazines also have peripheral vasodilating effects, and chlorpromazine inhibits shivering. In many published series, phenothiazines are implicated in accidental hypothermia.

Although hypothermia-related deaths are preventable, more than 9000 deaths attributable to environmental hypothermia occurred in the United States from 1979 to 1990, and no trends toward improved survival were seen during that time (37). Risk of death from hypothermia is twice as high in persons aged 65 and older and five times higher in persons 75 and older than it is in younger persons, with mortality in some series almost 75 percent (40). In general, mortality is related more to the severity of underlying diseases than to the age of the patient or the magnitude of the decrease in core temperature, although core temperatures of 29.4°C (85°F) and lower impart a poor prognosis (41). Infection has consistently been found to be a major risk for mortality (36,40,42–44). Other underlying medical conditions associated with high mortality include hypoproteinemia, thrombocytopenia, and coagulopathies (40). The literature is inconsistent regarding prognostic significance of other comorbid conditions. In the winter of 1992 to 1993 in Chicago, risks for hypothermia-related deaths included age older than 65 years, homelessness, alcohol intoxication, and use of neuroleptics (37). Racial mortality differences were thought to be related to socioeconomic factors such as poor nutrition and lack of adequate shelter. The most common antecedent of hypothermia was chronic indoor cold stress, to which the frail elderly, the immobile, the chronically ill, and the impoverished populations are most vulnerable.

Pathophysiology

The skin is the first line of defense against hypothermia. Normally, skin thermoreceptors are stimulated by cold, which causes reflex vasoconstriction and a decrease in skin temperature to as low as environmental temperature in an attempt to maintain core body heat. In elderly persons, impaired vasoconstrictor response of the peripheral blood vessels lessens heat conservation, deficient skin temperature sensors fail to alert the hypothalamus to stimulate behavioral and endocrine thermogenic responses, and thinning of the skin and subcutaneous tissues reduces insulation. The muscular responses to cold of shivering, which is followed by vasodilation to shunt warmed blood from the muscles to the body core, are also blunted. Autonomic nervous system dysfunction causes both a decrease in resting peripheral blood flow and impaired vasoconstriction. Mobility disorders not only diminish thermogenesis from motor activity, but also hinder the elderly person's adaptive behavioral responses to cold environments.

Clinical Characteristics

The diagnosis of hypothermia is often missed or made late. A high index of suspicion is needed to diagnose hypothermia, which should be considered in the elderly patient who presents with coma, hypotension, or acute stroke. Early signs of hypothermia are palpably cool skin, apathy, incoordination, drowsiness, and slurred speech. Delirium is a common presentation in the elderly (45). Shivering initially causes a transient rise in pulse and blood pressure, which is followed by bradycardia and a progressive depression of the cardiovascular system. The diagnosis is confirmed by a core body temperature of 35°C (95°F) or lower, which requires use of a low-reading thermometer.

As the body temperature falls, a gradual change in some body function occurs (Table 52.4). BMR falls to 50 percent of normal at 28°C; this is associated with a decrease in oxygen requirement, falling cardiac output, and hypotension. CNS blood flow drops 6 percent to 7 percent for each 1°C drop in core temperature (38). At core temperatures lower than 30°C, pupils dilate, reflexes become hypoactive or absent, and muscle tone increases such that the affected person appears to be dead with rigor mortis at temperatures of 26°C to 28°C. Because of these findings and the possibility of successful resuscitation with recovery of neurologic function in hypothermic patients with cardiac arrest, the adage "No one is dead until warm" should be heeded (46).

Common complications of hypothermia include early acidosis, both respiratory from hypoventilation and metabolic from shivering-induced lactic acidosis, tissue hypoperfusion, and hypoxia. Cardiac complications include sinus bradycardia refractory to atropine at core temperatures lower than 35°C, slow atrial fibrillation and other atrial arrhythmias, and ventricular fibrillation or asystole. All arrhythmias are more common at temperatures lower than 29°C. Ventricular arrhythmias are easily induced by rescue and resuscitative efforts, and ventricular fibrillation often is refractory to defibrillation and cardioactive drugs at core temperatures lower than 30°C (38,47). Most deaths are from ventricular fibrillation (15). Severe hypotension is common at core temperatures lower than 28.9°C; hypotension disproportionate to the degree of hypothermia should suggest other etiologies, such as hypovolemia, sepsis, and drug overdose (36).

Other complications are atelectasis, decreased cough reflex, and cold-induced bronchorrhea, all of which contribute to a high risk of pneumonia. The kidneys respond to cold with diuresis (10). Hyperviscosity with cellular

Table 52.4. Clinical Manifestations of Hypothermia

Level	Core Temperature (°C)	Clinical Signs
Mild	36	Peripheral vasoconstriction; hypertension; shivering begins
	34–35	Maximum shivering thermogenesis
	33–34	Dysarthria; impaired coordination; ataxia; confusion; ileus; normal blood pressure; bradycardia; atrial arrhythmias
	32	Decreased respiratory rate, heart rate and blood pressure; cold diuresis; stupor
Moderate	31	Shivering extinguished; Osborn J waves on ECG; coma
	30	Atrial fibrillation; decreased insulin secretion; increased target cell resistance; pulse and cardiac output 2/3 normal
	29	Muscular rigidity; pupils dilated but reactive
	28	Increased risk of ventricular fibrillation; severe hypoventilation
Severe	27	Pupils nonreactive
	26	Loss of reflexes, unresponsive to pain
	24–25	Cerebral blood flow 1/3 normal; refractory arrhythmias; pulmonary edema; shock
	22	Maximum risk of ventricular fibrillation
	18–20	Cardiac standstill, flat EEG
	15.2	Lowest recorded survival of accidental hypothermia

EEG = electroencephalogram; ECG = electrocardiogram.

sequestration in the spleen, liver, and blood vessels causes leukopenia and thrombocytopenia, which together with cold-induced clotting abnormalities can cause bleeding complications (45). Hyperglycemia from inhibition of insulin release and peripheral insulin resistance occurs at core temperatures lower than 30°C; because these abnormalities correct with rewarming, and glycogen stores are depleted by shivering, patients are placed at risk of severe hypoglycemia if elevated blood sugars are treated with insulin. Gastrointestinal complications include ileus and decreased hepatic metabolism of drugs. The relationship of hyperamylasemia to hypothermia is unclear. However, hypothermia-induced pancreatitis is common in some series, and acute hemorrhagic pancreatitis has been noted in some fatalities (36).

Treatment

Hypothermia is a medical emergency that requires prompt treatment. Hypothermia is classified as mild for core temperatures between 32°C and 35°C, moderate for those between 28°C and 31.9°C, and severe for temperatures lower than 28°C. Patients whose initial core temperature is higher than 32.2°C (95°F) and those in a nonarrested cardiac rhythm are likely to do well (41,45), but those whose temperature is lower than 29.4°C (85°F) have a poorer prognosis, with low likelihood of regaining full neurologic recovery after cardiac arrest (47). Because of the high prevalence of serious underlying diseases, most elderly patients, even those with mild hypothermia, require hospitalization.

Choice of rewarming technique is controversial and hampered by the lack of randomized, controlled trials. Rewarming strategies should be guided by the severity of hypothermia and the experience of the treating institution. The optimal rate of rewarming shown to be safe in the elderly is 0.5°C to 1.25°C per hour (38).

Passive external rewarming (PER) is recommended for mild hypothermia; use of techniques of insulation in an ambient temperature exceeding 21°C with high humidity, can achieve rewarming of 0.5°C to 2°C per hour. Frail elderly patients with mild hypothermia may not be able to generate sufficient heat by these mechanisms, and most authorities recommend addition of active core rewarming (ACR) using heated, humidified oxygen for this group (9,10,48).

Active external rewarming (AER), using methods such as heated blankets or immersion in a hot water bath, has the potential disadvantage of "afterdrop," an additional fall in core temperature that occurs during the initial period of rewarming. This phenomenon is thought to increase the potential of fatal cardiac arrhythmias by influx of cold blood to the heart. Although afterdrop is less likely to occur in mild hypothermia and in persons in whom hypothermia developed gradually (as in a geriatric patient who was lying on the ground) (49,50), AER should generally be combined with core rewarming techniques (9). Application of heat to the person's thorax, groin, and neck areas rather than to the entire body is the preferred method of AER, in part because this procedure reduces the risk of worsening hypotension from peripheral vasodilation. This form of AER is recommended for victims not in cardiac arrest and who have core temperatures of 30°C to 34°C (48).

ACR avoids the complication of afterdrop and is recommended for persons with moderate to severe hypothermia. Patients who require mechanical ventilation can be rewarmed approximately 2.5°C/hr with a cascade nebulizer heated to 42°C; nonintubated patients can be rewarmed approximately 1°C/hr with use of a mask and cascade nebulizer heated to 45°C (9). Heated intravenous fluids are recommended as an adjunct measure to avoid further heat loss but are ineffective as a sole rewarming technique (47). Peritoneal lavage with warmed dialysate is recommended for persons with moderate hypothermia if rewarming is proceeding at less than 1°C/hr and for severe hypothermia in a person with nonarrest rhythm (48). Invasive rewarming methods such as femoral-femoral cardiopulmonary bypass (CPB) with a heat exchanger or continuous arteriovenous rewarming (CAVR) should be reserved for critically ill, hemodynamically unstable patients, and are the treatments of choice for patients with severe hypothermia complicated by cardiac arrest (41,46,48). Numerous cases of survivors with intact neurologic function after use of these techniques have been reported (46,51,52). In the Multicenter Hypothermia Study of 428 cases, aggressive rewarming techniques were equally well tolerated by all age groups (36).

Survival has not been demonstrated to improve with rapid rewarming in patients with mild or moderate hypothermia. On the other hand, because cardioversion is often ineffective at core temperatures lower than 32°C, some authorities recommend rapid rewarming for patients with moderate hypothermia and cardiac complications (48). Protocols for cardiopulmonary resuscitation (CPR) have been proposed by the Emergency Cardiac Care Committee of the American Heart Association (47). Care should be taken in the diagnosis of cardiac arrest,

because 30 to 45 seconds may be required to confirm pulselessness or severe bradycardia, for which CPR is indicated. Ventricular fibrillation can be treated in the field with as many as three shocks, but if it persists, further cardioversion attempts with defibrillation or medications should be postponed until the person's core temperature is higher than 30°C. Unnecessary manipulations can easily precipitate fatal arrhythmias, and the patient must be handled very gently. However, endotracheal intubation can be safely performed without increased risk of ventricular fibrillation or asystole (36,47,48), especially if the patient is first ventilated with 100 percent oxygen by bag-valve mask (18,47).

Other management considerations are influenced by the patient's underlying medical conditions and the suspected cause of the hypothermia. Sepsis should always be considered in the elderly patient, especially if the person has mild hypothermia. Elderly persons in whom hypothermia develops gradually are likely to suffer from glycogen depletion and hypovolemia (36). Emergency protocols for coma (dextrose, naloxone, thiamine) should be considered. Atrial arrhythmias are common in persons with core temperatures lower than 32°C and usually resolve spontaneously with rewarming.

Hyperthermia

A broad spectrum of heat-related illnesses is seen in the elderly, the most serious of which is heat stroke. As noted with hypothermia, the diagnosis may be overlooked if presenting symptoms are acute myocardial infarction, stroke, or shock.

Hyperthermia is defined as an elevation of body temperature above the set point controlled by the hypothalamus (53,54). Hyperthermia occurs when the peripheral mechanisms of vasodilation and sweating, impaired by disease or drugs or overwhelmed by external (environmental) or internal (metabolic) heat, are unable to maintain a body temperature that matches the set point. In contrast, fever occurs when the hypothalamic set point is elevated by the action of circulating pyrogenic cytokines, and intact peripheral mechanisms conserve and generate heat until the body temperature rises to the higher set point (54). Hyperthermia and fever can be difficult to distinguish clinically by degree of temperature elevation or its pattern (54); fever can be a predisposing factor for development of hyperthermia.

Epidemiology

Over 300 deaths a year are attributed to heat exposure in the United States; in the severe heat wave of 1980, 1700 heat-related deaths were reported (55). Eighty percent of heat-related illnesses occur in persons age 50 years and older. Incidence of heat-related deaths progressively increases with advancing age, with persons age 85 years and older at greatest risk (55). Heat waves are also associated with increased all-cause mortality in older persons. For example, the 1980 heat wave in Memphis, Tennessee was associated with increased total mortality, with almost all deaths occurring in persons older than 60 years of age (56), and the 1980 heat wave in Missouri resulted in increased all-cause mortality as high as 60 percent above baseline in persons age 65 years and older residing in Kansas City and St. Louis (57). Cardiovascular and cerebrovascular disease contribute prominently to the excess mortality seen in older persons during heat waves (56,58,59).

Heat stroke epidemics occur with prolonged exposure to environmental heat, especially when accompanied by high humidity. Risks for hyperthermia include low socioeconomic status and urban living. Analysis of heat stroke cases in the 1980 Missouri heat wave confirmed that inadequate ventilation and lack of air conditioning were significant risks for heat stroke deaths in the elderly, as was functional dependence, which increased the risk for both fatal and nonfatal heat stroke fivefold (60). A particularly vulnerable population is the institutionalized elderly. In the 1955 southern California heat wave, deaths among nursing home residents increased fourfold (15). In the summer of 1976, a nursing home in southeastern Florida experienced a breakdown in its air conditioning system; 24 percent of residents developed sudden onset of temperature elevation higher than 38.1°C without evidence of infection, and five residents whose temperatures ranged from 39.4°C to 41.3°C died (61).

Numerous preexisting conditions predispose to heat-related illness (Table 52.5). Any disease that impairs the cardiovascular response to heat stress may lessen heat tolerance and lead to heat stroke (62). Hypertension, diabetes, and cardiovascular disease, particularly coronary

Table 52.5. Conditions Predisposing to Heat Stroke

Lack of acclimatization
Impaired circulatory response
  Dehydration
  Congestive heart failure
Increased endogenous heat production
  Strenuous exercise
  Thyrotoxicosis
  Pheochromocytoma
Chronic disease
  Alcoholism
  Diabetes
  Obesity
  Dementia
Drugs impairing sweat production
  Diuretics
  Neuroleptics
  Tricyclic antidepressants
  Antihistamines, other anticholinergics
Drug withdrawal syndromes
  Barbiturates
  Ethanol
  Benzodiazepines
Increased hypothalamic thermal set point
  Infection with fever
  Intracranial bleed

artery disease and congestive heart failure, have been reported to increase risk of heat stroke, as have dementia, neurologic disorders and obesity (10,54,58,63,64). Epidemiologic analyses of heat stroke epidemics have also found alcoholism and use of antipsychotic and anticholinergic medications to be common risk factors for heat stroke (55,60,65).

Pathophysiology

Hyperthermia is caused by excessive environmental temperature, excessive heat production, impaired thermoregulation, or combinations of these factors. Classic (nonexertional) heat stroke primarily afflicts elderly and functionally impaired persons, and is caused by failure of thermoregulation. Typically, it occurs at environmental temperatures higher than 90°F and humidity of 60 percent and higher, usually after several consecutive days and nights of high temperatures. Under these conditions, sustained heat loss by radiation or convection is necessary, which requires a well-functioning cardiovascular system to continuously deliver heated blood to the body surface. However, at ambient temperatures of 29°C

(84.2°F) and higher, particularly with no air movement to facilitate heat dissipation by convection, heat loss by these means is limited. Sweating, which produces heat loss by vaporization of water from the body surface, becomes essential, but evaporation of sweat starts to decrease at relative humidity of 60 percent and stops when humidity is higher than 90 percent (66). Sweating mechanisms, at least in some elderly persons, are impaired from peripheral or central malfunction, or from the effects of medication. Dehydration and use of diuretics further limit heat dissipation because volume depletion causes vasoconstriction and decreased sweating. Also, some evidence suggests that intense sweating is not sustained in many cases of classic heat stroke; after 6 or more hours of profound sweating, sweat production abruptly ceases, body temperature escalates, and the heat stroke syndrome is suddenly manifested by coma or collapse (62).

In contrast to classic heat stroke, which typically occurs in the sedentary elder, exertional heat stroke is seen in persons performing vigorous exercise or heavy work under hot conditions. Resting heat production can generate a 0.8°C/hr rise of body temperature (62). With exercise, heat production can increase as much as tenfold and overwhelm the heat-dissipating capabilities of the unacclimatized person. Although most older persons with heat stroke develop classic or nonexertional heat stroke, older persons engaged in outdoor activities in hot weather (as in the annual Mecca pilgrimage) may develop exertional heat stroke (67). Although acclimatization may be more difficult to achieve in the older person (13), Yousef found that healthy, heat-acclimated men as old as 80 years of age demonstrated no loss of thermoregulatory response to heat during a desert walk (68).

Clinical Syndromes

A spectrum of heat-related disorders, such as prickly heat, heat edema, heat tetany, heat syncope, heat exhaustion, and heat stroke, may occur in conditions of excessive high temperatures. Symptoms range from rash to a mild transient syndrome of headache, dizziness, muscle cramps, and fatigue, to fullblown heat stroke.

Prickly heat (heat rash, miliaria rubra) is a pruritic, erythematous rash associated with a vesicular eruption caused by blockage of sweat pores. Loose, lightweight clothing and avoidance of use of body powders in warm environments can help prevent the condition. Because it damages the sweating mechanism, miliaria predisposes affected persons to heat exhaustion and heat stroke.

Heat edema is commonly seen in older persons, especially women, within the first few days of exposure to a warm environment. Hands and feet show a mild pitting edema. The condition is usually self-limited and requires no specific treatment.

Although heat tetany and cramps are most often seen in younger persons, healthy older persons who engage in vigorous exercise can develop these syndromes after sweat-producing exercise. Body temperature is usually normal. Symptoms are carpopedal spasm and large muscle cramping; treatment includes rest, removal to a cool environment, and fluid and electrolyte replenishment, intravenously if necessary.

Heat syncope results from vasodilation under warm conditions without compensatory tachycardia, and usually occurs in unacclimatized individuals. Use of beta blockers or peripheral arteriolar vasodilators predisposes elderly persons to heat syncope. Onset is sudden and the sufferer is cold, clammy, tachycardic, and has orthostatic hypotension. A variant of vasovagal syncope, the condition is self-limited, and the thermoregulatory system is otherwise maintained. Heat syncope can be confused with heat exhaustion and other cardiovascular causes of syncope. Treatment includes removal from the warm environment and positioning, either supine or with the feet elevated. Use of leg pressure stockings may help prevent heat syncope.

The clinical characteristics of heat exhaustion and heat stroke overlap. Although both manifest elevated core temperatures, in persons with heat exhaustion, core temperature is usually lower than that seen in persons with heat stroke, and mentation is often intact. Symptoms include weakness, dizziness, vertigo, headache, anorexia, nausea, vomiting, myalgias, faintness, and syncope. Heat exhaustion should be regarded as a diagnosis by exclusion and requires monitoring in the emergency or inpatient setting while the diagnosis of heat stroke is entertained. Heat exhaustion of the water depletion or hypernatremic type is particularly common in elderly persons treated with diuretics and in dependent, nursing facility residents who are not given adequate fluids.

Treatment consists of rest in a cool environment and gradual rehydration with intravenous fluids (0.9 percent sodium chloride).

In heat stroke, body temperature characteristically rises to 40°C (105°F) and higher. Temperatures of 41.1°C rectal are common, and temperatures as high as 44.4°C rectal (112°F–113°F) have been reported. The diagnosis of heat stroke should always be considered in the context of exposure to heat stress in persons with the triad of elevated core temperature, severe CNS dysfunction (psychosis, delirium, coma) and, in classic heat stroke, anhidrosis with hot, dry skin. Heat stress is usually environmental, but can be internal, as seen with delirium tremens. In both classic and exertional heat stroke, onset is sudden, accompanied by hyperventilation, tachycardia, and hypotension. Classic heat stroke may occur at lower temperatures in the elderly, and the physical examination may be misleading because underlying diseases and use of medications may blunt characteristic physical signs. Patients may have nonspecific symptoms such as malaise, dizziness, anorexia, and shortness of breath. CNS dysfunction ranges from mild irritability to delirium to seizures; progression is rapid from lethargy to stupor and coma. With the exception of cerebellar signs, a focal neurologic examination is uncommon and should raise the suspicion of an acute CNS event, such as hemorrhage. Classic heat stroke may lack prodromal symptoms—the first symptom may be coma or collapse.

As a person's core temperature rises, oxidative phosphorylation is uncoupled and leads to widespread breakdown of enzyme systems throughout the body. At core temperatures of 42°C (107.6°F), widespread organ failure results (9). Vascular endothelium, neurons, and hepatocytes are most susceptible to heat-related necrosis. Clinically, cerebral edema with coma, seizures, and diffuse neurologic deficits, particularly in the cerebellum, develop, which are proportionate to the duration and degree of hyperthermia (69). Thermal injury to vascular endothelium initiates a disseminated intravascular coagulation state (DIC), most commonly seen in persons with exertional heat stroke. Adult respiratory distress syndrome (ARDS) is sometimes seen in persons with DIC (70). Centrilobular hepatic necrosis is common, and hepatic failure is a fatal complication (67). Other complications are congestive heart failure, myocardial infarction, and cardiogenic shock. Myocardial ischemia is very common (71). Acute renal failure, rhabdomyolysis, and ARDS are more common in persons with exertional heat stroke (63) than in persons with classic heat stroke (Table 52.6) (72).

At initial core temperatures higher than 42°C, prognosis of classic heatstroke is poor (63,67,69), although normal recovery has been seen in patients with core temperatures of 43.9°C (67). Prognosis is correlated with the duration of severe hyperthermia, and cooling requiring longer than 1 hour leads to poorer outcomes (63,67,73,74). Clinical features portending a poor prognosis include severe hypotension, respiratory failure, ARDS, DIC, and seizures (63,67,73,74). Although metabolic acidosis is very common in persons with exertional heat

Table 52.6. Characteristics of the Two Types of Heat Stroke

	Classic	Exertional
Usual age group	Older	Younger
Epidemics	Yes	No
Functional status	Dependent	Healthy, independent
Predisposing illnesses	Chronic illness	Acute illness or none
Activity	Sedentary	Vigorous (e.g., marathon runners, military recruits)
Weather	Prolonged heat wave	Variable
Environment	Indoors without air conditioning	Outdoors
Sweating	Usually absent	Often present
Acid-base disturbance	Respiratory alkalosis	Lactic acidosis
Rhabdomyolysis	Rare	Common
Disseminated intravascular coagulation	Rare	Common, severe
Acute renal failure	Rare	Common

stroke, when metabolic acidosis is seen in persons with classic heat stroke, it is a marker of severity of illness and is associated with poorer outcomes (64). Coma has been reported to be a poor prognostic indicator; however, some patients have recovered completely despite earlier evidence of lack of brainstem function (67).

The differential diagnosis of heat stroke includes the neuroleptic malignant syndrome. Although usually seen in younger persons receiving neuroleptic medications, the syndrome has also been reported in a 65-year-old man with Alzheimer's disease who was given haloperidol for treatment of agitation and paranoia (75). Manifestations include extrapyramidal signs; altered consciousness and delirium; autonomic dysfunction with lability of blood pressure, tachycardia and pallor; and temperatures as high as 42°C (107.6°F). Neuroleptic malignant syndrome can be distinguished from heat stroke by onset within hours to days of initiating neuroleptic medication, rigidity (which precedes the development of hyperthermia), and, often, a profound diaphoresis (62,76). The syndrome is an idiosyncratic reaction to neuroleptic agents, and occurs in 0.2 percent of patients receiving these drugs, usually within the first month of treatment (54). It is more common with the use of high potency neuroleptics such as haloperidol. Complications include rhabdomyolysis, hypernatremic dehydration, and acute renal failure. Mortality is high, approximately 20 percent, even when the medication is withdrawn and intensive supportive measures are given.

Other considerations in the differential diagnosis of heat stroke include thyrotoxicosis, especially thyroid storm (62,77), infections, delirium tremens, and anticholinergic poisoning. Rarely, pheochromocytoma storm and stroke involving the brainstem, hypothalamus, or anterior pituitary can mimic heat stroke (62).

Treatment

Fullblown heatstroke requires emergency treatment with the goals of cardiovascular support and rapid, aggressive cooling. Various methods of cooling have been proposed. Historically, immersion in ice-water baths has been advocated, but this procedure has the disadvantages of causing vasoconstriction and shivering and impedes CPR, which could be necessary. Ice applications selectively applied to the patient's lateral thorax, groin, and neck can minimize clinically significant vasoconstriction and are effective cooling methods. The evaporation method, refined at the Makkah Body Cooling Unit, consists of a sling suspended over a tub of water with atomized 15°C water sprayed over the patient's body by a 45°C air current. Rapid heat loss without vasoconstriction or shivering can be achieved, and many authorities now recommend this approach (72,78). Modifications include external cooling by hosing down the person with tepid water while a fan blows over the person's body.

Shivering and seizures that occur with cooling are hypothesized to be secondary to vascular and CNS overcooling. Because overcooling is common in all methods (a 33% incidence was found in a 1992 meta-analysis of cooling studies) (79), continuous temperature monitoring is mandatory, and cooling measures should be discontinued at 39°C. Auditory canal temperatures may be preferable because rectal temperature changes can lag behind core temperature during periods of rapid cooling (79). Cooling should progress at 0.1°C/min or faster, with the goal of achieving core temperature of 38.5°C to 39°C within 1 hour (9,10,62,65,72). Monitoring for recurrence of hyperthermia for as long as 3 to 6 hours is necessary.

Often, hypotension will respond to cooling alone because the high-output cardiac failure and peripheral vasodilation characteristic of heat stroke cause extensive shifts of body fluids to the periphery, and cooling causes redistribution of fluids to the central circulation. Elderly patients with volume depletion or persistent hypotension may require central monitoring with a Swan-Ganz catheter. Vasopressors should be used with caution because vasoconstriction hinders cooling. The treatment of cooling-associated shivering is controversial. Chlorpromazine was extensively used in the past, but it has the disadvantages of slow onset, toxicity from hepatic dysfunction, reduction in the seizure threshold, and worsening of hypotension. Use of intravenous diazepam has been suggested, but can contribute to delirium in the elderly patient. Even with optimal treatment, mortality is at least 10 percent (54). Therefore, public health measures, such as emphasis on the importance that persons maintain adequate hydration and the necessity that persons rest in an air conditioned environment and reduce their activity during heat waves, are essential.

References

1. Darowski A, Weinberg JR, Guz A. Normal rectal, auditory canal, sublingual, and axillary temperatures in elderly afebrile patients in a warm environment. Age Ageing 1991;20:113–119.

2. Mackowiak PA, Wasserman SS, Levine MM. A critical appraisal of 98.6°F, the upper limit of normal body temperature, and other legacies of Carl Reinhold August Wunderlich. JAMA 1992;268:1578–1580.

3. Prinz PN, Christie C, Smallwood R, et al. Circadian temperature variation in healthy aged and in Alzheimer's disease. J Gerontol 1984;39:30–35.

4. Moe KE, Prinz PN, Vitiello MV, et al. Healthy elderly women and men have different entrained circadian temperature rhythms. J Am Geriatr Soc 1991;39:383–387.

5. Castle SC, Norman DC, Yeh M, et al. Fever response in elderly nursing home residents: are the older truly colder? J Am Geriatr Soc 1991;39:853–857.

6. Mitchell D, Laburn HP. Pathophysiology of temperature regulation. Physiologist 1985;28:507–517.

7. Castle SC, Toledo SD, Daskal SL, Norman DC. The equivalency of infrared tympanic membrane thermometry with standard thermometry in nursing home residents. J Am Geriatr Soc 1992;40:1212–1216.

8. Matz R. Hypothermia: mechanisms and countermeasures. Hosp Pract 1986;21:45–71.

9. Harchelroad F. Acute thermoregulatory disorders. Clin Geriatr Med 1993;9:621–639.

10. Brody GM. Hyperthermia and hypothermia in the elderly. Clin Geriatr Med 1994;10:213–229.

11. Allen J, Boyd K, Hawkins SA, Hadden DR. Poikilothermia in a 68-year-old female. Q J Med 1989;70:103–112.

12. Wagner JA, Robinson S, Marino RO. Age and temperature regulation of humans in neutral and cold environments. J Appl Phys 1974;37:562–569.

13. Collins KJ, Exton-Smith AN. Thermal homeostasis in old age. J Am Geriatr Soc 1983;31:519–524.

14. Tzankoff SP, Norris AH. Effect of muscle mass decrease on age-related BMR changes. J Appl Physiol 1977;43:1001–1006.

15. Wongsurawat N, Davis BB, Morley JE. Thermoregulatory failure in the elderly. J Am Geriatr Soc 1990;38:899–906.

16. Schwartz RS, Jaeger LF, Veith RC. The thermic effect of eating in older men: the importance of the sympathetic nervous system. Metabolism 1990;39:733–737.

17. Thörne A, Wahren J. Diminished meal-induced thermogenesis in elderly men. Clin Physiol 1990;10:427–437.

18. Moss J. Accidental severe hypothermia. Surg Gynecol Obstet 1986;162:501–513.

19. Collins KJ, Dore C, Exton-Smith AN, et al. Accidental hypothermia and impaired temperature homeostasis in the elderly. BMJ 1977;1:353–356.

20. MacMillan AL, Johnson RH, Corbett JL, et al. Temperature regulation in survivors of accidental hypothermia in the elderly. Lancet 1967;2:165–169.

21. Richardson D, Tyra J, McCray A. Attenuation of the cutaneous vasoconstrictor response to cold in elderly men. J Gerontol 1992;47:M211–M214.

22. Sagawa S, Shiraki K, Yousef MK, Kenju M. Sweating and cardiovascular responses of aged men to heat exposure. J Gerontol 43:M1–M8.

23. Crowe JP, Moore RE. Physiological and behavioral responses of aged men to passive heating. J Physiol 1973;235:43–45.

24. Fennel WH, Moore RE. Responses of aged men to passive heating. J Physiol 1973;231:118–119.

25. Miescher E, Fortney S. Responses to dehydration and rehydration during heat exposure in young and older men. Am J Physiol 1989;257:R1050–R1056.

26. Phillips P, Rolls B, Ledingham J, et al. Reduced thirst after water deprivation in healthy elderly men. N Engl J Med 1984;311:753–759.

27. Freinkel N, Metzger BE, Harris E, et al. The hypothermia of hypoglycemia. N Engl J Med 1972;287:841–845.

28. Sugarek NJ. Temperature lowering after iced water: enhanced effects in the elderly. J Am Geriatr Soc 1986;34:526–529.

29. Fox RH, Woodward PM, Exton-Smith AN, et al. Body temperatures in the elderly: a national study of physiological, social, and environmental conditions. BMJ 1973;1:200–206.

30. Keilson L, Lambert D, Fabian D, et al. Screening for hypothermia in the ambulatory elderly: the Maine experience. JAMA 1985;254:1781–1784.

31. Lloyd EL. Hypothesis: temperature recommendations for elderly people: are we wrong? Age Ageing 1990;19:264–267.

32. Lomax P. Drugs and body temperature. Int Rev Neurobiol 1970;12:1–43.

33. Olson KR, Benowitz NL. Environmental and drug-induced hyperthermia. Pathophysiology, recognition, and management. Emerg Med Clin North Am 1984;2:459–474.

34. Mann SC, Boger WP. Psychotropic drugs, summer heat and humidity, and hyperpyrexia: a danger restated. Am J Psychiatry 1978;135:1097–1100.

35. Centers for Disease Control and Prevention. Hypothermia-associated deaths–United States, 1968–1980. MMWR 1985;34:753–754.

36. Danzl DF, Pozos RS. Multicenter hypothermia study. Ann Emerg Med 1987;16:1042–1055.

37. Centers for Disease Control and Prevention. Hypothermia-related deaths–Cook County, Illinois, November 1992–March 1993. MMWR 1993;42:917–919.

38. Reuler JB. Hypothermia: pathophysiology, clinical settings, and management. Ann Intern Med 1978;89:519–527.

39. Neil HAW, Dawson JA, Baker JE. Risk of hypothermia in elderly patients with diabetes. BMJ 1986;293:416–418.

40. Kramer MR, Vandijk J, Rosin AJ. Mortality in elderly patients with thermoregulatory failure. Arch Intern Med 1989;149:1521–1523.

41. Hauty MG, Esrig BC, Hill JG, Long WB. Prognostic factors in severe accidental hypothermia: experience from the Mt. Hood tragedy. J Trauma 1987;10:1107–1112.

42. Darowski A, Najim Z, Weinberg JR, Guz A. Hypothermia and infection in elderly patients admitted to hospital. Age Ageing 1991;20:100–106.

43. Lewin S, Brettman LR, Holzman RS. Infections in hypothermic patients. Arch Intern Med 1981;141:920–925.

44. Morris DL, Chambers H, Morris MG, Sande M. Hemodynamic characteristics of patients with hypothermia due to occult infection and other causes. Ann Intern Med 1985;102:153–157.

45. Treatment of hypothermia. Med Lett Drugs Ther 1986;28: 123–124.

46. Gentilello LM, Cobean RA, Offner PJ, et al. Continuous arteriovenous rewarming: rapid reversal of hypothermia in critically ill patients. J Trauma 1992;32:316–327.

47. Emergency Cardiac Care Committee, American Heart Association. Guidelines for cardiopulmonary resuscitation and emergency cardiac care. Part IV. Special resuscitation situations. JAMA 1992;268:2242–2250.

48. Jolly BT, Ghezzi KT. Accidental hypothermia. Emerg Med Clin 1992;10:311–327.

49. Savard GK, Cooper KE, Veale WL, Malkinson TJ. Peripheral blood flow during rewarming from mild hypothermia in humans. J Appl Physiol 1985;58:4–13.

50. Webb P. After drop of body temperature during rewarming: an alternative explanation. J Appl Physiol 1986;60:385–390.

51. Maresca L, Vasko JS. Treatment of hypothermia by extracorporeal circulation and internal rewarming. J Trauma 1987;27:89–90.

52. Baumgartner FJ, Janusz MT, Jamieson WR, et al. Cardiopulmonary bypass for resuscitation of patients with accidental hypothermia and cardiac arrest. Can J Surg 1992;35:184–187.

53. Dinarello CA, Cannon JG, Wolff SM. New concepts on the pathogenesis of fever. Rev Infect Dis 1988;10:168–189.

54. Simon HB. Hyperthermia. N Engl J Med 1993;329:483–487.

55. Centers for Disease Control and Prevention. Heat-related deaths–United States, 1993. MMWR 1193;42:558–560.

56. Applegate WB, Runyon JW, Brasfield L, et al. Analysis of the 1980 heat wave in Memphis. J Am Geriatr Soc 1981;29:337–342.

57. Jones TS, Liang AP, Kilbourne EM, et al. Morbidity and mortality associated with the July 1980 heat wave in St Louis and Kansas City, Mo. JAMA 1982;247:3327–3331.

58. Knochel JP. Environmental heat illness: an eclectic review. Arch Intern Med 1974;133:841–861.

59. Fish PD, Bennett GC, Millard PH. Heatwave morbidity and mortality in old age. Age Ageing 1985;14:243–245.

60. Kilbourne EM, Choi K, Jones S, Thacker SB. Risk factors for heatstroke. JAMA 1982;247:3332–3336.

61. Sullivan-Bolyai JZ, Lumish RM, Smith EW, et al. Hyperpyrexia due to air-conditioning failure in a nursing home. Public Health Rep 1979;94:466–470.

62. Knochel JP. Heat stroke and related heat stress disorders. Dis Mon 1989;35:301–378.

63. Tucker LE, Stanford J, Graves B, et al. Classical heatstroke: clinical and laboratory assessment. South Med J 1985;78:20–25.

64. Hart GR, Anderson RJ, Crumpler CP, et al. Epidemic classical heat stroke: clinical characteristics and course of 28 patients. Medicine 1982;61:189–197.

65. Centers for Disease Control and Prevention. Heatstroke–United States, 1980. MMWR 1981;30:277–279.

66. Zelenak RR, Miller K. Heat stroke New Orleans Style. Am J Med Sci 1987;294:268–274.

67. Yaqub BA, Al-Harthi SS, Al-Orainey IO, et al. Heat stroke at the Mekkah pilgrimage: clinical characteristics and course of 30 patients. Q J Med 1986;59:532–539.

68. Yousef MK, Dill DB, Vitez TS, et al. Thermoregulatory responses to desert heat: age, race and sex. J Gerontol 1984;39:406–414.

69. Clowes GHA, O'Donnell TF. Heat stroke. N Engl J Med 1974;291:564–567.

70. El Kassimi FA, Al-Mashadani S, Abdullah AK, Akhtar J. Adult respiratory distress syndrome and disseminated intravascular coagulation complicating heatstroke. Chest 1986;90:571–574.

71. al-Harthi SS, Nouh MS, al-Arfaj H, et al. Non-invasive evaluation of cardiac abnormalities in heat stroke pilgrims. Int J Cardiol 1992;37:151–154.

72. Tek D, Olshaker JS. Heat illness. Emerg Med Clin 1992;10:299–310.

73. Yacub BA. Neurologic manifestations of heat stroke at the Mecca pilgrimage. Neurology 1987;37:1004–1006.

74. Vicario SJ, Okabajue R, Haltom T. Rapid cooling in classic heatstroke: effect on mortality rates. J Emerg Med 1986;4:394–398.

75. Serby M. Neuroleptic malignant syndrome in Alzheimer's disease. J Am Geriatr Soc 1986;34:895–896.

76. Lazarus A. Differentiating neuroleptic-related heatstroke from neuroleptic malignant syndrome. Psychosomatics 1989;30:454–456.

77. Simon HB, Daniels GH. Hormonal hyperthermia. Am J Med 1979;66:257–262.

78. Graham BS, Lichtenstein MJ, Hinson JM, Theil GB. Nonexertional heatstroke: physiologic management and cooling in 14 patients. Arch Intern Med 1986;146:87–90.

79. Ash CJ, Cook JR, McMurry TA, Auner CR. The use of rectal temperature to monitor heat stroke. Mo Med 1992;89:283–288.

Chapter 53
Hematologic Problems

Paul A. Seligman

All the soarings of my mind begin in my blood.
Rainer Maria Rilke
Wartime Letters, 1921

The biologic processes of aging are associated with a number of changes in the hematologic system. Aging may also lead to a higher incidence of neoplasia. However, in discussing hematologic and oncologic problems it is difficult to separate biology from the socioeconomic conditions complicating the lives of the elderly, and it is necessary to include both these factors when evaluating patients and considering treatment. For example, older persons tend to be relatively more anemic than are young adults, a circumstance that may be related to the effects of aging on bone marrow reserve. However, older persons who have higher intelligence, periodic health examinations, and adequate health care and who live at home and retain social activity tend to have higher hemoglobin levels [1], which indicates that socioeconomic conditions play an important role in influencing hemoglobin levels in the elderly. Similarly, various effects of aging can increase neoplastic potential, but socioeconomic factors such as neglect and poor nutritional status may further complicate the diagnosis and treatment of neoplastic disease in the elderly. Therefore, because so many factors are involved, each elderly patient must be considered as an individual as the physician determines how and to what extent a hematologic or oncologic problem will be investigated and treated.

Biologic Effects of Aging on Hematologic Function

Although some hematologic values such as hemoglobin (Hgb) level appear to be decreased in the elderly, there is controversy about whether the decreases are a result of the effects of aging on diminished bone marrow prolifera-tive capacity. It has been hypothesized that the bone marrow precursors for red cells, granulocytes, and platelets (noncommitted stem cells) have limited proliferative capacity and thus diminish as the patient gets older. This concept is supported by studies demonstrating that the extent of the hematopoietic bone marrow and percentage of active bone marrow at any one site steadily shrink with age [2]. However, these studies show great individual variation from patient to patient, and the average bone marrow cellularity in the anterior iliac crest drops only 33 percent during adult life (from about 60% at age 20 to about 40% at age 70) [2]. Because bone marrow reserves are probably not decreased in the elderly and aplastic anemia is not common in the aged [3], effects of aging on bone marrow proliferative capacity may occur but may not have clinical significance within the existing human life span. This controversy notwithstanding, some poorly defined factors are associated with the aging process and they must be considered when the physician evaluates hematologic laboratory data for elderly patients.

Although there have been conflicting reports [4,5], a number of studies have indicated that hemoglobin level decreases as a function of age [6–8]. However, as shown in Table 53.1, the average decline is not marked. Besides a decrease in stem cells, the decline in part may be explained by a relative decrease in erythropoietin response to anemia in elderly subjects [9]. However, the studies that show a drop in hemoglobin level in apparently physically well individuals may still not account for mild nutritional deficiency or other treatable causes for the anemia other than the mere biologic process of aging.

Total leukocyte count is decreased in elderly patients (Table 53.1), but the absolute number of granulocytes does not appear to change significantly in the elderly. Although, on the whole, older patients maintain an adequate leukocyte response to infection [10], reports have indicated that patients older than age 55 have a smaller

Table 53.1. Hematologic Values in the Elderly

Values	Hemoglobin (gm%) Mean (range, ± 2 SD)	Hematocrit (%) Mean (range, ± 2 SD)	Leukocyte Count/μL Mean (range, ± 2 SD)	Lymphocyte Count/μL Mean (range, ± 2 SD)
Normal adult	men–15.5 (13.3–17.7) women–13.7 (11.7–15.7)	men–46.0 (39.8–52.2) women–40.9 (34.9–46.9)	men–7250 (3900–10,600) women–7280 (3900– 11,000)	men and women–2500 (1000–4800)
Adults age 65+*	men–12.9 (9.9–15.9)	men–38.6 (29.8–47.4)	men and women–5280 (3130–8910)	men and women–1520 (600–3500)

*Most studies indicate hemoglobin levels are similar for both sexes older than age 65.
SOURCE: Williams WJ. Peripheral blood. In: Williams WJ, ed. Hematology. New York: McGraw-Hill, 1981:10–19; Smith J, Whitelow DM. Hemoglobin levels in aged men. Conn Med Assoc J 1971;105:816. Caird FI, Andrews GR, Gallie TB. The leukocyte count in old age. Age Ageing 1972;1:239

neutrophilic leukocytosis after the oral administration of prednisolone than do young adults (11); certain responses of neutrophils, such as reproduction of superoxide, may also be deficient (12). Other studies indicate that a leukocyte response in the elderly person with infection often results in an increase in the number of immature forms rather than an increase in the leukocyte count itself (13). Although the exact cause has not been explained, these studies indicate that the elderly have a mildly diminished granulocyte response to stress.

The slight decrease in the leukocyte count seen in persons older than 65 years of age is mainly caused by a decrease in the lymphocyte count, specifically a decrease in T lymphocytes (14). Therefore, it is not surprising that lymphocytes from elderly subjects have shown significantly less mitogenic response to plant mitogens and growth factors (15). B lymphocytes are normal in number in the peripheral blood, but lower immunoglobulin levels are seen in elderly subjects. The immunoglobulin G (IgG) antibody response to specific antigens is depressed, but this abnormality may be caused by immunoregulatory dysfunction of T cells (16). The exact mechanisms for the decrease in T lymphocytes and altered immunoglobulin response seen in elderly patients are unexplained.

No age-related changes in the platelet count have been seen (17), and there are no reports of platelet function abnormalities in the elderly. Although the elderly have a number of diseases such as including atherosclerosis, that are associated with increased thrombotic phenomena, definitive data are not available to indicate that the elderly have an acquired abnormality of the clotting system, which would result in an increase in thrombus formation.

Although not necessarily a hematologic value, the erythrocyte sedimentation rate (ESR) shows a progressive increase with age, and a decrease occurs in the percentage of elderly subjects who have ESRs that fall within the normal range (18). Thus, apparently healthy persons older than 70 years of age can have Westergren ESRs as high as 50mm/hr. The cause for the increase in the ESR is presently unknown, although a number of these elderly patients may have preclinical diseases associated with a rise in the sedimentation rate.

Anemia in the Elderly

Anemia is the most common hematologic problem encountered in the elderly. As shown in Table 53.1, a mild decrease in hemoglobin might be expected in elderly patients, but far too often mild and even moderate anemia (Hgb lower than 10gm/100mL) is ascribed to the biologic effects of aging, and a correctable cause for the anemia is not investigated. Particularly in patients with cardiac or pulmonary disorders, which lead to decreased tissue oxygen tension, raising the hemoglobin level (i.e., to 11–13gm/100mL) may lead to a significant improvement in both physical and mental function in the elderly. Although it is possible that a below-normal hemoglobin level may be caused by poorly defined factors, such as lack of bone marrow reserve or lack of activity in an elderly patient, a change in hemoglobin level of more than 1gm/100mL or a hemoglobin level below 11.5gm/100mL should be investigated extensively for a correctable cause.

Nutritional Anemias in the Elderly

Iron deficiency anemia is the most common cause of nutritional anemia in the elderly, as it is in other age groups.

In young adults, menstruating women have a much higher incidence of iron deficiency than do men, but there is almost an equal distribution of men and women with iron deficiency in the elderly population (19).

Several reports have indicated that even when patients have normal iron stores, serum iron and total iron-binding capacity (serum transferrin) are decreased in elderly patients (20). Whether these decreases are the result of the mild decrease in erythropoiesis seen in the elderly or are caused by factors such as chronic inflammation, the values indicate that for the elderly patient, on average, adequate iron is available for production of red cells. Elderly patients also tend to have poorer diets than those of younger adults (normal diets contain 6 mg of iron/1000 cal) and may not take in approximately 10 mg of dietary iron that is required to absorb 1 mg of iron needed daily by postmenopausal women and adult men (1). Iron absorption itself may be compromised in elderly patients because many aged patients have achlorhydria, which inhibits the absorption of the ferric form of iron found mainly in plant products.

Although any of these factors may complicate iron deficiency anemia in the aged, particularly in women who have decreased iron stores, the most common major cause for iron deficiency in the elderly individual, as in all other adult patients, is blood loss. Although acute blood loss from a duodenal ulcer, hemorrhoids, and postmenopausal bleeding may be obvious, chronic intermittent blood loss may be difficult to diagnose and may cause significant iron deficiency anemia. Even small losses of blood can result in significant loss of iron. For example, if 1 mL of packed red cells contains approximately 1 mg of iron, an average loss of 6 mL of packed red cells a day (12 mL of blood) results in a net loss of 5 mg of iron (i.e., 6 mg loss to 1 mg absorbed) a day if the patient is on a normal diet. Thus, a subject who loses this amount of blood can deplete even the normal 1 gm of iron stores and manifest iron deficiency anemia within 1 year of the initiation of blood loss. The gastrointestinal tract is by far the most common site of chronic blood loss in the elderly patient (19). Examples of gastrointestinal sites of chronic intermittent blood loss in the elderly patient include bleeding from internal hemorrhoids, colonic carcinoma, diverticula, and atrophic gastritis. Chronic aspirin or nonsteroidal anti-inflammatory drugs (NSAIDs) inges-

tion, a situation often encountered in the elderly patient, can result in significant enough blood loss to cause iron deficiency anemia (21).

Diagnosing iron deficiency anemia may be difficult in elderly patients. Classic hypochromic microcytic red cell indexes are not generally seen unless the patient's hemoglobin level is below 10 gm/100 mL, although the red blood cell distribution width (RDW) may be increased and an examination of the peripheral smear may show a population of hypochromic microcytic cells much earlier in the course of the anemia. Also, because elderly people tend to have lower transferrin levels in serum and often have associated chronic diseases that cause anemia, their transferrin saturation and serum ferritin levels may not be diagnostic for iron deficiency. Two recent analyses of anemic elderly documented that the best blood test for determining iron deficiency is the serum ferritin level. A serum ferritin of less than 18 ng/mL was diagnostic for iron deficiency and values between 18 and 45 ng/mL were highly suggestive of iron deficiency (22,23). Thus, ferritins that fall in the low normal range in the anemic elderly population provide probable diagnosis of iron deficiency. If, on the basis of this information, the clinician determines that an individual patient has iron deficiency, besides initiating adequate iron therapy the clinician should determine the source of the patient's blood loss.

Anemia of chronic disorders is characterized by normal iron stores, low or normal serum transferrin, and high serum ferritin (24,25). However, all these disorders are associated with low serum iron, which results in iron deficiency and diminished erythropoiesis (24). In the elderly, diseases that are associated with this rather poorly characterized abnormality include collagen vascular disease, chronic infections, and neoplasia. Although anemia from these conditions is usually not severe, it may be complicated by iron deficiency. Therefore, a bone marrow biopsy or clot section must often be performed to diagnose iron deficiency in the elderly patient. Absent bone marrow iron stores indicate that iron deficiency exists and necessitate a trial of iron therapy.

Oral iron therapy generally requires the patient to take 60 mg of elemental iron in the form of ferrous sulfate or ferrous fumerate three times a day. On this regimen, persons with moderate anemia (Hgb 8–10 gm/100 mL) should normalize hemoglobin level after 2 months of therapy. Reasons for failure to respond completely to oral iron therapy include poor compliance in taking the medication, poor iron absorption, or continued bleeding. In these patients, a trial of intravenous iron (iron dextran) is warranted (26), with appropriate precautions taken to minimize the frequency and extent of the associated hypersensitivity reactions (26). If a patient does not respond to intravenous iron therapy and does not have obvious active bleeding, another cause for the anemia should be considered, particularly if the patient has a chronic disorder. A search for a site of blood loss must be conducted in every elderly patient with iron deficiency anemia because the most important treatment for most patients is correction of the cause of the bleeding.

Cobalamin (vitamin B_{12}) is a nutrient that is synthesized by microorganisms and is found in trace amounts in humans (27). Although cobalamin acts as a coenzyme in at least two mammalian enzyme systems, it is still not known exactly how cobalamin deficiency causes megaloblastic anemia and neurologic abnormalities. Megaloblastic anemia is characterized by a hypercellular bone marrow associated with macrocytic anemia, pancytopenia, and abnormal neutrophil morphology (hypersegmented neutrophils). Neurologic disease is generally associated with abnormalities of the posterior spinal column but can be manifest clinically as any abnormality, including dementia and psychiatric problems (28). Pernicious anemia is a disease caused by a lack of intrinsic factor, the cobalamin-binding protein found in the stomach, and whose presence is essential for absorption of cobalamin (29). Lack of intrinsic factor is associated with gastric atrophy and achlorhydria. In patients with pernicious anemia, a Schilling test demonstrates poor absorption of free cobalamin but normal absorption of cobalamin when intrinsic factor is added. The incidence of pernicious anemia increases markedly after a person is 50 years of age and parallels the incidence of atrophic gastritis seen in the elderly population. An immunologic mechanism has been proposed for pernicious anemia because the disease is associated with serum antibodies directed against intrinsic factor and the gastric parietal cell and, in some cases, against thyroid cells (30).

Although the incidence of pernicious anemia associated with gastric atrophy, megaloblastic anemia, and neurologic diseases is relatively rare, a number of individuals with reduced intrinsic factor secretion and persistent low serum cobalamin levels but without anemia or central nervous system disorders have been described as having latent pernicious anemia. One study indicated that about 15 percent of nonanemic individuals older than age 65 have below normal serum cobalamin levels (31). Measuring physiologic substances such as methylmalonic acid and homocystine in serum (32) improves our understanding of the physiologic effects of cobalamin deficiency on the elderly patient. Use of these measurements has shown a high incidence of true deficiency of cobalamin in both well and hospitalized elderly patients (33,34). Even in patients without anemia, cobalamin therapy in these deficient patients caused a marked fall or complete correction of elevated methylmalonic acid and homocysteine levels. After these patients received 6 months of cobalamin treatment, the mean red cell volume fell significantly and in at least one patient was associated with marked improvement in neurologic abnormalities (34). Thus, elderly patients who are deficient in cobalamin but are not anemic should still be treated with cobalamin because their red cell production may be diminished in response to a stress such as bleeding, and even poorly defined abnormalities in neurologic loss may be improved.

Other causes for cobalamin deficiency can be seen in elderly patients. Achlorhydria associated with partial gastrectomy or atrophic gastritis with adequate amounts of intrinsic factor may be associated with cobalamin deficiency. The mechanism for cobalamin deficiency in these patients is related to the necessity for free acid in the stomach to release cobalamin from food so that it can be bound to intrinsic factor and absorbed. These patients take 10 years or longer to become deficient in cobalamin. The time interval is long compared with the 3 to 5 years for deficiency to develop in patients who lack intrinsic factor and who cannot absorb any endogenous cobalamin found in the gut. Usually patients with achlorhydria have a normal Schilling test because free cobalamin is easily absorbed. However, if the Schilling test is done with cobalamin bound to proteins (such as egg white protein) poor absorption is seen both with and without added intrinsic factor (35). These patients should be treated with cobalamin (i.e., 100 μg IM biweekly until values normalize, then a maintenance dose of 100 μg IM/month) in the same manner as patients with classic pernicious anemia. A response to cobalamin treatment is usually associated with a brisk reticulocytosis that peaks about 4 days after the initiation of therapy. As erythropoiesis normalizes, serum lactic dehydrogenase will fall within the normal range, and, more important, there may be a sudden drop in serum potassium to below normal levels (36). The latter complication may be particularly dangerous for elderly patients who have co-existent heart disease. Improvement of the neurologic disease often takes much longer than obtaining a hematologic response, and in some cases, neurologic abnormalities never completely normalize.

Folic acid (pteroylmonoglutamic acid) is the parent compound of a large number of related compounds, such as purine and pyrimidine synthesis, that act as coenzymes in a number of metabolic systems in animal cells (37). Folic acid deficiency causes megaloblastic anemia and pancytopenia that is indistinguishable from the clinical presentation of cobalamin deficiency. However, unlike cobalamin deficiency, folic acid deficiency by itself does not result in neurologic disease. Because the amount of folic acid in the diet is not greatly in excess of the nutritional requirement and because body folate stores are relatively low, folic acid deficiency develops within 2 to 3 months in persons taking an inadequate diet (38). The short time necessary to develop a deficient state is in contrast to the much longer time it takes to become cobalamin deficient. Because elderly persons' diets are frequently inadequate and often do not contain fresh vegetables or fruits, which have the highest amounts of folic acid, it is not surprising that the elderly develop nutritional deficiency of folates. Malabsorption caused by intestinal disease or alcohol intake, which interferes with the metabolism of folic acid (39), may also complicate folic acid deficiency in the elderly.

Folic acid deficiency is demonstrated by the finding of low serum folate value in a patient with macrocytic anemia. If the patient's diet is nutritionally inadequate, determining the red cell folate level, an assay that is said to provide a better assessment of tissue folic acid stores, may be helpful (40). Although patients require only about 50 μg of folic acid a day, treatment for folate deficiency generally consists of 1 or 2 mg of folic acid given orally daily. Persons who have megaloblastic anemia caused by folate deficiency respond with a peak reticulocytosis

about 4 days after the institution of therapy. Patients who have megaloblastic anemia and are cobalamin deficient or who have mixed deficiencies exhibit a hematologic response to milligram doses of folic acid; however, the folic acid therapy will not benefit neurologic disease. In fact, there have been reports that demonstrate that neurologic disease caused by cobalamin deficiency may be severely exacerbated when treatment with folic acid is instituted (41). Because elderly patients may have a number of problems that result in nutritional deficiency, it is not uncommon for these patients to have *combined* nutritional deficiency that results in anemia. Anemia caused by combined nutritional deficiencies may be difficult to characterize and often leads to a diagnostic and therapeutic approach of trial and error.

Cobalamin and folic acid deficiency not only are difficult to distinguish from each other but often appear concurrently. This situation may occur in a patient with long-standing cobalamin deficiency who either does not take in enough folic acid in the diet or has megaloblastic changes in the gastrointestinal tract that lead to malabsorption of folic acid. While waiting for results of the serum assays for cobalamin and folic acid, the physician should institute therapy with both nutrients because folic acid given alone in a cobalamin-deficient patient may exacerbate neurologic disease. Therapeutic trials with physiologic amounts of cobalamin and folic acid as a diagnostic test for a specific deficiency are no longer in vogue because serum radiodilution assays can be performed much more rapidly than was possible in the past.

Folic acid or cobalamin deficiency may be complicated by iron deficiency. For example, a patient may have macrocytic anemia, a low serum folate, and a normal serum iron. The patient may respond partially to folate but will remain anemic, although the macrocytic indexes are not seen. Often a repeat serum iron determination will be lower than the initial value (42), presumably because the iron is utilized for erythropoiesis when folic acid therapy is initiated. The patient may then show an increase in hemoglobin when treated with iron therapy. As with other patients who have iron deficiency, these patients should be investigated for blood loss. Conversely, other patients with obvious iron deficiency should be treated accordingly. Sometimes a clue to this form of mixed nutritional deficiency is the finding of many hypersegmented neutrophils on the peripheral smear, although there is still controversy about whether iron deficiency alone can cause this abnormality (43).

Other Causes of Anemia Seen in the Elderly

Hemolytic anemia is not a common finding in elderly patients. In anemic, geriatric hospitalized patients, less than 1 percent had definite evidence of hemolysis (44). However, some specific considerations exist for patients who develop hemolysis in old age. First, because hemolysis may co-exist with nutritional deficiency, an elderly patient may not show the same degree of compensatory erythropoiesis as that shown by a younger patient with hemolysis; thus, the reticulocyte count may be lower than expected. Also, when hemolytic anemia is suspected in an elderly patient, associated diseases that produce hemolysis should be considered.

Although idiopathic autoimmune hemolytic anemia of the warm antibody type is not more prevalent in the elderly, secondary causes for this form of immune hemolysis are significantly increased in people older than age 45 (45). Drug-induced immune hemolytic anemia is commonly seen in the elderly, particularly that associated with alpha-methyldopa and penicillin-like drugs. Autoimmune hemolysis secondary to a lymphoproliferative neoplasia or collagen vascular disease should always be considered in the elderly, especially because hemolysis may be the first clinical presentation of the disease. Cold antibodies, generally immunoglobulin M (IgM), that cause cold agglutinin disease are particularly common in a person's seventh and eighth decades of life. Although hemolytic anemia is not usually clinically significant when cold agglutinins are present, it can sometimes be extremely severe (46), and, as with warm antibody hemolysis, the patient may have an associated disease, such as a malignancy.

Hereditary hemolytic anemias caused by hemoglobinopathies or enzyme deficiencies are rarely diagnosed for the first time in an elderly patient. Hereditary spherocytosis, on the other hand, is not uncommonly diagnosed in older patients (47). Sometimes these patients present with gallbladder disease (bilirubin stones) and have mild hemolytic anemia, spherocytes on peripheral smear, and slight splenomegaly.

An ill-defined form of anemia classified as refractory or sideroblastic anemia is not uncommonly seen in older persons. This form of anemia, when associated with abnormalities of white cells and platelets, is termed *myelodysplastic syndrome* (44). The anemia is defined as refractory because specific therapy, such as nutritional supplementation, does not result in improvement. Most often, patients with myelodysplastic syndrome have macrocytic anemia and varying degrees of leukopenia and thrombocytopenia associated with a hypercellular bone marrow (48). Although familial or drug-induced sideroblastic anemia can be seen in persons of all ages, primary acquired idiopathic sideroblastic anemia is not frequently seen in patients older than 50 years of age (49) and clinically resembles refractory macrocytic anemia, except that ringed sideroblasts are seen in the bone marrow (49). Sometimes patients with refractory anemia, particularly the sideroblastic variety, respond to pharmacologic doses of folate, pyridoxine, or recombinant erythropoietin. Most often, however, elderly patients with refractory anemia require maintenance transfusion therapy. A variable number of these patients eventually develop acute granulocytic or monocytic leukemia. The prevalence of this form of anemia appears to be increasing; more than 5 percent of hospitalized anemic geriatric patients are now found to have some form of myelodysplastic syndrome.

General Considerations

Table 53.2 contains a review of some general considerations for approaching the diagnosis and treatment of anemia in an elderly patient. Although a number of differences exist in elderly patients compared with the young adult population, there are more similarities than differences, and a patient's old age should in no way negate the consideration of a reasonable investigation for a treatable cause of anemia.

Patients who have refractory anemia or severe anemia associated with nutritional deficiency or bleeding, may require transfusion therapy. Considerations for transfusion therapy are the same in the elderly as in younger adults. However, because the elderly often have severe cardiac or pulmonary disease, individual patients may require hemoglobin levels greater than the 10 or 11 gm/

Table 53.2. Anemia in the Elderly

Hyperproliferative Anemia	Hypoproliferative Anemia (low reticulocyte count)
With effective erythropoiesis (high reticulocyte count)	Iron deficiency (almost always caused by
Hemolytic anemia	blood loss)
Immune hemolysis secondary to	Anemia of chronic disorders
Drugs	Chronic infections
Neoplasia	Collagen vascular disease
Infections	Neoplasia
Collagen vascular disease	Anemia of chronic renal disease
Hereditary spherocytosis	Aplastic anemia
Hypersplenism secondary to	Idiopathic
Infections	Secondary to toxic substances
Collagen vascular disease	Hypothyroidism
Neoplasia	Pure red cell aplasia
Bleeding (acute)	
With ineffective erythropoiesis (normal or low reticulocyte count)	
Nutritional deficiency	
Cobalamin	
Folic acid	
Refractory macrocytic anemia (myelodysplastic disorder, sideroblastic anemia)	

100 mL that are anecdotally suggested as maintenance levels for patients receiving transfusion therapy. The appropriate level of hemoglobin in a patient should be assessed individually according to the symptomatology. Because many elderly patients have relative difficulty in accepting a fluid load, transfusions of aged patients should be carefully maintained. Specifically, patients with pernicious anemia often have low hemoglobin levels (less than 5 gm/100 mL), volume overload, high output cardiac failure, and underlying cardiac disease. Once the appropriate studies are done and the patient is started on cobalamin therapy, the patient may be slowly transfused with packed blood cells with careful observation for volume overload. However, most of these patients are well compensated, and although the level of the anemia may be worrisome, they do not require transfusion therapy because they begin to respond to cobalamin within a few days.

References

1. Talley L. Geriatric Nursing. In: Centrovoli O, Patrick M, eds. Nursing management for the elderly. Philadelphia: Lippincott, 1979:85.
2. Hartsock RJ, et al. Normal variation with aging of the amount of hematopoietic tissue in bone marrow from the anterior iliac crest. Am J Clin Pathol 1965;43:325–331.
3. Young N. Aplastic anemia: research themes, clinical issues. In: Brown EB, ed. Progress in hematology. X. vol. 11. New York: Grune & Stratton, 1981:1–42.
4. Purcell Y, Brozonic B. Red cell 2,3-diphosphoglycerate concentration in man decreases with age. Nature 1974;251:511.
5. Zauber NP, Zauber A. Hematological data of healthy very old people. JAMA 1987;257:2181.
6. Smith JS, Whitelow DM. Hemoglobin levels in the elderly. Can Med Assoc J 1971;105:816.
7. McLennan WJ, Andrews GR, MacLoed C, et al. Anemia in the elderly. Q J Med 1973;42:1.
8. Nilsson-Ehl H, Jagenburg R, Landahl S, Svanborg A. Decline of blood hemoglobin in the aged: a longitudinal study of an urban Swedish population from age 70 to 81. Br J Haematol 1989;71:437.
9. Nafziger J, Pailla K, Luciani L, et al. Decreased erythropoietin responsiveness to iron deficiency anemia in the elderly. Am J Hematol 1993;43:172–176.
10. Sorso RD, Hammer EA, Moore DL. Leukocyte and neutrophil counts in acute appendicitis. Am J Surg 1970;120:563.
11. Timaffy M. A comparative study of bone marrow function in young and old individuals. Gerontol Clin (Basel) 1962;4:13.
12. Nagel JE, Pyle RS, Chrest JF, Adler WH. Oxidative metabolism and bactericidal capacity of polymorphonuclear leukocytes from normal young and aged adults. J Gerontol 1982;37:529.
13. Thorbjarharson B, Loehr WJ. Acute appendicitis in patients over the age of sixty. Surg Gynecol Obstet 1967:125:1277.
14. Diaz-Jonanen E, Strickland RG, Williams RC. Studies of human lymphocytes in the newborn and the aged. Am J Med 1975;58:620.

15. Gillis S, Kozak R, Durante M, et al. Immunologic studies of aging. J Clin Invest 1981;67:937–942.

16. Pahwa SG, Pahwa RN, Good R. Decreased in vitro humoral immune responses in aged humans. J Clin Invest 1981;67:1094–1102.

17. Shapleigh JB, Mayes S, Moore CV. Hematologic values in the aged. J Gerontol 1952;7:207.

18. Sharland DE. Erythrocyte sedimentation rate: the normal range in the elderly. J Am Geriatr Soc 1980;28:346.

19. Council on Foods and Nutrition. Iron deficiency in the United States. JAMA 1968;203:207–411.

20. Powell DEB, Thomas JH. The iron-binding capacity of serum in elderly hospital patients. Gerontol Clin (Basel) 1969;11:36.

21. Roth WA, Waldes-Dapener A, Pieses P, et al. Topical action of salicylates in gastrointestinal erosion and hemorrhage. Gastroenterology 1963;44:146.

22. Guyatt GH, Patterson C, Ali M, et al. Diagnosis of iron-deficiency anemia in the elderly. Am J Med 1990;88:205.

23. Joosten E, Hiele M, Ghoos Y, et al. Diagnosis of iron-deficiency anemia in a hospitalized geriatric population. Am J Med 1991;90:653.

24. Cartwright GE. The anemia of chronic disorders. Semin Hematol 1966;3:351.

25. Lipschitz DA, Cook JP, Finch CA. A clinical evaluation of serum ferritin as an index of iron stores. N Engl J Med 1974;290:1213.

26. Hamstra RD, Block M, Schocket A. Intravenous iron dextran in clinical medicine. JAMA 1980;243:1726–1731.

27. Allen RH. The plasma transport of vitamin B_{12}. Br J Haematol 1976;33:161–171.

28. Shulman R. Psychiatric aspects of pernicious anemia. BMJ 1967;3:366.

29. Castle WB. Current concepts of pernicious anemia. Am J Med 1970;48:541–548.

30. Doniach D, Reitt IM. An evaluation of gastric and thyroid autoimmunity in relation to hematologic disorders. Semin Hematol 1964;1:313.

31. Elwood PC, Shinton NK, Wilson CID, et al. Haemoglobin, vitamin B_{12}, and folate levels in the elderly. Br J Haematol 1971;21:557.

32. Stabler SP, Marcell PD, Podell ER, et al. Elevation of total homocysteine in the serum of patients with cobalamin or folate deficiency detected by capillary gas chromatography/mass spectrometry. J Clin Invest 1988;81:466–474.

33. Joosten E, van den Berg A, Riezler R, et al. Metabolic evidence that deficiencies of vitamin B-12 (cobalamin), folate, and vitamin B-6 occur commonly in elderly people. Am J Clin Nutr 1993;58:468.

34. Pennypacker LC, Allen RH, Kelly JP, et al. High prevalence of cobalamin deficiency in elderly outpatients. J Am Geriatr Soc 1992;40:1197.

35. Doscherholman A, Swaim WR. Impaired assimilation of egg Co^{57}-vitamin B_{12} in patients with hypochlorhydria and achlorhydria and after gastric resection. Gastroenterology 1973;64:913–919.

36. Lawson DH. Early mortality in the megaloblastic anemias. Q J Med 1972;41:1.

37. Huennekens FM. Folic acid coenzymes in the biosynthesis of purines and pyrimidines. Vitam Horm 1968;26:375–386.

38. Herbert V. Minimal daily adult folate requirement. Arch Intern Med 1962;110:649–659.

39. Sullivan LW, Herbert V. Suppression of hematopoiesis by ethanol. J Clin Invest 1964;43:2048.

40. Schreiber C, Waxman S. Measurement of red cell folate level by ^{3}H-pteroylglutamic acid radioassay. Br J Hematol 1974;27:551.

41. Israels MCG, Wilkinson JF. Risk of neurological complications in pernicious anemia treated with folic acid. BMJ 1949;2:1072.

42. Hawkins CF. Value of serum iron levels in assessing effect of hematinics in the macrocytic anemias. BMJ 1955;1:383.

43. Beard ME, Weintraub LR. Hypersegmented granulocytes in iron deficiency anemia. Br J Hematol 1969;16:161.

44. Joosten E, Pelemans V, Hiele L, et al. Prevalence and causes of anaemia in a geriatric hospitalized population. Gerontology 1992;38:111–117.

45. Dacie JV, Worlledge SM. Autoimmune hemolytic anemias. Prog Hematol 1965;6:82.

46. Schubothe H. The cold hemagglutinin disease. Semin Hematol 1966;3:27.

47. Race RR. On the inheritance and linkage relations of alcoholic jaundice. Ann Eugen 1942;11:365–373.

48. Vilter RW, Janold T, Will JJ, et al. Refractory anemia with hyperplastic bone marrow. Blood 1960;15:1.

49. Kuscher JP, Lee GR, Wintrobe MM, et al. Idiopathic refractory sideroblastic anemia. Medicine 1971;50:139.

Chapter 54
Geriatric Oncology

Steven W. Andresen

The most important thing in illness is never to lose heart.

V. I. Lenin

Cancer is a major health problem and cause of death in the geriatric population. Much epidemiologic information is available concerning cancer incidence and mortality (Figures 54.1, 54.2, Tables 54.1, 54.2 (1)). Fifty percent of all cancers and more than 60 percent of cancer deaths occur in patients older than 65 years of age (1). As this segment of the United States population grows, the approach to the diagnosis and treatment of cancer in the elderly will assume increasing importance.

Numerous current studies address the problems unique to geriatric oncology. Cancer is diagnosed at a later stage in elderly persons compared with the time of diagnosis for younger persons (2). The presence of comorbid conditions in the older patient often masks recognition of early symptoms and delays evaluation of treatment (3). Further, elderly patients may be less likely to receive specific antineoplastic treatment once the diagnosis of malignancy has been made (3–8). This information is clinically useful when coupled with the knowledge of specific disease processes, diagnosis, and therapy.

This chapter provides information to strengthen the way health care is provided to the elderly patient with cancer.

Molecular Basis of Cancer

The development of neoplasia is a multistep process (Figure 54.3). During the first step, initiation, exposure to a carcinogen produces damage to cellular DNA and, consequently, produces an altered genetic message. Potential initiating agents include viruses, physical agents, and chemicals. The cell may attempt to reverse the genetic aberration, but, if not successful, fixation of damage occurs.

The second phase, promotion, begins when genetic damage is no longer reversible (9). Transformation in the phenotype of the cell as the result of genetic change, produces progressive molecular and biochemical anomalies and ultimately results in cell surface antigenic changes. Accordingly, altered interactions with host cells and clonal expansion occurs. Promoters alone do not produce neoplasia, but exposure of initiated cells to these agents (which include certain drugs, hormones, and alcohol) enhances the process of carcinogenesis (Table 54.3). As a consequence of continued promotion, which may occur over years, histologic changes occur and, at a cellular level, can be microscopically identified as premalignant. Examples of premalignant states include oral leukoplakia, cervical dysplasia, colonic polyps, and actinic keratoses.

About the time of conversion to premalignancy, the third phase of carcinogenesis, progression, occurs. During this phase, premalignant cells progress to become frankly malignant. Interestingly, progression is infrequent and not inevitable. Spontaneous regressions occur. Little is known about this phase of carcinogenesis, but premalignant cells apparently remain more or less responsive to host regulation. With ongoing progression, the cell becomes frankly malignant and develops the potential to be locally invasive and perhaps metastasize. At this time, further genetic aberrations occur and the cell becomes poorly responsive to host regulation and acquires an autonomous nature.

Classes of genes most likely to be the molecular targets for this development of neoplasia include proto-oncogenes (10), cellular oncogenes (11), and tumor suppressor genes (12). As proto-oncogenes and cellular oncogenes occur normally in the genetic material of cells, they must be activated during the process of carcinogenesis (Figure 54.4).

The incidence of cancer increases exponentially with

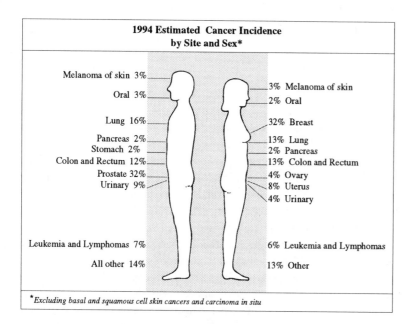

Fig. 54.1. 1994 estimated cancer incidence by site and sex, excluding basal and squamous cell skin cancers and carcinoma in situ. (Reproduced by permission from Boring CC, Squires TS, Tong T, Montgomery S. Cancer Statistics. CA Cancer J Clin 1994;44:7–26.)

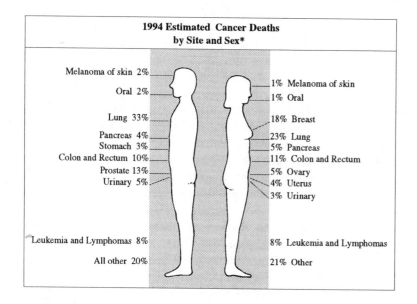

Fig. 54.2. 1994 estimated cancer deaths by site and sex. (Reproduced by permission from Boring CC, Squires TS, Tong T, Montgomery S. Cancer Statistics. CA Cancer J Clin 1994;44:7–26.)

advancing age (13). Proposed explanations for the increase include decreased immune surveillance, different susceptibility to carcinogens, prolonged exposure to carcinogens, and alterations in DNA repair mechanisms. Whatever the mechanism, strategies designed to affect the aging rate may lead to a large reduction in cancer incidence.

Cancer Prevention

Ideally, primary prevention of cancer would involve repair of genetic abnormalities that occur during the phase of initiation. Deletions of tumor suppressor genes have been identified in many common cancers. In hereditary retinoblastoma, a portion of chromosome 13p is deleted.

Table 54.1. Mortality for the Five Leading Cancer Sites for Males by Age Group, United States, 1990

55–74 yr	75+ yr
All cancer 141,787	All cancer 94,739
Lung 56,225	Lung 25,770
Colon and Rectum 14,190	Prostate 19,622
Prostate 12,423	Colon and Rectum 11,842
Pancreas 6771	Pancreas 4128
Non-Hodgkin's lymphomas 4516	Bladder 3694

Reproduced by permission from Boring CC, Squires TS, Tong T, Montgomery S. Cancer Statistics. CA Cancer J Clin 1994;44:7–26.

Table 54.2. Mortality for the Five Leading Cancer Sites for Females by Age Group, United States, 1990

55–74 yr	75+ yr
All cancer 110,545	All cancer 93,235
Lung 29,729	Colon and Rectum 15,524
Breast 20,096	Lung 14,924
Colon and Rectum 11,205	Breast 13,458
Ovary 6575	Pancreas 6376
Pancreas 5674	Ovary 4310

Reproduced by permission from Boring CC, Squires TS, Tong T, Montgomery S. Cancer Statistics. CA Cancer J Clin 1994;44:7–26.

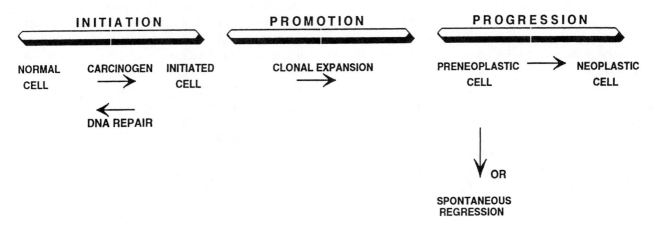

Fig. 54.3. Carcinogenesis: a multistep process.

Table 54.3. Promoters and Their Associated Malignancies

Promoter	Malignancy
Estrogen	Endometrium
Alcohol	Oropharynx, Larynx, Esophagus
Immunosuppressive agents	Lymphomas

Recently, this anomaly has been repaired by delivery of the intact gene utilizing a retroviral vector. With refinement in the current science of gene therapy, this type of approach may have a major role in cancer prevention. The elimination of smoking and use of sunscreens are examples of primary preventive practices which would have an enormous effect on cancer incidence. The use of anti-

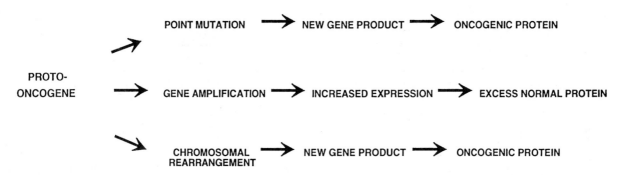

Fig. 54.4. Potential mechanisms of proto-oncogene activation.

initiators such as beta-carotene, selenium, vitamin E, and soybean extract is being studied. As oxidized molecules are involved in the process of initiation, use of reducing agents such as vitamin C may be found to be helpful.

Secondary prevention involves decreasing the exposure to promoting agents such as aniline dyes, fat, and hormones and other agents that lead to the development of the premalignant state. Strategies that reduce exposure to promoters, for example the use of dietary fiber, may be effective in secondary prevention.

Once the histologic changes of preneoplasia occur, tertiary interventions are required. This may take the form of surgical ablation in the setting of skin, oral cavity, and cervical lesions. The use of antiproliferative compounds or agents that promote differentiation (e.g., retinoids) may suppress the transformation of cells from a preneoplastic to a frankly malignant state. Recently, several studies have demonstrated the ability of transretinoic acid to induce terminal differentiation in leukemic blasts, and clinical responses in patients with acute promyelocytic leukemia have been seen. This approach is being studied in other settings, for example, in patients with preneoplastic oral lesions. As preneoplastic cells retain, to some extent, responsiveness to host regulatory mechanisms, the augmentation of host immune defenses may prove helpful in tertiary prevention. Current studies of biologic response modifying agents such as the interleukins may provide information concerning their use in this setting. The results of recent chemoprevention studies, such as the use of tamoxifen to prevent breast cancer in those at high risk of developing the disease, will provide valuable information concerning this modality in

tertiary prevention. As with other major human diseases, the most effective therapy of cancer will ultimately be through prevention.

Cancer Screening

There is evidence that, for some malignancies, early detection reduces mortality. Physicians are not only responsible for the diagnosis and treatment of disease but also for the detection of early asymptomatic disorders at a time when treatment may significantly reduce morbidity and mortality. Cancer screening has yet to be fully integrated into the daily practice of most physicians. Major problems appear to be a lack of awareness on the part of physicians concerning the value of screening and poor compliance by patients. Screening is a joint responsibility. As the elderly are at highest risk for developing cancer, and, second to heart disease, cancer is the most common cause of death (14), cancer screening could have significant impact on this segment of the population. It is estimated that approximately 90 percent of the elderly population see a physician at least every 2 years. However, one study demonstrated that only about 10 percent of physicians follow regular screening guidelines. One survey demonstrated that approximately 25 percent of elderly females have never had a Pap smear (15). It is apparent that many physicians are not aggressive in using preventive medicine techniques in the elderly.

The general population, and the elderly in particular, may believe that cancer is always incurable, which may foster a reluctance to participate in screening procedures. Loss of independence, the fear of chronic debilitating disease, and the fear of ultimately becoming a burden to one's family are likely reasons why elderly patients do not seek screening measures in the absence of symptoms. Many physicians avoid screening practices in the elderly because they believe they may upset or embarrass the patient (16).

For successful screening, a healthy open relationship is needed between physician and patient. The health care provider must have adequate knowledge of cancer screening techniques and be able to communicate their importance to their elderly population (Table 54.4) (See also Chapter 5).

Table 54.4. ACS Guidelines for the Early Detection of Cancer in People Without Symptoms

Age 20–40 yr	Age 40+ yr
Should include the procedures listed below plus health counseling (such as tips on quitting cigarettes) and examinations for cancers of the thyroid, testes, prostate, mouth, ovaries, skin, and lymph nodes. Some people are at higher risk for certain cancers and may need to have tests more frequently.	Should inlude the procedures listed below plus health counseling (such as tips on quitting cigarettes) and examinations for cancers of the thyroid, testes, prostate, mouth, ovaries, skin, and lymph nodes. Some people are at higher risk for certain cancers and may need to have tests more frequently.

Breast
Examination by doctor every 3 years
Self-examination every month
One baseline breast x-ray between ages 35 and 40
Higher risk for breast cancer:
    Personal or family history of breast cancer,
    never had children, first child after 30
	Breast
	Examination by doctor every year
	Self-examination every month
	Breast x-ray every year after 50
	Between ages 40 and 50, breast x-ray every 1–2 years
	Higher risk for breast cancer:
	    Personal or family history of breast cancer,
	    never had children, first child after 30

Uterus Pelvic examination every 3 years	Uterus Pelvic examination every year

Cervix
Pap test–after two initial negative tests 1 year apart–at least every 3 years, includes women under 20 if they are at high risk
Higher risk for cervical cancer:
    Early age at first intercourse, multiple
    sex partners
	Cervix
	Pap test–after two initial negative tests 1 year apart–at least every 3 years
	Higher risk for cervical cancer:
	    Early age at first intercourse, multiple
	    sex partners

Endometrium
Endometrial tissue sample at menopause if at high risk
Higher risk for endometrial cancer:
    Infertility, obesity, failure of ovulation, abnormal uterine bleeding,
      estrogen therapy	

Colon and Rectum
Digital rectal examination every year after age 40
Stool blood test every year after age 50
Proctoscopic examination–after two initial negative tests 1 year apart–every
    3–5 years after age 50
Higher risk for colorectal cancer:
    Personal or family history of colon or rectal cancer, personal or family
      history of polyps in the colon or rectum, ulcerative colitis	

SOURCES: ACS = American Cancer Society.
Reproduced by permission from American Cancer Society. Publication 84-20M-No. 5005, 1984.

Principles of Cancer Therapy

Surgical Oncology

The radical surgical procedures used by William Halsted and his contemporaries at the turn of the century are now less often necessary. Screening techniques have made earlier diagnosis possible. Accordingly, small tumors are more common and more conservative surgical approaches may be used. In addition, combined modality therapy—use of surgery, radiotherapy, and chemotherapy—can lessen the need for radical surgery. The benefit of surgical cancer therapy to elderly patients is, in general, no different than that for younger patients. Stage-for-stage management does not change much for the older person, and responses to therapy and survival are similar. Associated medical illnesses make side effects and complications of therapy greater in the elderly; however, preoperative screening should identify those not fit for standard procedures, and alternative plans may be considered.

Breast-conserving cancer operations are as important for the elderly patient as they are for younger patients. The older woman is no less concerned with her physical appearance, self esteem, or sexuality than is the younger patient. The elderly patient chooses a breast-sparing operation with the same frequency as that of younger women. It remains important that other treatment modalities such as radiation therapy, hormonal therapy, or chemotherapy be considered when clinically indicated in the older patient.

Radical prostatectomy is the therapy of choice in early stages of prostate cancer. This approach is currently under question and if significant co-morbid illnesses exist, irradiation or expectant observation may be the best approach.

As more older patients are screened for rectal cancer, smaller lesions have been found. This makes possible the use of sphincter-saving operations such as electrocoagulation. Local excision and irradiation may also prove beneficial in some settings (17,18). Patients whose cancers are high enough to permit anterior resection may avoid abdominoperineal resection, which eliminates the need for colostomy, a difficult situation for the elderly patient with co-morbid illness to manage (19).

Cancers of the head and neck area are frequently man-aged today with a combined modality approach, often beginning initially with chemotherapy and then proceeding to surgery, irradiation, or both. Although difficult and fraught with the potential for multiple complications, many elderly patients can be successfully carried through this type of therapy.

Although, as a group, sarcomas are uncommon malignancies, the malignant fibrous histiocytoma occurs with some regularity in the elderly. When this tumor occurs on an extremity, amputation has been considered the best surgical approach. However, recent evidence suggests that, for many patients, wide excision followed by postoperative irradiation may be a significant treatment option and result in equivalent survival. This is particularly important for elderly patients because they are less able to adapt to the prostheses used and to undergo the rigors of modern physical therapy.

The endoscopic use of laser for photocoagulation has been very helpful in the local control of obstructing lesions of the upper and lower gastrointestinal tract and lung. Although this cannot offer therapy with curative intent, the patient who is not considered a candidate for a more extensive surgical procedure may achieve significant palliation through this form of therapy.

Cancer Chemotherapy in the Elderly Patient

The use of pharmacologic agents for antineoplastic therapy has produced significant benefit in many forms of malignancy. Although much additional information is needed, the potential for chemotherapy-related toxicity is greater in the elderly patient.

Pharmacokinetic changes related to aging may enhance the toxicity of chemotherapeutic agents. Organ system dysfunction or decreased reserve may also contribute to this problem (20). Because the glomerular filtration rate (GFR) declines with age, renal excretion of drugs decreases. This enhances the potential toxicity of chemotherapy. However, when dosage adjustments are made on the basis of decreased GFR, toxicity is decreased but therapeutic benefit is not diminished (21). Aging may impair hepatic metabolism of drugs secondary to decreased hepatic blood flow or reduced activity of enzymes. However, this decrease may not significantly alter the metabolism of chemotherapeutic agents (22).

Although poorly studied from a clinical standpoint,

primary drug resistance to chemotherapy may be more common in the elderly. Transmembrane transport may be altered by the synthesis of abnormal proteins, which becomes more common with cellular aging. Cellular hypoxia and enhanced mechanisms of DNA repair are more prevalent in the aged cell and are also associated with increasing resistance to chemotherapeutic agents (20).

Myelotoxicity is a very common problem with the administration of cancer chemotherapy. Hematopoietic recovery from anticancer agents is in large part produced by self renewal of multipotential hematopoietic stem cells. In the older patient decreased numbers of multipotential stem cells may exist (23). Potential depletion may produce decreased tolerance to agents with marrow toxicity. However, the availability and sensitivity to hematopoietic growth factors is retained in the elderly (24).

Inflammation of mucosal membranes, common with many chemotherapeutic agents, is more frequent and more severe in the elderly population. This may be related to depletion of mucosal stem cells.

Less acute nausea and vomiting is experienced by elderly patients than by younger patients. Delayed nausea and vomiting is the form most commonly seen in the geriatric population.

Anthracycline antibiotics, such as doxorubicin, are associated with cardiotoxicity, which is enhanced in elderly patients. Aging is known to cause a decrease in cardiac muscle fibers, which likely leads to enhancement of toxicity. The neurotoxicity seen with the administration of the vinca alkaloids such as vincristine and the quaternary ammonium compounds such as cisplatinum is more common and more severe in the elderly (25).

Administration of hormonal agents is well tolerated in the geriatric population. Tamoxifen and megestrol acetate are commonly used in patients with breast cancer. Tamoxifen may be rarely associated with deep vein thrombosis and, with long-term use, the potential development of endometrial cancer and cataracts (26). Megestrol acetate is infrequently associated with toxicity, but fluid retention, deep vein thrombosis, and weight gain may be seen. The antiandrogens, such as cyproterotene and flutamide, are commonly used in patients with prostate cancer (27). They are well tolerated by the elderly. Toxicity from cyproterotene includes weight gain, deep vein thrombosis, and impotence. Diarrhea and gynecomastia can occur with flutamide. Luteinizing hormone-releasing hormone (LHRH) analogues are also effective in patients with prostate cancer and are well tolerated. The main toxicity of these agents is impotence and hot flashes.

The use of biologic response modifying agents, such as recombinant alpha interferon, is becoming more common. Interferon is active at low doses for hairy cell leukemia and many of the myeloproliferative disorders. Very little toxicity is seen at lower doses. At higher doses, interferon is effective for lymphoproliferative disorders, melanoma, and acquired immunodeficiency syndrome (AIDS)-related Kaposi's sarcoma. Higher doses are associated with significant constitutional symptoms, hematopoietic toxicity, and neuropathy. Elderly patients treated with interferon as part of the therapy for metastatic large bowel cancer were shown to develop a peculiar dementia syndrome (28).

In summary, although there may be an excess of potential toxicity with the use of cancer chemotherapeutic agents in the elderly, when these agents are clinically indicated, most patients will benefit from such therapy. The physician must weigh the potential risks and benefits of such therapy and specifically define treatment goals. The chemosensitivity of the neoplasm, extent of disease, and physical condition of the patient are all factors that determine whether therapy is potentially curative, aimed at prolongation of survival, or palliative in nature. The patient's attitude and expectations concerning therapy are of the utmost importance, and particularly when treatment is palliative in nature, should be the primary determinant in management.

Specific Neoplasia

Lung Cancer

Despite public education concerning smoking and attempts to improve early detection, lung cancer remains the leading cause of cancer-related deaths in the United States. At present, its incidence continues to increase and cure rates remain low. Lung cancers are divided into two groups: non-small-cell (NSCC) and small-cell cancer (SCC). Surgery remains the principal modality of therapy for NSCC; however, most patients are not candidates for an operation because of advanced disease at diagnosis. There is evidence that NSCC presents at a less advanced state in the elderly (29), possibly because the number of squamous cell cancers increases with age. This type of malignancy may be more amenable to resection because it is more likely to be detected at an earlier stage.

Patients with advanced local regional disease, those with metastatic disease, and those with medical contraindications to surgery may be considered for irradiation. Patients without extensive local disease may obtain prolonged, disease-free survival with this modality. For other patients, substantial palliative benefit often results. Irradiation may also be helpful in those who develop central nervous system or skeletal metastasis. Bronchoscopically applied laser or endobronchial irradiation may also reduce tumor mass and enhance palliation. To date, the use of combination chemotherapy for NSCC of the lung has failed to demonstrate a substantive benefit.

SCC of the lung is a systemic disease with metastatic disease commonly present at the time of initial diagnosis. Although a tumor may be responsive to chemotherapy and radiation, most patients die with this illness; long-term survival is less than 10 percent. Chemotherapy is the initial treatment modality. Irradiation to the mediastinum, brain, or both is commonly prescribed. Although radiation to these areas decreases the incidence of local failure, it is difficult to demonstrate a survival advantage with this approach. As in NSCC of this malignancy, irradiation is commonly given to areas of skeletal or central nervous system metastases for palliation.

Epidemiologic evidence suggests that cessation of smoking in the elderly decreases the risk of cancer and may approximate the risk of a nonsmoker within 10 years of cessation (30). At present, no specific recommendation for screening can be made for lung cancers, but a periodic chest radiograph for the patient who continues to smoke does not seem unreasonable.

Colorectal Cancer

Colorectal carcinoma is the second most common malignancy affecting men and women in the United States. A diet high in saturated fats and low in fiber may predis-
pose to this malignancy. In addition, ulcerative colitis and familial polyposis syndromes greatly increase the risk of this malignancy. The incidence of colorectal cancer increases with age and peaks in persons 80 years of age and older. Colorectal cancer is diagnosed at a similar stage in both the elderly and younger patients. A major problem is that early signs and symptoms of this malignancy may be minimal or nonspecific and similar to complaints common in older patients. Accordingly, in the elderly new symptoms such as constipation, anorexia, or weight loss should be investigated.

Screening for colorectal cancer is important because localized lesions detected at an early stage may be curable. Digital rectal examination, stools for occult blood, barium enema, sigmoidoscopy, and colonoscopy are tests commonly used in screening. Unfortunately, because of the intermittent nature of bleeding in these malignancies, stools for occult blood are not always positive. Colonoscopy remains the most accurate diagnostic test. Patients with large bowel symptoms or bleeding should undergo colonoscopy. If negative, and symptoms persist, a double contrast barium enema should be performed. The tests are commonly complementary. Unfortunately, when symptoms are present, lesions are generally fairly advanced.

Local electrocoagulation or local excision with endocavitary radiation may offer a high rate of control for patients with small rectal cancers close to the anus (18). It may be possible to avoid abdominoperineal resection in the elderly patients with a rectal cancer if the lesions are high enough to permit anterior resection, which avoids the necessity for colostomy.

Surgical resection is the only potential cure for carcinomas of the large bowel in all but early rectal cancers. Although 70 percent to 80 percent of patients have lesions potentially resectable for cure, approximately 50 percent of these patients eventually die of recurrent disease. Approximately 30 percent of patients present with metastatic disease, usually to liver or lung. For patients with metastatic disease, palliative resection of the primary lesion may be helpful to treat or prevent obstructive symptoms or bleeding. Surgical procedures involve removal of the primary tumor with significant lateral margins as well as regional lymph nodes and lymphatic channels. Staging and recommendations for adjuvant therapy are derived from the extent of penetration through the bowel wall and the extent of lymph node involvement.

Because most recurrences happen within 2 years of surgery, frequent follow-up during this period is indicated. Re-evaluation should be performed at 3-month intervals for 2 years, at 4-month intervals the third year, and at 6-month intervals until 5 years have elapsed. Yearly examinations are then adequate. Carcinoembryonic antigen (CEA) levels should be determined at each visit, colonoscopy at intervals of 6 to 12 months for 2 to 3 years, and then every 2 to 3 years. Chest x-rays should be obtained at six-month intervals for 2 years and then yearly. In some patients with recurrent disease, resection of solitary hepatic or pulmonary metastases may be considered, which may result in prolonged disease-free survival.

Approximately 15 percent to 20 percent of patients with colon cancer present with disease that does not extend through the bowel wall. Most of these patients are cured with resection. Approximately 50 percent of patients present with disease that has extended through the bowel wall or has involved regional lymph nodes. In approximately half these patients the tumor will recur. At present, data suggest that the use of 5-fluorouracil (5-FU) and levamisole as adjuvant therapy produces a survival benefit for this population of patients. Adjuvant pelvic irradiation, generally in combination with chemotherapy with 5-FU, seems to decrease the rate of local recurrence of rectal cancers and likely provides a survival benefit.

Patients with metastatic disease may respond to chemotherapy with 5-FU in combination with calcium leucovorin. Approximately 20 percent of patients respond, and the response generally lasts 6 to 12 months. Some studies have suggested that there is an additional benefit to combining interferon to this combination, but use of interferon has been associated with a peculiar dementia in the elderly (28). Although local perfusion of an organ such as the liver with chemotherapy enhances response rates, at present a survival advantage has not been demonstrated. Isolated skeletal or brain metastases may be approached with irradiation, which produces significant palliative benefit. The results of therapy for patients with metastatic colorectal cancer is unsatisfactory at present. Patients should be encouraged to consider hospice care and should be offered the opportunity to participate in clinical trials.

Pancreatic Cancer

Carcinoma of the pancreas is increasing in frequency in the United States. The high mortality rate from this tumor is related to the fact that most tumors are locally advanced and unresectable at diagnosis. Despite the use of combined modality therapy of surgery, radiation, and chemotherapy, less than 5 percent of patients with pancreatic cancer survive as long as 5 years. Anorexia, weight loss, pain, or jaundice are the most frequent symptoms at presentation. Abdominal ultrasound or computed tomography (CT) are the usual diagnostic radiographic procedures. A CT scan-guided needle biopsy most frequently provides the diagnosis.

If disease is localized, surgical resection offers potentially curative treatment. Most frequently, however, extensive local disease renders a complete excision impossible and biopsy, perhaps with a bypass procedure such as choledochojejunostomy, is all that is performed. For patients who have unresectable disease, radiation, often combined with 5-FU chemotherapy, may provide a palliative benefit. Studies are ongoing concerning the potential benefit of techniques such as intraoperative irradiation. At present, there is no documented survival benefit for use of adjuvant chemotherapy or irradiation therapy in patients with pancreatic cancer.

Patients with recurrent local or metastatic disease to the liver may be considered for systemic therapy. Standard chemotherapeutic agents have not provided a survival advantage for patients with this neoplasm. Patients in this clinical situation should be encouraged to consider participation in clinical trials. If this is not possible, the use of supportive measures without specific antineoplastic therapy may be the most reasonable approach for many patients.

Cancer of the Esophagus

This year, more than 10,000 Americans will be diagnosed with cancer of the esophagus and over 9000 will die of the disease. Most patients present with a history of dysphagia lasting several months. Extensive involvement of the esophagus is usually present, and many patients have lymph node metastases. Cough, hoarseness, or aspiration are late signs of locally advanced disease. Metastasis to cervical lymph nodes or liver are present at diagnosis in some patients. More than 90 percent of malignancies of the esophagus are squamous cell cancers; the remaining are adenocarcinomas. The peak incidence of this malignancy is in persons from age 50 to 70 years.

Surgical resection provides the only potential route for cure for patients with this neoplasm. Unfortunately, of those having an operation, only about 4 percent survive as long as 5 years (31). Because of this poor result, present approaches often involve the use of radiation, chemotherapy, or both as part of primary multimodality therapy. Primary irradiation may be considered for patients who are medically inoperable or who have unresectable disease. Again, this is often in combination with chemotherapy.

Postoperative adjuvant irradiation may provide a survival benefit, but improvement appears to be limited. Most patients whose lymph nodes are found to be positive at operation have recurrence despite postoperative irradiation. This technique may be of most benefit for patients whose lymph nodes are negative (32). Intraluminal irradiation, hyperfractionation, and the use of agents such as 5-FU are currently under study.

Significant palliation for the patient who has unresectable disease or who has a local recurrence after primary therapy may be provided with intraluminal endoscopic laser. Cisplatinum-based combination chemotherapy has been used as part of a primary multimodality approach and in patients with recurrent or metastatic disease. Despite measurable responses, a survival benefit has yet to be demonstrated. Patients who are candidates for systemic therapy should be encouraged to consider participation in clinical trials.

Cancers of the Head and Neck

This year more than 40,000 patients will be diagnosed with a carcinoma of the upper aerodigestive tract. Most of these malignancies will be squamous cell carcinomas associated with such risk factors as tobacco (carcinogen) and alcohol (promoter) use. Oral cancers may be preceded by precursor lesions such as leukoplakia and/or erythroplakia. Laryngeal cancers account for approximately 30 percent of head and neck cancers. These are more difficult to detect by physical examination, but are often detected at an early stage by their interference with vocal cord function. Cancers of the head and neck infrequently metastasize. When they do cause death, it is be-

cause of failure of local control. Proper staging is critical to define the therapeutic approach and involves the use of various endoscopic techniques, CT, and magnetic resonance imaging (MRI).

The optimal therapy for this disorder requires the use of a multidisciplinary approach. Although surgery and radiation have been considered the cornerstones of such therapy, the recent use of chemotherapy appears to enhance the therapeutic response (33). The potential advantage of incorporating the use of systemic agents in initial therapy is to increase the rate of local control and, potentially, the overall rate of cure through the sterilization of distant metastases. The overall impact of this multimodal approach remains to be identified. The toxicity of this therapy is considerable but manageable. Patients with recurrent disease or those medically unfit for the standard multidisciplinary approaches, may achieve significant benefit with radiation therapy techniques or supportive care measures.

Breast Cancer

Breast cancer increases in incidence with advancing age. Most breast cancers are detected by physical examination, either by the patient or a physician. A steady increase in lesions diagnosed by mammography is occurring. Although advances in detection and treatment have been made, the overall mortality rate has not changed appreciably during the past decade (34). Risk factors for breast cancer include a family history of breast cancer, previous breast cancer, other breast disease, previous ovarian or endometrial cancer, menarche before age 12, menopause after age 50, or a first pregnancy after age 30 (35).

Elderly women are more reluctant than are younger women to examine their breasts. In addition, they are more likely to have their health care provided by physicians who take a less aggressive approach to screening (36). Breast self examination has been found to be less effective in women older than age 60, perhaps because of inadequate training, a lack of physical ability to perform the procedure, and changes in breast tissue with age. The loss of fatty tissue that occurs with age may make interpretation of mammographic findings more difficult and decrease the visualization of smaller tumors. Needle biopsy of a palpable mass is the most common method of diagnosis of breast cancer. Subtle mammographic signs of cancer, such as fine microcalcifications, may be biopsied by fine-needle localization under mammographic control. In addition to pathologic review, tissue should be sent for estrogen and progesterone receptors and for studies of tumor cell DNA ploidy and S-phase fraction with flow cytometry.

Modified radical mastectomy with axillary lymph node dissection is the most common surgical procedure for early breast cancer because it provides a more pleasing cosmetic result than the old radical procedure and the two operations result in equivalent survival.

Breast-conserving surgical techniques such as lumpectomy, partial mastectomy, and segmental mastectomy are becoming more frequent. These techniques involve local excision sufficiently wide so that the tumor is removed with adequate margins. In addition, an axillary dissection is also performed. The tumor must be small enough so that adequate margins can be obtained and a reasonable cosmetic result achievable to utilize this technique. Radiation therapy is administered to the remaining breast tissue. Contraindications to breast-conserving surgery are a tumor greater than 5 inches in size, a poorly defined tumor, a large tumor in a small breast, multiple malignant tumors within the breast, and malignancy involving the skin or chest wall musculature.

Locally advanced cancers that are not technically resectable often are approached initially with chemotherapy followed by modified radical mastectomy. A less than satisfactory result to chemotherapy may suggest that radiation is a better approach than surgery.

Patients with inflammatory carcinoma present with a breast that is erythematous and indurated. Pain may be present. Pathologically, the tumor is associated with lymphatic spread, which may reach the dermal region. Metastatic disease is not infrequently noted. The initial therapy involves chemotherapy followed by mastectomy, radiation therapy, or both.

The use of adjuvant systemic therapy with use of hormonal agents or chemotherapy has provided a survival benefit for some subsets of patients with breast cancer. Therapeutic decisions concerning the use of these agents are made on an individual basis and take into consideration axillary nodal involvement, whether the patient is pre- or postmenopausal, and estrogen and progesterone receptor status. Other features that are helpful in making this decision include tumor size, nuclear grade, DNA ploidy, and growth fraction.

In general, premenopausal women with positive lymph nodes benefit from adjuvant chemotherapy. For the premenopausal patient with negative axillary nodal involvement, therapy must be individualized because studies do not clearly demonstrate a benefit for chemotherapy. Patients with negative hormone receptors, large tumors, high nuclear grade, those with a high growth fraction, or combination of these factors may be considered for chemotherapy.

The postmenopausal woman with positive axillary nodal involvement and positive estrogen receptor levels should receive tamoxifen. Although data are unclear at present, postmenopausal women with positive axillary nodes and negative hormone receptors may be considered for chemotherapy. The postmenopausal woman with negative nodes, particularly if estrogen receptor is positive, may not benefit from additional adjuvant therapy. Nevertheless, some data suggest that adjuvant hormonal therapy may benefit these patients. In the node-negative patient, if poor prognostic factors are present (large tumor size, high nuclear grade or high growth fraction), chemotherapy may be considered. Treatment decisions must be based on individual situations (Table 54.5). The main role of the medical oncologist is to provide accurate information and help the patient make an informed decision.

Unfortunately, metastatic breast cancer is not curable with standard treatment techniques. All current therapy is palliative. The approach to the patient with metastatic disease must therefore be individualized. Patients with asymptomatic, nonvisceral, and nonlife-threatening disease should initially receive endocrine therapy irrespective of hormone receptor status. If liver or pulmonary lesions are asymptomatic, not rapidly progressing, and not life-threatening, these also may be approached with initial endocrine therapy. Approximately 20 percent of patients whose tumors are known to be estrogen-receptor-negative may respond to initial endocrine therapy. Patients who have progressed during initial endocrine therapy may respond to second- and, possibly, third-line agents. Those whose tumors are refractory to endocrine therapy or who have symptomatic or rapidly progressive visceral disease should be considered for

Table 54.5. Adjuvant Therapy in Elderly Women with Breast Cancer

Axillary Lymph Nodes	Receptor Status	Tumor Size (•)	Poor Prognostic Factors*	Treatment
None	+ or −	<1	+ or −	None or tamoxifen
None	+ or −	>1	−	Tamoxifen
None	+ or −	>1	+	Tamoxifen +/− chemotherapy
1–3	+	<1	−	Tamoxifen
1–3	+ or −	>1	+	Tamoxifen +/− chemotherapy
>4	+ or −	>1	+	Tamoxifen +/− chemotherapy

*High nuclear grade; high S-phase fraction; large tumor size.

Table 54.6. Treatment Options for the Elderly Woman with Metastatic Breast Cancer

As all therapy is palliative, quality of life is the major consideration.

Unless metastases are rapidly progressive, visceral, or life-threatening, initial therapy in all patients should be endocrine therapy, irrespective of receptor status.

Patients who progress during initial endocrine therapy may respond to second- and, possibly, third-line hormonal agents.

Patients whose tumors are refractory to endocrine therapy or who have symptomatic, life threatening, or visceral disease should be considered for chemotherapy, the intensity of which should be determined on the basis of performance status and major organ system function.

In addition to systemic therapy, palliative irradiation to the central nervous system or painful skeletal metastasis is often helpful.

chemotherapy. Various regimens of differing intensity are available and the specific program should be selected on the basis of performance status and major organ system function. Response rates to chemotherapy approach 50 percent to 60 percent, with response durations lasting approximately 12 to 18 months. Second- and third-line salvage chemotherapeutic regimens are available, but they possess a lower order of activity and, often, excessive toxicity. Other hormonal agents available for clinical use include megesterol acetate, diethylstilbestrol (DES), testosterone, and aminoglutethamide (Table 54.6). The use of palliative irradiation for chest wall, skeletal, or central nervous system metastasis often provides significant palliative benefit.

Although breast cancer is controllable for significant periods of time with use of the modalities noted above, most patients eventually die of the disease. Adequate use of supportive measures such as pain control and treatment of psychological problems is very important.

Cancer of the Prostate

More than 100,000 new cases of prostate cancer will be diagnosed this year, and approximately 30,000 individu-

als will die from the disorder. It is estimated that approximately 50 percent of American males older than 50 years of age have a focus of adenocarcinoma within their prostate glands. However, most do not develop a clinically important cancer.

Most men with cancer of the prostate present with obstructive voiding symptoms or an abnormal digital rectal exam. Approximately 10 percent have symptomatic metastatic disease, for example, skeletal pain. Once the diagnosis is suspected, a needle biopsy should be performed to ascertain information concerning staging and the grade of the tumor.

Serum prostatic acid phosphatase (PAP) and serum prostatic-specific antigen (PSA) are used diagnostically to assess the possibility of metastatic disease and for follow-up subsequent to definitive therapy. Other staging studies such as chest x-ray, bone scan, and CT scan of the abdomen and pelvis to look for lymphadenopathy are commonly performed.

Although prostatic cancer is a major cause of death in older men, in many patients the cancer remains dormant for extensive periods of time and death occurs from other causes. Accordingly, immediate therapy for all prostate cancers is not necessary. For instance, in patients with stage A-1 disease, that is patients found to have a single focus of adenocarcinoma discovered at the time of transurethral prostatectomy for benign hyperplasia, the prognosis is so good that it is difficult to show a benefit with therapy. In patients with asymptomatic metastatic disease, there is no evidence that systemic therapy prolongs survival. Thus, a period of expectant observation is a reasonable option.

Patients with disease localized to the gland itself may be offered radical prostatectomy or irradiation. Management decisions related to these options must consider the patient's overall medical health. Patients with symptomatic metastatic disease most frequently receive hormonal therapy. Options within this type of management include castration, LHRH analogues such as leuprolide and antiandrogens such as flutamide (37). In addition, areas of painful skeletal metastatic disease are well treated with local palliative radiation therapy. At present, the use of systemic chemotherapeutic agents has not been helpful.

Metastatic Cancer of Unknown Primary Site

Patients with a metastatic carcinoma and no definable primary site are relatively common and account for approximately 10 percent of all patients with cancer. A typical patient develops symptoms at a metastatic site and radiographic abnormality and a biopsy subsequently reveals cancer. However, history and physical examination, laboratory studies, and radiographic procedures fail to demonstrate the primary neoplasm.

Some subgroups of patients with this entity have treatable and perhaps curable disease; others, however, have unresponsive neoplasms. Approximately 75 percent of carcinomas of unknown primary site are adenocarcinomas. Most patients are elderly and are found to have diffuse metastatic disease. Despite extensive evaluation, a primary site is determined in only about 10 percent of patients. The most common primary sites are gastrointestinal and lung. Biopsy specimens from men should be stained for prostatic acid phosphatase and PSA. Specimens from women should be evaluated for estrogen and progesterone receptors. Helpful radiologic studies include chest x-ray, mammograms in females, and CT scans of the abdomen, chest, and

pelvis. Other radiographic procedures may be used if the patient's history or physical examination suggest an abnormality.

Women who have axillary nodal metastasis may be treated as having a potential breast cancer. Women with peritoneal carcinomatosis may be treated as patients with ovarian malignancies. Men with diffuse skeletal metastasis may benefit from therapy used for prostatic carcinoma. However, most patients do not fit into any of these categories. The survival rate is very poor for this group of patients, generally a matter of months.

For most patients with a metastatic, well-differentiated adenocarcinoma of unknown primary site, treatment with a variety of chemotherapeutic agents produces an exceedingly low response rate. Responses are generally partial and short term. In the appropriate clinical setting, a trial of such therapy may be reasonable, but usually symptomatic or palliative care should be the main thrust of therapy, particularly for the debilitated or elderly patient.

Patients with poorly differentiated carcinomas or adenocarcinomas form a separate subgroup of patients with malignancies of unknown primary site. These patients are generally younger, give a history of rapid progression, and have mid-line involvement, such as the mediastinum and retroperitoneum. Special pathologic studies such as immunoperoxidase staining and electron microscopy may identify specific malignancies in this subgroup of patients. Measurement of serum tumor markers such as human chorionic gonadotropin (HCG) and alpha fetal protein (AFP) is essential for these patients because elevations of such markers may suggest the presence of a germ cell tumor. Despite extensive pathologic study and evaluation of serum markers, most patients with poorly differentiated carcinomas will not have a more specific diagnosis made. Nevertheless, some may respond exceedingly well to systemic chemotherapeutic programs that use cisplatinum-based regimens (37). Some patients who respond may have prolonged, disease-free survival.

Non-Hodgkin's Lymphoma

The non-Hodgkin's lymphomas are a diverse group of malignancies with clinical courses that vary according to histologic subtype. A working formulation has been developed to classify histologic subtypes by prognosis. Three grades—low, intermediate, and high—correlate with favorable, intermediate, and unfavorable prognoses.

Of the approximate 30,000 new cases of lymphoma seen yearly in the United States, approximately 40 percent are low-grade lymphomas, and of these, the follicular, small-cleaved cell (FSCL) is the most common. The median age at diagnosis is in persons 50 to 60 years of age. Patients generally present with slowly progressive enlargement of lymph nodes. Most patients have extensive nodal disease and frequent involvement of the bone marrow. Although initially indolent, these histologies tend to become more aggressive over time and approximately 25 percent undergo a histologic transformation to an intermediate- or high-grade lymphoma. The median survival time of this subgroup of lymphomas is approximately 7 years.

Staging studies include routine laboratory tests, chest radiograph, CT scan of the abdomen and pelvis, and bone marrow aspirate and biopsy. Treatment decisions are based on the presence of symptoms, tempo of progression, and the patient's overall medical condition. At the present time, although these neoplasms are generally responsive to chemotherapy or irradiation, curative therapy is not available. The asymptomatic patient with slowly progressive disease and no evidence of significant organ system dysfunction should be observed over time. When therapy becomes indicated, generally as a result of the development of symptoms or evidence of organ system dysfunction, relatively nontoxic chemotherapy with oral alkylating agents or parenteral chemotherapeutic regimens may be used. Often, intermittent courses of chemotherapy may control the disease for a significant period of time (38). Localized diseased areas that produce a problem can frequently be treated with irradiation. Over time, the neoplasm becomes less and less sensitive to specific therapy and causes death. Not infrequently, however, the elderly patient with this subtype of lymphoma dies from causes unrelated to the neoplasm.

Diffuse, large-cell lymphoma (DLCL) is the most common of the intermediate-grade lymphomas. DLCL is an aggressive lymphoma and requires the prompt initiation of therapy. Staging studies are similar to those used for indolent lymphomas. Intermediate-grade lymphomas more frequently present in a localized early stage than do indolent lymphomas.

In contrast to indolent, low-grade lymphomas, curative therapy is potentially available for intermediate-grade lymphomas. Chemotherapy is the most frequently used modality for these lymphomas. Patients with localized stage I or stage II disease may be treated with irradiation, but, at the present time, chemotherapy is also recommended. For those patients with stage III or IV disease, aggressive systemic chemotherapy is used. With modern day regimens, approximately 50 percent of patients enter a complete response and, of these, about 80 percent achieve long-term remission. Numerous studies suggest that older patients can achieve a complete remission. Chemotherapy doses should not be reduced simply on the basis of the patient's age. Nevertheless, treatment-related toxicity may be increased, and the overall medical status of the patient needs to be considered before these regimens are used (39–41).

Hodgkin's Disease

Most patients with Hodgkin's lymphoma present with lymphadenopathy. Alternatively, a patient may present with constitutional (B) symptoms such as fever, night sweats, or weight loss. Lymph node biopsy reveals the diagnosis and the histologic subtype, such as lymphocyte predominance, nodular sclerosing, mixed cellularity, and lymphocyte-depleted. These subtypes present with more advanced disease in this order, and a significant worsening of prognosis is related to the advanced stage. The histology itself does not portend poor prognosis.

Staging studies include patient history and physical examination and, routine laboratory studies such as sedimentation rate, bilateral bone marrow biopsies, CT scanning of the chest, abdomen, and pelvis, lymphangiogram, and, potentially, a staging laparotomy.

Patients with stage I and stage II disease most often are treated with irradiation. Chemotherapy as a primary modality of therapy is considered for patients with bulky stage II disease or for patients with constitutional symptoms. Most patients with stage III or IV disease are treated with chemotherapy.

Patients older than 60 years of age often present with advanced disease and other medical problems that interfere with proper staging and treatment. Even when stratified by stage, constitutional symptoms, and treatment, older patients demonstrate poor 5-year survival (42).

Nevertheless, a poor prognosis should not be assumed for all elderly patients, particularly those with early stage disease (43).

The elderly patient who cannot be approached with modern irradiation techniques or combination chemotherapy may achieve a significant response and clinical benefit by the judicious use of local irradiation or relatively nontoxic chemotherapeutic agents.

Chronic Lymphocytic Leukemia

Chronic lymphocytic leukemia (CLL) is the most common leukemia in the elderly population. Like indolent lymphomas, CLL is a slowly progressive, lymphoid malignancy. The diagnosis is most frequently made on the observation of an asymptomatic lymphocytosis, which may or may not be associated with other abnormalities of the blood count. Alternatively, lymphadenopathy or splenomegaly may be the initial finding.

As with indolent non-Hodgkin's lymphomas, CLL responds very well to therapy; however, curative treatment is not yet available. Because CLL is slowly progressive, a period of watchful observation is frequently the initial management of choice. Indications for therapy include progressive, disease-related symptoms, progressive anemia or thrombocytopenia, bulky adenopathy that is painful, cosmetically unpleasant, or interferes with organ system function, progressive splenomegaly, or a white blood cell count larger than 150,000. All these indications relate to a progressive increase in tumor burden. In addition, recurrent sepsis associated with hypogammaglobulinemia or disease-related autoimmune hemolysis are other indications for treatment.

Initially, patients respond well to the use of the oral alkylating agent chlorambucil used as a single agent or in combination with prednisone. Alternatively, cyclophosphamide may be used for the unusual patient who does not tolerate chlorambucil, the patient who no longer responds to this agent, or in whom thrombocytopenia is a particular problem. Cyclophosphamide is relatively platelet-sparing (44). Fludarabine has high efficacy in patients with CLL refractory to chlorambucil or cyclophosphamide (45).

Transfusions of red blood cells and platelets may be helpful for patients with CLL who develop progressive marrow failure or pure red cell aplasia. Infusions of gamma globulin may be helpful to the patient with hypogammaglobulinemia and recurrent bacterial infections.

Ultimately, death occurs from an infectious or bleeding complication. Richter's syndrome, the transformation of CLL to large-cell lymphoma, is an unusual event. On rare occasions, CLL may transform into a prolymphocytic form of leukemia. Both these transformations respond poorly to therapy.

Acute Non-Lymphocytic Leukemia

Patients with acute non-lymphocytic leukemia (ANLL) most commonly present with symptoms referable to an excess of leukemic blasts in the peripheral blood, or symptomatic anemia, thrombocytopenia, or infections related to leukopenia. Most studies indicate that the elderly do not fare well with modern antileukemic therapy. This may be as a result of poor prognostic features, such as an antecedent hematologic disorder such as myelodysplasia, and the fact that poor prognostic cytogenetic abnormalities are more frequently present in the elderly population (46). In addition, comorbid conditions such as cardiovascular and pulmonary disease complicate induction therapy. Use of full-dose induction regimens results in an excess of early death among the elderly. Attenuated induction programs may be the treatment of choice for the elderly (47,48).

The most reasonable approach is to individualize the intensity of induction chemotherapy for the elderly patient with ANLL. Those with a good performance status and absence of comorbid conditions may benefit from full-dose induction therapy. Alternatively, the frail, elderly patient with significant cardiopulmonary disease may be best served with supportive or palliative therapy.

Multiple Myeloma

Multiple myeloma, a plasma cell neoplasm, increases in incidence with age. Patients may present with symptoms related to skeletal destruction, bone marrow failure with attendant anemia or thrombocytopenia, or as a consequence of the attendant dysproteinemia, which may cause renal failure, a coagulopathy, hyperviscosity, or amyloidosis. Severe infection related to altered humoral immunity may also be present.

Clinical staging which quantitates tumor burden uses such measurements as the degree of anemia, the presence of renal failure or hypercalcemia, number of lytic lesions, and the quantity of paraprotein. In addition, sophisticated scientific techniques such as thymidine labeling and the use of β_2-microglobulin may also correlate with tumor burden.

Patients with symptomatic multiple myeloma frequently respond well to chemotherapy with melphalan in combination with prednisone. The use of intensive multidrug regimens remains controversial. For patients who respond, discontinuing therapy at 1 to 2 years is reasonable. Some studies suggested that elderly patients had response and survival rates equivalent to younger patients (49), but recent studies suggest that survival in the elderly may be poorer than that for younger patients (50,51). Intensive adriamycin-based chemotherapeutic regimens are available for patients who have not responded or who have relapsed during primary therapy. These regimens may be too intense for the elderly; however, this has not been adequately studied.

Patients with indolent or smoldering myeloma, that is, patients who are asymptomatic and lack hematologic, biochemical, or evidence of disease, may be followed with expectant observation. Treatment can be considered if there is evidence of progression.

References

1. Yancik R. Frame of reference: old age as the context for the prevention and treatment of cancer. In: Yancik R, ed. Perspectives on prevention and treatment of cancer in the elderly. New York: Raven Press, 1983:5–17.
2. Goodwin JS, Samet JM, Key CR, et al. Stage of diagnosis of cancer varies with the age of the patient. J Am Geriatr Soc 1986;34:20–26.
3. Greenfield S, Blanco DM, Elashoff RM, Ganz PA. Patterns of care related to age of breast cancer patient. JAMA 1987;257:2766–2770.
4. Samet J, Key C, Hunt C, Goodwin JS. Choice of cancer therapy varies with the age of the patient. JAMA 1986;255:3385–3390.
5. Mor V, Guadagnoli E, Silliman RA, et al. Influence of old age, performance status, medical, and psychosocial status on management of cancer patients. In: Yancik R, Yates J, eds. Cancer in the elderly. New York: Springer, 1989:127–148.
6. Bergman L, Dekker G, van Leeuwen FE, et al. The effect of age on treatment choice and survival in elderly breast cancer patients. Cancer 1991;67:2227–2234.
7. Silliman RA, Guadagnoli E, Weitberg AB, Mor V. Age as a predictor of diagnostic and initial treatment intensity in newly diagnosed breast cancer patients. J Gerontol 1989;44:M46–M50.
8. Goodwin JS, Hunt WC, Same MS, Same JM. Determinants of cancer therapy in elderly patients. Cancer 1993;72:594–601.
9. Pitot HC. The molecular biology of carcinogenesis. Cancer 1993;72:962–970.
10. Temin HM. On the origin of RNA tumor viruses. Annu Rev Genet 1974;8:155–177.
11. Garrett CT. Oncogenes. Clin Chim Acta 1986;156:1–40.
12. Marshall CJ. Tumor suppressor genes. Cell 1991;64:313–326.
13. Dix D. The role of aging in cancer incidence: an epidemiological study. J Gerontol 1989;44:10–18.
14. List ND. Perspectives in cancer screening in the elderly. Clin Geriatr Med 1987;3:433–445.
15. Mandelblatt J, Gopaul I, Wistreich M. Gynecological care of elderly women: another look at Papanicolaou smear testing. JAMA 1986;256:367–371.
16. 1989 Survey of physicians' attitudes and practices in early cancer detection. Cancer 1990;40:77–101.
17. Hoekstra HJ, Verschueren RCJ, Oldhoff J, et al. Palliative and curative electrocoagulation for rectal cancer: experience and results. Cancer 1985;55:210–213.
18. Harms BA, Starling JA. Current status of sphincter preservation in rectal cancer. Oncology 1990;4:53–60.
19. Minsky BD, Cohen AM. Conservative management of invasive rectal cancer: alternative to abdomino-perineal resection. Oncology 1989;3:137–142.
20. Balducci L, Parker M, Sexton W, et al. Pharmacology of antineoplastic agents in elderly patients. Semin Oncol 1989;16:76–84.
21. Gelman RS, Taylor SG. Cyclophosphamide, methotrexate, and 5-fluorouracil chemotherapy in women more than 65 years old with advanced breast cancer: the elimination of age trends in toxicity by using doses based on creatinine clearance. J Clin Oncol 1984;2:1406–1414.
22. Balducci L, Phillips DM, Davis KM, et al. Systemic treatment of cancer in the elderly. Arch Gerontol Geriatr 1988;7:115–150.
23. Lipschitz DA, Udupa KB. Age and the hematopoietic system. J Am Geriatr Soc 1986;30:448–454.
24. Shank WA Jr, Balducci L. Hemopoietic growth factors in older cancer patients. J Am Geriatr Soc 1992;40:151–154.
25. Harris R. Cardiovascular diseases of the elderly. Med Clin North Am 1983;67:379–394.
26. Love RR. Tamoxifen therapy in primary breast cancer: biology, efficacy and side effects. J Clin Oncol 1989;7:803–810.
27. Balducci L, Parker M, Hescock H, et al. Systemic management of prostate cancer. An annotated review. Am J Med Sci 1990;299:185–192.
28. Wadler S, Schwartz EL, Goldman M, et al. Fluorouracil and recombinant alpha 2A-interferon: An active regimen against advanced colorectal carcinoma. J Clin Oncol 1989;7:1775–1789.

29. Yancik R, Ries LG. Epidemiological features of cancer in the elderly. In: Zenser TV, Coes RM, eds. Cancer and aging: progress in research and treatment. New York: Springer, 1989:95–103.

30. Public Health Service. The health consequences of smoking: cancer and chronic lung disease in the workplace. Publ. DHEW (PHS) 85-50207. Washington, DC: Department of Health and Human Services, 1985.

31. Earlam R, Cunha-Melo JR. Esophageal squamous cell carcinoma: a critical surgical review of surgery. Br J Surg 1980;67:381–390.

32. Earlam R, Cunha-Melo JR. Esophageal squamous cell carcinoma: a critical review of radiotherapy. Br J Surg 1980;67:457–461.

33. Erwin TM, Clark JR, Weichselbaum RR. Multidisciplinary treatment of advanced squamous cell carcinomas of the head and neck. Semin Oncol 1985;12:71–78.

34. Lawrence RS. The role of physicians in promoting health. Health Aff 1990;9:122–132.

35. McLellen GL. Screening and early diagnosis of breast cancer. J Fam Pract 1988;26:561–568.

36. Stomberg M. Early detection of cancer in the elderly: problems and solutions. Int J Nurs Stud 1989;16:139–156.

37. Hainsworth JD, Dial TW, Greco FA. Curative combination chemotherapy for patients with advanced poorly differentiated carcinoma of unknown primary site. Am J Clin Oncol 1988;11:138.

38. Portlock CS. Management of the low-grade non-Hodgkin's lymphomas. Semin Oncol 1990;17:51–59.

39. Dixon D, et al. Effect of age on therapeutic outcome in advanced diffuse histiocytic lymphoma. The Southwest Oncology Group Experience. J Clin Oncol 1986;4:295–305.

40. Voss JM, Armitage JO, et al. The importance of age in survival of patients treated with chemotherapy for aggressive non-Hodgkin's lymphoma. J Clin Oncol 1988;6:1838–1844.

41. O'Reilly S, Klimo P, Conners J. Low-dose ACOP-B and VABE: weekly chemotherapy for elderly patients with advanced-stage diffuse large cell lymphoma. J Clin Oncol 1991;9:741–747.

42. Walker A, et al. Survival of the older patient compared with the younger patient with Hodgkin's disease. Cancer 1990;65:1635–1640.

43. Austin-Seymour M, Hoppe R, et al. Hodgkin's disease in patients over 60 years old. Ann Intern Med 1984;100:13–18.

44. Foon KA, Rai KR, Gale RP. Chronic lymphocytic leukemia: new insights into biology and therapy. Ann Intern Med 1990;113:525–539.

45. Keating MJ, Kantarjian H, Talpaz M, et al. Fludarabine: a new agent with major activity against chronic lymphocytic leukemia. Blood 1989;74:19–25.

46. Champlin RE, et al. Treatment of acute myelogenous leukemia in the elderly. Semin Oncol 1989;16:51–56.

47. Yates J, Glidewell O, Wiernik PA, et al. Cytosine arabinoside with daunorubicin or adriamycin for therapy of acute myelocytic leukemia. A CALGB study. Blood 1982;60:454–462.

48. Kahn SB, Begg C, et al. Full dose versus attenuated dose daunorubicin, cytosine arabinoside, and 6-thioguanine in the treatment of acute nonlymphocytic leukemia in the elderly. J Clin Oncol 1984;2:865–870.

49. Cohen HJ, Bartolucci A. Age and the treatment of multiple myeloma. Am J Med 1985;79:316–324.

50. Froom P, et al. Multiple myeloma in the geriatric patient. Cancer 1990;66:965–967.

51. Alexanian R. Ten-year survival in multiple myeloma. Arch Intern Med 1985;145:2073–2074.

Chapter 55
Diabetes Mellitus and Dyslipidemia Disorders in the Elderly

Fred D. Hofeldt

Although the world is full of suffering, it is full also of the overcoming of it.

Helen Keller
Optimism, 1903

Diabetes Mellitus

Diabetes mellitus is a common medical condition of the elderly (1–6) and is seen in nearly 20 percent of persons older than 85 years of age. The incidence of diabetes in the elderly is three times greater than that of the general population. In American, Finnish, and New Zealand populations, the prevalence of frank diabetes in the elderly older than 65 years of age is approximately 10 percent, an additional 5 percent to 10 percent are diabetic by oral glucose tolerance testing, and an additional 15 to 20 percent have impaired carbohydrate tolerance. Diabetes is seen more commonly in elderly black and Mexican American populations. The prevalence of diabetes in the elderly is predicted to increase by 44 percent during the next 20 years. Estimated costs for health care services for the diabetic population are $5.2 billion annually (7). The expenditures per capita for medical care is 50 percent higher for elderly diabetic patients than expenditures for elderly nondiabetic patients. More than 80 percent of the health care is provided by general and family physicians and internists (7).

The most common type of diabetes in the elderly is type II, non-insulin-dependent diabetes mellitus (NIDDM), which has a hereditary association, is aggravated by obesity and diabetogenic drugs, and often responds to diet or antihyperglycemic drug therapy. Eight to 10 percent of elderly diabetic patients have insulin-dependent diabetes mellitus (IDDM), which includes both juvenile and adult-onset type I IDDM. These patients are best identified by low basal and nonresponsive postglucagon C-peptide measurements (8,9).

Associated with aging itself is an age-related deterioration in carbohydrate tolerance (10–12) that significantly affects about 20 percent of the elderly and as much as 50 percent of those with physical inactivity, poor dietary composition (13,14), or obesity. Hemoglobin A_1C increases with age, mainly as a reflection of elevated postprandial glucose levels, as fasting glucose values change little with aging. Aging is associated with a change in body composition—an increase in adipose mass. Upper body segment obesity with excessive adipose accumulation in the neck, shoulders, and abdomen has been associated with a higher risk of diabetes mellitus for men and women compared with lower body segment obesity involving the hips or thighs (15–18).

Studies of the age-related deterioration in carbohydrate tolerance implicate an acquired state of insulin resistance. Earlier studies (19) of elderly humans did not show decreased insulin secretion, in contrast to studies of aging animals, which suggests that there is decreased insulin secretion per beta cell with an age-related impairment of glucose-induced margination of secretory vesicles at the beta cell plasma membrane (20). Recent reports, however, describe an age-related decline in B-cell function in men (13,21–23). The major alteration associated with hyperglycemia of aging is peripheral changes in insulin metabolism and action. These changes include a decreased metabolic clearance rate of insulin and defective insulin action in promoting glucose transport, primarily in muscle. Most studies report that the number of insulin receptors on target tissues are not decreased; basal hepatic glucose production remains normal, but its suppression by insulin is delayed in elderly patients (10,11,23,24). Fink et al (25,26) showed insulin resistance is caused by a postreceptor defect in insulin action in elderly patients. The defect exists in elderly patients even when their carbohydrate tolerance is normal, which suggests a decreased number of glucose transporters (24).

The carbohydrate intolerance of aging can be readily distinguished from diabetes mellitus. The criteria established by the National Diabetes Data Group for diabetes mellitus is so generous that it need not be modified for elderly patients (27). Because very little change occurs in fasting glucose values with aging, the finding of fasting glucose values larger than 140 mg/dL (7.8 mmol/liter) on two occasions establishes the diagnosis of diabetes mellitus in the elderly. Symptoms of hyperglycemia are usually also present. A glucose tolerance test rarely needs to be performed in elderly patients to establish the diagnosis of diabetes mellitus. Elderly type II diabetic patients manifest the same metabolic defects as those seen in adult-onset type II patients, namely, peripheral insulin resistance, increased fasting hepatic glucose production, and a delayed but enhanced insulin secretion to an oral glucose stimulus at fasting glucose values of 140 to 160 mg/dL (7.8–8.9 mmol/liter) but glucotoxicity and beta cell desensitization at higher fasting glucose levels (28–31).

Diabetes mellitus and aging share certain similarities, and as such, diabetes mellitus is considered a model for premature aging (32–34). With aging, there is a progressive increase in capillary basement membrane thickening, which is also seen in patients with long-standing diabetes mellitus, especially if hyperglycemia is not controlled. Atherosclerotic complications occur commonly in elderly patients and prematurely in diabetic patients. Increased collagen cross-linking and resistance to collagenase digestion is seen with aging and at an earlier age in patients with diabetes mellitus. These changes in collagen have some common biophysical and biochemical properties, but the underlying molecular process is different (35). Human skin fibroblasts, when maintained in tissue culture, have a finite in vitro lifespan. With increasing donor age of these fibroblasts, there is decreased cell replication. A marked reduction in the replication lifespan of fibroblasts is seen in patients with diabetes mellitus. Increased oxidative stress and free radical production occurs with aging, and poor diabetic control, and are related to diabetic complications (36,37). Hence, the combination of diabetes plus aging leads to a functional age greater than chronologic age in the diabetic individual. It has been estimated that the chronologic age of the diabetic patient plus the years of duration of diabetes is an assessment of the functional (physiologic) age.

The presentation of diabetes mellitus in the elderly may be typical, with the usual symptoms of hyperglycemia (i.e., polyuria, nocturia, polydipsia, weight loss) or its presentation may be atypical and confused with other age-prevalent issues (38). The diabetic state may be precipitated by stress, infection process, myocardial infarction, or stroke or may be an incidental finding during evaluation for other complaints involving the eyes, central nervous system (CNS), sexual dysfunction, or atherosclerotic complication. Some cases are diagnosed during routine physical examinations or diabetic screening programs.

Aging, with its physiologic deterioration and changes in nutritional status (39–42), makes the elderly diabetic patient difficult to manage. These changes include alterations in memory, hearing, and vision; muscle weakness and incoordination; arthritis; and absent teeth or loose dentures. There may also be insufficient financial resources, lack of support systems, an absent spouse, poor health care communications, and insufficient patient-provider relationships. Older patients may be housebound, which is associated with reduced social contacts, reduced physical activity, and inadequate diet. Functional impairment is common among the elderly. In a survey of institutionalized elderly patients (43), mental impairment was seen in 32 percent, malnutrition in 39 percent, visual impairment in 23 percent, gait disturbances in 39 percent, and incontinence in 29 percent.

With aging, there is a decrease in the metabolic rate (44) that results in a reduced caloric requirement of approximately 500 kilocalorie (kcal) per day. The reduced metabolic rate is a result of changes in the resting or basal metabolic rate and physical activity. The major decrease in energy expenditure occurs because of reduced activity (45–47). Even though the principles of dietary management for elderly diabetic patients are the same as those for younger patients, dietary recommendations need to be individualized to recognize the patient's food preferences, ethnic background, financial resources, nutritional state, and support systems (48–51). Emphasis should focus on avoiding hypoglycemia; if unrecognized, hypoglycemia may accelerate mental deterioration (51,52). Overweight patients should be prescribed a 1200 to 1500 kcal diet. Many older diabetic patients are of ideal or less than ideal body weight and need approximately

25 kcal/kg body weight. Meals should be proportioned into three equal feedings, and snacks are advised for insulin-treated patients. Avoidance of a high-fat diet, as advocated by the American Diabetes Association (46,48–50), addresses the issue of a co-existing lipid disorder. Increasing dietary fiber content to 40 gm/day assists in digestive function and has a beneficial effect on carbohydrate intolerance and hyperlipidemia. Fructose can be used as a sugar substitute, as long as its caloric content is realized (53).

The diet of elderly persons is influenced by altered food preference caused by aging, changes in taste and smell perception, difficulty in swallowing (a result of loss of salivary secretions), loose dentures or missing teeth, and altered gastrointestinal function with constipation, bloating, abdominal gas, and discomfort. There is a decreased perception of thirst, which makes elderly persons more prone to dehydration. Preparing foods may be difficult because of diminished vision, incapacitating arthritis, tremor, and musculoskeletal weakness. House-boundness and poor food selection contribute to a monotonous diet. Elderly people comprise one of the poorer socioeconomic groups, with 20 percent existing at or below the poverty level.

Excessive alcohol ingestion, which is common in retired elderly persons, can lead to worsening carbohydrate tolerance and can potentiate hypoglycemia (54). Approximately 4 percent to 8 percent of elderly patients are alcoholics (55).

A regular exercise program can be prescribed after a thorough physical or medical evaluation that notes limiting complications, glucose control, and cardiovascular response to an exercise stress test (45–47). Exercise may be limited by the physical, mental, and neuromuscular deterioration accompanying aging and by the tendency of elderly persons toward inactivity and houseboundness. For many elderly patients, it is important simply to promote walking or prescribe a walking-exercise program (45–47). Attention must also be given to household hazards that may lead to falls and injury.

Most elderly diabetic patients respond to oral hypoglycemics (56–58). The major class of drugs used to lower blood glucose in type II diabetic patients is the sulfonylureas. In 1956, the first agent, tolbutamide, was released for clinical use in the United States. In subsequent years, additional oral hypoglycemic agents such as chlorpropamide, acetohexamide, and tolazamide were effectively used in the management of adults with diabetes. These agents have been called the first-generation sulfonylureas. Newer, second-generation agents available in the United States are glyburide and glipizide. The choice of an oral agent depends on its metabolic characteristics, such as its hepatic metabolism, the toxicity of its metabolic by-products, and their accumulation in patients with renal disease. Mild renal impairment occurs with aging with nearly a 30 percent decline in creatinine clearance in older subjects (see also Chapters 8 and 49). In elderly patients, an estimation of creatinine clearance can be obtained by use of the Cockcroft-Gault equation:

$$\frac{(140-age) \times weight\ (kg)}{72 \times serum\ creatinine}$$

The formula is corrected for elderly women by multiplying by 0.85.

Of the first-generation sulfonylurea agents, tolbutamide has been the agent of choice because of its short half-life, its hepatic metabolism to inactive compounds, and the safety associated with a wide dosage range from 0.25 to 3.0 gm daily.

The second-generation sulfonylureas have fewer side effects because of their nonionic binding to serum proteins, their less active or inactive metabolites, and a significant decrease in water retention. First-generation oral agents are characterized by ionic binding to serum proteins and can be displaced or can displace similar acidic drugs, such as phenylbutazone, warfarin, and salicylates. An increase in the level of free sulfonylureas that cause hypoglycemia can occur in ill patients who continue medication when food intake is limited and are ingesting other medications such as aspirin.

The elderly commonly receive polymedication and consume a number of over-the-counter medications, shared medications, and self-prescribed medications. Fewer drug interactions occur with the nonionic binding, second-generation sulfonylureas. The second-generation sulfonylureas are metabolized to less active compounds, especially glipizide, which has inactive metabolites. These agents have a very potent effect in lowering blood glucose levels and should be prescribed to the elderly with mild diabetes at the lowest possible daily dose (i.e.,

1.25 mg for glyburide or 2.5 mg for glipizide) with careful glucose monitoring before any increase in dose. Micronized glyburide tablets provide serum concentrations higher than nonmicronized tablets and must be prescribed with caution and careful titration for glucose control. Table 55.1 lists various oral agents as well as those preferred for elderly patients. With acute stress, a mild, non-insulin-requiring, elderly diabetic patient may experience sudden metabolic decompensation with progression to severe hyperglycemia (59,60), hyperosmolar dehydration or coma, or even diabetic ketoacidosis. The impaired thirst mechanisms accompanying aging contribute to the dehydration. Hence, insulin therapy may be required for the acute illness. The newly released oral medications Metformin and Acarbose are also helpful in elderly diabetic patients.

Insulin treatment is required for symptomatic elderly patients (51,61,62). About 30 percent of insulin-requiring, elderly type II diabetic patients can be treated with one injection of intermediate-acting insulin daily. A reasonable starting dose for insulin is 0.5 U/kg. If short-acting insulin is needed, premixed insulin preparations are ideal because they are easier for older patients to draw the correct dose. Obesity is associated with insulin resistance and increases insulin requirements, which leads to more intensified insulin programs such as the split-mix use of neutral protamine Hagedorn (NPH) and regular insulin before breakfast and NPH and regular insulin before sup-per. With split-mix regimens, two-thirds of the insulin dose is given in the morning before breakfast and the remainder before supper. Usually 4 to 16 units of preprandial regular insulin are sufficient when the patient mixes the insulin. Lente-regular insulin combinations should be avoided because mixing causes loss of the short-acting insulin activity.

A blood glucose measuring meter is very useful for elderly patients. A well-instituted home glucose monitoring (HGM) program improves compliance and provides guidelines for altering therapy (61–63). Urine testing is rarely sufficient and should be discarded. Insulin-treated patients require more frequent HGM determinations, which are done by checking a fasting glucose value and a glucose profile (before lunch, at midday, and at bedtime), which should be done at least twice during the week and once on the weekend. For patients treated with diet or oral agents, a fasting HGM value performed once on a weekday and once on the weekend may be sufficient. Many times it is difficult for elderly patients to test at more frequent intervals because of the complexity of their life situation and their physical impairment caused by the aging process.

The treatment goal is to relieve symptoms (64–66) such as polyuria, polydipsia, decreased visual acuity, fatigue, weight loss, general malaise, vaginitis, or recurring urinary tract infections. Lowering blood glucose to levels below the renal threshold is sufficient to relieve

Table 55.1. Comparison of Oral Hypoglycemic agents

Drug	Daily Dose Range (mg)	Tablet Size (mg)	Administration (times/day)	Metabolism
First-generation				
Tolbutamide*	500–3000	250, 500	2–4	Liver to inactive metabolites; short half-life (4 hr)
Tolazamide	100–1000	100, 250, 500	1–2	Liver to metabolites with hypoglycemic activity; medium half-life (7 hr)
Acetohexamide	500–1500	250, 500	1–2	Short half-life (2 hr) but liver metabolites have 6-hr half-life
Chlorpropamide	100–750	100, 250	1	Renal excretion of unmetabolized drug; long half-life (36 hr)
Second-generation				
Glyburide	1.25–20.0	1.25, 2.5, 5.0	1–2	Liver to weakly active metabolites; medium half-life (10 hr)
Glipizide*	2.5–40.0	5, 10	1–2	Liver to inactive metabolites; short half-life (4 hr)
Micronized glyburide	0.75–12.0	1.5, 3.0	1	Metabolism similar to glyburide; elderly may have higher blood levels

*Ideal agent for elderly patients.

glycosuria and nocturia. With aging, the renal tubular glucose reabsorption threshold may increase from 180 mg/dL to approximately 260 mg/dL, which allows the patient to be asymptomatic at higher glucose values. The accepted glucose profile for the elderly diabetic is maintenance of a fasting plasma glucose level at or less than 150 mg/dL (8.4 mmol/liter), and a plasma glucose profile less than 200 mg/dL (11.1 mmol/liter). Measurements of hemoglobulin A_1C or its equivalent at 6-month intervals establishes the degree of overall glucose control; fructosamine as a monitoring tool is unreliable because low albumin states alter its value.

Hypoglycemia

Of special concern in the elderly diabetic patients is hypoglycemia, which can go unrecognized (51,52,66,67). Hypoglycemia is potentiated by alcohol, malnutrition, beta blockers and angiotensin-converting enzyme (ACE) inhibitors (68,69). Hypoglycemia is a myocardial stressor and may unmask subclinical coronary artery disease or cerebral vascular insufficiency. Hypoglycemia is particularly dangerous for the patient with autonomic neuropathy, in whom there is a deficient counterregulatory hormonal response of glucagon and catecholamines to the hypoglycemia, and hypoglycemic unawareness exists. Autonomic neuropathy may also cause a decrease in gastric emptying and gastrointestinal motility, which affects the absorption of nutrients. Hypoglycemia may be associated with other medical illnesses, such as disorders of the gastrointestinal tract that cause failure of nutrient absorption, renal failure, chronic liver disease, hypopituitarism, hypothyroidism, and adrenal insufficiency. Hypothermia may be a clue to undiagnosed hypoglycemia. Because of the seriousness of hypoglycemia in elderly patients, the criteria for glucose control should be less strict (64–66).

Surgical Management

Diabetic patients undergoing surgical procedures need a very thorough preoperative assessment of their cardiopulmonary, hepatic, renal, and central nervous system functional reserve capacity (70,71). They need careful intraoperative and postoperative observation for complicating disorders of these vital organ systems, particularly complicating infection, hyponatremia, or hypernatremia

(70–74). The insulin-treated patient can be managed during surgery with the administration of one-half the usual NPH insulin dose given subcutaneously just before surgery with a saline 5% dextrose infusion at 125 mL/hr. The evening dose of NPH is not given on the day before surgery. Even better interoperative management is provided by a regular insulin infusion adjusted to maintain a blood glucose at 150 to 180 mg/dL (8.3–10 mmol/liter) during the operative procedure. Intraoperative hypoglycemia must be avoided. Postoperatively, the patient's blood sugar should be measured at 6-hour intervals and the patient should be treated with regular insulin doses until the patient resumes oral feeding, at which time the previous insulin program can be reinstituted. Immediately after surgery, while constant glucose solutions are infused, 4 to 16 units of regular insulin every 6 hours, adjusted by glucose measurement, are usually required.

Foot Care

Good foot care is essential for all diabetic patients (75–79), particularly the elderly patient in whom the aging process has led to poor foot sensation, foot deformities, and peripheral vascular insufficiency. These patients are prone to foot trauma, ulceration, and infection. Of note, 40 percent of elderly diabetic patients cannot reach their toes (79).

The patient's feet should be inspected at each office visit and also inspected daily by the patient to ensure the absence of any lesion. Patients should be taught how to inspect their feet and how to palpate the foot for pressure points, warm spots, or breaks in the skin. The feet should be kept dry and clean; they should be washed several times weekly to ensure good hygiene. Dry feet can best be treated by the application of a lanolin-containing preparation. Ideally, patients should wear well-fitted leather shoes that are supportive and comfortable. Walking barefooted should be avoided. Toenails should be neatly trimmed transversely and the nail edges filed carefully.

Pressure spots need to be evaluated for the need of a metatarsal bar. Trivial lesions may progress to chronic nonhealing wounds, gangrene, or deep infection. Foot ulcers are slow to heal because of atherosclerotic, microvascular disease and neuropathic-related complications. Superficial ulcers can be treated by the patient at home with local foot care, debridement, and oral antibiotics. When infection is present, limited walking is advocated for proper healing. Penetrating ulcers should be aggressively treated with hospitalization and intravenous antibiotics. These infections are usually polymicrobial. With proper attention to good foot care, the patient's quality of life is improved, morbidity is less, and amputation is avoided.

Atherosclerosis

Diabetic patients have more complicating atherosclerosis, compromising peripheral vascular disease, cerebral vascular disease, and arteriosclerotic coronary heart disease than do nondiabetic persons (80–82). These conditions are increased approximately two to three times for diabetic patients compared with the general population, especially for diabetic women.

Generalized atherosclerotic disease including coronary artery disease is seen in elderly subjects with syndrome X (83). This multimetabolic disease has insulin resistance and hyperinsulinemia as contributing factors to the atherosclerosis. These patients are identified by an increased waist-hip ratio (>1.0 in men and >0.8 in women) (84). The disease is associated with varying degrees of carbohydrate intolerance to frank diabetes, and a dyslipidemia characterized as an elevation in triglycerides and accompanying low high-density lipoprotein (HDL) levels. Other features of this syndrome are hypertension, physical inactivity, and hyperuricemia. The hyperinsulinemia of aging contributes to the occurrence of this syndrome in the elderly (18).

Macrovascular atherosclerotic disease is multifactorial and assessment requires consideration of the patient's family history for atherosclerotic disease and the presence of traditional risk factors such as dyslipidemia, diabetes, smoking, hypertension, postmenopausal status, and obesity (85). Coronary atherosclerosis occurs prematurely and is more severe in diabetic patients than in age-matched controls (86,87). Coronary atherosclerosis, although perceived to be a diffuse process in diabetic patients, may actually be focal and remedial to revascularization procedure (88). Diabetic patients may experience silent (painless) myocardial infarction more commonly than do nondiabetics (89–91). The fatality rate

is one to two times higher in the older diabetic patient than it is in the nondiabetic patient.

Peripheral vascular disease of the lower extremities contributes to disability with claudications, foot ulcerations, ischemia, and amputations. Diabetic patients with peripheral vascular disease and an ischemic extremity should be evaluated for small-vessel bypass surgery as a consideration for limb salvage (92). Cerebral vascular disease with stroke or transient ischemic attacks is more common in diabetic patients (89). When stroke occurs, the elderly diabetic patient is more likely to experience associated complications or death than when the same event occurs in the nondiabetic patient. This result appears to be related to the presence of underlying coronary artery disease in the diabetic patient.

Therapeutic approaches for atherosclerotic manifestations are symptomatic. Aspirin, 65 to 325 mg per day, may play a preventive role. Vascular surgery for coronary, peripheral, and cerebral vascular disease merits the same consideration as it does for nondiabetic persons, but carries additional risk for diabetic patients of any age, particularly the elderly, who may have compromised multisystem organ function reserve and advanced physiologic age. The mortality of diabetic patients receiving thrombolytic therapy is reduced the same as it is for nondiabetic patients, and the risk of bleeding or stroke is not increased (93). Intravenous dye contrast studies for diabetic patients need cautious consideration, and when performed, the patient should be well hydrated to avoid complications of renal insufficiency. Administration of mannitol may also be preventive. Although cessation of smoking and lowering of the blood pressure in hypertensive patients are recommended, there is no proof that altering any risk factors for atherosclerosis is beneficial to the elderly diabetic patient with established macrovascular disease. However, recent evidence in younger patients suggests that normalizing serum cholesterol may reduce incidence of coronary insufficiency and fatal myocardial infarction in both primary and secondary preventive studies (85,94,95) and possibly may reverse large vessel atherosclerosis and coronary artery stenosis (96).

Retinopathy

Diabetic retinopathy is less common in elderly patients

with type II diabetes than in patients with type I diabetes. However, diabetes continues to be the leading cause of blindness in the United States. In the elderly type II patient, visual loss may be caused by vascular insufficiency of the macular or proliferative retinopathy, which includes a moderate-to-severe neovascularization on or near the disc, with or without vitreous hemorrhage. Focal photocoagulation is of value in these conditions. The efficacy of photocoagulation in the treatment of background retinopathy has yet to be established. If loss of vision has occurred from a vitreous hemorrhage or retinal traction, vitrectomy may be helpful. Control of hypertension is recommended. Other preventive treatments of retinopathy are not well-established. The results of the Diabetes Control and Complication Trial (DCCT) Research Group has clearly established that hyperglycemia is an important factor in the retinopathy, neuropathy, and nephropathy seen in type I diabetes (97). Similarly, hyperglycemia in the elderly diabetic patient is associated with retinopathy (82).

Cataracts

There is an increased prevalence of cataracts in diabetic patients younger than 70 years of age. In patients older than age 70, cataracts are equally common in diabetic and nondiabetic patients. Patients with significant visual impairment from cataracts are surgical candidates if diabetic retinopathy is not severe enough to prevent useful vision.

Nephropathy

Diabetic nephropathy is more common in type I than in type II diabetes, but is the cause of end-stage renal disease in approximately 5 percent to 20 percent of type II diabetic patients. Nephropathy in most patients follows a slowly progressive course throughout many years and leads to mild renal insufficiency (98). However, an accelerated form of diabetic glomerulosclerosis may be superimposed, which leads to renal failure.

Proteinuria is the first manifestation of diabetic nephropathy and is detected by the finding of more than 15μg/min of urinary microalbumin (98,99). A sensitive radioimmunoassay is necessary to detect microalbuminuria (15–150μg/min) because the dipstick for protein will be negative. When microalbuminuria is present, the condition is termed incipient nephropathy.

Elderly patients with proteinuria or impaired renal function need to be evaluated for other forms of urinary tract disease such as obstructive uropathy, urinary tract infections, hypertensive nephropathy, and papillary necrosis. Diabetic nephropathy can be diagnosed clinically if there is persistent proteinuria, diabetic retinopathy, diabetes of more than 10-years' duration and no clinical or laboratory evidence of kidney or renal tract disease other than diabetic glomerulosclerosis.

For patients with declining renal function, control of hypertension and the use of low-protein diets (0.8 grams protein/kg body weight) may slow progression. Aggressive control of blood glucose is more important in arresting the progression of complications before clinical nephropathy occurs (i.e., microalbuminuria) (97). ACE inhibitors can reduce the severity of proteinuria in diabetic patients (100). With end-stage renal disease, the choice between hemodialysis, peritoneal dialysis, or no dialysis must be made on the basis of the needs of the individual, needs of the patient's family, community resources, and the medical team. Although renal transplantation has been performed in diabetic patients younger than 60 years of age, this is a less viable option in the elderly diabetic patient. As renal failure advances, there is a decrease in the insulin requirement.

Neuropathy

The etiology of the diabetic neuropathy is multifactorial: altered metabolism involving the sorbitol-myoinositol pathway may lead to axonal dysfunction or microvascular abnormalities with neural ischemia, and segmental demyelinization may occur. Neuropathy may affect the CNS and peripheral nervous system, isolated cranial or spinal nerves, or the autonomic nervous system. It may present as a specific neuropathic syndrome such as diabetic neuropathic cachexia or diabetic amyotrophy. The most common presentation is that of a symmetrical, bilateral, peripheral neuropathy with pain or paresthesia of the extremities, loss of Achilles reflex, and alterations on sensory testing.

Treatment of symptomatic peripheral neuropathy has been notoriously ineffective. Improved glycemic control is always advocated (101). Specific drug therapies have included supplemental B vitamins, oral pyridoxine, diphenylhydantoin, clonazepam, amitriptyline, imipramine, fluphenazine, carbamazepine, and mexiletine (101,102). The most effective combination is a tricyclic antidepressant and a phenothiazine; however, these drugs should be cautiously prescribed to the elderly patient because induced cardiac arrhythmias or oversedation can occur. CNS cognitive dysfunction, altered regional blood flow, and CNS atrophy as assessed by computed tomography (CT) have been noted to be present in poorly controlled elderly diabetics (103–106). These changes have been seen less commonly in diabetics with good control or on diet alone. When elderly diabetic patients are treated to improve glycemic control, there is improvement in selective areas of cognition (107). Coexisting depression should always be considered for the elderly patient.

Diabetic neuropathic cachexia is a syndrome characteristically seen in depressed, middle-aged-to-elderly males who have mild type II diabetes (108). The syndrome presents with profound weight loss, cachexia, and severe pain of the extremities, with a bilateral symmetrical neuropathy. These patients frequently are evaluated for occult malignancy or radiculoneuropathy. Spontaneous recovery is the rule, but the course is shortened with amitriptyline, 10 to 50mg at bedtime and fluphenazine, 1mg two or three times a day.

Diabetic amyotrophy is a disorder characterized by progressive weakness and wasting of the pelvic girdle and thigh muscles and is associated with severe pain. There is little or no sensory involvement. This syndrome is also associated with mild diabetes and usually spontaneously resolves within 1 year.

Autonomic neuropathy has many manifestations in the elderly diabetic patient, including impotence, neurogenic bladder, disordered gastrointestinal motility, gastroparesis, orthostatic hypotension, or altered autonomic cardiac function. In evaluating the neurogenic bladder, one must rule out obstructive uropathy (109). Neurogenic bladder may improve with frequent voiding, application of suprapubic pressure, and bethanechol chloride, 10 to 50mg three or four times a day. Gastroparesis diabeticorum may respond to metoclopramide, 5 to 15mg four times a day (30 minutes before each meal and at bedtime), or erythromycin (110). Frequent small feedings of liquid or semisolid food and application of abdominal (stomach) pressure while the patient is up-

right may be beneficial. Diabetic diarrhea may be neuropathic or caused by small bowel bacterial overgrowth or pancreatic insufficiency. Tetracycline, 250mg four times a day for 7 to 10 days, can be empirically tried. Metoclopramide, 5 to 15mg four times a day, or clonidine, 0.05mg twice a day may be helpful.

Patients with orthostatic hypotension should be evaluated for anemia and volume depletion. Sudden postural changes should be avoided by these patients. Orthostatic hypotension may respond if the patient wears elastic stockings, eats a high-sodium diet; or if the patient is prescribed 9-alpha-fluorohydrocortisone (0.05 to 0.2 mg daily), clonidine, or erythropoietin (111).

Cardiovascular autonomic neuropathy with cardiac denervation is manifest as a fixed tachycardia, loss of cardiac deceleration to single deep breath, loss of cardiac responsiveness to Valsalva maneuver, and sudden death. When autonomic cardiovascular reflexes are absent, the diabetic patient is at risk for sudden cardiopulmonary death after minor or major surgical procedures.

Impotence occurs in 50 percent of diabetic men and has multiple etiologies, such as deteriorating marital relationships, performance anxiety, associated endocrinopathy (e.g., hypogonadism, hypopituitarism, hypothyroidism), vascular insufficiency, drug or alcohol usage, or diabetic autonomic neuropathy (112). Impotence may be precipitated by initiating antihypertensive therapy. Testosterone treatment is effective only for patients with hypogonadism. Some neuropathic patients may respond to bethanechol chloride, 10 to 50 mg three times a day. Patients unable to perform adequately sexually after treatment of their medical condition should be advised of alternative methods of treatment for impotence (vacuum pump, penile injection, penile prosthesis) or alternative methods of sexual fulfillment and gratification. In some cases, an affectionate, caring companionship needs to be established, along with supportive counseling.

Hypertension

As discussed earlier, diabetic hypertension may present as part of the multimetabolic syndrome X with associated hyperinsulinemia. In this syndrome, a close association exists among obesity, aging, hypertension, hyperinsulinemia, increased sympathetic drive, and enhanced renal sodium reabsorption (113). Diabetic hypertension has been characterized as a volume-expanded state (114). A sodium-restricted diet and weight loss may be helpful. When nonpharmacologic therapy fails, lipid-neutral antihypertensive drugs should be considered. Because of their beneficial effect on the diabetic kidney, ACE inhibitors are recommended as initial therapy for white patients or for patients with diabetic proteinuria or microalbuminuria. ACE inhibitors may also improve metabolic control (68,115,116). Because type II diabetic black patients have salt-sensitive hypertension, calcium channel blockers frequently are the initial drug of choice for these patients. Alternately, first-line agents might include alpha-adrenergic receptor blockers and thiazide diuretics in low doses (i.e., hydrochlorothiazide, 25 mg/ day, or chlorthalidone, 25 mg/day). Indapamide is a reasonable choice when a diuretic agent is desired. With more severe forms of hypertension, multiple agents such as beta-adrenergic blocking agents and vasodilators such as hydralazine or minoxidil may be required to control blood pressure.

Dyslipidemia

Sufficient evidence is available to implicate the dyslipidemias (disorders resulting in high cholesterol, high triglyceride, or low HDL cholesterol) in promoting the atherosclerotic process that results in clinically significant coronary artery disease, cerebral vascular disease, and peripheral vascular disease (117–120). The association of dyslipidemia with atherosclerosis in the elderly is complex because multiple other etiologies contribute to the atherosclerosis, including genetics, hypertension, smoking, hyperinsulinism, obesity (especially abdominal obesity), dyslipidemia, lack of physical activity, diabetes, and renal disease. Epidemiologic studies consistently relate the incidence and complications of coronary artery disease positively to total cholesterol but more specifically to low-density lipoprotein (LDL) cholesterol, with a less positive association with hypertriglyceridemia. Low HDL levels correlate inversely with coronary artery disease and LDL/HDL ratio correlate positively (117–119). In evaluating the dyslipidemic disorder, attention should be given to age-related lipid values (121–124).

Plasma cholesterol increases with age in both sexes until approximately age 60, when cholesterol values in

men plateau or slightly decrease. Women show a later plateau or continued rise (124). Mean total LDL cholesterol and HDL cholesterol are higher in women than elderly men (121, 122). In the eighth and ninth decades of life, reductions in total plasma cholesterol are probably accounted for by reductions in LDL cholesterol while HDL cholesterol remains stable. Octogenarians may also have lower levels of plasma cholesterol because disease processes and death remove from the population those individuals having high LDL cholesterol and lower HDL cholesterol and coronary artery disease (121).

Plasma triglyceride levels increase in both sexes with aging, with a plateau occurring in men at age 50 to 60 years, after a decline with further aging; in elderly women, the plateau may occur later, with a fall in later years. Lipoprotein lipase activity is decreased with aging, which accounts for some of the changes in plasma triglyceride levels. In the elderly, triglyceride concentration is positively associated with obesity (in women), central fat or abdominal obesity, glucose intolerance, use of beta blockers (in men) and use of estrogen in women.

Fasting free fatty acids are unaltered with aging. LDL degradation in peripheral tissue is decreased with aging as is the rate of conversion of cholesterol to bile acids (124). Tissue content of cholesterol and cholesterol ester increases with age. The activity of 3-hydroxy-3-methylglutaryl coenzyme-A (HMG-CoA) reductase (the rate-limiting enzyme for cholesterol synthesis) is normal in the elderly.

Lipoprotein (a) may not be a significant risk factor for coronary artery disease, especially in the elderly (125,126). The Honolulu Health Study (127) reported an association between elevated total cholesterol and LDL cholesterol and the occurrence of coronary artery disease in the elderly. However, the 30-year follow-up data from the Framingham Study (128), which evaluated the relationship between initial cholesterol measurements to cardiovascular disease mortality, concluded that, for persons younger than 50 years of age, cholesterol levels are directly related with the 30-year overall and cardiovascular disease mortality. For persons age 50 and older, there was no increase or overall change in mortality as related to high or low serum cholesterol levels. For persons older than age 50, the association of mortality with cholesterol values was believed to be compounded by individuals whose cholesterol levels were falling perhaps because of a disease process that leads to death. A similar explanation of a J- or U-shaped distribution between total cholesterol and mortality was seen by other investigators (129,130).

In agreement with the Honolulu Health Study were the findings from the Whitehall civil servants followed for 18 years. In the Whitehall Study (131), plasma cholesterol concentrations continued to predict coronary artery disease in elderly people. In addition, the study concluded that reducing plasma cholesterol concentrations in middle-aged men may influence the risk of death from coronary artery disease in older age. In long-lived individuals (>85 years of age), those free of atherosclerotic vascular disease had lower cholesterol values and more favorable overall lipid profiles (132).

The risk factors for coronary heart disease for elderly men are increasing age, hypertension, family history, low HDL, obesity, carbohydrate intolerance, and physical inactivity (132–135). For elderly women, the risk factors include increasing age, years of education, elevated serum triglycerides, low HDL levels, small atherosclerotic LDL particles, hypertension, obesity (especially abdominal obesity), carbohydrate intolerance, cigarette smoking, and low exercise levels.

Of recent note is the high incidence of coronary artery disease in women and the poor prognosis observed after myocardial infarction. This was initially described in the Framingham Study (136), in which it was noted that the risk of death after first myocardial infarction within 1 year was 23 percent for men and 45 percent for women. A second myocardial infarction occurred in 13 percent of men and 40 percent of women within 5 years of the first myocardial infarction. Women with coronary artery disease may have delay in diagnosis and referral for coronary artery bypass surgery (137–141). Estrogen replacement therapy (142–145) improves the lipid profile by lowering LDL cholesterol and raising HDL levels, but may have a worsening effect by increasing triglyceride values. The effect on serum triglyceride may not be seen with the estrogen transdermal delivery system. In addition to its cardioprotective effects on serum lipids, estrogen has a coronary relaxing effect through vasodilatation or increased levels of vasodilatory prostaglandins and calcitonin-related peptide.

During the past 30 years, there has been a decline in incidence of coronary artery disease and its mortality in the American population (146,147). This may be a result of the impact of lifestyle modification reducing cardiovascular risk factors early in younger individuals. There has been 15 percent to 20 percent decline in death rates from coronary heart disease in persons older than 75 years of age. The National Health and Nutrition Examination Surveys I, II, and III (NHANES I–III) has shown declining mean levels for total cholesterol and LDL cholesterol in the American population. This decline has occurred across the entire distribution of serum cholesterol levels and in all age-sex groups. HDL cholesterol and very low LDL (VLDL) cholesterol levels have not changed. This suggests that public health programs designed to reduce cholesterol levels are successful.

Absolute incidence rates of coronary heart disease are increased in elderly individuals. Despite the fact that the relative risk of coronary heart disease conferred by an elevated cholesterol is weaker in the elderly than it is in younger and middle-aged adults, high cholesterol levels lead to more coronary heart disease events in the elderly (148). The recent recommendations of the Second Report of the National Cholesterol Education Program Expert Panel (NCEP) (148) concluded that "while there are limiting clinical trials available in the elderly population, extrapolation of data from trials showing reduction in coronary heart disease risk in middle-aged patients seems reasonable." Angiographic studies (96) show that even advanced coronary atherosclerosis responds to cholesterol-lowering treatment. These considerations suggest that substantial benefit in coronary heart disease risk reduction for the elderly patients may be achieved by cholesterol lowering. Inasmuch as atherosclerosis is an ongoing, metabolically active degenerative pathological process, its occurrence in the elderly with vasoocclusive disease is not pathologically different than that occurring in nonelderly persons.

The NCEP Adult Treatment Panel II guidelines recommend for screening patients at risk for coronary artery disease caused by dyslipidemic conditions, both total cholesterol and HDL cholesterol be measured. Certainly, random, nonfasting, nonage-adjusted, nonsex-adjusted cholesterol screening led to abnormal NCEP values in 70 percent to 80 percent of elderly subjects (142). Fewer patients will be overscreened when a fasting lipid profile is ordered rather than a nonfasting total cholesterol measurement (143). The current Adult Panel II NCEP risk assessment based upon risk factors other than LDL include men older than 45 years of age, women older than 55 years of age, and women with premature menopause without estrogen replacement therapy. A family history for premature coronary artery disease is defined as a myocardial infarction or sudden death before 55 years of age in father or other male first-degree relative or before 65 years of age in mother or other female first-degree relative. Other risk factors include current cigarette smoking, hypertension, low HDL cholesterol 35 mg/dL (0.9 mmol/liter), and diabetes mellitus. A negative risk factors is now defined for coronary artery disease and includes HDL cholesterol greater than 60 mg/dL (1.6 mmol/liter). When this finding occurs, one may subtract one other risk factor in risk factor assessment. Two risk factor for established coronary artery disease places the individual at high risk.

Hypercholesterolemia in the elderly patient may occur on a genetic basis but is more likely to be sporadic and acquired. It can occur in association with hypothyroidism, nephrotic syndrome, obstructive liver disease, and diabetes mellitus. Hypercholesterolemia in the elderly is significant when it is associated with a personal history of atherosclerotic disease. Recently, several secondary prevention studies have shown the impact of lifestyle modification, diets, or pharmacologic cholesterol-lowering intervention in retarding progression or allowing regression of the ongoing atherosclerotic process (94,96,148). Within 1 to 2 years of secondary prevention therapy, beneficial effects have been noted. The treatment of these dyslipidemic disorders in the elderly must be approached from the standpoint of the multiple contributing factors to the atherosclerotic process such as obesity, smoking, diabetes mellitus, and hypertension. It is prudent to screen elderly individuals for hypercholesterolemia according to NCEP guidelines and to treat those individuals at risk initially with diet (144,145).

The elderly are a heterogenous group of individuals who differ widely in their abilities to function physically, behaviorally, cognitively, and emotionally. Not all elderly patients qualify for pharmacologic cholesterol-lowering therapy (146–149). Diet modification can serve all elderly patients as primary intervention for lowering cholesterol,

and early estrogen replacement therapy in women, when not contraindicated, is also preventive. Exercise and dietary modification are the first steps in treatment. The diet should consist of a step I prudent diet for 3 to 6 months and advance to a step II diet, which further restricts saturated fat and total cholesterol content. Use of monounsaturated fats, such as olive oil and canola oil, are effective in reducing cholesterol levels and in raising HDL levels. The use of soluble fiber-containing foods, such as oatmeal and oat bran, are beneficial. Diet modifications may lead to a 10 percent to 15 percent reduction in plasma cholesterol levels and may normalize mildly elevated cholesterol values.

Clinical assessment for drug intervention (149,150) should be individualized. The working or lively retired, physically and emotionally active, apparently disease-free elderly individual, especially persons with occlusive atherosclerotic disease, can be targeted for therapy along the current recommended NCEP guidelines. When prescribing drug therapy, the physician should consider the usual adverse effects associated with the use of lipid-lowering drugs along with the patient's renal and hepatic function.

Drugs used for treating the hyperlipidemic disorders are shown in Table 55.2. The primary cholesterol-lowering agents are the bile absorption resins (cholestyramine, colestipol), nicotinic acid, HMG-CoA reductase inhibitors, and probucol. Nicotinic acid may worsen diabetic control. Gemfibrozil lowers cholesterol levels, particularly in patients with a combined dyslipidemia consisting of elevated VLDL triglycerides and LDL cholesterol. It is debatable at this time whether an isolated low HDL cholesterol value needs treatment. However, a consideration of HDL cholesterol levels

Table 55.2. Dietary Treatment

Dietary Component	STEP I	STEP II
Fat (percent of calories)	<30	<30
Saturated fatty acids (percent of calories)	8–10	<7
Monounsaturated fatty acids (percent of calories)	15	15
Polyunsaturated fatty acids (percent of calories)	10	10
Carbohydrate (percent of calories)	≥55	≥55
Protein (percent of calories)	15	15
Cholesterol (mg/day)	<300	<200
Calories to maintain weight	+	+

Table 55.3. Hypolipidemic Drugs

Generic	Trade Name(s)	Dose	Side Effects
Cholestyramine	Questran	16–24 gm/day	GI upset
Colestipol	Colestid	15–30 gm/day	Constipation, interference with absorption of fat-soluble vitamin A, D, E and with other drugs
Nicotine acid (niacin)	Nicobid, Nico-400, Nicolar	2–6 gm/day	Flushing and pruritus, hyperuricemia, hyperglycemia, hepatitis, dermatitis
Probucol	Lorelco	1 gm/day	Few except minor GI symptoms
Clofibrate	Atromid-S	2 gm/day	Few except minor GI symptoms
Gemfibrozil	Lopid	1.2 gm/day	Few except minor GI symptoms
HMG-CoA reductase inhibitors			
Lovastatin	Mevacor	10–80 mg/day	Few, watch liver function tests, myalgias, myositis
Pravastatin	Pravachol	5–40 mg/day at bedtime	Few, watch liver function tests, myalgias, myositis
Simvastatin	Zocor	10–40 mg/day	Few, watch liver function tests, myalgias, myositis
Fluvastatin	Lescol	20–40 mg/day	Few, watch liver function tests, myalgias, myositis

GI = gastrointestinal; HMG-CoA = 3-hydroxy-3-methylglutaryl coenzyme A.

should be taken into consideration when one is making the choice of drug therapy. The drugs that elevate HDL levels are gemfibrozil, nicotinic acid, estrogens, and HMG-CoA reductase inhibitors. The vast experience with HMG-CoA reductase inhibitors indicate they are effective and well tolerated (150,151). Individual therapy should be determined by selection of appropriate candidates, application of clinical judgment on the patient's overall health status, assessment of a risk-benefit ratio, drug side effects profile, expense, and long-term goals anticipated (145–151). For patients with established atherosclerosis, the goal of therapy is an LDL level of 100 mg/dL or less (2.6 mmol/liter).

Elderly patients with chylomicronemia syndrome have severe hypertriglyceridemia (values exceeding 1000 mg/dL). These persons experience more morbidity and mortality from recurrent pancreatitis than younger patients—hence, the importance of treating this syndrome. The chylomicronemia syndrome is associated with eruptive xanthomas of the skin, lipemia retinalis, and pancreatitis. Peripheral neuropathy and dementia may also be seen. This syndrome usually results from the combination of a genetic disorder of VLDL metabolism plus a secondary cause of hypertriglyceridemia or two secondary causes of hypertriglyceridemia simultaneously (152).

In patients with acute pancreatitis, the hypertriglyceridemia levels resolve rapidly when the patient's oral lipid intake is restricted. Secondary causes, such as hypothyroidism, diabetes mellitus, drugs, nephrotic syndrome, uremia, obesity, estrogens, glucocorticoid excess, hepatocellular liver disease, and alcoholism, should be sought. If the secondary causes cannot be identified or effectively treated, clofibrate, gemfibrozil, or nicotinic acid may be necessary (Table 55.3). Dietary approach to treating hypertriglyceride disorders consists of weight reduction, avoidance of alcohol, and progressive fat restriction, especially if chylomicronemia is present. Fish oils are useful in treating hypertriglyceridemia but may aggravate hyperglycemia in diabetic patients.

The incidence of diabetic dyslipidemia approximates 70 percent in diabetic population (153,154). In diabetic patients, elevated triglycerides may be an additive risk factor for the progression of atherosclerosis, particularly peripheral vascular disease. Improved diabetic control is advocated for the treatment of diabetic dyslipidemia; however, in most instances, both a lipid-lowering diet and drug therapy are required to treat the accompanying lipid disorder effectively.

Long-term intervention studies of dyslipidemia treatment in elderly patients are not available but are needed to clarify the issues of aggressive management of dyslipidemia and to determine the impact of risk-factor modification on atherosclerosis.

References

1. Wilson PWF, Anderson KM, Kannel WB. Epidemiology of diabetes in the elderly. Am J Med 1986;80:3–9.

2. Wingard DL, Sinsheimer P, Barrett-Connor E, McPhillips JB. Community-based study of prevalence of NIDDM in older adults. Diabetes Care 1990;13(suppl 2):3–8.

3. Mykkänen L, Laakso M, Pyörälä K. Asymptomatic hyperglycemia and atherosclerotic vascular disease in the elderly. Diabetes Care 1992;15:1020–1030.

4. Lintott CJ, Hanger GC, Scott RS, et al. Prevalence of diabetes mellitus in an ambulant elderly New Zealand population. Diabetes Res Clin Pract 1992;16:131–136.

5. Aronow WS, Kronzon I. Prevalence of coronary risk factors in the elderly blacks and whites. J Am Geriatr Soc 1991;39:567–570.

6. Harris MI. Epidemiology of diabetes mellitus among the elderly in the United States. Clin Geriatr Med 1990;6:703–719.

7. Weinberger M, Cowper PA, Kirkman MS, Vinicor F. Economic impact of diabetes mellitus in the elderly. Clin Geriatr Med 1990;6:959–970.

8. Madshad S. Classification of diabetes in older adults. Diabetes Care 1990;13(suppl 2):93–96.

9. Seclén-Santisteban S, Alvarez-Huaman RI, Chantnes-Antoranz MT. Diabetes mellitus in the elderly: a study on its clinical presentation, C-peptide reserve and immunogenetic markers of insulin dependence. Rev Clin Esp 1993;192:162–168.

10. DeFronzo RA. Glucose intolerance and aging. Diabetes Care 1981;4:493–501.

11. Raven GM, Raven EP. Age, glucose intolerance and NIDDM. J Am Geriatr Soc 1985;33:286–290.

12. Broughton DL, Webster J, Taylor R. Insulin sensitivity and secretion in healthy elderly human subjects with "abnormal" glucose tolerance. Eur J Clin Invest 1992;22:285–290.

13. Chen M, Bergman RN, Porte D Jr. Insulin resistance and B-cell dysfunction in aging: the importance of dietary carbohydrate. J Clin Endocrinol Metab 1988;67:951–957.

14. Feskens EJM, Bowles CH, Kromhout D. Inverse association between fish intake and risk of glucose intolerance in normoglycemic elderly men and women. Diabetes Care 1991;14:935–941.

15. Mykkänen L, Laako M, Penttilä I, Pyörälä K. Asymptomatic hyperglycemia and cardiovascular risk factors in the elderly. Atherosclerosis 1991;88:153–161.

16. Coon PJ, Rogus EM, Drinkwater D, et al. Role of body fat distribution in the decline in insulin sensitivity and glucose tolerance with age. J Clin Endocrinol Metab 1992;75:1125–1132.

17. Mykkänen L, Kuusisto J, Pyörälä K, Laakso M. Cardiovascular disease risk factors as predictor of type 2 (non-insulin-dependent) diabetes mellitus in elderly subjects. Diabetologia 1993;36:553–559.

18. Kohrt WM, Kirwan JP, Staten MA, et al. Insulin resistance in aging is related to abdominal obesity. Diabetes 1993;42:273–

281.

19. Palmer JP, Ensinck JW. Acute-phase insulin secretion and glucose tolerance in young and aged normal men and diabetic patients. J Clin Endocrinol Metab 1975;41:498–593.

20. Draznin B, Steinberg JP, Leitner JW, Sussman KE. The nature of insulin secretory defect in aging rats. Diabetes 1985;34:1168–1173.

21. Chen M, Bergman RN, Pacini G, Porte D Jr. Pathogenesis of age-related glucose intolerance in man: insulin resistance and decreased B-cell function. J Clin Endocrinol Metab 1985;60:13–20.

22. Jackson RA, Hawa MI, Roshania RD, et al. Influence of aging on hepatic and peripheral glucose metabolism in humans. Diabetes 1988;37:119–129.

23. Kahn SE, Larson VG, Schwartz RS, et al. Exercise training delineates the importance of B-cell dysfunction to glucose intolerance of human aging. J Clin Endocrinol Metab 1992;74:1336–1342.

24. Jackson RA. Mechanisms of age-related glucose intolerance. Diabetes Care 1990;13(suppl 2):9–19.

25. Fink RI, Kolterman OG, Griffin J, Olefsky JM. Mechanism of insulin resistance in aging. J Clin Invest 1983;71:1523–1535.

26. Fink RI, Kolterman OG, Kao M, Olefsky JM. The role of the glucose transport system in the postreceptor defect in insulin action associated with human aging. J Clin Endocrinol Metab 1984;58:721–725.

27. National Diabetes Data Group. Classification and diagnosis of diabetes mellitus and other categories of glucose intolerance. Diabetes 1979;28:1039–1057.

28. Olefsky JM, Kolterman OG. Mechanisms of insulin resistance in obesity and non-insulin dependent (Type II diabetes). Am J Med 1981;70:151–168.

29. DeFronzo RA. New concepts in the pathogenesis and treatment of non-insulin-dependent diabetes mellitus. Am J Med 1983;74:52–81.

30. Truglia JA, Livingston JN, Lockwood DH. Insulin resistance: receptor and post-binding defects in human obesity and non-insulin dependent diabetes mellitus. Am J Med 1985;79:13–22.

31. DeFronzo RA. The triumvirate: B-cell, muscle, liver. Diabetes 1988;37:667–687.

32. Kent S. Is diabetes a form of accelerated aging? Geriatrics 1976;31:140–151.

33. Monnier VM, Sell DR, Nagaraj RH, et al. Maillard reaction-mediated molecular damage to extracellular matrix and other tissue proteins in diabetes, aging and uremia diabetes. Diabetes 1992;41(suppl 2):36–41.

34. Stout RW. Diabetes, atherosclerosis and aging. Diabetes Care 1990;12(suppl 2):20–23.

35. James VJ, Delbridge L, McLennon SV, Yue DK. Use of x-ray diffraction in study of human diabetic and aging collagen. Diabetes 1991;40:391–394.

36. Mooradian AD. Increased serum conjugated dienes in elderly diabetic patients. J Am Geriatr Soc 1991;39:571–574.

37. Paolisso G, D'Amore A, DiMaro G, et al. Evidence for a relationship between free radicals and insulin action in the

elderly. Metabolism 1993;42:659–663.

38. Gambent SR. Atypical presentation of diabetes in the elderly. Clin Geriatr Med 1990;6:721–729.

39. Morley JE. Nutritional status of the elderly. Am J Med 1986;81:679–695.

40. Young EA. Nutrition, aging and the aged. Med Clin North Am 1983;67:295–313.

41. Anderson LA. Health-care communication and selected psychosocial correlates of adherence in diabetic management. Diabetes Care 1990;13(suppl 2):66–76.

42. Morley JE, Kaiser FE. Unique aspects of diabetes mellitus in the elderly. Clin Geriatr Med 1990;13(suppl 2):86–92.

43. Pinholt EM, Kronke K, Hanley JF, et al. Functional assessment of the elderly. Arch Intern Med 1987;147:484–488.

44. McGandy RB. Nutrient intake and energy expenditure in men of different age. J Gerontol 1966;21:581–587.

45. Richter EA, Ruderman HB, Schneider SH. Diabetes and exercise. Am J Med 1981;70:201–208.

46. Goldberg AP, Coon PJ. Non-insulin dependent diabetes mellitus in the elderly; influence of obesity and physical inactivity. Endocrin Metab Clin 1987;16:843–865.

47. Schwartz RS. Exercise training in treatment of diabetes mellitus in elderly patients. Diabetes Care 1990;34(suppl 2):77–85.

48. Vinik AI, Franz SJ, Crapo PA, et al. Nutritional recommendation and principles for individuals. Diabetes Care 1987;10:126–132.

49. Reed RL, Mooradian AD. Nutritional status and dietary management of elderly diabetic patients. Clin Geriatr Med 1990;6:883–901.

50. Henry RR, Edelman SV. Advances in treatment of type II diabetes mellitus in the elderly. Geriatrics 1992;47:24–30.

51. Pegg A, Fitzgerald F, Wise D, et al. A community-based study of diabetes-related skills and knowledge in elderly people with insulin-requiring diabetes. Diabet Med 1991;8:778–781.

52. Stepka M, Rogala H, Czyzyk A. Hypoglycemia: a major problem in the management of diabetes in the elderly. Aging 1993;5:117–121.

53. Osei K, Falko J, Bossetti BM, Holland GC. Metabolic effects of fructose as a natural sweetener in the physiologic meals of ambulatory obese patients with type II diabetes. Am J Med 1987;83:249–255.

54. Boden G, Chen X, Desantis R, et al. Effects of ethanol on carbohydrate metabolism in the elderly. Diabetes 1993;42:28–34.

55. Hurt RD, Finlayson RE, Morse RM, Davis LJ. Alcoholism in elderly persons. Mayo Clinic Proc 1988;63:753–768.

56. Halter JB, Morrow LA. Use of sulfonylurea drugs in elderly patients. Diabetes Care 1990;13(suppl 2):86–92.

57. Gerich JE. Oral hypoglycemic agents. New Engl J Med 1990;321:1231–1245.

58. Lun WS. Use of oral hypoglycemic agents in the elderly. Pract Diabetol 1993;12:10–13.

59. Meneilly GS, Tessier D, Dawson K. Alterations in glucose metabolism in the elderly patient with diabetes. Diabetes

60. Ferner RE, Ashworth L, Tronier B, Alberti KGMM. Effects of short-term hyperglycemia on insulin secretion in normal humans. Am J Physiol 1986;250:E655–E661.

61. Hofeldt FD. The office management of diabetes mellitus. Mod Med 1990;58:36–58.

62. Hofeldt FD. Managing diabetes mellitus in the aged. Geriatr Consult 1991;10:23–26.

63. Gilden JL, Casia C, Hendryx M, Singh SP. Effects of self-monitoring of blood glucose and quality of life in elderly diabetic patients. J Am Geriatr Soc 1990;38:511–515.

64. Nathan DM. Insulin treatment in the elderly diabetic patient. Clin Geriatr Med 1990;6:923–931.

65. Froom J. Glycemic control in elderly people with diabetes. Clin Geriatr Med 1990;6:933–941.

66. Walter RM. Hypoglycemia: still a risk in the elderly. Geriatrics 1990;45:74–75.

67. Thomson FJ, Masson EA, Leeming JT, Boulten AJ. Lack of knowledge of symptoms of hypoglycemia by elderly diabetic patients. Age Ageing 1991;20:404–406.

68. Watson N, Sandler M. Effects of captopril on glucose tolerance in elderly patients with congestive cardiac failure. Curr Med Res Opin 1991;12:374–378.

69. Arauz-Pacheco C, Ramirez LC, Rios JM, Raskin P. Hypoglycemia induced by angiotensin-converting enzyme inhibitor in patients with non-insulin dependent diabetes receiving sulfonylurea therapy. Am J Med 1990;89:811–813.

70. Nolan TE. Surgery in the elderly. Postgrad Med 1992;91:199–202.

71. Gavin LA. Perioperative management of the diabetic patient. Endocrinol Metab Clin North Am 1992;21:457–475.

72. Phillips PA, Rolls BJ, Ledingham TGG, et al. Reduced thirst after water deprivation in healthy elderly men. N Engl J Med 1984;311:753–759.

73. Beck LH, Lavizzo-Mourey R. Geriatric hyponatremia. Ann Intern Med 1987;107:768.

74. Snyder NA, Feigel DW, Arieff AJ. Hypernatremia in elderly patients. Ann Intern Med 1987;107:309–319.

75. Bessman AN, Kasim S. Managing foot infections in the older diabetic patient. Geriatrics 1985;40:54–63.

76. Wheat LJ, Allen SD, Henry M, et al. Diabetic foot infections. Arch Intern Med 1986;146:1935–1940.

77. Edmonds ME. The diabetic foot pathophysiology and treatment. Clin Endocrinol Metab 1986;15:889–916.

78. Lipsky BA, Percoraro RE, Ahroni JH. Foot ulceration and infections in elderly diabetics. Clin Geriatr Med 1990;6:747–769.

79. Thomson FJ, Masson EA. Can elderly diabetic patients cooperate with routine foot care? Age Ageing 1992;21:333–337.

80. Wingard DL, Barrett-Connor EL, Scheidt-Nave C, McPhillips JB. Prevalence of cardiovascular and renal complications in older adults with normal or impaired glucose tolerance of NIDDM. Diabetes Care 1993;16:1022–1025.

81. Minaker KL. What diabetologists should know about elderly patients. Diabetes Care 1990;13(suppl 2):34–46.

82. Cohen DL, Neil HAW, Thorogood M, Mann JI. A

population-based study of the incidence of complications associated with type 2 diabetes in the elderly. Diabet Med 1991;8:928–933.

83. Karain JH. Type II diabetes and syndrome X. Endocrinol Metab Clin North Am 1992;21:329–350.

84. Björntorp P. Regional patterns of fat distribution. Ann Intern Med 1985;103:994–995.

85. Expert Panel on Detection, Evaluation and Treatment of High Blood Cholesterol in Adults. Summary of the second National Cholesterol Education Program (NCEP) Expert Panel on detection, evaluation, and treatment of high blood cholesterol in adults. JAMA 1993;269:3015–3023.

86. Minaker KL. Aging and diabetes mellitus as risk factors for vascular disease. Am J Med 1987;82(suppl 113):47–53.

87. Aronow WS, Sterling WS, Etienne F, et al. Risk factors for coronary artery disease in persons older than 62 years in a long-term health care facility. Am J Cardiol 1986;57:518–520.

88. Fein FS, Scheuer J. Heart disease in diabetes. Rifkin H, Ponte D, eds. Diabetes mellitus: theory and practice. 4th ed. New York: Elsevier, 1990:812–823.

89. Kuebler TW, Bendick PJ, Fineberg SE, et al. Diabetes mellitus and cerebrovascular disease of carotid artery and associated risk factors in 482 adult diabetic patients. Diabetes Care 1983;6:274–278.

90. Nakagawa S, Mitamura H, Kimura M. Characteristics of acute myocardial infarction, preinfarct angina and post infarction angina in patients with diabetes mellitus. J Cardiol 1992;22:11–20.

91. Aronow WS, Mercando AD, Epstein S. Prevalence of silent myocardial ischemia detected by 24-hour ambulatory electrocardiography and its association with new coronary events at 40-month follow up in elderly diabetic and nondiabetic patients with coronary artery disease. Am J Cardiol 1992;15:553–556.

92. Quinones-Baldrich WJ, Colburn MD, Ahn SS, et al. Very distal bypass for salvage of the severely ischemic extremity. Am J Surg 1993;166:117–123.

93. Barbash GI, White HD, Modan M, Van de Werf F. Significance of diabetes mellitus in patients with acute myocardial infarction receiving thrombolytic therapy. J Am Coll Cardiol 1993;22:707–713.

94. Report of the National Cholesterol Education Program, Expert Panel on Detection, Evaluation and Treatment of High Blood Cholesterol in Adults. Arch Intern Med 1988;148:36–69.

95. Dutfield GM, Lewis B, Miller NE, et al. Treatment of hyperlipidemia retards progression of symptomatic femoral atherosclerosis. Lancet 1983;2:639–641.

96. Blankenhorn DH, Hodis HN. Arterial imaging and atherosclerosis reversal. Atheroscler Thromb 1994;14:177–192.

97. Diabetes Control and Complication Trial Research Group. The effect of intensive treatment of diabetes on the development and progression of long-term complications in insulin-dependent diabetes mellitus. N Engl J Med 1993;329:977–986.

98. Iqbal Z, Meguira S, Feiedman EA. Geriatric diabetic nephropathy: an analysis of renal referral in patients age 60 or older. Am J Kidney Dis 1990;16:312–316.

99. Veberta G, Keen H. The patterns of proteinuria in diabetes mellitus. Diabetes 1984;33:686–692.

100. Lewis EJ, Hunsicker LG, Bain RP, Rohde RD. The effect of angiotensin-converting enzyme inhibitor on diabetic nephropathy. New Engl J Med 1993;329:1456–1462.

101. Riddle MC. Diabetic neuropathies in the elderly: management update. Geriatrics 1990;45:32–36.

102. Dejgard A, Petersen P, Kastrup J. Mexiletine for treatment of chronic painful diabetic neuropathy. Lancet 1988;2:9–11.

103. Pfeifer MA, Ross DR, Schrage JP, et al. A highly successful and novel model for treatment of chronic painful diabetic peripheral neuropathy. Diabetes Care 1993;16:1103–1115.

104. U'Ren RC, Riddle MC, Lezak MD, Bennington-Davis M. The mental efficiency of the elderly patient with type II diabetes mellitus. J Am Geriatr Soc 1990;38:505–510.

105. Tun PA, Nathan DM, Perlmuter LC. Cognitive and affective disorder in elderly diabetics. Clin Geriatr Med 1990;6:731–746.

106. Soininen H, Puranen M, Helkala EL, et al. Diabetes mellitus and brain atrophy. A computed tomograph study in an elderly population. Neurobiol Aging 1992;13:717–721.

107. Meneilly GS, Cheung E, Tessier D, et al. The effects of improved glycemic control on cognitive function in the elderly patient with diabetes. J Gerontol 1993;48:M117–M121.

108. Gade GN, Hofeldt FD, Treece GL. Diabetic neuropathic cachexia. JAMA 1980;243:1160–1161.

109. Starer P, Libow L. Cystometric evaluation of bladder dysfunction in elderly diabetic patients. Arch Intern Med 1990;150:810–813.

110. Janssens J, Peeters TL, Vantrappen G, et al. Improvement of gastric emptying in diabetic gastroparesis by erythromycin. N Engl J Med 1990;322:1028–1031.

111. Hoeldtke RD, Streeten DH. Treatment of orthostatic hypotension with erythropoietin. N Engl J Med 1993;329:611–615.

112. Whitehead ED, Klyde BJ. Diabetes-related impotence in the elderly. Clin Geriatr Med 1990;6:771–795.

113. Modan M, Halkin H. Hyperinsulinemia or increased sympathetic drive as links for obesity and hypertension. Diabetes Care 1991;14:470–487.

114. Stein PP, Black HR. Drug treatment of hypertension in patients with diabetes mellitus. Diabetes Care 1991;14:425–448.

115. Paolisso G, Gambardella A, Verza M, Varricchio M. Quinapril reduces arterial blood pressure and improves metabolic control. Diabetes Metab 1990;16:264–265.

116. Torlone E, Britta M, Rambotti AM, et al. Improved insulin action and glycemia control after long-term angiotensin-converting enzyme inhibitor in subjects with arterial hypertension and type II diabetes. Diabetes Care 1993;16:

1347–1355.

117. Casteli WP, Garrison RJ, Wilson PWF, et al. Incidence of coronary heart disease and lipoprotein cholesterol: the Framingham study. JAMA 1986;256:2835–2838.

118. Martin MJ, Hulley SB, Browner WS, et al. Serum cholesterol, blood pressure and mortality: implications from a cohort of 361,662 men (MRFITT). Lancet 1986;2:933–936.

119. Stamier J, Wentworth D, Neaton JD. Is relationship between serum cholesterol and risk of premature death from coronary heart disease continuous and graded (MRFITT). JAMA 1986;256:2823–2828.

120. Kannel WB. Lipids, diabetes and coronary artery disease. Am Heart J 1985;110:1100–1107.

121. Nicholsen J, Gartside PS, Siegel M, et al. Lipid and lipoprotein distributions in octo- and nonagenarians. Metabolism 1979;28:51–56.

122. Ettinger WH, Wahl PW, Kuller LH, et al. Lipoprotein lipids in older people: results from the cardiovascular health study. Circulation 1992;86:858–869.

123. Kreisberg RA, Kasim S. Cholesterol metabolism and aging. Am J Med 1987;82(suppl B):54–60.

125. Bertolotti M, Abate N, Bertolotti S, et al. The effect of aging on cholesterol alpha-hydroxylation in humans. J Lipid Res 1993;34:1001–1007.

126. Ridker PM, Hennekens CH, Stampfer MJ. A prospective study of lipoprotein (a) and the risk of myocardial infarction. JAMA 1993;270:2195–2199.

127. Simons L, Friedlander Y, Simons J, McCallum J. Lipoprotein (a) is not associated with coronary heart disease in the elderly. Atherosclerosis 1993;99:87–95.

128. Benfante R, Reed D. Is elevated serum cholesterol level a risk factor for coronary heart disease in the elderly. JAMA 1990;263:393–396.

129. Anderson KM, Castelli WP, Levy D. Cholesterol and mortality: 30 years of follow-up from the Framingham study. JAMA 1987;257:2176–2180.

130. Fletcher AE, Bulpitt CJ. Epidemiological aspects of cardiovascular disease in the elderly. J Hypertens 1992;10(suppl 1):551–558.

131. Nikkilä M, Heikkinen J. Serum cholesterol, high-density lipoprotein cholesterol and five-year survival in elderly people. Age Ageing 1990;19:403–408.

132. Shipley MJ, Pocock SJ, Marmot MG. Does plasma cholesterol concentration predict mortality from coronary heart disease in elderly people: 18-year follow-up in White-Hall Study. BMJ 1991;303:89–92.

133. Hermann W, Hanf S, Lindhofer HG. Lipoprotein as coronary risk or non-risk indicators in elderly people. Z Gerontol 1990;23:338–344.

134. Simons LA, Friedlander Y, McCallum J, et al. The Dubbo study of the health of elderly: correlates of coronary heart disease at study entry. J Am Geriatr Soc 1991;39:584–590.

135. Mykkänen L, Laakso M, Pyörälä K. Association of obesity and distribution of obesity with glucose tolerance and cardiovascular risk factors in the elderly. Int J Obes 1992;16:695–704.

136. Kannel WB, Sorlie P, McNamara PM. Prognosis after initial myocardial infarction: the Framingham study. Am J Cardiol 1979;44:53–59.

137. Caspensen CJ, Bloemberg BP, Saris WH, et al. The prevalence of selected physical activities and their relationship with coronary heart disease risk factors in elderly men: the Zutphen study. Am J Epidemiol 1991;133:1078–1092.

138. Greenland P, Reicher-Reiss H, Goldbourt U, et al. In-hospital and 1-year mortality in 1524 women after myocardial infarction. Comparison with 4315 men. Circulation 1991;83:484–491.

139. Mansan JE, Colditz GA, Stampfer MJ, et al. A prospective study of obesity and risk of coronary heart disease in women. N Engl J Med 1990;322:882–889.

140. Wing RR, Matthew KA, Kullen LH, et al. Waist to hip ratio in middle-age women. Associations with behavioral, psychosocial factors and with changes in cardiovascular risk factors. Artheroscler Thromb 1991;11:1250–1257.

141. Selby JV, Austin MA, Newman B, et al. LDL subclass phenotypes and the insulin resistance syndrome in women. Circulation 1993;88:381–387.

142. Khan SS, Nessim S, Gray R, et al. Increased mortality of women in coronary artery bypass surgery. Ann Intern Med 1990;112:561–567.

143. Petticrew M, McKee M, Jones J. Coronary artery surgery: are women discriminated against? BMJ 1993;306:1164–1166.

144. Sullivan JM, Vander-Zwagg R, Lemp GF, et al. Postmenopausal estrogen use and coronary atherosclerosis. Ann Intern Med 1988;108:358–363.

145. Stampfer MJ, Colditz GA, Willett WC, et al. Postmenopausal estrogen therapy and cardiovascular disease. N Engl J Med 1991;325:756–762.

146. Rosano GMC, Sarrel PM, Poole-Wilson PA, Collins P. Beneficial effects of oestrogen on exercise-induced myocardial ischemia in women with coronary artery disease. Lancet 1993;342:133–136.

147. Garry PJ, Hunt WC, Koehler KM, et al. Longitudinal study of dietary intakes and pleasure lipids in healthy elderly men and women. Am J Clin Nutr 1992;55:682–688.

148. Johnson CL, Rifkind BM, Sempos CT, et al. Declining serum total cholesterol levels among US adults. JAMA 1993;269:3002–3008.

149. Expert Panel. Summary of the second report of the National Cholesterol Education Program (NCEP), Expert panel on detection, evaluation and treatment of high blood cholesterol in adults (Adult Treatment Panel II). JAMA 1993;269:3015–3023.

150. Fritzsche V, Tracy T, Speirs J, Glueck CJ. Cholesterol screening in 5,719 self-referred elderly subjects. J Gerontol 1990;45:M198–M202.

151. Kligman EW, Watkins AJ. Screening for coronary heart disease risk in the elderly. Am J Prev Med 1991;7:263–267.

152. Myrianthopoulos M. Dietary treatment of hyperlipidemic in the elderly. Clin Geriatr Med 1987;3:343–359.

153. Luepker RV. Dyslipoproteinemia in the elderly. Endocrinol

Metab Clin North Am 1990;19:451–462.

154. Bilheimen DW. Clinical considerations regarding treatment of hypercholesterolemia in the elderly. Atherosclerosis 1991;91(suppl 1):S35–S57.

155. Denke MA, Grundy SM. Hypercholesterolemia in elderly persons. Ann Intern Med 1990;112:780–792.

156. Kirby B. Lipoproteins in the elderly. J Int Med Res 1991;19:425–432.

157. Antonicelli R, Lipponi G, Cadeddu G, Gaetti R. Hypercholesterolemia in the aged: rational approach to the problem. Clin Ther 1990;134:173–180.

158. Denke MS. Drug treatment of hyperlipidemia in elderly patients. Curr Opin Lipidol 1993;4:56–62.

159. Antonicelli R, Onorato G, Pagelli P, et al. Simvastatin in the treatment of hypercholesterolemia in elderly. Clin Ther 1990;12:165–171.

160. Chait A, Brunzeil JD. Severe hypertriglyceridemia role of familial and acquired disorders. Metabolism 1983;32:209–214.

161. Hannah J, Harper P. Nonpharmacologic treatment of diabetic dyslipidemia. Diabetes Spectrum 1993;6:289–309, 365–388.

162. Dunn FL. Management of hyperlipidemia in diabetes mellitus. Endocrinol Metab Clin North Am 1992;21:395–414.

Chapter 56
Geriatric Dermatology

James E. Fitzpatrick and Milton J. Schleve

I promise to keep on living as though I expected to live forever. Nobody grows old by merely living a number of years. People grow old only by deserting their ideals. Years may wrinkle the skin, but to give up interest wrinkles the soul.

Douglas MacArthur
New York Times, June, 1984

Survey studies have shown that inflammatory skin diseases and cutaneous tumors are more common in the elderly than they are in the general population. The largest survey, done between 1971 and 1974, revealed that among patients aged 65 to 74 years, 410,000 individuals had a total burden of 655,000 significant skin problems (1). Extrapolation of these data suggests that the burden of significant skin disorders is likely to be higher in patients even older.

Aging of the skin affects the patient both functionally and cosmetically; however, it is the cosmetic change that is usually most disturbing to patients. The appearance of our exposed skin and hair defines our society's perception of our age. Billions of dollars are spent annually by the pharmaceutical and cosmetic industries to lure the aging population to buy products that will retard skin aging or make us appear younger. Even the medical profession offers treatments and surgical procedures that alter appearance.

The perceived aging of the skin and its appendages are caused by both intrinsic and extrinsic mechanisms. It is the perception of the lay public and many health care professionals that intrinsic aging (Table 56.1) has the most profound effect on appearance; however, extrinsic factors are far more important (2). The most important extrinsic factors are ultraviolet radiation from the sun or artificial sources (tanning parlors) and smoking. Ultraviolet radiation produces numerous adverse affects on skin associated with aging, such as epidermal atrophy (often most pronounced over the backs of hands), solar elastosis

causes yellow, wrinkled, leathery skin (Figure 56.1), structurally abnormal blood vessels (telangiectasia and senile purpura), and dyspigmentation (lentigo senilis, liver spots).

Several surveys document the most common skin diseases in the elderly. The most common complaint is pruritus, which may affect as much as 29 percent of the geriatric population, and the most common dermatoses are solar elastosis, xerosis, dermatophytosis, senile purpura, contact dermatitis, and seborrheic dermatitis. The most common benign skin tumors are seborrheic keratoses, cherry hemangiomas, nevi, acrochordons, and sebaceous hyperplasia. Actinic keratosis and Bowen's disease are the most common premalignant skin lesions, with the former being one of the most common reasons for patients to visit a dermatologist. The most common malignant skin tumor is basal cell carcinoma, followed by squamous cell carcinoma and malignant melanoma.

Common Inflammatory Skin Disorders

Xerosis

Xerosis is the most common dermatosis in the geriatric population. The stratum corneum has numerous abnormalities with aging, such as decreased water content, increased profillaggrin, and amino acids, which produce an altered skin surface contour that is clinically perceived as dry skin or xerosis. Clinical studies have also shown a direct correlation between the degree of xerosis and the degree of pruritus in the elderly (3).

Clinically, xerosis appears as a fine, white scale that is usually most prominent on the extensor aspects of the extremities. If the scales are large, an inherited or acquired ichthyosis should be considered. Xerotic skin is susceptible to cracking, which may allow irritants such as soap to produce an inflammatory reaction called erythema craquelé.

The treatment of xerosis consists of the removal of irritants, especially highly alkaline soaps and replacement with soaps that have a neutral pH. Evidence suggests that older persons bathe more frequently and longer, and this might contribute to xerosis. Patients should be encouraged to modify their bathing routine. Severe cases should be treated with emollients, which are best used after hydration of the skin. The most severe cases may require

treatment with emollients that contain lactic acid or one of its salts. These emollients are highly effective, but they are expensive and may produce a burning sensation in some patients.

Seborrheic Dermatitis

Seborrheic dermatitis is a common disorder of the elderly. The pathogenesis is uncertain, but recent studies have suggested that seborrheic dermatitis may be caused by a host response to *Malassezia ovalis* (*Pityrosporum ovale*), a lipophilic yeast that is found in large numbers in the hair follicle and skin surface (4). Clinically, seborrheic dermatitis is characterized by erythema and scale that may have a yellow, greasy appearance. Seborrheic dermatitis may be asymptomatic or produce variable pruritus. The distribution of the lesions tends to parallel areas of high sebaceous gland activity, such as the scalp, ears, eyebrows, sides of the nose, and anogenital area. Occasional cases may demonstrate extensive involvement.

Seborrheic dermatitis is treatable but not curable. The scalp and other hairy areas are best treated with topical keratolytics, tar shampoos, and shampoos that contain cytostatic agents, such as zinc pyrithione and selenium sulfide, or keratolytics, such as salicylic acid. Recalcitrant cases may require the addition of topical hydrocortisone lotions or solutions. Glabrous (nonhairy) areas, such as

Table 56.1. Important Intrinsic Structural Changes of Aged Skin

Keratinocytes
  Decreased numbers
  Retraction of rete ridges
  Weakened dermoepidermal junction
Melanocytes
  Decreased numbers
Langerhans cells
  Decreased numbers
Dermis
  Decreased collagen
  Loss of ground substance
  Decreased elastin
  Abnormal elastic fibers
Adnexal structures
  Depigmented hair (canities)
  Loss of terminal hairs (androgenetic alopecia)
  Fewer sweat glands
  Sebaceous gland hyperplasia

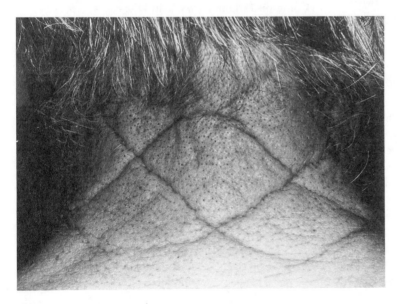

Fig. 56.1. Severe solar damage of the back of the neck manifesting as leathery, yellowish, wrinkled skin.

primary lesion is a poorly demarcated erythema with variable scale that is frequently associated with reddish-brown puncta and dilated superficial veins. Secondary changes, including ulcerations, excoriations, and infection, are common.

The mainstay of therapy for stasis dermatitis is treatment of the underlying defect of venous hypertension by elevation of the legs and use of supportive stockings. More severe cases may require surgical treatment (ligation and stripping of the superficial veins and/or ligation of the perforator veins). Sclerotherapy of selected perforators has also been reported to be useful. The dermatitis can be treated with mild to moderate potency topical corticosteroids. Secondary infections should be treated with appropriate oral antibiotics. The management of stasis ulcers is somewhat controversial, but occlusive dressings are useful in promoting re-epithelialization.

Autoimmune Bullous Disorders

Bullous Pemphigoid

Bullous pemphigoid is an uncommon, autoimmmune blistering disease in which antibodies are directed against antigens in the basement membrane zone between the epidermis and dermis. Clinically, the primary lesions appear as pruritic urticarial plaques or tense blisters that have a predilection for the lower legs (Figure 56.4) although any site, including oral mucosa, may be involved. The diagnosis is established by biopsy and direct immunofluorescent studies that demonstrate a linear deposition of immunoglobulin G (IgG) and serum protein complement (C3) along the basement membrane zone (8).

Mild cases of bullous pemphigoid may respond to potent topical corticosteroids, but most cases ultimately require oral prednisone, usually titered to disease activity. Dapsone and immunosuppressive drugs are occasionally used for their steroid-sparing effect. Most cases of bullous pemphigoid remit spontaneously.

Pemphigus Vulgaris

Pemphigus vulgaris is another autoimmune blistering disease that may affect the geriatric age group although the peak incidence is in the 40- to 60-year-old age group. Clinically, it is easily confused with bullous pemphigoid, but the pathogenesis is different in that antibodies are

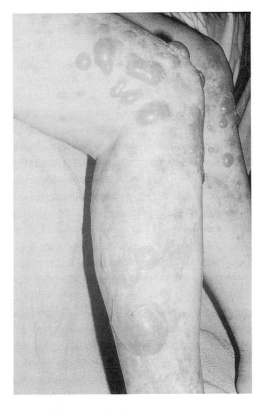

Fig. 56.4. Severe bullous pemphigoid demonstrating numerous tense bullae.

directed against one or more antigens in the intercellular substance between keratinocytes, which ultimately leads to a loss of cohesion between keratinocytes and produces blisters within the epidermis.

The primary lesions in pemphigus vulgaris are large flaccid blisters that easily break and produce erythematous denuded areas that may become extensive. In contrast to bullous pemphigoid, the oral mucosa is frequently involved and may be the only site involved at the time of initial presentation. Diagnosis of untreated pemphigus vulgaris is important because the mortality rate for untreated disease is high. The diagnosis is established by biopsy that demonstrates an intra-epidermal blister with acantholytic cells and direct immunofluorescence that demonstrates antibodies directed against the intracellular space.

The mainstay of therapy for pemphigus vulgaris is oral corticosteroids, often in initial doses as high as 100 to 200 mg per day. Because most patients require long-term therapy, adjunctive therapies, such as methotrexate, cyclophosphamide, azathioprine, gold, and plasmapheresis, are frequently added.

Common Infections of the Skin

Dermatophytosis

Fungal infections of the skin are very common in the elderly population—one study demonstrated an incidence of 79 percent. The most commonly affected sites are the feet (tinea pedis), nails (tinea unguium), hands (tinea manum), and, in men, the groin (tinea cruris). The most common organism in the elderly is *Trichophyton rubrum*, an anthropophilic organism acquired by person-to-person contact or from fomites.

Tinea manum and tinea pedis present as either focal or diffuse scaling with variable erythema of the palmar and plantar surfaces. Pruritus is a variable feature, but older patients frequently complain that they have "dry" feet or hands. In severe inflammatory cases, bullae may be present. Tinea unguium (onychomycosis) typically presents as subungual hyperkeratosis that thickens and may grossly deform the nail. The diagnosis is usually established by the clinical presentation and demonstration of organisms by light microscopy examination of scrapings that have been treated with potassium hydroxide (KOH) or fungal culture.

Dermatophytosis of the skin can usually be treated with the topical application of imidazoles (miconazole, ketoconazole, spectazole, oxiconazole, clotrimazole), ciclopirox olamine, or allylamines (naftifine, terbinafine). More extensive or recalcitrant cases may require treatment with oral griseofulvin or ketoconazole. Onychomycosis is especially resistant to topical or oral therapy, although intraconazole, fluconazole, and oral terbinafine have shown promise. Severe cases of onychomycosis may require surgical removal of the nail (9).

Candidiasis

Candidiasis is frequent mucocutaneous mycosis caused by the opportunistic yeast, *Candida albicans*. Infections are more common in diabetic, immunocompromised, and obese patients. The most common sites affected are the oral mucosa (thrush), corners of the mouth (perlèche), body folds (intertrigo), periungual tissue (paronychia), interdigital spaces (erosio interdigitalis blastomycetica), and the anogenital region. On cutaneous surfaces, candi-

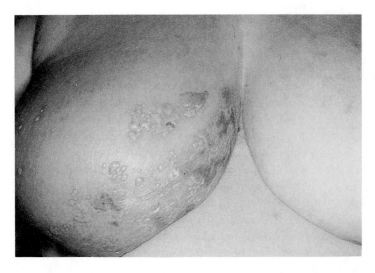

Fig. 56.5. Herpes zoster demonstrating grouped vesicles in a unilateral dermatomal distribution.

diasis produces primary lesions that are erythematous and frequently have smaller satellite lesions. Small pustules are frequently present. The diagnosis is established by clinical presentation, demonstration of yeast and pseudohyphae by KOH examination, or by culture.

Mild cases are easily treated with topical preparations, such as topical imidazoles (miconazole, ketoconazole, spectazole, oxiconazole, clotrimazole), ciclopirox olamine, or nystatin. Recalcitrant or severe cases may require treatment with oral ketoconazole, itraconazole, or fluconazole.

Herpes Zoster (Shingles)

Herpes zoster is a viral infection caused by the reactivation of latent varicella-zoster virus that has been dormant in the dorsal sensory ganglia. It is increasingly common with advancing age; most cases occur in patients older than 50 years. Most patients are normal. Herpes zoster is more common and more severe in immunocompromised patients (10).

Before the onset of clinical lesions, patients may complain of a prodrome consisting of neuralgic pain of the affected dermatome. Within days, the primary lesions, consisting of grouped vesicles on an erythematous base arranged in a dermatomal distribution, become apparent (Figure 56.5). The most commonly affected dermatomes are C-2, L-2, and the fifth cranial nerve. The lesions crust and may heal with scarring. Patients older than 55 years of age are particularly prone to be left with postherpetic neuralgia. The diagnosis is established by clinical presentation, Tzanck preparation, or viral culture.

Oral acyclovir or famacyclovir are the treatment of choice for early herpes zoster. During the acute phase of illness, oral narcotic analgesics may be required for symptomatic relief. The use of oral prednisone for the prevention of postherpetic neuralgia remains controversial.

Benign Tumors

The appearance of most benign skin tumors starts in middle age. Because skin tumors rarely disappear spontaneously, they increase in number as people age. The most common skin tumors are skin tags, seborrheic keratoses, cherry hemangiomas, sebaceous hyperplasia, venous lakes, melanocytic nevi, and lentigines.

Skin Tags (Acrochordons)

Skin tags are very common cutaneous growths that usually begin in middle-aged persons. Clinically, they are pedunculated, soft, 1 mm to 1 cm or larger, flesh-colored to brown growths that have a predilection for areas subject to friction, such as the neck, axillae, groin, and beneath the breasts. Patients often request removal of skin tags for cosmetic reasons or because the tumors have become infarcted secondary to becoming twisted. Treatment is easily accomplished by scissor excision, electrosurgery, or cryotherapy; all these procedures can be performed without anesthesia.

Seborrheic Keratoses

Seborrheic keratoses typically appear in a person's fifth decade of life, but they may appear earlier. By the seventh decade, most individuals have one or more lesions. Clinically, the lesions are 3 mm to 2 cm exophytic growths that appear to be "stuck on" to the skin like candle wax. The surface may be either smooth or verrucous. Seborrheic keratoses are usually tan, brown, gray, or black in color, although yellow and pink variants exist. They are most often located on the back, but can be seen anywhere except the palmar and plantar surfaces. Clinical variants of seborrheic keratoses include stucco keratoses and dermatosis papulosa nigra. Stucco keratoses are 1 to 5 mm, white to skin-colored growths on the lower legs and dorsum of the feet. Dermatosis papulosa nigra refers to 1 to 3 mm dark brown to black lesions that appear on the face of dark-skinned individuals.

Because seborrheic keratoses are so common, they are often not treated unless irritated or cosmetically objectionable. Treatment options include curettage, cryotherapy, scissor excision, or electrosurgery. Cryotherapy should be used with caution in dark-skinned individuals because it may produce hyperpigmentation.

Cherry Hemangiomas

Cherry hemangiomas are 1 to 5 mm benign vascular neoplasms that are commonly seen on the trunk of middle-aged and elderly persons. They are deep red to purple in color and may regress in persons of extreme age. They have no potential for malignant transformation and demonstrate little tendency to bleed unless traumatized.

Treatment is usually not indicated, but they are easily removed by electrosurgery or cryotherapy.

Sebaceous Hyperplasia

The face is the usual site of this common sebaceous tumor, which typically develops in middle-aged and elderly persons. Sebaceous hyperplasia is often multiple but may be solitary. The individual lesions are typically 1 to 3 mm papules with a distinct yellow color and a central follicular pore. This may give the tumor an annular appearance and may be confused with a basal cell carcinoma. Histologically, this tumor is composed of mature sebaceous glands arranged around a central pore. Treatment is usually not necessary, but when requested, cryotherapy or very light electrosurgery is effective.

Venous Lakes

Venous lakes are collections of dilated venules that occur on the lips, ears, and faces of the elderly. Clinically, they are deep purple or blue papules that are soft and compressible. They rarely exceed 5 mm in diameter. They may mimic melanotic lesions and are occasionally excised to exclude malignant melanoma. Removal, when desired, is usually accomplished under local anesthesia with electrosurgery.

Melanocytic Nevi (Moles)

Most nevi develop during the first two decades of a person's life, which gives the average, young white adult about 20 lesions. Melanocytic nevi are commonly referred to as "moles." They are subdivided into junctional, compound, and intradermal categories on the basis of histologic criteria. Junctional nevi are typically 1 to 10 mm tan to black macules. Compound nevi are similar, but are usually of a palpable thickness. Intradermal nevi are more elevated, and through maturation they can lose their pigment and become skin-colored. Melanocytic nevi are best removed by superficial shave biopsy or excision. All biopsied nevi should be submitted for histologic examination to ensure that they are benign.

Lentigines

Lentigines may arise in any age group but when acquired by the elderly, they are referred to as lentigo senilis or solar lentigo ("liver spots"). Histologically, they demon-strate variable epidermal hyperplasia associated with increased numbers of melanocytes and increased melanin in the basal keratinocytes. Clinically, they are tan to brown macules that are most common on sun-exposed skin, with a predilection for the dorsum of the hands and the face. Lentigines may be clinically indistinguishable from freckles. They can be removed by cryotherapy, peeling agents, and certain lasers, but they may reappear with further exposure to sunlight.

Premalignant and Malignant Tumors

Solar irradiation (UVB), especially in the 290 to 320 nm range, contributes significantly to the development of many changes in the skin previously considered to be age-dependent. These changes include wrinkling, atrophy, irregular pigmentation, lentigines, freckles, and precancerous keratoses (11). In addition, most squamous cell carcinomas, basal cell carcinomas, and malignant melanomas are induced by solar irradiation (12). All three cancers occur more often in fair-skinned people with light eyes (grey, blue, green) who burn easily and rarely tan. Skin cancer is rare in dark-skinned individuals. Many of the sequelae of solar irradiation can be prevented by the use of sunscreens and avoidance of the sun. Overzealous programs of sun avoidance, however, may conflict with a healthy outdoor lifestyle, so care should be taken to not turn the elderly into "sun cripples." People who are consciously protecting themselves from the sun or who normally receive little sun exposure should augment their diets with 200 IU per day of vitamin D (13).

Actinic Keratoses (Solar Keratoses)

Actinic keratoses are seen predominantly after middle age in fair-skinned people (14). They are particularly common on the dorsum of the hands and arms, on the face, and on the scalp of bald men. The primary lesions are skin-colored to red, scaly, and may range in size from a few millimeters to more than 4 cm (Figure 56.6). These lesions are occasionally precursors to squamous cell carcinomas of a slow-growing type that rarely metastasize. Actinic cheilitis is a term applied to actinic keratoses that are found on the lips, especially the lower lip. The border of the lip may often become indistinct and be chronically rough and scaly.

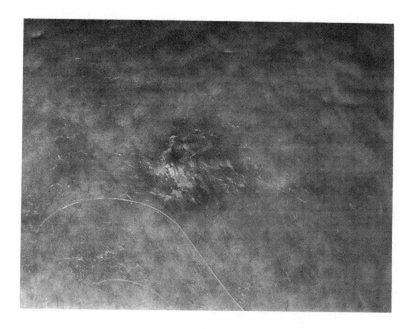

Fig. 56.6. Actinic keratosis demonstrating erythematous plaque with overlying scale.

Solitary keratoses can be treated with cryotherapy or curettage. Large areas of actinic damage are most easily treated using 5-fluorouracil cream, masoprocol cream, chemical peels, or dermabrasion. Carbon dioxide (CO_2) lasers work especially well for actinic cheilitis. Sun protection using clothing and adequate sun screen can help prevent new lesions.

Bowen's Disease (Squamous Cell Carcinoma in situ)

Bowen's disease is synonymous with squamous cell carcinoma in situ of the skin. Histologically, it demonstrates full thickness cytological atypia of the keratinocytes in contrast to actinic keratosis in which the atypia is confined to the lower portions of the epidermis. Bowen's disease may occur on sun-exposed or covered skin as well as mucosal surfaces. Clinically, the primary lesion is a scaly, irregular, erythematous plaque that is well-demarcated. On mucosal surfaces, it is known as erythroplasia of Queyrat and the lesions are erythematous and sharply demarcated, with a velvety surface.

Because atypical cells may extend down hair follicles and sweat ducts in Bowen's disease, surgical treatment is the treatment of choice for small lesions. Destruction of lesions in nonhairy areas with CO_2 laser, cryotherapy, curettage, or topical 5-fluorouracil (especially for genital lesions) is usually effective. Recurrent lesions can be treated with Moh's micrographic surgery.

Keratoacanthoma

Keratoacanthoma is a rapidly growing tumor usually found on sun-exposed surfaces of middle-aged and elderly persons (15). It begins as an erythematous, dome-shaped papule that enlarges to 1 to 3 cm in diameter during several weeks and develops a keratin-filled central crater (Figure 56.7). Schwartz, in his recent review of this tumor, stated that "It may be viewed as an aborted cancer that only rarely progresses into an aggressive squamous cell carcinoma" (16). After several months, the lesions usually involute spontaneously, often leaving a scar. Rarely, multiple keratoacanthomas may be present, either with classic morphology and clinical course or as small, persistent lesions. Predilection for the latter variant is often inherited in an autosomal dominant fashion.

Keratoacanthomas can resemble several other lesions, such as hypertrophic actinic keratosis, verruca vulgaris, and squamous cell carcinoma. Keratoacanthomas should be excised entirely or incised through the center of the lesion to include fat and normal skin and should be submitted for histology. It is important that adequate tissue be submitted for histologic evaluation because small bi-

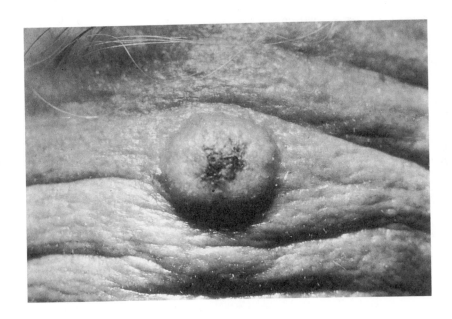

Fig. 56.7. Keratoacanthoma demonstrating characteristic crateriform appearance with central keratin plug.

opsies are very difficult to differentiate from squamous cell carcinomas.

Keratoacanthomas respond to multiple forms of treatment, including excision, curettage and electro-desiccation, radiotherapy, cryotherapy, intralesional 5-fluorouracil, and interferon α-2a (17).

Squamous Cell Carcinoma

Squamous cell carcinoma is the second most common form of skin cancer. It occurs most often in the fair-skinned individuals who have had significant sun exposure and are past middle age. Squamous cell carcinomas usually arise in sun-exposed skin, sometimes from preexisting actinic keratoses. With the exception of those occurring on the lips, which have a 12 percent to 14 percent rate of metastasis, actinically-induced squamous cell carcinomas rarely metastasize. Metastases are much more likely to occur in areas of late-radiation dermatitis, scars, and chronic ulcers.

Clinically, early squamous cell carcinomas are ill-defined, erythematous areas of induration and scaling that may be difficult to differentiate from hypertrophic actinic keratoses. The surface is often friable and may bleed easily. With continued growth, the tumor may appear nodular or verrucous, and it frequently becomes ulcerated (Figure 56.8).

Treatment is determined by the size, location, and type of skin from which the tumor arises. For small cancers (less than 1 cm) on sun-damaged skin, simple excision with histopathologic margin control often suffices. For larger tumors, and for tumors arising on the lips, in scars, and in irradiated skin, more radical surgery is necessary.

Basal Cell Carcinoma

Basal cell carcinoma is the most common form of skin cancer (18). It occurs predominantly in fair-skinned individuals on sun-exposed surfaces, especially the face, but it may also be seen in scars, in irradiated skin, and after chronic arsenic exposure. Basal cell carcinomas usually begin as small, pearly, translucent nodules with prominent telangiectasias; however, they may be quite subtle, presenting as small areas of induration, atrophy, or superficial ulcers with crust formation (Figure 56.9). They typically enlarge by peripheral extension and may reach several centimeters in diameter. Basal cell carcinomas rarely metastasize, but they are invasive and locally destructive. Some basal cell carcinomas have an infiltrative histology (morpheaform basal cell carcinomas), which can predispose to residual tumor and recurrence.

The treatment of basal cell carcinoma depends on the tumor size, site, and histologic pattern. Treatment modalities include curettage and electrodesiccation, exci-

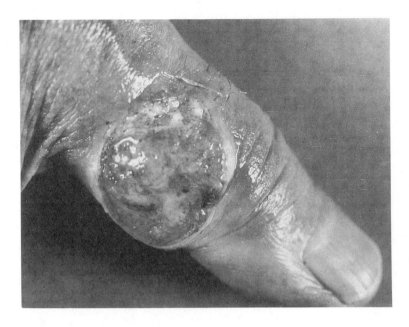

Fig. 56.8. Ulcerated squamous cell carcinoma of the thumb.

sion, irradiation, cryosurgery, and Moh's micrographic surgery. Moh's micrographic surgery is usually the treatment of choice for large tumors, recurrent tumors, infiltrative tumors, and tumors at certain sites (e.g., tip of the nose).

Lentigo Maligna (Hutchinson's Freckle)

Lentigo maligna is usually a large, hyperpigmented macule with an irregular border situated most commonly on the sun-damaged skin of the elderly. The most common site is the face although it can occur at other sites. Lentigo malignas characteristically demonstrate slow growth and may attain a diameter of several centimeters. Approximately one-third of lentigo malignas develop into lentigo maligna melanomas (19). The treatment of choice is surgical excision, but other modalities are sometimes used.

Malignant Melanoma

Malignant melanomas are seen most commonly in fair-skinned individuals with light hair and eyes. As with basal cell carcinomas and squamous cell carcinomas, exposure to ultraviolet light is considered to be an important etiologic factor. Malignant melanoma is one of the most rapidly increasing cancers in the world, with an 83 percent increase in incidence during the past 7 years (20).

From an incidence of 1 in 1500 in 1930, incidence has increased to 1 in 135 in 1987, and is expected to reach an incidence of 1 in 90 by the year 2000.

There are four major types of malignant melanoma that arise in the skin: 1) lentigo maligna melanoma arising in a lentigo maligna, 2) superficial spreading melanoma, 3) nodular melanoma, and 4) acral-lentiginous melanoma. Superficial spreading melanomas are the most common form of melanoma and constitute about 70 percent of all cases. Clinically and histologically, malignant melanoma is characterized by a superficial growth phase that may last for several years before a nodule (vertical growth phase) develops. In general, the horizontal growth phase is of shorter duration than that of lentigo maligna. Nodular melanomas are rapidly growing tumors that enter vertical growth phase without a preexisting radial growth phase. Acral lentiginous melanoma occurs on the palms, soles, nail beds, mucocutaneous junctions, and some mucosal surfaces.

The distinguishing features of malignant melanoma are asymmetry; irregular borders; irregular pigment with shades of white, tan, brown, gray, blue, and black; and size usually 6mm or larger (Figure 56.10), although melanomas as small as 3mm have been documented. Nodular melanomas can be amelanotic from inception.

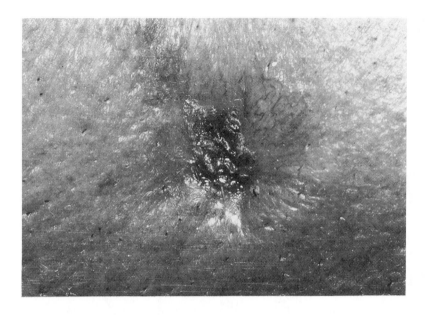

Fig. 56.9. Ulcerated basal cell carcinoma demonstrating indurated pearly border with telangiectatic vessels.

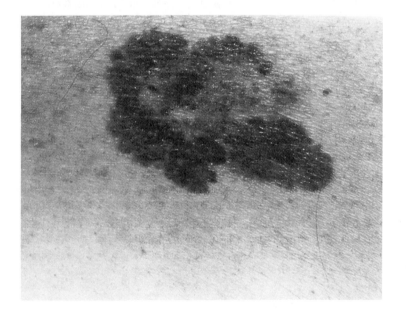

Fig. 56.10. Superficial spreading malignant melanoma demonstrating large size, irregular border, and variegation of color.

Because virtually all malignant melanomas have a preinvasive phase in which tumor cells are confined to the epidermis, with small chance of metastasis, the key to survival is early detection and removal. Valuable prognostic information can be obtained by histopathologic determination of the tumor depth (Breslow level) and mitotic rate; thus, whenever possible, the entire lesion should be excised for diagnosis. The treatment of primary malignant melanoma is by surgical excision. There is a growing body of evidence suggesting that wide surgical margins (i.e., 5 cm) do not improve survival. For this reason, many dermatologists and surgeons are opting for

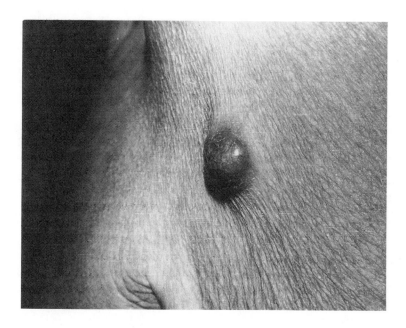

Fig. 56.11. Squamous cell carcinoma of the lung presenting as a firm dermal nodule of the upper shoulder.

conservative excisions, which result in reduced morbidity and improved cosmesis (21,22).

Metastatic Tumors

Skin metastases are the presenting sign in less than 1 percent of internal malignancies. Frequently, skin metastases grow rapidly and present as red nodules (Figure 56.11) or subcutaneous masses. The tumor can arise by direct extension to the skin, as a local metastasis, or as a distant metastasis (23). Conversely, metastatic lesions can appear many years after treatment of the primary cancer. This occurrence is usually a poor prognostic sign. Tumors that commonly spread to the skin are those of breast, lung, gastric, renal, ovarian, and malignant melanoma.

Acknowledgement. The opinions or assertions contained herein are the views of the authors and are not to be considered as reflecting the views of the Department of the Army or the Department of Defense. This is a U.S. government work and is in the public domain.

References

1. Johnson MLT. Skin conditions and related needs for medical care among persons 1–74 years. United States, 1971–1974. Vital and Health Statistics. Series 11. National Health Survey, No. 212. DHEW Publication No. (PHS)79-1660. Hyattsville, MD: Department of Health, Education, and Welfare, 1978.
2. Lavker RM, Zheng P, Dong G. Morphology of the aged skin. Dermatol Clin 1986;4:379–389.
3. Long CC, Marks R. Stratum corneum changes in patients with senile pruritus. J Am Acad Dermatol 1992;27:560–564.
4. Jacobs PH. Seborrheic dermatitis: causes and management. Cutis 1988;41:182–186.
5. Sibenge S, Gawkrodger DJ. Rosacea: a study of clinical patterns, blood flow, and the role of *Demodex folliculorum*. J Am Acad Dermatol 1992;26:590–593.
6. Cappiello RA, Espinoza LR, Adelman H, et al. Cholesterol embolism: a pseudovasculitis syndrome. Semin Arthritis Rheum 1989;18:240–246.
7. Fitzpatrick JE. Stasis ulcers: update on a common geriatric problem. Geriatrics 1989;44:19–31.
8. Anhalt GJ, Morrison LH. Pemphigoid: bullous, gestational, and cicatricial. Curr Prob Dermatol 1989;1:125–156.
9. Lesher JL Jr, Smith, JG Jr. Antifungal agents in dermatology. J Am Acad Dermatol 1987;17:383–394.
10. Huff JC. Herpes zoster. Curr Prob Dermatol 1988;1:5–40.
11. Forbes PD, Davies RE, Urbach F. Aging, environmental influences, and photocarcinogenesis. J Invest Dermatol 1979;73:131–134.
12. Kripke ML. Carcinogenesis: Ultraviolet radiation. In: Fitzpatrick TB, Eisen AZ, Wolff K, et al, eds. Dermatology in general medicine. 4th ed. New York: McGraw-Hill, 1993:797.
13. Prystowsky JH. Photoprotection and the vitamin D status of the elderly. Arch Dermatol 1988;124:1844–1848.
14. Gilchrest BA. Age associated changes in the skin: overview and clinical relevance. J Am Geriatric Soc 1982;30:139–142.

15. Rook A, Whister I. Keratoacanthoma: a thirty-year retrospect. Br J Dermatol 1979;100:41–47.

16. Schwartz RA. Keratoacanthoma. J Am Acad Dermatol 1994;30:1–19.

17. Grob JJ, Suzini F, Richard MA, et al. Large keratoacanthomas treated with intralesional interferon α-2a. J Am Acad Dermatol 1993;29:237–241.

18. Mackie RM. Tumor of the skin. In: Rook A, Wildinson DS, Ebling FJG, et al, eds. Textbook of dermatology. Oxford: Blackwell, 1986:2375.

19. Wayte DM, Helwig EB. Melanotic freckle of Hutchinson. Cancer 1968;21:893–911.

20. Rigel DS. What's new in malignant melanoma? Presented at the Symposium of Cutaneous Tumors, Annual Meeting of the American Academy of Dermatology, San Antonio, December 7, 1987.

21. Day CL, Mihm MG Jr, Sober AJ, et al. Correspondence on width of excision for melanoma. N Engl J Med 1982;307:440–444.

22. Lang NP, Stair JM, Degges RD, et al. Melanoma today does not require radical surgery. Am J Surg 1984;148:723–726.

23. Lookingbill DP, Spangler N, Sexton FM. Skin involvement as the presenting sign of internal carcinoma: a retrospective study of 7316 cancer patients. J Am Acad Dermatol 1990;22:19–26.

Appendix

Table A1. Diagnostic Clinic Assessment: Folstein Mini-mental State

Maximum score	Score	Category
		Orientation
5	_____	What is the (year) (season) (date) (day) (month)
5	_____	Where are we (state) (county) (town) (hospital) (floor)
		Registration
3	_____	Repeat three objects named. Trials.
		Attention and calculation
5	_____	Serial 7s
3	_____	Recall
9	_____	Language
		Name a pencil and a watch. (2)
		Repeat the following: "No, ifs, ands, or buts." (1)
		Follow a three-stage command. (3)
		Read and obey: "close your eyes." (1)
		Write a sentence. (1)
		Copy the following design. (1)
30	_____	Total_____

Reproduced by permission from Folstein MF, et al. Mini-mental state: a practical method of grading the cognitive state of the patient for the physician. J Psychiatr Res 1975;12:189.

Table A2. Hearing Handicap Inventory for the Elderly–Screening Version

Does a hearing problem cause you to feel embarrassed when you meet new people?
Does a hearing problem cause you to feel frustrated when talking to members of your family?
Do you have difficulty hearing when someone speaks in a whisper?
Do you feel handicapped by a hearing problem?
Does a hearing problem cause you difficulty when visiting friends, relatives, or neighbors?
Does a hearing problem cause you to attend religious services less often than you would like?
Does a hearing problem cause you to have arguments with family members?
Does a hearing problem cause you to have difficulty when listening to television or radio?
Do you feel that any difficulty with your hearing limits/hampers your personal or social life?
Does a hearing problem cause you difficulty when in a restaurant with relatives or friends?

Table A3. Determine Your Nutritional Health

The Warning Signs of poor nutritional health are often overlooked. Use this checklist to find out if you or someone you know is at nutritional risk.

Read the statements below. Circle the number in the yes column for those that apply to you or someone you know. For each yes answer, score the number in the box. Total your nutritional score.

	YES
I have an illness or condition that made me change the kind and/or amount of food I eat.	2
I eat fewer than 2 meals per day.	3
I eat few fruits or vegetables, or milk products.	2
I have 3 or more drinks of beer, liquor or wine almost every day.	2
I have tooth or mouth problems that make it hard for me to eat.	2
I don't always have enough money to buy the food I need.	4
I eat alone most of the time.	1
I take 3 or more different prescribed or over-the-counter drugs a day.	1
Without wanting to, I have lost or gained 10 pounds in the last 6 months.	2
I am not always physically able to shop, cook and/or feed myself.	2
TOTAL	

Total Your Nutritional Score. If it's —

0–2 Good! Recheck your nutritional score in 6 months.

3–5 You are at moderate nutritional risk. See what can be done to improve your eating habits and lifestyle. Your office on aging, senior nutrition program, senior citizens center or health department can help. Recheck your nutritional score in 3 months.

6 or more You are at high nutritional risk. Bring this checklist the next time you see your doctor, dietitian or other qualified health or social service professional. Talk with them about any problems you may have. Ask for help to improve your nutritional health.

These materials developed and distributed by the Nutrition Screening Initiative, a project of:

AMERICAN ACADEMY OF FAMILY PHYSICIANS
THE AMERICAN DIETETIC ASSOCIAION
NATIONAL COUNCIL ON THE AGING, INC.

Remember that warning signs suggest risk, but do not represent diagnosis of any condition.

Table A4. Geriatric Depression Scale (short form)

Choose the best answer for how you felt over the past week.

1. Are you basically satisfied with your life?	yes/no
2. Have you dropped many of your activities and interests?	yes/no
3. Do you feel that your life is empty?	yes/no
4. Do you often get bored?	yes/no
5. Are you in good spirits most of the time?	yes/no
6. Are you afraid that something bad is going to happen to you?	yes/no
7. Do you feel happy most of the time?	yes/no
8. Do you often feel helpless?	yes/no
9. Do you prefer to stay at home, rather than going out and doing new things?	yes/no
10. Do you feel you have more problems with memory than most?	yes/no
11. Do you think it is wonderful to be alive now?	yes/no
12. Do you feel pretty worthless the way you are now?	yes/no
13. Do you feel full of energy?	yes/no
14. Do you feel that your situation is hopeless?	yes/no
15. Do you think that most people are better off than you are?	yes/no

This is the scoring for the scale. One point for each of these answers. Cut-off: normal (0–5), above 5 suggests depression.

1. no	6. yes	11. no
2. yes	7. no	12. yes
3. yes	8. yes	13. no
4. yes	9. yes	14. yes
5. no	10. yes	15. yes

SOURCE: Courtesy of Jerome A. Yesavage, MD.

Table A5. Performance-Oriented Assessment of Mobility

BALANCE

Chair

Instructions: Place a hard armless chair against a wall. The following maneuvers are tested.

1. Sitting down
   0 = unable without help *or* collapses (plops) into chair *or* lands off center of chair
   1 = able *and* does not meet criteria for 0 *or* 2
   2 = sits in a smooth, safe motion *and* ends with buttocks against back of chair *and* thighs centered on chair

2. Sitting balance
   0 = unable to maintain position (marked slide forward *or* leans forward *or* to side)
   1 = leans in chair slightly *or* slight increased distance from buttocks to back of chair
   2 = steady, safe, upright

3. Arising
   0 = unable without help *or* loses balance *or* requires > three attempts
   1 = able but requires three attempts
   2 = able in ≤ two attempts

4. Immediate standing balance (first five seconds)
   0 = unsteady, marked staggering, moves feet, marked trunk sway *or* grabs object for support
   1 = steady but uses walker *or* cane *or* mild staggering but catches self without grabbing object
   2 = steady without walker *or* cane *or* other support

Stand

5a. Side-by-side standing balance
   0 = unable *or* unsteady *or* holds ≤ three seconds
   1 = able *but* uses cane, walker *or* other support *or* holds for 4–9 seconds
   2 = narrow stance without support for 10 seconds

5b. Timing ___ . _ seconds

6. Pull test (subject at maximum position attained in #5, examiner stands behind *and* exerts mild pull back at waist)
   0 = begins to fall
   1 = takes more than two steps back
   2 = fewer than two steps backward *and* steady

7a. Able to stand on right leg unsupported
   0 = unable *or* holds onto any objects *or* able for < three seconds
   1 = able for three *or* four seconds
   2 = able for five seconds

7b. Timing ___ . _ seconds

8a. Able to stand on left leg unsupported
   0 = unable *or* holds onto any object *or* able for < three seconds
   1 = able for three *or* four seconds
   2 = able for five seconds

8b. Timing ___ . _ seconds

BALANCE (*continued*)
9a. Semitandem stand
0 = unable to stand with one foot half in front of other with feet touching *or* begins to fall *or* holds for ≤ three seconds
1 = able for four to nine seconds
2 = able to semitandem stand for ten seconds
9b. Timing ___ . _ seconds
10a. Tandem stand
0 = unable to stand with one foot in front of other *or* begins to fall *or* holds for ≤ three seconds
1 = able for four to nine seconds
2 = able to tandem stand for ten seconds
10b. Timing ___ . _ seconds
11. Bending over (to pick up a pen off floor)
0 = unable *or* is unsteady
1 = able, but requires more than one attempt to get up
2 = able *and* is steady
12. Toe stand
0 = unable
1 = able but < three seconds
2 = able for three seconds
13. Heel stand
0 = unable
1 = able but < three seconds
2 = able for three seconds

Bed *or* Couch
14. Stand to sit
0 = unable without help *or* collapses (plops) onto bed *or* falls back onto side *or* lands close to edge of bed
1 = able *and* does not meet criteria for 0 *or* 2
2 = able in a smooth motion *and* ends with buttocks away from edge of bed
15. Sit to lie
0 = unable without help *or* lands close to edge of bed *or* > three attempts
1 = able but requires three attempts
2 = able in ≤ two attempts
16. Lie to sit
0 = unable without help *or* ≥ three attempts *or* ends close to edge
1 = able but requires three attempts (falls back, *or* getting legs over)
2 = able in ≤ two attempts
17. Sit to stand
0 = unable without help *or* loses balance *or* requires > three attempts
1 = able but requires three attempts
2 = able in ≤ two attempts

Possible score: 36 [18 not included in scoring]
18. Was the transfer to *and* from:
1 = bed
2 = couch

GAIT
Instructions: Subject stands with examiner. Walks down 10 foot walkway (measured). Ask subject to walk down walkway, turn, *and* walk back. Subject should use customary walking aid.

Bare Floor (flat, even surface)
1. Type of surface: 1 = linoleum/tile; 2 = wood; 3 = cement/concrete; 4 = other —— [not included in scoring]
2. Initiation of gait (immediately after told to "go")
0 = any hesitancy *or* multiple attempts to start
1 = no hesitancy
3. Path (estimated in relation to *tape measure*). Observe excursion of foot closest to tape measure over middle 8 feet of course.
0 = marked deviation

Index

Note: Page numbers in *italics* refer to illustrations; page numbers followed by t refer to tables.